‘All manner of ingenuity and industry’

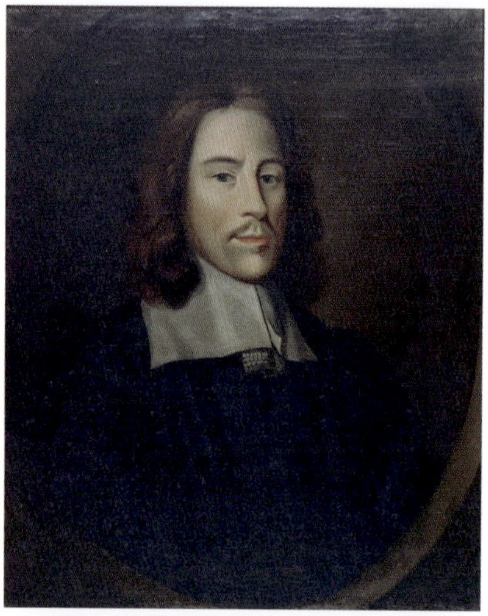

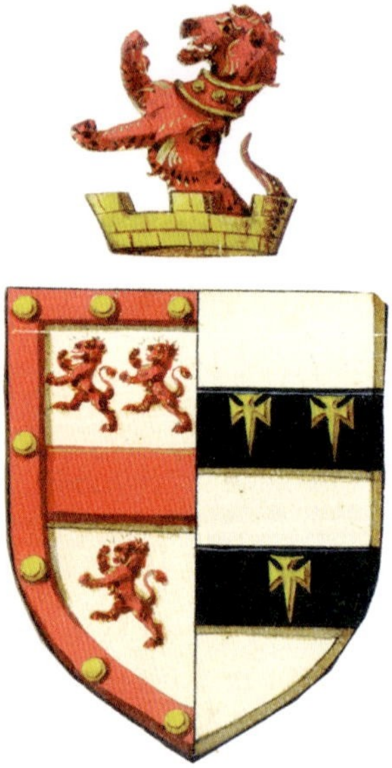

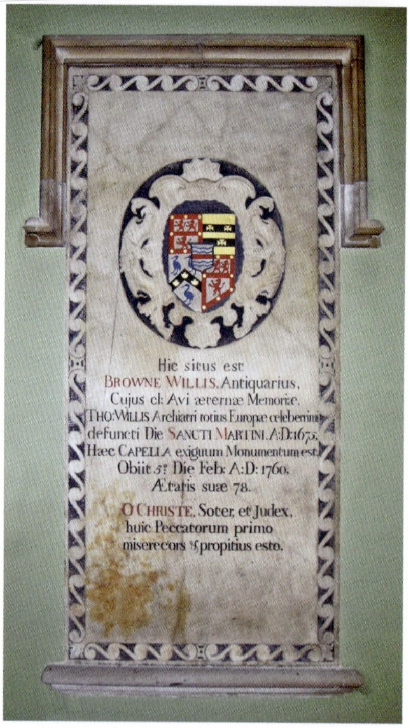

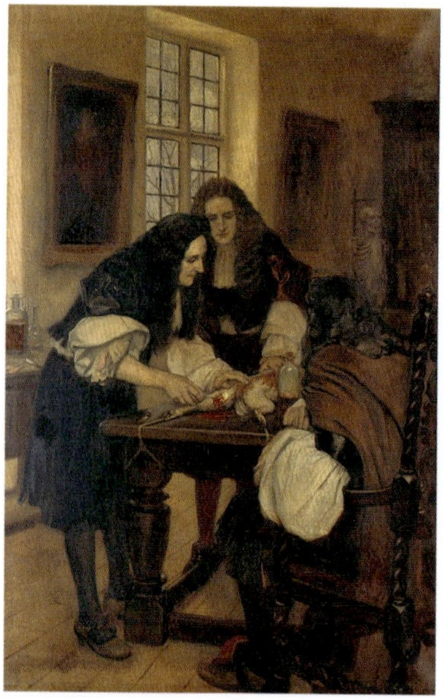

Portrait of Thomas Willis (© Bodleian Libraries, the University of Oxford)

The Coat of Arms of Thomas Willis impaled with those of the Fell family (Reproduced courtesy of Willis Fleming Historical Trust)

Memorial stone to Browne Willis and his grandfather Thomas Willis (Reproduced courtesy of St. Martin's Church, Fenny Stratford)

Christopher Wren demonstrating to Dr Willis a method for introducing drugs into a vein (With permission from Wellcome Collections).

‘All manner of ingenuity and industry’

A bio-bibliography of Dr Thomas Willis 1621–1675

ALASTAIR COMPSTON
Professor emeritus of neurology, University of Cambridge

OXFORD
UNIVERSITY PRESS

OXFORD
UNIVERSITY PRESS

Great Clarendon Street, Oxford, OX2 6DP,
United Kingdom

Oxford University Press is a department of the University of Oxford.
It furthers the University's objective of excellence in research, scholarship, and education by publishing worldwide. Oxford is a registered trade mark of Oxford University Press in the UK and in certain other countries

First Edition published in 2021

Impression: 1

Published in the United States of America by Oxford University Press
198 Madison Avenue, New York, NY 10016, United States of America

British Library Cataloguing in Publication Data

Data available

Library of Congress Control Number: 2020950907

ISBN 978–0–19–879539–1

DOI: 10.1093/med/9780198795391.001.0001

Printed in Great Britain by
Bell & Bain Ltd., Glasgow

Dedication

To the many nameless artisans who produced the books described herein and those who, at one time or another, have turned their pages

Acknowledgements

Many people helped with the preparation of this book. Roger Gaskell (Blaen Onneu) was a constant source of guidance on the principles of bibliography; his sharp eye detected many features of the books that are described; he answered endless questions based on his knowledge of books and their structure; and he and Lucy provided much hospitality during working visits to their home in the Brecon Beacons. The defects and errors that remain are despite his patience and expertise. Jan van Gijn (Utrecht) accepted the challenge of translating from Latin those parts of the text that were not available from other sources; he read and improved several chapters; and he and Carien were generous in making their home a base for visits to libraries in The Netherlands. Robin Compston (London) gave generously of his time and skill as a photographer in capturing the many images that appear in the book, and others that could not be accommodated. Juliet Compston (Cambridge) provided encouragement and support throughout; and, with a watchful eye, proofread the final manuscript.

John Wing (Bickley) kept in touch with the project over a period of ten years and gave unrestricted access to his unpublished bibliography of Thomas Willis (1962). Philip Oldfield (Harrogate) was equally generous in making available his unpublished bibliography of *De anima brutorum* (1991); he read and made useful amendments to selected chapters. Harry Willis Fleming (Montrose) discussed his illustrious ancestor and supplemented the accounts of Thomas and Browne Willis with important details from the Willis Fleming Historical Trust. Katrina Dedman (Cambridge) was tireless in searching out and making available articles and other printed material, and in providing typed copy of some starting material for the book.

John Cornwell (Cambridge), Christopher Ellis (Solihul), Mordechai Feingold (Pasadena), John Trevor Hughes (Oxford), Jurg Kesselring (Bern), and Simon Shorvon (London) read and commented constructively on chapters, each of which benefitted from their expertise.

Those who provided answers to specific questions, or other invaluable help, include: Stephen Andersen (New College, Oxford), Alex Bamji (University of Leeds); Charlotte Berry (Magdalen College, Oxford); Evanthe Blandy (London); Grace Bottomley (Eton College); Hans Brandhorst (Leiden University); Father Victor Bullock (St Martin's Church, Fenny Stratford); Polly Compston (Cambridge); Judith Curthoys (Christ Church, Oxford); Robert Evans (Oriel College, Oxford); Sam Hill (Oxford), Paul Hoftijzer (Leiden University); Sheila Markham (Sheila Markham Rare Books); Colin Mumford (Edinburgh, Scotland); Tom Piper (London); Goran Proot (Folger Shakespeare Library); James Raven (Magdalen College, Cambridge); Julian Reid (Corpus Christi College, Oxford); and Jennifer Thorp (New College, Oxford).

Apart from unnamed desk staff at the Wellcome Library, Bodleian Library, British Library, and the Royal Society of Medicine Library, others provided access to individual books and helped with enquires, some straightforward others much more complex, relating to individual items in the bibliography: Caitlin Angelone (College of Physicians of Philadelphia); Katie Birkwood (Royal College of Physicians of London); Stephen Greenberg (US National Library of Medicine, Bethesda); William Hale (Cambridge University Library); Francesca Heaney (Wadham College, Oxford); Petra Hofmann (St John's College, Oxford);

James Freeman (Cambridge University Library); Tim Kirtley (Wadham College, Oxford); Stephanie Krauss (Countway Library, Boston); Gaye Morgan (All Souls College, Oxford); Keith Moore (Royal Society); Stephen Tabor (Huntington Library, San Marino); Jaap de Vreugd (Leiden University Library); Anita Weaver (Huntington Library, San Marino); Claire Welford-Elkin (Cambridge University Library); and Yvonne de Wit (Amsterdam University Library).

It has been a pleasure to work with Peter Stevenson and Rachel Goldsworthy (Oxford University Press), both of whom provided constant encouragement and much flexibility as the book evolved from its original modest outline to the print and e-book versions now published; with Anya Hastwell (London) during copy-editing; Ruth Martin (Gers) in preparation of the index; and, especially, with Julia Turner (Charleston) who nurtured the manuscript and illustrations through the many stages of production. Their efforts are all the more appreciated for having been completed on schedule over a nine-month period when work was necessarily home-based and all communication remote.

Contents

Illustrations

Chapter 4

Chapter 9

Chapter 10

Chapter 11

Chapter 12

Chapter 13

Chapter 14

Chapter 15

Introduction

This is a book about books: those written by Thomas Willis and those that were informed or influenced by his work. It celebrates the quatercentenary of his birth on 27 January 1621.[1]

When Thomas Willis died in 1675, aged 54, he left a body of work on the structure and function of 'humane bodies', important especially for his contributions to knowledge on the 'brain and nervous stock', and a fine reputation as a physician. Willis is remembered for several reasons. As a physician working in and around Oxford whose studies, originally in chemistry from March 1637, were interrupted by the Civil War during which he served the Royalist cause, Willis's work in the 1650s provides an example of rural medical practice in early modern England. As a member of the Philosophical Club that met in Oxford from the 1640s, he was central to the move from classical scholasticism to accounts of medical science based on observation and experiment. As Sedleian professor of natural philosophy in Oxford (1660–1675), the surviving records of his lectures provide an example of pedagogy in medicine at that time.

After moving to London in 1667, and already elected a Fellow of the Royal Society although never much involved in its affairs, Willis interacted with a community of scientists and physicians who transformed ideas on human anatomy and physiology relating to respiration, muscular movement, and the nervous system. Despite a busy clinical practice, Willis found time to write three thousand pages of printed text on anatomy and physiology, clinical medicine, and therapeutics which, although not always acknowledged as such, are now recognized as wise, original, and influential.[2]

Between 1659 and 1675, Willis wrote fourteen treatises of varying length. The first thirteen originally appeared in six books, the last published in two parts, printed in Latin. The fourteenth treatise was published posthumously and in English. Willis started with *Diatribæ duæ medico-philosophicæ* (1659) which, despite the title, contained three treatises. The first provides an account of fermentation as the basis of life but a process prone to disorder and therefore also representing an ubiquitous mechanism of disease. Often dismissed as plain wrong, it takes little imagination to see in Willis's concept a formulation of present day biochemistry and metabolism. Because fermentation depended on heat, it was logical that the second treatise dealt with fevers. A short treatise on urines, one of the earliest essays on biomarkers in disease, was included in the volume. Over the next thirteen years, the emphasis of Willis's work was on the brain, nerves, and muscle in health and disease as set out in *Cerebri anatome* (1664: two treatises), *Pathologiæ cerebri* (1667: two treatises), *Affectionum quæ dicuntur hystericæ et hypochondriacæ* (1670: three treatises), and *De anima brutorum* (1672: two parts in one treatise). Willis died a few days before publication of the second part of his last work, on the treatment of disease, *Pharmaceutice rationalis* (1674 and 1675: two treatises) in which he rehearsed and explained in more detail his ideas on how to manage and treat diseases resulting from perturbations of fermentation.

[1] In line with the Julian calendar used at the time, Willis's birthday lies before Lady day (25 March) and so might be denoted as 27 January $\frac{1620}{1621}$.

[2] With preliminaries and end-matter: original editions, 2976 pages mainly in quarto; *Opera omnia*, 1576 pages in quarto; English translations, 1210 pages in folio.

A start was made on translating all Willis's works into English under the licensing of Roger L'Estrange (1616–1704) in 1679 (*Pharmaceutice rationalis*), followed by *The remaining medical works* (apart from *Affectionum quæ dicuntur hystericæ et hypochondriacæ*) translated by Samuel Pordage (1633–1691) in 1681 and, with *Two discourses concerning the soul of brutes* appearing in 1683, the project to publish *Dr Willis's practice of physic* was eventually concluded in 1684. Aside from the many descriptions of anatomy and clinical disorders of the nervous system, *Cerebri anatome* and *De anima brutorum* are additionally important for their anatomical illustrations; and other plate leaves were included in *De motu musculari* (part of *Affectionum quæ dicuntur hystericæ et hypochondriacæ*, 1670) and both parts of *Pharmaceutice rationalisis* (1675, 1675). The illustrators were Christopher Wren (1632–1723) and Richard Lower (1631–1691), Edmund King (1630–1709) and, perhaps, Willis himself.

Although planned for some time, this book has had a slow gestation. At the request of the Master and Fellows, an exhibition was held in the newly opened quincentenary library at Jesus College, Cambridge, between October and December 1997 displaying twenty-eight items from the now much larger collection on which the bibliography is largely based. This was accompanied by an illustrated catalogue, 'Dr Thomas Willis and the Origins of Clinical Neuroscience'. In 2000, thirty-five years after publishing the tercentenary edition of *The anatomy of the brain* (1965), the late William Feindel (1918–2014) suggested a book based on *De anima brutorum*: he was to write on the anatomy, Philip Oldfield would deal with the bibliography, and the present author was to tackle the clinical neurology. A start was made by copying and annotating the English text of *Two discourses concerning the soul of brutes* (1683). But knowing little of Willis's iatrochemical principles, it proved hard going and the project never materialized. In the years before his death in 2014, Dr Feindel was busy with the second volume of the history of the Montréal Neurological Institute and work related to the Osler Library. A start was made on the book as it has now materialized in the form of extended notes made for the Fitz-Patrick lecture delivered to the Royal College of Physicians on 29 March 2010: 'Dr Thomas Willis' works: "The most learned Dr Christopher Wren; and the inward dens of the Brain"'; and the 'Willis lecture', of the same title, given in Montréal on 14 February 2011 at the invitation of Dr Feindel. The thrust of those lectures, aimed primarily at physicians, was that, structured around the works of Thomas Willis, no two copies of a book published in the late seventeenth century are necessarily identical because of stop-press changes and the variable distribution of printed sheets to binders and booksellers. It made sense also to say something of the man and his times, but there was little in these lectures on the scientific and medical content of his treatises. After an interval of several years, and with the perceived leisure of retirement from neurological medicine, a much fuller account of the lecture has now been written. This was done, working more or less full-time, between August 2017 and July 2020. During that period, the shape changed but not the original perspective on the life of an eminent clinician scientist, the circles in which he moved, and the books he wrote.

The eighteen chapters are in four sections. Chapter 1 is biographical; chapters 2, 3, and 4 describe aspects of the history of the book and illustration relevant to Willis's printed works; chapters 5–14 provide bibliographical details of Willis's treatises printed in Latin, English, Dutch, and French between 1659 and 1721; and chapters 15–18 describe the content of Willis's works and their contribution to medical science. Each chapter is complete in itself with minimal cross-referencing.[3] The book is aimed at readers who have an interest in

[3] Dates of birth and death of named individuals are given at first mention in each chapter, where known (*c.*, circa; b., born; d., died; fl., flourished; and nd, no date). Citations are given in full at first listing but shortened for subsequent mention of the same source. For printed books, the distinction between whether a named individual was primarily engaged in printing or selling copies, or did both, is occasionally blurred. Prefaced by the term 'Impensis' (at the expense of) or 'Apud' (at the shop of), a much larger group was involved in producing books

bibliography, the history of the book, and medical history especially as it relates to the brain and nervous system. It is recognized that some readers will already be well informed on the content of particular parts.

The biographical account of Thomas Willis is culled from various sources, as described, but without original research or identification of new archival material. No claim is made to having provided a comprehensive summary of the literature relating to Thomas Willis and his contemporaries written from the perspective of the history and philosophy of science. With few exceptions, recent scholarship on Thomas Willis and his times has not rigorously been included. Those who have written on Willis, the people with whom he interacted, and the institutions with which he was associated will understandably be disappointed not to find their work cited. This is not to undermine the authority of their scholarship. Even with filters, an internet search on Thomas Willis yields several million hits, very many of which merely mention him in passing. In not exploring the entirety of the recent literature, inevitably some original and important analyses have been overlooked.

The details of book production in the late seventeenth century are focused mainly on the individuals who produced Willis's works. Many were artisans who by nature of plying the trades of printing, publishing, and selling books were not necessarily distinguished and are now forgotten. The work involved in setting these texts, and printing with the hand press, was prodigious. A physician not trained in history and with an amateur knowledge of the history of the book treads warily on this topic. If some of the details seem elementary, it is hoped that experts will acknowledge that other readers will not be familiar with how books were produced in the seventeenth century. Authorities on book history will readily identify material that ought to have been mentioned in addition to the sources that are cited. But perhaps even the experts will not have considered all the details of printing and illustration that make up the account of those who produced the one hundred and three volumes described, or the illustrations and ornaments used by individual printers in Oxford, London, and continental Europe to decorate these works.

With chapters 5–14, the author is, in one sense, on slightly firmer ground but, in another, taking risks. The amateur who compiles a bibliography needs to explain why. Finding that there is no standard work in a particular field of interest, or the available descriptions leave open questions relating to copies at hand, the bibliophile creates a list of items in the collection or needing to be found. The principles of descriptive bibliography and history of the book are then learned. These self-taught amateurs may bring the rigour of another academic discipline to their private study of books but they proceed cautiously in the unfamiliar world of bibliography.

The amateur bibliographer is mindful of the cautionary advice of professionals. In *Principles of bibliographical description* (1949), Fredson Bowers (1905–1991) warns that bibliography requires a purpose over and above slavish listing. It must be competent and, since the existing systems work well, there is no place for ignoring accepted uses of symbols and methodology. Eccentricity and personal prejudice are unwelcome. Bibliographies should be worthy of the name or not done at all. In writing the bibliography of a single author, Bowers proposes listing editions for each title rather than a chronological account of the books irrespective of subject matter. Bibliography is not concerned with textual value or

than the individuals designated 'Typis' (printed by) or 'Ex officina' (from the workshop of) on the title pages. For seventeenth- and eighteenth-century books, the number identified on the title page may go well into double figures. For these reasons, only the place of publication is given for book titles. It follows that, for example, 'Oxford' is not invariably the University Press but may refer to other publishers based in or around the city.

factual correctness of the information printed. Modern studies place more emphasis than Bowers on binding, aspects of provenance and other markings which show in what way, and by whom, the printed sheets in a particular copy were subsequently used.

Central to this book is a copy-specific bibliography of items published from 1659–1721. These dates are boundaries for the printing of Thomas Willis's first book and the final issue of his last treatise or collected works in that period. There were no further printings of Willis's treatises until the twentieth century. As explained in chapter 4, apart from a listing of editions of *Cerebri anatome* (1965), there is no complete bibliography of Thomas Willis. There are two important unpublished manuscripts: one, by HJR Wing (former librarian of Christ Church, Oxford), lists all the writings; and the other, by Philip Oldfield, formerly of the Rare Books Library, University of Toronto, deals only with *De anima brutorum*. In a letter dated 14 March 2015, replying to an invitation to coauthor this book, Mr Wing declined but released the copyright of his bibliography, subject to approval from the Department of Information Studies, University of London. In correspondence dated 9 March 2015, Philip Oldfield, also agreed to make his text available without restriction. In the event, although both bibliographies were much used, each served mainly as a point of reference and all the bibliographic descriptions in this book are based on direct scrutiny of individual copies.

Eighty-five of the one hundred and three entries for the bibliography use copies in the author's collection, sometimes one of several for that item. These were acquired through the antiquarian book trade or, occasionally, as gifts between 1982 and 2021. The bibliography has been supplemented, where necessary, from institutional resources: Wellcome Library, five (**1I**, **IK1**, **7B**, **10A2.c2**, **10A2.c3**), British Library, two (**1D2**, **2F**), Royal Society of Medicine, three (**7A4**, **8D**, **10A4**), Bodleian Library, three (**1A1.c1**, **1A1.c2**, **10A3.c2**), Cambridge University Library, one (**4C**), St. John's College, Oxford, one (**1A2**), and Wadham College, Oxford, one (**6B1**). Two books are known only from copies held outside the United Kingdom: one in the University of Leiden (**1A3**), and one in the Huntington Library (**9C**).

As one justification for private collecting, it may be worth adding that this bibliography could not have been written without repeated access to individual copies, some handled many times each day away from the watchful eye of diligent librarians fretting over the rapid turning of leaves and the painstaking unfolding of large illustrations, many already torn and fragile. Also clear to anyone trying to resolve the architecture and status of a particular copy is the importance of original binding and end-papers, and manuscript ownership entries. Pleasant as it is to have a pristine copy, the archaeology of a book is often more important than its appearance. It is also self-evident that, especially with library visits restricted during the difficulties of 2020 and 2021, the availability of e-book copies and other internet sources enabled a great deal of archival searching and checking that would otherwise not have been possible. In the event, the brief periods of access and their kindness in dealing with questions by correspondence or telephone calls, allowed library staff to answer most enquiries. The very few loose ends which could not be resolved during the Covid-19 pandemic are listed in the footnotes for individual chapters.

Since no attempt has been made to identify page-by-page textual alterations and other variations that distinguish one copy from another, it follows that this is not a descriptive bibliography but, rather, a bibliographical catalogue. Nevertheless, several differences between copies of the books described in detail, some already noted and others newly identified, are listed. In providing a physical description of the structure, contents, and illustrations of these copies, others can add further comparisons and detect as yet unrecorded variants requiring more detailed investigation. Whilst confidence can be placed in those listed, it is inevitable that errors of transcription and omission of details within the categories under consideration will have escaped repeated checking.

Bibliography is not primarily concerned with the factual content of the printed page or the advancement of knowledge, nor does it provide textual and literary criticism. The accounts of Willis's contributions to knowledge are considered in chapters 15–18 under the general headings of medical chemistry; anatomy and physiology of the brain; neurological and psychiatric conditions; and therapeutics and general medical disorders. Although some secondary sources have been consulted, as listed, it is again important to make clear that those who have written recently on the works of Thomas Willis will be disappointed not to have their analyses cited. Important critiques will undoubtedly have been overlooked, to the detriment of this book and the annoyance of their authors. Because it would lengthen the book and directly help relatively few readers, quotations in the original Latin have not usually been transcribed. Nor has assistance been taken in order to provide new translations of all passages quoted in English. Rather, in most instances, the versions printed in the contemporary licensing to Roger L'Estrange and the translations of Samuel Pordage have been used, retaining their rich language and use of metaphor and analogy even if this strays from the original Latin text and is considered inaccurate by experts in the classics. Occasionally, texts offered by recent commentators—notably Hansruedi Isler (1934–2019), Edwin Clarke (1919–1996) and Charles O'Malley (1907–1970), and Kenneth Dewhurst (1919–1984) assisted by Leofranc Holford-Stevens and Alastair McCann—who have translated key passages have been preferred. The original Latin is provided, and kindly translated by Jan van Gijn, for selected extracts that are considered of particular importance and which have not previously been made available in English.

Whilst the transcriptions retain the spelling and punctuation as printed, a few truncated words are completed in order to retain the sense and syntax of individual quotes. Names are as written by Willis. Elsewhere an arbitrary position has been taken on individuals who are variously spelled: *inter alia* James Allestry or Allestree; William Crook or Crooke; Anne Greene or Green; James Flesher or Fletcher; John Martyn or Martin; Gerbrandt Schaghen or Schagen. Readers will detect some inconsistency in use of the long 's', i.e. 'ſ': this has usually been retained in the longer Latin and some English transcriptions but not in the shorter quotes, even if this typography is not as originally printed. The many footnotes mainly refer readers to the English translations of Willis's works, not the original editions. To save space, abbreviations of the Latin or English titles are often used. Since these translations retain the structure of the original chapters and their paragraph breaks, it is easy to locate the appropriate Latin text should that be preferred. Because it appears that the seventeenth-century English texts were translated and set down without any attempt at editing, the content of Willis's treatises is often re-ordered so as to maintain the narrative and avoid confusion arising from the many repetitions, contradictions, and erratic presentation of his ideas. Illustrations relating to the printed works are taken from the author's copies. A few attractive printers' ornaments which would otherwise have been included, could not be accessed during the restrictions of 2020–2021. The plate leaves retain three-dimensional features such as creases, warping, and offsetting, together with blemishes. Their sizes are not strictly comparable but the original dimensions for each are given.

Although not first to use the word, the detailed study of 'neurologie' begins with the writings of Thomas Willis, and he respected the etymology of the term by always referring to νευρολογία. The subsequent accumulation of knowledge concerning structure and function of the brain and nervous stock is not the purpose of this book. Rather, the aim is to see Willis's writings as instrumental in the evolution of knowledge defining the brain as a system for sensing the external and internal environment, integrating responses through voluntary and involuntary actions, and learning from those experiences to initiate behaviour and interact socially with other nervous systems. No claim is made for authority with respect to a new interpretation of the history of seventeenth-century medicine. The intention is to put the reader in the presence of Thomas Willis, hearing his voice and whimsical turns of phrase (in translation), knowing that he has a particular view on physiology and mechanisms of disease, and is a man not shy about stating his opinions and disdain for those who practised medicine without respect for observation and the evaluation of evidence. The sense is of standing alongside Willis as he goes about his work in the houses of the sick—listening, examining, opining, explaining, and treating his often illustrious patients surrounded by the odours, sights, and drama of domestic medicine, and the often perilous plights of his trusting patients.

Apart from a few lapses when the urge proved too great, the danger of holding a retrospective diagnostic clinic in which Willis's patients are assigned diseases recognized in twenty-first-century clinical neurology and medicine has been resisted. It may be harsh that those who have succumbed to this temptation are occasionally reprimanded. That said, the commentary and many quotations are chosen in the expectation that readers familiar with the nosology and phenomenology of medicine will readily reach their own conclusions on what Willis is describing. And they also will be astonished by the range and prescience of his descriptions and witty asides. To the informed reader, hardly a single page does not contain an observation that resonates with the symptoms, signs, and mechanisms of disease encountered by any general physician, neurologist, gastroenterologist, or specialist in respiratory medicine working in any one of the last four centuries.

Horseheath, Cambridge
27 January 2021

1

'In the tents of the King as well as the Muses'

The life and reputation of Thomas Willis

Acknowledged as a distinguished physician with successful practices in Oxford and London; fourth incumbent of the Sedleian professorship of Natural Philosophy in Oxford; prominent among scientists and physicians who transformed ideas on human anatomy and physiology relating to respiration, muscular movement, and the nervous system; and the author of fourteen treatises, Thomas Willis might reasonably have gone to his grave in Westminster Abbey knowing that he was revered by his contemporaries and confident that posterity would continue to celebrate his manifold achievements. In 2021, the 400th anniversary of his birth, although his writings are considered not always free from speculation, Thomas Willis is recognized as someone who replaced theoretical dogma in medicine with empirical wisdom based on observation of the human body in health and disease. Willis thought about different bodily structures and their functions, but his abiding interest was the 'brain and nervous stock' and he is unambiguously the founder of clinical neuroscience (see: Figure 1).[1]

In the immediate shock of his death on 11 November 1675, Willis's brother-in-law, John Fell (1625–1686), added a postscript to the preliminary pages of what now became the posthumously published second part of *Pharmaceutice rationalis*.[2] Fell explains that whilst the text was being printed, the news arrived that Willis had died. There was still time to amend the preliminaries. Fell is unambiguous in his praise. He laments a person 'equally Good and Learned ... [and] also exercised himself in the Practice of Piety who was most conversant ... in Physick'. His eulogy concludes with a summary of Willis's courage in adversity, modesty, temperance, forgiving nature, loyalty to the Crown, devotion to the Church, ingenuity in his work, diligence in his studies, and precision in his speech. Death came when, 'being near Fifty seven years of Age' (a miscalculation by Fell), at the beginning of November 1675 he developed a cough, from which followed pleurisy and pneumonia

[1] The account that follows is necessarily derivative. Anyone writing on Willis starts with the contemporary accounts of Fell, John Aubrey (1626–1697), and Anthony Wood (1632–1695). There are two full-length more recent biographies: J Trevor Hughes, *Thomas Willis 1621–1675. His life and work*, London (1991), reprinted with minor amendments, Oxford (2009); and Hansruedi Isler, *Thomas Willis. Ein Wegbereiter der Modernen Medizin 1621–1675*, Stuttgart (1965) translated as *Thomas Willis 1621–1675. Doctor and scientist*, New York (1968). Others who have researched aspects of Willis's life and writings include Charles Symonds (1890–1978), Alfred Meyer (1895–1990), William Feindel (1918–2014), Kenneth Dewhurst (1919–1984), Raymond Hierons (1921–2001), John Wing, Robert Frank, and Robert Martensen (1947–2013). Hughes and Frank, in particular, have used documentary sources in Oxford and London and theirs are the definitive accounts of the man and his family; Hughes, Isler, Frank, and Martensen have read the treatises and analysed their contributions. Dewhurst has located and made available important contemporary archival resources, especially the lectures and casebook; and Feindel, Harold Denham (1917–1999), HJR Wing, and Philip Oldfield have considered the bibliography of one or more of the printed books. These and many others who have written on Willis are acknowledged in the text and footnotes that follow.

[2] John Fell, *Pharmaceutice rationalis, sive diatriba de medicamentorum operationibus in humano corpore, pars secunda*, Oxford (1675): pages [12–17]; translated by Samuel Pordage (1633–1691) in *Pharmaceutice rationalis or an exercitation of the operations of medicines in humane bodies.* The second part, London (1679): pages [6–8].

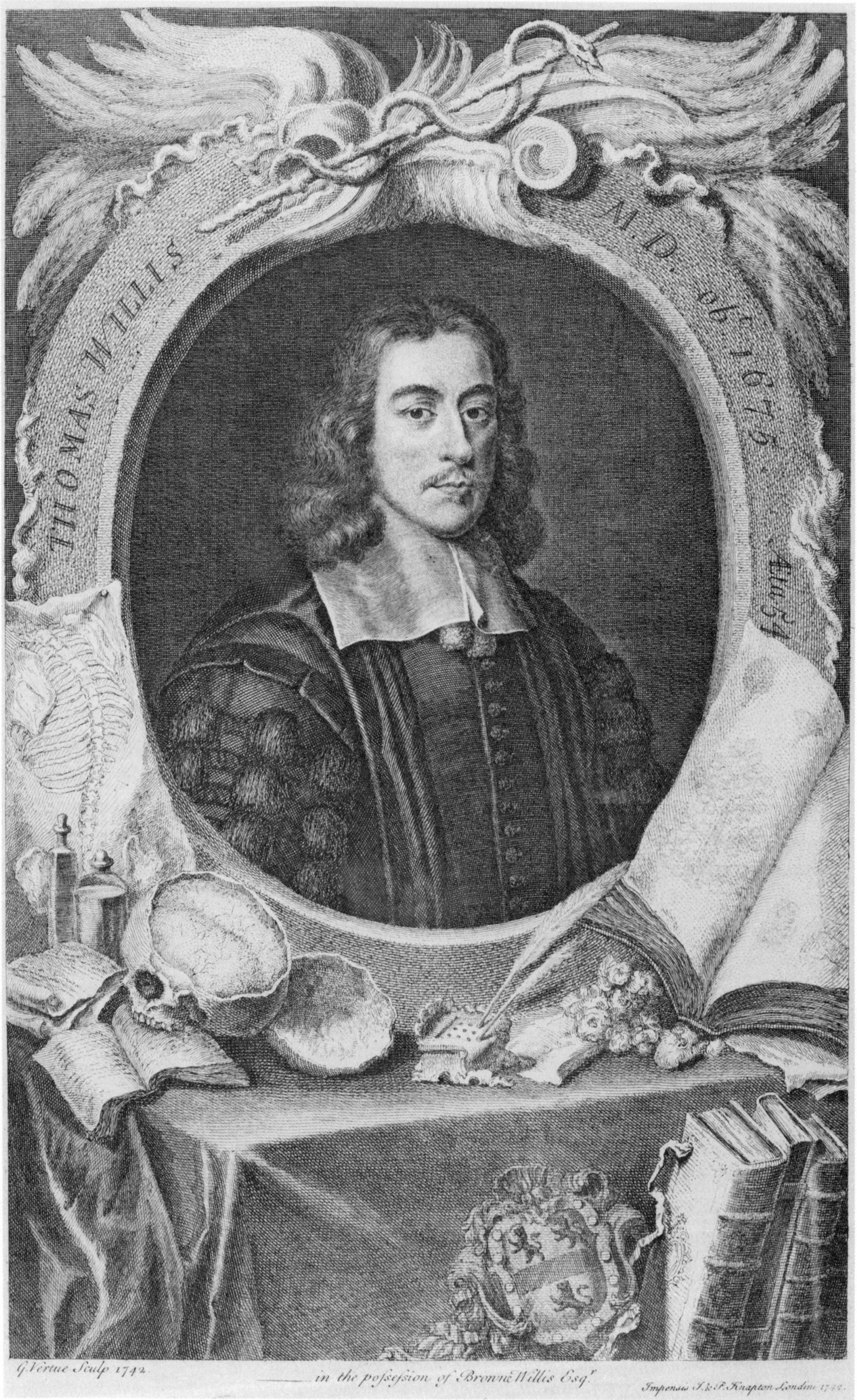

Figure 1 Portrait of Thomas Willis engraved by George Vertue, 1742, commissioned by Browne Willis for £21 and published in Thomas Birch *Heads of various illustrious persons of Great Britain* (1743–1751).

unresponsive to bleeding and other remedies. Realizing that the illness would prove fatal, Willis settled his affairs, took the 'Viaticum of the Holy Eucharist... commended his pious Soul to God, having his senses entire to the last breath, and finisht his most exemplary Life with the like Death'.

Also printed in the preliminary pages of *Pharmaceutice rationalis* part 2 (1675), and already planned—but not reproduced by the first translator[3] or Samuel Pordage in the 1679 and 1684 editions in English—is a celebration in verse by Gul. [William] Dawkins (nd):

AUTORI CLARISSSIMO, nec non mihi (de quo jure glorior) AMICISSIMO, in illius Pharmaceutices Rationalis *Partem utramque*

Carmen Gratulatorium.

SEcula ſollicitos ſuderunt anxia queſtus,
Demirata diu, cur tot Medicina per annos
Nondum ætatem habuit, nondum matura Hymenæas
Accendit pro more faces, nec robore crevit
Firmo, nec ſtabilem ſolidæ rationis ad uſum
Pertigerit, ſed adhuc rudis, infans, brutaque manſit.
Scilicet Egregium nondum Illi fata dederunt
WILLISIUM, Illo, Illo ſub vindice floſque, vigorq;
Seraque Phœbœæ perfectio contigit Arti.
Illa prius riſu potuit cognoſcere Matrem
Naturam, blandamque Patri tibi, Phœbe, ſalutem
Dicere, ſed proprio pede non ſtetit, omnia cæcis
Fortunæ auſpiciis, caſuque edocta Magiſtro
Crediderat, vario ſucceſſum errore requirens;
Et ſua per mediam librans veſtigia noctem,
Miſcuit incertis temeraria pocula ſatis:
Dum tibi ſuccurit, medicaſque accommodat ultro
Languenti *Medicina* manus, dum diſcutit umbras,
Admittitque Diem late, nova lumina pandens
WILLISIUS; Lynceus, Phœbeius, intima doctus
Corporis humani penetralia, doctus in illis
Quaque viâ tacito ſerpent Medicamina greſſu;
Quoq; modo herbarum hinc, hinc vis contraria morbi
Bella ſalutiſero movet inteſtina tumultu.
  Olim cum vulgo Medicus ſimul ipſe profano,
Ignarus propriæ ſtupuit Magnalia dextræ.
Et ſtetit ad dubois cæci medicaminis hauſtus,
Vota tibi, Fortuna, ferens, atque anxius hæſit,
Vilibus an lateat tam ſacra potentia ſuccis.
Tandem aliquando datur rerum cauſaſque modoſque,
Sympathiaſque fugaſque diu per opaca latentes

[3] The book was '*Licensed, October* 31. 1678. R. L'Estrange'. This has been taken to indicate that the translator was Sir Roger L'Estrange (1616–1704).

Mechanice explorare, & fida indagine rerum
Deprenſas, facilem mirâ arte reſolvere in uſum.
Quippe volubilium vaga copia Particularum,
Exercet medicas in fluxo corpore vires:
Exileſque atomi, naturæ, artiſque Miniſtræ
Proripiunt agili, ſeſe hinc, ſeſe inde volatu:
Inque ſinus refugos, diverſaque clauſtra receptæ
Exagitant varios partier, reprimuntque tumultus.
Nunc ſuccum à ſtomacho nimis indignante repoſcunt
Morbificum, liquidæ profluis nunc ductibus alvi
Præcipitant denſo glomeratas agimine fæces.
Diverſoque modo morborum ſemina pellunt,
Hinc dum conſtringunt fibras, atque inde relaxant.
Nunc patulas ſubeunt venas, atque agmine facto,
Purpureo rabiem torrenti, æstuſque remittunt;
Efferveſcentem veluti Sal miſſus in Ollam,
Æquora prætumidis inducit priſtina lymphis.
Nunc in ſtagnanti glaciali frigore Maſſâ,
Nativos reparant curſus, tepidoſque fluores:
Sic aqua liberior limoſæ immiſſa paludi,
Continuum jugi deducit flumine rivum.
Nunc vitæ penetrant ſedes, & perpetis arcem
Lampadis, irriguos quæ dat per membra calores.
Lucida nunc agilis ſubeunt confinia ſenſus,
Spirituumque vagis miſcent commercia turmis.
Nunc præcluſa diu vitæ ſpiracula, rupto
Expurgant aditu, tabiſque repoſta futuræ
Semina, diffiſſis depellunt undique rimis,
Diſtentoſque replent leni ſpiramine folles.
Nunc in ſanguiferas Jecoris penetrare cavernas,
Et male ceſſantem gaudent urgere laborem.
Vel cute ſtagnantes ſatagunt depellere lymphas,
Aut relevare gravem membrorum tabe lienum.
Sic ſub mille viis actæ, ſub mille figuris
Extrudunt morbos partier, pariterque repullunt.
Harum agiles motus, veſtigiaque abdita noſſe,
Quaſque habeant vires, ac *quare* dicere, & *unde*,
Hic labor, Hoc opus eſt, ſtudiumque & cura Sagacis
WILLISII, cujus maturâ ope, vindiciiſque
Conſcia Virtutis propriæ *Medicina* triumphat,
Nec veram, Ratio ſi deſit, ſe putat Artem.
Illa ſui certos præbet Mortalibus uſus,
Dum Methodum ſequitur facto & ratione probatam.
  Interea meritâ veheris ſuper æthera famâ,
  Naturæ interpres fidus, Phœbique Sacerdos,
  Abbrevians artem pariter, vitamque perennans.

Gul. Dawkins.

TO THE VERY FAMOUS AUTHOR, and to me (of which I am deservedly proud) A VERY GOOD FRIEND, for both parts of his Rational Pharmaceutics.[4]

The centuries, worried, poured restless plaints
In lasting marvel why Medicine in so many years
Has not come of age, why it has not yet kindled
Traditional bridal torches, nor grown to strength
In full, and has not reached the balanced use
Of solid reason, but stayed crude, childlike and lazy.
Of course fate had not yet given it the outstanding
WILLIS; with him, him as champion, bloom and force
And late fulfilment have come upon Apollo's Art.
Before, it could by laughing recognise Mother
Nature, and neatly greet you, her father, Phoebus
But could not stand on its own feet, entrusting all
To blind fortune and chance, instructed by the Master,
Seeking success through manifold errors;
And with tottering steps in the deep of night
It mixed audacious drinks, with uncertain results:
When he joins your side and freely places healing
Hands on ailing *Medicina*, while chasing darkness,
Lets in the Day, widely spreading new light
WILLIS; keen-sighted, Apollinic, versed in deep
Secrets of the human body, learned in ways
And paths where Medicines sneak in silence;
Now with herbs, then force countering illness
Moves the fine bowels with salubrious turmoil.
Of old, when the Doctor, like common folk,
Ignorant of proper skill, was baffled by Creation;
And faced perilous draughts of unknown drugs,
Sending pleas to you, Fortune, and clinging to hope
That such divine force might hide in simple juices.
At last there is a time that matter, its reasons and ways,
And sympathies and pursuits, long hiding in shade
Is explored with tools, and by faithful scrutiny
Mastered, allowing smooth practice by wondrous art.
Indeed a roaming swarm of volatile particles
Employs medical forces in the fluid body:
Tiny atoms, Servants of nature and art,
Rush nimbly hither and thither in their flight:
Penetrating distant nooks and sundry barriers
They rouse in one place, repress riot in another.
Now they reclaim from a ruffled stomach noxious
Juice, then they halt fluid rushing down bowels

[4] Translation by Jan van Gijn, 7 April 2018.

And deliver compact stools in orderly fashion.
In various ways they dispel the seeds of illness,
Here by tightening fibres, there by relaxing them.
Some force entry into veins, and in closed ranks
They curb rage and frenzy in the purple spate,
Like Salt, put in a bubbling cooking Pot,
Reduces swollen water to its former calm.
Now they return Matter, frozen by chill,
To its natural course and balmy flow:
As water freely added to a muddy swamp
Shows the safe bank by its steady stream.
Then they enter life's seat, fortress of enduring
Light, providing limbs with liquid warmth.
Or they pass glassy borders of nimble sense
And sort out traffic of spirits in wandering throngs.
Now life's airways, blocked since long, with cracked
Windpipe; they purge the hidden seeds of future
Ills, expel them far and wide from foetid fissures,
While they refill exhausted bellows with mild air.
Then they slink into the blood-filled spongy liver,
And joyfully attack the evil marring its task.
Or struggle to remove stagnant fluids from the skin
Or relieve the spleen, heavy with body's waste.
So by a thousand routes, by a thousand ways,
They draw diseases out as well as chase them
To know their sprightly moves, their hidden tracks,
What forces they have, to say *why* and *whence*,
This is the labour, task, the zeal and concern of Keen
WILLIS, through whose timely help and protection
Medicine triumphs, conscious of intrinsic merit,
And does not judge itself an Art if Reason is missing.
Its art provides trusted practices to Mortals,
If it follows a Method proved by fact and reason.
Meanwhile you wander in the sky by rightful fame,
Star interpreter of Nature, Priest of Apollo,
Shortening the art while also prolonging life.

Gul. Dawkins.

For anyone familiar with Willis's treatises, this was a neat and lyrical summary of his ideas on the particulate basis of fermentation, the circulation of blood nourished by digestion and respiration to the various organs, but especially those concerned with bodily movements, the removal of waste, and both the mechanisms and treatment of disease. It celebrated the transformation of ideas that his work had enabled. But since Willis's unexpected death had delayed the printing of *Pharmaceutice rationalis* part 2 in order to accommodate John Fell's notice, and although the dedicatory epistle was already written and not to be wasted, William Dawkins took the opportunity to add his own more sober posthumous thoughts on Willis within the hastily rearranged preliminaries:

QUERELA LIBRI POSTHUMI DE OBITU AUTORIS.

QUiſquis es, O ſicci procul abſint Lector ocelli;
Tingatur lacrymis pagina quæque tuis.
Geſtiet haſce pati charta officioſa lituras,
Deflens WILLISSII fata inopina ſui.
Scilicet hinc almæ vocor ad conſortia lucis,
Ut videam Dominum non ſupereſſe meum?
Perſonet ingratus noſtris vagitibus Orbis,
Diſcat & à nobis funera tanta queri.
Credideris Lector ſcripta immortalia volvens,
Quod potuit fato jura dediſſe ſuo.
Quanquam mille aditus latè panduntur in Orcum,
Mille ſagax vitæ repperit ille vias.
Cæſaris ad magni ritum, contra agmina mortis,
Pugnavit totos Marte favente dies.
Cumque hoſti intentum premeret nox ſera, redegit
Pernox ſucceſſus victor in acta ſuos.
Viderat autumno quot reſtituiſſet in illo,
Spargebat ſegnis quo pituita neces.
Indoluit *Fatum*: jamque æmula regna timebat,
Atque novus pallor Mortis in ore fuit.
Portitor infernus raptos fleviſſe trientes
Creditur, & vacuam deſeruiſſe ratem.
Tandem adit immites Mors indignata ſorores,
Nilque agimus, clamat, ſoſpite WILLISIO.
Quin hunc pallentes propere damnemus ad umbras,
Non aliter regni robora ſalva mei.
Annuerat truculenta trias, mora nulla ſecuta eſt,
Concita per medium tranſit arundo latus.
Invida *Phœbigenam* ſic dextera miſit in Orcum,
Cum medica fatum perdomuiſſet ope.
Sic etiam *Eurypylus* ſtraviſſe *Machaona* fertur,
Auſus adoratum contemerare caput.
Hac ſed flebilior nulla unquam victima, nunquam
Intravit Stygias ſanctior umbra domos.
Aurea præreptum *Cythereïa* flevit *Adonin*:
Heu mage WILLISIUM flet Medicina ſuum.
Extinctum magicæ reſonabant *Memnona* chordæ,
His at in exequiis carmina ſurda tacent.
Orphea Calliope mœſtis eſt queſta Camœnis,
Non patitur blandos noſtra querela modos.
Interea dictis *Libitina* abſiſte ſuperbis,
Luctibus hæc olim gaudia ſæva lues.
Poſthuma perpetuis reparantur prælia Chartis,
Et nova jam vindex Pagina bella geret.

Gul. Dawkins. MED. B.

LAMENTING IN A POSTHUMOUS BOOK ITS AUTHOR'S DEATH[5]

Whoever you are, Reader, let dry eyelets be far away;
   Let every page be stained with your tears,
The paper will welcome the task of bearing these blotches
   Bewailing WILLIS's unexpected fate.
Forsooth, am I called away to the sphere of propitious light
   To see that my Master is no longer alive?
Let the ungrateful Globe resound with laments,
   Let it also learn from us to mourn such great losses.
Reader, studying the immortal texts, could you believe
   That fate has rightfully treated him.
Though a thousand doors to Death are wide open,
   He cleverly found a thousand paths to life.
Like a great king he fought the ranks of death,
   All his life, with Victory on his side.
Though cruel darkness hovered, intent on its prey, he gained
   His successes throughout the night, victorious in actions.
He had seen how much he had put right in that autumn
   In which stagnant phlegm sprinkled deaths around.
Fate smarted: now she feared her reign was challenged,
   And even more pallid became the face of Death.
The underworld's ferryman bewailed his lost fees, so
   It is said, and he would have deserted his raft.
In the end Death calls upon her merciless sisters,
   Crying: we're useless, as long as WILLIS is alive.
We must speedily banish him to the pale shades,
   In no other way the power of my reign is safe.
The grim trio assented and no time was lost,
   An arrow, shot through the sky, pierces his side.
By envious hand she sent *Apollo*'s son to the Underworld,
   Though he had vanquished fate with medical aid.
Similarly, it is said, *Eurypylus* has slain *Machaon*,
   Daring to defile the worshipped face.
But no victim has ever been more deplored, never
   A more hallowed shade has crossed the river of Death.
Golden *Aphrodite* wept over her lost *Adonis*:
   O, Medicine weeps even more over her WILLIS.
Magic chords resounded in dead Memnon's statue,
   But in his remains mute songs remain silent.
Calliope, mother of *Orpheus*, grieved with sad songs,
   Our lamentation does not fit with melodies.
Meanwhile, Libitina, desist from proud statements,
   Once you will atone for these wild joys with grief.

[5] Translated by Jan van Gijn, 13 November 2019.

Posthumous battles will be resumed by Paper,
And each new Page will again engage in war.
Gul. Dawkins. MED. B.

From these accounts it might have seemed that Willis's reputation was ensured and no word of criticism would be uttered. But this was not to be. After his death, aged 54, Thomas Willis soon proved victim to waspish criticism. Loyal efforts were made to perpetuate his memory and elevate the reputation but it was not until the twentieth century that his originality and contributions were unreservedly acknowledged. Why, when the modern placement of Thomas Willis is in the first rank of clinician scientists to the extent that he has been dubbed the 'Harvey of the nervous system'[6] did his early reputation falter? After Fell, and over the next 66 years, three people in particular wrote contrasting accounts of Willis as entries in biographical encyclopaedia: Aubrey, who was factual and complimentary;[7] Wood who, rich in Oxonian waspishness, was not;[8] and Willis's grandson, Browne Willis (1682–1760) who, coming after the others, sought to set the record straight.

Wood's biography of Willis went through three iterations. First published in 1690, and reprinted without alteration other than to abbreviations and punctuation in 1721, further material relating to his grandfather was made available by Browne Willis through his account in the *General dictionary* and from a letter written in 1725 found inserted into Bishop Kennett's (1660–1728) copy of the 1690 edition of Wood's book.[9] With these additions, a final version of the entry appeared in the 1813 edition of *Athenæ Oxoniensis*, in which the letter to Kennett was printed in full.[10] It did not take long for the tone of Wood's book to be challenged, his love for gossip displacing discretion, so that a copy of the second volume was burned in public by order of the vice-chancellor, Henry Aldrich (1647–1710), and Wood was expelled from the University of Oxford.[11] Understandably, Browne Willis preferred the opinion of Fell to that of Wood: 'Bpp. Fell says much more of his charity, but as he knew

6 See: W Russell Brain, 'The concept of hysteria in the time of William Harvey', *Proceedings of the Royal Society of Medicine* 1963: 56; 317–24.

7 See: [John Aubrey] *'Brief lives', chiefly of contemporaries, set down by John Aubrey, between the years 1669 and 1696*, volume 2, Ed. Andrew Clark, Oxford (1898): pages 302–4; and John Aubrey. *Brief lives with an apparatus for the lives of our English mathematical writers*. Ed. Kate Bennett, Oxford (2015): pages 550–1 (volume 1) with notes on the edited entry at pages 1477–81 (volume 2).

8 See: [Anthony Wood] *Athenæ Oxoniensis. An exact history of all the writers and bishops who have had their education in the most ancient and famous University of Oxford, from the fifteenth year of King Henry the Seventh, Dom. 1500, to the end of the year 1690. Representing the birth, fortune, preferment, and death of all those authors and prelates, the great accidents of their lives, and the fate and character of their writings. To which are added, the Fasti or Annals, of the said University, for the same time*, volume 1. London (1690): pages 402–3, entries 364–5; *Athenæ Oxoniensis*, volume 2, London (1721): pages 549–52, entry 408; and *Athenæ Oxoniensis*, volume 3, London, and Oxford (1817) [1813–1820]: pages 1048–53, entry 550.

9 See: [Browne Willis], 'Willis (Thomas)'. In: [John Bernard, Thomas Birch, John Locke, and other hands] *A general dictionary, historical and critical: in which a new and accurate translation of that celebrated Mr. Bayle with the corrections and observations printed in the late edition at Paris, is included; and interspersed with several thousand lives never before published. The whole containing the history of the most illustrious persons of all ages and nations, particularly those of Great Britain and Ireland, distinguished by their rank, actions, learning and other accomplishments*, volume X, London (1741): pages 171–5. The essay has a hand sign indicating that it is new and signed 'T'. Everything suggests that it is by Browne Willis, as confirmed in his correspondence with Philip Morant, see next. This copy was owned by Richard Gough (1735–1809) and bequeathed with most of his books to the Bodleian Library. See: *The Gentleman's Magazine* 1 February 1831: page 564.

10 See: Wood (1817): footnote 3, pages 1048–50.

11 See: Sir Charles Symonds, 'The circle of Willis'. The Harveian oration delivered at the Royal College of Physicians of London on 18 October 1954, reprinted from the *British Medical Journal* for 15 January, London (1955): pages 1–16.

him near 30 years, your lordship will give him leave to know him better than A. Wood'. This swipe at Wood apart, the letter to Kennett mainly corrects or provides fresh information on aspects of Willis's life. Later, on 11 February 1756, Browne Willis wrote to Reverend Philip Morant (1700–1770) expressing pleasure that Morant was engaged in a biography of Thomas Willis and wishing that he might help but, being over 73 years old, he had written what he could about his most learned and excellent grandfather in the tenth volume of the *General dictionary*. The difficulty with Anthony Wood he put down to 'dissention among servants setting them at variance'. With the subsequent full rehabilitation of Willis's reputation, the tables have turned and it is now the verdict on Wood that is qualified:[12]

> Although unrivalled as Oxford's greatest antiquarian and diarist ... [he was] ... never anything but a fierce hater, with very little sense of humour, a great capacity for making himself and all around him both disagreeable and miserable.

Thomas Willis in Oxford: 1621–1666

Thomas Willis was born on 27 January 1621 at Great Bedwyn, Wiltshire, a village on the edge of the forest at Savernake that prospered through the wool trade and had a population at the time of *c.*2000 (see: Figure 2). His baptism was recorded in the Church register on 14 February:[13]

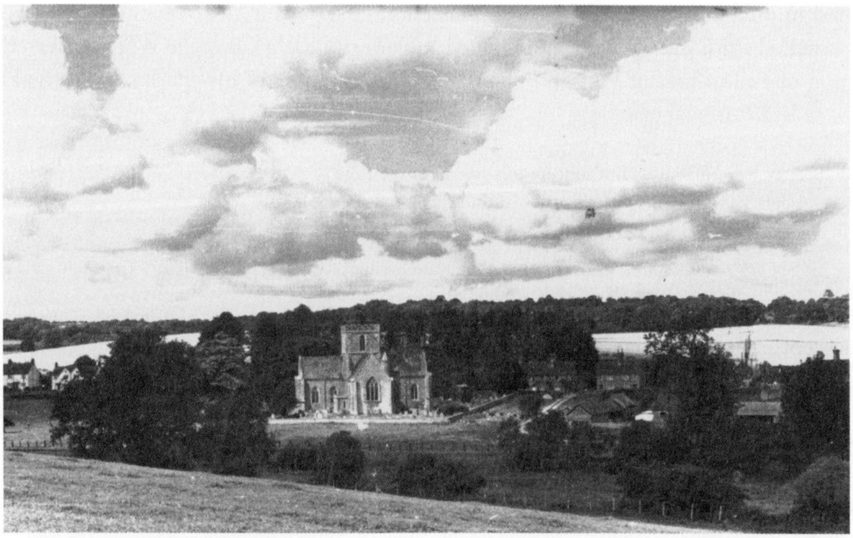

Figure 2 Great Bedwyn, Wiltshire; the birthplace of Thomas Willis. From a postcard purchased in the village by Raymond Hierons, *c.*1960.

[12] Cited from earlier sources in William Feindel, 'The life of Thomas Willis'. In: *The anatomy of the brain and nerves*, volume 1, Montreal (1965): page 7. See also: William Feindel, 'The beginnings of neurology: Thomas Willis and his circle of friends'. In: Ed. F Clifford Rose, *A short history of neurology. The British contribution 1660–1910*, Oxford (1999): pages 1–18.

[13] See: Hughes (1991): page 5. This was prior to Lady Day (25 March) allowing the year of his birth sometimes to be misquoted, according to the Julian calendar, as 1620.

> *Thomas Wyllis the sonne of Thomas Willis and Rachell his wyffe was baptised the xiiij day of February anno predicto.*

Trevor Hughes found the entry to be damaged. At some point, chemicals had been applied causing the page to darken and become barely legible, and with Browne Willis having added to the original wording:

> NB. He was the most Famous Physitian in the World in his tyme & dying Nov. the 11th 1675 in the 54th year of his age, was buried in Westminster Abbey.

Thomas was the eldest son of Thomas Willis (1575–1643) about whom opinions differed as to his education and social standing.[14] For Fell, Willis's father was Master of Arts in the University of Oxford and, whatever his subsequent occupation, could rest comfortably in his grave 'being enough deserving of the World, who begat such a Son'. Aubrey has it from Thomas Willis 'himself' that his father 'was steward to Sir Walter Smyth ... and had been sometime a scholar at St. John's College in Oxford'. Later he adds: 'His father was steward to Sir John (I thinke) Smyth and had a little estate at Ivy Hinksey'. This is corrected in footnote 4 (presumably by Andrew Clark) to 'Sir Walter Smith of Great Bedwyn, Wilts.[15] The older Thomas Willis may also have served as a menial butler to Sir George Stonehouse of Radley (1603–1675).[16] Always ready to disparage Willis, according to Wood his father was:

> Sometime a retainer to *S. John's* Coll. (but no Graduate) afterwards Bailiff or Steward to Sir *Walt. Smith* of *Bedwyn*, and in his last days a constant Inhabitant of N. Henxsey ... Which last Thomas Willis was Son of another Thomas, a Taylor, as I have been informed, who mostly lived at *Kennington* near *Abingdon* also.

Browne Willis rehearsed the matter of his great-grandfather's education and occupation in his letter to Kennett, putting right the family history[17] and, in passing, making clear his feelings about Wood:

> I most readily obey your lordshipp's commands in communicating something of my good grandfather Dr. Willis. A. Wood, who was his next neighbour in St. John Baptist's parish Oxon, and had a disagreement with the family, says several things untrue of his descent ... what is delivered as hear-say by Mr Wood concerning our author's ancestors and extraction, may be justly questioned ... By an ancient deed I have ... wee were an yeoman family at Church Hanborough in Oxfordshire about the beginning of queen Elizabeth's reign ... [but] can't find so much a name of a Willis, till some years after 1600 and not Thomas Willis in any of these places till about 1630 ... In Great Bedwin register, co. Wilts, ... I met with several Willis's before 1620 and an entry of the birth of my good grandfather, who is the last of the name of Willis born there.

[14] See: Andrew Hegarty, *A biographical register of St John's College, Oxford, 1555–1660*, Martlesham (2011): pages 488–9 for biographical details of Thomas Willis's father in connection with St John's College.

[15] See: Aubrey (1898): pages 302–4; and Bennett [Aubrey] (2015): page 550 and 1478.

[16] See: Hughes (1991); and Robert Martensen, 'Willis, Thomas (1621–1675)'. *Oxford dictionary of national biography* (2004a), https://doi.org/10.1093/ref:odnb/29587 citing Bodl. Oxf., MS Aubrey 12, fol. 294*r*, which is footnote ** in Aubrey (1898).

[17] Browne Willis acknowledged that the name Willis was not to be found in the registers of Hinksey, 'wherefore the pedigree seems to want foundation'. See: Additional manuscripts 37222 (f 114–5, f127–8, and f 139), British Library, transcribed by Raymond Hierons.

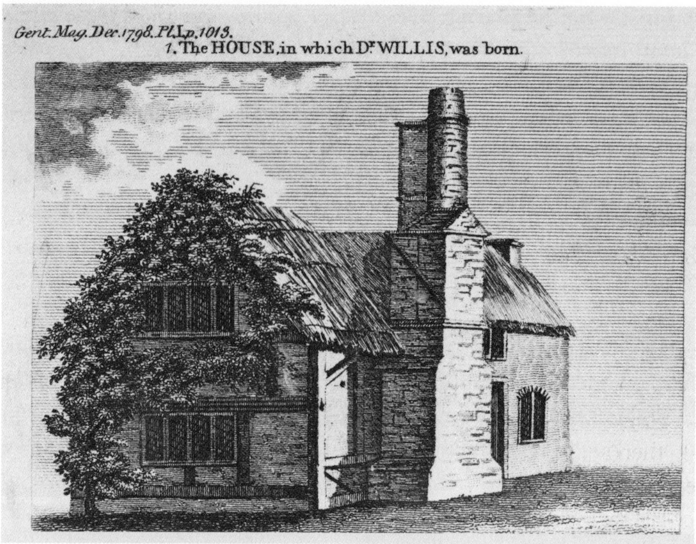

Figure 3 'The HOUSE in which Dr WILLIS, was born.' *Gentleman's Magazine* December 1798. Pl.1, page 1019.

Trevor Hughes examined original local county records and established that the family came from the adjacent villages of Church Handborough and Long Handborough, each on land owned by St John's College, Oxford. Francis Willis (d.1597: also Wyllys), president of the College from 1577 to 1590, may have been a relative. If we are left unsure of the education and occupations of Thomas Willis's ancestors, we do know that Willis's mother was Rachel (née Howell: d.1631) and she married Thomas in *c.*1600.[18]

In April 1969, realizing that his own country house at Ham was only 5 miles away and learning that the house where Willis lived as a child (originally Ivy Cottage but later renamed The Castle) still existed, Charles Symonds paid a visit (see: Figure 3).[19] The owner, Mr Sherwill Thomas (nd), showed a cutting from the *Gentleman's Magazine* referring to the house in Farm Lane:[20]

> Remarkable for its antique appearance, being almost overgrown with ivy, and having a cylindrical stone chimney to which another of brick had been added in which that illustrious physician, Dr Willis, was born and where there is a print of the Doctor in the house said… to have been left there by his grandson, Browne Willis.

The house was presumed originally to have been part of a larger monastic building since the beams and chimney were inappropriately large. Rachel inherited land (50 to 75 acres) at North Hinksey[21] but she soon died and was buried on 5 July 1631 in the parish church of St Lawrence where the stone marking her grave is still present. Willis's father then married

[18] She was said to be descended from William Wykeham (1320–1404), Bishop of Winchester and Chancellor of England, who founded New College, Oxford (1379) and Winchester College (1382).

[19] See: Sir Charles Symonds and William Feindel, 'Birthplace of Thomas Willis', *British Medical Journal* 1969: 3 (13 September); 648–9.

[20] See: 'The house in which Dr Willis was born', *Gentleman's Magazine* (December 1798): plate X, page 1013.

[21] This was visited by Trevor Hughes and described in much architectural detail. See: Hughes (1991): pages 8–9.

a widow, Elizabeth (also known as Magdalene) Ruffin (nd), whose five children joined the household. Willis's father moved later to Ferry Cottage, North Hinksey, near Oxford, where he died from camp fever shortly before the first siege of Oxford in the Civil War (1642–1651). This was followed 10 days later by the death of Elizabeth, Willis's stepmother, leaving Thomas, then aged around 20 years, responsible for his siblings.

The subsequent history of the family is well documented.[22] All first-born sons of the Willis family were named Thomas, down to Browne Willis's grandson and heir (Thomas Willis: 1738–1762) who was unmarried. His interests passed to Thomas's half-brother, John Willis (1749–1802) who also died without issue. By private act in 1767, John took on the name of Fleming, being the grandparental surname of Browne Willis's wife Katherine (née Eliot: 1686–1724), Thomas Fleming (1609–1638). The line descended through the family of Browne Willis's younger son, Henry Willis (1713–1747). By a further private act of 1813, the surname Willis Fleming was taken by Henry's grandson John Fleming Barton Willis (1781–1844), thereafter John Willis Fleming. The surname survives by direct descent through five further generations to Thomas Willis Fleming (b.1958), now the senior representative of the family, and the direct descendant of Dr Thomas Willis in the male line through ten generations.

Willis attended Edward Sylvester's (*c.*1586–1653) school at 135 High Street in Oxford, also known as Sylvester's Academy, 'where he ayred his muse and made good exercise' and was 'bred in grammar learning'.[23] Browne Willis learned from local villagers that Thomas gave to the poor the food he carried to school in the walk across Botley water meadows until observed by his parents who declared that 'this boy will starve himself and would latterly make him eat his meat at home before he went to schoole'. Willis was admitted as a battler at Christ Church. Strictly, a student supplied with provisions from the buttery who paid only for what he consumed, this was one of the third rank of '*pauperes scholares, mediastini*', also described as sizars or servitors and ranking below gentlemen commoners. Servitors had menial duties and were required to serve the gentlemen commoners, clean their shoes, and wait at table:[24]

> The difference, Sir, between us Serviters, and Gentlemen Commoners is this, that we are men of Wit, and no Fortune, and they are Men of Fortune and no Wit.

Willis was under the patronage of Dr Thomas Iles (d.1649), one of the canons of Christ Church. Iles's wife knew about physic and surgery and suggested various remedies. Aubrey writes that:[25]

> Tom Willis ... wore a blew livery-cloake and studied at the lower end of the Hall by the Hall-dore, was pretty handy, and his Mistresse would oftentimes have him to assist her in making of Medicines, this did him no hurt and allured him on.

[22] See: Willis Fleming Historical Trust http://www.willisfleming.org.uk/; and Harry Willis Fleming: personal communication, 21 June 2020.

[23] See: Wood, volume 2, (1692): column 703; and Bennett [Aubrey] (2015): page 1479. Sylvester was educated at Balliol College and gave private tuition in Latin and Greek. He was the 'common drudge' of the University charged with editing 'Latin sermons of certain dull Theologists' before these were delivered at St Mary's Church. Students in divinity, law, and physics hosted an annual feast at which Sylvester presided.

[24] See: lines in a play by Thomas Baker, *An act at Oxford*, London (1704), although usually attributed to Samuel Johnson (1709–1784).

[25] Hughes (1991): page 9 makes the point that the limited information on Willis's education comes from John Aubrey. See: Bennett [Aubrey] (2015): page 551 and page 1481 for discussion that the Hall-dore was furthest from the high-table and close to the kitchens. The blue cloak was worn by those in receipt of charitable education.

Willis was grateful for this help and his grandson, Browne Willis, erected a monument in memory of Thomas Iles at Christ Church in 1759:[26]

> MS THOMAS ILES STP. Hujus Ædis Canonici; Qui obijt 20 Iunii 1649: Cuius intèr Encomia non hoc erat minimum, Quod ſub ejus Auſpiciis ac Patrocinio Academicæ Eruditionis Elementa Hâc in Æde hauſerat THOMAS WILLIS MD Literato in Orbe Notiſſimus Uiro De ipſius Avo, etiam̃que de Patriâ Optimè merito Hoc parentavit MNEMOSYNON BW: LL.D.

Willis matriculated on 3 March 1636/7. Aubrey says that he studied:[27]

> Chymistry in Peckwater Inne chamber ... he was in those dayes very Mathematicall, and I have heard him say his genius lay more to Mathematiques than Chymistry.

All students were required to take a course in Liberal Arts in order to qualify for the degree of Master of Arts, as determined by the constitution of the University of Oxford in 1636. The university statutes required instruction in grammar, rhetoric, logic, politics, economics, and ethics using Greek and Latin texts. A dominant source of information was Aristotle (385–323 BC). This curriculum was adapted by the tutor and College to which the student was attached and extended beyond the humanities to include mathematics, astronomy, and science. Dewhurst and Trevor Hughes assume that Willis followed these courses but also gained some knowledge of medicine.[28] Willis graduated Bachelor of Arts on 19 June 1639 and Master of Arts on 18 June 1642. This latter degree was awarded following four days of examination which concluded with a discussion on various topics in St Mary's Church.[29]

Eleven days before Willis graduated, parliament had delivered nineteen propositions to Charles I (1600–1649), which he rejected, leading to the Civil War. Oxford became the Royalist headquarters after Charles's retreat from the battle of Edgehill (23 October 1642) until the city surrendered to Thomas Fairfax (1612–1671) in June 1646.[30] As a Royalist, Willis was 'harassed by the Incursions of the Rebels' operating from a nearby garrison that threatened to raid the house in Hinksey where he was then living. Fell wrote that Willis:

[26] See: Hughes (1991): page 10. Some details that follow are taken from Raymond Hierons, *The man and his personalites*, an unpublished typescript with manuscript annotations by Hierons headed 'I wrote this over 30 years ago and never completed it'. See also: Sir Charles Symonds, 'Thomas Willis F.R.S. (1621–1675)', *Notes and Records of the Royal Society of London* 1960: 15; 91–7, reproduced in *The Royal Society. Its origins and founders*. Ed. Sir Harold Hartley F.R.S., London (1960): pages 91–7.

[27] See: Bennett [Aubrey] (2015): page 550. Trevor Hughes has examined the University of Oxford records and considers that the correct date is 1638.

[28] See: Kenneth Dewhurst, *Thomas Willis as a physician*, Los Angeles (1964): pages 1–20; Dr Kenneth Dewhurst, 'Willis in Oxford: some new MSS'. In: Commemoration of the Septencentenary of Merton College, Oxford, *Proceedings of the Royal Society of Medicine* 1964: 57; 682–7; and Kenneth Dewhurst, 'Thomas Willis and the foundations of British neurology'. In Ed. F Clifford Rose and WF Bynum, *Historical aspects of the neurosciences. A festschrift for Macdonald Critchley*, New York (1982): pages 327–46.

[29] John Ward (1629–1681), a contemporary of Willis, was required to debate whether the delights of summer were more numerous than those of winter: summer was favoured after 15 minutes exchange in Latin. See: D'Arcy Power, 'John Ward and his diary', *Transactions of the Medical Society of London* 1917: 40; 1–26; reprinted in Sir D'Arcy Power *Selected writings*, Oxford (1931): pages 172–200; and Robert Frank, 'The John Ward diaries: mirror of seventeenth century science and medicine', *Journal of the History of Medicine and Allied Sciences* 1974: 29; 147–79.

[30] St Mary's College, now Frewin Hall and part of Brasenose College, was (from 1644 to 1646) the royal army's only medical facility in the city; see: Jessie Childs, *London Review of Books* 3 January 2019, page 25, citing Eds. David Appelby and Andrew Hopper, *Battle-scarred: mortality, medical care and military welfare in the British civil wars*, Manchester (2018).

> Returned to the Tents of the King as well of the Muses ... listing himself a Souldier in the University Legions, he received Pay for some years; until the Cause of the Best Prince being overcome, Cromwell's Tyranny afforded to this wretched Nation a Peace more cruel than any War.

The University legion consisted of 600 students under arms. Willis was involved in defence of the city entrance at Magdalen College Grove from assault by a Parliamentary battery on Headington Hill; but he may also have been posted to the Royal Garrison at Wallingford Castle.[31] Wood writes that those who enlisted soon became:

> Much debauched and idle by their bearing arms and keeping company with rude soldiers ... gaming, drinking, swearing, etc ... they were so guilty of those vices, that those that were looked upon as good wits ... were by strange inventions (not now to be named) to entice them to drinking and to be drunk, totally lost and rendered useless.

As his grandson made clear, Willis resisted such degenerate behaviour and did not ignore his studies:

> He among the Scholars that were then remaining, bore Arms in [the King's] defence, and all the time that he could obtain, he bestowed on his beloved Study of Physic.

With religious activities suppressed, and his experience with Mrs Iles at Christ Church expanded through concern with the issues of camp fever, Willis veered away from the obligation for ordination on members of the university and turned to medicine. Qualification could only be conferred by examination in the universities of Oxford or Cambridge, or patronage granted by the king or Archbishop of Canterbury. Although there was no actual requirement for attendance and tuition could be obtained in continental Europe, Willis did study at Oxford in line with the Caroline code instituted under revised statutes drafted by William Laud (1573–1645), Archbishop of Canterbury. Students were required to attend twice weekly lectures. The lecturer spoke slowly in Latin for 45 minutes so that notes could be taken and questions asked before the hour was up. There was a 10s fine on the lecturer for noncompliance and 4d on students who did not attend. Instruction was by the regius professor of medicine, the two lecturers in medicine attached to Merton College, and the Tomlins reader in anatomy (to which the regius professor might be appointed).[32] The last was significant for what followed since the terms of the lectureship required that a 'sounde body' of a person executed after the Lent Assizes in Oxford be dissected annually by a surgeon who demonstrated the different parts and their 'site, nature, use and office'. The student also had to participate in two public discussions and deliver six one-hour lectures on Galen. In principle, the course lasted 14 years: four to graduate Bachelor of Arts, three more to become Master of Arts; four to qualify as Bachelor of Medicine, and four for a doctorate. This extended course might be shortened on request for those who had studied away from Oxford.

[31] A full account of the role played by Willis in the Civil War is given by Kenneth Dewhurst, *Willis's Oxford casebook (1650–1652)*, Oxford (1981): pages 5–21.

[32] See: HM Sinclair and AHT Robb-Smith, *A short history of anatomical teaching in Oxford*, Oxford (1950): pages 10–15 for details based on their catalogue for an exhibition held at the Radcliffe Science Library from 20 February to 29 July 1950.

Willis's teachers were few but there was an undercurrent of new learning influenced by the writings of Francis Bacon (1561–1626), William Gilbert (1544–1603), and William Harvey (1578–1657) who was attached to the Royal household in Oxford when King Charles I took up residence at Christ Church. Harvey remained in Oxford between 1642 and 1646, becoming warden of Merton College in 1645.[33] Harvey visited George Bathurst (d.1645 whilst defending Faringdon), father of Willis's friend Ralph Bathurst (1620–1704) who 'had a henne to hatch eggs in his chamber ... [so that he and Harvey] daily opened [the eggs] to discern the progress'. Later Willis referred to 'our most famous Harvey [who] hath laid the Circulation of the Blood as a new Foundation in medicine'. Willis may have been present when Harvey demonstrated circulation of the blood in a live dog; and Willis was not alone in building the entire edifice of his own ideas on the fact that the blood is changed by nutrition and respiration, and that it circulates. Another influence was William Petty (1623–1687), a physician scientist close to Willis in years, and deputy to Sir Thomas Clayton (1612–1693) the son of Sir Thomas Clayton (1575–1647) who recommended Willis's graduation as a physician. Both Claytons were appointed regius professor of medicine in Oxford (1611–1647; and 1647–1665, respectively). The younger Clayton was considered the worst regius in the entire history of the University, described by Wood as 'posses'd with a timorous and effeminate Humour [who] could never endure the sight of a mangled or bloody body'.[34] In the event, with interruptions from the Civil War, Willis studied for only four and a half years, graduating Bachelor of Medicine on 8 December 1646. Without the intervention of Thomas Clayton before Cromwell's troops arrived in Oxford, this might never have happened.

After qualification in medicine but still without much experience, Willis 'fell to the practice of it and every Monday kept Abingdon market', sharing a horse with Dr Richard Lydall (1621–1704: later warden of Merton College) and where he was also joined by Ralph Bathurst, ordained in 1644 but turning to medicine during the Civil War.[35] These physicians competed against unlicensed practitioners wielding 'a sword in a blind man's hand'. Petty described Willis 'casting waters', a reference to the prescribing of medicines based on examination of the urine without the patient necessarily being present. Presumably this is where Willis first tasted the sweetness of diabetic urine. This practice did not always serve him well. On 1 August 1650, the son of widow Wise of Stadhampton brought a sample of his sick mother's urine which Willis found to be red, thick, and turbid. He suspected that it was menstrual fluid 'but there was no one who could tell me for sure'. Prescribing a light emetic, to treat Mrs Wise's headaches and abdominal pain, within two days the patient had developed unmistakeable signs of smallpox.[36]

In the thirteen years after medical qualification and throughout the Commonwealth period (1649–1660), Willis continued his practice and taught anatomy in the university despite Oxford being held by Cromwell's troops. He moved to the parish of St John the Baptist living, from 1657, at Beam Hall opposite Merton College. Beam Hall originally referred to what are now numbers 3 and 4 Merton Street, with number 3 (at present

[33] See: Hughes (1991): pages 14–17.

[34] See: Gunther *Early medical and biological science*, London (1926): pages 88–90 for reproduction of a contemporary derogatory rhyme popular amongst students that derided Clayton's squeamishness when dissecting corpses taken from the gibbet, and his lectures: 'Hee trembled more to reade, I hope / Then the fellow did when hee came to the rope / etc.'

[35] See: Bennett [Aubrey] (2015): page 1479 for discussion of the need for newly qualified medical practitioners to ply for trade in markets; and William Petty's claim that whilst he was 'at the top of practice at Oliver's Court, when Dr Willis was casting waters at Abingdon Market' in 1656, later acknowledging that, even by 1652, Willis's practice was larger than his own.

[36] See: Dewhurst (1981): page 43.

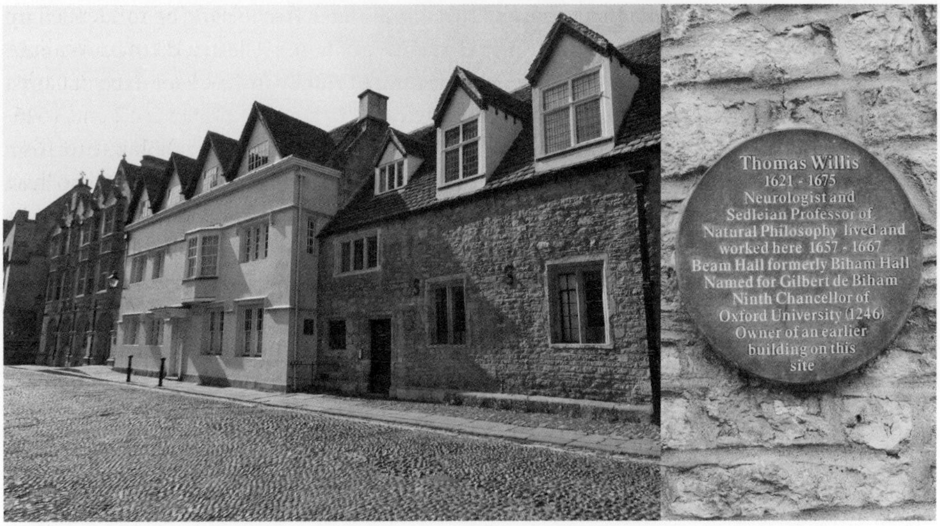
Thomas Willis
1621 - 1675
Neurologist and
Sedleian Professor of
Natural Philosophy lived and
worked here 1657 - 1667
Beam Hall formerly Biham Hall
Named for Gilbert de Biham
Ninth Chancellor of
Oxford University (1246)
Owner of an earlier
building on this
site

Figure 4 Numbers 3 and 4, Merton Street, with the plaque in memory of Thomas Willis identifying Beam Hall, formerly Biham Hall, placed on number 4.

the lodgings of the president of Corpus Christi College) serving as the main house, and number 4 forming the kitchen and service area. These were separated into two dwellings at some point during the twentieth century, perhaps restoring an earlier arrangement. The plaque identifying the house where Thomas Willis lived is placed on number 4, whereas he actually lived at number 3 Merton Street providing space for his family and household, including a coachman, valet, three other servants, and an apothecary (see: Figure 4). The site originally accommodated a building bought by Gilbert de Biham (nd), chancellor of the University in 1246. Biham subsequently became the owner of number 3, from William de Bosco (nk: later also chancellor of the University), in 1248. When this building was demolished, the space was known, for a while, as Beam Hall Garden. Both sites were purchased by Corpus Christi College in 1553 from whom Willis leased the replacement buildings. It is number 4 that members of the College, past and present, know as 'Beam Hall'. This corruption in name is thought to have occurred during the Latinate period in Oxford when phonetic spellings were often adopted. The existing plaque in memory of Willis was recently revised to reflect the earlier history.[37]

The buildings that comprised Beam Hall amounted to a substantial property. In 1665, Willis had to pay eight shillings 'hearth tax' based on two shillings for each fireplace. In 1667, he was required to pay poll tax: £5 for being a physician, two shillings in the pound for his practice and 20 shillings for every £100 income. There was no escape for Willis since, as commissioner for the parish of St Michael, his brother John was responsible for levying the taxes. Given that all Anglican rituals were prohibited by the puritans, 'even to the danger of his life', Willis used 'part of his House for Holy uses [holding] Assemblies, and Publick Prayers, and other Offices of Piety ... according to the Rites of the Church of England'. There

[37] Details provided by Alastair Buchan following the initiative of Valentine Cunningham, fellow of Corpus Christi College, Oxford, in 2014. Subsequent clarification of the use of 3 and 4 Merton Street was provided by Julian Reid, archivist to Corpus Christi and Merton Colleges. To the right of Beam/Biham Hall are the Merton College stables and Postmaster's Hall where Anthony à Wood lived (and which also has a plaque in his memory).

were present, amongst others, John Dolben (1625–1686: later, Archbishop of York), Richard Allestry (1619–1681: later provost of Eton, and a relative of James Allestry, d.1670, who published several of Willis's books), and John Fell (his future brother-in-law, later dean of Christ Church and vice-chancellor of the University of Oxford).[38]

As his reputation increased, Willis became wealthy and, by 1659, he was able to buy from Aubrey the Manor House of Burlton Court in Burghill, Herefordshire, set in 240 acres, even though it was occupied by tenants. It may have been sold to cover Aubrey's debts and the costs of a lawsuit. This did not stop Willis from haggling over the price of £1200.[39] But Willis could afford to pay since his income, £300 per annum, was the highest for any physician in Oxford in that year, and he also had accumulated £300 capital. He was generous to his family, as Anthony Wood conceded:

> When he came into business tis certain he maintained his brother and sisters. He paid several debts of his brother William, who dyed fellow of Trinity College, Oxford, as I find by his account and Mr Benson his nephew, archdeacon of Hereford, who dyed a non-juror aged about 86 last year, told me. He had several sisters well married, and a puritanical brother one John Willis[40] a good attorney, chapter clerk of Christ Church college who drew up all the leases &c. of that college.

Willis's clinical casework

Willis made clear that he did not find the existing literature sufficient for the practice of medicine. In the 1650s, his preferred method for learning about disease was to study patients. The preface to his treatise on fevers (1659) makes this clear:

> Altho that I know well enough, I have not obtained it, yet I will freely profess, that I have aimed at this Mark; and perhaps I may have deserved some praise, even in failing in these sort of Adventures; for after I had not found in Books, what might satisfy a mind desirous of Truth, I resolved with my self, to search into living and breathing Examples: and therefore sitting oftentimes by the Sick, I was wont carefully to search out their Cases, to weigh all the Symptoms, and to put them, with exact Diaries of the Diseases, into writing; then diligently to meditate on these, and to compare some with others; and then began to adapt general Notions from particular Events.

[38] Footnote 4 (page 1050) to the 1813 edition of *Athenæ Oxoniensis* indicates that a copy of *Prayers or intercessions for their use, who mourn in secret for the publique calamaties of the Nation. With an anniversary prayer for the 30 of January* (1650) previously owned by Mary Cary had an inscription in Browne Willis's hand: 'N.B. I was informed by the rev. Mr. Roper of St John's College in Cambridge, that these are the prayers which were used in Dr. Willis's oratory, during the former rebellion. J.C. May 25, 1729'. William Osler (1849–1919) suggests that a picture hanging in the hall of Christ Church, in his day, showing Dolben, Allestry, and Fell with a copy of the liturgy open in front of them was painted in Willis's house at Beam Hall.

[39] See: Dewhurst (1964) citing John Aubrey, Bodleian Library MS: 1662, f254, and 255r. Dewhurst (1981): page 3 has the cost as £1900 with Willis negotiating for time to come up with the final £300.

[40] Browne Willis (1741) writes that John had a daughter Margaret who married George Cooper, of the parish of Holywell in Oxford. They had a son also George Cooper (1696–1763) who matriculated at New College on 20 August 1715, aged 19. He became a fellow of the college in 1717 but was required to relinquish that fellowship in 1736, upon marriage. He had graduated in medicine (1725) and practised as a physician in Oxford and Bedford. Thomas Willis's uncle (John), the brother of his father, moved to Liverpool where he and his own son Thomas were wealthy merchants. Dates for these family members have not been found. Wood's details on the relationship of Mr Benson to Willis, and his age at death, appear incorrect.

Much can be gleaned about the patients Willis saw from his treatises, most of which are illustrated by case reports. The correspondence of Aubrey, Richard Lower (1631–1691) and Robert Boyle (1627–1691) provides another source of information. Some of Willis's surviving letters describe his cases.[41] In 1664/5 Willis wrote to Dr Nathaniel Hodges (1629–1688) explaining that although he had not seen the patient, he was concerned that his earlier speculations had been unsatisfactory and he was loath to recommend treatment 'in soe pertinacious a disease as hers'. Nonetheless, he advised purging, induced vomiting, an abdominal foment, and the pills and liquor that (evidently) he and Hodges had previously discussed. Much is given on the timing of these remedies with respect to intake of food and fluids. Willis suggests that the mineral water he has obtained locally[42] may be sufficient without needing to send to Tunbridge for medicinal water. Several letters involve correspondence with Dr Higgs (nd) of Coventry (see: Figure 5). Some are evidently in Willis's hand and others dictated to an amanuensis. These letters date from 1666 to 1672 by which time Willis was based in London.[43] Some of the handwriting is similar to that in the Oxford casebook despite the interval of 15 years. In an undated fragment, Willis recounts that:

> After I parted from you [presumably Dr Higgs] and was come to Banbury, I met with a messenger to carry me back to Warwick, where I am now lately arrived, Mrs Childe has had 2 fitts since we left it. Besides ye remedy we directed her and meanwhile other remedies are sent in and commended from severall hands. I shall leave it wholly to my Lord and Ladies to admit or not from them. I shall motion that when I get home tomorrow you may be sent for, and Mr Cooke[44] shall give you an account of what has been done.
>
> I have met with a Gentlewoman that is of kin to my wife, Mrs Grandy who has desired my advice, and after I had mentioned to her all I would have done in her case, shee told mee at last that that shee had bin yor patient whereupon I replied that what I had prescribed should be showed to you, and if there should be occasion that wee might meet to consult together.
>
> Besides general remedies for the [undecipherable] use: I think it is necessary something be done in order to her frequent miscarriages shee has had, and in particular in order to a hurt she had 10 months since by a fall, which made her miscarry, Mrs Childe was much bruised, and ever since shee has had a paine in her body, on one side with some other symptoms that imply shee has had some hurt on ye body of ye womb which will not easily be remedied . . . [letter curtailed here].

41 Writing from the reading room of the British Museum on 21 March 1961, Elizabeth Palmer, of 132 Harley St, London, W1, wrote to Raymond Hierons explaining that she had found three letters from Browne Willis to Philip Morant; a long letter in Latin from Willis to an unknown correspondent (MS ADD 34727); two in English to Dr Hodges (Sloane MS 810 f229) and Mr White (Sloane MS 1513 f1), respectively; and case notes, with a commentary by Henry Power, both in Latin, on Mr Richard Fincham. Raymond Hierons remained sceptical about the authenticity of the letter to Mr White given the subject matter and style. However, Willis undoubtedly did correspond with a Mr White (see next).

42 This is the famous water from the stream at East Throp that Willis discovered with Lower (see next).

43 The thirteen letters at St John's College Library, Oxford, are referred to by kind permission of Dr Petra Hofmann. Three are written by Willis, two in English and one in Latin. Those presumed to have been written by an amanuensis are scribbled with many abbreviations and largely undecipherable, other than getting a general sense of offering advice to Dr Higgs on management.

44 Presumably this is James Cooke (1614–1694) who practised at Warwick and wrote *Mellificium Chirurgiæ: or the marrow of chirurgery, much enlarged to which is now added anatomy illustrated with twelve brass cuts and also the marrow of physic both in the newest way*, London (1676). The leaf endorsing the work before the title page reads: 'Having perused Mr. *James Cook's* Marrow of Chirurgery, I cannot but well approve it; and think it may prove a very useful Book. The Author I know to be skilful in his Profession. *Tho. Willis*. M.O *Sept*. 25. 1675.'

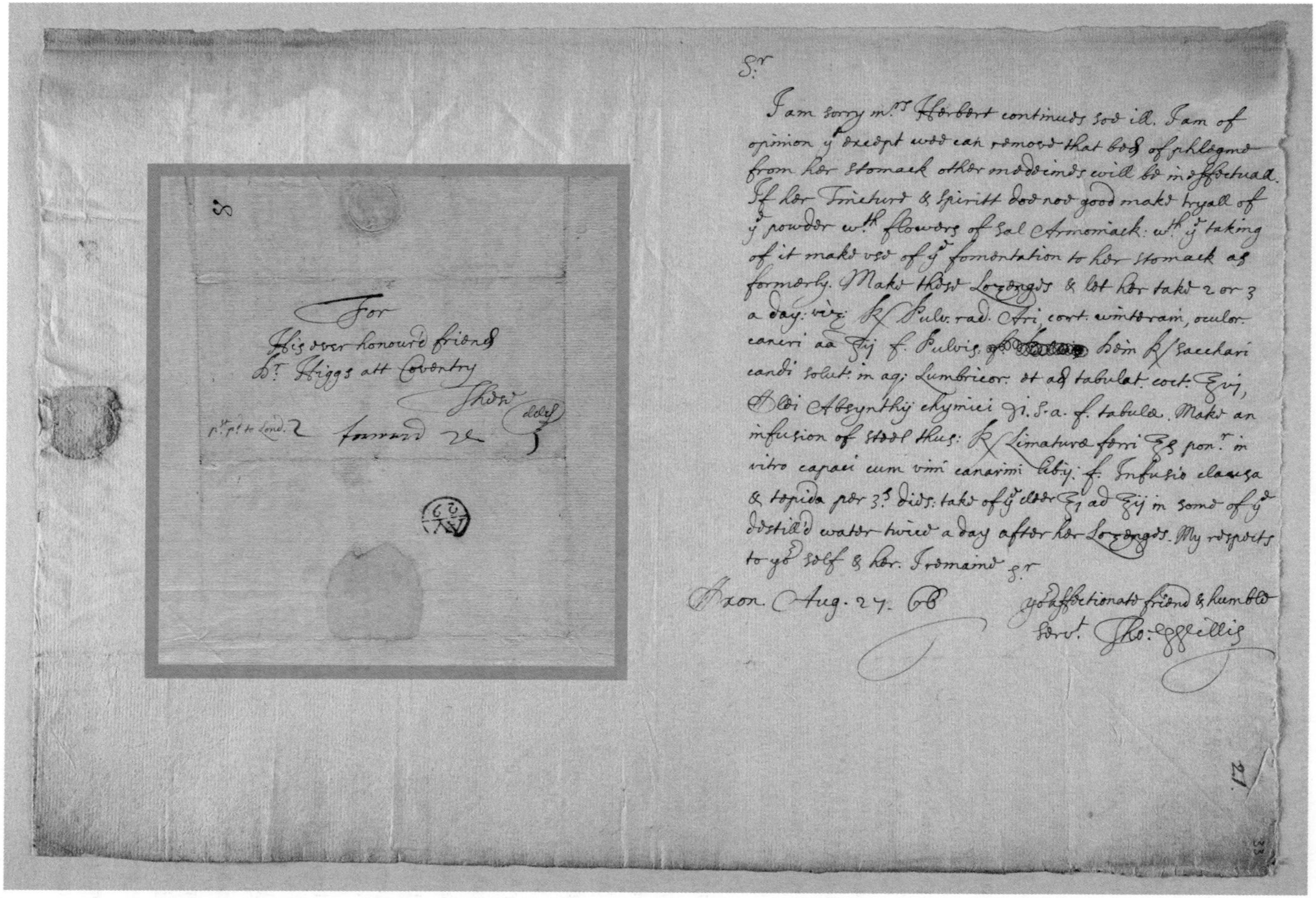

Figure 5 Manuscript letter in the hand of Thomas Willis to Dr Higgs at Coventry dated 27 August 1666.

By permission of the President and the Fellows of St John's College, Oxford.

The other letters, apparently following earlier correspondence, relate to a variety of patients and mostly contain suggestions on purges, vomits, and bleeding, and frequency and timing of medicines needed to deal with symptoms that are not described. In his own handwriting on 27 August 1666, Willis writes expressing regret that 'Mrs Herbert continues so ill but confident that the body of phlegm can be removed from her stomack'. There follows a long list of remedies, including lozenges to be taken three times each day followed by distilled water, and fomentations that Willis recommends with the warning that all other medicines will be ineffectual.

On 29 March 1669, Willis writes to Mr White, a patient but also someone to whom, apparently, he felt an obligation for past services:

> I have sent you a Truss for the falling out of the fundament. A . . . patient of mine has used it with very much benefit these many yeeres, you may easily guess at the use of it. The waistband is to goe about the middle, the points are to truss it to your dublet. If you must wear it in the night, the clasp-holes are to bee fitted to claspes, that are to be on the corners of a canvas wastrobe: but if you need it not in the night you may take all those eyes or claspholes off: The button is to bee on the fundament to keep it up, the bag is for the members, the two straps are to come up on each thigh, and the clasp-holes to fit to the claspes on the waistband. If in anything else I may serve you, bee assured I shall most readily do it, being mindful of that great obligation you have formerly laid on mee, I desire yr. prayers for me and mine and remain Sir, Yr. most obliged friend and humble servant T.W.

The undated letter to an unknown correspondent, written in Latin,[45] concerns 'a maiden of a good family' who has endured 'inveterate and herculean disease' without response to various remedies. Willis advises acid waters, baths, and fomentations to aid the mixing of the blood and humours, and to align the diastasis of her viscera. Should this fail, 'we must go from the camp of Apollo to that of Christ'. Moving on to a second case, a noble lady, Willis feels bound to ask whether she might have contracted the disease from her husband, rather than the more sinister explanation that she has a cancerous growth of the womb? In either case, she has a settling down of hot blood and acrid humours in the uterus leading to inflammation and pain. What must not be done is to use cathartics or evacuants that will drive waste products to the site of disease and stir up those that are stagnating in the womb. The answer is a gentle enema and phlebotomy. Rather more elaborate is the recommendation that she should sit on a stool with a hole through which vapours of his medicinal concoction can waft the affected parts. And there is advice on a rigid milk-based diet. He ends:

> I leave it to your discretion to decide which of these is appropriate to her acute disease and agree with her temperament, constitution and strength. Indeed all these I submit with a consciousness of my deep affection and duty towards you. Commend me to the suffering lady. Dr . . . [indecipherable] . . . Dr Millington and Mr Lower send you greetings, etc.

These surviving letters (and others that may be found) give no more than a glimpse of Willis's activities as a physician. Rather more is learned from the surviving manuscript of a casebook for 1650–1652, one of at least three known to have been kept in his lifetime. This was bought by the Wellcome Trust in December 1961 from Mr Richard Hatchwell (1927–2009)

[45] Translated by Elizabeth Palmer and sent to Raymond Hierons, thanking him for a cheque ('I don't feel worth all that') on 11 May 1961.

of Malmesbury, Wiltshire, a well-known dealer in antiquarian books. It came from the library at Llantarth Court near Abergavenny in South Wales, when the building passed from private ownership to become a boys' preparatory school. Almost certainly, the manuscript was originally in the possession of Browne Willis.[46] The fate of the other two is unknown. Inscribed in the Wellcome manuscript (788A) is:

> Liber Manuscriptus Clarissimi Doctor Thome Willis Medici Insign ... Two of these MSS of Dr Willis Lent Dr Chace abt. 5 years agoe and not returned 1737.

Stephen Chace (1677–1742) leased the estate at Great Brickhill from Browne Willis and acted as physician to the Willis family. Chace studied first at Magdalen Hall, Oxford, graduating in medicine on 27 April 1703, and then Merton College where he became doctor of medicine on 30 December 1713. He was elected a Fellow of the Royal College of Physicians (23 March 1719: where he was censor in 1722), and of the Royal Society (30 November 1724).[47] Despite such distinction, he seems to have been rather casual with respect to other people's possessions.

The entries are in Latin and Dewhurst considers that the leather bound manuscript is in the handwriting of Thomas Willis (see: Figures 6–7).[48] The back free endpaper does contain signed text matching that on various letters signed by Willis. The 'd' and 'f' have the same unusual loops and flourishes, as does the circle placed under Willis's name. But similarities are less apparent when comparing the main text with examples of Willis's script. Here, although some are similar, the shapes of several characters differ and the size of the handwriting is generally smaller. The probability that Thomas Willis used an amanuensis to take notes would not be unusual, as made clear by Wood.

In the period covered by Willis's casebook he was meeting with others interested in natural philosophy in Oxford. Insistence on 'palpable and visible experience' was beginning to permeate the thoughts and discussions of students; and, as apothecaries and physicians, chemical treatments were starting to replace botanical remedies. Before long, Willis was prominent amongst practitioners known as chymists or spagyrists and, later, iatrochemists. Such was his influence that the group was later referred to as 'Willisians' and he was described, as early as 1650, by Aubrey as 'oure Chymist'.[49] In speculating on the nature of disease, Willis was aligning the Galenic principles that he had been taught prior to graduation in 1646 with concepts beginning to take shape in the minds of iatrochemists. His analyses

[46] Kenneth Dewhurst (1981): page 63 speculates that this found its way to Abergavenny, 15 miles from Burghill, near Hereford, when Browne Willis sold Burlton Court. Harry Willis Fleming corresponded with Richard Hatchwell in 2006 on details of the purchase. Although the casebook came from Llanarth Court, Mr Hatchwell was not the bidder but learned of the earlier provenance when he acquired the casebook. That its location near Abergavenny has to do with the proximity of Burlton Court remains speculative. See: Sheila Markham, *A second book of booksellers*, London (2014): pages 44–52 for details of an interview in which Mr Hatchwell makes no reference to Willis's casebook among the items that passed through his hands and which he found memorable during a long career in the book trade; Sheila Markham confirms that the casebook was not mentioned during their conversation.

[47] See: William Munk, *The roll of the Royal College of Physicians of London*, volume 2, 1701–1800, London (1878): page 64.

[48] The translations are by Dewhurst assisted by Leofranc Holford-Strevens and Alastair McCann (nd); and in writing his commentaries, Dewhurst used the copy of *Dr Willis's practice of physick* (1684) previously owned by Edwin Clarke (now **9E.c2**). Documents which are considered to be in Willis's hand show at least three different scripts, making it difficult to distinguish the writing of an amanuensis from that of Willis himself. The most reliable example is likely to be Willis's name in the register of the Royal Society; see: [Anon] *The signatures in the first journal-book and the charter-book of the Royal Society*, London (1936): page 6.

[49] See: Bennett [Aubrey] (2015): page 1477; and Martensen (2004a): https://doi.org/10.1093/ref:odnb/29587.

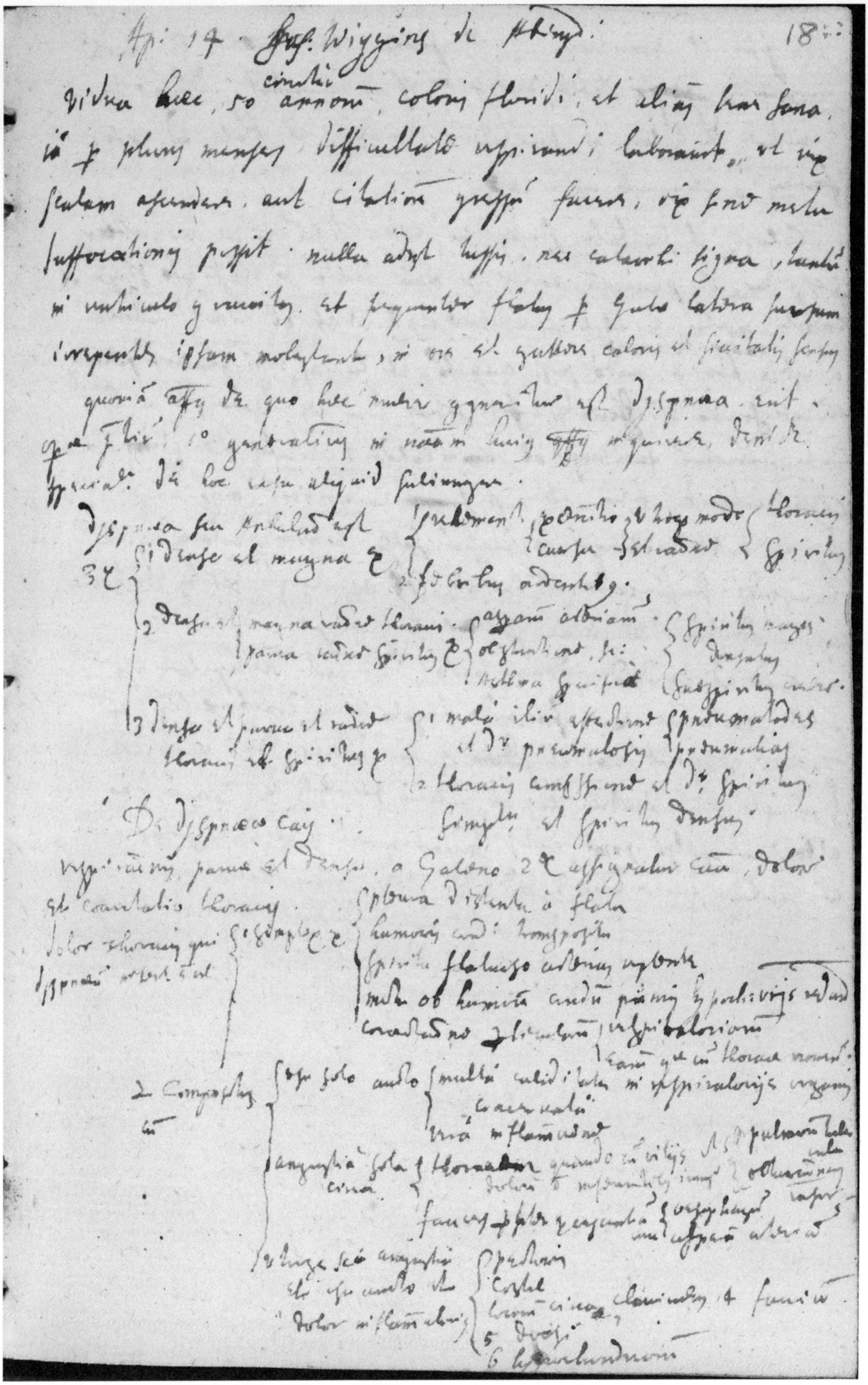

Figure 6 Manuscript leaf from Thomas Willis's casebook.
With permission from Wellcome Collection.

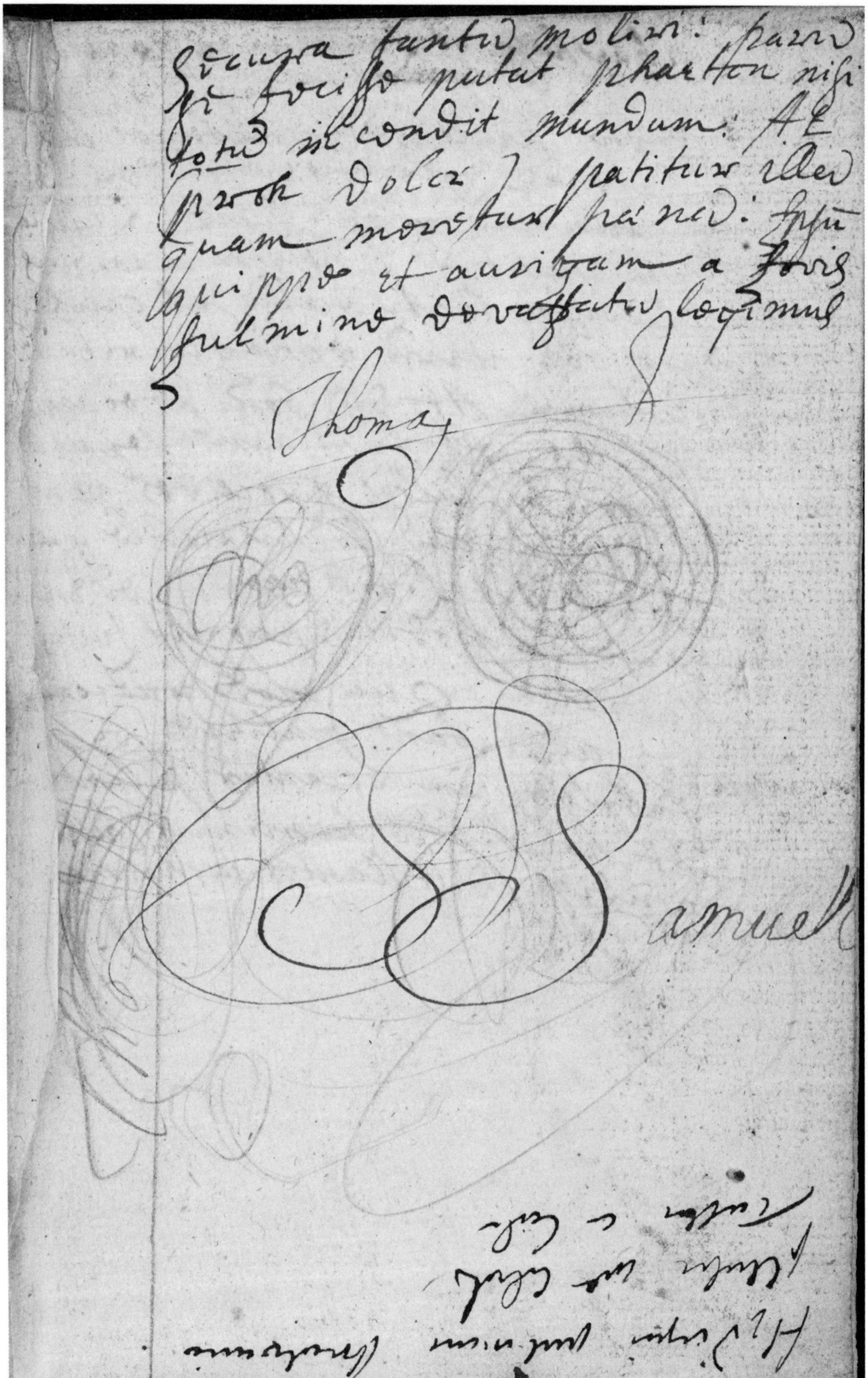

Figure 7 Manuscript entries on back free endpaper from Thomas Willis's casebook.
With permission from Wellcome Collection.

of these cases and suggestions on disease mechanisms were eventually summarized in *De fermentatione*, written by 1656, and *De febribus* and *De urinis* published with that treatise in 1659.[50] To the modern reader his formulations seem archaic, and less authoritative than the anatomical descriptions published between 1664 and 1672. But, in the 1650s, Willis was starting the transition from slavish adherence to classical doctrines to a new mechanistic chemical approach based on observation and interpretation, no longer shackled by ancient dogma. Moreover, in documenting these fifty cases directly or through his amanuensis, Willis demonstrates that he had already developed a reasonably standard method for clinical observation and description.[51]

Most of the patients are named, often with a brief demographic statement. Many come from wealthy families or are relatives of Willis. Robert Wyld (1595–1650), aged 55 (but described as 40), the brother of Willis's mother-in-law and whose son Thomas (1623–1669) studied with him at Christ Church, 'pisses bloody urine' and is dead within a few months of Willis's second consultation. John Finmore (d.1683), from a Royalist family with Christ Church connections, suffers repeatedly from discharging tumours (lymph glands) on his neck but recovers with treatment. E. Willis (presumed to be a relative), aged 50, has swollen lymph nodes and develops an ulcerated lesion of the elbow, with itch and scab formation. He is cured by three exposures to *aqua vitrolica*.

The documented symptoms are limited in scope and relate mainly to respiration, appetite, activity of the bowel and bladder, and the appearance of their effluents, pain, weakness, and altered mental function. Signs reflect what can easily be observed: fever, patterns of respiration and the pulse, frequency of excretion, material emitted from the throat and various orifices, the appearance of the pudenda, swellings, and skin eruptions. Fluids—especially urine, sweat, and semen—might be tasted. Invasive examination is also carried out by a surgeon [usually William Day (nd)], who insets his finger in the anus or introduces a catheter into the bladder. Not every patient is seen personally: Widow Wise of Stadham is one of many treated on the basis of examining her urine.[52]

Mr Hobbs of Marcham has dry skin lesions that itch and bleed when scratched. S. Wilkins, a blacksmith aged 34, has fever, headache, giddiness, and swollen glands in his neck with gastric and urinary symptoms. He recovers with purges, bleeding, and the use of diaphoretics. Robert Finer (aged 34) of Sunningwell has hip pain which responds to heat and other local measures. A. Smith of Freeland has self-medicated with a drug designed to act as a cathartic but, after also developing scabs and itching treated with a mercurial ointment, has a respiratory illness followed by paralysis 'now of this, now of that part', and constipation. Within a few days, excretion is induced and gradually he recovers. M. Stenning develops acute urinary retention after a long journey on horseback. After four days, temporary relief is obtained from catheterization but the procedure is followed by rigors and loin pain; gradually but intermittently he is able to pass cloudy urine and after three weeks has gradually recovered. Mr Barker of Wickham has dark urine and pale stools followed by jaundice from which he recovers.

[50] See: chapter 15 for more detailed discussion of Willis on medical chemistry.

[51] In extensive footnotes, Kenneth Dewhurst (1981) adds a commentary and hazards a diagnosis in each case. His analysis of the cases by system, diagnosis and where the patient lived, showing the range of Willis's practice, is summarized in a table at page 157. Imposing the nosology of modern medicine on seventeenth-century cases is notoriously risky; without wishing to be uncharitable, several of Dewhurst's suggestions do seem slightly wide of the mark. The index is useful and takes readers to the account of each named case.

[52] This is the case of smallpox mentioned by Petty with respect to Willis 'casting waters' and working as a 'piss prophet' at Abingdon (see earlier).

Many of the patients are children. The infant son of William Phelps of Warborough and Willis's sister, hence his nephew, is seen aged 10 months, and again at 3 years, with fever and respiratory symptoms. Mrs Phelps begs Willis to administer a vomit dissolved in cooked plums. The child recovers for a while but relapses briefly three years later after eating unripe fruit. After purging, he passes several worms and recovers.[53] The three-year-old son of Mr Wise of Dorchester-on-Thames has an acute gastrointestinal condition, with fever, from which he recovers. After being unwell for several months, the four-year-old son of Mrs Dapwell of Abingdon becomes weak with fever and develops swellings on his chest, abdomen, and limbs. He has headache, respiratory difficulties, and altered posture. The case is complex with more than one condition present. The problem is due to morbid humours from the head accumulating in the chest; and those from the spleen and liver retained in the abdomen. Despite the benefit of Willis's many and varied remedies, within five days the child is dead. The son of F. Symms, aged 5, develops difficulty with speaking and swallowing. These symptoms persist and he has dyspnoea with stridor. The prognosis does not seem good. Henry Jones, the eight year old son of Walter (1605–1672) and his wife, Willis's sister-in-law, has generalized oedema and reduction in urine output but nonetheless recovers.[54] The son of F. Pordings of Clifton, aged 10, develops a tumour of the humerus and elbow which ulcerates and suppurates. A surgeon explores the lesion and finds necrotic bone. Jon Dew, aged 10, from a puritan family but with Royalist connections, suffers renal colic and passes several small stones. He recovers after purging, application of leeches, and exposure to various medicines including feverfew and opiates. Anne Mason, aged 16, has a subacute abdominal illness with a superficial abscess that discharges, but she lapses into coma with convulsions and dies, the agonal illness lasting seven days.[55] Maria Rowney, a virgin aged 17 with delayed menarche, the daughter of Thomas Rowney (d.1665), an Oxford lawyer whose wife was godmother to Anthony Wood and whose family gave land on which the Radcliffe Infirmary was built, loses her appetite and craves salt; she falls when standing presumably due to faints, but the illness is self-limiting with recovery attributed to Willis's remedies. The infant daughter of F. Bodily appears to have measles but this develops into swellings in the axilla and neck which become gangrenous and discharge, associated with convulsions and drowsiness. Matters are not helped by the grieving mother since, reverting to Galenic formulations, Willis considers her milk to be tainted with melancholic juice or black bile. He does not relate the outcome.

There are psychiatric cases. After her husband's death, widow Badcocke of East Hagbourne has a prolonged grief reaction characterized by headache, anorexia, and lassitude. The wife of H. Bolt of Eaton, near Abingdon, aged 45, develops mania and has to be restrained in bed. She screams and cries out but does not respond to Willis's treatments and is dead within 48 hours. T. Rome of Freeland, prone to melancholy since the death of his brothers from that condition, has a productive cough with haemoptysis, and breathlessness on exertion. The diagnosis is ulcer of the lungs and treatment is purging and bleeding with remedies to dry

[53] This is one of the nephews who received a legacy of £10 in Willis's will.

[54] Later, Henry Jones matriculated at Christ Church, Oxford (1668), was ordained and became rector of Sunningwell in Berkshire until 1700, when he resigned his position, being a non-juror, although he qualified again for the position in 1706. He died in 1707. As his nephew, Henry inherited many of John Fell's manuscripts and much of Henry's own collection eventually came to the Bodleian Library.

[55] See: Dewhurst (1981): page 91, endnote 2, for the suggestion that she was the daughter of William Mason who completed buildings for the University of Oxford, including the Selden End of the Bodleian Library, in 1635 for the sum of £4216, citing Andrew Clark, *The life and times of Anthony Wood, antiquary, at Oxford, 1632–1695, described by himself*, volume 4, Oxford (1895): pages 53–5.

the ulcer. He must eat a roasted apple stuffed with frankincense, olibanum, and sugar candy baked on ashes each night, and live off chicken and turtle as a tisane or in broth. Mr Everard is constitutionally melancholic, with hypochondriasis induced by excessive studying, abdominal complaints, and vapours striking his brain preventing concentration and acting as a prelude to phantasy. When the wind is from the south, or the weather cloudy, Everard feels serum moving in his head.

Willis records past medical history or aetiological factors that he considers to be relevant. For women: virginity, menstrual activity, childbirth, and any tendency to hysterical or hypochondriacal passions are noted. G.H., aged 40, dies from pneumonia brought on by menstruation. Late in pregnancy, and with dietary idiosyncrasies, Mrs Falkam has fever, sweats, and rigors with altered respiration. She recovers from this presumed tertian fever (malaria). Pl. N, a virgin aged 26, has *fluor albus* (vaginal discharge) and irregular menstrual periods. Management is by diverting the impurities and bad chemistry accumulating in her uterus to the bowels or bladder. Mrs Terry has puerperal sepsis, the outcome of which is not recorded although the report stops at a point where the prognosis seems poor. The wife of Thomas Pierce of Thame, aged 50, has severe bouts of wandering pains, with restlessness, or involuntary movements, and fever. Everything resolves with the onset of her irregular menstrual periods, releasing the presumed ill humours. S. Willmot, perhaps related to the Oxford bookseller John Wilmot (fl. 1637–1665) of Abingdon, aged 40, has recurrent haemorrhoids after each childbirth. The wife of Francis Day of Wallingford has lower abdominal pain radiating to the back, with colic and melaena. This is due to accumulation of malignant and poisonous humours which must be evacuated from her uterus.

The daughter of F., a virgin of good family, aged 20, has dysmenorrhoea with each menstrual cycle but is better if she exercises by riding a horse or rapid walking. She is managed by purging with senna dissolved in milky beer when each menstrual flux is expected. Mrs White of Pusey, the vicar's wife, has puerperal productive cough and breathlessness attributed by another of her brothers, a doctor, and empiric women to phthisis. Treatment is with various expectorants and although she survives, the child dies a few years later. Miss Anne Parratt of Northleigh, a virgin with small and discoloured menstrual periods and the sister of Richard Lydall's second wife, has productive cough with wheezing and breathlessness on exercise. At her suggestion, a change of air by a visit to Cornwall is proposed. Although this illness recovers, Anne dies two years later. Mrs Herne of Abingdon is nursing her fourteen-month-old child but has a productive cough, breathlessness, anorexia, and lassitude. She improves, temporarily, with the resumption of menstruation. In the same note, Willis discusses gonorrhoea and the nature of the discharge in women and men that follows impure intercourse, the unnamed case in question being unable to walk due to the pain in her pudenda. The discharge leads to extreme emaciation and consumption of the body, as in those who have intercourse immoderately; and infertility is a common consequence of the condition.

The wife of Dr N.D., prone to hysteric and hypochondriacal states, has crusting scabs on her face and abdominal pain 'such as that of a wild animal running from the side to the ilium'. Mrs Jennings, of a good family, subject to hysteric passions, has episodes of burning pain in the thoracic spine radiating both to her head and legs. Willis asks rhetorically what is it that the viscera communicate and what is the influence of the uterus on the rest of the body? Another Mrs Jennings of Clifton Hampden near Abingdon, also victim of hysteria and hypochondriasis, sweats, shakes and swoons before developing pustules that discharge bloody material. This crusts and is accompanied by severe pain in the right arm made worse by movement. She recovers but has a further episode three months later.

For men, excessive use of alcohol may be relevant. Eustace, aged 35, drinks too much and feels unwell the next day, so takes more beer to effect a cure but develops fever and abdominal pains. These recover when he passes large quantities of urine. H.A., from a good family and a close acquaintance of Willis, has a urethral stricture and gonorrhoea, aggravated by excessive drinking of wine and riding too often on horseback. F. Edwards, a man of rank, also drinks too much thick beer that is going sweet, and develops respiratory symptoms with headache and night sweats. He has burning pain in the extremities and generalized weakness with difficulty swallowing, inability to speak clearly and cloudy urine. Within a month of the consultation, he is dead. Abel Paine, given to inebriation and continuous drinking, is emaciated, anorectic and with persistent cough and breathlessness. Willis diagnoses morbus gallicus (syphilis) but two of Abel's brothers have died of phthisis. W.K. cannot tolerate his beer but this seems unrelated to his complaint of genital pruritus to the extent of self-inflicted excoriation, presumed to be scabies.

Influenced by Harvey, Willis's formulations on mechanisms mainly involve the blood and its circulation. Almost 10 years before publishing his first treatise, he is thinking in terms of the five chemical constituents: spirit, sulphur, and salt with water and earth binding them together. Modified in response to differing amounts of heat from fermentation, these elements compete in his analyses with the four humours: blood, yellow bile, black bile, and phlegm. And Willis's focus is already on the organs that later dominated his writings. At fault are usually the intestines, liver, spleen, kidneys, lungs, and the uterus. In the case of Jaf. Wiggins, a widow, with breathlessness on exertion, Willis sets out an elaborate table classifying dyspnoea in the Galenic tradition. More generally, his position is that with illness the natural temper of the organs is disturbed, the spirits and humours having accumulated in inappropriate places. Thus, enlarged glands in the neck result from abnormal humours draining from the head failing, as normally occurs, to be excreted through the skin as sweat. Treatment might be through raising a blister allowing the noxious material to escape. W.W. has a chronic infected ulcer of the foot with erosion of the underlying bone. Management to date has included tying a tight ligature around the knee to reduce the discharge. Willis plans to remove the ichor (discharge) derived from the blood and containing unhelpful secretions, by bandaging with material soaked in (Jean) Fernel's (1497–1558) ulcer waters, and then to keep the lesion clean and dry so as to aid regeneration of the tissues. Much blame is attached to the stomach and spleen which, performing inadequately, allow 'tartarean feculencie' to pass to the kidney and bladder where, adequate mixing of the various components failing to take place due to continual descent of a sharp humour, the result is stone in the bladder, disruption of urination, and urethral discharge. Based on what the patient vomits or passes, Willis often proposes that an 'abscess', in or near the belly but internal, has ruptured. This is usually fatal. When no other explanation is forthcoming, Willis proposes:[56]

> Dissolution of the humours and vapours arising from the blood and filthy excrements, which are infected sometimes with a sulphurous, sometimes with a vitriolic, nitrous or aluminous quality. And also these humours in the body ferment, coagulate, dissolve and undergo various agitations ... and if we plough with this calf the enigma of these prodigious conditions may perhaps, in some way, be solved.

It does not sound promising. Willis's treatments are based on correcting the altered chemistry of the blood and humours; removing ill-digested material by purges, emetics, sudorifics,

[56] See: Dewhurst (1981): page 98, relating to the wife of Dr N.D. (see earlier).

or bleeding; and using his own receipts or remedies made up by apothecaries. Caution is needed since treatment may disturb the peccant (faulty) material and worsen the condition. Often a country woman or an 'empiric' has seen the patient before Willis and confused matters through the injudicious use of her quack remedies. As early as 1650, Willis is using the medicines to which he remained faithful up to his death in 1675 and which are listed and rationalized in his last two treatises, *Pharmaceutice rationalis* parts 1 and 2. Many and varied herbal remedies are described in the casebook but also with less obvious materials such as extracts of insects and vertebrates, powder of burnt hare, spirits of billy-goats' blood, newly drawn bee-stings, as well as the milk of asses, mineral waters, beer and wine, lithotryptic measures, opiates, bezoar and other pharmaceuticals, and much cupping, leaching, and bleeding. Willis prescribes salts of tartar, antimony, and iron taken in the slime of worms as aqua lumbricorum or aqua limacum composite. He uses higher doses of quicksilver than colleagues such as William Conyers (1622–1665) in patients afflicted with iliac passions (intestinal obstruction).

Willis did well in his practice, Seth Ward (1617–1689: later, Bishop of Exeter) reporting that: 'he had rich peeces of plate presented to him as well as great fees'. From Ward we learn that:[57]

> Dr. Willis imparts his receipts chiefly to 2 Apothecaries in Oxford as farre as I can perceive, Mr. Hazlewood and Mr. Crosse. Hee hath a syrup of sulphur wch hee makes much use of. Itt is his owne composition and no Apothecarie hath itt or knows itt but ye two aforementioned. Itt may be taken and is so usually with a Liquorish stick. It is a compound not above 4*d*. an ounce, but it is most used in Colds and distempers of the Lungs . . . Two ounces and a half of quicksilver given by Dr. Conyers to a patient yt was troubled with ye Iliack passion. Itt is very good for yt distemper. Dr. Willis uses to give more: ye more you give ye less is ye danger. Itt does by its own weight passe quickly. Doe but mix itt with a plaister and heat itt a little and presently itt flies away, but boyling hurts itt not at all.

When the outlook seems obvious, Willis is not afraid to confirm the prognosis. Ward reports that Willis had treated Stephen Toone (1636–1681), an Oxford apothecary, with strangulated hernia:

> Stephen Toon's rupture was laid open, as ye phrase is, and caused a peristaltic motion of ye guts. At last eased by a plaister and a grain of laudanum wch Dr. Willis said hee was too weak to take, the Dr. left him with these words: 'Stephen, God comfort ye'.

Despite, or perhaps because of, these comforting words Toone lived happily in Oxford until 1681. Willis could also be inventive as in the case of a 'certain man of Oxford' who vomited after eating and was fitted with an oesophageal stent.[58]

In the casebook, outcome is judged by the disappearance of visible signs of disease, increase in number and appearance of excretions by the bowel and bladder, recovery, and the resumption of normal life or, not infrequently, death after which post-mortem examination is sometimes carried out. Mr Capell is confused and drowsy with palpitations and bouts of fever probably due to malaria; he recovers with induced vomiting, purging, and leeches

[57] See: D'Arcy Power, *Selected writings 1877–1930*, Oxford (1931): pages 190–1.

[58] See: Thomas Willis, *Pharmaceutice rationalis* part 1 (1679): page 23; and chapter 18 for a description of this case.

applied to his haemorrhoids. Mrs Hill has fever, haemoptysis, cough, and chest pain but is fully cured after purging: 'she had 16 stools with great euphoria and completely recovered'. However, her treatment was distinctly gentle compared with Francis Day who, after purging, passed 200 stools in 24 hours. Even so, Ward is of the opinion that, compared to other practitioners, 'Dr Willis his purges, generally very gentle: hee advised pulp of Tamarinds to one yt was hot and hectique'. [59] Less happily, J. Bird (aged *c.*20) dies from pneumonia brought on by ploughing in a biting north wind. The wife of J. Sterne has gastrointestinal symptoms with pale blood-stained stools and fever. As she deteriorates, William Petty is consulted but to no avail and, breathless and increasingly weak, she dies within two weeks from presentation. F. Symmons dies soon after developing pain in the right side with inability to move. The autopsy shows that his lungs are floating in fluid contained within the thorax which coalesces on heating into a foul-smelling coagulum 'like flour porridge and white of egg'.

The Oxford casebook is important not only as a record of medicine as practised in the 1650s in rural Oxfordshire, but because it illustrates the early phases of Willis's convergence of classical humoral doctrines into concepts that shaped his ideas on fermentation in explaining human physiology and, when perturbed, a generic mechanism of disease. Although later much concerned with anatomical studies, the principles of iatrochemistry remained central to his formulations on function of the nervous system and muscle.

Willis's Oxford lectures

At the Restoration in 1660, Willis was appointed Sedleian professor of Natural Philosophy in the University of Oxford and a student of Christ Church. He was the fourth incumbent of the professorship, replacing Joshua Crosse (*c.*1614–1676) who had held the position for twelve years (1648–1660) after John Edwards (1600–*c.*1655) was removed from office by the parliamentarians. Crosse was himself expelled from the University by the Commissioners for Charles II (1630–1685), allegedly for embezzlement. The first Sedleian professor was Edward Lapworth (1574–1636), appointed in the year of Willis's birth. The professorship had been endowed by Sir William Sedley (*c.*1558–1619) and sustained by income from the purchase of an estate at Waddesdon, Buckinghamshire. The requirement was to study and teach medicine and experimental philosophy. Willis's salary was approximately £120 per annum. After his election, on 30 October 1660, Willis received his doctorate of medicine. People who had served the Royalist cause and were close to Willis also took up influential positions: John Fell became dean of Christ Church (from 1660) and vice-chancellor of the University (1666–1669);[60] and Gilbert Sheldon (1598–1677) was appointed Bishop of London (1660) and Archbishop of Canterbury (from 1663 until his death). Willis first acknowledged the patronage from Sheldon in his dedication to the

[59] See: Dewhurst (1981): page 166 and endnote 58 citing transcript of John Ward's diaries, volume 4, page 868.

[60] As is well known, in 1680 Fell required a student, Tom Brown (1663–1704), to translate the 32nd epigram from Martial, 'Non amo te, Sabidi / nec possum dicere quare / Hoc tantum possum dicere / non amo te'. Brown suggested; 'I do not like thee, Doctor Fell, / The reason why—I cannot tell; / But this I know, and know full well, / I do not like thee, Doctor Fell'. Other versions, naming Tom as Browne, lack prosody: 'I do not love you, Doctor Fell, / But why—I cannot tell; / But this I know full well, / I do not love you, Doctor Fell'. Whatever he wrote, the poke at Fell seems harsh since the exercise was a condition of pardon for Brown who otherwise faced expulsion from the University.

third edition of *Diatribæ duæ* (1662) within the preliminaries of *De fermentatione*. In the English translation (1681):

> It was by your means (most Noble Prelate) that I obtained the Votes in this Famous University for the place of Sidly Professor for how small soever my merits might seem they were helped by the greatness and weight of your opinion.

Yet more adulatory was the dedication to Sheldon in the preliminaries of *Cerebri anatome* (1664) which preceded Willis's cleverly worded explanation of how, in placing his attempts to 'unlock the secret places on Mans Mind, and to look into the living and breathing Chapel of the Deity' at the 'most holy Altar of Your Grace', he had avoided 'the School-house of Atheism'. In the English translation (1681):

> Once more your Sidley Professor and your Servant (the more happy Title) flings himself at Your feet, with this only Ambition, that he might render something of Thanks for your Kindness and benefits.

The homage to Sheldon was further developed in *De anima brutorum* (1672) making clear, in the English translation (1683), that:

> The Academical Readings by a necessitated Duty belong to you, for that I received them from your Favours; and indeed, neither had ever seen the Light, not perhaps my self had ever been in the number of Authors, unless I had been made at first, your Sidlie Professor at Oxford.

Dedicating books to Gilbert Sheldon was wise since, although Willis was unlikely to be guilty of sectarianism, the Act of Uniformity (1662) required adherence to liturgy and governance under the direction of Sheldon, as archbishop, despite the unsuccessful efforts of Charles II to introduce freedoms at the time he was nurturing the Royal Society. Tightening his grip, in 1665, Sheldon instructed all bishops to:[61]

> Certify me, the names sirnames, Degrees and qualities of all Practicers of Physick within their respective dioceses: In what towns villages or Places they live; whether licensed & by whom; & how they appear affected to His Ma(jesty) gouerm't & ye Doctrine and Discipline of ye church of Engl'd.

Later Sheldon meted out the same restrictions on ministers and printers. But he did well not to antagonize Willis since, in the same year, he suffered apoplexy and became Willis's patient.[62] The duties of the Sedleian professor were clear:[63]

> The Reader of the Lecture is according to the Statutes to read in full term, on Wednesdays and Saturdays at eight of the clock in the morning, either Aristotle's *Physics* or his book *de Cœlo et Mundo* or that *de Meteroris* or his *Parvu Naturalia*, as also his book *de Anima*, and those of *Generation and Corruption*.

[61] See: Robert Martensen, *The brain takes shape. An early history*, Oxford (2004b): page 112.
[62] See: chapter 17 citing *Two discourses concerning the soul of brutes* (1683): page 160.
[63] See: Hughes (1991): page 30.

By his own account, 1660 marks the time at which Willis began to study the anatomy of the brain and nerves. The question has been raised as to whether, rather than a scientist driven by curiosity, Willis studied human anatomy merely in order to advance the teleological argument that mind and body are designed simply to enable the worship of God:[64]

> His aim was not merely to produce a straightforwardly 'scientific' theory of the brain and nerves. Instead, Willis turned to anatomy in order to defend the Restoration church and to provide his allies with evidence from which they might more effectively defend their shared conviction that we were all embodied, impassioned and fallible human beings ... His anatomical predecessors were actively opposed to the kind of research Willis so boldly published in the 1660s. They explicitly refused to engage in the kind of speculations that Willis aimed to substantiate in his neurology.

The argument offered by Louis Caron sees Willis, bruised by the Civil War and resistant to insistence of the Long Parliament on nonconformist religious practices, regarding adherence to the Christian liturgy as fundamental to lasting peace.[65] According to this analysis, Willis set out to show that structure and function in the brain and nervous stock enable the postures and practices of religious ceremony: bowing and kneeling and involuntary repression of urges in order to temper behavioural excess and maintain divine practice. It is an interesting analysis but one that is not without counterarguments.

It would be common ground that Willis was pious and a practising Christian who adhered to the liturgy of the Anglican Church. He entered Oxford University to study religion before converting to medicine. He was courageous in enabling others to worship in secret during the Civil War. He provided financial support for the church and its members whilst living in St Martin's Lane, London. As mentioned, he dedicated several books to Archbishop Sheldon. People who argued for strict adherence to practices set down in the *Book of Common Prayer* quoted Willis. One of these, Henry Hammond (1605–1660) who held strong views on human agency, sin, and morality and articulated a view that aligned spirit, soul, and body with Willis's rational and corporeal souls, respectively, named Willis in his will 'as friend and physician'.[66] Willis's grandson founded a church at Fenny Stratford in his memory. Willis makes repeated reference to divine creativity in his books.

Evidence for the conventional view that Willis was interested in structure and function of the brain, including the nature of mental processes, *per se*, is compelling. In pursuing his work, both for personal reasons and political expediency, Willis was at pains not to undermine religion or challenge the doctrines of the church. There was room for both in studying the wondrous arrangements of particles, organs, and beasts that God had created. Anatomy was a valid method available to natural philosophers for understanding the interplay between structure and function; and when contemplating digestion, respiration, blood, the circulation, excretion, and movement, why not also think about mind and the soul?

[64] See: Louis Caron, 'Thomas Willis, the restoration and the first works of neurology', *Medical History* 2015; 59: 525–53 for this suggestion and supporting evidence.

[65] See: Joanna Collicut, 'The scientific study of religion'. In: Eds. Alasdair Coles and Joanna Collicut, *Neurology and religion*, Cambridge (2020): pages 6–11 for evidence that theologians have also thought about Willis and religion. Canon Joanna Collicut judges Willis to have taken an unsatisfactory position in resolving his personal and political dilemma on the nature of the human soul by adopting the empirical solution that many functions of the mind previously considered immaterial, and designated corporeal or sensitive, have their basis in the substance of the brain working in parallel with a rational soul that exists after death.

[66] See: Caron (2015): section III, pages 533–41, for a detailed account of religious views at the time Willis was studying anatomy; and the case for mutual interaction of his ideas and those of philosophers and the religious community during the Long Parliament and after the Restoration.

Willis began as a chemist and his natural philosophy was rooted in fermentation and the ramifications thereof for the physiology and pathology of several organs other than those needed to consider and practice the worship of God. When his university education ended, unlike several of his contemporaries in Oxford who were also engaged in natural philosophy, Willis did not settle for the usual default position of ordination. It was natural that he should pay obeisance to Gilbert Sheldon, a man of influence and one to be feared, who had secured the Sedleian professorship of Natural Philosophy for Willis. All books needed a wealthy or influential sponsor in order to defray or avoid the costs of publication. Willis was intimate with a community that valued epistemology based on evidence and he kept the company of many who had no strong religious beliefs. He had ready access to humane bodies and confessed to being 'addicted to the opening of heads'. He was not the first to consider the nature of mental processes and mind.

Willis's books were popular and widely read amongst scientists and physicians and not only by theologians and philosophers. He mentions God but does not proselytize religiosity. He does not write on the anatomy or physiology of kneeling and postures of the clergy and congregation engaging in worship. Despite its concern with the corporeal and rational souls, his anatomy of the brain considers many functions other than mental processes. It is no fault of Willis that others, such as Henry More (1614–1687), took Willis's observations to extremes in anatomizing the mechanics of Christian worship. Whereas others may have used the discoveries as ammunition in favour of a selfish God who created bodies in order to be worshipped, that does not indict Willis for studying the structure of the brain simply in order to defend restoration of the Church after 1660.[67]

Willis gave three series of lectures as Sedleian professor. It is assumed that the first dealt mainly with the issues of fermentation and chemistry that had occupied his thoughts during the 1650s. Details are lost but, more generally, Edward Bagshaw (1629–1671) explains that deviating from the 1636 statutes on the content had become less easy with the swing away from Baconian philosophy back to traditional doctrines:[68]

> [Aristotle] has driven out all other philosophers, and rules supreme, especially in Christ Church. Here a temple and altar have been erected to the Stagyrite as a philosophical deity, to whom also festive days are consecrated and solemn pomp and annual panegyric dedicated. Here he walks and enjoys his praise as if he were loci genius.

Reflecting on Willis's teaching, Robert Plot (1640–1696) praised many discoveries in anatomy, but it was 'too difficult a task to give just account how far *Physick*, Anatomy, Chymistry, and Philosophy, stand indebted to him for their Improvements'. He records that:[69]

> in Natural Philosophy, the famous Dr Willis ... Sidleyan Professor ... in this University, first taught us, that the Generations, Perfections, and Corruptions of Natural Bodies,

[67] See: Caron (2015): page 552 and footnote 128 for the occasional slip of the historian straying into science, reminiscent of the much paraded hazards of the physician straying into history, in making the point that there is no connection between the intercostal nerve and the heart. Willis's 'intercostal' nerve is today's 'sympathetic' outflow and, with his 'wandring' nerve (now named the 'vagus'), part of the autonomic nervous system and therefore intimately involved in rhythmic activity and involuntary responses of the thoracic and abdominal organs.

[68] See: Kenneth Dewhurst, *Thomas Willis's Oxford lectures*, Oxford (1980): page 40 and note 23 citing Edward Bagshaw, *Exercitationes duæ; altera theologica de presbyteris et episcopis; altera academica de philosophia veterum ejusque usu una cum duabus orationibus ejusdem argumenti*, London (1661): page 147.

[69] See: Robert Plot, *The natural history of Oxford-shire*. Oxford (1677): pages 301–7, paragraphs numbered 215–34.

> whether Mineral, Vegetable, or Animal; and so like-wise of Bodies Artificial, do depend upon Fermentation, raised from the different Proportions and Motions of the Spiriti, Sulphur, Salt, water, and Earth, which he did constitute the ultimate sensible Principles of mixed Bodies.

This adaptation of Aristotelian wisdom, unchallenged for nearly twelve centuries, may have been part of Willis's university teaching or delivered in a more private setting. At one level, he was loyal to the older doctrines of medicine, being the last English physician to quote with approval the practice of John of Gaddeson (1280–1361).[70]

Much more can be learned from the notes taken down by two who attended the second and third courses which mainly mark Willis's emerging interest in the brain and its disorders: Richard Lower, between 1661 and 1662, and John Locke (1632–1704), in 1663 or 1664.[71] Together, they provide details of thirty-eight lectures, from approximately fifty that Willis may have been required to deliver between 1660 and 1667 (with an interval in 1665 when the Royal court moved from London to Oxford in order to escape the plague and took over the Court of Chancery).

The lectures attended by Lower are instructive with respect to Willis's evolving views on fermentation and chemistry, some years after he had first published on the topic in 1659.[72] He considers four classes of living creatures: plants and worms; insects; animals with a primitive circulation; and warm-blooded highly developed species. As to their physiology, the four humours of the ancients are not altogether disregarded, but the properties of circulating blood are related to heat resulting from fermentation of the five chemical particles. Like a lamp which requires fuel, space in which to burn, and removal of its soot, the blood is fuel, the heart is the burner, and space provided by the lungs and other vents. Any one of these elements or systems may be deranged and the cause of disease. The blood may be insufficient, as in haemorrhage, or burned out through fever. The heart may receive too little or too much blood; or fail to propel the fluid if it congeals and the spirits that move the heart under influence of the nerves falter. The flame may be extinguished if ventilation is prevented, congested, or obstructed. Heated spirits reaching the brain may be deficient, too plentiful, or otherwise perturbed. The theory and hypotheses are supplemented by clinical observations and evidence from autopsies, performed either soon after death or when the corpses were not so fresh.

But Willis had other ideas and was not to be constrained. His instructions insisted upon 'not that which was most true, but what was most convenient, and what was rather desired

[70] See: Norman Moore, 'WILLIS, Thomas, M.D. (1621–1675)', *Dictionary of National Biography*, Volume 62, London (1900): pages 25–6.

[71] See: Dewhurst (1980), which is based on John Locke's commonplace book (Bodleian Library, Locke f 19: pp 1–68), and material located in Robert Boyle's papers, library of the Royal Society (Boyle papers, volume XIX, ff 1–35). In 'Thomas Willis and his circle: brain and mind in seventeenth century medicine', Ed. GS Rousseau, *The languages of psyche*, Berkeley (1990): page 122, footnote 58, Robert Frank explains that it was he who, in 1969, identified Lower as the author of information on Willis's lectures in the Boyle papers. Dewhurst (1980) argues persuasively that Lower and Locke were present at the second, and Locke also at the third, series of lectures and made notes rather than summarizing what either knew to be Willis's ideas at some later date. Dewhurst suggests that there are no notes on the lectures from 1660 because these merely reiterated material already printed in *Diatribæ duæ* (1659). As with the casebook, Dewhurst was helped by Leofranc Holford-Strevens and Alastair McCann in translating the Latin texts. These are mainly based on Locke's notebook supplemented by Lower's versions where these differ or are more extensive. Dewhurst has cross-referenced each lecture to the text of *Dr Willis's practice of physick* using the copy owned by Edwin Clarke (now **9E.c2**).

[72] At the risk of transposing twenty-first century ideas onto Willis's explanations, these lectures can easily be aligned with the principles of modern cell and molecular biology, metabolic processes, and system-based medicine.

than what was known'. He started to question the authority of the Aristotelean formalists, agonizing that his lectures had 'a certain Poetical Philosophy and Physick neatly wrought with Novity and Conjectures' but were too faithful to the 'received Opinions of others'. Therefore Willis began to ignore the statutory instructions moving to his own theories on the senses, faculties and affections of the soul, and the anatomy of the nervous system.[73] This appealed to his audience and Willis attracted 'an unusual number of auditors'. Needing a strong foundation for his work on the nervous system, Willis studied anatomy and carried out experiments, validating his conclusions by clinical examples, where possible. Plot explained that:

> Dr Willis's Method of dissecting the Brain, (wherein he had the Assistance of the deservedly famous Sir Christopher Wren, Dr. Millington, etc.) is new, and most natural, and so exact, that there is scarce anyone part in it but what has receiv'd considerable advancements ... Several Things he observ'd very considerable in Fowls. Some parts of Animals he more exactly trac'd by the Help of Glasses as the Kidneys, the Plexus in the Brain, etc. ... The nerves he found to have little veins and Arteries in them.

Locke's notes headed 'Willis Praelector' make clear the emerging interest in the brain and nerves, and mental functions or 'psychologia'. Many concepts embedded in modern brain science are recognizable: chemical properties and conduction using a finite number of shared transmitters; different roles for the parenchyma and ventricles; classification of the cranial nerves; afferent and efferent pathways for sensation and movement; connectivity and reciprocal innervation; the integration of agonists and antagonists; proprioception and stereognosis; reflex activity and autonomic function; learning and plasticity; the localization of function and the site of disease; the concept of biological psychiatry including hysteria and hypochondriasis as brain disorders; hereditary factors in disease; comparative anatomy; and the adverse effects of alcohol. The lectures on convulsions, epilepsy, and hysteria rehearse concepts subsequently more fully elaborated in *Pathologiæ cerebri* (1667); and those on lethargy, coma, delirium, mania, stupidity, and imbecility anticipated ideas expanded in *De anima brutorum* (1672).

The two most extensively documented lectures are on the cerebrum and cerebellum, respectively. The *succus nervosus* is made in grey matter from the five particles in fermented blood delivered in the cerebral arteries. It diffuses through white matter, forging pathways and leaving traces that serve as retrievable memories. The corpus callosum binds the two halves of the brain and provides passages for the diffusion of spirits during movement. Sensation is registered in the striate bodies. The optic nerves are connected at the chiasm in order to bind the images from each eye. Brain function results from the expansion of spirits stimulating excitement in neighbouring parts. The lateral and third ventricles act as sumps for waste material. They drain through the infundibulum to the pituitary and from there to the palate, or via the mammillary bodies and cribriform plate to the nose, seeping like fluid through a cloth. The fourth ventricle is different. Protected by the pineal gland, cranial nerves originate in (or adjacent to) this ventricle and project to the head and thoracic and abdominal organs.

To a greater extent than in the treatises that followed, apart from the second part of *De anima brutoum* (1672), Willis is concerned in his lectures more with physiology and the nature of emotions and perceptions than with structure of the brain. The Oxonian students

[73] Dewhurst (1980): page 41 points out that the lectures reverted back to Aristotelean doctrines after 1667 when Willis moved to London and George Hooper (1640–1727) was appointed.

are told that when, by its movement or shape, an external object excites the spirits, sensation is conveyed to the cerebrum. But if the brain is deficient, or intent on some other duty as in meditation or grief, arrival is suspended and the sensation not registered. Imagination occurs when sensation excites spirits present in the medulla oblongata into movement. Ideas result from permeation of this material into the cerebral 'orbits' (spheres of influence). Memory is a recurrence of prior events involving agitation of spirits in preformed tracts.[74] Phantasy occurs when this movement is disordered. Pleasure is the sensation of agreeable dances of spirits moving from the nerves to the medulla where locally stored material joins in the titillation. Joy and sadness reflect expansion and stasis of the nervous spirits, respectively. Melancholy is persistent sadness, the imagination magnifying small objects like a microscope and giving them greater importance than they deserve, due to spirits permeating newly carved aberrant pathways.[75] Movement of spirits within the brain reawakens past experience as when the memory of food produces reflex salivation 'as though keen to meet a pleasant guest'. Pain is external, through pulling apart of the nervous spirits following stimulation, or internal from disordered motion occurring without provocation. Pain persists from failure to expel disordered spirits through the lungs or skin pores as vapours and sweats. Movement is the opposite of sensation, initiated in the cerebrum with spirits passing along nerves and exciting muscles to expand and shorten thereby drawing together the structures to which they are attached. This much is logical but Willis is already formulating novel ideas on voluntary movement and the cerebrum, the role of the cerebellum in reflective (or involuntary) movement, and on the cranial and spinal nerves.[76]

The structure of the cerebellum, generally less variable in size between species than the cerebrum, serves its purpose as the organ responsible for involuntary rhythmic movements such as those of the heart and lungs. It is connected to the medulla by the middle and inferior peduncles and is the origin of several cranial nerves. The fifth (now the seventh) emerges from the medulla so that it can gather the nervous spirits in passing, as does the seventh (now the eighth) which has two parts, one receiving sounds and the other echoing these into speech. Sound passes both to the cerebrum and the cerebellum where traces are stored and related to preexisting schemata. Because the cerebellum is more easily excavated with pores to accommodate these spirits than the cerebrum, people with 'musical ears' learn a tune easily and can rehearse the melody, but others scarcely at all even though not deficient in properties of the cerebrum such as memory and imagination. The cerebellum is also responsible for the repetition of learned skilled movements such as playing the lute—difficult to perform without practice but once acquired carried out perfectly and without conscious effort. The eighth (now the tenth) cranial nerve, connected to another originating in the upper spinal cord (now the eleventh or accessory nerve), projects to the viscera and organizes 'the beat of the heart, respiration, the concoction in the stomach, the grasping of food and its protrusion into the intestines, and the propulsion of chyle into the *venæ lacteae*'.

[74] See: Dewhurst (1980): pages 130–4, and chapter 17, for elaboration of the importance to Willis of the concepts of localization and pathways in formulating ideas on neurological and psychological disease. For example, in mania, those who recover have retained the old pores of the brain with no new orbits formed, whereas mania becomes chronic when 'a miasma' is left behind after each episode in aberrant pathways and passages of the brain.

[75] In the context of melancholy, Willis introduces two bizarre conditions to his attentive students, lycanthropy and metamorphosis, but he considers these too complex for further discussion. Dewhurst (1980): page 130, footnotes 7 and 8 explains that these are forms of delusional insanity in which the victim believes that he has been turned into a wolf and may have murdered or eaten children; or transformed into a dog, wolf, or some other animal.

[76] The text that follows is based on Willis's lectures and, whilst somewhat different in emphasis, covers the same ground as set out in more detail in chapters 16–18.

These structures move without the will but the cerebrum nonetheless registers their activities. Reciprocal flow of spirits between the cerebrum and cerebellum underlies physical expression of the emotions through movements and behaviour: searching for sustenance in response to hunger and satisfying thirst, often without awareness and by 'natural motion'; coughing or changes in temperature and colour of the skin, as in babies livid with rage; laughing and crying through alternating tension and relaxation in the diaphragm to the extent that other movements are interrupted; or carrying a heavy weight causing people to hold their breath and keep the chest full of air at the height of the struggle by diverting spirits away from the diaphragm. The movement of these spirits between the cerebellum and cerebrum traverses the protuberances of the midbrain, the *nates* and *testes* (superior and inferior colliculi) from which nerves (designated 'pathetic') that move the face and eyes in response to emotion take their origin.

Muscle fibres are lakes where the spirits rest until activated. They contain nervous juice but also have an independent source of vital spirits carried directly through the arteries. Both lie quiet until aroused by a command from the brain through the cranial and spinal nerves serving as a channel for the flow of nervous spirit. This explains why a nerve, exposed and touched, responds by vermicular motion and causes the muscle to which it is attached to expand and contract. The failure of spirits to flow into muscles from nerves that are 'griped, contracted and wrinkled', for any one of several reasons, leads to paralysis. With fault in the medulla, this results in paraplegia or hemiplegia depending on the site and extent. More restricted weakness results from effects centred on the individual nerves. Willis argues that the ambiguity whereby sensation may be preserved, in part or in whole, in the context of paralysis is explained on the basis that fewer spirits are required for sensation than movement. The spirits for each move through different pathways in the spinal medulla; and structures enabling the five senses respond only to specific stimuli.

Sleep allows the blood to rest and leaves the replenished nervous spirits ready to flow into the nerves on waking. Even during sleep, the nervous spirits may diffuse to the cerebrum resulting in nocturnal speech and walking, and induce phantasies and memories in dreams as the spirits 'go over the tracks and orbits marked out in the circuits of the brain, moving around in a varied and irregular manner'. Nightmares occur when this traffic reaches the cerebellum and involuntary movements erupt. For gravitational reasons, these disturbances of sleep are more likely to occur when lying on the back. Waste material escapes during sleep through sweating. Sleeping with the mouth agape and yawning on waking remove 'soot' through the breath. Some people are phlegmatic and sleep more readily because their blood is serous and easily induces relaxation of spirits in the brain. Others, with spirits that are continually agitated and expanded, experience and tolerate prolonged wakefulness. Sleep occurs by habit at fixed times and cannot easily be resisted; it may be encouraged by physical and mental exercise, staying awake for long periods, and by soothing music and the murmur of water and the wind. Sleep is analogous to the weather. It combines unhealthy elements when humid and wet with their separation during dry seasons. It follows that people are drowsy and like to sleep in wet weather and when the wind is from the south.

Sleep deprivation inhibits digestion and leads to foul belching. Sleeping immediately after a meal or drinking newly brewed beer have the same effect. Sleep occurs after drunkenness because the nervous spirits are diluted by extraneous matter and the brain loses the tension of its waking state until such time as the noxious material is dispersed. It follows that narcotics are useful in inducing sleep when the brain is overheated. The amount that can be tolerated differs (dogs are tolerant whereas the same quantity given to a cat 'launches it at once into eternity') and habitual use lessens its force. Willis speaks of a woman in London who eventually required twelve grains of laudanum each night in order to quieten the hot spirits in her brain.

In his lectures and the published treatises, Willis uses the term convulsion to denote the failure of antagonist muscles to relax when the agonist contracts. This causes pain and spasm. He argues that the ancient explanation for convulsion based on saturation of the nerves is not correct. Rather, convulsion occurs when nervous spirits in the medulla are corrupted and in tumult. There follows 'leapings and contractions' of the muscles and other affected parts. Not only a manifestation of disease, 'drunkards become paralytic, and lechers fall into convulsions'. Women with hysterical disorders and retention of the menses have convulsive abdominal complaints that may extend to intestinal compression, incontinence of urine and faeces, or uterine prolapse. But after much common sense, Willis's remedy for fever-induced convulsions is to apply poultices of freshly chopped-up puppies or the young of doves to the feet and head, in order to soak away the abnormal spirits and encourage flow to the lymphatics for removal by sweating. By now, the attention of his listeners, sympathetic to the physiological formulations, may have started to wander.

Willis's concept of convulsion does incorporate epilepsy. Its many causes lead to turbulence of the nervous spirits, which boil over in the cerebral cortex swamping the medulla and from there being transmitted to the nerves and muscles. Convulsions originating in the cerebellum alter the pulse and respiration, the patients beating their breasts during the seizure so as to restore these activities, and with involuntary emission of urine and faeces. The presence of undigested material in the brain causes loss of awareness during, and altered memory after, the paroxysm. Eventually the morbid matter dissipates or is excreted from the foaming mouth of the person with epilepsy. Arthritis is a convulsion arising from the collision of salt in blood needed for bone and acid in the nervous juice leading to 'wonderful battles and ebulliations' of fermentation leaving gravel, tophi, and argillaceous (sedimentary) material in the joints.

One of Willis's less well-recognized contributions was to discard the view that—heralded by vertigo, blurred vision, and headaches—hysteria is not due to vapours emanating from the uterus or spleen but a convulsive disorder of the brain resulting in stimulation of nerves and much distemper of the abdominal organs. As for its treatment, in line with Willis's view that the brain and genital organs compete for nutrients needed to make their respective spirits, and at risk of endorsing promiscuity, he advises that 'in all these cases there is no more beneficial cure than to exercise venery, and thereby evacuate the head in a natural manner and the mind will then become clear and attentive once more'. Other approaches to management of hysteria include stimulating the nostrils with fumigators, which compete with the spirits migrating towards the brain, stimulating the navel and pudenda with musk, or bleeding to remove the abnormal spirit.

Three lectures are specifically devoted to remedies: purges, cordials, and narcotics. By the time he had written the two parts of *Pharmaceutice rationalis* (1674 and 1675), Willis had reorganized his thoughts on these and other classes of treatment, considerably expanding his pharmacopoeia and account of the principles underlying the choice and combination of remedies. In that context, these lectures can be regarded as preliminary by comparison with those containing his already well-formulated ideas on the nervous system.

The intellectual stimulation of being amongst the first to hear Willis's ideas articulated in these lectures must have been immense. Almost immediately, his students were able to read Willis's thoughts on the brain in *Cerebri anatome* (1664). By the time he wrote *De anima brutorum* (1672) these ideas had crystallized into Willis's concept of reflex movement and the role (in modern terminology) of the autonomic nervous system; and his explanation of treatments in the two parts of *Pharmaceutice rationalis* (1674, 1675). For all their whimsicality, spurious chemicals, and flighty hypotheses, by any analysis the lectures given between 1660 and 1667 are sufficiently full of wisdom and novelty to constitute vital transitional readings in the history of ideas relating to order and disorder in the nervous system, and a taster of the monographs that summarized Willis's views on the doctrine of the nerves, and mechanism based therapeutics.

Thomas Willis and the Oxford Philosophical Club

There is ambiguity, and a trace of rivalry, on whether credit for initiating meetings of scientists that culminated in formation of the Royal Society lies with the groups that gathered first in Oxford or in London. Their activities overlapped and several individuals, including Thomas Willis, were involved with both communities. Whereas his engagement with the Royal Society was at best occasional, Willis interacted closely with his colleagues in Oxford, providing leadership and hosting meetings at Beam Hall which had a chemical laboratory and dissecting facilities. Aubrey wrote that Willis was a 'leading and prime man in the Philosophical Club at Oxford'.

Meetings of natural philosophers at which Willis was present were first held at Trinity College in the 1640s. The group was referred to as the Oxford Experimental Club and from 1651, the Oxford Philosophical Club.[77] It was occasionally described by Boyle as the 'Invisible College'.[78] Wood writes that the group 'gave themselves the name of Virtuosi and pretended to go beyond all others in the University for knowledge', a stance that earned them some disapproval elsewhere in the University and, later, from critics such as Henry Stubbe (1632–1676). Aubrey writes of these 'ingeniose scholars' and how 'about these times experimentall philosophy first budded here and was first cultivated by these virtuosi in that darke time'. The participants, around a dozen men, four of whom were physicians and 'many other of the most inquisitive persons', included John Ward, Ralph Bathurst, William Petty, and Willis, 'then an eminent physician in Oxford', and 'divers others'.[79] Of these Ralph Bathurst in particular remained close to Willis throughout his career. When Bathurst died, his acquaintance John Evelyn (1620–1706) made an entry in his diary for 30 May 1704:[80]

> I think the oldest acquaintance now left me in the world. He was 86 years of age, stark blind, deafe, and memory lost, after having ben a person of admirable parts and learning. This is a serious alarm to me. God grant that I may profit by it. He built a very handsome Chapel to

[77] There is no consensus on the dates at which meetings were held in Oxford. Frank (1990): page 119 suggests that these were led by Bathurst and Lydall (1648–1649); Petty (1649–1652); Wilkins (*c.*1651–1657); Boyle (1657–1659, and 1664–1668); and Willis (*c.*1657–1667) at their various homes and other locations.

[78] See: Douglas McKie in Hartley (1960): pages 21–3.

[79] See: Robert Frank, *Harvey and the Oxford physiologists*, Berkeley (1980): pages 53–5, and table 3, pages 63–89 for an excellent description of the various experimental clubs in Oxford and a full list of participants throughout the entire period. Despite their close relationship, John Fell was no admirer of the Royal Society or its predecessors, regarding experimental philosophy as a threat to religion and authority, and to the reputation of the University. See: Adrian Tinniswood, *His invention so fertile. A life of Sir Christopher Wren*, London (2001): page 76 and endnote 13, page 390.

[80] See: John Evelyn, *The diary of John Evelyn Esquire F.R.S.* Ed. William Bray, London (1818, printed *c.*1930): pages 742–3.

> the College [Trinity, Oxford], and his own tomb. He gave a legacy of money, and the third part of his library, to his nephew Dr. Bohun, who went hence to his funeral.

As the group began to formalize its activities, the club met in Petty's rooms at Buckley Hall (107 High Street) where discussions were held and simple experiments carried out. The emphasis was more on mathematics and astronomy than medical sciences and natural philosophy. In time, through its warden, Wilkins, meetings were held at Wadham College which offered access to scientific instruments for 'making chymicall experiments'.[81] On 25 January and 5 April 1649, Lydall informed Aubrey that:[82]

> Mr Batthurst saieth that your two boxes shall bee safe that hee will not forget ye aurum fulminans wch hee promised though hee deferre it because it is not yet prepared, Mr. Willis, our Chymist having beene long absent... [later] the aurum fulminans is now at least prepared as Mr Batthurst tells mee, but he could not meete with Mr. Willis since the arrival of your letter.

Seth Ward wrote in his diary that Willis was one of those who 'have joined together for the furnishing an elaboratory' at Wadham. Willis recorded his expenses 'laid out at Wadham Coll'. These are £21 18s 10d for previous expenditure and new costs for glassware and 'carriage ... of thinges from my Chamber' (£10 4s 8d), drugges from London (£1 19s 6d), carpentry, masonry, and other tradesmen (£6 7s 6d), and 'to old Watt for stilling fires' (£0 1s 6d). A separate account lists similar types of expenditure amounting to £3 16s 4d; and a third is for £2 17s 2d. But Willis needs an accountant since the items, chemical materials and labour services, add up to £2 19s 2d even without the purchase of 'hony', which is not costed.[83]

The Philosophical Club set rules written out by Gerard Langbaine (1609–1658) on 23 October 1651. Membership was by majority vote in a secret ballot which required a quorum of eleven. Subscriptions included provision for 'instruments in stock'. Meetings were held every Thursday before 2 pm with those who failed to attend for a period of six weeks deemed to have forfeited their membership. One person appointed for the day was expected to carry out an experiment, fined 2s 6d if he did not, and required to perform it at a later date appointed by the company.[84] Samuel Hartlib (1600–1662) noted that Willis was the member responsible for the Thursday experiment in November 1654:[85]

> Dr. Wellis of Dr Wilkins acquaintance a very experimenting ingenious gentleman communicating every weeke some experiment or other to Mr. Boyles chymical servant, who is a kind of cozen to him. Hee is a great Verulamian philosopher, from him all may bee had by means of Mr. Boyle.

Thus friendship and shared interests had by the early 1650s led to formation of a club in Oxford which met under defined rules and schedules. Those involved included Christopher Wren (1632–1723) and his cousin Mathew Wren (1629–1672), Robert Hooke (1635–1703)

[81] Although somewhat anachronistic, Wadham now has a 'Royal Society' room, opposite the porters' lodge, where small meetings are held.

[82] See: Bennett [Aubrey] (2015): page 1477; and Dewhurst (1981): page 30.

[83] These accounts are in Willis's handwriting on the rear endpapers of the casebook in the Wellcome Library.

[84] See: Douglas McKie in Hartley (1960): pages 25–6; and Dewhurst (1981): page 39, reference 43.

[85] See: Frank (1980): page 165 endnote 5, chapter 7; and Frank (1990): footnote 20 page 113, footnote 32 page 113.

and Lawrence Rooke (1622–1662) who, with John Wilkins (1614–1672), John Wallis (1616–1703), Jonathan Goddard (1617–1675), and Boyle were also at one time active in the London meetings. The participants were organized by Langbaine into three groups, representing the different areas of interest. The club was sensitive to the importance of books in the pursuit of knowledge. Seth Ward wrote of its purpose:[86]

> For what concerns our Clubb wch consists of about 30 persons we have (every one takeing a portion) gone over all or most of the heads of natural philosophy & mixt mathematics collecting onely an history of the phenomena out of such authors as we have in our library and sometimes trieing experiments as we had occasion and opportunity. Our first businesse is to gather together such things as are already discovered and to make a booke with a general index of them ... we have conceived it requisite to examine all the books of our public library ... and to make a catalogue or index of the matter and that very particularly in philosophy physic mathematics & indeed in all other facultyes.

As his assistant in chemistry in 1650, Hooke admired Willis to the extent that he was listed alongside Harvey, George Ent (1604–1689), and Francis Glisson (1597–1677) in the preface to *Micrographia* (1665) as the men responsible for prodigious advances in anatomy.[87] Geoffrey Keynes (1887–1982) suggests that the course of Hooke's life was determined by his meeting with Thomas Willis. In turn, Willis recommended Hooke to Boyle as his technical assistant. Hooke invented most of the instruments on which Boyle's own work depended.[88]

After Wilkins moved to Trinity College, Cambridge, in 1659 meetings were hosted by Robert Boyle at Deep Hall in the High Street and the group became the 'experimental philosophical clubbe'. Others who joined in that period included Stubbe, Robert Sharrock (1630–1684), Locke, David Thomas (1620–1689), Ralph Austen (1612–1672), Thomas Millington (1628–1714), Lower and Nathaniel Hodges (1629–1688). We learn something from an imaginary walk taken through Oxford in 1659 at the time Willis was living in Beam Hall and the people and places that shaped the activities and atmosphere of the place.[89] Trevor Hughes has compiled a list (with some duplications) of these and other individuals attached to Oxford Colleges who were close to Willis or contributed to the evolution of his work as physician and scientist, or who engaged with him professionally: he lists fifteen individuals including Wilkins, Rooke, Thomas Sprat (1635–1713), Seth Ward and Christopher Wren at Wadham; thirteen including Harvey, Goddard and Lydall at Merton; eleven including (apart from Willis himself) Richard Allestry (1619–1667), Hooke, Locke, Lower, Stubbe, and John Ward at Christ Church; eight including Aubrey and Ralph Bathurst at Trinity; and seven including Sheldon and Millington at All Souls; together with Petty (Brasenose), Wallis (Exeter) and Boyle who, as the son of the Earl of Cork (1566–1643), had independent means and needed no university attachment in Oxford.[90] The founder group started to disband

[86] See: William Poole, *Wadham College books in the age of John Wilkins (1614–1672)*, privately printed for Wadham College (2014): page 52.

[87] See: Allan Chapman and Cristina Neagu, *Robert Hooke's* Micrographia *and Christ Church science, 1650–1670*. An exhibition at Christ Church Upper Library (5 November 2015–20 January 2016): pages 1–26, for an account of Hooke's *Micrographia* and notes on his Oxford contemporaries, including Thomas Willis.

[88] See: Geoffrey Keynes, *A bibliography of Dr Robert Hooke*, Oxford (1960).

[89] See: Frank (1980): pages 60–2: this is reproduced in full by Hughes (1991): pages 22–4.

[90] See: Hughes (1991): page 47. Occasionally these colleagues made reference to Willis or his work: see, for example J Wallis, 'A relation of an accident of thunder and lightning at Oxford', *Philosophical Transactions of the Royal Society* (1666): 1; 222–6, in which Wallis describes the episode on 10 May 1666 when a Wadham College

when Wren and Rooke and then Boyle left Oxford, in or before 1659. For a while, Willis provided continuity from the earlier meetings. But although still in Oxford, his interest may have waned and Willis rarely if ever attended meetings in the 1660s before he also moved to London in 1667. Meetings which provided teaching and research as well as functioning as a club for dining and discussion continued in the Ashmolean theatre under the leadership of Wallis and Robert Plot. But activity gradually reduced as members moved elsewhere and after 1690, the era of seventeenth century scientific societies dedicated to natural philosophy in Oxford came to a close.

The episode of Anne Greene

We learn something of the methods used by members of the Philosophical club, and its successors, from the case of Anne Greene (also known as Anne Green: 1628–1665). Until the Anatomy Act of 1832 the victims of capital punishment were the only legitimate source of bodies for dissection. On 14 December 1650, Petty and Willis secured for their anatomical demonstration the body of Anne who had just been hanged by Jack Ketch (d.1686) in the Oxford Parks for the murder of her child following conviction by Serjeant Upton Croke (1593–1670).[91] Under the 1636 charter issued by Charles I, the Tomlins reader could command the body of anyone executed within 21 miles of Oxford. This meant that Petty, who held the position and was required to demonstrate a 'sounde' body of one such victim of jurisprudence dissected by a 'chirurgeon' every spring after the Lent Assizes had access to Anne's fresh corpse. She was taken to Petty's lodgings in Catte St, off the High Street and next to All Souls College, which he shared with Richard Tillyard (d.1693). They found, however, that 'some vital heat still remained' and so set to and after much perseverance restored her to life (see: Figure 8). As always, accounts differ slightly in terms of detail. Wood writes:[92]

> Anno Domini 1650 happened that memorable accident and experiment of the reviving of Nan Greene, a servant maid who was hang'd in the Castle of Oxon for murdering her bastard child. After she had suffer'd the Law, she was cut downe and carried away in order to be anatomiz'd by some young physitians.

A modern rendering of the story tells that in the confusion of finding her alive, those present wrenched open her clenched teeth, poured in 'hot and cordiall spirits', rubbed her down, bled her of five ounces, tickled her throat with a feather, worked in oils and other medicaments, and 'put her to bed to a warme woman'. However a lusty fellow had 'stamped on her breast and stomach severall times with all the force he could', thereby inadvertently resuscitating Anne, her survival being helped by the fact that it was December, and she was hypothermic.[93] Seth Ward described the episode as 'true natural Magick ... applying agent

undergraduate was struck by lightning whilst on the river Isis and killed instantly. Willis carried out an autopsy and apart from superficial burns found no internal injuries.

[91] Opinions differ on whether the execution took place in the Parks or Castle [Yard].

[92] See: Wood, volume 1 (1813): page xviii.

[93] See: William Feindel, 'Thomas Willis (1621–1675)—the founder of neurology', *Canadian Medical Association Journal* 1962; 87: 289–96. For a modern fictional rendering of the event, see: Iain Pears, *An instance of the fingerpost*, London (1997). Narrated by a series of observers, Sarah Blundy is hanged for the murder of Dr Grove of New

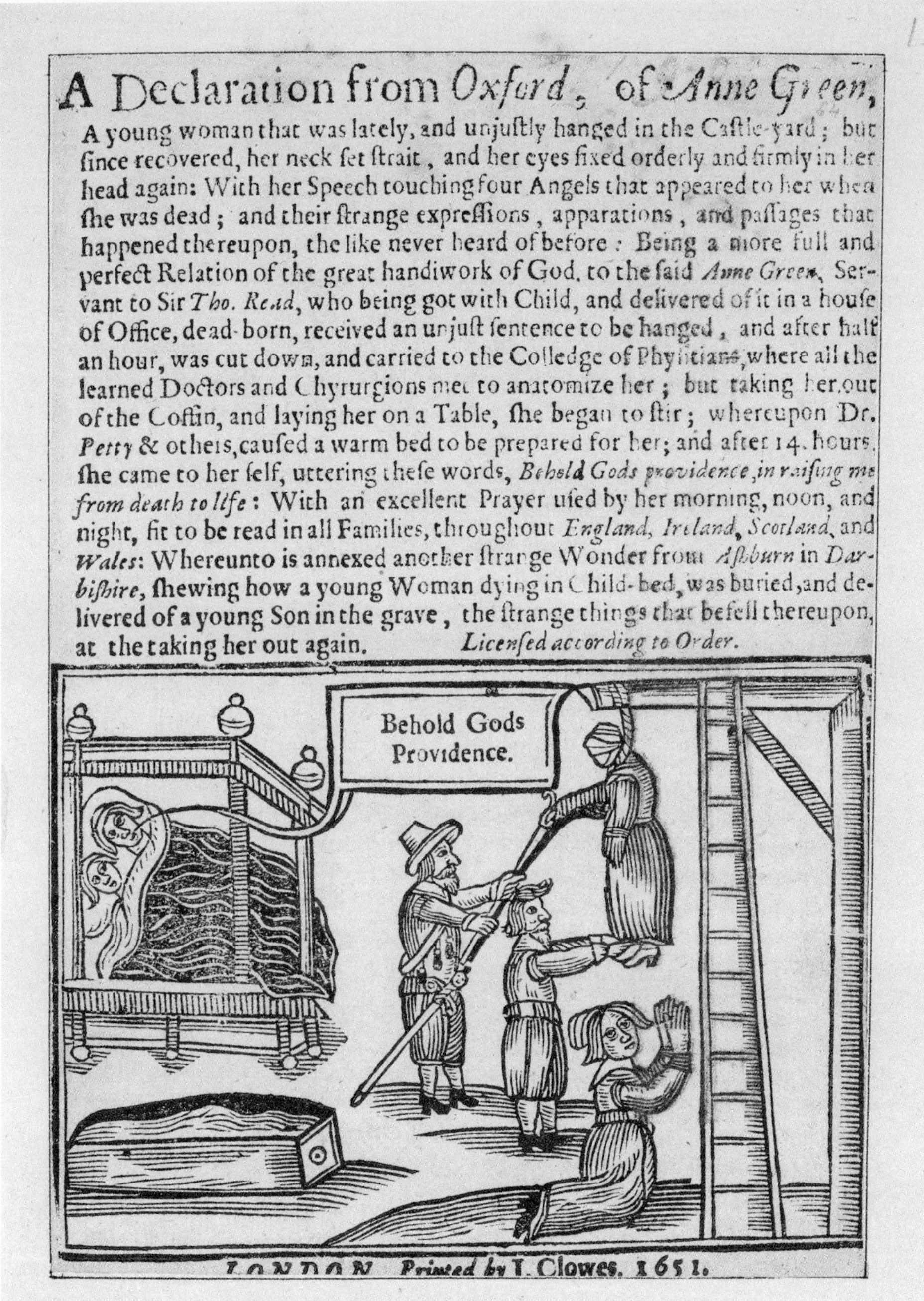

A Declaration from *Oxford*, of *Anne Green*,

A young woman that was lately, and unjuſtly hanged in the Caſtle-yard; but ſince recovered, her neck ſet ſtrait, and her eyes fixed orderly and firmly in her head again: With her Speech touching four Angels that appeared to her when ſhe was dead; and their ſtrange expreſſions, apparations, and paſſages that happened thereupon, the like never heard of before: Being a more full and perfect Relation of the great handiwork of God, to the ſaid *Anne Green*, Servant to Sir *Tho. Read*, who being got with Child, and delivered of it in a houſe of Office, dead-born, received an unjuſt ſentence to be hanged, and after half an hour, was cut down, and carried to the Colledge of Phyſitians, where all the learned Doctors and Chyrurgions met to anatomize her; but taking her out of the Coffin, and laying her on a Table, ſhe began to ſtir; whereupon Dr. *Petty* & others, cauſed a warm bed to be prepared for her; and after 14. hours, ſhe came to her ſelf, uttering theſe words, *Behold Gods providence, in raiſing me from death to life*: With an excellent Prayer uſed by her morning, noon, and night, fit to be read in all Families, throughout *England*, *Ireland*, *Scotland*, and *Wales*: Whereunto is annexed another ſtrange Wonder from *Aſhburn* in *Darbiſhire*, ſhewing how a young Woman dying in Child-bed, was buried, and delivered of a young Son in the grave, the ſtrange things that befell thereupon, at the taking her out again. *Licenſed according to Order.*

LONDON *Printed by* T. Clowes. 1651.

Figure 8 Contemporary depiction of the story of Anne Greene. Printed by T. Clowes, London, 1651.

College and found to be breathing as Lower and Locke proceed to the dissection; she is discretely removed from the premises and another corpse is substituted and mutilated so as not to offend the baying crowds. Many familiar names and places feature but of Willis there is only passing mention.

and Materiall causes to produce effects'.[94] Contemporary details are provided by Richard Watkins (nd: 1651):[95]

> In the House of Sir *Thomas Read* at *Dunstew* in *Oxfordshire*, there lived a Maid named *Anne Greene*, born at *Steeple-Barton* in the same County, being about twenty-two Years of Age, of a middle Stature, strong, fleshie, and of an indifferent good Feature: Who being (as she said) often sollicitied by faire Promises and other amorous Enticements of Mr *Jeffery Read* Grandchild to the said Sir *Thomas*, a youth of about sixteen or seventeen Years of Age, but of a forward Growth and Stature, at last consented to satisfy his unlawfull Pleasure. By which Act (as it afterward appeared) she conceived, and was delivered of a Man-child: Which being never made knowne, and the Infant found dead in the House of Office, caused a suspicion, that she, being the Mother had Murthered it, and thrown it there, on purpose to conceal both it and her Shame together... She was at a Sessions held in *Oxford*, arraigned, condemned, and on *Saturday* the 14th of *December* last, brought forth to the Place of Execution: Where after singing of a Psalme and something said in Justification of herself, as to the fact for which she was to suffer and touching the Lewdness of the Family wherein she had lately lived, she was turn'd off the Ladder, hanging by the Neck for the Space of almost halfe an Hour; some of her Friends in the meantime thumping her on the Breast, others hanging with all their Weight upon her Leggs, sometimes lifting her up, and then pulling her downe again with a sudden Jerke, thereby the sooner to dispatch her out of her only Paine, insomuch that the Under-Sherriff fearing lest thereby they should breake the Rope, forbad them to do so any longer. At length, when everyone thought she was dead, the Body was taken downe, and put into a Coffin, was carried thence into a private House, where some Physicians had appointed to make a Dissection. The Coffin being open she was observed to breath and in breathing (the passage of her Throat being straightened) obscurely to rattle: Which being perceived by a lusty Fellow who stood by, he (thinking to do an Act of Charity, in ridding her out of the small Reliques of a painful Life) stamped several Times on her breast and Stomach with all the force he could. Immediately after, there came in Dr *Petty* of *Brasen-nose* Colledge, our Anatomy-Professor, and Mr *Thomas Willis* of *Christ-Church*, at whose coming, which was about Nine a-Clock in the Morning, she yet persisted to rattle as before; laying all this while stretched out in the Coffin, in a cold room and Season of the Year. They perceiving some Life in her, as well for Humanity as their Profession-sake, fell presently to act in order to her recovery...
>
> ... About this Time came in Mr *Bathurst* of *Trinity Colledge*, and Mr *Clerke* of *Magdalen Colledge*, whose Advice and Endeavours were then, and all the Time afterwards concurrent with those of the other two above mentioned.[96] While the physicians were thus busy in recovering her to Life, the Under-Sherriff was soliciting the Governor, and the rest of the Justices of the Peace, for the obtaining her Reprieve; that in case she should, for that present, be recovered fully to Life, she might not be had back again to Execution.

[94] See: Seth Ward and John Wilkins *Vindicæ academiarum, containing some briefe animadversions upon Mr Webster's book stiled the examination of academies*, Oxford (1654), cited in Martensen (2004b): page 176.

[95] See: Richard Watkins, *Newes from the dead, or, a true and exact narration of the miraculous deliverance of Anne Greene: who being executed at Oxford Decemb. 14, 1650, afterwards revived and is now perfectly recovered: together with the manner of her suffering and the particular meanes used for her recovery*, Oxford (1651).

[96] A former owner has annotated the copy of Watkins's book held by the Wellcome Library in the margin: 'and Mr Conyers of St John's'

All contemporary accounts of the episode are thought to originate with William Petty since they differ in no material respect from his own 'History of the Magdalen (or the raising of Anne Greene)'. This is number 126 of his medical papers written in Latin and unpublished until the twentieth century.[97] Petty's account emphasizes the attempts to accelerate her death on the gallows by dragging on Anne's legs, beating her breasts, 'and moreover a souldier did the same severall tymes with the butt end of his musquett'. On arrival at the place for dissection, at 9 am, he writes that signs of life were detected which led to the stamping on her breasts and stomach by a lusty fellow: 'presently after myselfe and Mr. Willis came in, and found her yet to rattle a little as before notwithstanding the said latter strokes'. It was at this point that matters changed to efforts aimed at restoring not extinguishing life. Petty emphasizes the contribution made by bleeding: but 'as soon as her arme was bound . . . shee suddenly bent it, as if it had been contracted by a convulsion fit. The vayne being cut, she bled so freely that having bled 5 ounces, when we desired to stop, wee could not easily'. For a while, her pulse remained slow but Anne recovered with the practical measures well described by others. Petty's account provides details, not otherwise available, of the medications that he and Willis administered, immediately and over the next few days. These included cordials (rainwater and cinnamon in equal parts one ounce and Acetosella, a preparation of sorrel, four ounces); anointing the neck wound with turpentine and stimulating the nasal mucosa with oil of cloves; plasters to her breasts; and a healing and odiferous enema which 'came away' after some hours with the addition of a candle end by way of a suppository followed later by insertion of allum. When she started to respond, Petty and Willis rebled Anne and gave a lemon julep and syrup of tamarind. They left her at 9pm and during the late evening, Anne began to speak.

They returned early next day and had lucid conversations with Anne. Her sore throat was treated with a poultice. She was restless but settled that evening with a clyster (enema) which was imperfectly given due to the 'women's unhandiness'. A cataplasme (poultice) was applied to her temples. Now eating bread soaked in water and drinking 'small beere', after two days (16 December), Anne 'made some water but had no stoole' until the following day. When others were not present, Petty and Willis asked what Anne could recall of the past few days. The answer was nothing beyond taking off her bodice which had cost 5 shillings, and giving this to her mother, on the morning of the execution. Later she did remember seeing the executioner. By 17 December, Anne had a slow and irregular pulse and she was dizzy on standing in order to have her bed made. The tip of her tongue was numb. Unguents were applied to her sore and blistered skin, and further bleedings carried out. By 25 December, Anne had residual bruises but was otherwise well recovered.

Many curious people came to gaze at Anne and before long they were charged for the pleasure which earned her several pounds 'whereby the Apothecaries Bill, and other Necessaries for her Diet and Lodging, were discharged, but some Overplus remained towards the sueing out her Pardon'. Petty wrote out Anne's petition submitted to the Privy Council on the grounds that she had a spontaneous miscarriage at 18 weeks of a foetus dead at birth, and therefore the harsh sentence she received was undeserved. Petty also retained the 'certificates' that 'wee the physicians' submitted confirming details of the miraculous event. In this he makes clear that, on the testimony of the midwife, the foetus was not only aborted or stillborn but also so deformed and stunted as be of uncertain sex and never

[97] See: [William Petty] *The Petty papers. Some unpublished writings of Sir William Petty. Edited from the Bowood papers by the Marquis of Lansdowne*, volume 2, London (1927): pages 155, 157–67; and Dewhurst (1980): page 7 and page 30, note 39.

capable of life. It was more 'a lump of flesh than a mature and onely formed child'. Almost certainly, Anne had not even known that she was pregnant. His further pleading, with paragraphs crossed through which, on rereading, might not have strengthened her case, argues for a full pardon, not least because of her subsequent ordeal, repentance of having submitted to fornication, and the unanimous desire for clemency of the many good people who came 'to behold and admire this signall act of Providence'.

Anne was duly pardoned and became something of a circus act being exhibited laid in her coffin in the room where she was to have been dissected and requiring 'guards to control the crowd' when 'multitudes flooded daily to see her'. Her father continued to collect the fees. Eventually she was sent home with her coffin as a 'Trophey of her wonderful preservation'. According to Evelyn, 'the young scholars joined and made a little portion', and married her to a man in Steeple Barton by whom Anne had three children during the remaining 15 years of her life after this unhappy but profitable episode. It is a matter of irony that Sir Thomas Reade (*c.*1575–1650), her 'Grand Prosecutor', learning of her recovery died three days after Anne's execution but no one of the contemporary commentators made anything of this in terms of divine retribution. *Newes from the dead* (1651) concludes with nineteen verses, some in Latin with English translations.[98] Amongst these poets is William Willis (1631–1662), Thomas's brother:

In Puellam ſuſpenſam, & dein à Medicis Anatomiam Cadaveris aggreſſuris, in Vitam revocatam.

DUM Mors & Medici conſpirant fœdere certo,
Ambrorum ut telis una puella cadat;
Funi ut ſuccedat Ferrum, & ſuſpenſa ſecetur;
En Ferrum & Funis, bina venena, juvant.
Unâ mulctatam, geminâ dum morte parabant
Afficere, in vitam fit rediviva novam.
Naturæ in leges, ac Gentis jura, triumphans
Eluſit Fati Judicis atque, minas.
Nec Medici hoc, Sceleton faciunt, exangue Cadaver,
Quid magis eſt, vivum cedit in Automaton.
Guil. Willis Æd. Ch. Comm.

To a girl who was hung and subsequently brought back to life by the physicians who were about to dissect her cadaver.[99]

While Death and Doctors connive in a joint plan
So that one girl succumbs through instruments of both;
Knife succeeding the rope, dissection the hanging;
Behold, Rope and Knife, both lethal, rejoice.

[98] The authors are: H.B. [Henry Berkenhead] Coll. Om. Anim.; *Hen. Perin*, Gen. Com. of Trin. Coll.; *J. Hutton*, Fell. of New-Coll.; *Geo. Lee*, Coll. Reg. Commensalis.; *Jos. Williamson*, du Coll. de la Reyne.; *John Watkins* Gen. Com. of Q. Coll.; *Rob. Mathew* of New Coll.; *Guil. Fitz-Gerald* ex Æd. Ch.; Guil. Willis Æd. Ch. Comm.; *Rob. Sharrock* of New Coll.; *Dan Danvers* Coll. Trin. Alumnus.; *Jo. Aylmer* School of New Coll.; *Peter Killigrew*, Gen. Com. of Qu. Coll.; *Guil. Miles*, Nov. Coll.; *Rich. Glid*, New Coll.; *Geo Davenant*, Com. Of Q. Coll.; H. Davenant, Com. Coll. Reg.; *John Dwight*, Ch. Ch.; *Tho. Ireland*, Ch. Ch.; *Ed. Norreys*, Eq. Aur. fil. Coll. Reg.; *Edwin Skrymsher*, Armig. fil. Nat. Max. Coll. Trin.; *Christ Wren*, Gent. Com. of Wad. Coll.; *Car. Forster*, Eq. Aur. fil. Coll. Trin.; and *Kingsmill Lucy*, Gent. Com. of Ch. Ch.

[99] Translation by Jan van Gijn, 13 November 2019.

While both in unison prepared the condemned
For death, she can return to a new life.
Victorious over Nature's laws or Mankind's rules
She escaped the threats of Fate and Justice.
Physicians do not turn a bloodless Corpse into a Skeleton,
What is more, it yields a living Creature.
Guil. Willis Æd. Ch. Comm.

Christopher Wren also contributed a verse that bore passing reference to Anne Greene:

WOnder of higheſt Art! he who will reach
A Strain for thee, had need his Muſe should *ſtretch*
Till flying to the Shades, ſhe learn what Vein
Of *Orpheus* call'd *Eurydice* again:
Or learn of her *Apollo*, till ſhe can,
As well as Singer, prove Phyſician.
And then ſhe may, without *Suſpension*, ſing;
And, authorized, harp upon thy *String*.
Diſcordant String! for ſure thy Soul (unkind
To its own Bowels Iſſue) could not find
One Breaſt in Conſort to its jarring Stroke
'Mongſt piteous Female Organs, therefore broke
Tranſlation's due Law, from Fate repriev'd,
And ſtruck a Unison to her ſelf, and liv'd.
Was't this? or was it that the *Goatiſh* Flow
Of thy adult'rous Veins (from thence let go
By ſecond *Æſculapius* his Hand)
Diſſolv'd the *Parcæ*'s Adamantine Band,
And made thee, Artiſt's Glory, Shame of Fate
Triumph of Nature, *Virbius*'s Mate
Chriſt. Wren, Gent. Com. Of Wad. Coll.

And Kingsmill Lucy (*c.*1592–1667), of Christ Church, contributed lines that end with a much quoted and witty couplet:

To the happy Instruments *of the Executed* Maid's *Recovery.*

OXFORD (the Art's Metropolis) ne'er knew
A rarer Feat than was perform'd by you
Brave *Æſculapian* Friends! whoſe Art could give,
After the Execution, a Reprieve.
And yet 'twas timely too; for tho' grim Death
Had ſeiz'd the Paſſage of her vital Breath,
Yet you a new one made: And the ſame Vein
Which let out Blood, receiv'd in Life again.
The Soul, which is in every Part intire,
Can, undiſcern'd by you, to none retire:
Since you no leſs the Track of Souls do know,

Than that of Lev'rets in new-fallen Snow.
Others can by their Chymiftry reduce
A Plant or Flower from its Duft or Juice;
But your fublimer Art hath done much more,
While human Souls you from their Urns reftore.
Yet though your Skill and Pity could difpence
More Days to her beguiled Innocence;
No Art removes a ruin'd Virgin's Shame,
Unlefs revived fhe, be not the fame.
Thus 'tis more eafy to recal the dead
Than to reftore a once-loft Maidenhead.

The students who rallied to her cause were equally direct in a popular rhyme that went:

Anne Greene was a slippery quean
In vain did the jury detect her:-
She cheated Jack Ketch, and then the vile wretch
Scap'd the knife of the learned dissector

There are two other contemporary accounts of this episode each of which acquits Anne of the putative crime: W Burdet's (nd) *A wonder of wonders*; and Anon, *A declaration from Oxford*, both published as eight page pamphlets by John Clowes (fl. 1647–1660) London (1651). As Burdet has it:

> A wonder of wonders. Being a faithful narrative and true relation of one Anne Green, servant to Sir Tho. Reed in Oxfordshire, who being got with child by a gentleman, her child falling from her in the house or office, being but a span long, and dead born, was condemned on the 14. of December last, and hanged in the castle-yard in Oxford, for the space of half an hour, receiving many great and heavy blowes on the brests, by the but end of the souldiers muskets, and being pul'd down by the leggs, and was afterwards beg'd for an anatomy, by the physicians, and carried to Mr. Clarkes house, an apothecary, where in the presence of many learned chyrurgions, she breathed, and began to stir; insomuch, that Dr. Petty caused a warm bed to be prepared for her, let her blood, and applyed oyls to her, so that in 14 hours she recovered, and the first words she spake were these; behold Gods providence! Behold his miraculous and loving kindness! With the manner of her tryal, her speech and confession at the gallowes; and a declaration of the souldiery touching her recovery. Witnessed by Dr. Petty, and licensed according to order.

The anonymous version also published in 1651 reads:[100]

> A declaration from Oxford, of Anne Green a young woman that was lately, and unjustly hanged in the Castle-yard; but since recovered, her neck set strait, and her eyes fixed orderly and firmly in her head again: with her speech touching four angels that appeared to her when she was dead; and their strange expressions, apparations, and passages that happened thereupon, the like never heard of before: being a more full and perfect relation of the great handiwork of God, to the said Anne Green, servant to Sir Tho. Read, who

[100] See: Huntington Library, #123781; https://catalog.huntington.org/search?/X+A+declaration+from+Oxford.

being got with child, and delivered of it in a house of office, dead born, received an unjust sentence to be hanged, and after half an hour, was cut down, and carried to the colledge of physitians, where all the learned doctors and chyrurgions met to anatomize her; but... she began to stir; ... and after 14 hours, she came to her self, ... Whereunto is annexed another strange wonder from Ashburn in Darbishire, shewing how a young woman dying in child-bed, was buried, and delivered of a young son in the grave.

John Evelyn also gives a retrospective account of the episode in his diary for 22 March 1674. Dining with Seth Ward (now Bishop of Salisbury) and Petty, Evelyn wrote:[101]

> Sir William [Petty] was the sonn of a mean man some where in Sussex, and sent from Schole to Oxon, where he studied Philosophy, but was most eminent in Mathematics and Mechanics; proceeded Dr. of Physick, as was grown famous, as for his learning so for his recovering a poor wench that had been hanged for felony; and her body having ben begged (as the custom is) for the anatomie lecture, he bled her, put her to bed to a warm woman, and with spirits and other meanes restored her to life. The young scholars joyn'd and made her a little portion, and married her to a man who had severall children by her, she living 15 yeares after, as I have been assur'd. Sir William came from Oxon, to be tutor to a neighbour of mine; thence, when the rebells were dividing their conquests in Ireland, he was emply'd by them to measure and set out the land, which he did on an easy contract, so much per acre. This he effected so exactly, that it not only furnished him with a greate sum of money, but enabled him to purchase an estate worth £4000 a yeare. He afterwards married the daughter of Sir Hardresse Waller; she was an extraordinary witt as well as beauty, and a prudent woman.

Joseph Morgan prefaces the reprinting of *Newes from the dead* (1732) with an editorial comment:

> [The following remarkable Piece needs no better Recommendation than that of the ingenious Mr. Richard Glid, of New-College in Oxford, wherewith he concludes his Verses, on the Subject, hereunto (among the many other good Copies) annexed: And that one of these Pamphlets was lately sold for a Guinea. Nor can any Part of the Story itself be disputed, being quoted and confirmed by so many credible Writers, as Dr. Plott, in his Natural History of Oxfordshire; Dr. Derham, in his Phisico-Theologica, &c, which last affirms his having seen this Woman, alive and well, many Years after, and that she had divers Children. – In a small Octavo, I have by me, intitled Britain's Triumphs, &c. Printed in 1656, the Author, having given the Substance of the whole Fact, concludes thus. 'In short Space she perfectly recovered; upon which first her Reprieve and then her Pardon was procured. After this, she (as upon the Gallows) still insisted upon her Innocency and Integrity, in relation to the Fact, for which she was condemned. And, indeed, this was

[101] See: John Evelyn (1818, printed *c.*1930): page 475. In footnote 2, the editor, William Bray, draws attention to *Newes from the dead* but without identifying the author, citing the second impression (Oxford, with additions, 1651) and specifying the verses including that by 'Christopher Wren, the famous architect, then of Wadham College ... [and] Dr. Ralph Bathurst (the last under other names)'. Bray identifies a further printing of the pamphlet: see [Richard Watkins] 'News from the dead: or a true and exact narration of the miraculous deliverance of Anne Greene'. In: Joseph Morgan, *Phoenix Britannicus: being a miscellaneous collection of scarce and curious tracts, historical, political, biographical, satirical, critical, characteristical, &c. Prose and verse. Only to be found in the cabinets of the curious. Interspersed with choice pieces from original Mss*, volume I (all printed), containing numbers I, II, III, IV, V, and VI, London (1732): pages 233–48.

looked upon as a special Providence of God, thus to deliver her, who, in the Judgments of those who understood the Business was deemed guiltless. Herein did the Hand of God wonderfully appear, in detecting the unadvised Actings of Men, and in shewing us the Danger we are in, when we are swayed, either by Passion or Prejudice, against the Meanest of his Creatures'. – This Abridgement of the Narrative is introduced with these Words: – 'During which Interval, there happened as remarkable an Accident in England, as any Story can parallel; which, for the Strangeness and Rarity thereof, may well merit my Pains to recite, and the Reader's Patience to peruse' – N.B. I deviate nothing from the Original, only in putting the Copies of Verses after the Story, whereas in my Copy, they are prefixed, and in a few Literal Errors].

Thomas Willis and the Royal Society

'A Colledge for the promoting of Physico-Mathematicall Experimental Learning' was founded on 28 November 1660 by twelve individuals who met at 3pm after a lecture by Christopher Wren at Gresham College in London.[102] Thomas Willis was not present. The twelve suggested a further forty-one names for inclusion in their Society, not listed alphabetically, of which Willis is number 30.[103] He received the invitation to participate on 30 January 1661. The founders agreed to meet weekly and 'put downe ten shillings ... and one shilling weekly whether present or absent'. The initiative met with the approval of King Charles II. Before long eighty-five individuals had signed the form of obligation. On 12 December 1660, it was agreed that the membership of the Society be limited to fifty-five but with barons, Fellows of the Royal College of Physicians, and professors of Mathematics, Physic, and Natural Philosophy based in Oxford or Cambridge all eligible as supernumeraries. John Wilkins acted initially as chairman until (Sir) Robert Moray (*c.*1608–1673) was appointed on 6 March 1661. Two rooms at Gresham College were set aside for meetings and accommodating books and other material accumulated by the members. An important function of the Society was to perform experiments. In October 1661, King Charles was elected to the fellowship and, in that year, John Evelyn referred to 'The Royal Society' in the dedication of his translation of a book by Gabriel Nauté (1600–1653), his suggestion being acknowledged gratefully by the 'philosophic assembly'.[104]

The Society received its Royal Charter from the King on 15 July 1662, being renamed the Royal Society for improving Natural Knowledge. The charter was modified on 22 April 1663 and a further version issued in 1669. By then, the Royal Society had moved from Gresham College to Arundel House, at the invitation of Henry Howard, 6th Duke of Norfolk (1628–1684), who bequeathed the library created by his grandfather, Philip Howard, 1st Earl of Arundel (1557–1595). With sales, purchases, and donations this became a significant scientific library. None of Willis's research was first published in *Philsophical Transactions*

[102] These were: Lord Brouncker (1620–1684), Mr Boyle, Mr Bruce (1626–1685), Sir Robert Moray, Sir Paule Neile (*c.*1613–*c.*1686), Dr Wilkins, Dr Goddard, Dr Petty, Mr Ball (*c.*1638–1675), Mr Rooke, Mr Wren, and Mr Hill (1633–1721).

[103] Fifteen of the 41 were physicians, a representation that the Royal Society has not since maintained.

[104] See: Gabriel Naudé, *Instructions concerning erecting of a library presented to my lord, the President De Mesme by Gabriel Naudeus; and now interpreted by Jo. Evelyn, Esquire*, London (1661). Robert Harrison, 'The Royal Society'. In: *The Encyclopaedia Britannica*, Cambridge (1911): pages 791–3 points out that when, on 1 December 1690, Evelyn was himself elected president he declined: 'Having been chosen President of the Royal Society I desired to decline it, and with greate difficulty devolv'd the election on Sir Robert Southwell, Secretary of State to King William in Ireland. See: Evelyn (1818, printed *c.*1930): page 684.

but the Society did receive copies of all his published works and most were reviewed in the journal.[105]

However, despite being amongst the original 53 names and with his fellowship confirmed at the meeting on 18 November 1663, Willis was not admitted to the Royal Society until 24 October 1667. The delay was explained in the journal book:

> Dr Willis was chosen, having been forgot to be chosen again at the time when, upon the renewall of the charter, the Council, according to the power granted them therein, did receive and admitt into the Society such persons as had been elected Fellows afore upon the first charter.

Admitted on the same day was Henry, 2nd Earl of Peterborough (1621–1697). The signature book of the Royal Society shows Willis's name on page 6, the same as Petty and Boyle; with Hooke, Bathurst, Walter Charleton (1619–1707), Aubrey and Wren signed on page 5, and Lower on page 7. In the tercentenary celebration of the Society, biographies are provided on twelve founders and nine others roughly in the order that they contributed to early activities of the Society. After King Charles II, Willis is number five, preceded by John Wilkins, John Wallis, Jonathan Goddard, and William Petty.[106] From this it would appear that Thomas Willis was prominent in the origins of the Society and active in its initial meetings.

Although the most reliable source of information on how the Royal Society came about and who was involved is likely to be from those who were there, such accounts may favour the loyalties felt by the author of a particular account.[107] No one was impartial. Wallis writes that, in about 1645, whilst living in London and at a time when academic life was disrupted in 'both Universities' (Oxford and Cambridge), he became involved with a group interested in natural philosophy or in that branch which came to be known as experimental philosophy. Wallis left two accounts which differ somewhat in detail.[108]

The group in London met at the same time each week to discuss and carry out experiments. According to Wallis the initial suggestion had come from Theodore Haak (1605–1690: a German then resident in London) and the participants initially included Wilkins, Goddard, Ent, Glisson, Charles Scarburgh (1615–1694), and Christopher Merrett (1614–1695), all of whom were physicians, and Samuel Foster (d.1653), an astronomer. Meetings were often held at Goddard's lodgings since he had an operator skilled in grinding glass for making microscopes and telescopes. The group also met at the Mitre in Wood Street, The Bull Head in Cheapside, at Gresham College after the Wednesday and Thursday lectures of Wren and Rooke, and at Foster's home. 'Usually … there joined with them several eminent persons of their common acquaintance'. Others prominent in the early discussions included

[105] Despite this claim, the Society now has a relatively incomplete collection of Willis's works.

[106] See: *The Royal Society. Its origins and founders*. Ed. Sir Harold Hartley F.R.S., London (1960): pages 91–7.

[107] For assessment of the early history of the Royal Society, see Charles Webster, 'The origins of the Royal Society', *History of Science* 1967: 6; 106–28.

[108] See: John Wallis, *A defence of the Royal Society, and the Philosophical Transactions*, London (1678). A later and somewhat abbreviated version appears as: John Wallis, 'Account of some passages of his own life addressed to Dr Thomas Smith and dated from Oxford, 29 January 1696–7', published in the appendix to the preface of *Peter Langtoft's Chronicle*, volume 1 (of 2). Ed: Thomas Hearne, Oxford (1725): pages clxi–clxiv. In *The Royal Society. Its origins and founders* (1960): pages 14–16, Douglas McKie draws attention to differences in these accounts with the omission of Scarburgh from those who first met and the addition of Haak to that list; the probability that meetings started before 1645 and without Wallis's involvement; and the contested view on whether the origins of the Royal Society date from the meetings in London, or Oxford as argued by Thomas Sprat.

Brouncker, Neile, Evelyn, Nathaniel Henshaw (1628–1673), Henry Slingsby (*c.*1621–1688), Timothy Clarke (d.1672),[109] Ball, Hill, William Croone (1633–1684), 'and diverse other gentleman, whose inclinations lay the same way'. Mention of divinity, state affairs, and current news was prohibited. Legitimate topics included physic and anatomy: 'We there discoursed the Circulation of the Blood, the Valves in the Veins. Scientific discussion combined with friendship and conviviality'.

The situation changed in 1648–1649 when Wilkins, Wallis, and Goddard moved to Oxford, allowing Wallis to make the point that the London group was the originator of societies dedicated to natural philosophy. These three:

> Continued such meetings ... and brought those Studies into fashion there; meeting first at Dr Petty's lodgings in an apothecarie's house because of the convenience of inspecting Drugs when the occasion arose.

Whether the Royal Society can be said to have started with the meetings in London that Wallis narrated, or those in Oxford, is disputed. Thomas Sprat wrote the first full history of the Society under the guidance of John Wilkins.[110] The book was a manifesto of the Society's aims and methods and primarily aimed at the King in the (unrealized) hope that he would fund their future activities. Sprat wrote three parts to his book: a history of success and failure in ancient and modern philosophy so 'we may better shew, what is to be expected from these new Undertakers, and what mov'd them, to enter upon a way of Inquiry, different from that, on which the former have proceeded'; a narrative of what happened in the first few years; and a defence of the '*Advantage* and *Innocence*' of the work in the eyes of all professions and of religion. It was in this last respect that, not for the first time, Henry Stubbe took exception to views of the Royal Society and favoured Oxford for the initiative in forming a scientific society.[111]

> It was therefore, some space after the end of the Civil Wars at *Oxford*, in *Dr Wilkins* his lodgings, in *Wadham College*, which was then the place of Resort for Virtuous and Learned Men, that the first meetings were made, which laid the foundation of all this that follow'd ...The principal, and most consistent of them, were Doctor *Seth Ward*, the present Lord Bishop of *Exeter*, Mr. *Boyl*, Dr. *Wilkins*, Sir *William Petty*, Mr. *Mathew Wren*, Dr. *Wallis*, Dr. *Goddard*, Dr. *Willis*, Dr. *Bathurst*, Dr. *Christopher Wren*, Mr. *Rook*: besides several others, who joyn'd themselves to them, upon occasions ... For such a candid, and unpassionate company, as that was, and for such a gloomy season, what could have been a fitter subject to pitch upon, than *Natural Philosophy*.

[109] See: Adrian Tinniswood, *His invention so fertile. A life of Sir Christopher Wren*, London (2002): page 139 for details of Clarke taking up the method of injecting the veins of animals and being pressed by Lord Brouncker to submit a manuscript to the *Philosophical Transactions*. He delayed, saying that he intended to finish the piece but never did.

[110] See: Thomas Sprat, *The history of the Royal-Society of London for the improving of natural knowledge*, London (1667).

[111] See: [Henry Stubbe] *A censure upon certaine passages contained in the history of the Royal Society as being destructive to the established religion and church of England*, London (1670) for comments on this quote from Sprat (1667). Stubbe objects to passages in Sprat's book at pages 349, 355, 362, 414, and 415, citing the offending passages that reflect ideas of the 'Virtuoso' and explaining why these are contrary to faith and scripture, 'congeries of grosse untruths', and an '*Humour* that hath generally possessed the *Gallantilloes* of this age whereby they endeavour to recommend themselves as *agreeable company* to the *empty* or *lesse serious* part of mankind'.

Sprat does not doubt the sequence of events. After describing how the meetings were held in Oxford 'as frequent as their affairs permitted: their proceedings rather by action … no Rules nor Method fix'd', he makes clear that after 1658 when several of the group were 'called away to several parts of the Nation and the greatest number of them coming to London, they usually met at Gresham College after the Wednesdays, and Thursdays lectures of Dr. Wren, and Mr. Rook'. Thereafter Wallis and Sprat are agreed in listing those who were most prominent in the London meetings. For Sprat it was the mix of different professions which avoided any one subject in particular overweighing another, 'or making the *Oracle* onely speak their *private* fence', that made for success. In documenting the various bodies that had endorsed the founding and activities of the Society, Sprat mentions physicians. Without providing names, he writes:[112]

> Of our *Physicians*, many of the most judicious, have contributed their *purses*, their *bands*, their *judgments*, their *writings*. This they have done, though they have also in *London*, a Colledge peculiar to their *Profession*; which ever since its first foundation, for the space of a hundred and fifty years, has given the world a succession of the most eminent *Physicians* of *Europe*. In *that* they confine themselves to the advancement of *Physick*: But in *this*, they have also with great zeal, and ability, promoted this *universal inspection*, into all *Natural knowledge*. For without danger of flattery, I will declare of the *English Physicians*, that no part of the world exceeds them, not only in the skill of their own *Art*, but in *general Learning*: and of very many of that profession I will affirm that *All Apollo is their own*, as it was said by the best *Poet* of this Age, of one of the most excellent of their number.

But the evidence shows that relying on contemporary historians—Wallis and Sprat—is unwise. Each had his own reasons for promoting the case either for the group that met in London or in Oxford as primarily responsible for the evolution of what became the Royal Society of London. Wallis was keen to reduce the significance of Wilkins and adjusted the history in favour of London. Sprat was irritated by the nascent Royal Society and so batted for Oxford. The story is set out by Mordechai Feingold who traces the origin of the rival claims to the seemingly irrelevant matter of advice given to two deaf boys (Alexander Popham and Daniel Whaley) by William Holder (1616–1698) and John Wallis; and the differing accounts of their successful ministrations to the young lads, respectively.[113] Because these appeared in *Philosophical Transactions*, officers of the Royal Society were necessarily caught up in the dispute. Council was required to arbitrate, exposing rifts between Brouncker and Oldenburg that ultimately led to the foundation president's departure from office.

Holder took the opportunity of a lull in publication of *Philosophical Transactions* to give his version on how to improve speech in deaf children, mentioning in passing the origins of the Royal Society:[114]

> Some years immediately before His Majesties happy Restauration, divers ingenious persons in Oxford used to meet at the Lodgings of that excellent Person, and zealous promoter

[112] The poem refers to Abraham Cowley (1618–1667), 'Upon Dr Harvey'. In: *Verses on several occasions*, London (1663): pages 18–21. Stubbe (1670) reproduces some of Cowley's verse but not this piece on the merits of physicians.

[113] See: Mordechai Feingold, 'The origins of the Royal Society revisited', In: Eds. Margaret Pelling and Scott Mandelbrote, *The practice of reform in health, medicine, and science, 1500–2000, Essays for Charles Webster*, Aldershot (2005): pages 167–83.

[114] See: William Holder, *Supplement to the Philosophical Transactions of July 1670 with some reflexions on Dr John Wallis his letter there inferred*, London (1678): page 4.

> of Learning, the late Bishop of Chester, Dr. Wilkins, then Warden of Wadham College, where they diligently conferred about Researches and Experiments in Nature, and indeed laid the first Ground and Foundation of the Royal Society.

In his own first account of the paediatric speech defects, Wallis massaged events relating to the Royal Society so as to make clear his own position, subtly replacing 'some years immediately' with 'in that time, *viz.* in the Year 1659' and paraphrasing Holder as having written:[115]

> Divers ingenious persons in *Oxford* used to meet at the Lodgings of Dr. *Wilkins* ['that excellent Person, and zealous promoter of Learning, the late Bishop of *Chester*' is silently omitted], then Warden of *Wadham* College, where they diligently conferred about Researches and Experiments in Nature, and indeed laid the first Ground and Foundation of the Royal Society.

After stating that meetings started in London around 1645 before moving to Oxford, he explains that, from 1648 or 1649, some of the pioneers gathered in both cities and others newly joined one or other including Ward, Petty, Bathurst, and Willis in Oxford. Wallis accepts that after Petty had left for Ireland, the Oxford meetings did continue at Wadham, hosted by Wilkins, but emphasizes that these soon lapsed and the momentum was maintained at Gresham College in London. As for the significant involvement of physicians, the point was simply that, with no appeal from ordination or other intellectual pursuits that proved insufficient to support a living, taking up medicine proved to be an easy default profession:[116]

> Walter Charleton took the view that: 'our late Warrs and Schisms, having almost wholly discouraged men from the study of theologie; and brought the Civil Law into contempt: the major part of young Schollers in our Universities addict themselves to Physick'; and Ralph Bathurst reminded Seth Ward in 1664 that he had turned to medicine twenty years earlier to 'serve for a livelihood, (as indeed I never desired to have it, being only my refuge in bad times, and not my primitive designe)'. Other individuals who turned to science or medicine rather than to church or state included Seth Ward, Thomas Willis, and John Wallis, to name only those who left direct testimony of the fact.

In the event, natural philosophy and the practice of medicine proved attractive in their own rights, and therefore a not infrequent qualification amongst former members of the Oxford Philosophical Club who joined the Royal Society. But for all this swapping of affiliations, Willis remains largely absent from the records of the early history of the Royal Society.[117] Others were more committed. In his affirmation of the Royal Charter, the first president, Viscount Brouncker listed the twenty-one members of the inaugural Council of whom five, besides himself, were physicians: Kenelm Digby (1603–1665),[118] Petty, Clarke, Ent, and Goddard. One-fifth of the first 425 Fellows of the Royal Society (to 1687) were physicians, and the Royal Society had initially considered having its assembly in the College at Amen

[115] See: Wallis (1678): pages 7–8.

[116] See: Feingold (2005): pages 182–3.

[117] It follows that Willis's inclusion so prominently in the list of founders of the Royal Society of London leans less on Wallis than Sprat, whose account of the Oxford Philosophical Club hosted by Wilkins at Wadham may say more about the Oxford College that Sprat attended than the historical facts.

[118] John Evelyn had views on Kenelm Digby, noting in his diary for 18 June 1670 that 'Lord Stafford (*c.*1648–1719) rose in some distress from the table at dinner because there were roses placed around the table during discert because he had an antipathie to them which as Sir Kenelm Digby tells us, laying but a rose on her [Lady Selenger]

Corner with physicians elected on the same terms as noblemen.[119] But despite overlap of their fellowships, the Royal Society prioritized the scientific work of its fellows, including that of physicians, and sought international engagement, a stance that the College did not match.[120] In the event, the Society was not much concerned with the practice of medicine. That remained the business of the College of Physicians. In so far as it took a stance, and as might be expected from the interests of several founding fellows, the Royal Society aligned itself more with the iatrochemists than traditional Galenist physicians. Henry Stubbe makes clear that 'at first they would have incorporated the *Colledge of Physicians* into *their Society*: but that the *prudent* and *grave* did decline: then they promoted the *Anti-Colledge* of *Pseudo-Chymists*, encouraging *Odowde* and his *ignorant Adherents* in opposition to the *Physicians*'.[121] Despite his lack of attention to its activities, involvement in the emerging discipline of iatrochemistry did nevertheless single out Willis as the leading scientific physician of that period and one who was comfortable with the emerging style of the Royal Society.

Philipp Sachs (1627–1672), one of four physicians who cofounded the 'Academia Naturae Curiosorum' (Academy of the Curious as to Nature; now the National Academy of Sciences Leopoldina) in the imperial city of Schweinfurt on 1 January 1652, asked the secretary of the Royal Society, Henry Oldenburg, to encourage English and other European physicians to participate in its activities. Perhaps he had the ulterior motive of asking Willis to divulge, 'under pledge of secrecy', the nature of his means of dissolving various chemicals into fluids.[122] Willis was not compliant and made clear that he had no intention of revealing his methods.

The style of those associated with the Royal Society was to reject scholasticism and the dogma of ancient teachings and, in their natural philosophy, take the observations of the senses as the most reliable route to wisdom. Knowledge was a construct based on truth resulting from inductive and deductive reasoning which, ideally verified through experiment, was formulated as language and in images and communicated in groups.[123] Reluctant to extol the virtues of individuals, Sprat singles out Christopher Wren for particular praise, and Sprat is one of very few intimate enough to address him as 'Kit Wren' rather than 'Doctor Wren':[124]

> I must break this Law, in the particular case of Dr Christopher Wren ... For in turning over the Registers of the Society, I perceiv'd that many excellent things, whose first invention ought

cheeke when she was asleepe, it raised a blister; but Sir Kenelm was a teller of strange things'. See: John Evelyn (1818, printed *c.*1930): page 436.

[119] See: Sir George Clark, *A history of the Royal College of Physicians of London*, volume 1, Oxford (1964): pages 309–12.

[120] A Rupert Hall singles out the support for scientific work offered by the Royal Society to Thomas Willis; see: 'Medicine and the Royal Society'. In: Ed. Allen G Debus, *Medicine in seventeenth century England. A symposium held at UCLA in honor of C.D. O'Malley*, Berkeley (1974): pages 421–52.

[121] See: Stubbe's *Campanella revived* (1670) quoted in Henry Thomas, 'The Society of Chemycial Physitians. An echo of the great plague of London, 1665'. In: Ed. E Ashworth Underwood, *Science, medicine and history. Essays on the evolution of scientific thought written in honour of Charles Singer* volume 2, Oxford (1953): page 64. 'Odowde' is Thomas O'Dowd (d.1665, of the plague) who published *The poor man's physician* (1665).

[122] See: Thomas Willis, *The remaining medical works*, London (1681): page 35.

[123] See: Alexander Wragge-Morley, *Aesthetic science. Representing nature in the Royal Society of London, 1650–1720*, Chicago (2020) for discussion of aesthetics and communication as motivation for the work of Fellows of the Royal Society who wrote on natural history and anatomy.

[124] See: Sprat (1667): pages 311 and 317–8, cited by Tinniswood (2002): pages 81–2 and endnotes 24 and 25, page 390. See also: Tinniswood (2002): pages 336–7 for discussion of Wren (as surveyor general of the King's works) being asked, after Sprat's death, to provide a detailed account of building works carried out on the palace at Rochester during his tenure as bishop, and other recommendations of which only work on the transept porch was eventually carried out (in 1722); and page 83 for the remarks on 'Kit Wren'.

> to be ascrib'd to him, were casually omitted. This moves me ... to give this separate Account of his endeavours, in promoting the Design of the Royal Society, in the small time wherein he has had the opportunity of attending it ... For there is a peculiar reverence due to so much excellence cover'd with so much modesty. And it is not Flattery but honesty, to give him his just praise; who is so far from usurping the fame of other men, that he endeavours with all care to conceal his own.

Although in his diary Evelyn notes many ecclesiastical activities of Thomas Sprat during his tenure as Bishop of Rochester (1684–1713), the only entry of substance is a note for 13 September 1688: 'Dr Sprat, Bishop of Rochester, wrote a very honest and handsome letter to the Commissioners Ecclesiastical, excusing himselfe from sitting any longer among them, he by no means approving of their prosecuting the Cleargy who refus'd to reade the Declaration for liberty of conscience, in prejudice of the Church of England'.[125] Nowhere does Evelyn refer to his engraved title page that is found in some copies of Sprat's history, considerably enhancing its value to collectors. The allegorical image depicts Viscount Brouncker pointing to the Latin inscription identifying 'Charles II Founder and Patron of the Royal Society'. Charles is depicted as a classical bust wreathed by an allegorical figure of Fame; and Francis Bacon, 1st Viscount St Alban (1561–1626), philosopher and Lord Chancellor, designated 'ARTIVM INSTAVRATOR' (renewer of arts), is gesturing towards an array of scientific instruments. The plate is engraved by Wenceslaus Hollar (1607–1677) after Evelyn's design.

This illustrious frontispiece is the subject of a recent monograph.[126] Because it is so often lacking, the type disproportionately large, the leaf on which it is printed an awkward fit other than in the large paper copies, and the engraving bound between the leaf bearing the Society's coat of arms and the title page, the suggestion is that it was never intended for Sprat's book but part of a separate work that never materialized, John Beale's (1608–1683) defence of the Royal Society. Beale started to write his book when Sprat failed to deliver a manuscript on schedule. Beale's interest in the orchards of Herefordshire may have commended him to Evelyn who had written *Sylva, or a discourse on forest-trees* (1664) to which Beale contributed a section on cider apples. In the event, Sprat did deliver and, with some reluctance, Beale abandoned his book sometime between April and July 1667. But by now the Evelyn frontispiece was ready and not to be wasted, so it was decided to insert the available plate leaves in copies of Sprat's book. Michael Hunter (and Jim Bennett on the instruments) has analysed every aspect of the engraved frontispiece and the significance, political and allegorical, of its various parts. Of interest is the identification of books depicted on the left side. These are thought to include works by William Harvey, Evelyn, Nicolaus Copernicus (1473–1543), Christopher Merrett, Francis Bacon, Robert Boyle, and William Gilbert. These largely reflect the intellectual origins and work of the most prominent early Fellows of the Royal Society. Given his lack of involvement, it is unsurprising that Thomas Willis is not represented but the omission of Robert Hooke is less easily explained.[127]

[125] See: John Evelyn (1818, printed *c.*1930): page 655.

[126] See: Michael Hunter, *The image of restoration science. The frontispiece to Thomas Sprat's* History of the Royal Society *(1667)*, London (2017).

[127] See: Hunter (2017): pages 128–43 for details of the subsequent history of the plate into the twentieth century and the possibility that, now lost, it was sacrificed for scrap metal in the First World War.

Fellows of the Royal Society dined regularly at the Pontac's Head tavern in Abchurch Lane kept by François-Auguste Pontac (1636–1694);[128] and, after 1660, in celebration of their anniversary on St Andrew's Day (November 30th) annually they elected the Council and office bearers. Apart from these formal occasions, a few Fellows would have 'Club suppers' after a meeting of the Society for ordinary business. This became the Royal Society (Dining) Club. Although there is no mention of Thomas Willis having been a member of this closely related but independent group, Samuel Pepys (1633–1703) attended a dinner on 21 November 1667 at the tavern in St Clement's Churchyard with John Creed (d.1701), Wilkins, Daniel Whistler (1619–1684), Mr Floyd (nd: 'Secretary to the Lords Commissioners of Prizes') and 'other brave men'. Wilkins discussed an experiment about to be performed by Gresham College philosophers in which the blood of a sheep was to be transfused 'into the body of a poor debauched man'.[129] We know from Thomas Birch (1705–1666) that Willis contributed to this discussion, as recorded on 19 December 1667; and he may have been one of the 'brave men' who attended this (and other) Club dinners.[130]

Even after he moved to London in 1667, Willis still took rather little part in the proceedings of the Royal Society, Dr Edmund King (1629–1709) apparently making up for him, despite the statute that fines would be paid for nonattendance. In a letter to Oldenburg (see: Figure 9):[131]

> 'Recd Dec^{r}: 12: 1667. Sir. I am again hinder'd from waiting on y^{r} Royall Society and giving an account of those powders you left wth mee. But pleas'd to present my service to my Lord President and the company wth my sense in brief of those materialls. The powder that is to make the spaw water is dithor grisiolum martis at y^{r} best or what I rather think only common English copras dried and powder'd. This I shall make out when I come. For y^{r} other powders such of t'em being a sundrae Calx of minerall water evapourated, there is not use of t'em nor any thing worth enquiry to be insisted on about any of t'em. This is all at present from y^{r} most humble serv^{t}: Thomas Willis.

Willis did have some influence at the Society and, on 11 January 1668, it was resolved that his opinion, amongst others, be solicited about buying Chelsea College. Willis accumulated debts to the Society. On 22 October 1673, he was among 18 who were in arrears and asked to comply with the new form of obligation. By 28 January 1675, he still had not signed the new bond and further application was made. But he was not alone. On 24 June 1675 Lower was among five due for expulsion from the Society, including Henry Slingsby, one of the founders, for being in debt and unwilling to sign the obligation. In the end, the Society grew weary and, on 21 October 1675, recorded that Willis

[128] The Pontac's Head was active from 1666 to 1780, although François-Auguste, the son of Lord Arnaud de Pontaca, had returned to France in 1689. Dinner cost one or two guineas including a bottle of Haut Brion, from the family vineyard in Bordeaux, at two shillings. This, or the Royal Oak, in Lombard Street, is where Samuel Pepys was introduced to the better red wines.

[129] See: Sir Archibald Geikie, *Annals of the Royal Society Club. The record of a London dining-club in the eighteenth & nineteenth centuries*, London (1917): pages 1–4.

[130] Not every person who attended the Royal Society Club was a Fellow of the Royal Society; and by no means was every Fellow of the Society necessarily elected to the Dining Club (as at present).

[131] See: Royal Society Library. MS W 3, no. 9; and *The Correspondence of Henry Oldenburg*, volume IV (1667–1668). Eds. A. Rupert Hall and Marie Boas Hall, Madison (1967): page 33.

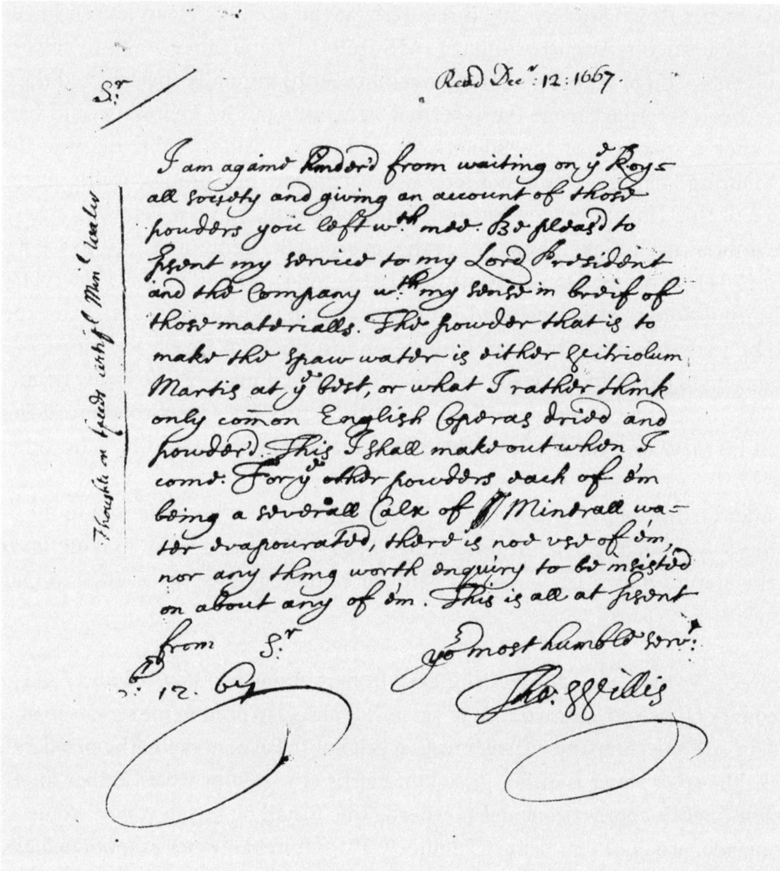

Read Dec.r: 12: 1667.

Sr

I am againe hindred from waiting on ye Royall Society and giving an account of those powders you left wth mee. Be pleasd to present my service to my Lord President and the Company wth my sense in breif of those materialls. The powder that is to make the spaw water is either Vitriolum Martis at ye best, or what I rather think only comon English Coperas dried and powderd. This I shall make out when I come. For ye other powders each of em being a severall Calx of Minerall water evapourated, there is noe use of em, nor any thing worth enquiry to be insisted on about any of em. This is all at present from Sr

yor most humble servt:
Tho: Willis

Figure 9 Manuscript letter in the hand of Thomas Willis to Henry Oldenburg dated 12 December 1667.

would no longer be asked to sign the bond. That did not prevent it being minuted on 29 November 1675 that:

> It be recommended to the care of Dr King to solicit the executors of the will of the late dr Willis for the payment of his arrears to the Society, amounting to twenty pounds and eleven shillings, as appeared from the treasurer's book.

Money matters apart, the records of the Royal Society make occasional reference to Willis.[132] On 27 January 1664, Charleton was ordered to form a committee:

> Made up of all physicians who were Fellows to order and manage dissections for the Society upon every execution day, and therein to divide the work among themselves, and give notice of what parts they intend chiefly to dissect . . . and Dr Goddard was appointed to take good care of the performance of this.

[132] For details of Thomas Willis and records of the Royal Society, see Thomas Birch, *The history of the Royal Society of London for Improving of Natural Knowledge*, London (1756): volume I, page 376; volume II, pages 217, 225, 227, 239, and 425, and volume III, pages 95, 178, 224, 228, 231, and 242.

On 12 December 1667, in a letter to Oldenburg, Willis:

> Sent (as he had been desired to do) his thoughts of a powder for making artificial spa-water; as also some extracts of St Vincent's water sent to the president by Mr Speed; in which paper he observed, that the powder was either vitriolum Martis at best, or, as he rather thought, only common English copper as dried and powdered; and that with regard to the extracts, each of them being a several calx of mineral water evaporated, there was no use of them, nor anything worth inquiry to be insisted on about any of them. But the Doctor referring the Society to what he should make out when he should come himself, the consideration of this particular was deferred till that time.

Of more significance are references to the first human blood transfusion in 1667. After the experimental work in dogs and when discussion turned to using this technique on patients in London hospitals, Willis suggested that the experiment 'might be proper to make use of in rotten sheep'. It is unclear whether this was intended as disparaging or a cautionary next step in moving towards human transfusions.[133] It is noticeable that no obituary of Willis was published by the Royal Society, and no notice of his life appeared in the records before 1960.

Thomas Willis and domestic life in Oxford and London

On the 7 April 1657 Willis married Mary Fell (*c.*1630–1670), daughter of Samuel Fell (1584–1649) at St Michael's at the North Gate, Oxford. The ceremony was conducted by 'Richard Phiullpott, J[ustice of the] P[eace] for Countie of Hereford', with John Dolben (1625–1686) of York, and Richard Allestry of Eton, reading the liturgy. The record describes the groom as 'Willis Thomas Mr. Bachelor of Physick at Christ-Church Oxford' and the bride as 'Fell Mary Mrs. of Hereford, Herefords, spinster'. Their acquaintance went back several years. Samuel Fell was an academic and theologian appointed a canon (1619) and, subsequently, dean (1638) of Christ Church, and professor of divinity in the University and vice-chancellor. He was also rector of Sunningwell, a village outside Oxford, where he died allegedly of shock three days after King Charles I, whom he had served loyally, was beheaded. Fell's tombstone dated 2 February 1649 is placed to the left of the altar.[134] He had married Margaret, daughter of Thomas Wylde (nd), in 1624. Their first three children died in childhood and are buried at Sunningwell; and Margaret died in 1653.[135]

Wood writes that, some years earlier (3 April 1648) at the time Samuel Fell as a Royalist was removed from Christ Church, the Provost Marshall and University visitors arrived at the deanery to evict Mrs Fell and the children. She refused to leave even after the doors were

[133] See chapter 16 for discussion of Willis's early involvement with the technique of intravenous infusion in his studies on the anatomy and physiology of the brain.

[134] See: Robert Evans, 'Fell (i) and Fell (ii)'. In *Tales from God's acre*, privately published (2016): pages 29–31 and 64–5. Professor Evans points out that the date is 1648/9, presumably referring to the Julian calender, and the mason carved 2 rather than 2nd, being illiterate and copying the more frequently used *n*[th].

[135] Robert Evans speculates that the silver chalice still used at Sunningwell church, dated 1660, was given in the year of restoration by John Fell in memory of the late King and his own father. One other daughter of Samuel and Margaret, Philippa, married Walter Jones (d.1657), also rector of Sunningwell, who neglected his flock and spent most of his time in London. See chapter 15 for details of Philip Fell (*c.*1632–1682) who wrote verse in Latin included in Willis's first book, *Diatribæ duæ*, and was an executor of Willis's will.

broken down. A guard was instructed to 'weary her out with noise, rudeness, smell of tobacco' but still the family would not budge. Eight days later:[136]

> In the morn, the Chancellor, the Visitors, certain Soldiers and a great rabble of people went to Christ Church, where forthwith entering Dr Fell's Lodgings (he being yet in safe custody at London) the Chancellor desired Mrs Fell to quit her Quarters, telling her that in so doing she would do God and her Country good service: but she refusing that kind proposal, had very ill language first given to her by him, and then she was carried into the Quadrangle in a chair by soldiers. Her children also were carried out upon boards, as 'twas reported.

Thomas and Mary had nine children, five of whom predeceased their father. Thomas, Anne, Jane, and Rachel survived to maturity.[137] Thomas was born 'in the great stone house against Mert. Coll[ege]' (Beam Hall) on 26 January 1658 and survived his parents. Wood mentions that Willis's first son was baptized: '1657/8, Jan. 26. Thomas son of Mr Thomas Willis a physician & Mary [Fell] his wife was born in the great stone house against Mert. Coll. church & afterwards bapt. in this par. Ant. a Wood'. Only Hutchinson amongst the early biographers, whilst leaning much on the narrative and anecdotes of Wood, appears also to have read the account left by Browne Willis, pointing out that Thomas, the son, 'falling into consumption, he [the father] sent him to Montpellier in France, for the recovery of his health, and it proved successful, Thomas returning to his studies at Westminster School'.[138] Later Thomas, the son, studied at Christ Church. He married Alice Browne in Westminster Abbey on 20 May 1681 and their son was Browne Willis. They lived in the manor of Fenny Stratford where one other of their sons, Thomas, died on 11 November 1699, by coincidence St Martin's Day the same as Thomas, his grandfather, 24 years earlier.

Samuel was born on 20 June 1660 but died in infancy, as did the next child, Mary, born on 1 January 1662 and living only until 1 September of that year. Another male, also named Samuel, lived only a few weeks and died on 11 April 1663. Katherine was born on 5 February 1663 and moved with the family to London but died as a child on 30 September 1667. She was buried in Westminster Abbey where her parents were later interred. Richard was born in Oxford on 20 January 1664 and lived for three years, being buried in Merton College. Anne (born 30 June 1665), and Jane (born 8 September 1666) were baptized in Oxford whereas the birth of Rachel, who was born in 1667, is not registered in the city providing some credence to the conclusion that the family moved to London in that year.[139]

It is unlikely that Willis had planned to move from Oxford since, on 11 April 1666 although living at Beam Hall, he took a forty year lease with Dr Peter Eliot (1618–1682) and a surgeon, Mr William Day (1604–1665), on the Angel, a coaching inn on the High Street at an annual rent of 70s. After Day's death, Willis and Eliot added Bostar Hall, also in the High Street (numbers 86 and 87), rented for 28s 4d per annum, as their premises for seeing patients. This meant that Willis and Eliot had a stake in almost half the High Street

[136] See: Anthony à Wood, *The history and antiquities of the University of Oxford by Anthony à Wood*, volume 2. Ed. John Glutch, Oxford (1796): pages 563–4; and [Anon] *The history of the visitations of the University of Oxford by a parliamentary commission in the year 1647, 1648 abridged from the annals of Anthony à Wood*, Oxford (1837): page 25.

[137] See: Hughes (1991): pages 97–8 for details of these siblings.

[138] See: Benjamin Hutchinson, *Biographia medicia or, historical and critical memoirs of the lives and writings of the most eminent medical characters*, volume II, London (1799): pages 481–5. Much of his account is taken from Anthony Wood and Browne Willis.

[139] See: Hughes (1991): page 99 for the suggestion that, born healthy, the children who died young were infected by one or other parent and died from acute miliary tuberculosis. Willis was liable to a chronic cough 'with abundant and thick spittle', and may also have had tuberculosis.

properties between Logic Lane and Eastgate. The location was convenient since it was close to where stagecoaches stopped on their way to the medicinal waters at Bath. But although he retained the appointment as Sedleian professor of Natural Philosophy in Oxford until his death in 1675, Willis went to live in London in 1667.[140] The reason may have been pressure from Sheldon, now Archbishop of Canterbury, and old Oxford friends who had themselves moved; and because London offered a better place in which to flourish and develop his clinical reputation. Anthony Wood considered that Willis: 'Became so noted and so infinitely resorted to in his practice that never any physician before went before him or got more money yearly than he'.

With this further prosperity, Willis acquired houses in St Martin's Lane (a coach house with stabling on the west side), a Norman mansion in Surrey, Hamm Court a house on the Thames at Chertsey (for £100 plus £18 annual rent and the price of a ton of wheat) and, bought from George Villiers, 2nd Duke of Buckingham (1628–1687), properties and land at Water Eaton with Bletchley and Fenny Stratford, together with Great Brickhill in West Bletchley thereby reuniting the manors into a single estate. Fell tells us that:

> It is incredible to relate, how soon, and with how great Commendations he grew famous, especially being so composed by Nature and Custom, that he could not recommend himself by words composed to deceive, or the cunning Arts of Mountebanks.

Willis was now a fashionable London doctor with a high clinical reputation. He was granted armorial bearings by the College of Arms (see: Figure 10). Whilst visiting Oxford, Lord Ashley (1621–1683) learned that his wife was ill and consulted Willis: 'One of the learnedest and most famous physicians in the world', whose prescription for treatment, made without visiting the patient, cured her Ladyship. King Charles II asked Willis to see his wife, Catherine of Braganza (1638–1705) who had miscarried. Gilbert Burnet, Bishop of Salisbury (1643–1715) recounted that:[141]

> The King told me she had been with child: and Willis the great physician told Doctor Lloyd, from whom I had it, that she had once miscarried of a child, which was so far advanced, that if it had been carefully look'd to, the sex might have been distinguished. But she proved a barren wife, and was a woman of a mean appearance, and of no agreeable temper: so that the King never considered her much ... For some time the King carried things decently and did not visit his mistress openly. But he grew weary of that restraint, and shook it off so entirely, that he had ever after that mistresses to the end of his life, to the great scandal of the world, and to the particular reproach of all that served about him in the Church. He usually came from his mistresses lodgings to Church, even on sacrament days.

Willis liked to reflect on the personality and style of his patients: 'a very honourable Old Gentleman dignified by many great Titles, himself being greater than all of them'; a man whose 'life was to be despaired of, to be long prolonged; yea, the Magistracy and Offices which he held, were fought for by others'; 'a certain cunning and crafty lawyer'. But his

[140] Opinions differ on the exact date: in his postscript to *Pharmaceutice rationalis*, part 2 (1675), John Fell (1675) writes 1667; Martensen (2004a) suggests 1666, even though Willis was still paying poll tax in Oxford in 1667; Raymond Hierons (unpublished manuscript) and Dewhurst (1664) go for 1668.

[141] See: Bishop Burnet, *History of his own time: from restoration of King Charles the Second to the treaty of peace at Utrecht in the reign of Queen Anne*, London (1857): page 154.

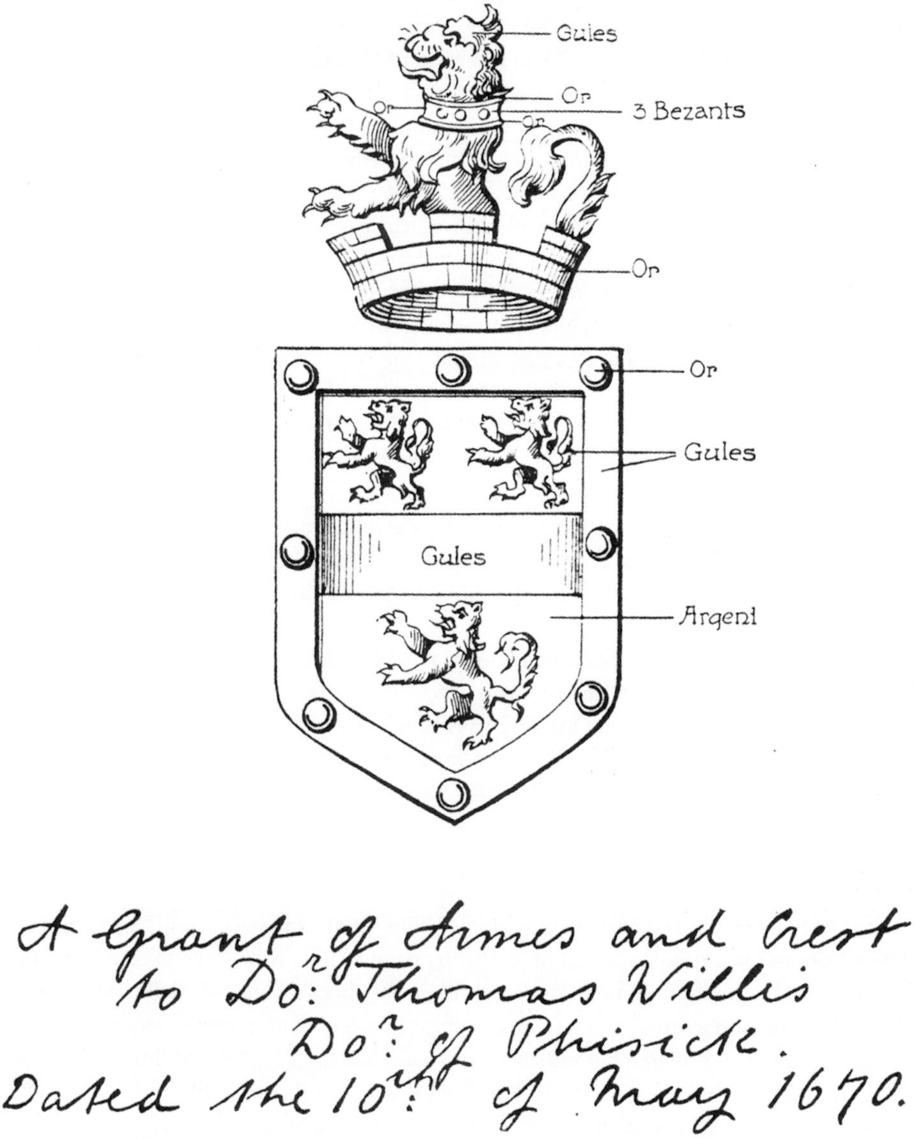

Figure 10 A coat of arms was granted to Thomas Willis on 10 May 1670. The grant remains in the collection of the Willis Fleming Historical Trust. Willis's arms comprise a horizontal band ('fess') between three rampant lions, all in red, on a white background. Around the shield runs a border, also in red, charged with eight gold discs ('bezants'). For the crest, the top half of a rampant lion in red emerges from a gold crown fashioned out of bricks ('mural crown'). The lion in the crest wears a collar of two narrow components ('collar gemelle') and this is charged with three bezants. Following his marriage to Mary Fell, Willis's arms (to the left) were represented alongside those of his wife's family on a single shield ('impaled'). The arms of Fell (to the right) place two black bars on a white background, the upper being charged with two gold crosses, the lower with one. The crosses have splayed ends, and a long pointed lower limb, referred to as 'formy fitchy' in heraldic terms. It is not known when and for whom this impaled shield was fashioned. Artwork for the image shown in the frontispiece was made for the Willis Fleming family, *c.*1825.
Reproduced courtesy of the Willis Fleming Historical Trust.

outspokenness was not always well received. Suspecting his wife of infidelity with the Duke of York (1633–1701: later King James II), the Earl of Southesk (*c.*1649–1688) acquired venereal disease and deliberately infected Anna, Countess of Southesk (nd) from where the condition eventually reached the Duchess of York accounting for ill-health in several of her children. Bishop Burnet wrote that:[142]

> The children were born with ulcers, or they broke out about them soon after, and sons died young and unhealthy. This has, as far as anything that could not be brought in the way of proof, prevailed to create a suspicion that so healthy a child as the pretended prince of Wales could neither be his, nor be born of any wife with whom he had lived long. The violent pain which his eldest daughter had in her eyes, and the gout which early seized our present queen, are thought the dregs of a tainted original. Willis, the great physician, being called to consult for one of his [the Duke of York] sons, gave as his opinion in the words 'mala stamina vitæ' [threads of the evils of life] which gave such offence that he was never called for afterwards.

Willis had a rival in Thomas Sydenham (1624–1689), based in Westminster, whom he had known in Oxford when they enlisted on opposite sides during the Civil War, and whose styles differed—Sydenham the practical clinician, Willis more bookish and enquiring of disease mechanisms and their anatomical basis. John Ward wrote that: 'Sydenham and some others in London say of Dr Willis that hee is an ingenious man but not a good physitian, and that hee does not understand the way of practice'.

Willis's former student John Locke was now based in the Strand. Richard Lower had also moved to London and settled in Hatton Garden, initially working with Willis, but as his own fame increased moving to Salisbury Court near Fleet Street, then Bow Street and King Street near Covent Garden, and in time supplanting Willis as 'most noted physician in Westminster and London, and no Man's Name was more cried up at Court than his'.[143]

The eight years before Willis died were busy not only with work as a physician but also writing. Again Fell relates that: 'though he spent whole dayes and nights in the care of the Sick, he was at leisure to adorn Art by composing Books ... [despite] a thousand Interruptions'. Whilst in London Willis wrote or completed the remaining nine treatises in five books, one in two parts, published during his lifetime or posthumously: *A plain and easie method* (1666, published 1691); *de morbis convulsivis, de Scorbuto* (as *Pathologiæ cerebri*: 1667); *Affectionum quæ dicuntur hystericæ et hypochondriacæ, de sanguinis accensione, de motu musculari* (1670); *De anima brutorum* (1672); and *Pharmaceutice rationalis* (part 1: 1674), and *Pharmaceutice rationalis* (part 2: 1675). Thomas Willis did not neglect his charitable work. He donated all fees earned on a Sunday (estimated at one

[142] Readers can be forgiven for pausing to work out the various relationships. The infected Duke of York, who became king, unwittingly passed on the venereal disorder to his wife and several of their children. The two Queens, Mary and Anne, survived but the story went that their younger half-brother, James the Old Pretender (1688-1766: sometime Prince of Wales), being unaffected, 'could neither be his, nor be born of any wife, with whom he had long lived'.

[143] Kenneth Franklin (1897–1966) describes Lower's last words quoting Cotton Mather (1663–1728): 'A Knight of my Acquaintance visiting the famous Dr Lower in his last Sickness ask'd him for the best Advice he could give, 'How to preserve his Health, and prolong his Life'; the Doctor only answered him, 'Don't eat too much'. After some other Discourse, the Knight not imagining that the Doctor had thoroughly answered his Enquiry, repeated it. The Doctor thereupon only repeated his Answer, 'Why Didn't I tell you; Don't eat too much!—And, further said not'. See: John Fulton, *A Bibliography of two Oxford physiologists: Richard Lower 1631–1691, John Mayow 1643–1679*, Oxford (1935): page 12.

tenth of his income) for distribution to the poor of the parish. Although Willis could afford to be generous, Fell relates that:

> One might easier have received from him, for a fit object of Charity, an hundred Crowns, than have extorted as many farthings from most others.

We learn from a conversation held a few days before his death that Willis refused to consider any sum of money his own until he had given to the poor, even at the expense of supporting his children. Symon Patrick (1626–1707), Bishop of Chichester, describes in his diary how he: [144]

> Met that great man Dr Willis; who understanding that I intended to return to London, and look after my parish, was wonderfully kind to me, and directed me how to order myself, and often in the time of the plague wrote to me, and sent me money to give to the poor.

Willis also continued his support of the Church in London. Not always able to attend parish services, he arranged for the schoolmaster who taught in the vestry room of St Martin's Church to read prayers twice daily: at 6am in summer and one hour later in winter, and at 5pm in the evening so that the ordinary working people could attend. In his will, Willis endowed the salary of a priest to provide the 'sacred offices of the Church' for those in the neighbourhood otherwise detained in commerce and trade. His faith was declared in several of Willis's treatises. The arterial circle at the base of the brain was evidence of the: 'Finger and Divine Workmanship of the Deity, a most strong and invincible Argument may be opposed to the most perverse Atheist'; the earthworm made him speculate that this 'Little living Creature, tho it be esteemed Vile and Contemptible, hath allotted to it vital organs, as also other Viscera and Members, made most admirable by a Divine Workmanship'; and 'The Physician, however Skilful he be, ought always to implore the help of the Heavenly Power, to be assisting to him'. Occasionally, as in the preface to *De anima brutorum* (1672), in the English translation, Willis expressed materialist views that went against the teachings of the Church: 'the Soul hath a material Subsistence, extended equally with the body ... it is found obnoxious also to preternatural Diseases and not seldom wants Medical help'.

Willis was not among those listed to be 'ordeyned' and appointed 'Doctors in Physicke the first and present Fellowes' in the charter of the College of Physicians ratified by King Charles II on 26 March 1663, as documented by Charles Goodall (1642–1712).[145] Feeling that a civil honour would reduce his earning capacity and make it difficult to support his family Willis is said, originally by Browne Willis, to have refused a knighthood from King Charles. Others took the view that the King did not take to Willis who he considered to have 'rid him of more of his subjects than any enemy army'. He was made an honorary Fellow of the Royal College of Physicians of London in December 1664.[146] Honorary fellowship was a category for doctors from the provinces, country physicians, or University teachers. They paid a higher fee (£20) and played no role in running the College. As with the Royal Society, it seems that

[144] See: Symon Patrick, *The works of Symon Patrick, D.D., sometime bishop of Ely*, volume 9. Ed. Rev. Alexander Taylor, Oxford (1858): pages 442–3.

[145] Charles Goodall, *The Royal College of Physicians of London founded and established by law; as appears by letters patents, acts of parliament, adjudged cases*, London (1684): pages 70–1.

[146] See: William Munk, *The roll of the Royal College of Physicians of London*. Volume 1, 1518 to 1700, London (1878): pages 338–42. Hughes (1991): page 90 has this as 1665.

Willis rarely attended not least because, for some years until the move to Warwick Lane, the College had no suitable premises following the Great Fire of London in 1666. With its espousal of new scientific ideas representing a threat to its own influence, the College considered involvement by Willis, Petty, Glisson, Goodall, and Millington in the Royal Society an act of betrayal at a time when restoration of the monarchy required undivided allegiance of physicians to their own College.[147] That this protectionist attitude was not reciprocated is seen in the categories of people eligible for Fellowship of the Royal Society and the account given by Sprat of its early history. As for his own style, Willis made clear in his preface to *De anima brutorum* (1672: English translation 1683) that:

> I speak not from the Tripos like an Oracle, nor from the Chair, but as one of a low form: I play not the Prophet, or Dictator, but the Philosopher, neither do I plant an Opinion, but propose an Hypothesis, and open my Judgment.

Willis probably had little time for leisure. In the preface to *Pharmaceutice rationalis* (part 2: 1675: English translation 1679), he writes:

> Since I first began to consider the Operations of Medicines in humane Bodies . . . I became affected with so vehement a desire of farther prosecuting that Speculation, that in all spare hours, (to wit, as frequently as I might be vacant from my practice) I could hardly intend or admit thoughts of any other thing: And that not so much that I might please others, as by often turning in my mind, and writing my Meditations of this Subject, I might be better instructed to prescribe to my Patients . . . I have not suffered my Faculties although small (as the Talent entrusted with me by God Almighty) to perish through sloth.

Willis's habits tended to abstemiousness and he considered, not unreasonably, many illnesses to be the result of overindulgence and the 'guzzling of strong wine'. The role of inebriation in causing disease often featured in his lectures.[148] More generally:

> Sometimes learned men, and very pretty ingenious women, to improve their fansie, and put themselves in a cheerful humour, do, by frequent sipping of Spirits and hot Waters, impair and oftentimes destroy their own health.

That said, his medicines were frequently dissolved in wine; and to prevent scurvy Willis recommended middling beer, mild and clear, altered with antiscorbutick ingredients. Willis did allow himself some pleasures and indulgencies: 'musick does not only affect the Phantasie with a certain delight, but besides chears a sad and sorrowful Heart; yea allays all turbulent Passions'. Coffee 'wonderfully clears and enlightens each part of the Soul, and disperses all the clouds of every Function':

> The use of Tobacco is not only good, but almost necessary for Souldiers or Seamen . . . where it agrees with them, as much as it makes them both undaunted in all dangers, and able to endure hunger, cold and labour . . . [although] . . . most men take too much of it.

[147] See: John Keevil, *The stranger's son*, London (1953): page 139.

[148] See chapter 18 for citations and many other examples of Willis's medicinal use of alcohol, coffee, and tobacco.

Aubrey describes Willis as being of middle height, with dark red brindle hair like a red pig, and a stammer. Wood rehearsed this caricature and added: 'a plain man, of no carriage, little discourse or complaisance and with no powers for appearing with advantage or brilliance in society'.[149]

When Willis's wife Mary became ill, and despite the accusation by Wood that 'the acquisition of riches being the predominant passion of his comfort', he was keen to take her and the surviving children to the countryside, in order to assist the recovery. But Mary refused 'preferring her children's increase in fortune, even before her own life itself'.[150] Willis may also have had medical reservations: 'London is not presently to be forsaken for all phthisical persons: for I have known ... many to have enjoyed their health much better in this smoaky air than in the Country'.[151] After being ill for four years, Mary died on 31 October 1670 from pulmonary tuberculosis and was buried in Westminster Abbey. As he tells us in the introduction, Willis absorbed his grief in writing *De anima brutorum* (1672):

> This difficult task, when at first denied leisure and retirement, it could not be performed; after the death of my Dear Wife, being lonely, with frequent and unseasonable Studies, that I might the less think on my Grief, I have at last finished this, according to my slender Capacity.

On 1 September 1672, Willis married Elizabeth Calley [sometimes Cawley, Cawly or Collier: 1644–1709, daughter of Mathew Nicholas (1594–1661), dean of Bristol and St Paul's, and his wife Elizabeth Foulkes of Bulwich (d.1673)] at Westminster Abbey. She was the widow of Sir William Calley (1602–1667) of Burderop Park, Wiltshire.[152] After Willis died in 1675, Elizabeth married Sir Thomas Mompesson (1630–1701) of Bathampton, Wiltshire. Widowed for the third time, she lived out her eight remaining years and was buried in Winchester Cathedral following her death on 29 November 1709. Willis's surviving family and descendants evidently disapproved of Elizabeth. When corresponding with Philip Morant concerning the latter's proposed but unrealized biography of Willis, pleading age and infirmity and referring Morant to the account already given in the *General dictionary*, Browne Willis preferred not to acknowledge the second Mrs Willis. On 11 June 1757, he writes:[153]

> As to marrying a second wife, that I think need not be mentioned; and concerning Her I can inform you very little. In the Register of Westminster Abbey is an entry in Sept. 1672 or 1673 of the marriage of Dr Thomas Willis and Mrs Elizabeth Colliar. But I think her name was Cawley, and so I remember to have heard ... what became of my grandfather's widow I know not, nor when she dyed.

On 28 March 1759 after pointing out that Willis left Elizabeth little in his will other than her own plate and belongings given to him as dowry on the marriage, Browne Willis adds:

149 See: Bennett [Aubrey] (2015): page 551; and chapter 3 for details of contemporary and later images of Thomas Willis.

150 See: [Anon] 'The life of Dr. Thomas Willis'. In: *Biographia Britannica*, Ed. Andrew Kippis with the assistance of Joseph Towers, volume VI, London (1747): pages 4291–7.

151 See: Thomas Willis, *Pharmaceutice rationalis* (1679): page 34.

152 See: Raymond Hierons archive, manuscript postcard sent to Box T. 32, *The Times*, by Donald Nicholas of Gatehampton Manor, Goring-on-Thames, Oxon, dated 12 September 1960.

153 See: Additional manuscripts 37222 (f 114–15, f127–8, and f 139), British Library: transcribed by Raymond Hierons.

> You call Dr Willis's 2nd wife Mrs Cawley, I was told she was a knight's Lady and a widow; and I asked you had rather … not take notice of his having a 2nd wife at all; For I heard she was for getting all she could from his Family.

As for Willis's surviving daughters—Anne, Jane, and Rachel—Browne Willis writes that Jane married Robert Symonds (nd), high sheriff of Hertfordshire[154] in the last year of the reign of King William III (1650–1702), and had one son, Thomas:

> Now of Pengethly near Rosse in that county, one of the most universal scholars of the age, eminently skilled in Physic and all other parts of learning, especially mathematics, so that his grandfather's genius will ever live in him.

Rachel, the younger daughter, married Roger Lingen (nd) of Radhook, and had a son, another Thomas, 'a gentleman of great estate, who, in 1735 was High Sheriff of Gloucestershire'. Of Anne, Browne Willis makes no mention.

Thomas Willis died from pneumonia at his house in St Martin's Lane on 11 November 1675, St Martin's day, after a short illness but according to Anthony Wood 'of drudgery in pursuit of lucre'. Pneumonia may have complicated influenza which bills of mortality suggest was epidemic during those weeks. Henry More wrote to Lady Conway (1631–1670): 'the famous physician Dr. Willis I hear is dead, and of a cold the Epidemicall disease of the City'. Lady Conway was a veteran patient of Willis. Her case was as famous as it was hopeless and neither Harvey, Kenelm Digby, Turquet de Mayerne (1573–1655), nor Boyle had managed to cure her of the headache which is fully described in *De anima brutorum* (1672).[155] Sir Thomas Browne (1605–1682) of Norwich wrote to his son Edward (1644–1708), discussing the composition of a pill: 'I have heard that Dr. Willis took it in his last sicknesse'.

Willis was attended during his last illness by Edmund King. The will, dated 10 November, the day before he died, was proved at London on 24 November 1674.[156] Willis required his body to be buried 'without any Pomp or Ostentation neere my wife and child in the Abbey Church at Westminster'. He left £20 to the poor of St Martin's in the Fields; and a further £20 to be paid annually as stipend for a priest, or 'a Scholemaster if he shall be in orders' on the requirement, as provided in Willis's lifetime, that he read the service of Common Prayer twice daily in that church. He left all his 'manors, lands, etc.' lately purchased from his Grace the Duke of Bucks in trust for a period of 99 years to Sir Lestrange Calthorpe (1624–1678), John Fell, George Benson (1613–1692), John Willis, and John Hemming,[157] and their executors, each of whom was to receive £20, to pay any debts and finance several beneficiaries. After 99 years, these estates were to pass in their entirety to the heirs of his only surviving son, Thomas.

Each of Willis's daughters was to receive £3000 on her twenty-first birthday or at marriage. His sister, Phelp, was bequeathed £20 per annum; her daughter, Mary, was left £100; and Phelp's two other sons, and the five children of his brother Thomas, £20 each to be paid

[154] He means Herefordshire where Robert Symonds was high sheriff in 1702 and after whom Symonds Yat (gate or pass) is named.

[155] See chapter 17 for details of Lady Conway's headaches.

[156] Raymond Hierons obtained a copy in manuscript; and a version was printed in *Wiltshire Notes and Queries*, Devizes (1917): pages 340–2. It is also reproduced in facsimile and text by Hughes (1991): pages 103–6.

[157] For a while John Hemming had lived at Beam Hall where he had a laboratory; see: Kenneth Dewhurst, *Richard Lower's* Vindicatio. *A defence of the experimental method*, Oxford (1983): page xiii.

on their twenty-first birthdays. £20 was to be distributed to those of his relatives deemed to be in need by the executors for a period of seven years. His wife received £100 and all the 'Plate and Goods which were hers before our marriage'. Legacies of £20 were left to 'my sister Willis' and John Fell. His sisters-in-law (but described in the will as 'sisters') Mrs Jones and Mrs Benson were asked to supervise the tuition and education of his children although not obviously with any financial provision being made. Each of his servants was to receive one year's salary and a 'legacy'. One, Thomas Bush (nd), was to work for Willis's son Thomas who inherited his father's estate in Hereford. The income from his properties in Bletchley was one of the bequests to be used in support of Thomas's daughters. The sole executors of the will were 'Mr Philipp Fell, of Eaton Colledg, and Mr Hemyng, the Apothecary' who received £20 each. The will was 'signed, sealed and published in the presence of William Dawkins, Thomas Bush and Pe. Scrivener'. According to his wishes, Willis was buried in the north transept of Westminster Abbey, beneath the central aisle close to Solomon's Porch, near his first wife Mary. The funeral expenses were £470 14s 4d, which John Fell and Browne Willis considered excessive especially since this did not include the memorial tablet. Browne Willis, who was born seven years after the death of his grandfather suggests that the legacies comprised a total sum of £1528 with £237 in a box labelled 'for the poor'. Whilst he may have been referring to 'cash', by any reckoning the probate on Willis's estate was very considerably more than this modest sum.

By the 1960s, the place of burial and original stone were unknown to the vergers and not mentioned in printed guides to Westminster Abbey. William Feindel and Charles Symonds used the detailed history of Westminster Abbey to locate the large stone, measuring 1.2 by 1.8 metres directly in front of the gates leading to the Royal Chapels.[158] The surface was worn smooth with all inscriptions obliterated other than 'Tho. Willis' in the lower right hand corner. The details of texts engraved on the original and eventual slabs are not easy to trace. Browne Willis tells us that Thomas Willis wrote the original inscription starting: 'MARIA, Uxtr charisi, THO. WILLIS, M.D. … Anno Dom. 1667' when Mary and Katherine were buried in Westminster Abbey. Browne Willis then added: 'Hic etiam iacet præictus THO. WILLIS M.D. celeberrimus. Obiit Novemb. 11. 1675, aetatis 54'. Browne Willis mentions that John Le Neve (1679–1741) had partially documented the text in Westminster Abbey but adding somewhat cryptically: 'this gentleman lies buried in Westminster Abbey but (I think) no monument as yet erected for him'.[159] According to William Munk (1816–1898), the original read in full:[160]

> Siste, properes licet quisquis es, Viator | Ne posthac doleas te tanti viri sepulchrum imprudentem præteriisse | Cuius forsan beneficio debetur quod ipse ad sepulchrum | nondum perveneris | Magnus hoc tumulo Willisius conditur: | Celeberrimus ille Thomas Willisius, M.D. | ex Æde Christi Philosophiæ naturalis | in florentissima Oxoniensi Academia Professor, et non tantum | Carolo II do Rege sed et Europæ universæ, | Princeps

[158] See: William Feindel, 'Restoration of memorial to Dr. Thomas Willis (1621–1675) in Westminster Abbey', *British Medical Journal* 1962; i (February 24th): 552–3.

[159] See: John le Neve. *Monumenta Anglicana: being inscriptions on the monuments of several eminent persons deceased in or since the year 1650, to the end of the year 1679. Deduced into a series of time by way of annals*, volume 5, London (1718): N° 257, pages 117–18.

[160] See: William Munk (1868): pages 338–42. This is the source used for the entry on Willis in *Encyclopaedia Britannica*, eleventh edition (1911): page 687, columns 1 & 2, and from which 13 lines of Munk's text are reproduced. Some authors of articles in this edition are identified by initials and with a final listing in the last volume but the entry for Willis is not attributed.

Medicus. | Cujus laudes sane non capit sepulchrale marmor | Quibus orbis ipse vix sufficit. | In Arte Medica et Philosophia naturali | Exercenda, excolenda, promovenda quantopere inclaruerit | Norunt omnes tum exteri quam nostrates | Alterum testabuntur morbi innumeri mirum in modum profligati. | Alterum arte non mediocri facta experimenta | Utramque doctissimæ ipsius lucubrationes hodie attestantur | Neque minus in pietate suit insignis quam ingenio et eruditione. | Regi in nequissimis temporibus fidelis | Ecclesiæ etiam oppressæ obsequentissimus, | Quam non modo affectu dilexit, sed munificentiâ locupletavit | Fortunâ adversâ inconcussus: | Affluente eximie temperans. | In summâ doctrinæ gloriâ humilis et modestus. | Pecuniâ erogandâ in pauperes effusissimus | In suorum gratiam, frugi et providus | In se solummodo parcus. | Labori et vigiliis (heu! nimis) indulgens; | Quibus factum est ut aliorum vitam producendo suam | contraxerit | E vivis enim excessit pleuritide confectus | Anno Atatis 54. | Nati Christi, 1675.

[Halt, even if thou are in haste, whoever you are, Traveller | Do not afterwards regret the folly of having passed by the grave of such a great man. | To whom perhaps you owe the fact that you have not yet | reached the grave yourself | In this tomb the great Willis lies buried: | That most celebrated man Thomas Willis, M.D. | Professor of Natural History at Christ Church | of the highly famous University of Oxford, and not only | of King Charles II but of entire Europe | Chief Physician. | Whose tributes do not fit into sepulchral marble | For these even the globe will barely suffice. | The Art of Medicine and Natural Philosophy | How much he brightened them through practising, perfecting, furthering | Is known to all, abroad and at home | Countless diseases, conquered in wonderful manner, attest the former. | Experimental facts, obtained through extraordinary art, [attest] the latter | Today the wisest products of his midnight oil bear witness of both | And he was no less great in piety than in character and learning. | Loyal to the King in very miserable times | Also devoted to the beleaguered Church, | Which he not only cherished with love but also enriched with gifts | Undaunted by adversities of fate: | Outstanding in his restraint of excess. | Humble and modest in the greatest glory of the creed. | Most lavish in spending money for the poor | Virtuous and prudent on their behalf | Frugal only for himself. | Given to work and (Oh! too much) waking; | Through which it occurred that by extending the life of others | he shortened his own. | For, overwhelmed by pleurisy, he left the living | At the age of 54. | In the year 1675 A.D].[161]

Repair was not possible because the stone had been cracked, probably when debris fell from fire to the great central roof lantern in 1941. Therefore Feindel and Symonds started a Willis Memorial Fund through the Royal College of Physicians of London and the Canadian Neurological Society, which quickly reached its target of 200 guineas. With permission from the Receiver General of the Abbey a new memorial stone was cut, as with the original, from black Belgian marble, and dedicated on 1 September 1960 at a meeting of the Association of British Neurologists under the presidency of Sir Russell Brain (1895–1966). It was unveiled at a service conducted by Canon Fox (1888–1977)[162] who offered prayers (see: Figure 11):

[161] Translation by Jan van Gijn: 23 March 2018.

[162] Reverend Adam Fox is also buried in Westminster Abbey. He had wanted the inscription on his own grave, also on Belgian stone, to read: 'a fox gone to earth'; but the Abbey preferred the somewhat drier: 'Adam Fox 1883–1977 scholar of Winchester, Warden of Radley 1918–24, Dean of Divinity, Magdalen College 1929–1942,

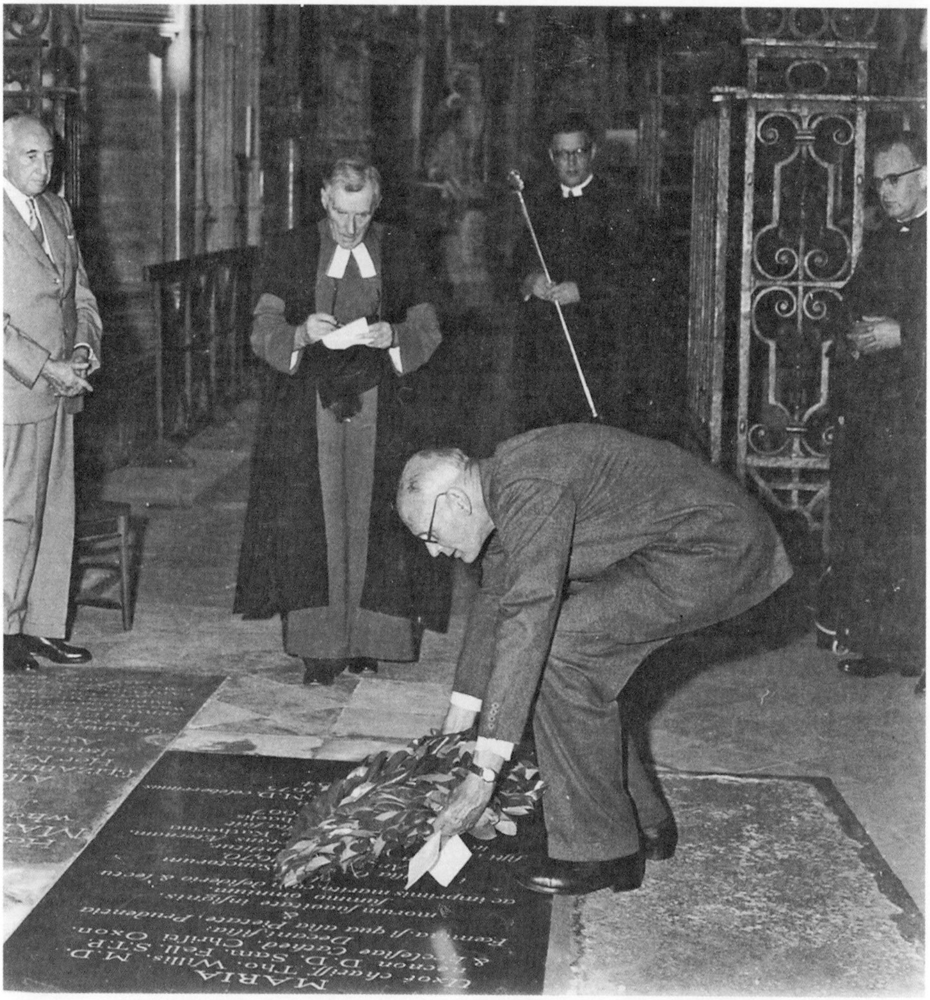

Figure 11 Sir Charles Symonds laying a wreath on the replacement tombstone of Thomas Willis in Westminster Abbey, under the supervision of Canon Fox, in September 1960. From the collection of William Feindel.

> In memory of the life and work of Thomas Willis, a pioneer in medicine and most worthy Christian man, as also for the long line of his successors who have increased our knowledge of the human frame, and the preservation of bodily and mental health.

Placing a wreath of laurel on the stone, Sir Charles Symonds said:

> It is fitting that the name of Thomas Willis should now again be graven as clearly in this Abbey as it is in the minds of his admirers, who to-day, nearly three hundred years after his death continue to draw inspiration from his work.

Professor of Poetry University of Oxford 1938–1943, Master of the Skinners' Company 1947–1948, Canon, archdeacon, and Sub-Dean of Westminster Abbey 1942–1963. Laetatus Sum'. The photograph of Canon Fox and Sir Charles Symonds shown in Figure 11 was reproduced with a brief note of the event in *The Times* for Saturday 2 September 1961.

The new inscription reads:

> MARIA | *Uxor chariſſ* Tho. Willis, M.D. | *necnon* D.D. Sam Fell S.T.P. | & *Eccleſia Cathed.* Chriſti Oxon | *Decani filia,* | *Femina ſi qua alia Pietate Prudentia* | *&* | *morum ſuavitate inſignis* | *ſummo omnium* | *ac imprimis marito, cum deſiderio & lectu* | *obiit* | *in vigilia Omnium Sanctorum* | *Anno Dom. 1670* | *Jamque hic conditur* | *fiſti illius auroram expectans Æternum* | *in eadem etiam humo* Katherina | *eorum filia, ſepulca fuit* | *poſridie* S. Michaelis | *Anno Dom. 1667* | *Hic etiam* | *jacet praedictus* Tho. Willis. M.D. *celeberrimus* | *obiit Nov. 11. 1675* | *a aetatis 54.*[163]

Canon Fox translated the wording as:

> Mary, very dear wife of Thomas Willis M.B. and also M.D., daughter of Samuel Fell, D.D. and Dean of Christ Church Cathedral Oxford, a woman, if ever there was one, distinguished for piety, good sense and sweetness of manners. She died to the great regret and grief of all, and especially of her husband, on the Eve of All Saints, A.D. 1670.
>
> And already lies there, expecting the eternal day-break of that feast, also in the same ground, Katherine, their daughter. She was buried on the day after Michaelmas, A.D. 1667.
>
> Here lies also the very celebrated Thomas Willis, M.D., aforesaid. He died November 11th, 1675, aged 54'.

Westminster Abbey now suggests:

> Mary, most beloved wife of Thomas Willis Doctor in Physick and daughter of Samuel Fell, D.D. and Dean of Christ Church in Oxford, valuable for piety, prudence and sweetness of manners, of all, but chiefly of her husband. She died loved and lamented on the vigil of All Saints 1670 and is buried here, expecting the eternal daybreak of that festival. In the same grave was buried their daughter Katherine, on the day after Michaelmas 1667. Here also lies the above mentioned Thomas Willis, most famous doctor of medicine, who died on the 11 November 1675 aged 54.

Thomas Willis and posterity

From the outset, Willis's clinical and scientific activities attracted controversy. At issue was whether he was the originator or merely the popularizer of work done with others, notably Lower and Wren. Aubrey writes of an occasion in about 1657 (Browne Willis puts this as April 1664) when Willis, on his way to see Lady Keyt (nd) at Brackley, Warwickshire, passed through Astrop, near King's Sutton, Northamptonshire, and noticed that the stones in the rill (stream) were discoloured in the tint of *Crocus martis* indicating the presence of iron. The

[163] The figure legend reproduced in Feindel (1962) reads: The new memorial stone to Thomas Willis and to his wife Mary and his daughter Katherine. (Photograph by A.F Brown.) Read 'luctu' for 'lectu', 'festi' for 'fisti', and postridie' for 'posridie'.

suggestion is that it was the thirst of Willis's horse that alerted him to the special aspects of the stream. Willis then:[164]

> getts Gaules, and putts some of the powder into the water, and immediately it turned blackish: then say'd he 'Ile not send my patients now so far as Tunbridge' and so in short time brought these waters into Vogue, and hath enriched a poore obscure village.

But Willis was not travelling alone and it has been suggested that Lower, not qualified as a physician until 1657, was responsible for the discovery. Lower had studied medicine after completing his Master of Arts degree at Christ Church in 1655. When they worked together and saw patients, Lower received half the fees charged by Willis, one of Locke's tutees paying £1 to Willis and 10s to Lower for a consultation.[165] Ward rehearses the allegation first made by Wood: 'Dr Lower found out ye famous well near King's Sutton though he was willing itt should goe under Dr Willis his name'. On this episode and the professional relationship between Willis and Lower, Wood had made clear that Lower:[166]

> Practiced that Faculty under Dr *Tho. Willis*, whom he helped, or rather instructed, in some parts of Anatomy, especially when he was meditating his book *De Cerebro*, as I have elsewhere told you. In *Apr.* 1664 he, in his Travels with the said Doctor to visit Patients, made a discovery of the medicinal Water at *East Throp* commonly *Alstrop* near *Kings-Sutton* in *Northamptonshire*, the Doctor being then, as usually, asleep or in a sleepy condition on Horseback. Afterwards, our Author *Lower* imparting his Discoveries to the Doctor, they in their return, or when they went that way again, made experiments of it, and thereupon understanding the virtue thereof, The Doctor commended the drinking of it to his Patients. Soon after the Water was contracted into a Well, and upon the said Commendations, 'twas yearly, as to this time it is, frequented by all sorts of People.

Wood is quoting more or less verbatim from Henry Stubbe who wrote several treatises aimed at discrediting the Fellows of the Royal Society:[167]

> Whatsoever there is in that piece [*Cerebri anatome*], which is Anatomical, the glory thereof belongs to Dr. Lower, whose indefatigable industry produced that elaborate Treatise; and any man that knows the great practice of that other Doctor [Willis], will grant, that although he could not want abilities, yet he wanted leisure to attend to such painful and tedious

[164] See: Bennett [Aubrey] (2015): pages 551 and 1480 for details from Aubrey's correspondence that Willis also claimed similar properties for a mineral spring at Wootton-Basset, but the Oxford scholars remained loyal to the 'famed' Astrop waters. The assumption is that by 'gaules', Willis means the excrescence on oak trees produced by infestation of insects, the powders of which he then mixed with the Astrop water.

[165] See: Frank (1980): page 180 for this and many biographical details of Lower in his excellent account of physiology in Oxford; and also Frank (1990): pages 107–46.

[166] See: [Anthony Wood] *Athenæ Oxoniensis*, volume 2, (1690): pages 651–2, entry 532.

[167] See: Henry Stubbe, *Legends no histories: or, a specimen of some animadversions upon the history of the Royal Society. wherein, besides the several errors against common literature, sundry mistakes about the making of salt-petre and gun-powder are detected, and rectified: whereunto are added two discourses … of Pietro Sardi, and … Nicolas Tartaglia … together with the Plus Ultra of Mr. Joseph Glanvill Reduced to a Non-plus, &c.*, part 2, London (1668): pages 95 and 178. The view that Lower was responsible for everything anatomical in Willis's works persisted into the twentieth century. Lower's biographer, Kenneth Franklin (1897–1966) initially held that opinion but, later acknowledged that he had been mistaken; see: KJ Franklin, 'The Work of Richard Lower (1631–1691)', *Proceedings of the Royal Society of Medicine* (1931): 25; 113–8; and Raymond Hierons and Alfred Meyer, 'Some priority questions arising from Thomas Willis' work on the brain', *Proceedings of the Royal Society of Medicine* (1962): 55; 287–92, at page 287.

> enquiries. Dr. Willis indeed candidly doth relinquish this honour to Dr. Lower … All that Dr. Willis contributed, that I hear, was the discourses and conjectures upon the Anatomical deductions of Dr. Lower, which as ingenious as they are, I am sure neither are, nor ever will, pass all for inventions.

Stubbe also commented, in the context of Boyle's work, which he had translated into Latin,[168] that 'Willis had used this to demonstrate many of the same conclusions'. Prompted in his criticism, apparently by Baldwin Hamey (1600–1676), Stubbe continues:

> I think myself obliged to adde one thing more where I speak as if Dr. Willis had had little to do in the discoveries of Dr. Lower about Anatomy: that although the great Physician had not leisure to attend the Anatomical Inquiries yet he did propose *new matter* for *improving the discoveries*, and put Dr. Lower upon continual investigation, thereby to see if Nature and his supposition did accord: and although that many did occur beyond his apprehension: yet was the grand occasion of that work, and in much the Author … thus much I thought fitting to annex, lest the Virtuosi should censure me as partial to my old School-fellow, Dr. Lower, or swayed by any regard than that of Truth.

The Royal Society itself noted the matter:[169]

> There is a certain gentleman, a florid writer, one of our royal collegiate, who intends to print shortly some paralipomena relating to the history of our Society … this author was evidently Mr Joseph Glanvill, rector of the Abbey Church at Bath … in his book Plus ultra … this treatise and Mr Sprat's History of the Royal Society gave great offence to Mr Henry Stubbe, the physician, of Warwick, who took occasion thence to attack that Society with uncommon virulence and scurrility of language, charing the members not only with bringing contempt upon ancient and solid learning, especially the Aristotelian philosophy, but likewise with undermining the universities, destroying the established religion, and introducing popery in its stead. These charges he attempts to support in his several pieces against Mr Sprat and Mr Glanvill.

These criticisms are at odds with the fact that Stubbe dedicated two of his books to Willis who he thanks for providing testimonials:[170]

> To my Learned Friend Dr. *Thomas Willis* Doctor of *Physick*, and Reader of *Natural Philosophy* in the University of *Oxon. When I first entered upon the practice of* Physick, *I had the honour of your* Testimonial*: and I now publickly acknowledge as well your* favours *as that* worth *which is* universally known, *and* admired. *Were I to celebrate your* Panegyrick, *I should no doubt to represent you as a* second to Harvey.

[168] See: Robert Boyle, 'A physico-chymical essay, containing an experiment with some considerations touching the different parts and reintegration of salt-petre'. In: *Certain physiological essays, written at distant times, and on several occasions*, London (1661): pages 107–35; and Frank (1980): page 123.

[169] See: Birch, volume 2 (1756): page 197 footnote.

[170] See: Henry Stubbe, *The Indian nectar, or, A discourse concerning chocolata the nature of cacao-nut and the other ingredients of that composition is examined and stated according to the judgment and experience of the Indian and Spanish writers … its effects as to its alimental and venereal quality as well as medicinal (especially in hypochondrial melancholy) are fully debated: together with a spagyrical analysis of the cacao-nut, performed by that excellent chymist Monsieur le Febure, chymist to His Majesty*, London (1662): page [3].

And, writing from Stratford upon Avon on 17 February 1665, Stubbe offers his book on therapeutics:[171]

> To his very worthy and Learned Friend Dr THOMAS WILLIS, Doctor in Physique, and Professor of Natural Phylosophy in OXFORD.

Willis acknowledged the contributions of Wren, Millington and Lower in the preface to *Cerebri anatome* (1664), one of two books published whilst still living in Oxford. Collectively he felt 'hem'd in by the plentiful assistances of the Illustrious Men'. Individually:

> And here I made use of the Labours of the most Learned Physician and highly skilful Anatomist, Doctor Richard Lower, for my help and Companion; the edge of whose Knife and Wit I willingly acknowledge to have been an help to me for the better searching out both the frame and offices of before hidden Bodies.

Lower himself defended his master's work against critics in his first publication which provides testimony of their harmonious relationship:[172]

> When set to embark on a controversy ... in which name not only of Willis, but even of Philosophy herself is in danger ... there was no ignoring insults that would allow ... honest effort to be brought to nought, and truth herself to be dishonoured.

Nonetheless the whiff of a strained relationship is detected by Hansruedi Isler (1934–2019) who senses reserve in a remark Lower included in *Tractatus de corde* (1669);[173] but, for all the stirring, Willis was at pains to acknowledge the collaboration and when Lower died in 1691, a broadsheet summarized their relationship:[174]

> ... When the learn'd WILLIS dy'd, he did impart
> His utmost Skill to thy capacious Heart.
> Full well he knew, there was no other Shrine
> So fit to keep his Treasure in, as thine.
> So the old Seer did to his Son dispense
> A double Portion of Prophetick Sense,
> When in his fiery Chair he mounted hence.
> WILLIS Expiring, joy'd in Thee, to find
> He'd such a Legacy for Human kind.
> A Legacy more valuable far,
> Than both the Indies and their Riches are.

[171] See: Henry Stubbe, *The miraculous conformist or an account of several marvailous cures performed by the stroaking of the hands of Mr Valentine Greatarick with a physical discourse thereupon, in a letter to the honourable Robert Boyle esq; with a letter relating some other of his miraculous cures, attested by E. Foxcroft M.A. and Fellow of King's College in Cambr:*, Oxford (1666).

[172] See: Richard Lower *Diatribæ Thomæ Willisii Doct. Med. & Profess. Oxon. De febribus vindicatio adversus Edmundum De Meara Ormoniensem Hibernum M.D.*, London (1665): page [4].

[173] See: Isler (1968): page 21 and endnote 170 presumably, as set out in chapter 15, referring to Lower distancing himself somewhat from Willis when explaining that any ambiguity expressed in the *Vindicatio* had arisen through relying too much on the authority and preconceived opinions of 'the learned Dr Willis'.

[174] See: Fulton (1935): facsimile inserted after page 32 of 'An elegy on the death of that learned and famous physician Dr. RICHARD LOWER', London (1691) taken from Bodleian Godw. Pamph. 2226.

They cannot to our Days one Minute give;
But Thousands by thy powerful Art still live....

An epigram written in verse by Nathaniel Williams (1656–1679), a Welshman who matriculated at Jesus College, Oxford, in 1672 and graduated Bachelor of Arts in 1676, appeared in the year that Willis died, ending with the lines:[175]

Thou knewst the wondrous art,
And order of each part,
In the whole lump, how every sense,
Contributes to the health's defense.
The severall, Channels which convey,
The vitall current every way,
Trackst wise Nature every where,
In every region, every sphere,
Fathomest the mistery
Of deepe Anatomy.
The unactive carcasse thou hadst preyd upon,
And stript it to a sceleton,
But now alas! The art is gone,
And now on thee,
The crawling Worms experience their Anatomy.

And for all his acerbic comments, Wood felt able to conclude:[176]

> Dr Willis left behind him the character of an orthodox, pious, and charitable physitian ... for his wonderful success and repute in his practice, the natural smoothness, pure elegancy, delightful, unaffected neatness of Latin stile, none scarce hath equall'd much less out-done him, how great soever. When at any time he is mention'd by authors (as he is very often) it is done in words expressing their highest esteem of his great worth and excellency, and placed still, as first in rank, among physicians. And further also, he hath laid a lasting foundation of a body of physic chiefly on hypotheses of his own framing.

But the most loyal voice came from Willis's grandson, Browne Willis, so named to honour his mother (Alice Browne) and patronymic name. On his grandfather, he wrote:[177]

> His merit gained the highest esteem among those of the first rank and fortune as well as genius and learning, which appears not only from common report, but likewise from various epistles of congratulation and consultation, which are now in the hands of his grandson Browne Willis Esq: But it would be needless as well as impossible to make a particular recital of the friends of that man, who never delivered an enemy ... tempering civil with divine matters ... he always afforded opportunities for the frequent calls of his profession, and was never wanting in his assistance to the poor or infirm in any capacity, or in giving

[175] See: Nathaniel Williams, *A pindarique elegie on the most learned and famous physitian Dr Willis*, Oxford (1675): stanza 6 of 12, each of 28 lines. A further edition, with a new title, appeared from Oxford in 1676 with the elegy at pages 98–108.
[176] See: Wood (1817): pages 1051–3.
[177] See: [Browne Willis] (1741): pages 171–5 (footnote 9); and Wood (1817): pages 1048–50.

> pleasure and satisfaction, to mankind in general. Considering then the many avocations, which a person of his disposition and extensive practice must necessarily have, we might reasonably conclude this to be full employment for the most active and robust constitution, did not his numerous writings above mentioned, those lasting monuments of an exalted genius, convince us, that human powers are not so limited as we are apt to imagine, but will, when duly exerted, overcome those difficulties, which seem even to men of common industry absolutely insupportable.

When his father died, Browne Willis, then aged 18 years, inherited in trust the remaining estate formed by his grandfather, thereby becoming lord of the manor of Fenny Stratford ('the marshy ford on a Roman road', Watling Street).[178] On reaching his maturity in 1703, Browne Willis resolved to commission the building of St Martin's parish church. The land was purchased from Mr Thomas Price on the site of the former Chantry Chapel of St Margaret and St Catherine for the nominal sum of 5s. Browne Willis was 'a man whose benefactions outran his resources' and fundraising started in 1721. He laid the foundation stone on 11 November 1724, and the requisite £1500 was achieved over the next nine years. The initial bricklaying was done by Daniel Eastment (d.1728). The original plan was modified in 1727 and the architect, Mr Edward Wing (nd) of Aynhoe near Brackley, was dismissed: 'he and his men drink ale more hours than work and that it was not worth twelve pence a day in the judgment of any man that understood work'. Wing was replaced by John Simmonds (nd), a local joiner. Donors included local gentry and the Universities of Oxford and Cambridge, the forty individuals and institutions who gave £10 or more having their coats of arms displayed on the ceiling of the chapel.[179]

With 'the whole of the work being happily finished', Richard Reynolds (1674–1743), Bishop of Lincoln, consecrated the church dedicated to St Martin of Tours (316–397), with its chapel in memory of Thomas Willis, on 29 May 1730. Browne Willis was pleased and considered St Martin's chapel to be 'his chiefist and most real worldly comfort and happiness'. He and Dr Martin Benson (1689–1752), rector of Bletchley and subsequently Bishop of Gloucester, each donated £100 to a fund from which to endow a curacy. This was also supported through income, eventually £18 per annum, mainly derived from a parcel of land, Parsons Piece, and (later) the adjacent farm.[180] From 1734, Browne Willis settled a rent charge of £1 on Benson, the churchwarden, and the overseer of the poor of Fenny Stratford. This allowed them to pay the curate of Fenny Stratford to deliver a sermon on St Martin's day (11 November), and the costs of a more extended celebration for the towns people. Browne

[178] See: British History Online https://www.british-history.ac.uk/vch/bucks/vol4/pp274-283 for details of 'Waterhall Farm, probably marking the site of the mansion of Waterhall, formerly belonging to the Lords Grey de Wilton. 'In 1711 Browne Willis, the eccentric Buckinghamshire antiquary, built a house on rising ground by Bletchley Church, which, as William Cole says "he very absurdly ... called ... Water Hall. He never lived there, and in 1780 it was put up for auction". Lipscomb says it was at some time purchased by Earl Spencer's steward, who pulled it entirely down. About 1862 there were remaining two portions of what might have been the out offices and a great portion of a moat still full of water. It was approached "by avenues of elm and lime trees from each side"'. The site of the Manor House is now known as Saffron Gardens.

[179] See: [Anon], *Saint Martin's parish church, Fenny Stratford. A short illustrated history*, Gloucester (nd): pages 1–34; revised by Edward Legg, privately published (1986). The names of those whose shields adorn the ceiling, including Christ Church, Corpus Christi, Brasenose and Jesus Colleges, Oxford, appear in the first pamphlet: pages 18–19. These are intact having been retouched by Dr William Bradbrook sometime before 1916; see: Henry Viets, 'A patronal festival for Thomas Willis (1621–75) with remarks by Sir William Osler, Bart., F.R.S.', *Annals of Medical History* 1917: 3; 118–24.

[180] The British History online archive mentions that through his charitable gifts and expenditure of £5000 on the building of Waterhall, Browne Willis was ruined and 'obliged towards the end of his days to dress meanly and to live in squalor, becoming very dirty and penurious, so that he was often taken for a beggar.'

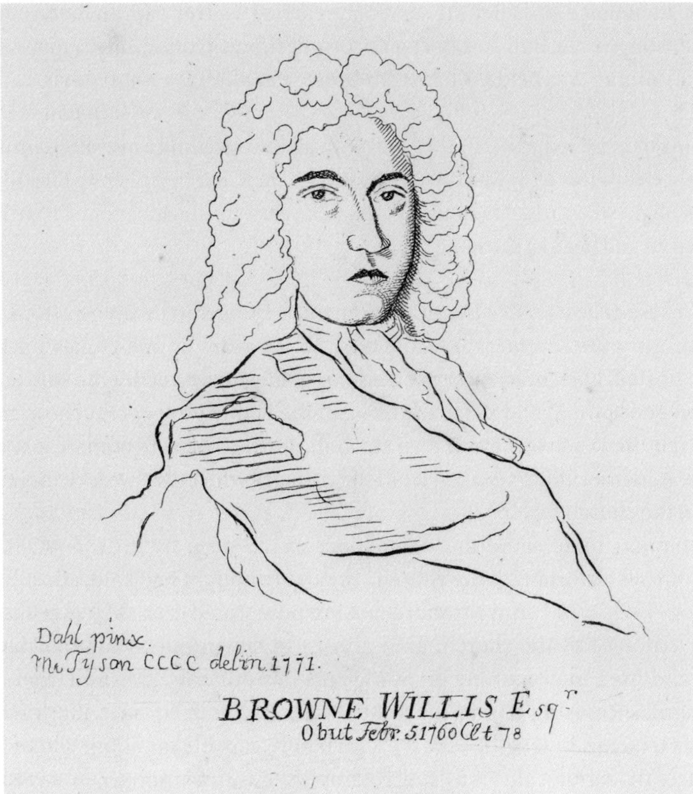

Figure 12 An engraving of Browne Willis by Mr Tyson 1771.
Reproduced courtesy of Father Bullock, St Martin's Church, Fenny Stratford.

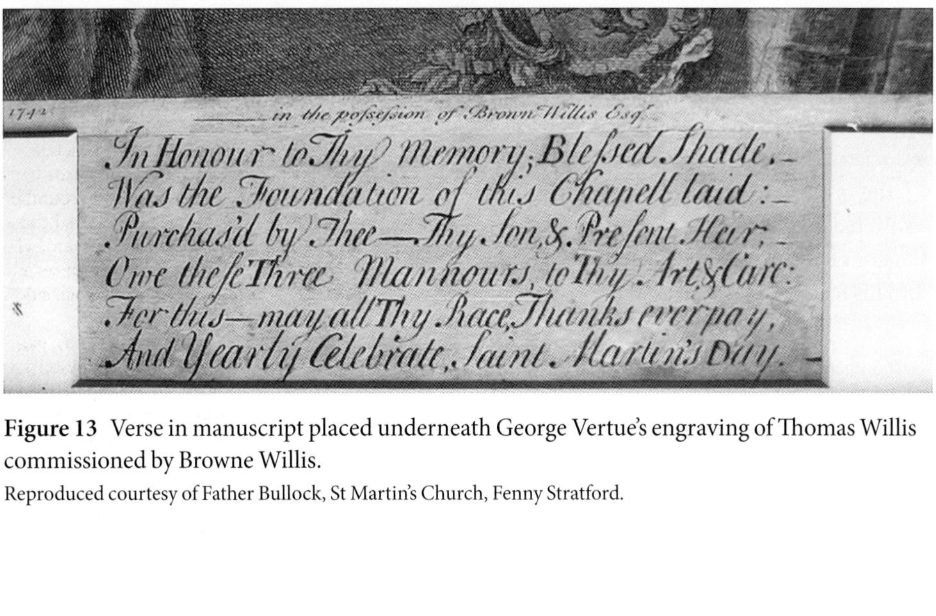

Figure 13 Verse in manuscript placed underneath George Vertue's engraving of Thomas Willis commissioned by Browne Willis.
Reproduced courtesy of Father Bullock, St Martin's Church, Fenny Stratford.

Willis was in attendance and after the service he carried a silver cup, an heirloom in the possession of Benson, to the Bull Inn, formerly Brotherhood House until suppressed in 1550, where a turkey dinner was held. At his death Browne Willis left a note:

> And I do make it my request that they will with all due solemnity ever keep up and see to the annual celebration of S. Martin's festival ... in the Church of Fenny Stratford, in the manner as I have solemnised it annually ... for 26 years, in all which time I have been constantly present and heard a sermon.

With the purchase of houses that became St Martin's Cottages in Fenny Stratford, by the early nineteenth century the revenue maintained an honorarium of one guinea for the sermon, dinner to be hosted, and the memory of Thomas Willis honoured by the sums of 2s for bell ringing, 6s on gunpowder, and 2s for the firing of the Fenny poppers.[181] Those attending the dinner were required each to 'pay his own alcoholic burden without compulsory aid from his companions'. A memorial stone taken from the cottages when they were demolished in 1915 was placed in the church tower.

The parishioners understand that the poppers were given by Browne Willis but this is disputed by official historians of the church. They were bought and sold, adorning the doorways of various houses in Fenny Stratford, but are now stored on a shelf over the inner door of the tower entrance to the church. They consist of six gunmetal cannonades filled with gunpowder and fired in synchrony on St Martin's day at noon, 2pm and 4pm by the vicar and town dignitaries using a long rod heated in the church furnace. Each weighs 8.5kg, and measures 6 inches in length, with a 1¾ inch bore capable of taking ¼lb of gunpowder. In the nineteenth century, this was supplied by Pacey's, ironmonger in Aylesbury Street. Enthusiasm sometimes exceeded caution. In 1857 (opinions on the date differ somewhat), the poppers were detonated in a field, Bull Close, and partially demolished the roof of the Bull and Butcher; and, on another occasion, the church clock tower. One popper had to be replaced by Barwell and Co., at the Eagle foundry in Northampton. Temporary cessation of the ceremony in 1905 on the basis of 'health and safety' by the vicar of St Martin's led to complaints and the poppers were soon reinstated although silenced again for seven years during and after the Second World War. The inhabitants of Fenny Stratford have been happy to fire the poppers on occasions other than St Martin's day: the death of Queen Victoria, on 1 January 2000, and to mark the late Queen Mother's 100th birthday on 4 August 2000. Filmed for the BBC in 1953 for the series 'England in November', the exact location of the Fenny Poppers has moved in recent years but this happy event, now in its 287th year survives and is associated with the Fenny Poppers festival held annually in August.

The orator on 14 November 1916 (the 183rd) was Sir William Osler (1849–1919) who exhibited his copy of *Dr Willis's practice of physick*.[182] Osler took as his text 'Willis the Anatomist'. He rehearsed the then familiar Oxonian line that whilst the anatomy of Willis and his friends was good, the therapeutic medicine was awful:[183]

[181] See: William Feindel 'Fenny Poppers: a quaint celebration for Dr. Thomas Willis', *Canadian Medical Association Journal* 1969: 101; 447–9.

[182] See: [William Osler] *Bibliotheca Osleriana*, Oxford (1929): page 384, #4248. Entries 4248–51 are works by Willis. Five books might be considered a surprisingly poor representation. Item 4248 has the note: 'Inserted: (i) 'A patronal festival for Thomas Willis ... with remarks by Sir William Osler' by Henry Viets, with portraits &c.; repr. Fr. Annals. Med. Hist., New York, 1917, I, pp 118–24; (ii) programmes and newspaper reports of this festival at Fenny Stratford in 1916; (iii) autogr. Letter from Dr. Bradbrook (cf. nos 4386–87); and (iv) a note on some Willis MSS. in the Bodleian'. William Feindel gave the 2002 address at the Fenny Poppers dinner.

[183] See: Mark Gardiner, 'An Osler centenary', *The Osler Library Newsletter* 2017: 126; 2–4.

> His 'Pharmaceutica rationale' is as dead as Willis. It gives me a shudder to think of the constitutions our ancestors had, and how they withstood the assaults of the apothecary. Willis did two things; he made himself a good scientific man as far as the science of that day went, and he made himself a first class practitioner, and those two sides of the man are presented in his works … Since I had your kind invitation I have had to read Willis's large book through, from which I got a great deal of information I did not want and have refrained from giving to you … Willis was a great and a good man … and the 15th Psalm the Chairman has read at the service is most appropriate. It just suited him. There are many good descriptions of the upright, righteous man, but none better than that … which fits Willis to a 't'.

Osler described the occasion in a letter to Fielding Garrison (1870–1935) mentioning that he had: [184]

> Talked about old Thomas … it was a most interesting occasion, and the 'Poppers' were popped at intervals throughout the day in honour of Thomas and his grandson, the famous antiquary.

The marble memorial to Thomas and Browne Willis at St Martin's Fenny Stratford reads (see: Frontispiece):[185]

> Hic situs est | BROWNE WILLIS, Antiquarius, | Cujus cl: Avi æternæ Memoriæ, | THO: WILLIS Archiatri totius Europæ celeberimi | defuncti Die Sancti Martini. A:D: 1675, | Hæc CAPELLA exigiuum Monumentum est, | Obiit 5°. Die Feb: A:D: 1760, | Ætatis suæ 78. | O CHRISTE, Soter, et Judex, | huic Peccatorum primo | misercors & propitus esto.*
>
> [Here lies Browne Willis, Antiquarian, to whose grandfather Tho. Willis, of everlasting memory, a leading physician renowned throughout Europe, and who died on St Martin's Day, A.D. 1675, this Chapel is a small memorial. He expired on the 3rd of February, A.D 1760, in his 78th year. O Christ, Saviour and Judge, be pitiful and merciful to this man, outstanding amongst us sinners.]

Together with a pen and ink sketch of Browne Willis given by Rev FF Field, rector of Woughton (fl.1894), a copy of the engraving of Thomas Willis by George Vertue (1684–1756) commissioned by Browne Willis at a cost of £21 and given by him on 11 November 1730 hangs in the Browne Willis chapel (see Figures 12–13). This has the inscription:

> Thos. Willis, M.D. obit 1675, Avus D. J. T. S. die Sancti Martini
>
> In Honour to thy Memory; Blessed Shade,
> Was the Foundation of this Chapell laid:

[184] See: Harvey Cushing, *The life of Sir William Osler*, volume 2, Oxford (1925): page 542.

[185] The memorial stone is now on the east wall in the north-east corner of the Browne Willis chapel, St. Martin's Church, Fenny Stratford. It was restored in 1957 under the supervision of Mr E Clive Rouse with support from the Buckinghamshire Archaeological Society.

* Underlined text originally printed in red.

> Purchas'd by Thee – Thy Son and Present Heir,
> Owe these Three Mannours to Thy Art and Care:
> For this – may all Thy Race Thanks ever pay,
> And Yearly Celebrate Saint Martin's Day.

It might have been expected that, after Anthony Wood, Browne Willis had put the record straight; and he would have been encouraged by John Freind (1675–1728) who had already declared (in the context of opinions on apoplexy):[186]

> I take notice of this. Because it is exactly the notion of the famous Dr Willis, the first inventor of the nervous system: who wou'd have the difference between the *Cerebum* and *Cerebellum,* as to their several uses, to consist in this, that the former is concern'd in animal or voluntary motion, and the latter in vital or involuntary.

But the reputation of Thomas Willis was still not entirely secure. At the end of the eighteenth century, Benjamin Hutchinson (nd) restated the essential facts of Thomas Willis's life and works, citing the *General dictionary* and Derham's (1657–1735) *Physico-theology* (1713), but in one important respect deviating from Browne Willis:[187]

> It will be agreed with Wood that WILLIS hath founded a body of physic, chiefly on hypotheses of his own framing; but it will not be agreed that this foundation will be lasting. The truth is, nothing could be more unfortunate than this method of proceeding of Dr WILLIS; who, instead of deducing real knowledge from observation and experiment, exercised himself in framing theories. Hence it is, that, while his books shew the greatest ingenuity and learning, very little knowledge is to be drawn from them, very little use to be made of them. And perhaps no writings, which are so admirably executed, and prove such uncommon talents to have been in the writer, were ever so soon laid aside and neglected as the work of Dr WILLIS.

Hutchinson then backs off slightly:

> It is not to be imagined, in the mean time, that there are not many curious things to be found in the works of this ingenious and able physician, or that he contributed nothing to the promotion of real knowledge; very far otherwise.

But the damage was done. William Munk largely reiterated Hutchinson's negative opinion although it was he who reproduced the extended wording on the memorial stone in Westminster Abbey, not otherwise available in its entirety.[188] Michael Foster (1836–1907) was vituperative in his dismissal of Willis:[189]

> Love of truth was in him less potent than love of fame ... Mixing with and ... in daily intercourse with the band of exact inquirers, who at Oxford and in London were striving to

[186] See: John Freind, *The history of physick from the time of Galen, to the beginning of the sixteenth century chiefly with regard to practice. In a discourse written to Doctor Mead*, part 2, London (1726): pages 315–16.

[187] See: Benjamin Hutchinson, *Biographia medicia*, etc., volume 2, London (1799): pages 481–5.

[188] See: William Munk, volume 1 (1878): pages 338–42.

[189] See: Michael Foster, *Lectures on the history of physiology*, Cambridge (1901): pages 268–80 at pages 270–1.

> establish the new philosophy and advance by experiment natural knowledge, Willis caught up their phrases and thinking himself one of them, attempted to expound in their fashion the physiology of the nervous system ... Willis's mind was of the rhetorical sort, he loved words as words, looked upon an illustration as an argument, and when he had discovered an analogy thought he had found a proof ... the views which he put forward ... do not of themselves form any real solid contribution to knowledge.

And so it went on into the twentieth century. FJ (Francis Joseph) Cole (1872–1959), in 1944:[190]

> It seems certain that the observational basis of these researches was not supplied by Willis himself, and that his own part lay in providing the ideas and plans which animated the labours of his more objective collaborators, and in discussing the results with them before drafting the letterpress. He cannot be said to have achieved his ambition in making himself clear to the meanest capacity. His language is often involved, in spite of the elegant Latin in which it is cast, and is not more comprehensible by a tendency to practise the subtleties of speculative disputation born of the Schoolmen, which is what Willis calls 'philosophising'. Neither has he the gift of clear and intelligible expression, but if we must admit the impossibility of discriminating the parts taken by various members of the company in formulating the text, we may suspect that this task was mainly, if not entirely, the prerogative of their pontifical leader.

And Cecilia Mettler (1909–1943):[191]

> Thomas Willis ... had one of the most fashionable practices in London. He was something of a dandy and, while neither original nor erudite, he had the good fortune to secure the help of two men ... in the preparation of the work on which his reputation as an anatomist is based ... while his philosophic and physiologic opinions were of very poor quality ... his work in clinical medicine is of a higher calibre.

But others had read the treatises more thoroughly and formed their own opinions, defending Willis against 'charges of dishonesty, plagiarism, dandyism, vanity, pomposity, and verbosity'.[192] One of the earliest to express admiration in the modern era was Victor Horsley (1857–1916):[193]

> Willis's researches on the central nervous system ... exhibit such an extraordinary grasp of the function ... of the brain and nervous system ... his remarks are almost invariably logical and accurate deductions from the actual facts which he observed ... he throws over the teachings of the Greek and Roman schools, which fell into the very natural but profound mistake of regarding the peripheral phenomena in the heart as the index of

[190] See: FJ Cole *A history of comparative anatomy*, London (1954): pages 222–31, for his analysis of *De anima brutorum*.

[191] Cecilia Mettler and Fred Mettler (editor), *History of medicine*, Philadelphia (1947): pages 66–7.

[192] See: Dewhurst (1983): pages 291–301.

[193] Victor Horsley *The structure and functions of the brain and spinal cord. Being the Fullerian lectures for 1891*, Lecture I, London (1892): pages 15–23. Horsley writes that it is 206 years since Willis's researches were published in his native language. Since that would be 1685, he might have been using *The London practice of physick* but that omits much of the work on structure and function of the brain, so Horsley is presumably one year out.

> local psychical changes, instead of mere secondary indications of central ones ... he first clearly enunciated ... the greatest advance gained in psychology ever since it became a science ... the localisation of function to distinct parts of the nervous system ... the reason why the cortex ... is thrown into convolutions, or 'cranklings' as he calls them.

Horsley then explains that, with others, Willis correctly relocated ideas on the ventricle as the place where spirits are produced to the substance of the brain, relegating the cavities of the brain to 'jakes' or 'sinks' that collect debris. Although correct in arguing that forces originate in the cortex and pass through the brain and spinal cord to the nerves, he argues that Willis is wrong in supposing that the responsible 'spirits' enter and leave the nerves through tiny pores throughout their course. But his admiration resumes with Willis's description that the 'cerebel[lum]' is the source of involuntary actions and 'passions'. And Willis clearly expressed the concept of the reflex in his account of lower animals lacking a developed brain:

> So long, therefore, they being destitute of the internal principle of motion, move themselves all members only as they are excited from the impulse of the external object, and so sensation preceding motion is in some manner the cause of it.

Fielding Garrison (1870–1935) also credited Willis, 'the most brilliant of the chemiatrists', with overturning the medieval cell doctrine that assigned functions to the cerebrospinal fluid in the ventricles.[194] Garrison argued that although Willis reasoned correctly that the cerebrum is the organ of thought, wrongly he assumed that the fatal character of lesions of the cerebellum identifies this structure as the centre of vital functions and the controller of involuntary mechanisms such as the beat of the heart and the movements of the lungs, stomach and intestines. Willis also went astray in assigning perception to the corpora striata, imagination to the corpus callosum, memory to the cerebral gyri, and instinct to the midbrain. It took the work of Albrecht von Haller (1708–1777) to displace Willis's localization of involuntary movement and replace this with the doctrine of irritability.[195]

Leonard Guthrie (1858–1918) took a similar position on Willis's contributions, pausing to accept that he was helped by Lower, 'an honest, able seeker of truth, but too tactless and unworldly to secure riches'. Guthrie lists as Willis's contributions: anatomy of the brain, its ganglia and circulation; the concept of afferent and efferent pathways; localization of function; the ventricles as lymph spaces not the source of animal spirits; and the cerebellum as the organ of involuntary action.[196] But these descriptions, important in their time, were later displaced or modified and all were surpassed by Willis's highly original ideas on reflex function:

[194] See: Fielding H Garrison, 'History of neurology'. In: Charles L Dana, *Textbook of neurology*, New York (1925): (10th edition) pages xxxiii–iv. Very little of substance is added to Garrison's account in the much expanded version, Lawrence McHenry *Garrison's History of neurology revised and enlarged with a bibliography of classical, original and standard works,* Illinois (1969): pages 55–8, with almost no mention of Willis's other treatises.

[195] See: Albrecht von Haller, *Dissertation on the sensible and irritable parts of animals*, London (1755): pages 1–73; although there is frequent reference to Robert Whytt (1714–1766) and to selected physicians of the seventeenth century, Haller does not mention Willis; and his name is also missing from the preface written by Samuel Tissot (1728–1797), see pages i–xxxii.

[196] Leonard Guthrie, *The history of neurology. The Fitz-Patrick lectures on the history of medicine, delivered at the Royal College of Physicians in the years 1907, 1908*, Lecture II, London (1921): pages 137–40.

> An object driving the animal spirits inwards, and modifying them in a certain peculiar manner, gives rise to sensation, and that the same animal spirits, in that they rebound from within outwards in a reflected wave as it were, call forth local movements.

For John Fulton (1899–1960):[197]

> Thomas Willis is a much underrated contributor to physiological literature. His methods of experiment and his process of reasoning were at times erratic, and did not conform with the standards set by some of his contemporaries such as Boyle and Lower. Yet Willis had wide clinical experience, he recorded what he saw and he frequently gave evidence of penetrating vision ... Much given to speculation he often weakened the value of his arguments, but this should not prevent us from recognising the nature of his achievement.

Harvey Cushing (1869–1939) concluded his Lister address to the Royal College of Surgeons in July 1930 on the pituitary by quoting Willis (who was actually describing the '*rete mirabile, a divine artifice*' and its function):[198]

> There is nothing in the whole fabric of an animal body more worthy of admiration ... nothing can be conceived as more skilful, and nothing which argues more forcefully the providence of a divine Author.

Omitted from the original edition of Webb Haymaker's (1902–1984) *The founders of neurology* (1953), there is an entry by William Feindel in the second edition that rehearses the well-known facts emphasizing contributions to knowledge of the cerebral vasculature.[199] But Willis's reputation as the founder of clinical neuroscience had already been proposed in Sir Charles Symonds's 1954 Harveian Oration on *The circle of Willis*.[200] Symonds emphasizes the physiological interpretation of Willis's anatomical observations, and points out the episode of headache which may have heralded the moment of carotid occlusion. Drawing on the example of Thomas Willis, Symonds introduces his Harveian Oration with a definition and defence of the clinical scientist, caught between research ambition and the pressures of clinical duties, with no time to reflect and a lack of training in laboratory methods. He argues for the appointment of clinicians to senior research posts: 'Every case he sees ... must become for the moment a personal issue wherein he has to acknowledge defeat. He is very often made to feel uncomfortable'. Geoffrey Keynes, who applauded Willis's description of myasthenia gravis, a disease to which Keynes contributed through the use of thymectomy, wrote:[201]

> Willis was one of the most important medical writers of the seventeenth century. He did not make any single forward step in science to compare with Harvey's demonstration of the circulation, but he covered a very wide field of observation in physiology, anatomy,

197 See: John F Fulton, *Selected readings in the history of physiology*, Illinois (1930): pages 194–5.

198 See: John Fulton *Harvey Cushing, a biography*, Illinois (1946): page 593; and Harvey Cushing 'Neurohypophysial mechanisms from a clinical standpoint', *Lancet* 1930: ii; 119–27 and 175–84.

199 See: William Feindel, 'Thomas Willis (1621–1675)'. In: *The founders of neurology*, Illinois (1970): pages 91–5.

200 See: Symonds (1954).

201 See: Geoffrey Keynes, 'The history of myasthenia gravis', *Medical History* 1961: 5; 313–26; adapted and reprinted in *Myasthenia gravis*, Ed. Raymond Greene, London (1969): pages 1–13. His comment on 'three folio volumes in 1683' is surprisingly inaccurate for such a dedicated bibliophile.

> and neurology, including mental disorders. He was distinguished even among the early fellows of the Royal Society. Everyone knows the implications of the 'circle of Willis', an eponym which I trust will never be done away with by any modern improver of nomenclature. It is less well known that he first distinguished true diabetes mellitus, and showed that the polyuria was not due to any disease of the kidney. He even anticipated the recognition of hormones in the circulation by his suggestion that the phenomena of puberty were due to a ferment distributed through the body from the genitals ... Unfortunately all his writings were composed and published in Latin. An English translation was published in three folio volumes in 1683, but these books are hard to come by and are insufficiently well known. They are packed with shrewd observations – along with much nonsense, it must be admitted.

By 1981 Willis's reputation was not in doubt when John ('Jerry') Spillane (1909–1985) wrote 'Willis and the nervous system', a long and analytical chapter on the man and his contributions to medicine and the nervous system and, taken from Willis, entitled his book *The doctrine of the nerves*.[202] The ample justification for that endorsement is set in chapters 16 and 17.

[202] See: John D Spillane, *The doctrine of the* nerves, London (1981): pages 53–107 in which he draws upon the writings of Feindel and Symonds, Hansruedi Isler's biography and the work of Hierons and Meyer. Spillane's copy of the English edition of Isler's monograph is heavily annotated with underlining, some corrections, and tick-marks against the references he had also consulted. By contrast, Raymond Hierons's copy of the German edition is pristine and unmarked (or unread). Thereafter, with the notable exceptions of the work of Robert Frank, Robert Martensen, and John Trevor Hughes, the only account of the life and work of Thomas Willis is Carl Zimmer, *Soul made flesh*, London (2004). Several much shorter biographical essays have been written since 1900: HG Anderson, 'The life of Thomas Willis, MD (being the Wix prize essay, 1921)', *St. Bartholomew's Hospital Journal* 1920–1: 28; 170–3; William Miller, 'Thomas Willis (1621–1675)', *Bulletin of the Society of Medical History of Chicago* 1923–1925: 3; 215–32; Humphry Rolleston, 'Thomas Willis', *Medical Life* 1934: 41; 177–91; Robert Dow, 'Thomas Willis (1621–1675) as a comparative neurologist', *Annals of Medical History* 1940: 2; 181–94; and Walter Wells, 'Dr. Thomas Willis (1621–1675): a great seventeenth century anatomist and clinician who anticipated many modern discoveries', *The Laryngoscope* 1949: 59; 287–305. See also a little known account of Thomas Willis: Alasdair Coles, *The neurophysiology and psychology of Thomas Willis (1621–1675) submitted for the Jane Willis Kirkaldy prize 1988*, University of Oxford: typescript (nd): pages 1–60. Jane Willis Kirkaldy (1869–1932) was a graduate in natural sciences and a science educator in Oxford unrelated by descent to Thomas Willis. There have been many articles on Willis's contributions to medicine and neurology, of which some are listed in chapters 15–18 dealing with the individual treatises.

2

'Setting down experiments of the sciences'

Printing and the works of Thomas Willis

Readership on science and medicine in the seventeenth century was largely confined to scholars and physicians. Usually written in Latin, most books served as a repository of knowledge that reflected the classical teachings. It took time for the observation of natural phenomena to replace the slavish rehearsal of scholastic dogma. There was reluctance to examine Francis Bacon's (1561–1626) book of nature—'that universal and publick Manuscript, that lies expans'd unto the Eyes of all'—and for natural philosophy based on experiment to replace the 'dust of yellowed parchments'. But change was underway and physicians were advised that 'the sick should be the doctor's books'.[1]

Thomas Willis as a reader

Thomas Willis occasionally mentions other authors. He draws on the ancients and moderns, physicians and chemists, and philosophers and theologians. At a superficial count he names 107 authors usually by Latin surname, variously spelled, and without providing details. Many of his authorities are identifiable. Others on whom he relied are no longer recognizable. Most of his references are to the ancients. Some are contemporary writers from continental Europe. A few are physicians with whom Willis was acquainted.

The person most often cited is Hippocrates (*c.*460–*c.*370 BC) but Willis also makes repeated reference to Aristotle (384–322 BC), Aulus Cornelius Celsus (*c.*25 BC–*c.*50 AD), Democritus (*c.*460–*c.*370 BC), Claudius Galen (*c.*130–210 AD), and Plato (*c.*428–348 BC). From this it is apparent that, as with other physicians of his time, Willis began with the classical doctrines of digestion, respiration, blood, and excretion as central to the 'oeconomy' of animal and human life. Organs functioned through activity of the four humours and the properties of vital and animal spirits. The atomic materials on which they depended were the physical embodiment of divine creation. The soul was immaterial and recycled from one body to another. But ideas were moving away from the heart as the centre of all things physiological towards a growing awareness of the importance of the brain.[2]

The list of writers closer to his own lifetime mentioned by Willis is indicative of his interest in alchemy and iatrochemistry. Further thought was being given to details of the particulate nature of organic matter. With knowledge on the circulation of the blood after 1628, a more interactive model of digestion, respiration, and excretion was

[1] See: Elizabeth L Eisenstein, *The printing revolution in early modern Europe*, Cambridge (1983): pages 91–106; and 187–95.

[2] See: Carl Zimmer *Soul made flesh*, London (2004) for a useful summary of people and teachings in the biological and physical sciences from antiquity to the mid-seventeenth century that shaped the evolution of methods of enquiry and attitudes forming the basis for Willis's ideas on structure and function of 'humane bodies' in health and disease.

emerging. Epistemology was increasingly based more on inductive Baconian and deductive Cartesian reasoning than scholasticism. Freedom of thought not fully constrained by doctrines of the church could be contemplated. Natural philosophers were beginning to consider mind based on a hierarchy of rational and vegetative souls. The shift towards materialism could be sensed in the metaphor of the body as a mighty building with component parts to which Willis often returned.

Comfortable with these challenges to the ancient doctrines, Willis refers often in his writings to René Descartes (1596–1650), William Harvey (1578–1657), Gabriel Fallopius (1523–1562), Jean Fernel (1497–1558), Pierre Gassendi (1592–1655), and Daniel Sennert (1572–1637); and occasionally to Francis Bacon (1561–1626), Francis Glisson (1597–1677), Jean Baptist van Helmont (1580–1644), Johannes Heurnius (1543–1601), Gregor Horstius (1578–1636), Théodore de Mayerne (1573–1655), Paracelsus (named at birth Philippus Aureolus Theophrastus Bombastus von Hohenheim: 1493–1541), Carolus Piso (1563–1633), and Lazare Rivière (Riverius: 1589–1655). Conspicuously absent from the list is Andreas Vesalius (1514–1564) and any mention of *De humani corporis fabrica libri septem* (1543).

Of those writing later in the seventeenth century, several of whom were Willis's near contemporaries, he mentions (not always with admiration) Thomas Bartholin (1616–1680), Robert Boyle (1627–1691), Frederik Deckers (1648–1720), Kenelm Digby (1603–1665), George Ent (1604–1689), Henry Hammond (1605–1660), Nathanael Highmore (1613–1685), Marcello Malpighi (1628–1694), Walter Needham (*c.*1631–1691), Prosper Martianus (nd), Konrad Schneider (1614–1680), Sylvius (Franciscus de le Boë: 1614–1672), Nicolas Steno (1638–1686), and Johann Wepfer (1620–1695). Within this list it is reasonable to assume that Willis was referring, inter alia, to Descartes' *Discourse de la method* (1637), *Principia philosophiæ* (1644), *Meditationes de prima philosophia* (1641) and *Les passions de l'ame* (1649); Digby's *Two treatises in the one of which, the nature of bodies; in the other, the nature of mans sovle; is looked into* (1644); Harvey's *Exercitatio anatomica de motu cordis et sanguinis in animalibus* (1628); Highmore's *Corporis humani disquisitio anatomica* (1651) and *Exercitationes duæ quaram prior de passione hysterica: altera de affectione hypochondriaca* (1660); Steno's *De musculis et glandulis observationum specimen* (1664), *Discours de Monsieur Stenon sur l'anatomie du cerveau a Messieurs de l'Assemblée, qui se fait chez Monsieur Thevenot* (1669), and *Elementorum myologiæ specimen* (1667); and Wepfer's *Observationes anatomicæ ex cadaveribus eorum quos sustulit apoplexia cum exercitatione de eius loco affecto* (1658). But since Willis almost never provides a citation, these attributions remain speculative.

By the late 1650s Willis felt that his own ideas were ready to be set down. Focusing on structure and function, the phenomenology of order and disorder especially in the brain and nervous stock, and mechanism-based therapeutics, a single theme runs through the fourteen treatises. Although an easy target for his critics, without an appreciation of the principles set out in *De fermentatione* (1659) the other works cannot easily be appreciated. Willis's writings from 1659 to 1675 are all grounded in the doctrine of iatrochemistry. Nutrition provides particles which are enkindled through interaction with air. The fermented blood is circulated to organs where it is further changed both in health and disease into vital spirits. Waste is removed. The aberrant state of the blood and animal spirits provides a rational basis for treatment. Willis was not the first to jettison Galenic principles and articulate the principles of iatrochemistry, but no one had previously extended particulate theory to the entirety of health and disease and set out ideas in such a comprehensive series of printed books, all linked by a common intellectual thread.

The London book trade in the seventeenth century

Although he worked in Oxford, Willis first turned to London printers for publication of his treatises. To some extent he had little choice, since navigating the restrictive practices of getting a manuscript printed and sold was no easy matter.

Much can be learned of the book trade with which Willis interacted from the contemporary account by Joseph Moxon (1627–1691). Written in English and first published in 24 parts, the second volume of *Mechanick exercises on the whole art of printing* (1683–1685) is the first detailed account of early modern printing.[3] Moxon observed book production whilst living in Holland for six years from the age of 11 where his father, John (nd), was involved in publishing seditious religious material. For three years after their return to London in 1646, father and son printed books from Cornhill 'at the sign of the *Atlas*' before Joseph took to the manufacture of globes and mathematical instruments. When the shop was lost in the fire of London, Joseph Moxon started cutting type. Boyle was one of several existing or future fellows of the Royal Society, including Robert Hooke (1635–1703) and John Mayow (1640–1679), with whom Moxon interacted. They discussed letter cutting and the mixing of metals for this and other purposes. This was a merry crowd: Hooke records that, on 2 April 1677, 'Wild, Aubrey, Merret, Moxon, &c. here to see comet but missd it. Drank 2 bottle of claret. Shewd them repository'.[4] The happy outcome for Moxon was that he was himself elected to fellowship of the Royal Society on 30 November 1678, proposed by George Ent with twenty-seven votes in favour and four against.[5]

Drawing on Moxon's knowledge of mathematics, sympathy with natural philosophy, and connections with the Royal Society, Moxon described the master printer as the soul of the enterprise with workmen as members of a subservient body. Printing was both a craft and a science. Type founding was architectural with the proportions of individual letters mathematically determined. The press was an instrument designed on the principles of mechanics and geometry, not a haphazard construction emerging from the brutish efforts of artisans. Moxon's epitome of a fine press was that built by Willem Blaeu (1571–1638). On bookselling, Moxon had nothing to say. He could afford to ignore that business not least since, writing in the 1680s, the difficulties that had beset the book trade over the previous century had largely settled.

In 1586, the Star Chamber decreed that printing should be limited to London and the Universities of Oxford and Cambridge.[6] The intention to publish a book and therefore stake a claim to ownership of rights was made through entries in the *Stationers' Register* (from 1557) and the *Term Catalogue* (from 1668).[7] The addresses of those who sold Willis's books in London are indicative of how bookselling spread from space between the buttresses of

[3] See: Joseph Moxon, *Mechanick exercises: or, the doctrine of handy-works. Applied to the art of printing. The second volume* (1683–1684). Eds. Herbert Davis and Harry Carter, London (1958). Published in parts, the first was priced at 6d but the rest appeared irregularly thereafter and sales were poor. Parts 1–3 were reprinted in 1684 and bound with the original unsold sheets.

[4] See: Moxon (1958): page xliv.

[5] Amongst eight elected on the same day were John Mayow (1640–1679), and Edmund Halley (1656–1742) afterwards Astronomer Royal.

[6] According to Henry R Plomer *A short history of English printing 1476–1898*, London (1900): pages 122–53, presses were active in York, Tavistock [Dan Thomas Rycharde (nd)], St Albans [John Herford (nd)], Bristol, Ipswich [Anthony Scoloker (d.1593), John Overton (nd), and John Oswen (fl.1548–53) who later printed in Worcester, Canterbury [John Mychell (d.1556)], and Norwich [Anthony de Solempne (*nk*)]. Several secret presses functioned elsewhere.

[7] These notices subsequently appeared in the *Booksellers of London* list (from 1709), the *Gentleman's Magazine* (from 1731) and the *English Catalogue of Books* (from 1835).

St Paul's Cathedral and the churchyard, into alleyways, lanes, and streets such as Paternoster Row, nearby coffee houses and taverns, and the Inns of Court and Stationers' Hall. With expansion of the city of London in the seventeenth century, and the division of individual wards or districts, 'within' and 'without' in printers and booksellers addresses referred to premises that lay inside or outside the old London wall and its seven original gates.[8] Several printers with whom Thomas Willis worked came from families that had started their businesses early in the seventeenth century. For example, George Eld (d.1624) was succeeded by Miles Fletcher or Flesher (fl.1611–1664: d.1664). Thomas Snodham (d.1625) inherited the business of Thomas East (*c.*1540–1609) on whose death the rights passed to William Stansby (1572–1638). That material went first to William Lee (fl.1640–1646) for £165 and then to Thomas Harper (d.1656).[9]

At the time Willis was beginning his studies in Oxford, a decree by the Star Chamber (1637) restricted the licensing of books to named individuals. Their endorsement therefore had to be secured (in principle) by aspiring authors: the Lord Chief Justice for law; various Secretaries of State for history; the Earl Marshall for heraldry; and the Archbishop of Canterbury, Bishop of London, or Chancellors of the Universities of Oxford and Cambridge for all other subjects. Catalogues and consignments from abroad were not to be distributed unless authorized. All books had now unambiguously to display the names of author, printer, and bookseller. Restrictions were imposed on those who cast type and the number of presses that any one printer might acquire was limited.[10]

With outbreak of the Civil War in 1642, book production, always eclipsed for quality by continental printers, declined further. Old type was reused even if worn and breaking. Sloppy workmanship characterized the trade. The freedom of printers was constrained by government, which sought to restrict subject matter. However the thirst for 'print' was not easily assuaged and, despite restrictions, secret presses and other businesses emerged. Sensing that it was losing control, the long parliament tightened its grip. Printers were required to lodge £300 as surety against providing 'scandalous or seditious' material, especially polemic pamphlets.[11] Penalties were not trivial: a fine of 40 shillings or 40 days' imprisonment for writing an offending pamphlet; 20s or 20 days, with forfeiture of his press for the printer; 10s or 10 days in prison for the bookseller; and a whipping for the street hawker.[12] Magistrates were entitled to open any package that might contain material violating these stringent laws. But the trade was not to be discouraged and, on the list from 1649 to 1650 of individuals who took over from existing printers in London or the two Universities, are James Fletcher (d.1670) and Thomas Harper, each based in Little Britain, and Thomas Roycroft (1637–1677) from Doctors' Commons. These were the individuals to whom Willis turned for the publication of *Diatribæ*

[8] See: James Raven, *Bookscape. Geographies of printing and publishing in London before 1800*, London (2014): pages 31–7.

[9] See: Plomer (1900): page 269.

[10] See: Ian Gadd, 'The press and the London book trade'. In: Ed. Ian Gadd *The history of Oxford University Press volume 1: beginnings to 1780*, Oxford (2013): pages 575–7, for an account of how the Stationers' Company exercised control but nonetheless served the interests of publishers by ensuring that printed material was genuinely original to the author—directly or through assignment, purchase, or inheritance—thereby establishing rights of 'copy'. Apprentices were bound to members and, after a period of several years, released to ply their trade without being constrained by the Stationers' authority and the requirement to be on the register. See: Nicholas Barker, 'The old English letter foundrie's. In: Eds. John Barnard and DFM McKenzie, *The Cambridge history of the book in Britain.* Volume IV (1557–1695), Cambridge (2002): pages 602–19, for a detailed account of type foundries and craftsmen in the seventeenth century.

[11] See: Plomer (1900): page 193.

[12] See: Henry R Plomer, *A dictionary of the booksellers and printers who were at work in England, Scotland and Ireland from 1641 to 1667*, Oxford (1907, new edition 1968): pages xi–xxiii.

duæ medico-philosophicæ, his first book, in 1659.[13] Roycroft had used type from the approved foundries, some characters originally cut by John Day (1522–1584) in the sixteenth century, for printing the London polyglot bible (1657) prepared by Brian Walton (1600–1661), Bishop of Chester. During the Civil War, he fled from London to Oxford where the idea of the bible developed.[14] Given these connections, it seems likely that Bishop Walton knew Willis and may have made the introduction to Roycroft. But this was a printer not free from controversy. Roycroft was among eleven individuals who, in 1660 or 1661, drew up a petition claiming that, in the interests of cheapening costs for the privileged few, the Stationers' Company had become nothing more than the stooge of booksellers engaged in producing inferior material.[15] Moreover, these petitioners argued that, compared with the excessive profits retained by booksellers, printers had been left impecunious. The dissident printers proposed forming an independent 'Companie of printers'. Everything was explained in their manifesto: *A brief discourse concerning printers and printing* (1663). Various events then unfolded in parallel.

By act of parliament dated 15 August 1663, Sir Roger L'Estrange (1616–1704), later associated with licensing the English translation of Willis's *Pharmaceutice rationalis* into English (1679), was granted sole responsibility for authorizing the printing of books other than works relating to the state, divinity, physic, philosophy, arts, and sciences for which rights had already been assigned by letters patent from the King. Although nominally answerable to the secretary of state and government, L'Estrange acted independently. Following the Printing Act of 1662, which again sought to restrict seditious and treasonable books and regulate presses, L'Estrange's report, *Considerations and proposals in order to the regulation of the press* (1663), advised reducing the number of printers from sixty to twenty, with attrition of their 160 apprentices and a large number of journeymen. The death penalty was imposed on printers who transgressed. This was no idle threat. First to suffer that fate was John Twyn (*c.*1616–1664) who, despite claiming that he had innocently printed a pamphlet arguing for deposition of the King and overthrow of the government without reading the text, was found guilty and executed at Tyburn in 1664.[16] Members of the jury that returned the verdict included Willis's printers, James Fletcher and Thomas Roycroft. L'Estrange had a wide circle of acquaintances. In his diary for 7 May 1685, John Evelyn (1620–1706) wrote:[17]

> Mr. Roger L'Estrange (a gentleman who I had long known, and a person of excellent parts abating some affections) appearing first against the Dissenters in several Tracts, had now

[13] See: Plomer (1900): page 194 for details of this transition. Bernard Alsop (1616–1653), Richard Bishop (fl.1631–1653), and Thomas Harper survived although three others were represented by their family successors: Elizabeth Purslowe (fl.1633–1646) for her husband Thomas (d.1632); Gertrude Dawson (fl.1649–1661) succeeding her husband John (fl.1634–1648); and James Fletcher in place of his father Miles.

[14] See: Nicholas Barker, 'The Polyglot Bible'. In: Barnard and McKenzie (2002): page 651. The six volumes appeared rapidly between 1654 and 1657. Costing £2700 to print, the book was sold by subscription and realized £9000 even before going to press. The nine languages were: Hebrew, Latin, Greek, Chaldean, Syriac, Arabic, Samaritan, Persian, and Ethiopic. Roycroft was dubbed 'Orientalium Typographus Regius'. Unsold sheets were lost with much of his stock in the fire of 1666.

[15] Another was John Hayes (fl.1658–1666: d.1705) who printed William Croone's (1633–1684) *De ratione motus musculorum*, London (1664). Hayes's books were seized on the edict of Sir Roger L'Estrange after the pamphlet relating to the 'Companie of printers' appeared. Details of these events affecting the London book trade are taken from Plomer (1900): pages 199–209.

[16] See: Michael Treadwell, 'The stationers and the printing acts at the end of the seventeenth century'. In: Barnard and McKenzie (2002): page 776, for details of two others: Simon Dover (d.1664: fl.1660–1664) and Thomas Brewster (d.1664: fl.1649–1664) were found guilty of printing outlawed material but, again, argued that booksellers did not read the books they produced, and thereby escaped the death penalty. However, as late as 1693, the Jacobite printer William Anderton (1663–1693) was tried and executed for treason, perhaps in order to reassure government that they had means other than licensing to control what was printed.

[17] See: John Evelyn, *The diary of John Evelyn Esquire F.R.S.* Ed. William Bray, London (1818, printed ca.1930): page 598.

> for some yeares turn'd his style against those whom (by way of hateful distinction) they call'd Whiggs and Trimmers, under the title of Observator, which came out 3 or 4 days every weeke, in which sheets, under pretence to serve the Church of England, he gave suspicion of gratifying another party, by several passages which rather kept up animosities than appeas'd them, especially now that nobody gave the least occasion ... [and in a footnote to page 598] In the first Dutch war, whilst Mr Evelyn was one of the Commissioners for sick and wounded, Mr L'Estrange in his Gazette mentioned the barbarous usage of the Dutch prisoners of war; Mr Evelyn wrote him a very spirited letter, desiring that the Dutch Ambassador (who was then in England) and his friends would visit the prisoners, and examine their provisions; and he desir'd Mr. L'Estrange would publish his vindication in his next number.

It was in this climate of suspicion that the Royal Society sought to publish material relating to natural philosophy and experimental science, allowing individuals not present at its demonstrations to read about the work.[18] In this way the Society started to wrestle scientific publication away from the grip of the Stationers' Company, initiating the culture of publishing short reports in a scientific journal rather than as pamphlets and treatises. All work written by Fellows, and those who aspired to the fellowship, was presented to the Society at its weekly meetings, reviewed, and registered in the contents of *Philosophical Transactions of the Royal Society*.

With thirty-three publications to date, John Martyn (1618–1678) and James Allestry (d.1670) already had a reputation for producing excellent scientific books. The first and second charters, of 1662 and 1663, allowed the Royal Society to select an official printer without interference from the Stationers' Company. Following a meeting on 28 October 1663, Martyn and Allestry were appointed by the president, Viscount Brouncker (1627–1688), with exclusive rights to all material relating to the Society but subject to statutes drafted by John Wilkins (1614–1672) and Jonathan Goddard (1617–1675).[19] These stipulated accuracy of the printing, the number of copies and format of each issue or volume, the quality of the paper and illustrations, and the price. Council had to approve reprinting full text or summaries, and any proposed translations. Well-bound copies of each work were to be presented to the King, Earl of Clarendon, Lord Chancellor, and the president and library of the Royal Society.

Martyn and Allestry agreed these terms and were sworn in on 9 November 1663.[20] They produced a first issue on 6 March 1665, and completed publication of the first volume of *Philosophical Transactions* for 1665 / 1666 from their premises: John Martyn at 'The Bell a little without Temple Bar' and James Allestry at 'Duck Lane'.[21] Much of their unsold stock

[18] The details that follow on printers to the Royal Society are taken from Leona Rostenberg, 'John Martyn, Printer to the Royal Society', *Papers of the Bibliographical Society of America* (1952): 46; 1–32; and Charles Rivington, 'Early printers to the Royal Society 1663–1708', *Notes and Records of the Royal Society of London* (1984): 39; 1–27. Although described as 'printers', Martyn and Allestry were publishers for whom books were printed by various individuals, including Thomas Roycroft.

[19] See: Rostenberg (1952): page 7 and footnote 20 for a list of sixteen scientific books produced for the Royal Society by Martyn (with and without Allestry); and pages 28–9 for an account of how Robert Hooke (1635–1703), who brokered the arrangement, rewarded himself by visits to Martyn's premises at The Bell indulging his bibliophilic habit, browsing freely and purchasing material 'on approval', much of which was returned when he had read the books. Other copies were retained before settling his account several weeks later, and not without amending the totals to his own advantage.

[20] See: Rostenberg (1952): page 10 for details of how Martyn also agreed to make available extra copies for Fellows and others who might be interested, although not without payment: 'what copies of Signor Malpighi's *De formatione pulli in ovo* [1673] the printer would not furnish for the author gratis should be paid for by the Society who has lately ordered 30 copies of it to be sent to him in Bologna'.

[21] A single issue cost between 6d and 1s; the bound volumes for the year ranged from 7s to 8s 6d.

was lost when Martyn's premises were destroyed in the fire of London. This and the plague led to further disruption in publishing issues of *Philosophical Transactions*, some of which were produced by other London printers and by Richard Davis (fl.1646–1688) in Oxford. Davis had been appointed casually by (Sir) Robert Moray (*c.*1608–1673) over dinner with Robert Boyle and John Wallis (1616–1703). But Moray was slightly dissatisfied with the quality of the work, and Davis did not sell as many copies as he had anticipated. The officers of the Society were concerned that Martyn and Allestry were in collusion with Davis and exercising a cartel on pricing. Relationships between Martyn and Henry Oldenburg (1619–1677) soured. Martyn considered the secretary 'of peculiar temperament which prevented him from agreeing well with others'. Oldenburg regarded Martyn as:

> Morose and fickle ... and mighty tedious ... an habituee of snuff ... Mr. Martyn deals very mercenarily with me knowing that others will hardly undertake the printing of these papers ... he hath constrained me to abate him the rate yet lower so that after the proportion he allows me, I shall hardly bring it to 30 pounds.

In the event, Martyn had to publish an apology in *Philosophical Transactions* for some of his remarks.[22] Confidence was eventually restored so that Martyn was entrusted with volumes 2 to 12 of *Philosophical Transactions*.[23] The printer from 1665 to 1669 was TN (Thomas Newcombe: fl.1649–1681 who owned the King's Printing House in the Savoy, employing seven compositors and five pressmen), followed by TR (Thomas Roycroft) for volumes from 1673 to 1676 when the journal temporarily lapsed.[24]

Printing in London suffered in 1665 and 1666. Eighty people associated with the trade died from plague. Eight London printers were ruined by the fire. The stationers and booksellers based around St Paul's Churchyard carried their stocks to St Faith's Church in the vaults under St Paul's for safety. One opened the door too soon and saw his books immediately burned. It is estimated that the loss of stock amounted to £150 000–£200 000. Undaunted, and although tenants not freeholders, many who lost premises in the fire of London rebuilt on the same footprint at their own expense and resumed business. Over time, premises which had originally clustered in Little Britain, St Paul's, and Paternoster Row became more widely distributed in the City of London, maintaining:[25]

> A plentiful and perpetual emporium of learned Authors ... where the learned seldom failed to meet with agreeable Conversation. And the booksellers themselves were knowing

[22] See: Rivington (1984): page 11, for an account of how when Richard Chiswell (1639–1711) was appointed as Martyn's successor in 1680, Council paused 'to peruse the Statute relating to the printer of the Society, and to draw up another patent for Mr Chiswell, in which the powers given to the printer may be less disadvantageous to the Society than (as by experience has been found) the patent given formerly to MARTYN and ALLESTEE appeared to be'.

[23] See: HR Plomer with the help of HG Aldis, ER McC. Dix, CJ Gray, and RB McKerrow, edited by Arundell Esdaile, *A dictionary of the booksellers and printers who were at work in England, Scotland and Ireland from 1668 to 1725*, Oxford (1922): page 153, for an account of Spencer Hickman (fl.1670–1672), publisher to the Royal Society, and a list of his books offered for sale in 1671 filling twenty-four pages but with no entry after the Hilary *Term Catalogue* of 1672. Martyn and Allestry and then Martyn alone remained as printer(s) to the Society until 1680, but Hickman was also so designated on 2 November 1671 having been apprenticed to Allestry. However this arrangement did not materialize perhaps because Hickman died in or about 1672, soon after Allestry. Another who had a loose connection with the Royal Society was Octavian Pulleyn (the younger: fl.1664–1667).

[24] Rostenberg (1952): page 17 suggests that the interval was from January 1679 to January 1683.

[25] See: Raven (2014): pages 16 and 70–72, also quoting Roger North, *The life of the honourable Sir Dudley North, Knt. commissioner of the customs, and afterwards of the Treasury to his majesty King Charles the second. And of the honourable and Reverend Dr. John North, master of Trinity College in Cambridge, and Greek professor, prebend of Westminster, and sometime clerk of the Closet to the same King Charles the second. By the honourable Roger North, Esq*, London (1744): page 241.

> and conversible Men, with whom for the sake of bookish Knowledge, the greatest Wits were pleased to converse.

Increasingly free from legislation, Fletcher acquired five presses and had fifteen employees, and Roycroft four presses and twelve workmen.[26] Not all books printed by these leading members of the trade were identified as their work but 'Roycroft, we know, was employed by all those who wanted the best possible work'.[27] Type was produced by three main foundries: Joseph Moxon; Joseph Andrews (nd) and Robert Andrews (1650–1735); James Grover (after 1676); and Thomas Grover (d.1728).[28]

Martyn and Allestry (with Thomas Dicas: fl.1660–1669) sold Thomas Willis's *Diatribæ duæ medico-philosophicæ*, printed by Roycroft, in 1659, 1660 and 1662 (**1A1, 1A2, 1B, 1C**, and **1D2**). Martyn also sold the 1677 edition, printed by T.R (Roycroft), after Allestry had died (**1I**). The quarto and octavo editions of *Cerebri anatome* (1664) were printed by Fletcher and Roycroft, respectively, each on behalf of Martyn and Allestry (**2A**, **2B**). Unsold sheets from 1664 that escaped the fire were assigned by Martyn's widow, Sarah (nd), to Robert Scott (1632–1710) in 1683.[29] Although a founding Fellow of the Royal Society, well acquainted with its printers and listing his fellowship on the title pages of books published after 1667 (starting with *Pathologiæ cerebri*: **3A**), nothing original by Thomas Willis was printed for the Royal Society. Reviews were published of four volumes containing eight of his fourteen treatises published between 1667 and 1675. Nor was much interest shown in *Philosophical Transactions* on the brain and nervous stock or any other of the topics that directly engaged Willis. Samuel Mihles (nd) abstracted all contributions to the journal relating to the practice of physic and surgery to the middle of the eighteenth century of which, from amongst Willis's contemporaries, one paper by Richard Lower (1631–1691) is included. Mihles's documentation may have been selective but there is only a single article relating to the brain published in the journal during Willis's lifetime (the last issue being number 122 in volume 10 for 16 March 1675).[30] More informative with respect to possible reading of *Philosophical Transactions* by Willis and his circle is the list published by James Briggs (nd) in 1818 on anatomical, medical, chirurgical, and physiological

[26] See: Roger L'Estrange, *A survey of the printing presses with the names and numbers of apprentices, officers, and workmen belonging to every particular press. Taken 29 July 1668*, London (1668); and Plomer (1900): pages 225–7 for details of two others active on this scale, Thomas Newcomb (fl.1649–1681) and John Maycocke (nd).

[27] See: Plomer (1900): pages 209–10.

[28] The number of printers authorized by the Stationers' Company had increased to 59 by 1662, subsequently falling to 33 with 82 presses (1668) and 55 with 145 presses (1685 / 6).

[29] See: Rostenberg (1952): page 20, footnote 59 for details of the full list: 'Order Book; the following pre-Fire imprints were consigned by Mrs. Martyn to Scott: *Italian English Dictionary* (1654), Claude Mauger, *French Grammar* (1656), Gilbert Clark, *De flenitudine mundi* (1660), Pietro Maria Canepari, *De atramentis* (1660), Jeremy Taylor, *The Worthy Communicant* (1660), Francis Hall, *Tractatus de Corforum insefarabilitate* (1661), John Evelyn, *Sylva* (1664), Thomas Willis, *Cerebri anatome* (1664), *Philosophical Transactions* (1665, 1666), Robert Hooke, *Micrografhia* (1665). This may explain why copies of the quarto edition are still not especially scarce although increasingly expensive in the antiquarian book trade.

[30] See: [Samuel Mihles], *Medical essays and observations relating to the practice of physic and surgery: abridg'd from the Philosophical Transactions, from their first publication down to the present time. The Latin papers are English'd, some occasional remarks are made, and the whole illustrated with necessary copper-plates*, 2 volumes, London (1745). The paper by Richard Lower is: 'The manner of respiration', *Philosophical Transactions* (11 November 1666), number 29: page 544 (see chapter 18 for discussion of its importance). The neurological paper is: M. Denys, 'An odd foetus without a brain', *Philosophical Transactions* (1673); number 99: page 6157.

papers including the early work on transfusion and papers by Boyle and by Hooke on respiration.[31]

The Oxford book trade in the seventeenth century

One person closely identified with printing in late seventeenth century Oxford has special significance for Thomas Willis. His brother-in-law, John Fell (1625–1686) was instrumental in establishing the University press and may have been responsible for ensuring that the quarto editions of *Pathologiæ cerebri* (1667: **3A**), *De anima brutorum* (1672: **5A**) and *Pharmaceutice rationalis* (1674 and 1675: **6A** and **6E**) were first printed in Oxford.

Printing in Oxford was active between 1478 and 1486, resumed briefly in 1517, and flourished after 1584 when Joseph Barnes (1550–1618) was appointed printer to the University with the imprimatur of the Star Chamber.[32] As in so many matters, the other University was slow to follow.[33] Barnes remained active as printer, bookseller, and wine merchant until 1617. Thereafter, printing in Oxford was largely the responsibility of the Lichfield family.[34] The publications were learned and the rights protected, especially for printing of manuscripts owned by individuals or Colleges of the University. As in London, surety against publishing seditious material required £300 deposit, and this encouraged the University not to meddle with material other than that on academic subjects. Matters were overseen by a delegate of eminent scholars from 1633. But progress towards a successful and fully independent press as part of the University paused after 1642 when the exiled King pushed for the printing of material sympathetic to his cause. Leonard Lichfield II found himself employed but not adequately reimbursed either by the University or Charles I. On the latter's recommendation, Henry Hall (1606–*c.*1681) was appointed printer to the University on 21 November 1644 working from premises off the High Street, east of Queen's Lane.[35] In March 1653, new delegates were appointed now including names with whom Thomas Willis was in close contact: John Wilkins, Jonathan Goddard, Joshua Crosse, and Ralph Bathurst (1620–1704).

Medical books were not prominent in the publications from Oxford. Most were imported from the major European centres.[36] Those within the University writing on medicine usually dealt with the London book trade. The most significant exception in the early seventeenth

[31] See: [James Briggs], *An index to the anatomical, medical, chirurgical and physiological papers contained in the Transactions of the Royal Society of London from the commencement of that work to the end of the year 1817, chronically and alphabetically arranged,* London (1818).

[32] See: Kristian Jensen, 'Printing at Oxford in its European context 1478–1584'. In: Gadd (2013): pages 40–8.

[33] Plomer (1900) lists nine books printed in Cambridge between 1517 and 1519 by John Lair de Siberch [(1476–1554, bound by Nicholas Spierinck (d.1546)]; and from 1583 when Thomas was appointed University printer. His activities were disparaged, Thomas being declared 'vtterlie ignoraunte in printinge'. For other details of the book trade in Cambridge, see also: Jensen (2013): page 43; SH Steinberg *Five hundred years of printing*, London (1955, new edition 1996): page 115; and Howard M Nixon, *Five centuries of English bookbinding*, London (1978): page 26.

[34] See Jason Peacey, 'Printers to the University 1584–1658'. In: Gadd (2013): page 69. Barnes worked with John Lichfield I (fl.1617–1635), William Wrench (nd: from 1617), and James Short (nd: from 1618 to 1624). From 1624, the printers were Lichfield and William Turner (d.1643). They fell out and worked independently from 1627 until Lichfield retired in 1635. The Lichfield dynasty was continued by John's son, Leonard I (1604–1657), his son Leonard II (ca.1637–1686: fl.1657–1686), and daughter-in-law Anne (d.1671). Leonard III (d.1744) continued printing in Oxford from 1686 to 1740. See: Gordon Goodwin, *Dictionary of National Biography, 1885–1900*, volume 33 (1893): pages 220–1 for details of Solodell Lichfield (d.1671) who did not join his siblings in the book trade 'and was good for nothing but for eating, drinking, smoaking, and punning'.

[35] The original choice had been William Hall (thought to be Henry's son) who had worked for the Lichfields in the 1620s.

[36] See: Peter Murray Jones, 'The learned press: law and medicine'. In: Gadd (2013): pages 469–78 for the account that follows.

century was Robert Burton's (1577–1640) *The anatomy of melancholy, what it is. With all the kindes, causes, symptoms, prognostickes, and severall cures of it* (1621) printed by John Lichfield I and James Short (nd) for Henry Cripps (d.1661: fl.1620–1640 in Oxford and 1650–1661 in London). Listed on the London Stationers' Company register, partly assigned to Michael Sparke (d.1653) to prevent piracy, the subsequent seventeenth-century editions were printed from London, Edinburgh, and Oxford.[37] *The anatomy of melancholy* is much more than a medical account of mood for it is rich in philosophy, history, and literary references. Written in the vernacular, it was intended for general readership. It is unashamedly Royalist in its political opinions. It is a book that Thomas Willis must have known through the Christ Church connection, and he would have met Burton since they overlapped at the college from 1636 to 1640. For all these reasons, it is all the more surprising that Willis does not refer to Burton's book. The subject matter is close to Willis's ideas on psychology and the doctrine of the soul as set out in *De anima brutorum* (1672). Although more Galenic than iatrochemical in its allegiances, much of Burton's book had not dated and ulterior motives for omitting all mention of this already famous work cannot be excluded.[38]

Gazing out 'from my Studie in Christ-Church Oxon.', Democritus Junior (Robert Burton), scholar, mathematician, astrologer, vicar of St. Thomas Church (from 1616), and rector of Segrave, Leicester (from 1630) completed the book on 'Decembr. 5. 1620'. The 1628 edition (third) has an elaborate title page with eleven panels, engraved by Michel Le Blon (1587–1656). A rhyming description of this engraving, 'The argument of the Frontispiece', was added in 1632.[39] Burton suggests that old age is a disease, explaining in humoral terms that melancholy is the consequence of black bile, cold and dry, acting on the brain. Both physical and mental conditions might be responsible. 'Besides fear and sorrow, sharp belching, fulsome crudities, heat in the bowels, wind and rumblings in the guts, vehement gripings, pain in the belly and stomack' are indicative of flatulous melancholy. And yet, conversely, the 'body matters little ... deformities or imperfections of our bodies be they innate or accidental torture many men; yet this may comfort to them, that those imperfections of the body do not a whit blemish the soul, or hinder the operations of it, but rather help and much increase it'. Then there are hereditary tendencies: 'an inward bred cause of the Melancholy, is our temperature in whol or part, which wee receive from our parents, which Fernelius calls *præter naturam*, or unnatural, it being an hereditary disease'. Children born of parents in the decline of life are more predisposed to one of the forms of partial insanity than those born under other circumstances. But the main causes are psychological: 'such as have lived in action all their lives, had great, employment, much business, much command and many servants to oversee, and leave off exabrupt ... resign up all of a sudden ... are overcome with melancholy all of a sudden'. Sorrow and dejection are essential elements of melancholy involving powerful emotions linked to suspicion, mistrust, anxiety, and trepidation. Comorbidity includes obsession and compulsion: 'an individual ... dared not go over a bridge, come near a pool, rock, steep hill, lie in a chamber where cross beams were, for fear he be tempted to hang, drawn or precipitate himself. In a silent auditorium as at a sermon he [was] afraid he shall speak aloud at unawares, something indecent, unfit to be said'. Treatments included

[37] See: Matthew Kilburn, 'The learned press: history, languages, literature, and music'. In: Gadd (2013): page 446.

[38] Also not mentioned by Willis is Thomas Browne's (1605–1682) *Religio medici*, London (1642).

[39] Headed: 'Ten distinct Squares here seene apart / Are ioyn'd in one by Cutters art' the argument of the frontispiece has ten stanzas of eight lines in rhyming couplets describing (1) saturnism, (2) jealousy, (3) solitariness, (4) in-amorousness, (5) hypochondriasis, (6) superstitiousness, (7) madness, the uses of (8) borage and (9) hellebore, and (10) facial appearance, ending with 'And I for it will stand in view / thine to commande, reader, Adew'.

exercise, distraction, travel, purgatives, blood-letting, diet, sexual moderation, and music. Burton concludes: 'Be not solitary, be not idle' and 'given man's mortality and the mutability of things, only a great oaf would not meet life's changes and chances with sober sadness'. It has been suggested that Burton hanged himself in his rooms at Christ Church.[40]

In Willis's lifetime, enshrined in the statutes from 1634, the University recommitted itself to printing. Samuel Clarke (d.1669) was appointed headprinter (architypographicus) on 14 May 1658 to supervise 'embellishment and perfection' of the press work.[41] Meanwhile John Wallis, who did not trouble himself with details when recounting the history of the origins of the Royal Society, had written an 'inquiry' into the origins of printing including the dubious claim that:[42]

> Early, after the first Invention of printing, it was used in Oxon. And that the said University was possessed of this priviledg, not only before any other place in England, but also in Europe (Mentz and Harlem excepted).

This proposition was dutifully rehearsed in his preface by Moxon (1683):

> After these two places [Mentz and Harlem] it seems next to have been practiced at Oxford ... soon after William Caxton (the same I suppose who first brought it to Oxford) promoted it to London also.

In repeating this self-congratulatory Oxonian passage in *The history and art of printing* (1771), Philip Luckombe (1730–1803) attributed the (mis)information to 'the learned Dr Willis, of Oxford'. Willis may have had his faults but rewriting the history of printing is a charge on which he can reasonably be acquitted.

Preceded in his efforts by William Laud (1573–1645), for John Fell the work of the press was to be the supreme culmination of his life and, after his tenure as vice-chancellor (1666–1669), it occupied him from 5 October 1671 until his death in 1686.[43] Fell envisaged a press 'which I hope by God's blessing may not only prove usefull to us poor Scholars but reflect some reputation and advantage on the Publick.'[44] Fell had been close to the publication of books in Oxford since the late 1650s, and was completing biographies of his mentor Henry Hammond (1605–1660) and of Thomas Fuller (1608–1661). These books were printed by individuals, some of whom were also involved in publishing Thomas Willis's works.[45] Between 1669 and 1670, Fell was largely responsible for buying type foundry including punches, matrices, and founts of Roman, italic, oriental, Saxon, and black letter type as well as moulds and other printing materials from suppliers in Dordrecht (south Holland), whilst searching a definitive set and appropriate type founder in England. Fell entrusted Dr Thomas Marshall (1621–1685) to acquire materials from Christoffel van Dijck (1605–1669). However much of the type came originally from Frankfurt and France, and van Dijck died shortly before

[40] Much of this is reproduced from [Editorial], *Brain* 2010: 133; 3157–9.

[41] Clarke had assisted Brian Walton and Edmund Castell (1606–1686) in publishing the polyglot bible.

[42] See: Ian Gadd, 'Introduction'. In: Gadd (2013): page 7.

[43] See: Stanley Morison (1889–1967), *John Fell: the University press and the 'Fell' types*, Oxford (1967): page 47.

[44] See: Harry Carter. *A History of the Oxford University Press*, volume 1, To the year 1780. With an appendix listing the titles of books printed there, 1690–1780, Oxford (1975): page 51.

[45] See: Vivienne Larminie 'The Fell era 1658–1686'. In: Ed. Gadd (2013): pages 83–4, for details of John Fell's *The life of the most learned, reverend, and pious Dr H Hammond*, London (1661); and *The life of that reverend divine, and learned historian, Dr. Thomas Fuller*, London (1661).

Marshall arrived.[46] Francis Junius (1591–1677) supplemented Fell's materials in 1677 with a collection containing Runic, Gothic, Saxon, Icelandic, Danish, and Swedish type in addition to standard roman, italic, greek, and black letter.[47]

Christopher Wren's (1632–1723) Sheldonian Theatre was completed in 1668. The fresco on the north-northwest corner of the ceiling, 'Truth descending upon the arts and sciences' by Robert Streater (1621–1679), included an image of printing, and a bare breasted woman clutching a locked forme and case of type.[48] The building served several functions and John Hall (fl.1670–1707) insisted that a room be allocated for type setting and printing. This resulted in a wooden building being constructed next to the Theatre in 1670.[49] This is visible on Loggan's map of 1675.[50] After working in private premises, the press moved to the basement of the Sheldonian Theatre and printed first *An ode in praise of the theatre and its founder* (1669). Caught between a sense of responsibility for independence from the Stationers' Company and improved quality, and despite reluctance to be overcommitted on the work of printing in Oxford, Fell did gradually assume a dominant role in the University press. His concern was with the material that should be printed. Leonine Jenkins (1625–1685) was legal adviser, Thomas Yate (*c.*1604–1681) manager of the finances, and Sir Joseph Williamson (1633–1701) exercised influence and provided contacts. Their reputation was acknowledged outside Oxford to the extent that Moxon's authoritative account of printing was dedicated to Fell, Jenkins, and Williamson.[51] Materials and printed books were transported to and from London by road, the Thames only being navigable as far as Henley. Skilled tradesmen from London worked in Oxford when local business was slack. Since the time of Joseph Barnes, partial protection on rights had been achieved by surrogate placement of titles on the Stationers' Company register using members of the London book trade. In turn, so as to protect its own activities, the Stationers' Company paid an annual inducement to the University in Oxford not to publish material that the King's printer considered profitable to his own trade. Since the agreed sum did not always materialize, printers in Oxford felt entitled to break the terms of these restrictions. Fell and his colleagues sensed that they might print books for profit and, in this way, the ambitions of the press soon expanded. However the situation was unstable and deals were made and broken between printers in London and Oxford, and the University and Stationers' Company, which occasionally erupted into Chancery proceedings. Yate and Fell started an Oxford register but still aimed to keep some distance from the University lest it claimed ownership of all titles that they printed under its privilege or which they acquired from elsewhere.[52]

[46] See: Lotte Hellinga, 'The bookshop of the world: books and their makers as agents of cultural exchange'. In: Eds., Lotte Hellinga, Alastair Duke, Jacob Harskamp, and Theo Hermans, with Elaine Paintin, *The bookshop of the world*. 't Goy-Houten (2001): page 13.

[47] See: Martyn Ould, 'The workplace: places, procedures, and personnel 1668–1780'. In: Gadd (2013): pages 215–18; and HJR [John] Wing, 'Fell's friends and the Sheldonian press'. In: *Christ Church Library Newsletter* (2011–2012) volume 8, issues 1, 2, and 3: pages 17–20. Reverend (Charles Henry Olive) Daniel (1836–1919) developed a private press at Worcester College, Oxford, with typeface based on the recently rediscovered Fell type. Wing states that Dr Fell also set up his own type foundry at Christ Church in 1672.

[48] See: Gadd (2013): page 8.

[49] See: Vivienne Larmanie (2013): page 86 for the suggestion that printing was moved to a tenement, Tom Pun's House, converted to 'the little Print-House' prior to building the 'New Print-House' in 1672.

[50] It proved inadequate and was replaced by the Clarendon building, designed by Nicholas Hawksmoor (1661–1736) and completed in 1713.

[51] See: Gadd (2013): page 6 for the suggestion that in dedicating the first issue of the second volume (on printing) of *Mechanick exercises* (1683–1684) to people based in Oxford, Moxon aimed to marginalize the London book trade. Larminie (2013): page 90 explains that Yate made clear in his will that, despite being younger, Fell was the senior partner.

[52] See: Gadd (2013): page 579.

The booksellers Richard Davis and Robert Scott were active with Samuel Clarke in publishing books using loans with security from the University.[53] In June 1668, Thomas Roycroft offered Clarke a press but those more experienced in printing and publishing, including Scott, were unimpressed with the results.[54] Even when the printing of books became increasingly professional, marketing was less successful and copies remained expensive.[55] It was little wonder that Willis steered clear of Oxford in publishing his first two books. But he may then have felt more relaxed for, despite ambiguity on the title page, Willis's third book was printed in Oxford by William Hall on behalf of James Allestry (*Pathologiæ cerebri*, 1667: **3A**). In 1672, Fell listed the first of eight forthcoming publications from his list. Number seven was described as 'A treatise concerning the Soul (in Latin) to be printed in quarto'. This is *De anima brutorum* (1672: **5A**) considered to be the 'first considerable medical work for the Sheldonian press'. Although consignments usually went by wagon, in 1671 John Fell used the 'Flying coach' to send two books to the London bookseller Robert Scott.[56] It seems likely the goods included sheets for the London quarto issue of *De anima brutorum* (1672: **5A4** and **5A5**). Commercially the most successful of Thomas Willis's works to be printed in Oxford was *Pharmaceutice rationalis*, (1674 and 1675: **6A** and **6E**), some copies of the first part also being distributed by Scott (**6A2**). Both *De anima brutorum* (1672) and *Pharmaceutice rationalis* (1674 and 1675) were unusual amongst Oxford medical publications from that period in having engraved plates.

Although the interest in books on science and medicine from Oxford reduced after the 1670s, the press remained increasingly active and some publications are relevant to Thomas Willis. When Fell learned that Anthony Wood (1632–1695) was writing a biographical dictionary of Oxford educated alumni, he purchased the existing text in manuscript for £100, with a further £50 to be given on completion.[57] Fell arranged for this to be translated into Latin by Richard Peers (1645–1690: Christ Church; 'a sullen, dogged, clownish, perverse fellow') and Richard Reeve (1642–1693). They edited and constantly altered the text to please Fell, much to Wood's distress: 'Dr Fell (who printed the book at his owne charge) took so much libertie of putting in and out what he pleased, that the author was so far from dedicating or presenting the book to anyone, that he would scarce owne it'.[58] Fell considered

[53] See: Gadd (2013): pages 556 and 560, for an account of Davis publishing more than 200 books in Oxford over a period of 60 years from the late 1620s. In 1675 he was reprimanded by the University for overcharging when valuing or making inventories of books.

[54] See: Larminie (2013): page 83.

[55] See: David McKitterick, 'University printing at Oxford and Cambridge'. In: Barnard and McKenzie (2002): page 203, citing Carter (1975): pages 61 and 151.

[56] See: Gadd (2013): page 27 and footnote 85.

[57] See: Colin Franklin, 'Additions and expunctions: Anthony à Wood and Doctor Fell' *The Book Collector* 2017: pages 751–63 for the history of Fell's involvement with Wood's *Historia et antiquitates Universitatis Oxoniensis* (1674–1675) and a forensic account of the provenance of various copies.

[58] See: DK Money *Oxford Dictionary of National Biography* (2004: https://doi.org/10.1093/ref:odnb/21772) for details of Peers's education and work as a translator including how he crossed Anthony Wood to the extent that they often fought in the printing house at the Sheldonian theatre and in a local cookshop, Peers invariably emerging 'with a bloody nose or a black eye'. Eventually, Wood's position softened: '[Peers's] initial work was poor, but gradually improved by great diligence and observation, so that he became a compleat master of the Latin tongue, and what he did was excellent'. Richard Reeve's style was less colourful. Reeve studied at Trinity College, Oxford, where he became a servitor in 1661. Later, he was Usher and Master of Magdalen College School (1670–1673). Reappointed in 1668, he was prevented from taking office as a schoolmaster and imprisoned as a Catholic and Jesuit. Anthony Wood describes how, lame following palsy in childhood, Reeve 'was taken off from the rambles of the world, [spending] his time in studies and devotion' and Wood gives a detailed account of Reeve's translation of his manuscript, concluding that 'he meant well, I really think, both to me and in what else he gave offence . . . I shall never tax him unkindly for what he meant honestly': see John Rouse Bloxham, *A register of the Presidents, Fellows, Demies . . . and other members of Saint Mary Magdalen College in the University of Oxford*, volume III, Oxford (1863): pages 207–16.

that Wood's project would benefit from the set of engravings showing the internal and external architectural splendours of Oxford, and the street life of the City, scheduled for David Loggan's *Oxonia illustrata* (1675). These were added to some copies of Wood's *Historia Oxoniensis* (1674); and an engraved leaf inserted in Loggan's book cross-referencing the illustrations. Overall, Wood was unhappy with these reciprocal arrangements, annotating his own copy: 'Dr. F [edits] . . . I never wrote this . . . here and in 500 places more ye may see what mischief ye Translator hath done'. Wood was not alone since emendations to his text instigated by Fell also offended Thomas Hobbes (1588–1679).

When Yate died in 1681, he left to Fell as legatee and executor all monies owing to the press and Yate's share in the equipment and other interests.[59] At his own death in 1686, Fell had evidently felt reluctant to release his press to the University and initially left it in the hands of his executors—his nephew Thomas Willis [1658—1699: son of Thomas Willis and Mary née Fell (d.1670)] and John Cross (nd)—to continue the work using money and stock from his estate for the next four years. Having discharged their responsibilities, and judging that 'the interests of learning & Printing [were] encouraged in the said University' the executors relinquished the lease on the printing press to the University of Oxford in October 1690.[60]

Willis's English printers and booksellers

It is against this background that the biographical and other details are given, where known, of those entrusted with the printing and selling of Willis's treatises in his lifetime; and others who took over responsibility for the two posthumous works, the English translations, and the continental editions. The list is alphabetical. It is not surprising that, in piecing together the often scant information on these members of the book trade, dates and details differ between sources making it necessary to take a somewhat arbitrary position on which is most likely to be correct. Information on the English printers and booksellers is mainly taken from the dictionaries by Henry Plomer.[61] Two other sources, as indicated in the footnotes, are John Dunton's (1659–1733) *Life and errors* (1705)[62] and Richard Smyth's (1590–1675) *Obituary* (1849).[63]

[59] See: Larminie (2013): page 101 for an account of how, in order to realize the bequest, Fell had first to sue Yate's brother Jonathan.

[60] See: Larminie (2013): pages 103 and 109.

[61] See: Plomer (1907, reprinted 1968); Plomer (1922); and http://bbti.bodleian.ox.ac.uk/.

[62] See: John Dunton, *The life and errors of John Dunton: late citizen of London; written by himself in solitude. With an idea of a new life; wherein is shewn how he'd think, speak, and act, might he live over his days again*, London (1705); reprinted as [John Dunton), Ed. JBN [Nichols] *The life and errors of J. D. late Citizen of London, written by himself in solitude: with an idea of a new life; wherein is shewn how he'd think, speak, and act, might he live over his days again ... With the lives and characters of a thousand persons now living ... Digested into seven stages*, 2 volumes, London (1818).

[63] See: [Richard Smyth] *The obituary of Richard Smith, secondary of the Poultry Compter, London: being a catalogue of all such persons as he knew in their life: extending from A.D. 1627 to A.D. 1674.* Edited by Sir Henry Ellis, London (1849). Smyth did not publish his obituary and a single copy of the original manuscript, now lost, is in the British Library. This was entitled: *A catalogue of all such persons deceased whome I knew in their life time, wherein are set down the several years of our Lord, and the dayes of the month when every one of them dyed or were buried, from the year of our Lord M.DC.XXVIII. Successively.* Briefly a student in Oxford, Smyth 'spent all the time he could obtain from his employment in books' spending 'two-thirds of the time in his library' at home in Little Jewry, and later Moorfields, or wandering the streets of Little Britain where he bought 'books that were not every day brought into public light' and many manuscripts. He collated and read his books, and noted defects and differences between issues. At his death on 26 March 1675, aged 85, the books, which he had intended for a public library, were passed by the executrix, his eldest daughter Martha Hacker (nd: whose husband William Hacker, we are told by Smyth, was 'murdered beyond sea'), into the hands of Richard Chiswell (1639–1711) and sold at auction in May and June 1662. The catalogue, of which one marked up copy exists in the British Library, required

Given the close proximity of individual premises, and the many professional interactions, it is not surprising that dynasties evolved within the book trade. These were often maintained across transitional periods by the widows of recently deceased printers and booksellers until the next male relative assumed responsibility, or the business was sold. For example, James Fletcher, the son of Miles who worked as a printer in Little Britain from 1611 to 1664, was active, also in Little Britain, from 1652 to 1667. He married Elizabeth, a daughter of Cornelius Bee who was also a bookseller from the 'King's Armes in Little Britaine' from 1634 to 1671. Elizabeth Fletcher (fl.1670–1688) printed at Little Britain after her husband's death, and is identified as EF on imprints from 1670 to 1688. Her brother, Lancelot Toppyn (d.1646) was also a bookseller, and he married Anne, sister to Dixy Page (fl.1664–1668), another bookseller. When Bee died on 2 January 1672, he bequeathed his business to Elizabeth Fletcher and another daughter, Mrs Norwood. Bee's younger daughter married Nathaniel Hooke (d.1673), also of the bookselling dynasty, who had been Bee's servant. Finally, Hooke's own daughter married Samuel Browne (fl.1639–1665) who worked at shops in St Paul's Churchyard, from 1638 to 1643, The Hague (1643–1660), and back at St Paul's Cathedral until 1665, the year of his death.[64] Against this background, thirty-four individuals were involved with the production and sale of Thomas Willis's books in England.

James Allestry (d.1670: Allestrye or Allestree) [**1A1, 1A2, 1B, 1C, 1D2; 2A, 2B; 3A; 3B2; 4A**] was a London bookseller active from the Bell in St Paul's Churchyard between 1652 and 1664; the Rose and Crown, St Paul's Churchyard from 1664 to 1666; the Rose and Crown, Duck Lane from 1667 to 1669; and, finally, the Rose and Crown, St Paul's Churchyard, from 1669 to 1670, which he acquired from George Thomason (1627–1666) to whom Allestry was apprenticed between 1638 and 1647.[65]

The family was talented. James's son Jacob (1653–1686) wrote poetry. Richard Allestry (1619–1681), scholar of divinity, was James's brother (or cousin). Richard was a delegate of the University press in Oxford from 1673 and accepted the thirteen boxes of Gothic, Anglo-Saxon, and Runic type bequeathed by Francis Junius in 1679.

James Allestry's career as a bookseller began in 1652 when he set up in business with John Martyn. They were joined by Thomas Dicas in 1660 and, probably, Timothy Garthwaite (d.1669). Allestry's shop was large and frequently visited by wealthy patrons and scholars. He moved to the Rose and Crown in 1664 on his appointment as publisher to the Royal Society. Along with many others, Allestry's premises were destroyed in the fire of London[66] and he

404 pages in quarto. In his preface to the 1849 edition, Sir Henry Ellis (1777–1869) lists many items and the prices realized: several Caxton incunabula sold for between 2s 0d and 18s 0d [for a copy of *Godfrey of Bulloigne* (1481) previously owned by King Edward IV]. The only medical book is John Gerard's (1545–1612) *Herbal* (the 1636 folio edition, which sold for £2 12s 0d). Smyth wrote, also only in manuscript, 'Of the first invention of printing' (nd). An analysis of Smyth's *Obituary* emphasizing the social context and attitudes discernible in his brief comments on people, mostly of his acquaintance or family but including some prominent figures and notorious people not known to Smyth, and a useful appendix abstracting the entries that deal with printers and booksellers, is provided by Vanessa Harding, 'Mortality and the mental map of London: *Richard Smyth's* Obituary'. In: Eds. Robin Myers and Michael Harris, *Medicine, mortality and the book trade*, London (1998): pages 49–71.

[64] Although not explicit, these connections can be traced from the brief entries in Smyth (1849) and other sources.

[65] Smyth (1849): page 71 describes 'Geo, Thomasin' as dying on 10 April 1666, 'a poore man'. The editor, Sir Henry Ellis, has added a footnote: 'This was George Thomasin, who formed the singular Collection of Books, Tracts, and single Sheets, from 1640 to 1660, now preserved in the British Museum, and known by the name of the "King's Pamphlets". They were purchased and presented to the British Museum by His Majesty King Geo. III. in 1762.—Ed.'.

[66] Allestry did manage to salvage the printed sheets of Robert Hooke's *Micrographia* (1665) with its two colour printed title page and the engravings, apart from plate 5. The 1667 reissue using some original material had a black title page, and plate 5 reengraved as a mirror image of the original. Before the fire, Allestry and Martyn had issued

moved to Duck Lane during the rebuilding of St Paul's Churchyard, getting his business re-started by publishing Richard Allestry's sermons. James returned to St Paul's but died the following year on 3 November 1670.

Smyth (1849) notes: '*Die Jovis hora* 8ª *ante merid. obijt Jacob. Allestry, Bibliopola in Cœmiter. D. Pauli Lond. sepult. Lunæ* 7 *Nov. Fitz-Williams capellan. Episcop. Winton. concionem facit funebr*'. He also records that Allestry's wife had died on 26 February 1667 and was buried four days later in Little St Bartholomew's, near Smithfield: 'Dr Stillingfleet preached yᵉ sermon'.[67] The Rose and Crown, St Paul's Churchyard (number 58), with '"its double arch and two doors", presses, shelves, counting house, benches, tables and stools, and trade sign together with supporting iron work', was taken over by John Wyatt (fl.1690–1711) and Richard Chiswell.[68]

Thomas Basset (*c.*1637–1699) [**10A1, 10A2, 10A3**] sold books in London from premises at St Dunstan's Churchyard, Fleet St; the George near St Dunstan's; and Westminster Hall, between 1659 and 1693. One of his apprentices was Jacob Tonson (*c.*1655–1736: fl.1678–1698). Basset's main interest was in law books on which he produced a catalogue in 1673.

Jeremiah Battely (d.1737) [**7B**] worked as a bookseller from the Dove in Paternoster Row from 1717 to 1737. He published John Aubrey's *Miscellanies* (new edition with additions, 1721) in the same year as his edition of Willis's *A plain and easie method*.

J.B. (nd) [**9B**]. Three individuals with the initials JB were active in 1681: John Bagford (1650–1716), Joseph Bennett (fl.1675–1691) and John Bringhurst (fl.1680–1684), no one of whom is known to have worked with Thomas Dring, for whom one section of the third part of *The remaining medical works* entitled 'An essay of the pathology of the brain and nervous stock: in which convulsive diseases are treated of:' was printed.[69]

Arthur Bettesworth (d.1739) [**7B**] sold books from 1699 to 1738. His main interest was in divinity but he also dealt in novels. Bettesworth worked from the Red Lion on London Bridge (1699–1737) and 'like all booksellers on the Bridge, [he] dealt in some questionable literature'. However, Dunton writes of 'Genteel Bettisworth: his garb and gesture is free and natural, and his eyes sparkle like anything'.[70] Bettesworth also occupied number 27 Paternoster Row from 1726 to 1738, moving to number 32 from 1736 to 1738. He worked in partnership with Charles Hitch (1715–1764) of Paternoster Row, who married Bettesworth's daughter, Elizabeth (d.1777). Hitch continued the business at 32 Paternoster Row from 1739 to 1762; but Bettesworth had bequeathed copies of books to his son Thomas, who was then underage, and the residue of his share in the stock of the partnership to be divided between all his children equally.[71]

Samuel Carr (fl.1675–1685) [**1I**] was a bookseller in London from the King's Head, situated at the west end of St Paul's Churchyard, from 1675 to 1685.

Edward Castle (d.1727) [**10A4**] sold books from 1695 to 1717 from the Angel and Crown, St Paul's Churchyard; then near Scotland Yard-Gate in Whitehall; and finally against Scotland Yard near the Admiralty. His edition of *The London practice of physick* was listed in

the original edition but each kept 50% of the surviving sheets and sold their books from different addresses, both designating themselves 'printer to the Royal Society'.

[67] See: Smyth (1849): pages 77 and 89.
[68] See: Raven (2014): pages 44–5.
[69] See: Plomer (1922): pages 13–14, 30, and 49–50.
[70] See: Dunton (1818): page 355, although it is not certain that this is the same Bettesworth.
[71] See: HR Plomer, GH Bushnell, and ER McC. Dix, *A dictionary of the printers and booksellers who were at work in England, Scotland and Ireland from 1726 to 1775*, Oxford (1932, for 1930): page 24.

the *Term Catalogue* (1695: II; 552). He also produced John Aubrey's *Miscellanies* (1696) and (with A and J Churchill) an abridged version of John Locke's *Essay on human understanding* (1689, dated 1690). In 1717, he and William Castle (nd) were granted a patent for the sole furnishing with stationery of offices in His Majesty's Revenue.

Henry Clark (d.1691) [**9F**] was a printer based near St Paul's Wharf in Thames Street from 1687 to 1691.[72] He may have been related to Francis Clark (fl.1687–1688) who provided surety for a plea of debt brought against the printer Francis Leach (fl.1673–1707: described as 'blest with a constant trade ... the handsomest printer in London') by Mr Malthus whose works were printed by Henry Clark.[73] Dunton (1818) writes of 'Mr *Henry Clark*, chief Printer to Mr Malthus; and through his persuasions I engaged him upon business. He was extremely civil to the Booksellers, and very diligent and dispatchful in what he did. He was a man of great openness in his temper, and was very seldom afraid to speak the very sentiments of his mind. After Mr Clark's decease, his Widow managed the Trade, by Mr *Sedgwick* first, and afterwards (to no better purpose) by Mr *Barber*'.[74] Dunton bumped into Malthus at Gravesend in 1685 when Dunton was setting sail for America and Malthus to Holland describing the latter as being in 'circumstances something perplexed ... very unfortunate'. Some insight into his misfortune is provided by a later entry in which Dunton vilifies S[arah] Malthus (fl.1700–1706) 'that spiteful woman that hired these fellows to slander me. S. Malthus was the famous Publisher of Grub-street News', and with a tirade on her dishonesty. Dunton then offers some verse which includes the lines: 'Treat me then with abuse no more; / Lest what I made, I uncreate / Let Clark* they haughty looks adore / I knew thee in thy begging state'; and in a footnote: '*This is a printer in Thames-street, who was very zealous to oblige Malthus; but what he got by her (except an opportunity to trust her with twelve pounds) he that knows can tell'.[75] After Clark's death, his widow employed Mr Sedgwick (fl.*c.*1691) and then J Barber (1675–1740) to continue the business.

Robert Clavell (*c.*1633–1711) [**9A1**; **9B1**] was a London bookseller active from 1658 to 1711. He was based initially at the Stag's Head, near St Gregory's Church in St Paul's Churchyard; the Stag in Ivy Lane; and at the Peacock from 1674.[76] He was the son of Roger Clavell (nd), gentleman, of the Isle of Purbeck, Dorset, and was apprenticed to Richard Royston (fl.1629–1686) for seven years before starting his own business. Robert Clavell was master of the Stationers' Company in 1698 and 1699. With John Starkey (fl.1658–1689), Clavell founded and edited a bibliographic journal, *Mercurius Libraries* which started in 1668 and became the *Term Catalogue*. Dunton records that: 'Mr Robert Clavel is a great dealer, and has deservedly gained himself the reputation of a just man. Doctor, Bishop of Lincoln, used to call him "the honest Bookseller". He has been Master of the Company of Stationers; and perhaps the greatest unhappiness of his life was his being one of Alderman Cornish's jury'.[77] Henry Cornish (1659–1685) was convicted of high treason and executed in Cheapside 'much lamented by his Fellow Citizens, a man unjustly sacrificed'.

William Crook(e) (*c.*1639–1694) [**7A**, **10A1**, **10A2**, **10A3**] sold books from Three Bibles on Fleet St. from 1664–1665; and then at the Green Dragon without Temple Bar, close to

[72] These dates taken from Plomer (1922): page 72 must be wrong since H[enry] Clark participated in printing *Dr Willis's practice of physick* in 1684.

[73] This is Thomas Malthus, a London bookseller (fl.1682–*c.*1703). See Plomer (1922): pages 195–6.

[74] See: Dunton (1818): page 249.

[75] See: Dunton (1818): pages 460–1.

[76] See: James Raven (2014): page 155, who gives his address as Cross Key Court, Little Britain in 1673; and his activity as 1656–1711.

[77] See: Dunton (1818): page 207.

Devereux Court, being a passage into the Middle Temple, from 1667 to 1694. He was the son of Andrew Crooke (fl.1630–1674), who published Sir Thomas Browne's *Religio medici* (1642). Andrew completed his training in 1629 and, from 1630 to 1674 was a leading bookseller in London, starting with premises at the Green Dragon. He was master of the Stationers' Company in 1665 and 1666, and died intestate on 20 September 1674, lamented by Smyth 'being well the day before among his acquaintance in Little Britain'.[78] Administration of Andrew Crooke's affairs passed to his widow but the bookselling was taken over by William. He printed for Richard Flecknoe (1600–1678) and Thomas Hobbes. Dunton notes that: 'he was well acquainted with Mr Hobbes, and published many of his Books. He got a good estate by his Trade; and was a man of extraordinary sense, which he had the happiness of being able to express in words as manly and apposite as the sense included under them'.[79] Crooke died in 1694 and was succeeded by his widow, Elizabeth, who continued the business from 1694 to 1696 when the firm ceased trading. The stock was remaindered and sold by D Brown (fl.1672–1729) at the Black Swan and Bible without Temple Bar.

Edmund Curll (1675–1747) [**7B**] was a bookseller based both in London and Tunbridge Wells. Born in the west of England, Curll was apprenticed to Mr (Richard) Smith by Exeter Change (fl.1698–1720). Curll had several premises, starting in Covent Garden with a stall and shop, probably on a retail basis. His first book was published from the Peacock without Temple Bar, near St Clement's Church in the Strand (where he worked from 1706 to 1710). Curll moved to the Dial and Bible against St Dunstan's Church occupying premises, from 1709, previously held by Alexander Bosvill (fl.1696–1709), to be near Egbert Sanger (fl.1707–1711) with whom he was in partnership at that time. His next move was to the Temple Coffee House in Fleet Street (1710–1723). He was able to open branch shops on the Walk at Tunbridge Wells (1712) and Paternoster Row (1720). His London business moved to Catherine Street in the Strand (1723–1726);[80] next to Will's Coffee House in Bow Street, Covent Garden (1723–1726); Burleigh Street, the Strand (1733); and then the Pope's Head, Rose Street, Covent Garden (1735–1747). Over time, Curll functioned as bookseller, auctioneer, and publisher. He quarrelled with Alexander Pope (1688–1744) who laced Curll's drink with an emetic in the Swan Tavern, Fleet Street after which Curll published *A full and true account of a horrid and barbarous revenge by poison on the body of Mr Edmund Curll bookseller* (1716). Controversy dogged Curll who was twice reprimanded by the House of Lords for publishing piratical material, tossed in a blanket and beaten by Westminster scholars for a similar offence, fined for publishing immoral books,[81] imprisoned for five months, and later placed in the pillory at Charing Cross for printing material defamatory to the government. Edmund's son (d.1742) had a separate shop from which he managed his father's affairs whilst the latter was in conflict. All of this left Edmund dubbed 'dauntless Curll' or 'shameless Curll'. Some of his publications were judged bad even by the standards of the day, and others libellous. Troubled by few scruples, Curll was prodigiously active as a bookseller and his 1735 list contained *c.*200 items. Henry Plomer agrees with others that: 'Curll was ... an ungainly, awkward, white-faced man. His eyes were a light grey, large, projecting, gogle and purblind. He was splay-footed and baker-kneed. He ... was well acquainted with more than the title pages of books ... He was not an infidel ... He was a debauchee ... By filling his translations with

[78] See: Smyth (1849): page 103.
[79] See: Dunton (1818): page 215.
[80] Raven (2014): page 126, has this as 1720–1729.
[81] Foremost amongst these was *Eunuchism display'd* (1718). Curll's claim that he sold only one copy of *Venus in the cloister* (1728) seems overstated since the book was still in his list of publications available in 1735.

wretched notes, forged letters and bad pictures, he raised the price of a four shilling book to ten … He died at last as great a penitent … as ever expired'.[82] At his death in 1747, Curll added a codicil to his will: 'I have no relatives, my son is dead / He left no issue, and his wife's re-wed / Therefore no legacys at all I leave / But all I've got to my dear wife bequeathe'.

Richard Davis (1618–*c.*1693) [**5A, 5B1; 6I**] sold books in Oxford near Oriel College from 1646 to 1688. His list contributes to the bibliographic maze of the final signature of *De anima brutorum* (1672).[83] Richard Davis was one of 25 booksellers in Oxford and he had a stock of more than 30 000 volumes including 4000 in medicine and related subjects.[84]

Thomas Dicas (d.1669) [**1A1, 1A2, 1B, 1C, 1D2**] sold books from the Bell, and the Hen and Chickens, both in St Paul's Churchyard, from 1660 to 1669. He worked with James Allestry and John Martyn. Dicas died on 6 February 1669 'at midnight of a consumption, much indebted'[85] and letters of administration were taken out by the principal creditor, Thomas Johnson (fl.1642–1677). Dicas was briefly in partnership with Sir Thomas Davies (1631–1680) in 1656, publishing four books with him that year listed in the Stationers' Register.

Thomas Dring (*c.*1644–1695) [**9A, 9B, 9C, 9D, 9E, 9F; 10A2, 10A3**] sold books from the White Lion, Fleet Street; the Blue Anchor, Fleet Street, over against Fetter Lane (1673); the Harrow, Fleet Street (1674); and in Chancery Lane over against the Inner Temple Gate (1668–1694). He dealt in law, plays, romances, and general literature. He was the son of Thomas Dring (d.1668), a London bookseller working from the George in Fleet St. near St Dunstan's Church (1649–1668). The older Thomas Dring left small bequests to John Place (fl.1645–1686) and Thomas Bassett, the residue of the estate to his son Thomas, and the premises in Fleet St. to his younger son Joshua. Thomas Roycroft was a witness to the will dated 12 September 1668 and proved on 21 December. The younger Thomas Dring died in 1695 and the *Term Catalogue* for the Trinity term mentions that some of his stock was sold by Nathaniel Rolls (fl.1692–1696), Daniel Brown (fl.1672–1729), and John Walthoe (fl.1683–1690).

Elizabeth Fletcher (1642–1697: Flesher) [**5B1**] was the daughter of Cornelius Bee (d.1672), a bookseller at the 'King's Armes in Little Britaine' from 1634 to 1671 who suffered losses in the fire since, although Little Britain was spared, his stock was stored elsewhere. Bee died on 2 January 1672 bequeathing his business to Elizabeth and another daughter, Mrs Norwood. He was buried 'Jan. 4 at Great St Bartholomew's 'w^th^out a sermon, w^th^out wine or waffers, only gloves and rosmary; Dr Wells of Aldersgate read ye service. His younger daughter married to Nath. Hook, his servant'.[86] Elizabeth married James Fletcher, inheriting from him one of the largest printing establishments in England with five presses and thirteen workmen. After James's death in December 1670, Elizabeth printed at Little Britain. Of the 97 works she published, sixteen appear with her initials and the rest under her full name.

[82] See: Plomer (1922): pages 92–5.

[83] See: Plomer (1907): page 62 who omits this detail but refers his readers instead to the earlier list of classical, scientific, and religious works, together with one play, printed on the last leaf of Zacharius Bogan's *Meditations or the mirth of a Christian life* (1653).

[84] See: Robert Frank, *Harvey and the Oxford physiologists*, Berkeley (1980): page 46, and endnote 9 to chapter 3 at page 310 citing the auction catalogues of Davis's entire stock: *Catalogus in quævis lengua & facultate insignium tam antiquorum quam recentium librorum Richardi Davis bibliopolæ*, three parts, Oxford (1686–1688). These listed 80 000 volumes, a quantity rivalled only by the London booksellers Robert Scott and Richard Chiswell. The auction became the subject of a satyrical poem, entitled *Auctio Davisiana Oxonii habita*, London (1689) by George Smalridge (1662–1719), Bishop of Bristol. See: John Lawler, *Book auctions in England in the seventeenth century (1676-1700) with a chronological list of the book auctions of the period*, London (1898): pages 30–8.

[85] See: Smyth (1849): page 80.

[86] See: Smyth (1849): pages 93 and 99.

Elizabeth was succeeded in 1679 by her stepson Miles Fletcher; and her brother, Lancelot Toppyn (d.1646), also a bookseller, married Anne, sister to Dixy Page (fl.1664–1668), another bookseller.

James Fletcher (d.1670: Flesher) [**2A**] worked as a printer in Little Britain from 1652 to 1667. Through parentage and his marriage to Elizabeth Bee, James was part of a book trade dynasty. He was in business with his father Miles Fletcher (d.1664) who owned premises at Little Britain from 1611 to 1664, joining George Eld (d.1624) in 1617, and being granted the rights of master printer after petitioning the Archbishop of Canterbury in 1624. Later Miles worked with Robert Young (fl.1625–1643) and John Haviland (nd). They prospered, taking a share in the King's Printing House and absorbing the businesses of William Stansby, George Purslow (d.1632), and Edward Griffen (fl.1613–1638). Miles was master of the Stationers' Company in 1652, 1653, 1662, and 1663. In 1629, he had acquired the rights of publishing law books from John More (fl.1629–1661) for a fee of £60 per annum and a one-third share of the profits. In 1661, the Stationers' Company purchased the lease from Miles and James Fletcher for £2000. This did not stop their work and, in 1664, James and Miles were proceeded against for illegally printing law books, this licence having already been contested in the case of John Streater (1620–1677) who had been given special privileges under the terms of the 1662 printing act.[87] A specimen sheet of the polyglot bible was printed by James Fletcher and its conspectus produced by Roger Norton (d.1662). Norton's death on 1 April 1662 is recorded by Smyth: 'Mr Roger Norton, printer in Black ffriers, died, whose daughter my coz. Dr Tho. Clutterbuck marr[d]'.[88] At his death on 12 November 1664, apart from plate gifted to the Stationers' Company, Miles left his entire estate to James, who did not long survive him dying at Clerkenwell on 30 December 1670.

William Hall (fl.1656–1672) [**3A**] was a printer in Oxford from 1656 to 1672 and may have been related to Henry Hall who worked in the same city from 1642 to *c.*1679. Henry was apprenticed to William Turner and purchased his 'presses, letters and utensils' on Turner's death in 1643, replacing him as printer to the University in 1644. He was one of those bound over in 1649 for £300 not to publish seditious or unlicensed material. William was also printer to the University, with Henry Hall, in 1662.

Charles Harper (*c.*1643–1714) [**9A, 9B, 9C, 9D, 9E, 9F; 10A2, 10A3**] sold books from the Flower de Luce, a building at the corner of Fetter Lane and Fleet Street, occupied in the first quarter of the seventeenth century by the bookseller, John Hodgets (fl.1601–1625).[89] Harper's main topic of interest was divinity. He was a considerable figure in the Stationers' Company, serving as junior warden in 1699 and 1700 to the extent that Dunton wrote: 'I believe him an honest man, and a warm votary for High Church. He printed 'Mr Wesley's Life of Christ', and makes a considerable figure in the Stationers Company'.[90] Harper's will, dated 24 October 1711, left the stock to his son-in-law James Rawlins (d.1715).

John Hayes (fl.1658–1666) printed ('excudebat') William Croone's essay on muscular motion, to be sold by Samuel Thomson (fl.1664–1668). This was pirated by Caspar Commelin (see next) and Gerbrant Schagen (see next) for the Amsterdam editions of *Cerebri anatome*

[87] See: Michael Treadwell, 'The stationers and the printing acts at the end of the seventeenth century'. In: Barnard and McKenzie (2002): pages 755–76. Whereas many authorities, including Plomer (1907) give the date of Streater's death as 1687, Adrian Johns, *Oxford Dictionary of National Biography* (2004 and 2008) corrects this to 1677: https://doi.org/10.1093/ref:odnb/26656.

[88] See: Smyth (1849): page 55.

[89] See: HG Aldis, Robert Bowes, ER McC Dix, E Gordon Duff, Strickland Gibson, GJ Gray, RB McKerrow, Falcaner Madan, and HR Plomer, *A dictionary of printers and booksellers in England, Scotland and Ireland, and of foreign printers of English books 1557–1640*, London (1910): page 139.

[90] See: Dunton (1818): page 210.

[2C2, 2D, 2E]. Hayes printed at Little Wood Street in London from 1658 to 1666, and was probably a descendant of another publisher, Lawrence Hayes (fl.1617–1637),[91] who sold books up to 1637. John was one of the eleven who petitioned for a 'companie of printers' in 1661. He suffered under the malign influence of Roger L'Estrange and was one of many members of the book trade ruined in 1666 by the fire of London.

John Leigh (d.1685) [**9A, 9B, 9C, 9D, 9E, 9F**] sold books from the Blue Bell, Fleet Street, by Flying Horse Court; and then from Stationers' Hall from 1670 to 1685, when he died. His main interests were divinity and law. He was treasurer of the Stationers' Company in 1679.

Susanah Leigh (d.1692) [**10A2**] was the widow of John Leigh and active from 1687 to 1689. Her stock passed to Christopher Wilkinson (fl.1669–1693). Her name appears on only one edition of Thomas Willis's books, published in 1689, four years after the death of John Leigh.

Thomas Leigh (d.1704) [**10B**], the son of John and Susanah Leigh, was a bookseller at the Peacock near St Dunstan's Church in Fleet Street; and then from the Rose and Crown, St Paul's Churchyard working from 1695 to 1704.[92] He was associated at the Peacock with Roger Clavell who had advertised in the *Post-Boy* on 17 / 19 September 1695: 'If any person has any study of books, or library consisting either of divinity, law, history, physic, etc., to dispose of, if they please to send a catalogue of them to Roger Clavel at the Peacock near St Dunstan's Church in Fleet Street, they shall have the full value for them, and the cost of carriage paid'. Clavell was succeeded by Thomas Leigh who entered into partnership with Daniel Midwinter and Richard Chiswell at the Rose and Crown. Leigh seems to have stopped selling books from 1704, after which the business was continued by Midwinter.

A.M. (nd) [**9F**]: the identity of this printer identified only by initials and responsible with R.R for printing the third part of *Dr Willis's practice of physick* (1684) is unknown. R.R is presumably Robert Roberts. Based on Plomer (1907; 1922) and printers known to be active in 1685, one candidate might be Alexander Milbourn who printed in London from 1684 to 1693. With his brother E. Milbourn (fl.1684), and S. Hinch (fl.1684) and J. Mason (fl.1684),[93] Alexander printed a broadside at the Thames Frost Fair of 1684. At the Old Bailey sessions in April 1693, he was bound over for judgment at the next sitting for printing libellous material. Alexander's wife Elizabeth ran the business from 1708, which may be the year in which Alexander died, until *c.*1721.

John Martyn (also known as Martin: 1618–1680) [**1A1, 1A2, 1B, 1C, 1D2, 1I; 2A, 2B; 3D; 4C**] worked as a bookseller from the Bell in St Paul's Churchyard from 1649 to 1680. Martyn was apprenticed to Humphrey Robinson (fl.1624–1670) from 1635 to 1643. He received the freedom of the Stationers' Company and its livery in 1657, also serving as underwarden in 1678. He was in partnership with James Allestry and, after the fire of London, worked with him for the Royal Society. Dunton describes Martyn as: 'Printer for many years to the Royal Society. He managed all his affairs with discretion, was a thriving man in his trade, and made a very pious end'.[94] Martyn specialized in publishing medical and scientific material, producing 134 books in the 1670s of which 51 related to natural or physical sciences. He advertised

[91] See: Aldis (1910): page 133.

[92] Plomer (1922): page 187 lists his period of activity as 1698–1704 but this must be wrong since Leigh's issue of *The London practice of physick* appeared in 1695.

[93] See: Plomer (1922): pages 156 and 199 citing William Hazlitt (1778–1830), volume 2, *Essays*, page 681 (although it is unclear to which edition and, hence, collective title of the *Essays* this refers), indicating that these four printed a broadside in verse, *On the Royal martyr, King Charles I.*, 'Printed on the frozen Thames, January the 30th 1683 [ie 1684] by the loyal young printers, viz G. and A. Melbourn, S. Hinch, and J. Mason'. Plomer concludes that they were very likely not master printers.

[94] See: Dunton (1818): page 212.

his stock in sale catalogues printed independently or appended to his publications. Martyn also acted as an importer and dealer in second-hand books, attending auctions and sometimes buying entire libraries or listing desiderata for himself or individual customers. His prices were considered steep by collectors such as Robert Hooke and Samuel Pepys (1633–1703).[95] Martyn was buried in St Faith's under what became Sir Christopher Wren's new cathedral, where a monument shows him dressed in the gown of warden of the Stationers' Company, with his wife Sarah kneeling before a table piled with books.[96]

S. Martyn (Martin: nd) [**9B**]. Nothing is known of this publisher who may be Sarah, wife of John Martyn, or another relative.

Daniel Midwinter (fl.1698–1725) [**10B**] sold books from the Rose and Crown and the Three Crowns in St Paul's Churchyard from 1698 to 1725 in partnership with Thomas Leigh. Of this partnership, Dunton writes: 'Mr *Leigh* and Mr *Midwinter* are in topping business, and no way inferior to their known Predecessor for justice and industry, &c.'[97] Their first premises were previously occupied by Richard Chiswell. Midwinter moved to the Three Crowns after the partnership faltered in 1704. Midwinter was one of few booksellers simultaneously to have premises in two places where the trade was active—Little Britain and St Paul's Churchyard. He was succeeded by his son Daniel Midwinter II (d.1757) in 1725.

Charles Rivington (1688–1742) [**7B**] was a bookseller from Chesterfield, Derbyshire, who worked from the Bible and Crown, Paternoster Row, from 1711 to 1742, after an apprenticeship with Emanuel Matthews (fl.1700–1717), moving to the north side of St Paul's Churchyard in 1734.[98] He bought the business of Richard Chiswell, 'the Metropolitan of Booksellers', in 1711.[99] The Rivington business depended mainly on the publication of sermons and works on divinity. Rivington responded to the order from a clergyman for 35 000 copies of a sermon and, after selling 17, sent an invoice for £784 but later confessed that he had only printed 100. Later, he published *Pamela* (1740) for Samuel Richardson (1689–1761) which 'Pope asserted would do more good than twenty sermons'. When Charles died, Samuel Richardson acted as his executor and guardian of the six children by his wife Elle Pease (nd) of Durham. The business passed to his sons Charles, John, and James and remained active into the nineteenth century.[100]

Robert Roberts (d.1703) [**9F**] was a printer in London active from 1679 to *c.*1699. He is believed to be the R.R. who printed *A true relation of the cruelties lately acted by the rebels in Scotland* (1679) with A.M. This links A.M. and R.R. to the printing of *Dr Willis's practice of physick* (1684) one year earlier than his first appearance in the Michaelmas *Term Catalogue* (1685) as printer of Thieleman J van Braght's (1625–1664) *Mirror of martyrs* (1685). Dunton

95 See: Rostenberg (1952): pages 21 and 23–7.

96 Reproduced by Rivington (1984) as Figure 1, page 8.

97 See: Dunton (1818): page 207.

98 See: Raven (2014) page 45 for details. The house was designated number 62, where the firm remained until 1853 although other evidence suggests that it was number 64, a more prestigious location adjoining Canon Alley (despite also being known as Pissing Alley) with living quarters and steps down to the Cathedral precinct.

99 Correcting Plomer (1922): page 254, Raven (2014): page 44 points out that Rivington was apprenticed to Awnsham Churchill (fl.1681–1728), quoting Barbara Fitzpatrick in the *Oxford Dictionary of National Biography*, https://doi.org/10.1093/ref:odnb/70881; and that Chiswell's tenancy, stock and goodwill were bought from Benjamin Cowse (fl.1714–1723).

100 See: EC Bigmore and CWH Wyman, *A bibliography of printing*, volume 2, London (1880): pages 262–6, for an account of Charles Rivington and the publishing business he founded. John Rivington (d.1785) was succeeded by his widow Ann (1756–1841) who continued the business, taking John Marshall (nd) into partnership in 1786. The firm specialized in classical authors. Eventually the business passed into the hands of Richard Gilbert (1794–1852) who, in 1830, entered into partnership with William Rivington (1807–1888), great-grandson of the first Charles Rivington after which it was known as Gilbert & Rivington converting (in 1881) into a limited liability company, and retaining a high reputation for its oriental printing.

admired Roberts: 'He was master over himself; when he had a storm in his heart, he made all fair-weather in his face. He would look big, but I never found he was passionate, proud or vain. However he had this particular in him, that he never broke his word to a Book-seller. In twenty Books that he printed for me, he never disappointed me once, or exacted two-pence; so that what he left to his widow will wear well, for it was every penny honestly gotten.'[101]

Samuel Roycroft (1657–1717) [**3D; 4C**], the son of Thomas Roycroft, was appointed city printer in succession to Andrew Clark (d.1677/8) who had himself succeeded James Fletcher in 1677, the year in which James took over his late father's printing house in Bartholomew Close. Samuel Roycroft's business was largely based on printing tickets and bills, and other jobbing work.[102]

Thomas Roycroft (1637–1677) [**1A1, 1A2, 1B, 1C, 1D2, 1I; 2B**] printed from Bartholomew Close and Printing House, Charterhouse Yard, from 1651 to 1677. He was appointed the King's printer in the oriental languages on the accession of Charles II (1630–1685) and had a share in the King's printing house. Dunton acknowledges that he had forgotten to mention various individuals including 'noble Captain Roycroft, Printer to the Honorable City of London'.[103] Roycroft became master of the Stationers' Company in 1675. He died on 10 August 1677 and was buried in the church of St Bartholomew the Great.

Robert Scott (*c.*1632–1687) [**5A4, 5A5; 5B2, 6A2, 6B2**] sold books from number 50 Princes Arms, Little Britain, from 1661 to 1691.[104] He bought books in France, Germany, and Holland and had wealthy customers. In the 1670s he sold books to Sir Joseph Williamson, for £61, eleven of which were chained (for an extra 14s). Dr John North (1645–1683) built a competent library through dealing with Scott who he considered to be the greatest bookseller of his time. Scott also supplied books to, among others, Robert Hooke, Christopher Wren, and Samuel Pepys. Scott's brother-in-law was William Wells (see next) whose business he acquired in 1673. Scott also bought John Martyn's stock from his widow in 1681 but expressed some dissatisfaction with the deal, perhaps in order to have the price reduced. This seems disingenuous since thereby he acquired the works of Hooke, John Ray (1627–1705), John Evelyn, Marcello Malpighi, Willis, the *Philosophical Transactions*, William Shakespeare (1564–1616), Francis Beaumont (1585–1616), John Fletcher (1579–1625), and many others.[105] In 1677, Scott's shop was threatened with closure by L'Estrange for selling copies of *L'escole des filles* (1655), an erotic work published anonymously in Paris that Scott had bought from Jean Maximilian Lucas (see next) in Amsterdam, a charge which Scott considered to be 'illegal, unjustifiable and uncivil'. Dunton evidently took Scott's side: 'grave *Scot* ... is always for doing the fair thing'.[106] In 1683, Scott acquired the rights to several of Willis's works that had formerly belonged to John Martyn.[107] Growing old, sometime around 1685, Scott closed his shop and sank £10 000 into a partnership with Adiel Mill (fl.1687–1690) of St Paul's Churchyard, who advertised Scott's stock for sale in the London Gazette for 5–9 January 1687. Mill was executor of the will of Henry Hills (fl.1641–1689) when he died in France having left London abruptly after his premises were attacked on Hills's conversion to Catholicism. Mill's business failed and he became a debtor in Fleet Street for £30 000, as a result of which Scott eventually lost most of his investment. Nonetheless Mill seems to have

[101] See: Dunton (1818): page 244.
[102] See: Raven (2014): page 102.
[103] See: Dunton (1818): page 292.
[104] Raven (2014) has this as 1661–*c.*1687: page 153.
[105] See: Rostenberg (1952): page 31.
[106] See: Dunton (1818): page 268.
[107] See entry for 21 August 1683 in Liber F of the register of the Stationer's Company; and earlier.

remained active; and R.R printed *Votes of the house of Commons in Ireland* for Mill in 1692. By the time of his death, in 1710, Scott was the second most senior member of the Court of the Stationers' Company.

Sheldonian Theatre (fl.1674–1679) [**6A, 6B, 6E, 6F, 6I**] refers to John Fell and printers working in association with the University of Oxford.

Richard Wellington (d.1724) [**10A4**] was a bookseller based at the Lute, St Paul's Churchyard from 1693 to 1699 and then at the Dolphin and Crown, St Paul's Churchyard, until *c.*1709. With John Minshull (fl.1674–1712) of Chester, he fell out with the Stationers' Company in 1704 for importing and selling books on divinity without authorization. Dunton considered that Wellington: 'is industrious and indefatigable in his calling; has the intimate acquaintance of several excellent Pens, and therefore, can never want Copies; and trust him for managing and improving them. He has a pretty knack at keeping his word; and I expect to see him Master of the Company at least, if not a *gold* chain around his neck, before he died'.[108]

William Wells (d.1673) [**5A4, 5A5; 5B2**] was apprenticed until 1637, and then worked as a stationer and bookseller based at the Princes Arms, Little Britain, from 1641 to 1673. As an apprentice Robert Scott was turned over to Wells in 1651, and they were in partnership from 1661 publishing seventeen works together, eight of which appeared in 1672. Scott was executor for the will of his sister who had married Wells. He took action against the Stationers' Company in order to protect his £80 share of the stock left when Wells died two years later in 1673. Smyth records that 'Mr Wells, bookseller in Little Britain (my old acquaintance) died this Satterday (26 January 1673) morning. Buried at St Butolphs ext. Aldersgate. Jan. No sermon'.[109]

Willis's printers and booksellers in continental Europe

After the publication of Thomas Willis's books in England, each was reissued in Europe, usually in the original Latin. Six treatises were translated into Dutch: *De fermentatione* (**1H**); *De febribus* and *De urinis*, (**1J**); *De scorbuto*, (**3C**); and the two parts of *Pharmaceutice rationalis*, (**6H** and **6J**); and one into French: *De urinis*, (**1K**). The collected works were first printed outside England (entitled *Opera medica et physica* or *Opera omnia*: **8A–8I**). The printers and booksellers who made these books available from 1676 to 1721 were based in the Netherlands, France, Switzerland, and Italy.

Imported from Germany and Italy, and active from *c.*1470, print arrived early in the Low Countries of the Netherlands, Belgium, Luxembourg, and northwestern France.[110] As elsewhere, each of the trades was plied from the same premises. The type was originally black letter, the language Latin, and the subject matter religious other than in Leuven where schoolbooks and those on the classics and humanities were also published. The Dutch book trade succeeded because the country was prosperous, capital available at low interest rates, the people educated, materials readily available, skilled workers abundant, economic conditions favourable, and transport of materials and books by road and canal easily arranged. In the seventeenth century, the development of highly legible small roman type,

[108] Quoted by Plomer (1922): page 306, citing Dunton (1818): page 212.

[109] See: Smyth (1849): page 97.

[110] Details are mainly taken from Paul Hoftijzer, 'The history of the book in the Low Countries'. In: Eds. Michael F Suarez and HR Woodhuysen, *The Oxford companion to the book*, volume 1, Oxford (2010): pages 212–21; Paul Hoftijzer, 'The English book in the seventeenth-century Dutch republic', Hellinga et al (2001): pages 89–107; and PG Hoftijzer, 'British books abroad: the Continent'. In: Barnard and McKenzie (2002): pages 735–43.

cast by Christoffel van Dijck, allowed the printing of smaller formats which were then adopted in England.[111]

Dutch printers proved to be enterprising businessmen with a skilful workforce. In Antwerp, Christopher Plantin (1520–1589) had a type foundry, sixteen presses, and a bookshop with international customers. As political upheavals subsided, printing concentrated in several other cities including Amsterdam, Leiden, and Middelburg. The successors of several booksellers active in these cities in the period around 1600 were involved in printing the books of Thomas Willis: Louis Elsevier (fl.1580–1617) in Leiden; Jan van Waesberge (fl.1587–1625) in Rotterdam; and Jan Commelin in Amsterdam. Daniel Elsevier (1626–1680) led the second period of prominent Amsterdam booksellers; and the next generation included Elsevier's former assistant Hendrik Wetstein (1649–1726), and Johannes (1616–1681) and Gillis Janssonius van Waasberge (Waesberge: 1646–1708). French printers and booksellers worked in Amsterdam at the end of the century, especially the brothers Jean Pierre and Marc Huguetan (fl.1687–1703), descended from the Lyon bookselling dynasty. Their work was notable for the quality and scope of the publication list, with a partnership that may have been worth more than half a million guilders (= €5 000 000) and stocks distributed across Europe and into the Levant. But their unscrupulous business methods were not much liked by colleagues, one of whom complained that the Huguetans had twelve to thirteen printing presses at their disposal kept active 'without making any distinction whom they damage or where'.[112]

As in England, censorship of material perceived to be heretical influenced book production. Regulations were in place but rarely enforced and decrees against illicit and seditious books were ignored both by printers and authorities. Driven by commercial urge, printers did not lack courage.[113] Protestant texts printed in the Netherlands were smuggled in small boats to coastal towns in England. Spies were sent abroad to suppress this activity.[114]

Royalists moved to the Netherlands during the Civil War and some sold books. Samuel Browne (fl.1638–1665) produced political material in The Hague and his name was a convenient front for books apparently imported from Holland but, in fact, printed in London (the 'Latin trade').[115] As with the third edition of his brother Thomas Browne's (1605–1682) work *Religio medici* (1642), Samuel included an elaborate engraved allegorical title page in his copy of Nathanael Highmore's work on anatomy published from The Hague.[116] Browne stocked English books and, although he returned to England in 1662, the catalogue was taken over and developed by his son-in-law, Johannes de L'Escluse (nd). The issues for 1676 and 1677 contain items by Thomas Willis which are either the English or Dutch imprints in the

[111] The name was originally Elzevier but became Elsevier at some point in the seventeenth century.

[112] See: PG Hoftijzer, 'Dutch printing and bookselling in the Golden Age'. In: Eds. WJ Boo, Y Shirahata. *Two faces of the early modern world. The Netherlands and Japan in the seventeenth and eighteenth* centuries, Kyoto (2001): pages 59–67.

[113] See: Hoftijzer (2014): page 214 for an account of Adriaen van Berghen (fl.1500–1542) convicted for selling forbidden books in Antwerp in 1535 and banned from the city of Delft in 1542, whose initial mild sentence was overturned by the Court of Holland so that he was beheaded at the Hague.

[114] Reference is occasionally made to Richard Allestry having been a spy carrying messages to and from Charles II in the context of his frequent travels to France during the reformation: see *Dictionary of National Biography* (1885) volume 1: pages 324–5.

[115] See: Marika Keblusek, 'The exile experience: Royalist and Anglian book culture in the Low Countries'. In: Hellinga et al (2001): page 152; and Plomer (1900): page 36. Smyth (1849): page 66, records the death in August 1665 of 'Mr. Brown, once a bookseller at ye Hague, who married ye daughter of Mr Nath. Hall of ye Excheq^r, died at ye Pest house *ex peste*, about this time'. This connects Samuel Browne to the Cornelius Bee dynasty.

[116] See: Highmore (1651). This shows a series of panels depicting work in the autopsy theatre with Hippocrates and Galen tugging on each arm of a double-headed cadaver, whose thorax, abdomen, and arms are covered with explanatory text, and with Highmore attending quietly to their deliberations.

stated formats. Those offered in 1676 are: #59, 'Willis celebri Anatomiæ' (octavo); #93, 'Willis celebri Anatomiæ' (duodecimo); and #98, 'Willis pharmaceutice' (duodecimo). In 1677, the only item for sale is: #59, 'Willis celebri Anatomiæ' (octavo). An earlier De L'Escluse catalogue from 1674 has no books by Thomas Willis.[117] Two widows, Mercy Browning (fl.1675–1687) and Abigael May (nd), were especially active in this trade. In 1678, widow Browning had a shop full of English books. These were listed in her stock catalogue for 1685 containing 1400 titles that included works by Thomas Browne, Robert Burton, and Francis Bacon, and a section on physick.[118]

Unlike the Stationers' Company, privileges and licences were not rigorously patrolled in Holland and the main restriction lay with publishers' copyright rather than the exercise of political control. Inability to protect the cartel exercised by the Stationers' company encouraged continental booksellers to pirate titles and undercut prices. No sooner was a book published in England than Dutch booksellers produced Latin and French translations or reissued those already printed in Latin.[119] Aware that a number of his works had been translated and printed by Dutch firms, Robert Boyle complained to Henry Oldenburg that he might be suspected of having 'taken divers things from others, which indeed [they] borrowed of me'. Although not on the best of terms, Oldenburg had warned John Martyn that he should print a cheap version of *Philosophical Transactions* in Latin so that the Dutch did not take advantage of his enterprise. Inevitably, Martyn's work was pirated when a Latin edition of *Philosophical Transactions* did appear from Amsterdam.[120] But not all was underhand. In the early years of publication after 1666, issues of *Philosophical Transactions* advertising recently published scientific books were sent to Europe. In 1686, the secretary of the Society, John Hoskyns (1634–1705) wrote to Pierre Bayle (1647–1706), editor of the *Nouvelles de la republique des lettres* asking to exchange news of scientific books published in England and the continent pointing out that: 'l'Angleterre n'est pas précisément sans savants ... et l'on fait imprimer ici fort souvent des choses dont peut-être vous feriez cas et dont la connaissance ne vous vient que fort tard, quelquefois même point du tout'.[121] [England isn't exactly without scholars ... and we have books printed here that you probably wouldn't consider and the knowledge of which reaches you too late, and even sometimes not at all]. As Latin was gradually replaced by the vernacular, the limited ability of readers in continental Europe to understand English, and Dutch not being a language that was read outside Holland, reduced the risk of unauthorized publication in Holland towards the end of the seventeenth century.

After Guillaume Le Roy (fl.1473–1488), originally from Liege in Belgium, opened a printing press in Lyon in 1473, printing spread to around thirty French cities by 1500. Lyon was geographically well placed to benefit from trade with northern Italy and southern

[117] See: Hoftijzer (2001): page 97 and footnote 53, page 105, explaining that unique copies of *Catalogus variorum insignium librorum in omni facultate, & lingua præcipue Anglica officinæ Johannis de l'Escluse p. m.*, The Hague (1676 and 1677) are in the Herzog August Bibliothek, Wolfenbüttel.

[118] See: Hoftijzer (2001): pages 41–5.

[119] See: Hoftijzer (2001): pages 92–3, and footnote 20, page 103 drawing attention to the checklist of books, mainly pious tracts, translated from English to Dutch in the seventeenth century citing CW Schoneveld, *Intertraffic of the mind. Studies in seventeenth century Anglo-Dutch translation with a checklist of books translated from English into Dutch, 1600–1700*, Leiden (1983); and Schoneveld's disclaimer that with no pretensions to bibliographic expertise, he has merely compiled his list from random notes. Only one on the list is considered to be medical; #22: Anthony Chute, *Tabaco. The ... opinions of the ... best physitions* (1595), translated as *Korte beschrijvinge van het wonderlijcke kruyt tabacco*, Rotterdam (1623); also translated is William Salmon's *Pharmacopaeia Londinensis* (1678; Dutch edition published by Johannes ten Hoorn, 1696: #532); and works by Robert Boyle (##115–117), Thomas Browne (##135–137), Kenelm Digby (#217), and John Locke (#379).

[120] See: Hoftijzer (2001): pages 89–107.

[121] See: Hoftijzer (2002): page 743, citing HJ Reesink, *Angleterre et la litérature anglaise dans les trois plus anciens périodiques Français de Hollande de 1684 à 1709*, Paris (1931): page 79.

Germany. After Venice and Paris, Lyon was by the 1490s the third most important place for printing in Europe. In all three cities, printing in the vernacular occurred earlier than in countries with smaller reading populations. As in the Netherlands, this restricted sales of many scholarly books to a readership that remained familiar with Latin.[122] The family of Jean de Tournes (1504–1564) started printing in Lyon from 1542. His books were handsomely decorated with woodcut borders, initials, and other printers' ornaments. De Tournes was able to exercise some freedom with respect to publishing dissident religious material, and this tradition reached Geneva where de Tournes's son moved in 1585.[123] Geneva had benefited over Lyon from exiles arriving during the reformation including Jean Girard (d.1558), who printed John Calvin's (1509–1564) works. Despite the decline of Lyon with the expansion of printing in other European cities, the Huguetan family business started in Lyon by the first Jean-Antoine Huguetan (1567–1650) remained active through three generations to 1685. But as refugees following revocation of the edict of Nantes (1685), Jean Pierre Huguetan (nd) and his brother and Marc (d.1702) were amongst 200 000 Huguenots who fled, in their case to Amsterdam, taking with them highly skilled artisans.

After the printing of individual books in Subiaco and Rome, the book trade in Italy concentrated in Venice from 1469 before spreading to around eighty cities by 1500.[124] Venetian type was cut by skilled workers from France and Germany. Many of these books remained large in format and superficially luxurious although matched for aesthetics by the Aldine (Manutius Aldus: 1449–1515) copies printed in small format using roman, italic, and greek types. Elements such as the index and illustrations were introduced. As in the Netherlands, high-quality materials were available and communication made easy by canal and sea. Mules took books across the Alps to other European cities. Venice remained dominant until several factors heralded its decline in the seventeenth century: competition and religious oppression from Rome, reduction in European trade during the Thirty Years' War (1618–1648), and plague in 1630. But many luxuriously printed books, rich in decorations, were still printed into the eighteenth century.

Against this background, editions of Thomas Willis's books were published by twenty-three individuals working in the Netherlands (16) from 1659 to 1682; France (2) from 1676 to 1687; Switzerland (1) from 1676 to 1694; and Italy (4) from 1695 to 1721.

Joannes Blaeu (1596–1673) [**5B3**] variously known as Joan Blavius, Giovanni Blaeu, Joannes Blaeuw, or Blavii, Joan was the son of Willem Jansz Blaeu (1571–1638), founder of the famous Blaeu firm in Amsterdam. In 1638, Joan Blaeu inherited nine printing presses, each one named after the Muses, and six plate presses for producing maps and illustrations. Joan had become a doctor of law (1620) but left that profession to work with his father and, at least from 1638 to 1642, his brother Cornelis (1610–1648). He worked from an address at Het Water, from 1643 to 1658, where the sign on his shop was 'Vergulde zonnewyser'. The Short Title Catalogue for the Netherlands[125] lists 535 items from his shop of which *De anima brutorum* (1672) is number 512. Blaeu also published works by John Aubrey and Thomas Hobbes. Although a printer, Joan is now better remembered as a cartographer and for his

[122] See: Lukas Erne. In: Suarez and Woodhuysen, volume 1 (2010): pages 237–9.

[123] See: Vincent Giroud, 'The history of the book in France'. In: Suarez and Woodhuysen, volume 1 (2010): pages 199–211; and volume 2: page 1212.

[124] See Neil Harris, 'The history of the book in Italy'. In: Suarez and Woodhuysen, volume 1 (2010): pages 257–69.

[125] For a critical analysis of the merits and limitations of the Short-Title Catalogue for the Netherlands, see Andrew Pettegree and Arthur der Weduwen, 'What was published in the seventeenth-century Dutch Republic?', *Revue Historique* (2018): pages 1–27. The Short Title Catalogue is a dynamic structure with additions and deletions. Numbers given in the text that follows were on the website as of 27 January 2021. See: http://picarta.nl/.

publication of the *Atlas maior*, an eleven-volume atlas of the world (1662–1667), considered the best of its time.[126]

Caspar Commelin (1636–1693) [**2C2**, **2E1**] was a bookseller active in Amsterdam from 1659 to 1690. He descended from a famous publishing family, which had come to Leiden and Amsterdam from Heidelberg around 1600. The son of his first marriage, to Margrieta Heydanus (nd), was a renowned Dutch botanist (also Caspar Commelin or Commelijn: 1668–1731). Caspar, the printer, worked from addresses at de Calver-straet (1662), Het Water (1664–1668), where the sign on these premises was 'in de Waerheydt'; and de Harte-straat (1690) where the sign on his shop was 'Het Vergulde block'. Commelin was variously known as Gaspar Commelin, Casparus Commelyn, and Casparus Commelijn. The Short Title Catalogue for the Netherlands lists 47 items from his shop. *Cerebri anatome* (1664: **2C2**) is omitted. *Cerebri anatome* (1667: **2E1**) is number 23 (and repeated as 25). William Croone's *De ratione motus musculorum* (1664 and 1667) is listed as numbers 14 and 26; and Nathaniel Highmore's *Exercitationes duæ. quarum prior de passione hysterica: altera de affectione hypochondriaca* (1660) is number 2.

Cornelius Driehuysen (fl.1663–1671) [**4B**] was active in Leiden (1663–1671) as a small academic bookseller. He worked from an address in over d'Academie (1668–1671) with the signboard 'in de Laurier Boom' and a subsidiary notice 'insigni Apollinis Laurus'. Driehuysen was also known as C. Driehusius. He married Elysabeth Moyaert (nk) of Leiden in 1664. The Short Title Catalogue for the Netherlands lists 28 items from his shop of which *Affectionum quæ dicuntur hystericæ et hypochondriacæ pathologia spasmodica vindicata, contra responsionem epistolarem Nathanael Highmori*, published with Felicem Lopez, is number 24. The variant title page is not listed. Driehuysen also sold works by Francis Glisson (1597–1677) and John Mayow.

Daniel Elsevier (1626–1680)[127] [**3B1**, **3B3**]. Together with his uncle Louis, Daniel Elsevier (fl.Leiden 1652–1655; Amsterdam 1655–1681), grandson of Louis Elsevier (1540–1617) the founder, was responsible for the Amsterdam branch of the firm. Daniel was variously known as Daniel Elsevier, Daniel Elsvirius, or Daniel Elsevirius.[128] Based in Leiden and Amsterdam, the firm published around 100 books in Latin by English authors across the seventeenth century. Daniel Elsevier visited England 'on some small business with his correspondents in London of ye same profession'. He had been given a letter of introduction to Sir Joseph Williamson, a customer of Martyn, who probably introduced him to 'the master of The Bell'.[129] English booksellers, including George Thomason and Robert Scott, were also occasionally in Amsterdam.[130] As with other Dutch publishers, the business methods involved piracy with reprinting duodecimo issues of expensive English imprints previously in quarto or octavo format. Sometimes, as with Cornelius Bee's publication of Christoph Scheiner's (1573–1650) *Oculus hoc est: fundamentum opticum* (1652), Dutch publishers were merely acting as distributors and agents of English booksellers or exercising legitimate contracts in

[126] See: J Koeman, *Joan Blaeu and his grand atlas*, Amsterdam (1970).

[127] See: Bigmore and Wyman (1880): page 195 who give Daniel Elsevier's date of death as 1689.

[128] See: DW Davies, *The world of the Elzeviers 1580–1712*, The Hague (1960).

[129] See: Rostenberg (1952): page 26 and footnote 75, which reads, 'M. M. Kleerkooper, "Daniel Elseviers Betrekkingen met Engeland" in Tijd scrift voor Boek-en Bibliotheekivezen (1910), VIII, 117; Robinson, of. Cit., 352: "April 6, 1678, [Hooke] talked with Martin about Eljiver."'

[130] See: Frans Korsten, 'The Elseviers and England'. In: Hellinga (2001): pages 131, 132, 133, and footnotes 4, 5, 23, pages 138 and 139. In 1675 Daniel Elsevier reclaimed copies of Hugo Grotius's (1583–1645) *De veritate religionis Christianæ* (1650: issued by Daniel Elsevier in 1675) confiscated by customs officers. This was mentioned in a conversation with Fell in Oxford. On a later occasion, 11 April 1678, Daniel met Robert Hooke and Abraham Hill (1633–1721); and in 1679 he was pleased to drink the health of John Locke (1632–1704).

order to spread costs.[131] Authors were pleased to have their books accepted by the Elsevier firm: 'I have been made a part of the immortal republic. I have been received in the society of the demi-gods'.[132] Between 1665 and 1680, in line with the interests of Daniel, the Amsterdam press focused on scientific books. He published many issues of works by René Descartes, and books by John Aubrey, Robert Boyle, Richard Lower, and Thomas Hobbes. The Short Title Catalogue for the Netherlands lists 683 items from Daniel Elsevier's shop of which Willis's *Pathologiæ cerebri, et nervosi generis specimen* (1668 and 1670) are numbers 389 and 439, respectively. The 1634 stocklist of Abraham (1592–1652) and Bonaventura Elsevier (1583–1652) had listed only seven books in English compared with more than 500 in French. By 1674, Daniel Elsevier's 800 page catalogue listing 20 000 titles with a single page of nineteen English language books.[133] English booksellers scrutinized foreign trade catalogues. John Martyn had the large Elsevier general Catalogue of 1674, and it is quite possible that he met Elsevier since Martyn discussed the Dutch dealer with Hooke. The evidence supports the view that Daniel Elsevier's publication of medical books that had been first published by James Allestry and John Martyn was by agreement. Each (but not Robert Scott) was identified with claims to the estate of Daniel Elsevier when the business was taken over by his widow in 1680.

Wilhelm Goeree (1635–1711) [**1H, 3C, 6H, 6J**] traded under the names Wilhelmus Goeree I or Guilielmus Goeree. He worked from 1668 to 1678 in his native town, Middelburg in Zeeland, from op den Burght under the signboard 'in Cicero'. After 1680, Goeree sold books in Amsterdam from Het Rokin (1681–1683), and de tusschen de Keisers en Prince-gragt, Leydse-straet (1683–1690), using the same signboard. His wife Elizabeth Janssonius van Waasberge (1643–1683) came from another printing family with whom Goeree had professional connections. Goeree's shop in Middelburg served as a branch for the von Waasberge family firm, but conflict arose about inheritance after the death of his father-in-law, Johannes Janssonius van Waasberge, in 1681, leading to a break between Goeree and the van Waesberge family. Goeree continued to work independently but spent more time writing on the art of drawing than publishing books. His son Willem Goeree II (nd) was active as a bookseller in Amsterdam from 1700 to 1726. Allowing for the change in name, the Short Title Catalogue for the Netherlands lists 62 items from Goeree's shop of which Thomas Willis's *Nieuwe en geneeskundige verhandeling vande fermentatie* (1676) and *D'algemeene en bysondere wercking der genees-middelen in s'menschen lichaam* (1677) are numbers 17 and 18, respectively.[134]

Johannes ten Hoorn (fl.1671–1711) [**1J**] was active from 1671 to 1715 as a prolific Amsterdam bookseller with a varied list ranging from academic works, among which were many medical texts, to popular works in Dutch. He worked from 1671 to 1709 at an address over het Oud-zijds Heeren Logement with a signboard 'in den History-schryver' used from 1686 to 1706, and in 1708. He was variously known as Jan Klaesz ten Hoorn, Johannes ten Hoorn, Joan ten Hoorn, Jean ten Hoorn, Jan Claesz ten Hooren, Jan ten Hoorn, Jan Tenhoorn, Jan Claesen ten Hoorn, or (simply) J.C.T.H. The Short Title Catalogue for the Netherlands lists 342 items from his shop of which *Nieuwe verhandeling van de koorsen*

[131] See: Kobsten (2001): page 132.

[132] Quoted by James Waddell, *Times Literary Supplement* 3 May 2019: page 33, citing Andrew Pettegree and Arthur der Weduwen, *The bookshop of the world. Making and trading books in the Dutch Golden Age*, London (2019).

[133] See: Hoftijzer (2001): page 91 and endnote 12 page 103.

[134] The Short Title Catalogue for the Netherlands omits the second volume of the Dutch translation of *Pharmaceutice rationalis* published in 1681 from Goeree's Amsterdam address without Johannes van Waesbergen, both in the list for Goeree and the twenty-three items listed under Thomas Willis's works.

(1681) is number 78. He also published many editions of works by Descartes, and the writings of Kenelm Digby.

Laurent d'Houry (1644–1725) [**1K**] was active from 1665 to *c.*1716 as a French bookseller working with his father, Jean d'Houry (d.1678) from 1665 to 1678, and continuing the business alone until 1712. He was variously known as Laurent Dhoury and Laurent of Hourry. In 1708, Laurent d'Houry was prosecuted for having established a printing press in his house and forced to sell the equipment. In 1716, he was imprisoned in the Bastille on the complaint of John Dalrymple, 1st Earl of Stair (1685–1747), ambassador in Paris, for disrespect to James, prince of Wales (1688–1766), nicknamed the Old Pretender and recognized by Louis XIV (1638–1715) as the legitimate king. In his almanac, d'Houry had not named James as King of England and failed to mention the prince's father, James II (1633–1701), who had been exiled to St. Germain. Despite these transgressions, d'Houry was appointed deputy assistant to the Order of Printers of Paris in 1716. Laurent d'Houry's bookstore and printing house produced numerous medical works including the only issues of Thomas Willis's treatises translated into French. At his death in 1725, the firm was continued by his widow and son (Charles-Maurice: 1688–1755) and grandson (Laurent-Charles d'Houry: 1723–1786).

Jean-Antoine Huguetan (1647–*c.*1750) [**8A, 8D**] was the son and successor of Jean-Antoine Huguetan II (1615–1681) and grandson of the first Jean-Antoine Huguetan (1567–1650), who had established the firm of Lyonnaise booksellers based between 1649 and 1680 in the Rue Mercière with the signboard 'À la Sphère'.[135] Jean-Antoine Huguetan II sold the business to his sons in 1680 who, in 1685, moved to Amsterdam as Huguenot refugees, setting up one of the most active Dutch book piracy businesses. Apart from the book trade, these Huguetans became wealthy through commercial activities and banking. There are few publications listing their names, as most of the output appeared under false imprints. It is also possible that publications listing their names were printed by others. It is thought that Jean-Antoine Huguetan III did indeed live to be around 100 years old.[136] Since there is nothing to distinguish the printer of the 1681 edition of *Opera medica et physica*, by which time the business had passed to the sons, from that of 1676, it seems most likely that both were the work of Jean-Antoine Huguetan III and not his father.

Arnold Leers (1643–1701) [**6C, 6D, 6G**] was active at The Hague from 1670 to 1699. He is not to be confused with his father, Arnout Leers I (also known as Arnold Leers and Aernout Leers) who worked in Rotterdam (fl.1644–1674) or his younger brother Reinier Leers (1654–1714) who took over the Rotterdam business in 1676. Arnold Leers II, was variously known as Arnout Leers II, Arnoldus Leers, A. (de jonge) Leers, or A. (junior) Leers. He worked from a shop at de Hoogh-straet (1670–1685; and again in 1688 and 1693) and de Groote zael (1688–1689) and de Speuystraat (1691) with the signboard 'in Plutarchus' (1670–1689).[137] The Short Title Catalogue for the Netherlands lists 123 items from his shop of which the issues of Thomas Willis's *Pharmaceutice rationalis sive diatriba de medicamentorum operationibus in humano corpore* (1674, 1675, and 1677) are numbers 16, 21, and 25. He also published the works of William Harvey, John Mayow, Walter Charleton (1619–1707), and Francis Glisson.

[135] See: IH van Eeghen, 'Europese "libraires": de gebroeders Huguetan in Amsterdam (1686–1705)', *Documentatieblad werkgroep 18e Eeuw*, numbers 53 & 54 (1982): pages 1–9; and IH van Eeghen, *De Amsterdamse boekhande*, volume III, Amsterdam (1965): pages 167–79.

[136] The digital collections catalogue of the University of Leiden offers these dates, equating to 103 years old. Biographical details of this particular member of the Huguetan family are not otherwise easily found.

[137] See: EF Kossmann, *De boekhandel te 's-Gravenhage tot het eind van de achttiende eeuw*, The Hague (1937): pages 231–4.

Felicem Lopez (fl.1664–1693) [**4B**] succeeded to the academic publishing business of his father David Lopez de Haro (1602–1670) in Leiden. The firm was located opposite the University. Lopez is variously known as Felix Lopes de Haro, Felix Loopes de Haro, or Felix Lopez. He also was printer to the college for the education of poor students of theology with a Walloon background (people speaking a French dialect who live in southern and eastern Belgium and neighbouring parts of France). Lopez worked from a shop in Het Raapenburg, teegen over de Academie from 1679 to 1688.[138] The signboard is unknown. The Short Title Catalogue for the Netherlands lists 150 items from his shop of which *Affectionum quæ dicuntur hystericæ et hypochondriacæ pathologia spasmodica vindicata, contra responsionem epistolarem Nathanael Highmori* is number 37 and identical to Driehuysen number 24. The variant title page with Lopez first named is not listed. Working with Driehuysen, Lopez also printed works by Francis Glisson, John Mayow, and Walter Charleton.

Joannes Malachin (nd) [**8I**] No details are known other than that he printed at Venice and was active at least from 1721 to 1724. He was variously known as Joannes Malachinum, or Joannes Malachini.[139]

Johannes Maximilianus Lucas (*c.*1646–1697) [**2E2**] was a Huguenot printer born in Rouen and active in Amsterdam (1672–1673, 1676–1680, and 1691); in Leyden from 1674 to 1675; and in The Hague from 1681 to 1690. His shop in Amsterdam was in Kalvestraet by de Dam from 1679 to 1680.[140] He is also known as Joannem Maximilianum Lucas. The Short Title Catalogue for the Netherlands lists 11 items from his shop of which Thomas Willis's *Cerebri anatome, cui accessit nervorum descriptio et usus* (1676) is number 4. Also listed is William Croone's *De ratione motus musculorum* (1676) which was published separately, and not bound with the 1676 edition of *Cerebri anatome*, as number 5.

Julii de Maphæis (nd) [**8I**]: no details are known.

Mariae Ruinetti (nd) [**8H**]: No details are known other than that Giuseppe Maria Ruinetti was active in Venice in the last decades of the seventeenth century and at least until 1704.[141]

Gerbrandt Schagen (b.1633) [**1E, 1F; 2C1, 2D, 2G**] variously known as Gerbrandt Schaghen or Gerbrandt Schagen and active between 1659 and 1688, was one of many smaller Amsterdam booksellers.[142] Schagen worked from shops in Kalverstraet, tegen over't Weeshuys, over St. Lucyen-steegh, inde naast de keysers kroon (1660–1666, 1685–1688). The emphasis of his list was on theology and his signboard was 'in de Staten Bybel' (1685–1687).[143] The Short Title Catalogue for the Netherlands lists 52 items from his shop of which Thomas Willis's *Diatribæ duæ medico-philosophicæ* (1663 and 1669), *Cerebri anatome* (1664 and 1666) are numbers 14 and 30, and 17 and 24, respectively. The variant title pages are not registered, nor is the issue in Dutch of [William Croone] *De ratione motus musculorum* listed. Schagen did publish two other items of importance with respect to Willis: Lower's *Diatribæ Thomæ Willisii* (1666), number 21; and O'Meara's *Examen diatribæ Thomæ Willisii* (1667, title page 1666), number 28. Schagen also published various works of Thomas Sydenham (1624–1689) and Robert Boyle.

[138] See: Eds. PG Hoftijzer and TSJG Bögels, *David en Felix Lopez de Haro (1627–1694). Boekverkopers op het rapenburg over de academie* Bibliotheek der Rijksuniversiteit, Leiden (1985): pages 1-65.

[139] See: Mario Emilio Cozenza, *Bibliographical and bibliographical dictionary of the Italian printers, and of foreign printers in Italy from the introduction of the art of printing into Italy to 1800*, Boston (1968): page 376 column 2.

[140] See: van Eeghen, volume III (1965): pages 228–39.

[141] See: Cozenza (1968): page 545, column 3.

[142] See: van Eeghen, volume IV (1967): pages 88–9.

[143] See: MM Kleerkooper, *De boekhandel te Amsterdam voornamlijk in de 17e eeuw*. Bijdragen tot de geschiedenis van den Nederlandschen boekhandel, volume 1, The Hague (1914): pages 688–9.

Johannes à Someren (1632–1678) [5C] variously known as Johannem à Someren, Joannes von Sommern, Johan van Someren, Jan van Zomeren, or Johannes van Zomeren was a well-established Amsterdam bookseller, active from 1665 to 1678 with a large and varied list.[144] He worked from shops in de (Korte) Gasthuys Molen-steegh / de Nieuwezijds Moolen-steegh (1656–1659), den Dam (1661–1674), and de Calverstraet (1674–1678). His signboards were 'in de Witte klock' (1657–1659), and 'in Perkins' (1661–1678). The Short Title Catalogue for the Netherlands lists 181 items from his shop of which Thomas Willis's *De anima brutorum quæ vitalis ac sensitiva est, exercitationes duæ* (1674) is number 115.

Gasparis Storti (nd) [8F, 8H]: no details are known other than that he printed at Venice where individuals of the same name were active from, at least, 1681 to 1796.[145]

Samuel de Tournes (1628–1695) [8B, 8C, 8G] came from a family of long-established printers, publishers, and booksellers based in Geneva but originating from Lyons in 1542. Jean de Tournes I (1504–1564) passed the business to his son Jean de Tournes II (1539–1615), then to Samuel's father Jean de Tournes III (1593–1669) in 1615, and eventually to Samuel (fl.1653–1695) and his brother Jean Antoine (fl.1653–1673). Jean de Tournes III sold the original house at the sign of the Deux Vipères in rue Raisin, Lyon, to the printer and bookseller Guichard Julliéron (d.1627) in 1619. After Jean de Tournes III retired in 1653, Jean Antoine and Samuel worked together until *c.*1673 after which Samuel published books on his own. Samuel was variously known as Samuel De Tournes, Samuel of I Tournes, or Samuel of Tournes I. He maintained strong trade relations with the Dutch book trade. The business passed to his son, Samuel de Tournes II (1669–1752) who was active from *c.*1695 to *c.*1719.

Adriaan Vlacq (1600–1667) [1A3, 1D1] established himself in The Hague in 1651, where he continued work until his death in 1667. Vlacq is variously known as Adriaen Vlack and Adriaen Vlac. He worked from a shop at 's-Gravenhage from 1651 to 1667, and as a printer during part of that period.[146] The Short Title Catalogue for the Netherlands lists 211 items of which Thomas Willis's *Diatribæ duæ medico-philosophicæ* (1659 and 1662) are numbers 105 and 161. Vlacq had a background in mathematics and, whilst living in Holland during his twenties, became interested in ideas on calculation using tables of logarithms. With Ezechiel de Decker (1603–1643), he translated and published books on this topic by John Napier (1550–1617) and Henry Briggs (1561–1630). The explanation for why a Dutch publisher produced an edition of Willis's first book in the year of publication (1659)[147] may lie in the fact that, in 1632, Vlacq became a bookseller in London, but he left for Paris at the start of the Civil War in 1642. The dedication in a book published 10 years later suggests that he sympathized with the Royalist cause and this may have brought him into direct contact with Thomas Willis. He remained in Paris as a bookseller until 1648 when he returned to Holland and started his business. Not all his customers were satisfied. Robert Creighton (1593–1672), who exiled himself in Utrecht, exploited Vlacq's strong connections with the English book trade in order to publish his history of the council of Florence (1660)[148] when his preferred publisher, Samuel Browne, moved to Heidelberg (1655–1662). But Creighton

[144] See: van Eeghen, volume IV (1967): pages 128–31.

[145] See: Cozenza (1968): page 602 column 2. He may be the Gasparo Storti listed in HF Brown *The Venetian printing press*, London (1891) London: page 417, who came from a family of Venetian publishers active between 1653 and 1796 that included Francesco Storti (fl.1724) and Eredi di Francesco Storti (nd).

[146] See: EF Kossmann, *De boekhandel te 's-Gravenhage tot het eind van de achttiende eeuw*, The Hague (1937): pages 435–43.

[147] See: chapter 5 for discussion of whether Vlacq has priority for publishing the first issue.

[148] See: Robert Creighton, *Historia Unionis inter Graecos et Latinos sive Concilii Florentini exactissima narratio*, Hagæ-Comitis (1660).

was dissatisfied and wrote to other contacts in Holland complaining that the printer 'should be called "Slack" instead of Flack'. Later Creighton expostulated:[149]

> We have been five months at press and yet in all that time we have printed but two sections, so if this business continues the whole book with my additions and prefaces will come to three more years stay. I went to Vlacq's house yesterday as I daily did—2, 3 or 4 times a day—to see how they composed their letters, or what proofs they had for me to correct and I expostulated with him that I had been there twice or thrice and found nothing going on. He answered me: Who commanded me to do so? And in the end at a great passion he bullied me to get out of his house, or he would take an order with me. He is the most perverse ill nature that lives.

After Vlacq's death in 1667, the business continued through his son, Johannes, but he remained active only for one year.

Johannes Janssonius van Waasberge (*c.*1616–1681) **[1H]** was the son of the Rotterdam bookseller Johann van Waesberge (1588–1633), and son-in-law of the Amsterdam printer-librarian Johannes I Janssonius (1588–1664) whose name he adopted forming the Amsterdam business of Johannes Janssonius van Waasberge in 1664. The firm had branches in Germany and Scandinavia. van Waasberge worked in association with Elizaeus Weyerstraten (d.1667) from 1664 to 1667, then with his widow and heirs until 1671. Johannes Janssonius van Waasberge (fl.1662–1680) was variously known as Johannes van Waesberge, J. à Waesberge, J.J. Waesberge, J.J. van Waasberge, Johannes Waesberg, Waesbergen, and Johannes Jansonius.[150] He worked from a shop at Het Water (1660–1680), and in de Laurier (1660–1662), using the signboard 'in de Pas-kaert' (1670–1673). The Short Title Catalogue for the Netherlands lists 222 items from his shop of which Thomas Willis's *Nieuwe en geneeskundige verhandeling vande fermentatie* (1676) and *D'algemeene en bysondere wercking der genees-middelen in s'menschen lichaam* (volume 1, 1677) are numbers 197 and 203, respectively. On receiving a large parcel of scientific books in the 'Latin-trade' written by Martin Lister (1639–1712)[151] and Robert Boyle from Samuel Smith (fl.1681–1703) van Waasberge, who was meant to sell these at 10 stuivers (half a guilder), wrote to Smith on 5 January 1685:[152]

> La balle de livres nous envoyé par Jean Janssen Rouland nous avons reçu, et dans la meme balle une grande quantité de Lyster et Boyle, mais comme ces livres se trouvent fort chères il est à craindre qu'ils se ne débiteront et aussi qu'ils seront contrefait et imprimés icy, car un livre de 9 feuilles petit papeir mettre à 10 sols netto est impossible de le vendre icy et personne ne le prendra à un si haut prix; et si vous considerez votre avantage vous trouverez juste qu'un livre qu'on imprimeroit icy pur 2½ sols personne ne payera pour sept sols; et les hauts prix sont pour la pluspart les causes qu'on peut à peine débiter les livres imprimeés en Angleterre.
>
> [We received the package of books sent us by Jean Janssen Rouland, and contained in this package were many books by Lyster and Boyle, but as the books are extremely expensive,

[149] See Keblusek (2001): page 155, and footnote 26, page 158.

[150] See: van Eeghen, volume IV (1967): pages 153–67.

[151] See chapter 3 for discussion of the inclusion of two figures on the oyster from *De anima brutorum* (1672: Pl.20) in Lister's publication on shells.

[152] See: Hoftijzer (2001): page 92. Although other sources give the year of van Waasberge's death as 1681, Hoftijzer (2001): page 92 mentions letters to Smith dated January 1685.

> and possibly will not sell, they might be counterfeit and printed here. Offering a little book of 9 pages for 10 sols [sous] net price, would be impossible to sell here, and no one would buy it at that high price. If you are to make a deal, you would accept that no one will pay 7 sols for a book published here for 2½ sols. And, generally speaking, the high prices are the reason for which books printed in England can hardly be sold.]

Smith supplied other Dutch dealers but the scientific books moved slowly and Pieter van der Aa (fl.1682–1730) returned to Smith seven of twelve copies of Isaac Newton's (1643–1727) *Principia mathematica* (1687) because they would not sell.[153]

Hendrik Wetstein (1649–1726) [**2F**; **8E**] came from a distinguished Swiss family and was active as a publisher from 1675 to 1725. His father and brother both held professorships in Greek and theology, and his grandfather was an eminent politician. Wetstein was born in Basle and first apprenticed to Jean Hermann Widerhold (*c.*1635–1683) in Geneva, then Daniel Elsevier in Amsterdam from 1669 to 1676 and can be regarded as Elsevier's successor. He was variously known as Heinrich Wetstein, Henricus Wetstein, Johann Heinrich Wetstein, Johann Hendrik, J. Henr. Wetstenius, and Henri Vetstein. He worked from a shop at de Calverstraet from 1685 to 1695. The Short Title Catalogue for the Netherlands lists 437 items from his shop of which Thomas Willis's *Opera omnia* (1682) and *Cerebri anatome* (1683) are numbers and 28 and 40, respectively. Wetstein was one of several Dutch booksellers who favoured English books, especially on spiritualism, and he published Dutch translations of Jane Lead's (1623–1704) *The heavenly cloud* (1681) and *The revelation of revelations* (1683).[154]

Gisbertus à Zyll (fl.1645–1672) [**1G**] was a lesser Utrecht publisher, variously known as Gisb. Zylius, Gysbert van Zyll, and Gisbertus à Zijll. He worked from a shop in op de Gansemarckt, from 1656 to 1666, and in 's Konings-Bijbel, at least during 1664. The Short Title Catalogue for the Netherlands lists 194 items from his shop, of which the volume on urines containing Thomas Willis's treatise *De urinis* (1670) is number 185.

[153] See: Hoftijzer (2001): page 100.

[154] See: Hoftijzer (2001): page 98 and footnote 62, page 105 citing Schonveld (1983) numbers 374 and 375.

3

'To delineate with most skillful hands'

Illustration and the printed works of Thomas Willis

Adding decoration to leaves of the codex is as old as the art of writing itself. By the seventeenth century, many printed books incorporated ornaments cut in relief on wood or metal to heighten attractiveness of the letterpress.[1] Other images served as the printer's trademark on the title page. More elaborate was the allegorical engraved title page or frontispiece.[2] Chapters were opened with decorated capital initials. Blank spaces at the beginning and end of sections were filled with head and tailpieces or repeats of simple ornaments. Many represented nature—leaves, stems, sprays, and flowers—and were therefore designated fleurons.[3] Partly because the depth of the woodcut and the metal type for that leaf differed, these images were often printed separately but the engraved block could be locked into the forme and inked with the text for a single pull of the press. This had the advantage of evening up the contour of the sheet so that part of the paper, otherwise blank, did not sag and compromise the printing process.

Introduced in the fifteenth century and gradually replacing complex images on wood, intaglio involved scoring lines on the surface of a copper plate using a burin or etching with acid. These engravings from metal had to be printed on a rolling press, different from that used to print text and woodcuts. The plate was inked and the surface wiped clean before pressing the dampened paper onto the plate so that it was forced into the still inked grooves. It is thought that, in order to register image and text, the engraved plate was inked and placed face down, the reverse of the normal arrangement, after the text had been printed and dried.[4] Engravings bound in as separate plate leaves could be designed much more elaborately than images added to spaces on the printed page, allowing skilled draughtsman to explain and complement the written text. Intaglio provided the greater level of detail needed to illustrate works on science and medicine. Engraving also allowed the more frequent use of the author's portrait. Whereas the text sheets were printed in one or a few impressions before redistribution of standing type, engraved plates were stored and reused over time to provide new batches of illustrations as required. The stocks of each did not necessarily match. Plate leaves that were reprinted when needed for binding with existing text sheets often showed signs of wear, with cracks appearing over time.[5]

[1] See: Plomer HR, *A short history of English printing 1476–1898*, London (1900): pages 12–13, and 26.

[2] The first image of relevance to medicine was the frontispiece to Erhard Reuwich's (1445–1505) *Gart der Gesuntheit* (1485), printed in Mainz by Peter Shöffer (1425–1503), which depicts a group of thirteen physicians listening to the description by one of a flowered medicinal herb, several of the others not evidently attending and two engaged in a rival conversation.

[3] See: *The Book Collector* (2017): pages 711–12 for discussion of fleurons introduced by punch cutters in the mid-1520s being mistaken for vine leaves and their combination as more complex ornaments, citing Hendrik Vervliet, *Vine leaf ornaments in Renaissance typography*, New Castle and 't Het Goy (2012); and Hendrik Vervliet, *Granjon's flowers: an enquiry into Granjon's, Giolito's and de Tournes' ornaments, 1542–1586*, New Castle (2016).

[4] See: Roger Gaskell, 'Printing house and engraving shop: a mysterious collaboration'; and 'Printing house and engraving shop, part II', *The Book Collector* (2004) 53: 213–51, and (2018) 67: 788–97. Gaskell provides details on the costs of setting up copperplate printing houses, the wages paid to skilled workers and insights obtained from a recently rediscovered work in verse by J Hanckwitz, *An essay on engraving and copper-plate printing* (1732) in which the author and his colleague, Smutty Dick and Black Tom, go about their laborious work amidst the still prevalent view of printing as closely allied to Satanism.

[5] See chapter 6 for the example provided by the various issues of *Cerebri anatome* printed in England. A letter to the *Times Literary Supplement* by Ruthven Todd from 29 August 1968 (reprinted *From the Archives* on 14

Ornaments were used more frequently by continental printers than those based in England. Work from Italy and France was aesthetically and technically the most superior.[6] It follows that decorations on the printed page were used sparingly by English printers but indulged by those producing Willis's books in continental Europe. The ornaments included many fleurons, head and tailpieces, and an occasional printer's device. These continental books also added a large number of decorated initials. The background images bear no relationship to the printed text.[7] Some are simply decorative; others are allegorical, fantastic in their design, or apparently relating to a particular event of no relevance to the books in which they appear.[8] Some letters, especially those used by individuals based in the Netherlands, were shared. Many appear to come from the same woodcutter or type foundry. When worn and unfit for further use, a new version was produced that closely resembled the original piece but differing in terms of sophistication, level of detail or size. Some decorated initials made use of criblé and factotums.

Decorated title pages

The design of title pages in the seventeenth century sometimes incorporated a device above the names of those involved in printing or selling the book.[9] Being expensive to produce, sometimes a generic design was passed around within the book trade; or a nondescript fleuron or tailpiece that had no personal significance, used elsewhere in the same book, was reproduced on the title page. The high period for use of printers' devices came after the last quarter of the sixteenth century coinciding with the decline of woodcutting and introduction of designs engraved on metal.[10] As illustrated title pages became more elaborate, with text printed on scrolls supported by architectural borders and frames, a theatre with its actors and stage director was adopted for scientific books of the late seventeenth century.[11] English printers associated with the publication of Willis's books occasionally incorporated devices on their other titles, but rather few were used in his books which, in terms of ornaments, remain simple and relatively unadorned.

December 2018) makes the point that copper plates originally etched by William Blake (1757–1827) *c.*1825 for Dante's *Inferno* Canto XXII, later declared worn and unusable, yielded excellent prints in 1968 when gently cleaned of dried ink from the grooves and applied to paper of the correct type and dampness.

[6] See: Henry R Plomer, *English printers' ornaments*, London (1924): pages 17–29.

[7] A notable exception is the engraved title page or frontispiece to Schagen's edition of *Cerebri anatome* (1666: **2D**) which appears on the dust wrapper and as Figure 114.

[8] This is in marked contrast to the decorated initials in Vesalius's *De humani corporis fabrica libri septem*, Basel (1543). For an account see: Samuel W Lambert, 'The initial letters of the anatomical treatise, *De humani corporis fabrica*, of Vesalius'. In: *Three Vesalian essays*, New York (1952): pages 3–24 where the background scene to the letter is always medical in context and, in one notorious example, a scatological tease on the juxtaposed text relating to rectal muscles.

[9] See: Alastair Fowler *The mind of the book, pictorial title pages*, Oxford (2017) for a detailed discussion of decorated title pages.

[10] See: Ronald B McKerrow *Printers' & publishers devices*, London (1913) for explanation of the difficulty in distinguishing devices from ornaments and less personalized emblems, especially those cast in metal which could more easily be reproduced and exchanged, despite which he is criticised by Plomer (1924): page 85 for several misclassifications.

[11] See: Fowler (2017): page 22. The Tournes firm, then in Lyons, which later published Thomas Willis's *Opera omnia* (Geneva 1676–1695) used sophisticated engravings by Jean Duvet (1485–1562) and others. See also: Paul Goldman, 'The history of illustration and its technologies'. In: Eds. Michael F Suarez and HR Woodhuysen, *The Oxford companion to the book* (2010) volume 1: pages 137–45. SH Steinberg, *Five hundred years of printing*, London (1996): page 69 is particularly hostile to the innovation of baroque engraved title pages describing the first example printed in London (1545) as 'already as fully repulsive as this aberration was ever to be' and blaming Christopher Plantin (1520–1589) for spreading a European epidemic from the pocket Elsevier editions to more regal folios celebrating the reign of Louis XIV (1638–1715).

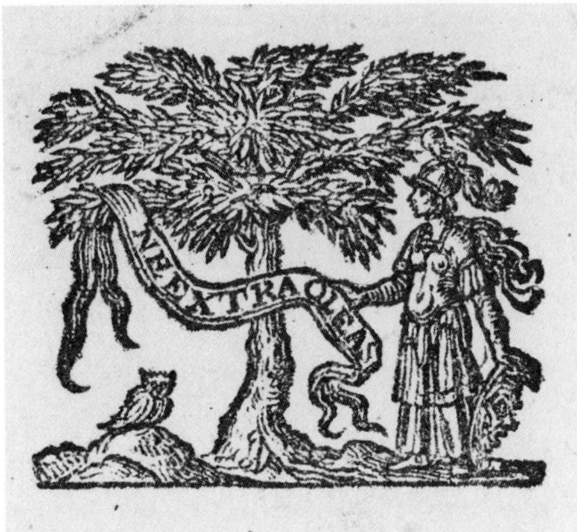

Figure 14 Printer's device used by Daniel Elsevier: *Pathologiæ cerebri*, Amsterdam, 1668 (Elsevier 1).

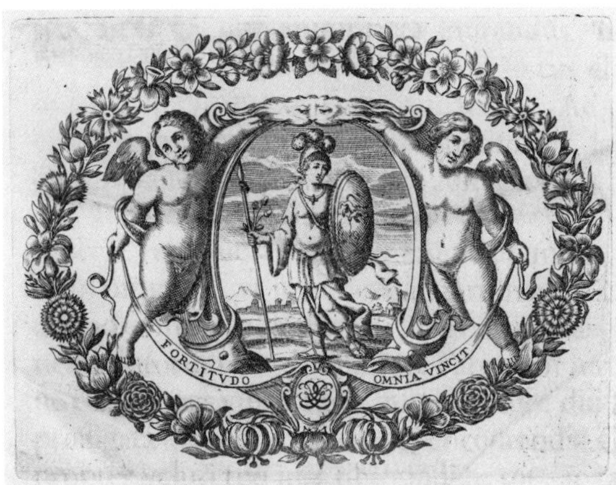

Figure 15 Printer's device used by Gasparis Storti: *Opera omnia*, Coloniæ, 1694 (Storti 1).

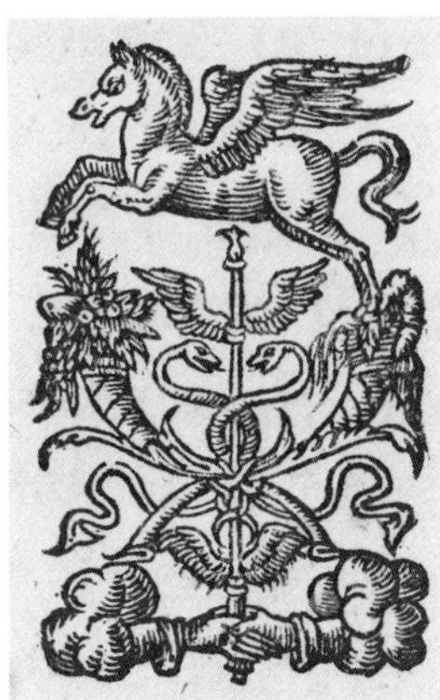

Figure 16 Printer's device used by Thomas Dring: *Pharmaceutice rationalis*, London, 1679 (Dring 3).

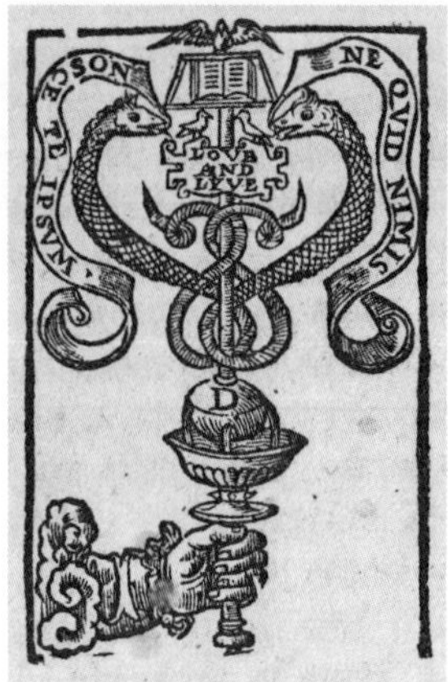

Figure 17 Printer's device used by Thomas Dring: *The remaining medical works*, London, 1681 (Dring 8).

The business of Thomas Harper (fl.1614–1656) whose (presumed) descendant Charles Harper (fl.1670–1709) printed books for Willis, used a device originally cut for Robert Waldegrave (*c.*1554–1603) around 1583 and still in use in the 1640s.[12] The device used by Henry Hall (fl.1642–1679) incorporated the arms of the University of Oxford on a shield within a rectangular frame with the motto 'SAPIENTA FELICITATIS' and 'ACADEMIA. OXONIENSIS' (Wisdom and Fortune, University of Oxford) which had belonged to William Turner (fl.1624–43) from 1628. A different device also showing the arms of the University of Oxford with the motto 'ACADEMIA OXONIENSIS SAPIENTIA ET FELICITATIS' was used in Oxford by Turner, passed to Hall in 1644 and used by him and Richard Davis (fl.1646–1688) at least until 1651.[13] In elaborate examples of Oxford printing, allegorical images and vignettes with explanatory verse were placed within compartments on the title page, as in Robert Burton's *Anatomy of melancholy* (1628). The Oxford printer did include a device showing the Sheldonian theatre in some issues of Willis's *Pharmaceutice rationalis* (1674, 1675, and 1679: **6A, 6E**, and **6I**). But in general, those who printed for Thomas Willis did not trouble themselves with these extravagances.

Consistent with the greater sophistication of other aspects of book design, title pages printed in continental Europe, often using black and red type, were generally more elaborate and attractive than those produced in England. The device of Henri Estienne (1460–1520), an olive tree with a falling branch combined with the figure of a man,[14] is recognizable in that used by Daniel Elsevier (1626–1680) in his printings of

[12] See: McKerrow (1913): page xxxiv.

[13] See: McKerrow (1913): page 153, #407; and page 159, #427.

[14] See: Fowler (2017): page 36. The tree refers to Israel and the church and the broken branch to unbelievers with the Gentile believers, the faithful, grafted on. This device was borrowed by John Wolfe (1548–1601) and later George and Elizabeth Purslowe (d.1632; and fl.1633–1646), John Norton (fl.1621–1645), and John Bill (1576–1630) allegedly by agreement with Paul Estienne (1566–1627) during a visit to London in 1594: see McKerrow (1913): pages xxv–vi.

Pathologiæ cerebri (1670: **3B1**, **3B3**). A more personalized device is used by Hendrik Wetstein (1649–1726) in his edition of the *Opera omnia* (1682: **8E**). But these are both surpassed by the extravagant devices used by Gaspar Storti (nd), Guiseppe Ruinetti (nd), and Joannes Malachin (nd) in the Venetian folio editions (1694, 1708, and 1720: **8F**, **8H**, and **8I**).

Leaving aside fleurons and tailpieces, nine printers used fourteen devices on the title pages of Thomas Willis's works. At first appearance, these are:[15]

> Commelin 1: *Cerebri anatome*, Amsterdam 1664 (**2C2**); Elsevier 1: *Pathologiæ cerebri*, Amsterdam 1668 (**3B1**); Fell 3: *Pharmaceutice rationalis*, part 1, Oxford 1674 (**6A**), Fell 9, part 2, Oxford 1675 (**6E**), and Fell 11: *Pharmaceutice rationalis* Oxford 1679 (**6I**); Huguetan 1: *Opera omnia*, Lyon 1676 (**8A**); Tournes 1: *Opera omnia*, Geneva 1676 (**8B**); Tournes 51 *Opera omnia*, Geneva 1680 (**8C**); Dring 3: *Pharmaceutice rationalis* London 1679 (**9A**); Dring 8: *The remaining medical works*, London 1681 (**9B**); Wetstein 1: *Opera omnia*, Amsterdam 1682 (**8E**); Wetstein 21: *Cerebri anatome*, Amsterdam 1683 (**2F**); Storti 1: *Opera omnia*, Coloniæ 1694 (**8F**): and Malachin 1 *Opera omnia*, Venice 1720 (**8I**).

Engraved frontispieces

Four editions of the printed works have engraved frontispieces, usually also duplicating details from the title page. The allegorical engraving (F.1a1) first included in *Diatribæ duæ medico-philosophicæ*, London 1660 (**1B**) is printed and bound at R11v, page [6] with oblique text: *Ita res accendunt lumina rebus* [In this way facts throw light on facts].[16] Surrounded by a black ruled border, two female figures, the one on the left robed, the figure on the right semi-clothed, set against an open room with chemist's earthenware and a retort in a garden with trees, are lighting torches held aloft using the sun's rays focused through a ring of glass. They stand on an architectural platform. The engraver is not identified. An explanatory poem is printed at R12r, page [7]:[17]

> ARtis *ope ætherios* Natura *exſuſcitat ignes*
> *Et cœlo attonitos, hac famulante vocat.*
> *Huic mox acceptas porrecta lampade flammas*
> *Reddit, & inde novum creſcit utrique jubar.*
> *Sic* lucem *unanimes* terris *tribuere* ſorores,
> *Et* lucem *unanimes ſic tribuere* ſibi.

[15] The numbers for each printer refer to the full list of their ornaments, detailed next. With later use, some engravings were in different states.

[16] The final line is a quotation from Titus Lucretius Carus (*c.*99–*c.*55 BC) *De rerum natura* Libri I, line 1117. This is variously translated. See: HAJ Munro, *On the nature of things*, Cambridge (1873): page 27 for 'in such wise things will light the torch for other things'; or WHD Rouse and MF Smith, *Lucretius de rerum natura*, London (1924): page 92 / 93, 'So clearly will truths kindle light for truths'.

[17] Translation by Jan van Gijn who points out this is literal, whereas a more felicitous reading might be: 'Nature helps Art to kindle her torch with sun rays and a magnifying glass. / The Art of Medicine uses the flame to recall the flame of life in people who seem dead / Medicine uses her torch to light the torch of Nature. / Now both ladies have a burning torch. / So the two sisters spread their light on earth / And to each other.'

By means of art Nature kindles celestial fires
And with her help she recalls the thunderstruck.
She soon returns the flames received from the extended torch
To her, and hence a new radiance grows from both.
So the sisters harmoniously distributed light to earth,
And so they harmoniously distribute it to themselves.

This is reproduced but printed with the poem at A1v, page [2] and the frontispiece at A2r, page [3] in the 'Editio Tertia' (1662: **1C**). The frontispiece is used in a new version (F.1b1) by Adriaan Vlacq (1600–1667) in the edition from The Hague printed with the frontispiece at A1r, page [1] and the poem at A1v, page [2] (1662: **1D1** and its London issue, **1D2**). This next appears, again reengraved, in the issue printed in Amsterdam by Gerbrand Schagen (b.1633) at A1r, page [1] (1663: **1E**; F.1c1). The obliquely printed text is present but the poem omitted. The image is reversed. The face of the sun is more evident; the foliage of the trees has changed; the face and proportions of the semi-clothed female figure are altered, as are the steps of the chemist's open room; the lines and cross-hatching are different; the border has gone and is replaced by a cartouche with the lettering AMSTELODAMI, | *Apud Gerbrandus Schagen*. This is reproduced by Schagen in the issue from Amsterdam (1669: **1F**; F.1c2) where he uses blank space on the architectural scroll to add the date *Anno* (left lower) and *1669* (right lower). A final printing of this frontispiece is at A2r, page [3] with the poem at A1v, page [2] in the London issue (1677: **1I**; F.1a1).[18]

Undoubtedly the most spectacular engraved title page relevant to Thomas Willis is that printed at A1r, page [1] in the Amsterdam issue of *Cerebri anatome* published by Schagen (1666; the image dated 1665: **2D**; F.2a1). Enclosed within a ruled border this has two main components. At the top are six surgical instruments in a cabinet surrounded by a frame scrolled on three sides and with an architectural border to the right. The instruments are scissors, saw, knife, clyster apparatus, retractor, and razor. These are flanked by a skeleton (left) and the skin of a headless figure. Below are a plant, a serpent, and a winged bird (presumably an owl). Further down are seven figures, six with hats and one wearing a skullcap, gathered around a dissecting table on which is placed a discretely robed corpse. The head is to the front and the prosector is holding a probe to the opened skull. Waiting at the foot of the table is a spotted dog (we can assume this to be a Dalmatian). The end of the table is lettered: CEREBRI | ANATOME | *Cui aceſſit* | NERVORUM | Deſcriptio & Usus | STUDIO THOMÆ WILLIS. The floor is tiled. Outside the border but as part of the plate is printed: AMSTELDOMI | Apud GERBRANDUM SCHAGEN. M. DC. LXV.

A preliminary sketch for this image is held in the prints and photographs collection of the history of medicine division of the National Library of Medicine.[19] The artist is unknown but the image has many similarities to the plate used for Francis Glisson's *Anatomia hepatis* (1665) published in Amsterdam by Johann Janssonius a Waasberge (1588–1664) and Elizaeus Weyerstraten (d.1677). Drawn in pencil, it measures 175 × 120 millimetres, with lines in ink and grey wash to the tonal areas. It is reversed with respect to the printed image. A window in the extreme upper left of the drawing has been removed and details of the

[18] See: chapter 5 for details of changes to accents on certain words in resetting the poem for these different editions.

[19] Details are taken from Ellen B Wells (edited by Dorothy M Schullian), 'Notes and Events', *Journal of the History of Medicine* (1967): pages 182–85.

cabinet are improved. The placing of the cadaver is unusual in that the head is foremost, an arrangement reproduced by Adriaan Backer (1635–1684) in 'The anatomy of Professor Fred. Ruysch' (1670). The figure in the skullcap is presumed to be Willis.[20] This image from 1665 therefore precedes the first known portrait engraved by David Loggan (1634–1692) printed in 1667. However William Feindel (1918–2014) does not agree. He considers that the prosector is Richard Lower (1631–1691) with Willis, the more commanding presence and elegantly dressed, to his left; John Hemming (nd), the apothecary, with notebook; the others, in no special order, being Christopher Wren (1632–1723), Thomas Millington (1628–1714), Edmund King (1630–1709), John Locke (1632–1704), and Robert Hooke (1635–1703).[21] The spotted dog refers to experimental work on vascular injection. The snake represents health and immortality and leads towards the owl, which may reflect wisdom or the mythical ability of the owl to sniff out the putrefaction of death.

Although this engraved frontispiece does not appear in any other printings of Thomas Willis's works, it may have been intended for the Schagen 1664 edition (**2C1**). In a notarized statement dated 30 June 1664, witnessed by Caspar Commelin (fl.1659–1690) and Michael de Groot (nd), Schagen commissioned Salomon Savry (1594–*c.*1665), who had worked in Oxford in the 1630s, to produce two copper engravings for *Cerebri anatome* over the next eight days in return for 15 guilders exclusive of materials. One is likely to have been the engraved frontispiece; and the other may have been the plate leaf found in Croone's *De ratione motus musculorum*.[22] Kenneth Russell (1911–1987) is of the opinion that the engraved frontispiece is called for in Schagen's 1664 issue of *Cerebri anatome* (**2C1**) but 'lacking' from the copy he examined in the Sydney University Library.[23] Ellen Wells writes that she contacted Harold Denham (1917–1999) who confirmed on 15 December 1966 that, in his opinion, the frontispiece was not intended for the 1664 issues.

The edition of *Pharmaceutice rationalis* (part 1) printed 'ex officinâ' (from the workshop) in The Hague by Arnold Leers (1643–1701: 1674, **6C**; F.3a1) has an allegorical engraved title page at *1r, page [1]. Within a ruled border, three figures are placed at the top. On the right is an unclothed female with a winged and starred headdress, standing in front of a skeleton, astride a plinth lettered DISTINCTI VERI (Distinct and True), which gesticulates at her. The figure is holding a burning lamp in her left hand and addressing a second, clothed, female who has a five pointed starred headdress containing letters. Her right hand is directed towards a third figure, who appears to be sick, with left hand pointing towards a caduceus. To the right of the lettering PHARMACEUTICE | RATIONALIS. | *Authore.* | Thom. Willis. M.D.|1674.|is Britannia seated with her head turned away and her sleeve engraved SOCIETAS REGII (Royal Society). On the right is a stone plinth engraved *Romeyn de Hoogh fecit 1674.* Romeyn de Hoogh (1645–1708) was a Dutch painter, sculptor and engraver who illustrated books and designed emblems. He was conspicuous for the complex arrangement of figures in his prints and, later in his career, considered by some to be risqué in his subject matter, reflecting his personal lifestyle. His satire depicting the efforts of William of Orange (1650–1702) at the end of the seventeenth century in relentless wars against the French

[20] See chapter 6 for Figure 113, showing the preliminary sketch; and Figure 114 and front cover of the dust wrapper for details of the printed version.

[21] See: William Feindel, 'The beginnings of neurology: Thomas Willis and his circle of friends'. In: Ed. F Clifford Rose, *A short history of neurology: the British contribution 1660–1910*, Oxford (1999): pages 1–18.

[22] See chapter 6 for other details of the commission to Savry and discussion of plates used by Schagen and Commelin.

[23] See: KF Russell, *British anatomy. 1525–1800*, Melbourne (1963): page 224 (item 870).

monarch Louis XIV (1638–1715) and his allies, depicted as a battle between liberty and religious despotism, is not without its admirers.[24]

An engraved allegorical title page is included at π2r, page [3] in the *Opera omnia* (1682) published in Amsterdam by Wetstein (**8E**; F4a1). The border is double-ruled. Set in a rural landscape is a castle wall with a five pointed star lettered SALUS (safety), surmounted by six stone figures on the crest, and with surrounding shrubs and trees. Two figures are standing on a stone column. One is a naked male, perhaps a satyr, with a bow and arrow standing next to a partially obscured figure with a long beard. Nine human figures are shown. The two on the extreme left are conversing with each other but not otherwise involved in the scene. An older man in robes is touching the arm of the central figure, female with one breast bared, who is turning the pages of a book supported on a round table with the pedestal formed by a child's skeleton at whose foot is placed a human tibia. An urn sprouting vegetation is alongside. In the female's left hand is a lancet with which she is dissecting an opened human head sitting on a stone plinth. Five figures are grouped to the right. A sick man is lying on a couch with one other speaking close to his ear and a second person touching his arm. One of the two remaining men gazes distractedly and the other is drawing a horizontal section of the brain with his right hand whilst gesturing with his left to the engraved title on the plinth, lettered TH | WILLIS | OPERA | OMNIA. At the bottom on a step leading up to the tiled floor is engraved *AMSELÆDAMI* | Apud HENRICUM WETSTENIUM | CIↃ IↃ CLXXXII. The artist and engraver are unknown. To summarize the details of these sparse but spectacular engravings:

F.1a1. Engraved allegorical frontispiece with oblique text: *Ita res accendunt lumina rebus*. 122 × 68 millimetres (plate marks), 117 × 65 millimetres (image). *Diatribæ duæ medico-philosophicæ*, London 1660 (**1B**); London 1662 (**1C**); London 1677 (**1I**); see: Figure 95.

F.1b1. Engraved allegorical frontispiece with oblique text: *Ita res accendunt lumina rebus* [diagonal, top left to bottom right]. 125 × 70 millimetres (plate marks), 116 × 65 millimetres (image). *Diatribæ duæ medico-philosophicæ*, The Hague 1662 (**1D**).

F.1c1. Engraved allegorical frontispiece with oblique text: *Ita res accendunt lumina rebus*; AMSTELODAMI, *Apud Gerbrandus Schagen*. 127 [cropped] × 66 millimetres (plate marks), 126 [cropped] × 65 millimetres (image). *Diatribæ duæ medico-philosophicæ*, Amsterdam 1663 (**1E**); see: Figure 96.

F.1c2. Engraved allegorical frontispiece with oblique text: *Ita res accendunt lumina rebus*; AMSTELODAMI, *Apud Gerbrandus Schagen, Anno 1669*. 131 [cropped] × 69 millimetres (plate marks), 126 [cropped] × 65 millimetres (image). *Diatribæ duæ medico-philosophicæ*, Amsterdam 1669 (**1F**).

F.2a1. Engraved title page: CEREBRI ANATOME *Cui acceſſit* NERVORUM Deſcriptio & Uſus STUDIO THOMÆ WILLIS. AMSTELODAMI Apud GERBRANDUM SCHAGEN. M. DC. LXV. 127 × 78 millimetres (plate marks), 115 × 75 millimetres (image). *Cerebri anatome*, Amsterdam 1666 (**2D**); see: Figure 114, and dust wrapper.

F.3a1. Allegorical engraved title page: PHARMACEUTICE RATIONALIS. *Authore*. Thom. Willis. M.D. *1674*. *Romeyn de Hoogh fecit 1674*. 123 × 66 millimetres (cropped)

[24] See: Arnold Houbraken, Romeyn de Hooghe (biography). In: *De groote schouburgh der Nederlantsche konstschilders en schilderessen*, Amsterdam (1718): pages 257–9; and Simon Schama, 'Liberty and laughter will live on', *Financial Times* (7 January 2015): page 1.

(plate marks), 121 × 67 millimetres (image). *Pharmaceutice rationalis*, The Hague 1674, 1675 (**6C, 6D**); see: Figure 137.

F.4a1. Allegorical engraved title page: TH WILLIS OPERA OMNIA *AMSTELÆDAMI* Apud HENRICUM WETSTENIUM CIↃ IↃ CLXXXII. 223 × 176 millimetres (plate marks), 220 × 168 millimetres (image). *Opera omnia*, Amsterdam 1682 (**8E**); see: Figure 149.

Portraits of Thomas Willis

Although crude by comparison with illuminated manuscripts, the practice of including an image of the author was maintained after the introduction of printing from woodcuts and metal engravings. Printed separately from the text leaves and bound within the preliminaries, these usually featured the author enclosed in an oval frame, the whole surrounded by a cartouche often with elaborate strapwork. The patron or printer might be named or even depicted as part of the engraving. Some images identified the artist and engraver. The tendency not to include portraits of authors until their collected works were published posthumously did not apply to Thomas Willis.

A plate leaf with his image was first printed by William Hall (fl.1656–1672) on behalf of James Allestry (d.1670) and bound before A1r, page [1] in the first edition of *Pathologiæ cerebri* (1667: **3A**; Pt.1a1). It shows Willis aged 45 dressed in a fine coat with white collar, trimmed moustache and hair to the shoulders, turned to his left with the eyes facing, surrounded by an oval frame within which is cross-hatching and horizontal lines outside. The expression is reflective and conveys the impression of authority. The engraving is signed *D: Loggan: delin: et sculpt* at the base on the left. Below is a border with vertical lines labelled *AETATIS SUÆ, 45*. There is the impression of exotropia on the right with a slight ptosis.[25] The plate was retained for copies printed in the first edition of *Affectionum quæ dicuntur hystericæ et hypochondriacæ* (1670: **4A**); and, despite the sheet size increased for folio format, in *The remaining medical works* (1681: **9B**) and the first two editions of *Dr Willis's practice of physick* (1681, 1684: **9C, 9E**).

David Loggan's image was reengraved for several of the books published after 1667. Some are faithful to the original, others more loosely based on Loggan but recognizable as having been copied from his original depiction. Loggan was born in Danzig, Poland, the only son of John Loggan (b.1608), a Scottish merchant.[26] He learned engraving in Poland from Willem Hondius (1598–1652) and Crispijn de Passe (*c.*1597–1670) in Amsterdam. Later, Loggan lived in London and established his reputation after portraying Oliver Cromwell (1599–1658), shortly before Cromwell's death. In the 1660s, Loggan become well known for his black lead portraits on vellum including a depiction of Charles II (1630–1685), architectural images such as the view of St Paul's Cathedral engraved for Daniel King (d.1664) in 1658, and book work including the title page to the *Book of common prayer* (1662) and plates for William Dugdale's (1605–1686) *Origines judiciales* (1666). Loggan moved to Oxford during the 1665 plague where his reputation for portraits led to an association with Anthony Wood (1632–1695), Elias Ashmole (1617–1692) and John Aubrey (1626–1697). Whilst living in

[25] Accounts of Thomas Willis make no mention of difficulty with vision or hints of a partial third cranial nerve palsy and this may merely be an artistic effect.

[26] The details that follow are taken from Geoffrey Tyack, 'David Loggan' *Oxford Dictionary of National Biography* (2004): https://doi.org/10.1093/ref:odnb/16945.

Holywell Street, in 1669, Loggan sold his rolling press to the University of Oxford. Through the influence of John Fell (1625–1686), Loggan was appointed engraver on 30 March 1669 with an annual retainer of 20*s*, and later made a member of the University.

Loggan is thought to have engraved the plates for *Cerebri anatome* (1664) and *De anima brutorum* (1672), and the three versions of the image showing the Sheldonian Theatre which appeared on the title pages of *Pharmaceutice rationalis* (1674–1679: **6A**, **6E**, **6I**). His engravings for *Oxonia illustrata* (1675), a set of aerial views of the Colleges, academic halls, and University buildings, with a map, originally intended for Wood's *The history and antiquities of the university of Oxford* (1674), was much admired. Loggan engraved Christopher Wren's design for the new library at Trinity College, Cambridge (1676) and that led to the production of *Cantabrigia illustrata* (1690). As a result, Loggan was also appointed engraver to the other University. George Vertue (1684–1756) noted that Loggan so 'hurt his sight in delineating of King's College Chappel . . . that he engraved but little afterwards'. This seems unduly pessimistic since Loggan moved back to London, living in Leicester Fields where he was a neigbour of Thomas Willis in St Martin's Lane, continuing to engrave portraits and images of books and furniture, and experimenting with mezzotints. Loggan was assisted by Robert White (1645–1703) who also depicted Willis, after Loggan's image. Despite his prominence, Loggan died in Leicester Fields with few assets and debts of £140. He was buried on 1 August 1692 at St Martin-in-the-Fields.

The Amsterdam and London issues of *Pathologiæ cerebri* published by Daniel Elsevier (1668, 1670: **3B1**, **3B3**) and James Allestry (1668: **3B2**) each have the Loggan portrait printed at *6v, page [12] (Pt.1b1). The arrangement is broadly similar to the 1667 version but the plate is reduced in size and reversed so that Willis points to the right with his head turned and facing. The frame is cropped on all four sides, the dress subtly different and Willis's expression now appears less settled and somewhat more quizzical. The apparent ptosis and exotropia are now on the left. Loggan's name and attribution as artist and sculptor are removed. The portrait is not included in the London (1678: **3D**) issue printed by Samuel Roycroft (1657–1717) for John Martyn (1618–1678).

A version of the Loggan portrait next appears in the *Opera medica & physica* published by Jean-Antoine Huguetan (1647–*c.*1750)[27] in Lyon (1676, 1681: **8A**, **8D**; Pt.1c1) printed at *1r, page [1]. The arrangement is familiar: Willis is turned to the right but his eyes are lowered and not engaging the reader. The drooping right eyelid and exotropia are apparent. The proportions of head and torso are changed, the head too small and short, the face more rounded, the chin less prominent, the right shoulder too large, and details of the dress recognizable but different from 1667. The oval frame has the lettering THOMAS WILLIS MEDIC. PROFESSOR. COLLEGII MED. LONDON. ET SOCIET. REG. SOCIVS, with a rosette fleuron separating SOCIVS from THOMAS. Underneath is ÆTATIS SVÆ, 45.

A new version of the Loggan image is engraved and printed as ¶4v but sometimes bound before ¶1r as page [2] in the *Opera omnia* published by Samuel de Tournes (1628–1695: 1676, **8B**; Pt.1d1). Willis is turned to the left with the eyes directed forwards, wearing the same gown with bands, tassel, and collar, albeit slightly altered. The drooping right eyelid and exotropia are apparent. There is cross-hatching within the oval frame and horizontal lines. It is signed *Fr: Diodati. Pin. ſcu.* Beneath a thin border of vertical lines is: THOMAS WILLIS, M. D. *Naturalis Philosophiæ Professor Oxoniensis, necnon Inclyti Medicinæ Collegii Londinensis, & Societatis Regiæ Socius* (unusually, the long *ſ* is not used). By comparison

[27] These dates seem improbable but several sources do state that Huguetan lived to 100 years old.

with the Geneva imprint (**8B1**), those from Coloniæ Allobrogum (**8B2**, **8B3**) show marked cracking suggesting that the Geneva issue came first.[28] The same image but with subtle alterations to the engraving is used by Tournes in his later issues (1680: **8C**, 1695: **8G**; Pt.1d2) by which time it is showing signs of wear. François Diodati (1647–1690) was a deafmute French-Swiss engraver and painter on enamel who also illustrated works by Robert Boyle (1627–1691).

The engraving printed by Wetstein at π1v, page [2] in *Opera omnia* (1682: **8E**; Pt.1e1) is closer to Loggan's original than most others in proportions of the head and torso, and facial expression, but has the eyes differently directed, again with apparent exotropia. Design of the oval frame and the background engraving are after Loggan. All lettering is omitted, leaving blank space under a three-stepped plinth for an entry in manuscript.[29] Also close to Loggan's original arrangement in terms of orientation, proportions, facial appearance, clothing, oval frame and background, but lettered *Thomas Willis M. D.* in the space within the lower border, is the version included in all but the last issue of *The London practice of physick* (1685–1692: **10A1**–**10A3**; Pt.1f1) and those of *A plain and easie method* printed in the sixteenth century (1691: **7A1**, **7A2**; Pt.1f1). This is signed *R. W. ſculp*. Robert White was active as a prolific portrait engraver from 1666 to 1702.[30] As with his tutor Loggan, White used black lead on vellum and produced work of high artistic merit and representational quality. He also engraved frontispieces, bookplates, almanacs, architectural views, and notices of public events. White illustrated Andrew Snape's (b.1644) *The anatomy of an horse* (1683) taking the images from earlier woodcuts. He worked from Bloomsbury Market charging between £4 and £30 depending on the size of the image and was assisted by his son, George (*c.*1684–1732). Nonetheless, Robert White died poor, perhaps through competition from mezzotint, which he tried himself. At his death in October 1703, the business was acquired by John King (fl.1698–*c.*1703).[31]

The portrait included in the *Opera omnia* printed by Storti (1694; **8F**), Ruinetti and Storti (1708; **8H**), and Malachin (1720, **8I**: Pt.1g1) follows Huguetan, although the proportions and facial expression are closer to Loggan. It differs in that the lettering around the frame has SOCI^{VS} for SOCIVS. The sleeves of Willis's coat are more finely elaborated and the dress extends lower. The engraving has *suor Isabella Piccini S'colpì* on the left end of the top shelf of the tiered plinth. Isabella (Elisabetta) Piccini (1644–1734) was descended from a family of Venetian graphic artists. She was trained by her father and uncle, Guglielmo (nd) and Jacopo (nd) who engraved reproductions of paintings by Titian (Tiziano Vecelli: 1488–1576) and Peter Paul Rubens (1577–1640). On Guglielmo's death, Elisabetta requested and was granted exclusive rights by the Doge of Venice to print certain engravings. In 1663 she joined the convent of Santa Croce in Venice and took the name of Sister Isabella (hence 'soror Isabella' on the portrait of Thomas Willis), with which she signed her work. All her income was distributed between the convent and her family. Isabella retained her obligations as a nun for the annual sum of 200 ducates. She paid the dowry for her sister Franceschina who entered a monastery in 1673 but later resigned in order to marry. Isabella was appointed abbess in 1718, aged 74, remaining in post until ten years before her death on 29 April 1734. Not surprisingly most of her work adorned religious texts, but Isabella also illustrated books on philosophy,

[28] See chapter 12 for further discussion of priority for the two 1676 editions.

[29] In the example used for this bibliography, a previous owner has added: *Thomas Willis, M. D.* Of two other copies, one has an ownership inscription and the other is left blank.

[30] The details that follow are taken from Antony Griffiths, 'Robert White', *Oxford Dictionary of National Biography* (2004): https://doi.org/10.1093/ref:odnb/29268.

[31] See: Plomer (1922): pages 179–80.

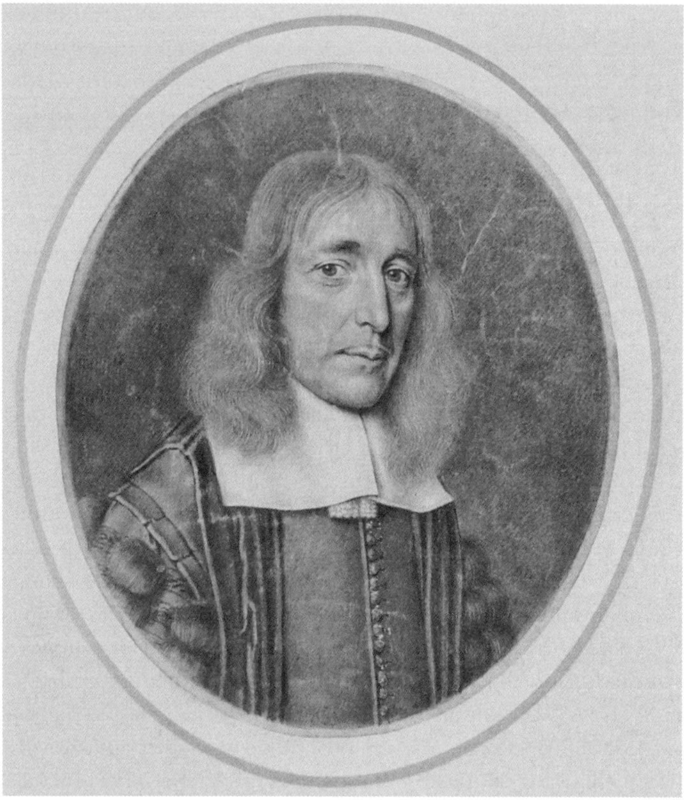

Figure 18 Drawing in graphite on vellum of Thomas Willis by David Loggan, 1667. Bequeathed to the Ashmolean Museum by Reverend William Bentinck L. Hawkins, 1894.

horses, and poetry, working closely with the firm of printers founded by Giovanni Antonio Remondini (b.1634) who worked in Bassano de Grappa from the mid-seventeenth century and distributed Isabella's prints throughout Europe.

Apart from portraits included in the printed works of Thomas Willis, a different version, also by Loggan and completed in 1667, drawn in black lead on vellum, is in the Ashmolean Museum.[32] This shows Willis turned to the left with head and eyes facing forwards. It measures 147 × 127 millimetres (oval). He is barely recognizable by comparison with the image by Loggan printed in 1667 (see: Figure 18). The brow, high cheekbones, and chin are less pronounced but the long nose, and his coat and collar, are as in the more familiar version. He looks weary. Two engraved images by William Read (nd) survive with copies in the Wellcome Library.[33] One shows the familiar hair, long nose, and moustache but the face is fuller, round, and shortened. Willis is turned to the left and with his gaze averted. He is

[32] See: http://collections.ashmolean.org/collection/search 'David Loggan AND Thomas Willis'.

[33] See: https://wellcomecollection.org/works/jx8t2awc; and https://wellcomecollection.org/works/vzajms6v. One is listed by Robert Martensen (2004). It is unclear whether these ever appeared in a printed book. The engraver may be William Read (fl.1824–1837); see: Renate Burgess, 'WILLIS, Thomas [1622–1675], In: *Portraits of doctors & scientists in the Wellcome Institute of the history of medicine*, London (1973): page 393, no. 3196.8; and page 451.

wearing the usual brocade coat with white collar indicating that this is copied from Loggan. The figure is unframed and set against a minimum of stippled background engraving. The image is signed *W Read Sc* set diagonally under the torso on the left, and entitled THOMAS WILLIS MD. The second, also attributed to Read, shows Willis turned to his right with the head and eyes forward but the gaze averted. The face is easily recognized, as are the coat and collar. There are widely spaced horizontal lines as background but nothing outside the single oval lined frame.

In 1742, George Vertue was commissioned by Browne Willis (1682–1760) for £21 to produce a new engraving (see: Figure 1). More elaborate than Loggan's this appeared, together with a short biography, in Thomas Birch's (1705–1766) *Heads of various illustrious persons of Great Britain* (1743–1751).[34] Willis is faithfully copied from the Loggan engraving with the same posture, hair, moustache, facial appearance, and dress. The text on the spandrel reads: THOMAS WILLIS M.D. ob^{t}. 1675. Æta. 54. Above the elaborate cartouche is a caduceus. Placed on a clothed table to the left are a human vertebral column and ribcage, a skull, two medicine bottles, and two open books. Central are feather quills, an inkstand, and paper. To the right is an opened copy of the 1679 English edition of *Pharmaceutice rationalis* showing various images taken from part 2 (Tabulæ II, III, and IV, but not in the arrangement as printed). Below the table are three unidentified books and the Willis coat of arms showing three lions rampant in an inverted triangular arrangement.[35] Beneath the image is printed: *G. Vertue Sculp 1742 ___ in the poſseſsion of Browne Willis Esq Impensis J. & P. Knapton Londini 1742*. The engraving measures 363 × 233 millimetres (plate marks); 343 × 219 millimetres (image). After Loggan, it is the most attractive image and richly allegorical in its arrangement of books and furniture. Apart from the various medical objects, Willis does not appear to have aged much in the nine years since his portrait was first done by Loggan.

A further version, anonymous but close to Loggan in posture and overall design, appeared in the *Universal Magazine* with the lettering: THO^{s}. WILLIS, M.D. | *Printed for J. Hinton at the Kings Arms Paternoster Row*. It measures 155 × 92 millimetres (see: Figure 19).[36] John Hinton (fl.1732–1781) sold books in Bow Street, Covent Garden, then from the King's Arms, St. Paul's Churchyard, Newgate Street near Warwick Lane, and later from the King's Arms, Paternoster Row. It is unclear whether the J. Hinton accused in 1739 of selling bogus issues of the *Craftsman* in Bow Street was a relative. Undoubtedly the Hintons were not above controversy and John appeared as plaintiff in an action against Alexander Donaldson (1727–1794) in Edinburgh in 1773 over copyright to the printing of Thomas Stackhouse's (1677–1752) Bible, the rights to which he had acquired by marrying the widow of the original holder, Stephen Austin (fl.1768–1776).[37] It was

[34] See plate preceding the biographical entry at volume 1, pages 119–20; further editions were published in 1756 and 1813.

[35] See chapter 1 for discussion of the genealogy of the family and the Willis coat of arms.

[36] This is undated but the issue of the *Universal Magazine of Knowledge and Pleasure* for July 1768, volume XLIII: pages 17–22 has a biographical essay on Thomas Willis largely based on the account in *The general dictionary* (1641: see chapter 1) and presumably also written, or authorized, by Browne Willis. 'DIRECTIONS to the BINDER for placing CUTS in this Forty-third VOLUME' in the index lists 'The Head of Dr Willis' at page 17. The online example of this volume has no engraving at page 17 or elsewhere in the file. The example illustrated (Figure 19) is from a contemporary print present in the archive formed by Raymond Hierons, the origin of which is unknown.

[37] See: HR Plomer, GH Bushnell and ER McC Dix, *A dictionary of the printers and booksellers who were at work in England, Scotland and Ireland from 1726 to 1775*, Oxford (1932, for 1930): pages 10 and 126.

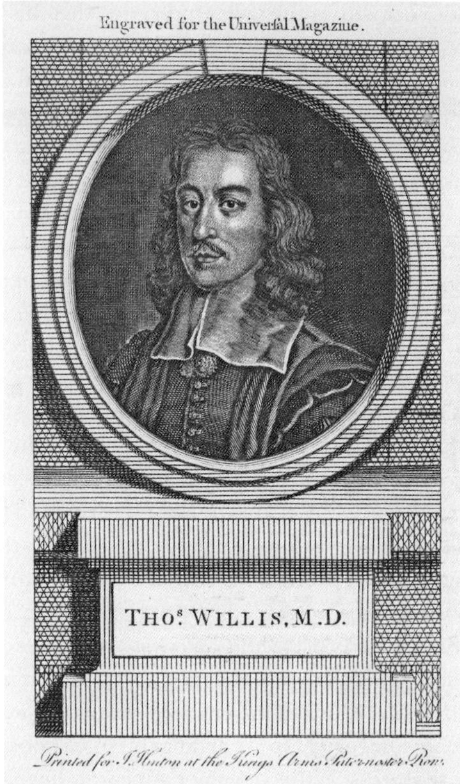

Figure 19 Portrait of Thomas Willis: the *Universal Magazine*, London, 1768.

presumably a son, also J. Hinton, who published the *Universal Magazine* from 1781 until his death on 21 May 1814.

There are two surviving oil paintings of Thomas Willis. One, attributed to John Wollaston (1710–1775), is now in the Lower Reading Room of the Bodleian Library.[38] This is oil on canvas measuring 740 × 620 millimetres, acquired as a gift from Humphrey Bartholomew (d.1764), a physician, in 1735. It shows Willis much as engraved by Loggan in terms of orientation, posture, facial appearance, hair and moustache, and dress (see: frontispiece). There is no hint of exotropia or ptosis. The portrait in the Royal College of Physicians of London is by an unknown artist (see: dust wrapper). It is oil on canvas measuring 749 × 622 millimetres, and shows Willis turned to the right, the head and grey eyes forward but the gaze averted, with dark brown hair and more luxuriant moustache than in other images, the black coat decorated with gold, white collar, and ribbed white cuffs. Willis is holding a partly rolled scroll marked 'Anatomy B . . .'. It is inscribed at the top: *THOMAS WILLIS MD, FRS Morum Suavitate insignis. Summo Omnium, ac imprimis merito* [Impressive by the sweetness of his manners. By the summit of all, and especially as deserved].[39] There is a record of a portrait

[38] See: Image No. BOD000067-01 (Lower as in upper, not Richard Lower).

[39] See: *The Royal College of Physicians of London. Portraits* (catalogue I). Eds. Gordon Wolstenholme, the portraits described by David Piper, London (1964): pages 444–5. This portrait was acquired by the College in 1911,

donated to the University of Oxford by Browne Willis in 1720, not that in the Bodleian, and one other believed to have been amongst his property in 1760, but both are now lost.[40] Robert Hooke (1635–1703) reported:[41]

> Saw Mr Dwight's English China, Dr Willis his head, A little boye with a hauke on his fist, Severall little Jarrs of severall colours all exceeding hard as a flint, very light, of very good shape. The performance very admirable and outdoing any European potters.

Unfortunately examples of this porcelain piece have not survived. To summarize the details of those portraits included in the printed works:

Pt.1a1. [Engraved portrait of Thomas Willis] *D: Loggan: delin: et sculpt | ÆTATIS SUÆ, 45*. 187 × 139 millimetres (plate marks), 184 × 135 millimetres (image). *Pathologiæ cerebri*, London 1667 (**3A**); *Affectionum quæ dicuntur hystericæ et hypochondriacæ*, London 1670 (**4A**); *The remaining medical works*, London 1681 (**9B**); *Dr Willis's practice of physick*, London 1681, 1684 (**9C, 9E**); see: Figure 118.

Pt.1b1. [Engraved portrait of Thomas Willis] *ÆTATIS SUÆ, 45*. 109 × 65 millimetres (plate marks), 107 × 64 millimetres (image). *Pathologiæ cerebri*, Amsterdam 1668, 1670; London 1668 (**3B**); see: Figure 119.

Pt.1c1. [Engraved portrait of Thomas Willis] THOMAS WILLIS MEDIC. PROFESSOR. COLLEGII MED. LONDON. ET SOCIET. REG. SOCIVS, with ÆTATIS SVAE, 45. 172 × 130 millimetres (plate marks), 168 × 127 millimetres (image). *Opera medica & physica*, Lyon 1676, 1681 (**8A, 8D**); see: Figure 147.

Pt.1d1. [Engraved portrait of Thomas Willis] THOMAS WILLIS, M. D. *Naturalis Philosophiæ Professor Oxoniensis, necnon Inclyti Medicinæ Collegii Londinensis, & Societatis Regiæ Socius*, [signed] *Fr: Diodati Pin. ſcu.* 205 × 153 millimetres (plate marks), 202 × 150 millimetres (image). *Opera omnia*, Geneva 1676 (**8B**); see: Figure 148.

Pt.1d2. [Engraved portrait of Thomas Willis] THOMAS WILLIS, M. D. *Naturalis Philosophiæ Professor Oxoniensis, necnon Inclyti Medicinæ Collegii Londinensis, & Societatis Regiæ Socius*, [signed] *Fr: Diodati Pin. ſcu.* 202 × 153 millimetres (plate marks), 202 × 150 millimetres (image). *Opera omnia*, Geneva 1680, 1695 (**8C, 8G**).

Pt.1e1. [Engraved portrait of Thomas Willis] [*Thomas Willis, M.D* added in manuscript]. 213 × 158 millimetres (plate marks), 204 × 154 millimetres (image). *Opera omnia*, Amsterdam 1682 (**8E**); see: Figure 150.

the earlier provenance being unknown. It is described as likely to have been made up posthumously from various images and, incorrectly, the editors state that the original engraving by Loggan appeared as a frontispiece to *Pharmaceutice rationalis (*1674), an error reproduced by Martenson (2004) who wrongly cites such copies in the British Library. Whoever transcribed the inscription on the portrait in the College of Physicians misread 'merito' for 'marito' thereby altering the meaning to the less likely 'Impressive by the sweetness of his manners. By the summit of all, and especially as spouse'.

[40] See: J Trevor Hughes, *Thomas Willis 1621–1675. His life and work*, London (1991): pages 108–9.

[41] See: Eds. Henry Robinson and Walter Adams, *The diary of Robert Hooke (1672–1680)*, London 1935: pages 86–7; and Dewhurst (1980): page 23 and endnote 141 at page 36. Despite the punctuation, Hooke is referring to several different pieces, one of which has Willis's head.

Pt.1f1. [Engraved portrait of Thomas Willis] *R. W. ſculp. Thomas Willis M. D.* 162 × 107 millimetres (plate marks), 150 × 95 millimetres (image). *London practice of physick*, London 1685, 1689, 1692 (**10A1–10A3**); *A plain and easie method*, London 1691, 1695 (**7A1, 7A2**); see: Figure 158.

Pt.1g1. [Engraved portrait of Thomas Willis] THOMAS WILLIS MEDIC. PROFESSOR. COLLEGII MED. LONDIN. ET SOCIET. REG. SOCI^{VS}, *suor Isabella Piccini scolpì*, AETATIS SVÆ. 45. 262 × 171 millimetres (plate marks), 258 × 167 millimetres (image). *Opera omnia*, Venice 1694, 1708, 1720 (**8F, 8H, 8I**); see: Figure 151.

Head and tailpieces

Most of those who printed Thomas Willis's treatises included decorations of one kind or another. With few exceptions, each printer used his or her own set of ornaments.[42] The same piece locked into a different forme may explain the repeated appearance of one design on different sheets within a single printed work. That some appear within a single signature indicates that, as with type letters and punctuation, indistinguishable copies of each were available.

Several books include headpieces at the start of new sections and tailpieces in blank space where a chapter ends.[43] Most headpieces are rectangular. Some are made up of individual fleurons differing in design or repeating the same motif, occasionally reversed and inverted, in order to create a larger and visually more interesting arrangement (see: Figure 31). Repeated use led to signs of wear, cracking, and broken corners. Sometimes a fragment was used, alone or in combination with another piece (see: Figure 24). Tailpieces are usually shaped as inverted triangles, or otherwise designed to provide visual symmetry with the textblock above.

These ornaments incorporated botanical items (stems and leaves, curved or intertwined, rosettes, individual flowers or sprays, acorns and fruit, corn stooks, garlands of fruit or flowers); furniture (urns, pedestals, plinths, baskets); vehicles (chariots); musical

Figure 20 *Dissertation sur les urines*, Paris, 1683 (D'Houry 2).

[42] One exception is the use of Thomas Roycroft's ornaments in the quarto edition of *Pathologiæ cerebri* (1667: **3A**), although he appears not to have been involved in the printing; see chapter 7 for details of the publication.

[43] Plomer (1924): page 55 makes the point that, whereas he was able to draw upon existing sources and collections in his chapter on borders, no such authority existed for consideration of ornaments used to fill blank spaces at breaks in the text of printed books, and he was required to break new ground.

Figure 21 *Opera omnia*, Lyon, 1676: (Huguetan 2).

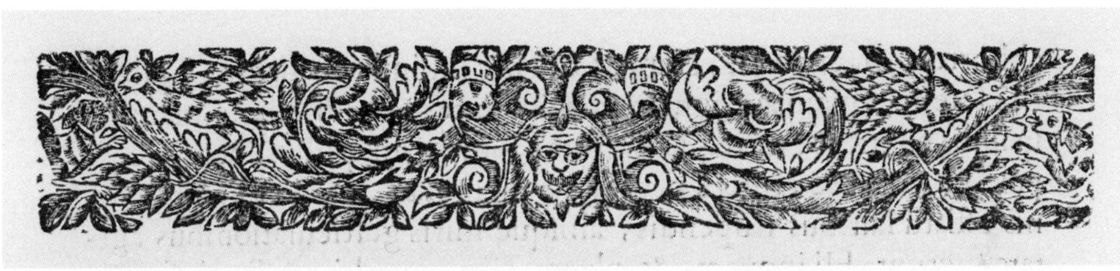

Figure 22 *Opera omnia*, Lyon, 1676: (Huguetan 4).

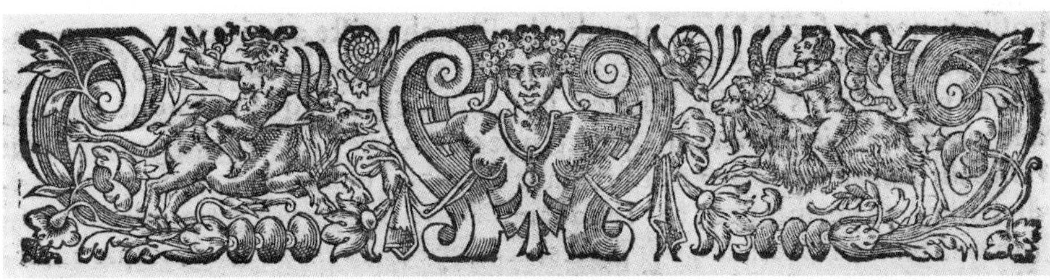

Figure 23 *Opera omnia*, Lyon, 1676: (Huguetan 41).

Figure 24 *Pharmaceutice rationalis* part 2, The Hague, 1677: (Leers 11: cut down and inverted).

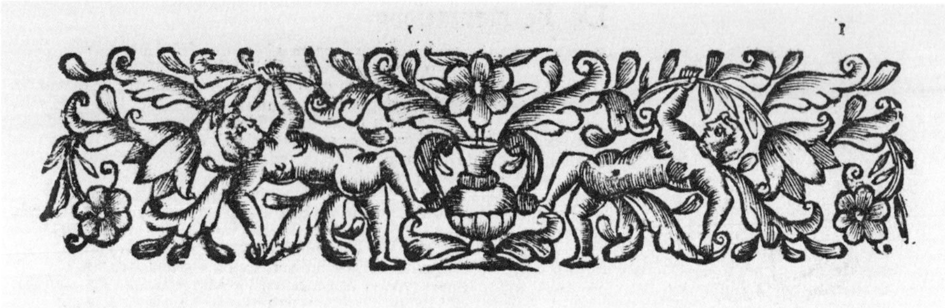

Figure 25 *Opera omnia*, Venice, 1720 (Malachin 4).

Figure 26 *Diatribæ duæ medico-philosophicæ*, London, 1662 (Roycroft 21).

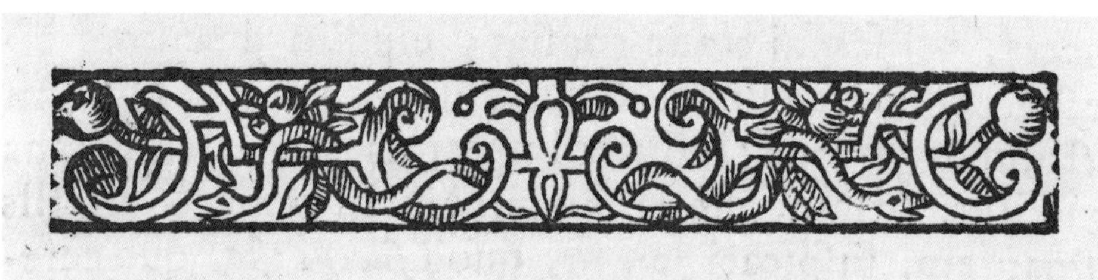

Figure 27 *Diatribæ duæ medico-philosophicæ*, London, 1662 (Roycroft 25).

Figure 28 *Pathologiæ cerebri*, London, 1678 (Roycroft 37).

Figure 29 *Pathologiæ cerebri*, London, 1678 (Roycroft 39).

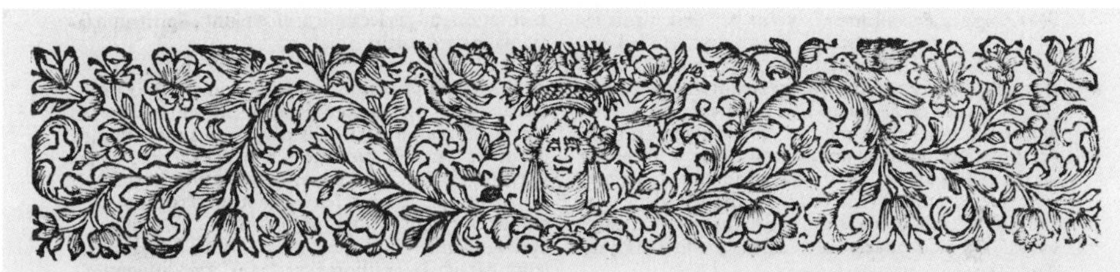

Figure 30 *Opera omnia*, Venice, 1708 (Ruinetti 11).

Figure 31 *Diatribæ duæ medico-philosophicæ*, Amsterdam, 1663 (Schagen 1 and 2).

Figure 32 *Diatribæ duæ medico-philosophicæ*, Amsterdam, 1663 (Schagen 9).

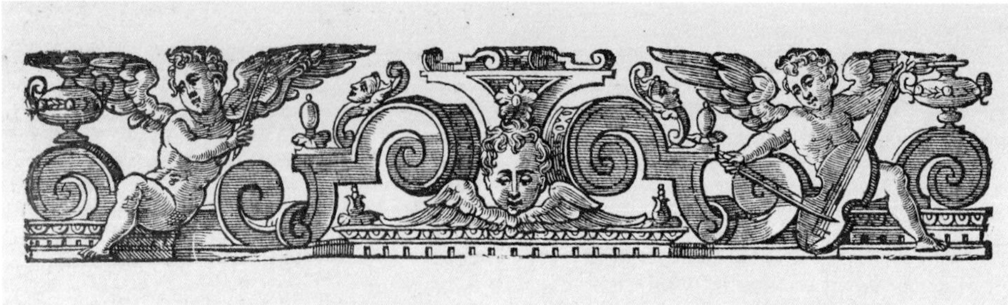

Figure 33 *Opera omnia*, Coloniæ, 1694 (Storti 12).

Figure 34 *Opera omnia*, Geneva, 1676: (Storti 25).

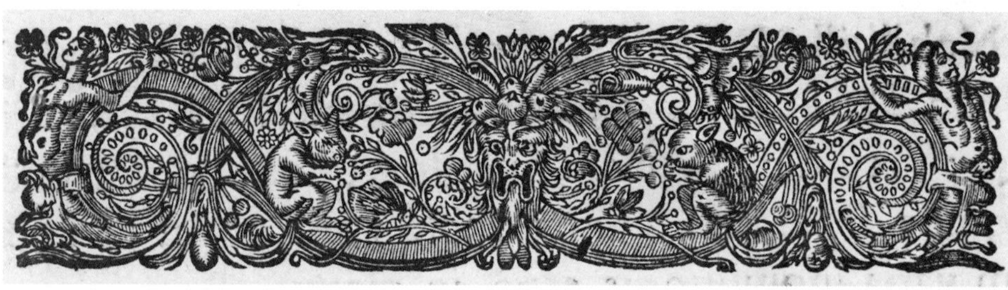

Figure 35 *Opera omnia*, Coloniæ, 1694 (Tournes 2).

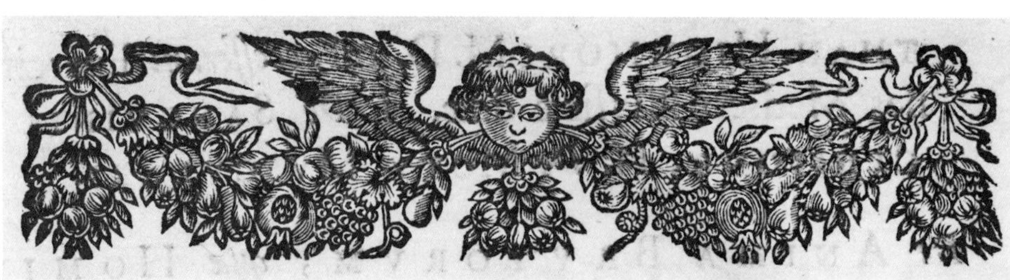

Figure 36 *Opera omnia*, Geneva, 1676: (Tournes 4).

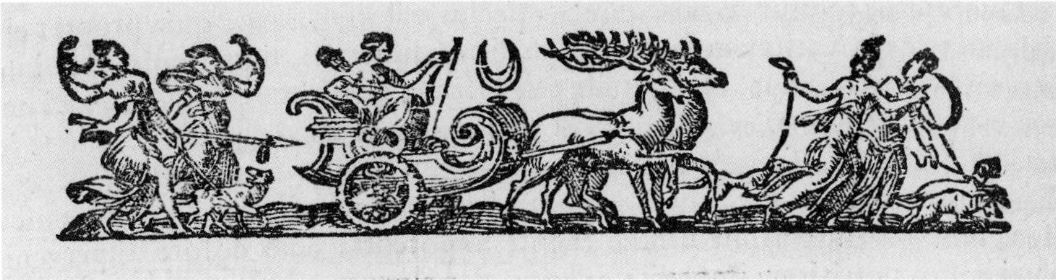

Figure 37 *Opera omnia*, Geneva, 1676: (Tournes 26).

Figure 38 *Opera omnia*, Geneva, 1676: (Tournes 35).

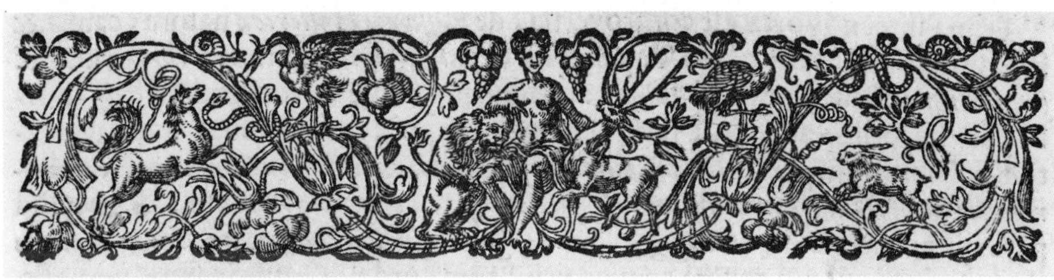

Figure 39 *Opera omnia*, Geneva, 1676: (Tournes 39).

instruments (harps, viols, flutes, and horns); animals and insects (squirrels, horses, hounds, hares, deer, lions, reindeer, dogs, bears, lambs, snails, snakes, locusts, and serpents); birds (ravens, doves, eagles, owls, peacocks, and swans); human figures (children and adult males and females); recognizable individuals (Minerva, Romulus and Remus, Bacchus, Neptune, and Adam and Eve); mythical creatures (cherubs, angels, and griffins); hybrid animal and human forms (mermaids and satyrs); national emblems (rose, thistle, and fleur-de-lys); shapes (rectangles, penwork, scrolls, strapwork, and arabesques); and borders (cartouche, lines, stipples, and dots).

Whilst many of the images are simply decorative, others are more informative even if their meaning is elusive, enigmatic, or private to the cutter and printer. Roycroft incorporated a deconstructed caduceus, and imaginary scenes of cherubs riding horses. In a background of stems, leaves, buds, bird, and squirrels, Huguetan included a human face, complete with moustache and pointed beard that may be a self-image. Later he used a design that incorporates stems, leaves, flowers, snails, unclothed males riding a bull and a goat, and a garlanded African female with one eye closed. Tournes had leaves, stems, flowers, with mermaids, squirrels eating nuts, a lion's head, four females with dogs on leashes, and a chariot pulled by reindeer. Storti used a figure playing the viol (held under the chin) and a violin. Wetstein had stems, flowers, hares, goats, men carrying bows and arrows, and a seated figure supporting peacocks.

As with other ornaments, individual tailpieces were shared. By way of example, one ornament was first used by Johannes van Ravenstein (fl.1659–1679) in 1670, and passed to Jacob de Jonge (fl.1657–1678) and then his widow (fl.1679–1684) before being linked to Wetstein from 1682.[44] It served both as a tailpiece and an 'ornament as printer's device' on the title page. The central motif is a 'house-mark' with lettering I D I which, although first used in books published by van Ravenstein, suggests Iacob De Ionge. The design incorporating a large diagonal cross and inverted triangle also appears in a headpiece used by Gerbrandt Schagen in 1663 (**1E**) and Hendrik Wetstein in 1682 (**8E**). This may simply be a printer's mark copied by engravers working on behalf of different printers, publishers, and booksellers. But if it has symbolic significance, the design may relate to alchemy.[45]

Ruinetti depicted urns, seated figures in a landscape with distant roofed building, and leaping harts. Arthur Bettesworth (d.1739) had stems, leaves, and flowers on a criblé background within an elaborate cartouche. Scientific books printed in Oxford after Willis's death, included head and tailpieces engraved by Michael Burghers (*c.*1647–1727) depicting Britannia with her shield and trident flanked by books and mathematical instruments.[46] This construction had already been incorporated in the allegorical engraved title page for Arnold Leers's editions of *Pharmaceutice rationalis* part 1 [**6C** and **6D**; F.3a1 (see earlier)]. Together, thirty-six headpieces are used by sixteen printers. At first appearance, these are:

> Allestry 2: *Affectionum quæ dicuntur hystericæ et hypochondriacæ*, London 1670 (**4A**); Bettesworth 1: *A plain and easie method*, London 1721 (**7B**); D'Houry 1 and 2: *Dissertastion sur les urines*, Paris 1683, 1687 (**1K1, 1K2**); Driehuysen 1: *Affectionum quæ dicuntur hystericæ et hypochondriacæ*, Leyden 1671 (**4B**); Fell 1: *De anima brutorum*, Oxford 1672 (**5A1**); Fell 4: *Pharmaceutice rationalis* (part 1), Oxford 1674 (**6A**); Goeree 5: *Nieuwe en Geneeskundige verhandeling vande fermentatie*, Middelburg and Amsterdam 1676 (**1H**); Huguetan 2, 4, 41 and 43: *Opera omnia*, Lyon 1676 (**8A**); Huguetan 55 and 82: *Opera omnia*, Lyon 1681 (**8D**); Leers 11: *Pharmaceutice rationalis* (part 2) The Hague 1677 (**6G**); Malachin 4: *Opera omnia*, Venice 1720 (**8I**); Roycroft 21 and 25: *Diatribæ duæ medico-philosophicæ*, London 1662 (**1C**); Roycroft 27: *Diatribæ duæ medico-philosophicæ*, London 1677 (**1I**); Roycroft 37 and 39: *Pathologiæ cerebri*, London 1668 (**3B2**); Ruinetti 4 and 11: *Opera omnia*, Venice 1708 (**8H**); Schagen 7 and 9: *Diatribæ duæ medico-philosophicæ*, Amsterdam 1663 (**1E**); Schagen 12: *Diatribæ duæ medico-philosophicæ*, Amsterdam 1669 (**1F**); Storti 12 and 25: *Opera omnia*, Coloniæ 1694 (**8F**); Tournes 2, 4, 26, 35 and 39: *Opera omnia*, Geneva 1676 (**8B**); Vlacq 1: *Diatribæ duæ medico-philosophicæ*, The Hague 1662 (**1D1**); and Wetstein 3 and 18: *Opera omnia*, Amsterdam 1682 (**8E**).

[44] See: P. van Huisstede and J. P. J. Brandhorst, *Dutch printers' devices 15th–17th century: a catalogue*, three volumes, Nieuwkoop (1999): volume 1, page 652; volume 2, pages 907 and 1155; and Arkyves-Brill: https://brill.com/view/db/arko.

[45] This suggestion was made in correspondence with Goran Proot, 17 June 2020.

[46] See: Plomer (1924): page 76.

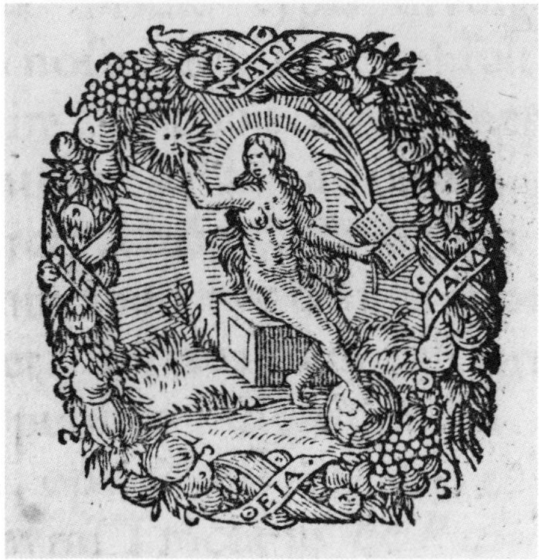

Figure 40 *Cerebri anatome*, Amsterdam, 1664 (Commelin 1).

Figure 41 *Dissertation sur les urines*, Paris, 1683 (D'Houry 4).

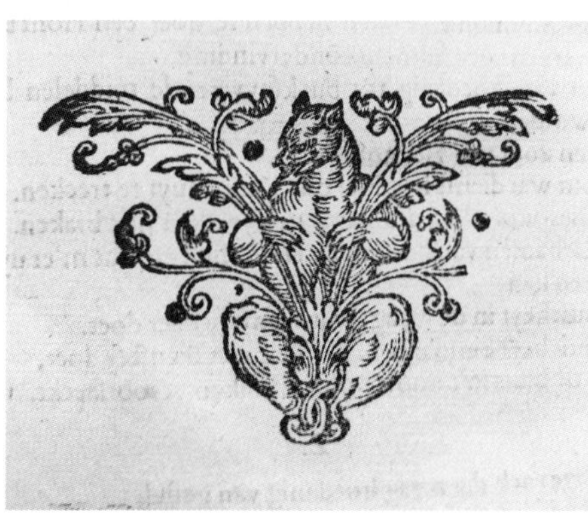

Figure 42 *Genees-middelen in s'menschen lichaam*, Middelburg and Amsterdam, 1677 (Goeree 12).

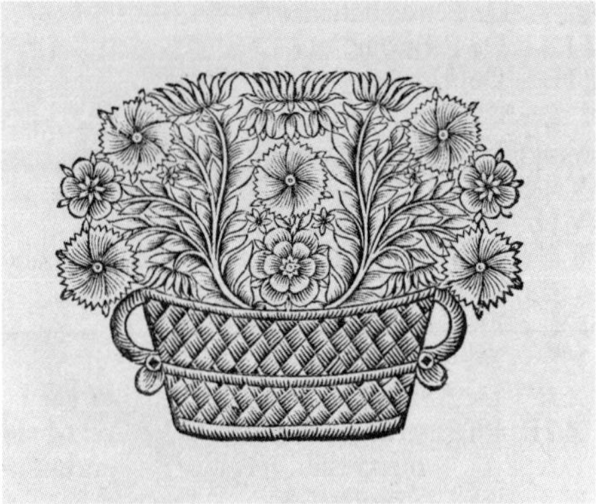

Figure 43 *Opera omnia*, Lyon, 1676 (Huguetan 8).

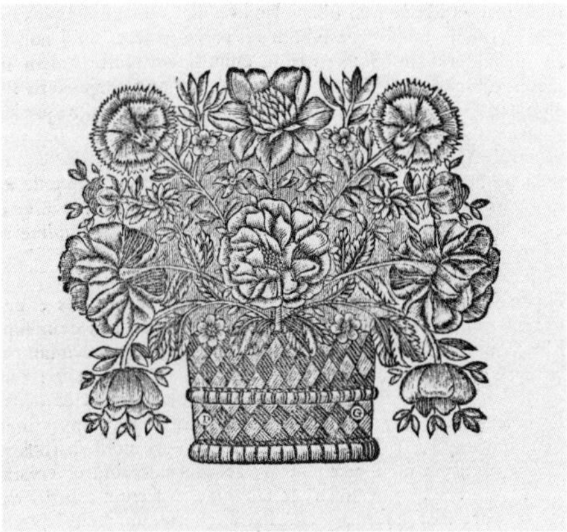

Figure 44 *Opera omnia*, Lyon, 1676 (Huguetan 29).

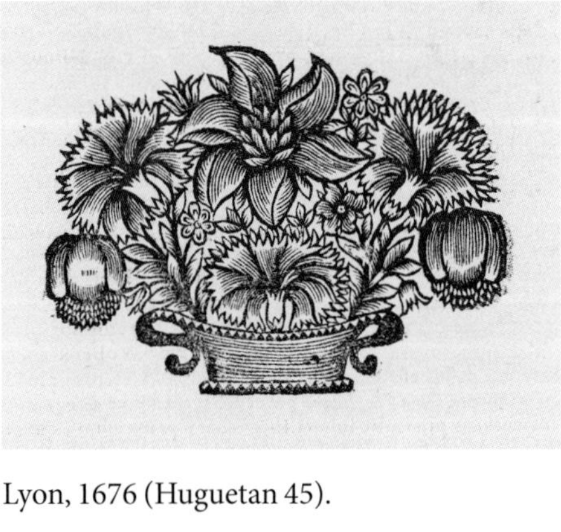

Figure 45 *Opera omnia*, Lyon, 1676 (Huguetan 45).

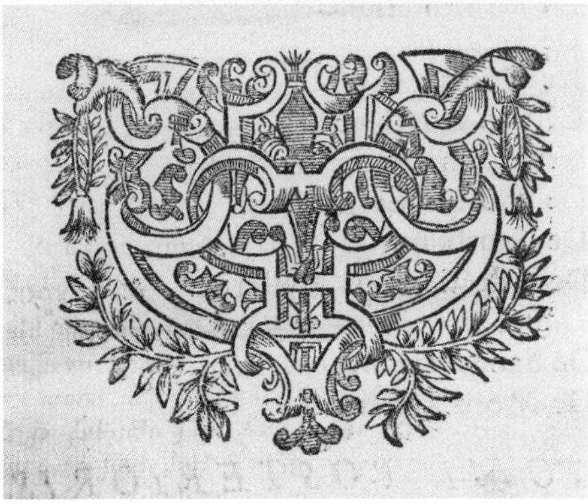

Figure 46 *Opera omnia*, Lyon, 1681 (Huguetan 57).

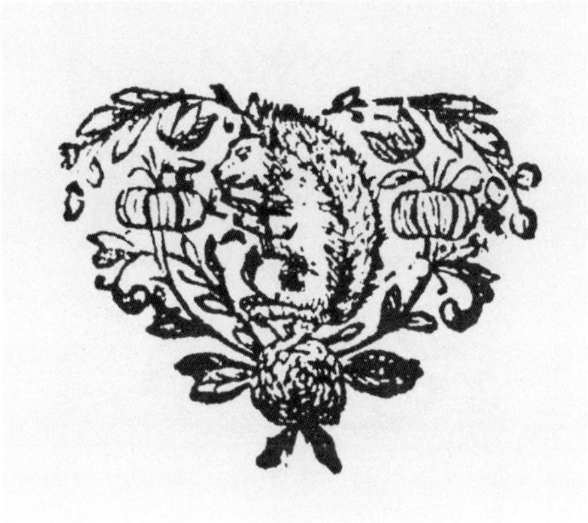

Figure 47 *Pharmaceutice rationalis* part 2, The Hague, 1677 (Leers 12).

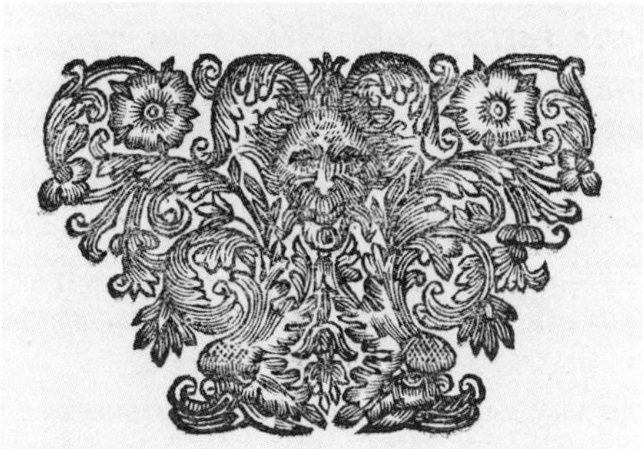

Figure 48 *Opera omnia*, Venice, 1720 (Malachin 3).

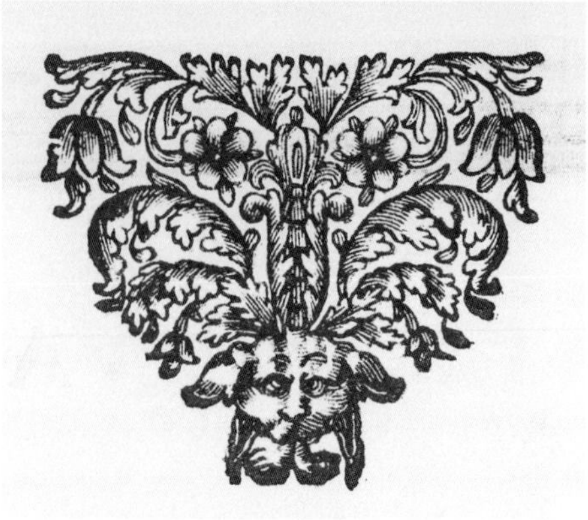

Figure 49 *Opera omnia*, Venice, 1708. (Ruinetti 3).

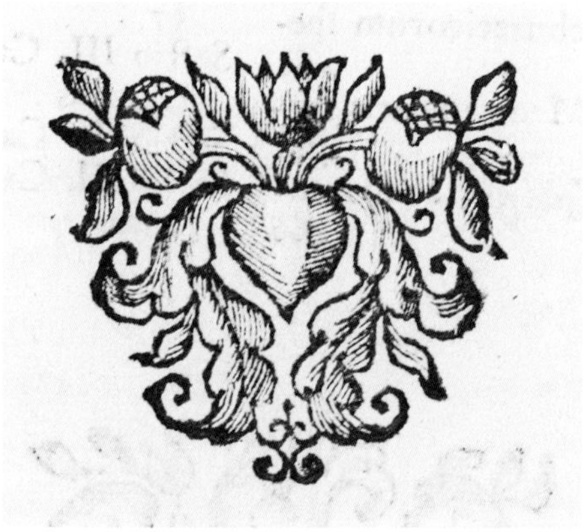

Figure 50 *Opera omnia*, Venice, 1708. (Ruinetti 10).

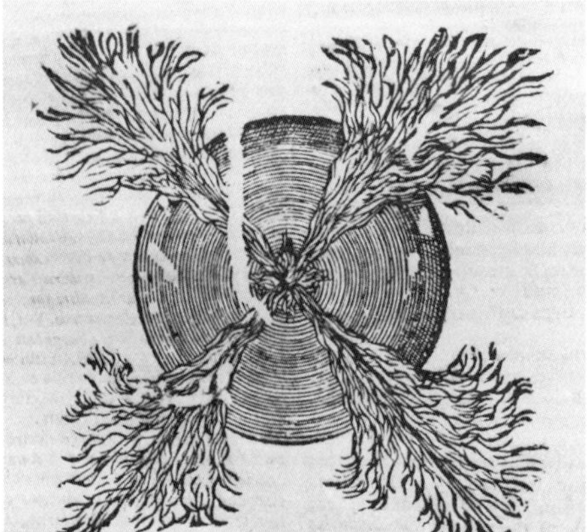

Figure 51 *Opera omnia*, Venice, 1708. (Ruinetti 14).

Figure 52 *Opera omnia*, Venice, 1708. (Ruinetti 18).

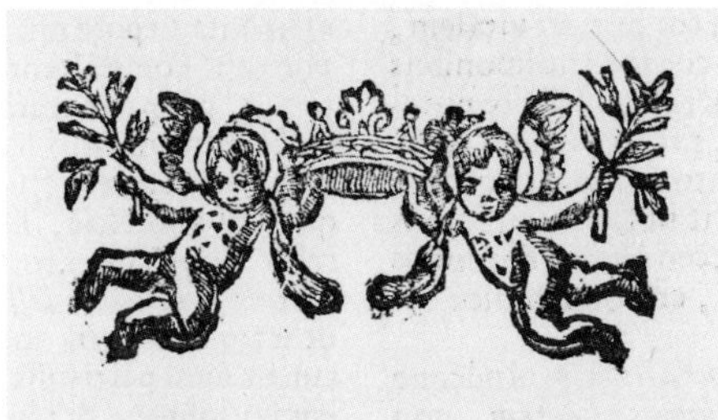

Figure 53 *Opera omnia*, Venice, 1708. (Ruinetti 24).

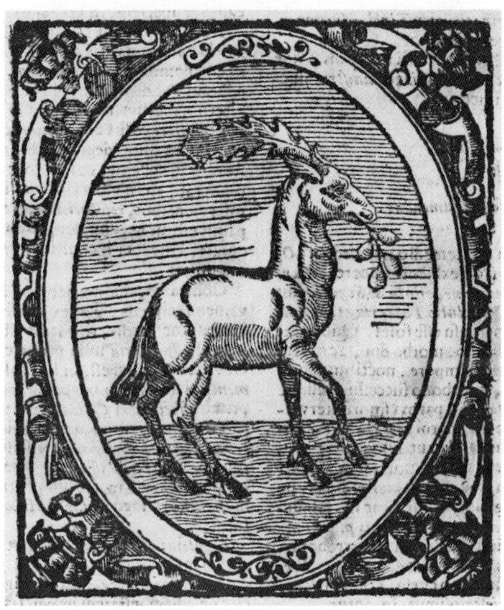

Figure 54 *Opera omnia*, Venice, 1708. (Ruinetti 28).

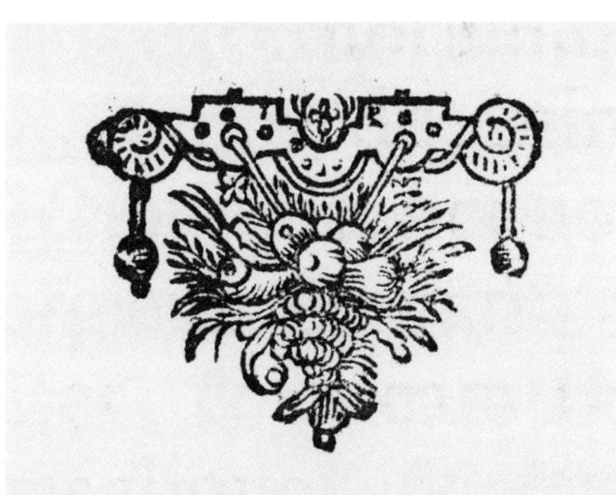

Figure 55 *Cerebri anatome*, Amsterdam, 1666 (Schagen 16).

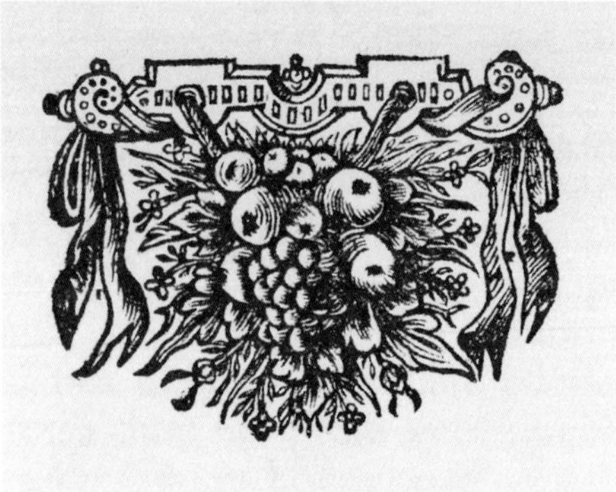

Figure 56 *Cerebri anatome*, Amsterdam, 1666 (Schagen 19).

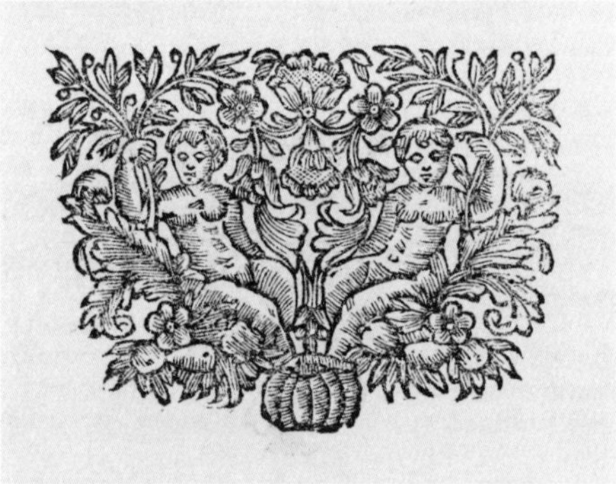

Figure 57 *Opera omnia*, Coloniæ, 1694 (Storti 11).

Figure 58 *Opera omnia*, Coloniæ, 1694 (Storti 17).

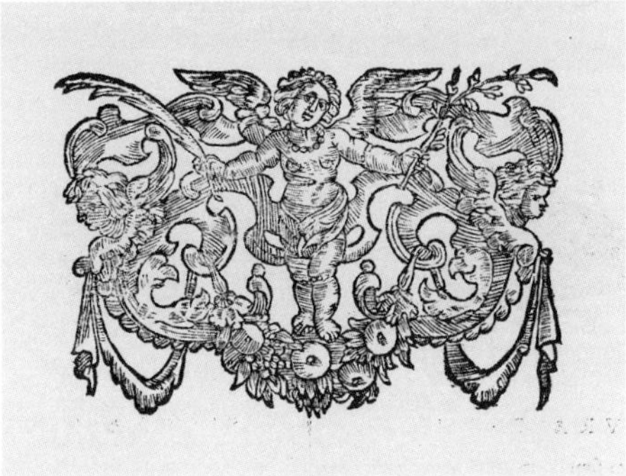

Figure 59 *Opera omnia*, Coloniæ, 1694 (Storti 24).

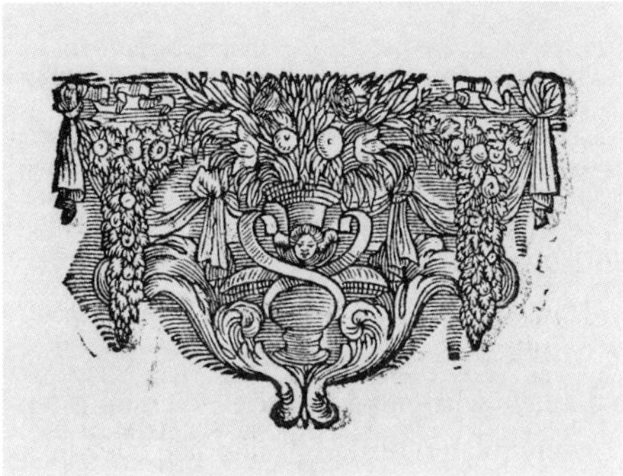

Figure 60 *Opera omnia*, Geneva, 1695 (Tournes 71).

Figure 61 *Opera omnia*, Amsterdam, 1682 (Wetstein 10).

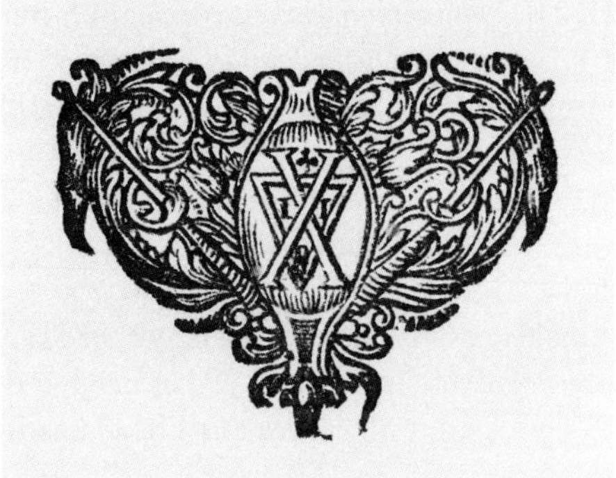

Figure 62 *Opera omnia*, Amsterdam, 1682 (Wetstein 19).

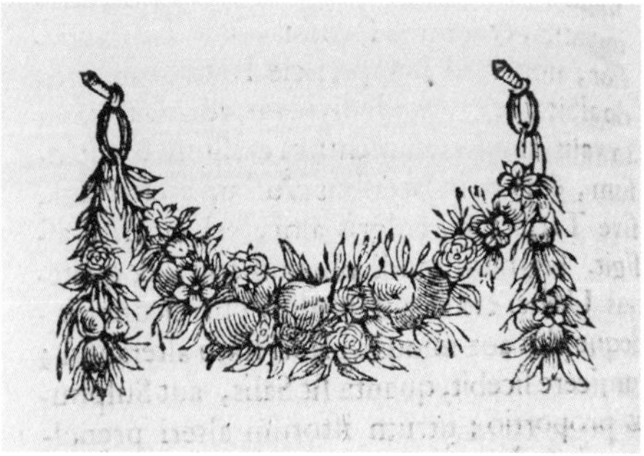

Figure 63 *De urinis*, Utrecht, 1670 (Zyll 1).

Tailpieces are generally less sophisticated than headpieces and rarely tell a story. Most printers of Thomas Willis's books settled for baskets of flowers, an inverted botanic design with garlands, or a collection of fleurons. But some were more inventive. Ruinetti used a sphere with flames, perhaps a bomb or firework. Leers included squirrels. Wetstein added a bear and serpents; and Goeree had previously used a bear clutching stems and leaves. Some incorporated animal faces in their design. Ruinetti surrounded a lion's head with leaves and flowers; another piece had a horse with leaves and berries of holly held in its mouth. Others worked in human faces. Storti used a face with headdress of leaves, an open mouth below two doves eating buds (used in two closely related designs), a female cherub, and Romulus and Remus. Wilhelm Goeree (1635–1711) depicted a mermaid. Ruinetti seemed particularly fond of angels. Together fifteen printers use sixty-three tailpieces. At first appearance, these are:

> Bettesworth 4: *A plain and easie method*, London 1721 (**7B**); D'Houry 4, 9: *Dissertation sur les urines*, Paris 1683 (**1K1**); Elsevier 4: *Pathologiæ cerebri*, Amsterdam 1668 (**3B1**); Goeree 3, 8: [*Diatribæ duæ medico-philosophicæ*], Middelburg and Amsterdam 1676 (**1H**); Goeree 9, 12, 14: [*Pharmaceutice rationalis* parts I and II] Middelburg and / or Amsterdam 1677 and 1681 (**6H, 6J**); Huguetan 8, 22, 25, 29, 45, 46, 49, 51: *Opera omnia*, Lyon 1676 (**8A**); Huguetan 57, 81: *Opera omnia*, Lyon 1681 (**8D**); Leers 1: *Pharmaceutice rationalis* (part 1). The Hague 1674 (**6C**); Leers 4, 6: *Pharmaceutice rationalis* (part 1) The Hague 1675 (**6D**); Leers 10, 12: *Pharmaceutice rationalis* (part 2), The Hague 1677 (**6G**); Lucas 1, 2: *Cerebri Anatome*, Amsterdam 1676 (**2E2**); Malachin 3, 6: *Opera omnia*, Venice 1720 (**8I**); Ruinetti 3, 6, 7, 8, 10, 14, 17, 18, 24, 28, 31, 34: *Opera omnia*, Venice 1708 (**8H**); Schagen 6, 11: *Diatribæ duæ medico-philosophicæ*, Amsterdam 1663 (**1E**); Schagen 16, 19: *Cerebri anatome*, Amsterdam 1666 (**2D**); Someren 4: *De anima brutorum*, Amsterdam 1674 (**5C**); Storti 4, 6, 7, 9, 11, 14, 17, 24: *Opera omnia*, Coloniæ 1694 (**8F**); Tournes 10, 17, 22: *Opera omnia*, Geneva 1676 (**8B**); Tournes 71: *Opera omnia*, Geneva 1695 (**8G**); Wetstein 5, 10, 13, 16, 19: *Opera omnia*, Amsterdam 1682 (**8E**); and Zyll 1: *De urinis*, Utrecht 1670 (**1G**).

Fleurons

By their nature, fleurons make less visual impact than other examples of printers' ornaments. Compared with the relatively infrequent use of head and tailpieces, the English printers of Thomas Willis's books did fill spaces and create headlines by inserting a row of fleurons made up of one or more designs arranged in combination. When two or more rows were created, one or another might be inverted to enhance the overall appearance. With more elaborate ornaments, rotation and inversion created a complex design that, at first glance, appeared to be a single unit; but the misalignment and slippage of individual fleurons, occasional overlapping and varying numbers in a given line indicate that these are composites made up of many individual parts. Common designs included flowers, leaves, acorns, urns, sprays, fleur-de-lys, rosettes, strapwork, scrolls, and badges over heraldic devices.

Because they were simple and easy to cast, it is not surprising that different printers used similar fleurons. Those present in the Dutch editions of Elsevier, Commelin, Cornelius Driehuysen (fl.1663–1671), Johannes ten Hoorn (fl.1671–1711), Leers, Vlacq, and Wetstein are similar in design. Vlacq, who had worked in England, incorporated designs closely resembling those used by Fell and by Johannes à Someren (1632–1678). Several used by Huguetan and Tournes were shared. Malachin used several ornaments and letters borrowed from Ruinetti and Storti. But there are as many subtle differences as there are superficial similarities and it is likely that each printer had his own set of designs even if these were reasonably faithful copies acquired from the same foundry. Together twelve printers used seventy-one fleurons, at first appearance, in the works of Thomas Willis:

> Allestry 1: *Cerebri anatome*, London 1664 (**2A**); Allestry 3: *Affectionum quæ dicuntur hystericæ et hypochondriacæ*, London 1670 (**4A**); Bettesworth 3: *A plain and easie method*, London 1721 (**7B**); D'Houry 5, 6, 8: *Dissertation sur les urines*, Paris 1683 (**1K1**); D'Houry 10, 11: *Dissertation sur les urines*, Paris 1687 (**1K2**); Dring 1: *Pharmaceutice rationalis* (English) London 1679 (**9A**); Dring 10: *Dr Willis's practice of physick*, London 1684 (**9F**); Fell 2: *De anima brutorum*, London 1672 (**5B**); Fell 7, 8: *Pharmaceutice rationalis*, Oxford 1674 (**6B**); Huguetan 6, 9, 10, 12, 27, 38: *Opera omnia*, Lyon 1676 (**8A**); Huguetan 58, 59, 80: *Opera omnia*, Lyon 1681 (**8D**); Roycroft 1, 2, 3, 4, 5, 6, 7, 8, 10: *Diatribæ duæ medico-philosophicæ*, London 1659 (**1A**); Roycroft 11, 12, 13, 14, 15, 16, 17, 18, 20: *Diatribæ duæ medico-philosophicæ*, London 1660 (**1B**); Roycroft 28: *Cerebri anatome*, London 1664 (**2B**); Roycroft 31, 32, 33, 34, 35, 36: *Pathologiæ cerebri*, London 1667 (**3A**); Schagen 1, 2: *Diatribæ duæ medico-philosophicæ*, Amsterdam 1663 (**1E**); Schagen 22: [*De ratione motus musculorum*]. Amsterdam 1667 (**2G**); Someren 1: *De anima brutorum*, Amsterdam 1674 (**5C**); Storti 20: *Opera omnia*, Coloniæ 1694 (**8F**); Tournes 7, 8, 11, 12, 18, 19, 31, 42: *Opera omnia*, Geneva 1676 (**8B**); Tournes 53 *Opera omnia*, Geneva 1680 (**8C**); Tournes 59, 61, 62, 64, 69, 72, 73, 74: *Opera omnia*, Geneva 1695 (**8G**); and Vlacq 2, 3: *Diatribæ duæ medico-philosophicæ*, The Hague 1662 (**1D1**).

Decorated initials

Dating from the mid-sixteenth century, the subject matter of historiated initials changed from ecclesiastical, classical, or heraldic subject matter to depictions of animal and human figures, lifelike and grotesque, set in rural scenes or on geometric backgrounds that lacked any apparent symbolism. Occasionally, the cutter worked into these capitalized letters some form of signature. Other letters were embedded in arabesques made up of spirals, vague shapes, and stipple work. Any capital letter could form the basis for decoration, the shape clearly determining the most felicitous design. As printing became increasingly industrial and suppliers of type served many clients, factotums were introduced, cut in wood and metal, which served as a template to which any letter could be added.

Decorated initials were used sparingly by the English printers of Thomas Willis's works but indulged by those producing these books in continental Europe.[47] Self-evidently, the letter to be initialled was determined by the first word of key sections but certain forms predominated: 'A', 'I', 'D', and 'T'. Most letters are open with a faint or bold shadow and relatively crude in design and cutting. A large proportion are simply placed on an arrangement of stems and leaves, without borders. The same initials are found in books issued by different printers, consistent with sharing or a common and relatively cheap source. Those used in the same book vary in quality and presumably come from more than one workshop. For example, Roycroft 9, 19, 22, 23, 24, 38, 40, and 41 are similar in design and likely to be from one source whereas 26 is entirely different and 29 and 30 much more sophisticated. Tournes used decorated initials of more than one style including a number with criblé markings indicating that these, at least, were cut on metal. Schagen's letters are on a dentelle background as are some used independently by Commelin. Presumably these came from the same source. Although not designed as such, palindromic initials, 'I', 'O', and 'N' were sometimes accidentally reversed or inverted for printing. Some printers seemed to be selective in their use: Dring much favoured the decorated initial 'T'.

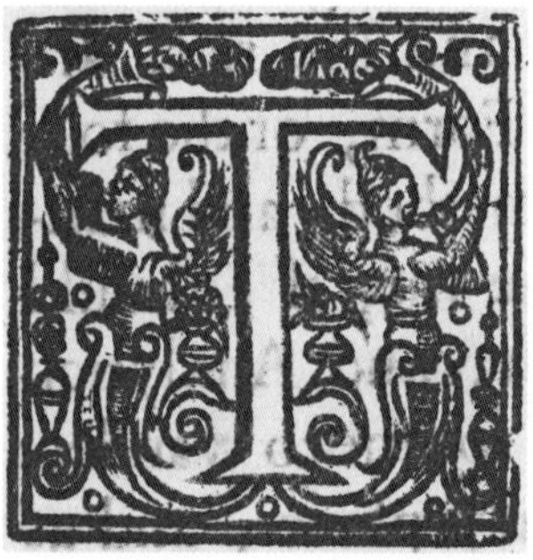

Figure 64 *The remaining medical works*, London, 1681 (Dring 5).

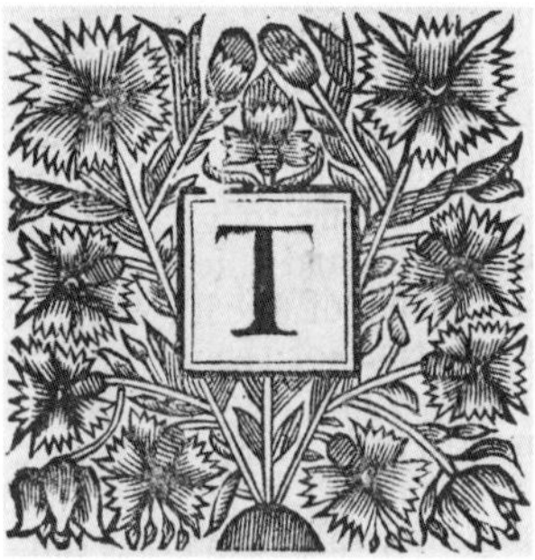

Figure 65 *The remaining medical works*, London, 1681 (Dring 11).

[47] Bold capitals in a type size greatly in excess of the remainder of the printed text are almost invariably present but excluded from this account of decorated capital initials.

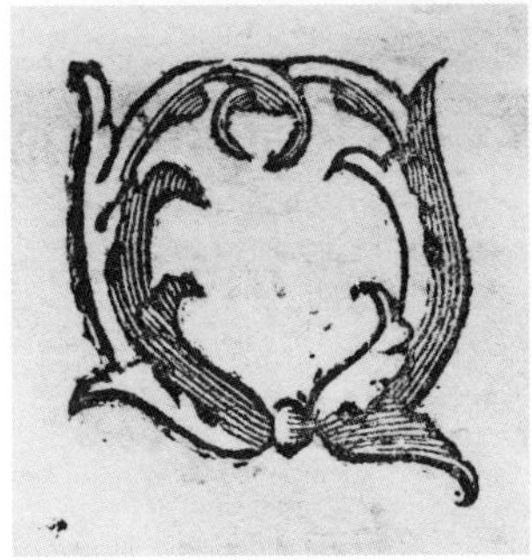

Figure 66 *Pharmaceutice rationalis* part 1, Oxford, 1674. (Fell 5).

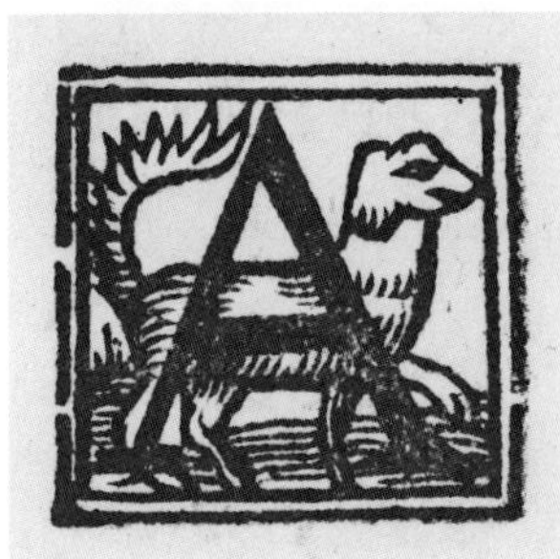

Figure 67 *Nieuwe en Geneeskundige verhandeling vande fermentatie*, Middelburg, 1676 (Goeree 1).

Figure 68 *Opera omnia*, Lyon, 1676 (Huguetan 16).

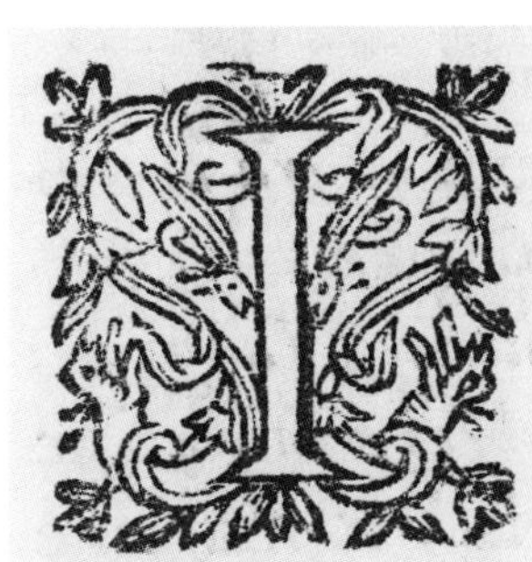

Figure 69 *Opera omnia*, Lyon, 1676 (Huguetan 26).

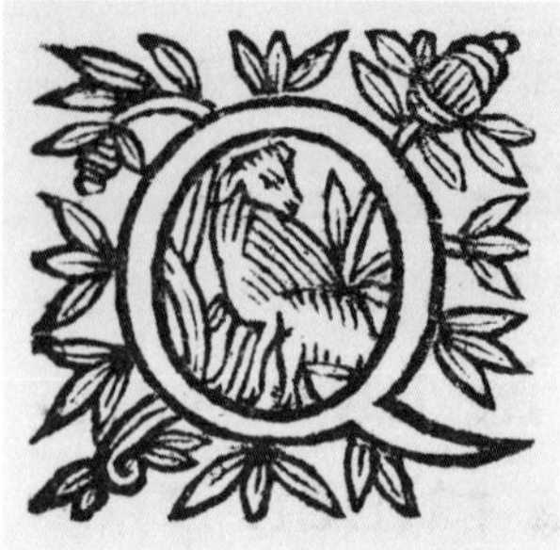

Figure 70 *Opera omnia*, Lyon, 1676 (Huguetan 33).

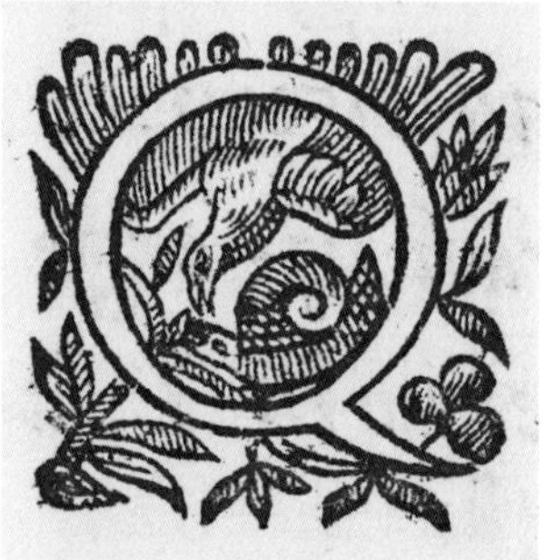

Figure 71 *Opera omnia*, Lyon, 1676 (Huguetan 36).

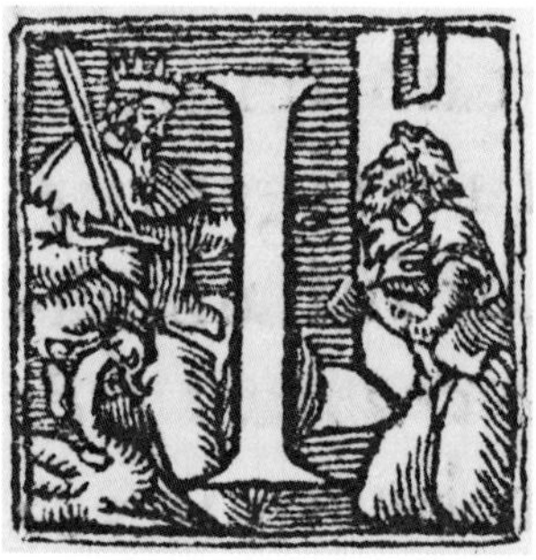

Figure 72 *Opera omnia*, Lyon, 1676 (Huguetan 44).

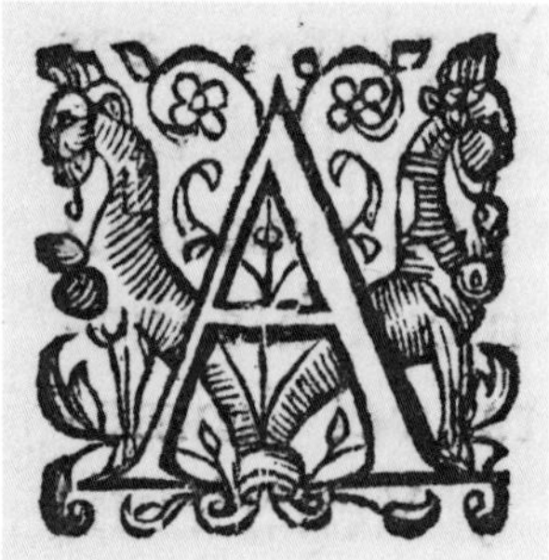

Figure 73 *Opera omnia*, Lyon, 1676 (Huguetan 48).

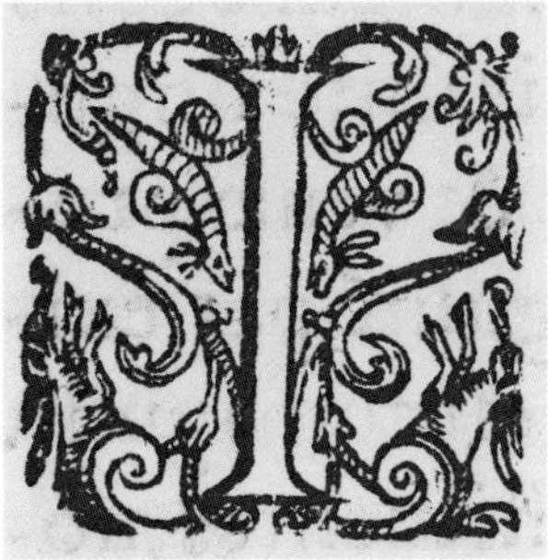

Figure 74 *Opera omnia*, Lyon, 1676 (Huguetan 52).

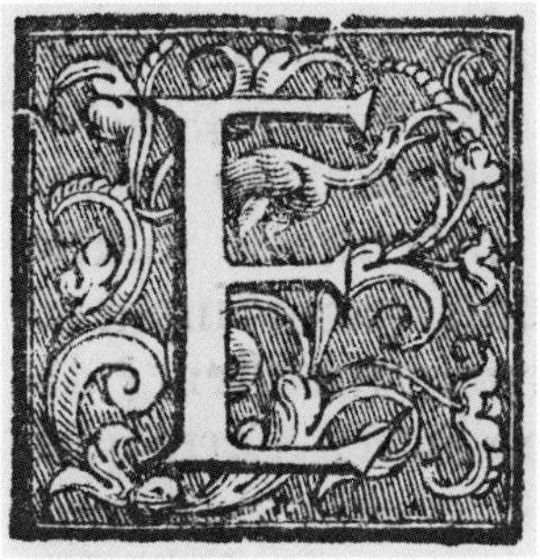

Figure 75 *Opera omnia*, Venice, 1720 (Malachin 9).

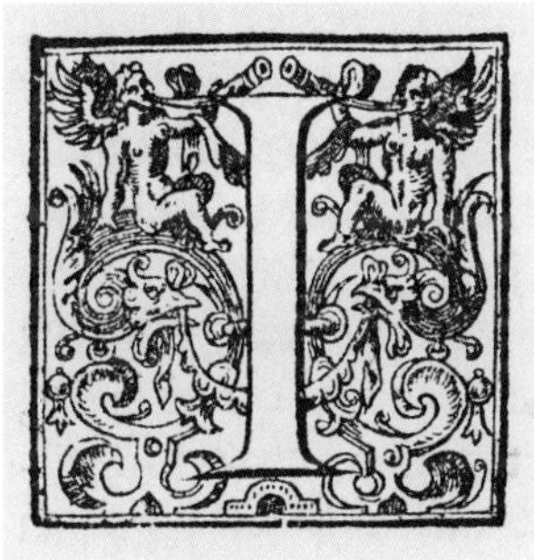

Figure 76 *Pathologiæ cerebri* London, 1667 (Roycroft 30).

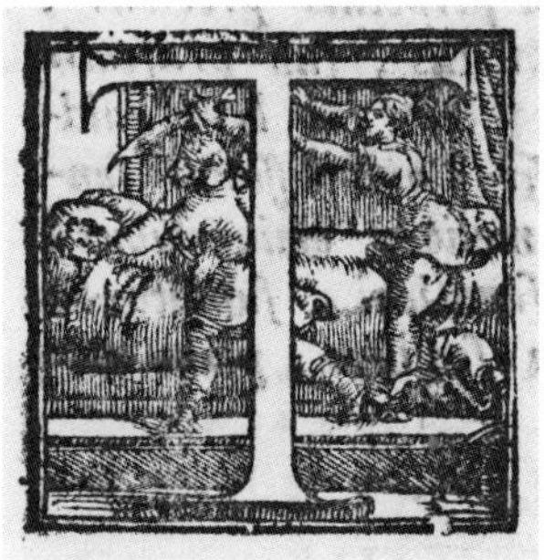

Figure 77 *Opera omnia*, Venice, 1708 (Ruinetti 5).

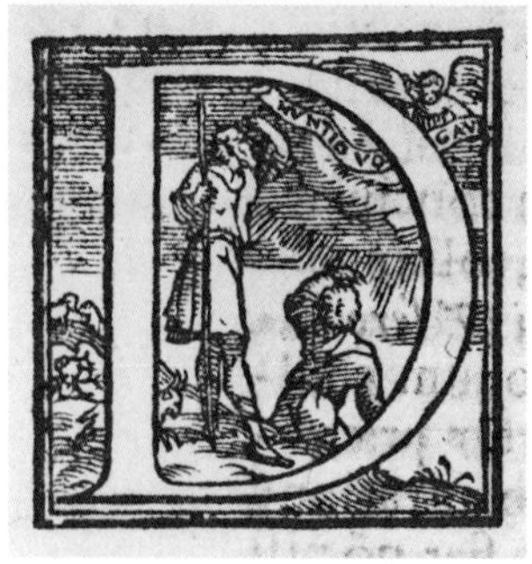

Figure 78 *Opera omnia*, Venice, 1708 (Ruinetti 13).

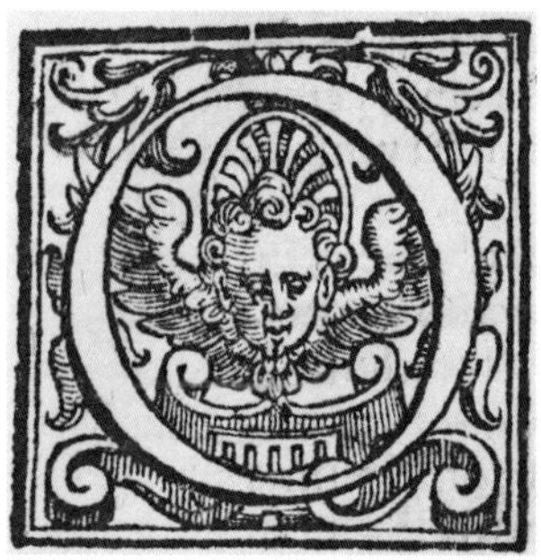

Figure 79 *Opera omnia*, Venice, 1708 (Ruinetti 15).

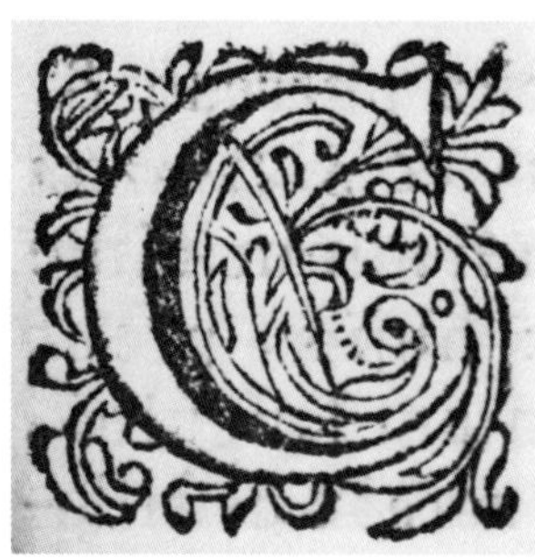

Figure 80 *Opera omnia*, Venice, 1708 (Schagen 10).

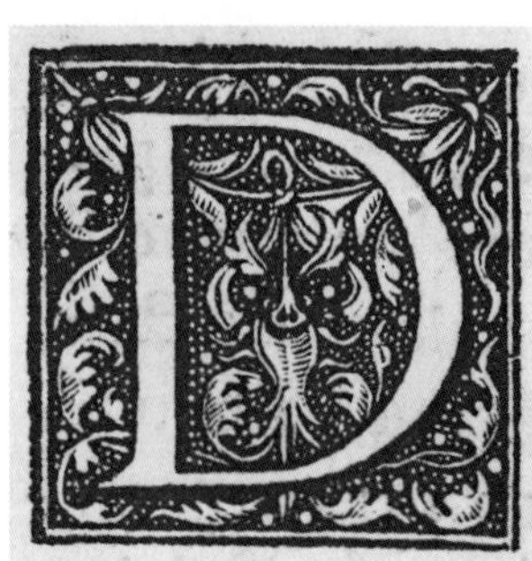

Figure 81 *Opera omnia*, Geneva, 1676 (Tournes 6).

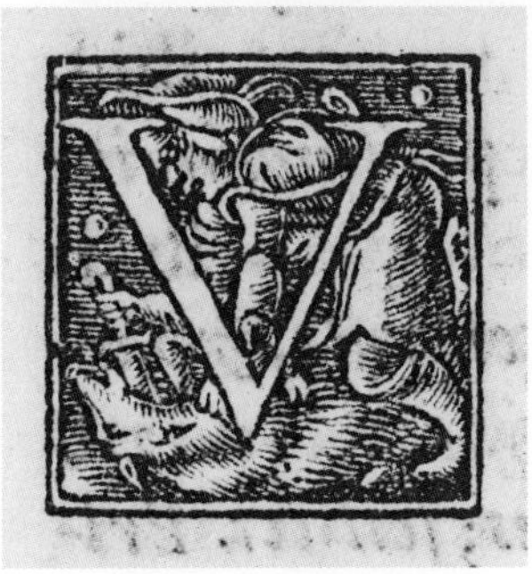

Figure 82 *Opera omnia*, Geneva, 1676 (Tournes 14).

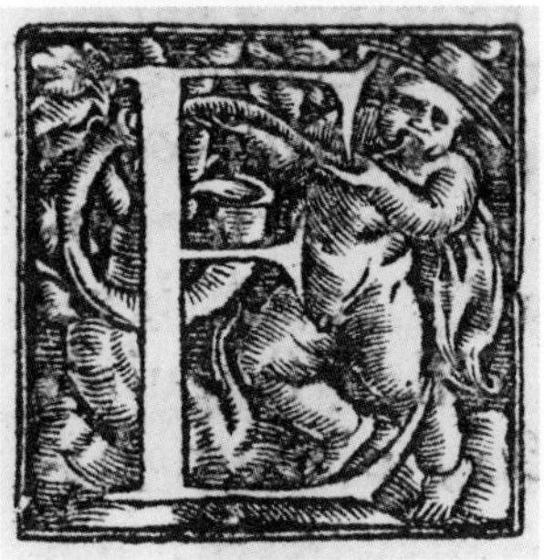

Figure 83 *Opera omnia*, Geneva, 1676 (Tournes 16).

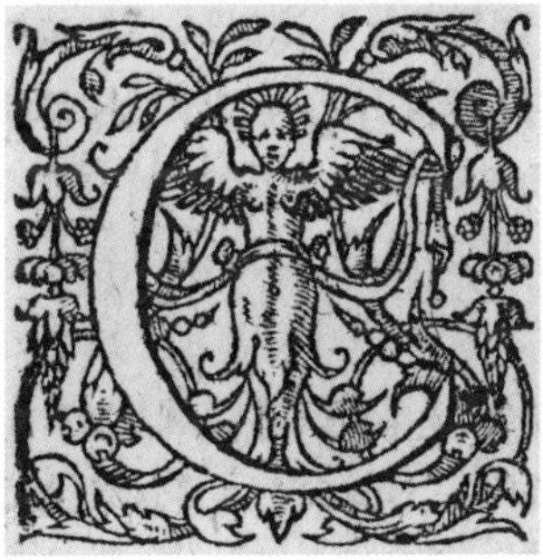

Figure 84 *Opera omnia*, Geneva, 1676 (Tournes 21).

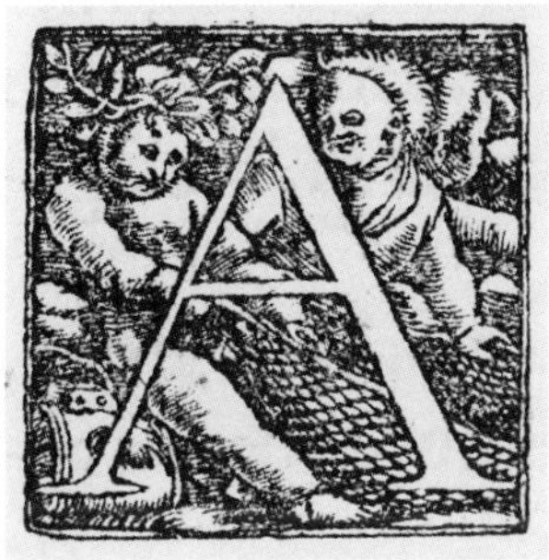

Figure 85 *Opera omnia*, Geneva, 1676 (Tournes 23).

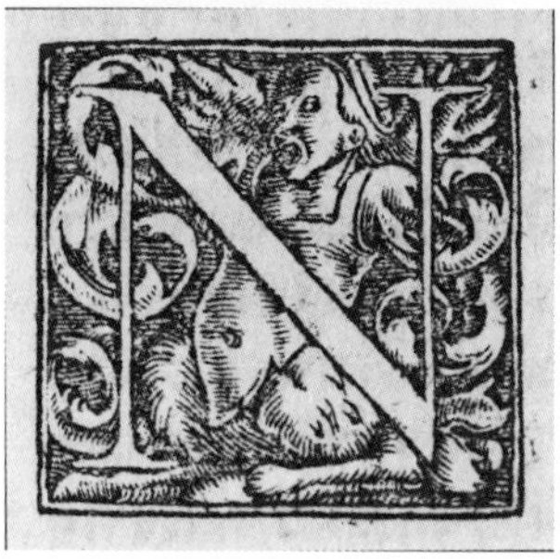

Figure 86 *Opera omnia*, Geneva, 1676 (Tournes 27).

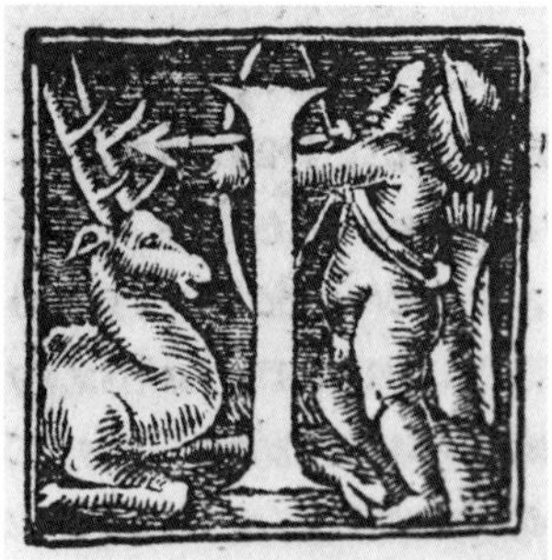

Figure 87 *Opera omnia*, Geneva, 1676 (Tournes 37).

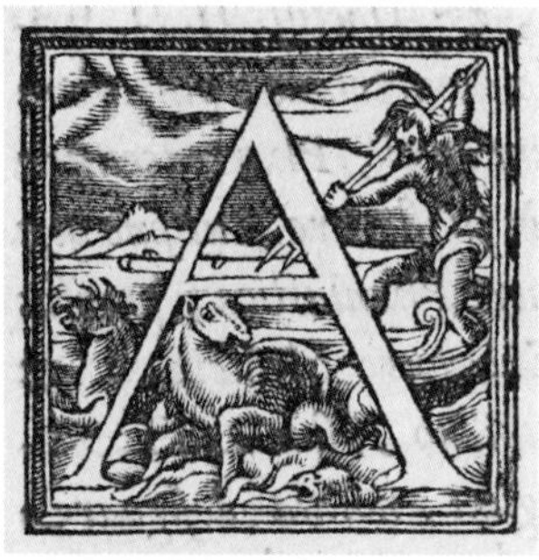

Figure 88 *Opera omnia*, Geneva, 1676 (Tournes 45).

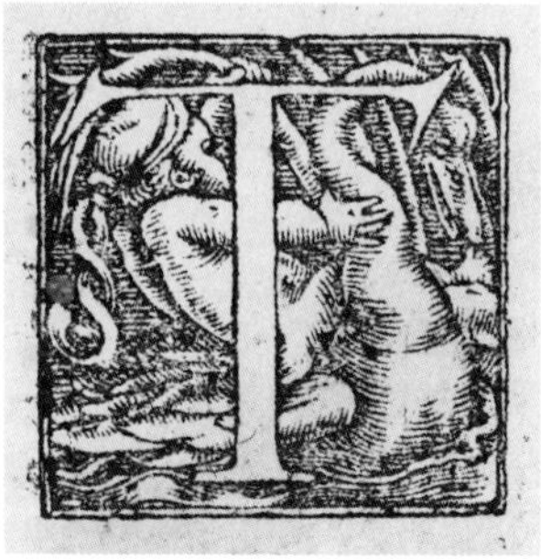

Figure 89 *Opera omnia*, Geneva, 1695 (Tournes 60).

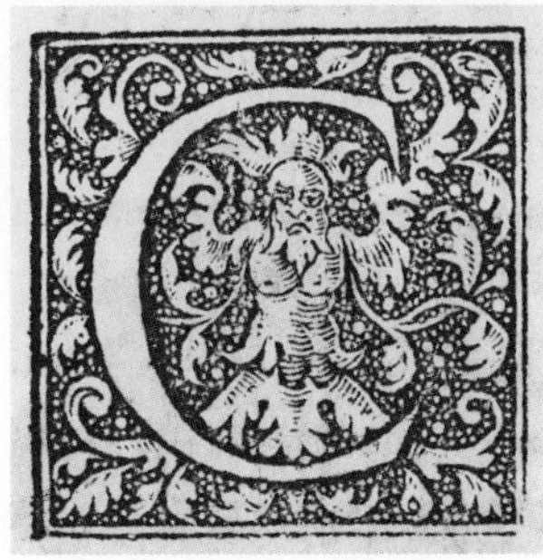

Figure 90 *Opera omnia*, Geneva, 1695 (Tournes 70).

Outstandingly the most interesting decorated initials are those with human and animal figures, realistic and mythical, engaged in various activities. The scenes are mainly rural and include hunting, fishing, blowing horns, conversation, a supplicant before his king, the slaughter of a cow, a man riding a swan, and contemplation of the heavens. The most extraordinary is Ruinetti 5 depicting what appears to be an imminent murder for adultery (see: Figure 77). The background to the initial 'T' shows a male figure poised to strike a person lying in bed with a raised dagger being restrained by a third, female, figure. Quite what real or imaginary episodes provoked the decision to illustrate such events is unclear but these images provide regular and not unwelcome distraction from the Latin text that follows. Together nineteen printers used 232 decorated initials in the works of Thomas Willis. At first appearance, these are:

Bettesworth 2: 'I', *A plain and easie method*, London 1721 (**7B**); Commelin 2 'P', 3 'D': *Cerebri anatome*, Amsterdam 1664 (**2C2**); Commelin 4 'A', 5 'I': *Cerebri anatome*, Amsterdam 1667 (**2E1**); D'Houry 3 'M', 7 'Q': *Dissertation sur les urines*, Paris 1683 (**1K1**); Driehuysen 2 'R', 3 'I': *Affectionum quæ dicuntur hystericæ et hypochondriacæ*, Leiden 1671 (**4B**); Dring 2 'W', 4 'T', 5 'T', 6 'T', 7 'T': *The remaining medical works*, London 1681 (**9B**); Dring 9 'I': *Concerning the soul of brutes*, London 1683 (**9D**); Dring 11 'T', 12 'T': *Dr Willis's practice of physick*, London 1684 (**9F**); Elsevier 2 'I', 3 'Q', 5 'I': *Pathologiæ cerebri*, Amsterdam 1668 (**3B1**); Fell 5 'Q', 6 'A': *Pharmaceutice rationalis* (part 1), Oxford 1674 (**6A**); Fell 10 'I': *Pharmaceutice rationalis* (part 2), Oxford 1675 (**6E**); Fell 12 'A': *Pharmaceutice rationalis* (parts 1 & 2), Oxford 1679 (**6I**); Goeree 1 'A', 2 'W', 4 'I', 6 'B', 7 B': *Nieuwe en Geneeskundige verhandeling vande fermentatie*, Middelburg and Amsterdam 1676 (**1H**); Goeree 10 'H', 11 'D': *Genees-middelen in s'menschen lichaam*, Middelburg and Amsterdam 1677 (**6H**); Goeree 13 'N', 15 'S', 16 'I': *Genees-middelen ontrent de deelen en sieketen des menschen lichaams*, Amsterdam 1681 (**6J**); Hoorn 1 'H', 2 'W': *Diatribæ duæ medico-philosophicæ*, Amsterdam 1681 (**1J**); Huguetan 3 'S', 5 'I', 7 'A', 11 'F', 13 'F', 14 'V' [U], 15 'C', 16 'V', 17 'Q', 18 'I', 19 'O', 20 'I', 21 'A', 23 'P', 24 'D', 26 'I', 28 'D', 30 'E', 31 'A', 32 'N', 33 'Q', 34 'R', 35 'A', 36 'Q', 37 'E', 39 'A', 40 'C', 42 'Q', 44 'I', 47 'M', 48 'A', 50 'A', 52 'I', 53 'H', 54 'A': *Opera omnia*, Lyon 1676 (**8A**); Huguetan 56 'A', 60 'F', 61 'F', 62 'V', 63 'Q', 64 'I', 65 'O', 66 'I', 67 'A', 68 'D', 69 'I', 70 'E', 71 'N', 72 'D', 73 'I', 74 'R', 75 'C', 76 'A', 77 'Q', 78 'I', 79 'E', 84 'M', 85 'A', 86 'A', 87 'H': *Opera omnia*, Lyon 1681 (**8D**); Leers 2 'Q', 3 'A': *Pharmaceutice rationalis* (part 1), The Hague 1674 (**6C**); Leers 5 'Q', 7 'A': *Pharmaceutice rationalis* (part 1), The Hague 1675 (**6D**); Leers 8 'A', 9 'D', 13 'I': *Pharmaceutice rationalis* (part 2), The Hague 1677 (**6G**); Malachin 2 'N', 5 'I', 7 'A', 8 'Q', 9 'E', 10 'D': *Opera omnia*, Venice 1720 (**8I**); Roycroft 9 'I', 19 'D', 22 'S', 23 'D', 24 'I': *Diatribæ duæ medico-philosophicæ* London 1659 (**1A**); Roycroft 26 'S': *Diatribæ duæ medico-philosophicæ*, London 1677 (**1I**); Roycroft 29 'N': *Cerebri anatome*, London 1664 (**2B**); Roycroft 30 'I': *Pathologiae cerebri*,

London 1667 (**3A**); Roycroft 38 'Q', 40 'I': *Pathologiæ cerebri*, London 1668 (**3B2**); Roycroft 41 'R': *Affectionum quæ dicuntur hystericæ et hypochondriacæ*, London 1678 (**4C**); Ruinetti 1 'C', 2 'S', 5 'T', 9 'D', 12 'I', 13 'D', 15 'O', 16 'A', 19 'D', 20 'Q', 21 'Q', 22 'R', 23 'I', 25 'C', 26 'E', 27 'Q', 29 'Q', 30 'A', 32 'A', 33 'I': *Opera omnia*, Venice 1708 (**8H**); Schagen 3 'D', 4 'D', 5 'I', 8 'E', 10 'C': *Diatribæ duæ medico-philosophicæ*, Amsterdam 1663 (**1E**); Schagen 13 'C': *Diatribæ duæ medico-philosophicæ*, Amsterdam 1669 (**1F**); Schagen 14 'A', 15 'N': *Cerebri anatome*, 1664 (**2C1**); Schagen 17 'A', 18 'N', 20 'P', 21 'D': *Cerebri anatome*, Amsterdam 1666 (**2D**); Someren 2 'Q', 3 'E', 5 'A': *De anima brutorum*, Amsterdam 1674 (**5C**); Storti 2 'C', 3 'S', 5 'T', 8 'C', 10 'D', 13 'I', 15 'O', 16 'A', 18 'D', 19 'Q', 21 'I', 22 'R', 23 'C', 26 'E', 27 'Q', 28 'A': *Opera omnia*, Coloniæ 1694 (**8F**); Tournes 3 'E', 5 'S', 6 'D', 9 'D', 13 'F', 14 'V', 15 'I', 16 'E', 20 'V', 21 'C', 23 'A', 24 'C', 25 'I', 27 'N', 28 'T', 29 'D', 30 'I', 32 'Q', 33 'Q', 34 'I', 36 'I', 37 'I', 38 'Q', 40 'R', 41 'I', 43 'C', 44 'A', 45 'A', 46 'M', 47 'A', 48 'A', 49 'O', 50 'A': *Opera omnia*, Geneva 1676 (**8B**); Tournes 52 'I', 54 'V', 55 'E', 56 'C', 57 'T', 58 'R': *Opera omnia*, Geneva 1680 (**8C**); Tournes 60 'T', 63 'D', 65 'D', 66 'F', 67 'E', 68 'V', 70 'C': *Opera omnia*, Geneva 1695 (**8G**); and Wetstein 2 'S', 4 'T', 6 'D', 7 'I', 8 'E', 9 'C', 11 'A', 12 'Q', 14 'A', 15 'R', 17 'Q', 20 'A': *Opera omnia*, Amsterdam 1682 (**8E**); Wetstein 22 'A', 23 'I', 24 'N': *Cerebri anatome*, Amsterdam 1683 (**2F**).

A descriptive list of printers' ornaments in the works of Thomas Willis

Allestry:

Allestry 1. *Cerebri anatome*, London quarto 1664: fleuron, fleur-de-lys; 5 × 4 millimetres

Allestry 2. *Affectionum quæ dicuntur hystericæ et hypochondriacæ*, London quarto 1670: relief, headpiece, stems, leaves, flowers and vase, no border; 21 × 85 millimetres

Allestry 3. *Affectionum quæ dicuntur hystericæ et hypochondriacæ*, London quarto 1670: fleuron, spray; 8 × 5 millimetres.

Bettesworth:

Bettesworth 1. *A plain and easie method*, London octavo 1721: relief, headpiece, stems, leaves, flowers, shaded design within a cartouche border; 27 × 69 millimetres

Bettesworth 2. *A plain and easie method*, London octavo 1721: relief, factotum, closed initial 'I', winged angel with spear and a horn, shaded design within a cartouche border; 33 × 34 millimetres

Bettesworth 3. *A plain and easie method*, London octavo 1721: relief, fleuron, scroll; 3 × 5 millimetres

Bettesworth 4. *A plain and easie method*, London octavo 1721: relief, tailpiece, inverted triangle, garland of stems and leaves, no border; 30 × 35 millimetres.

Commelin:

Commelin 1. *Cerebri anatome*, Amsterdam duodecimo 1664: relief, printer's device, garland of fruit lettered ΑΛΗ ΘΕΙΑ ΠΑΝΔΑ ΜΑΤΩΡ [ΑΛΗΘΕΙΑ ΠΑΝΔΑΜΑΤΩΡ; 'Truth, conqueror of all'], with 'Veritas' unclothed and seated with sun, globe, and book; 35 × 33 millimetres (see: Figure 40, where this is grouped with headpieces indicating the occasional ambiguity in classifying these ornaments; see footnote 10 earlier)

Commelin 2. *Cerebri anatome*, Amsterdam duodecimo 1664: relief, open shadowed initial 'P', dentelle background, no border; 13 × 13 millimetres
Commelin 3. *Cerebri anatome*, Amsterdam duodecimo 1664: relief, open shadowed initial 'D', dentelle background, no border; 13 × 13 millimetres
Commelin 4. *Cerebri anatome*, Amsterdam duodecimo 1667: relief, open shadowed initial 'A', leaf background, no border; 12 × 12 millimetres
Commelin 5. *Cerebri anatome*, Amsterdam duodecimo 1667: open shadowed initial 'I', leaf background, no border; 12 × 12 millimetres.

D'Houry:

D'Houry 1. *Dissertation sur les urines*, Paris octavo 1683: relief, headpiece, stems, leaves, and flowers, no border; 20 × 34 millimetres
D'Houry 2. *Dissertation sur les urines*, Paris octavo 1683: relief, headpiece, orbs on vertical plinths, leaves and flowers, no border; 13 × 57 millimetres (see: Figure 20)
D'Houry 3. *Dissertation sur les urines*, Paris octavo 1683: relief, factotum, closed initial 'M' inserted, circular stem with leaves, no border; 15 × 15 millimetres
D'Houry 4. *Dissertation sur les urines*, Paris octavo 1683: relief, tailpiece, intertwined stems, leaves, open book, empty shield, no border; 30 × 46 millimetres (see: Figure 41)
D'Houry 5. *Dissertation sur les urines*, Paris octavo 1683: relief, fleuron, spray; 6 × 4 millimetres
D'Houry 6. *Dissertation sur les urines*, Paris octavo 1683: relief, fleuron, spray; 6 × 4 millimetres
D'Houry 7. *Dissertation sur les urines*, Paris octavo 1683: relief, open shadowed initial 'Q', leaf background, no border; 15 × 16 millimetres
D'Houry 8. *Dissertation sur les urines*, Paris octavo 1683: relief, fleuron, spray; 6 × 6 millimetres
D'Houry 9. *Dissertation sur les urines*, Paris octavo 1683: tailpiece, urn, no border; 41 × 40 millimetres
D'Houry 10. *Dissertation sur les urines*, Paris octavo 1687: relief, fleuron, spray; 7 × 6 millimetres
D'Houry 11. *Dissertation sur les urines*, Paris octavo 1687: relief, fleuron, shield, and crossed lances; 6 × 6 millimetres.

Driehuysen:

Driehuysen 1. *Affectionum quæ dicuntur hystericæ et hypochondriacæ*, Leiden duodecimo 1671: headpiece, scrolls; 9 × 32 millimetres
Driehuysen 2. *Affectionum quæ dicuntur hystericæ et hypochondriacæ*, Leiden duodecimo 1671: relief, open shadowed initial 'R', leaf background, no border; 13 × 12 millimetres
Driehuysen 3. *Affectionum quæ dicuntur hystericæ et hypochondriacæ*, Leiden duodecimo 1671: relief, open shadowed initial 'I', leaf background, no border; 15 × 15 millimetres.

Dring:

Dring 1. *Pharmaceutice rationalis* (English), London folio 1679: relief, fleuron, strapwork, four pieces grouped into one overall design; 18 × 25 millimetres

Dring 2. *Pharmaceutice rationalis* (English), London folio 1679: relief, open shadowed initial 'W', stem and leaf background, no border; 30 × 32 millimetres

Dring 3. *Pharmaceutice rationalis* (English), London folio 1679: relief, printer's device, winged horse, flowers, cornucopia, caduceus held at the base by human hands, no border; 41 × 36 millimetres (see: Figure 16)

Dring 4. *The remaining medical works*, London folio 1681: relief, open shadowed initial 'T', stem and leaf background, no border; 31 × 32 millimetres

Dring 5. *The remaining medical works*, London folio 1681: relief, open shadowed initial 'T', winged angels holding branches aloft, coiffed hair background, double-lined border; 38 × 38 millimetres (see: Figure 64)

Dring 6. *The remaining medical works*, London folio 1681: relief, bordered initial 'T', factotum, single-lined surround, flowers, leaves, and stem background, no border; 35 × 36 millimetres

Dring 7. *The remaining medical works*, London folio 1681: relief, open shadowed initial 'T', stem and leaf background, no border; 32 × 31 millimetres

Dring 8. *The remaining medical works*, London folio 1681: relief, printer's device, caduceus held by one hand, with two birds and open book on lecturn surmounted by an eagle, lettered LOVE AND LIVE, and NE QVID NEMIS / NOSCE TE IPSVM [Nothing in excess / know thyself], single-lined border (not printed on the base); 56 × 36 millimetres (see: Figure 17)

Dring 9. *Two discourses concerning the soul of brutes*, London folio 1683: relief, open shadowed initial 'I', leaf background, no border; 28 × 28 millimetres

Dring 10. *Dr Willis's practice of physick*, London folio 1684 (1): relief, fleuron, urn, and flower; 14 × 8 millimetres

Dring 11. *Dr Willis's practice of physick*, London folio 1684 (2): relief, initial 'T', factotum, double-lined surround, stems and bud background, no border; 48 × 48 millimetres (see: Figure 65)

Dring 12. *Dr Willis's practice of physick*, London folio 1684 (2): relief, initial 'T', factotum, single-lined surround, stems and flower background, double-lined border; 48 × 48 millimetres.

Elsevier:

Elsevier 1. *Pathologiæ cerebri*, Amsterdam duodecimo 1668: relief, printer's device, Minerva, tree, owl and scroll lettered NE EXTRA OLEAS [Nothing but the olives];[48] 27 × 32 millimetres (see: Figure 14)

Elsevier 2. *Pathologiæ cerebri*, Amsterdam duodecimo 1668: relief, open shadowed initial 'I', leaf background, no border; 16 × 16 millimetres

Elsevier 3. *Pathologiæ cerebri*, Amsterdam duodecimo 1668: relief, open shadowed initial 'Q', leaf background, no border; 13 × 13 millimetres

[48] The original Elsevier printer's device is found in Domenicus Baudius, *De inducis brlli Belgici*, Elsevier, Leyden (1613); this was replaced by the emblem of the olive tree and vine, under it an old man gathering fruit and on the other side, on a scroll, the motto 'Non soleus'. See: EC Bigmore and CWH Wyman, *A bibliography of printing*, London (1880), volume 1: page 196: 'The adoption for their mark of the prolific vine—crowned by Grecian fable as the greatest blessing to mankind, and the gift of the wise Minerva—was very appropriate for a family so many in number and so multitudinous in words'. The symbolism and design of the version used by Elsevier in the 1660s, an olive tree with a falling branch combined with the figure of a man, closely resembles the device of Henri Estienne (1460–1520).

Elsevier 4. *Pathologiæ cerebri*, Amsterdam duodecimo 1668: relief, tailpiece, inverted triangle, stems, leaves and crowned face, no border; 20 × 30 millimetres
Elsevier 5. *Pathologiæ cerebri*, Amsterdam duodecimo 1668: relief, open shadowed initial 'I', leaf background, no border; 12 × 10 millimetres.

Fell (Sheldonian Theatre):

Fell 1. *De anima brutorum*, Oxford quarto 1672: engraving, headpiece, coat of arms of Bishop Sheldon, no border; 55 × 66 millimetres (plate marks, 60 × 72 millimetres)
Fell 2, *De anima brutorum*, London octavo 1672: fleuron, thistle; 7 × 4 millimetres
Fell 3. *Pharmaceutice rationalis* (part 1), Oxford quarto 1674: engraving, printer's device, Sheldonian theatre surrounded by railings with 14 burghers facing on plinths, single-lined border; 110 × 148 millimetres (plate marks 119 × 150 millimetres)
Fell 4. *Pharmaceutice rationalis* (part 1), Oxford quarto 1674: relief, headpiece, intertwined stems, leaves, and flowers, no border; 28 × 93 millimetres
Fell 5. *Pharmaceutice rationalis* (part 1), Oxford quarto 1674: relief, open, leaf design initial 'Q', no background or border; 20 × 19 millimetres (see: Figure 66)
Fell 6. *Pharmaceutice rationalis* (part 1), Oxford quarto 1674: relief, open, leaf design initial 'A', no background or border; 22 × 24 millimetres
Fell 7. *Pharmaceutice rationalis* (part 1), Oxford duodecimo 1674: fleuron, stems, and flower; 3 × 9 millimetres
Fell 8. *Pharmaceutice rationalis* (part 1), Oxford duodecimo 1674: fleuron, rosette; 3 × 2 millimetres
Fell 9. *Pharmaceutice rationalis* (part 2), Oxford quarto 1675: engraving, printer's device, Sheldonian theatre surrounded by railings with 14 burghers facing on plinths, single-lined border; 110 × 148 millimetres (plate marks 119 × 150 millimetres)
Fell 10. *Pharmaceutice rationalis* (part 2), Oxford quarto 1675: relief, open, leaf design initial 'I', no background or border; 21 × 10 millimetres
Fell 11. *Pharmaceutice rationalis* (parts 1 & 2), Oxford octavo 1679: engraving, printer's device, Sheldonian theatre surrounded by railings with 14 burghers facing on plinths, single-lined border; 56 × 53 millimetres (plate marks 59 × 52 millimetres)
Fell 12. *Pharmaceutice rationalis* (parts 1 & 2), Oxford octavo 1679: relief, open shadowed initial 'A', leaf and flower background, no border; 16 × 16 millimetres.

Goeree:

Goeree 1. *Nieuwe en geneeskundige verhandeling vande fermentatie*, Middelburg and Amsterdam octavo 1676: relief, closed initial 'A', wolf, double-lined border; 16 × 17 millimetres (see: Figure 67)
Goeree 2. *Nieuwe en geneeskundige verhandeling vande fermentatie*, Middelburg and Amsterdam octavo 1676: relief, open shadowed initial 'W' overlined (may be artefactual and not as cut), stem and leaf background, no border; 19 × 18 millimetres
Goeree 3. *Nieuwe en geneeskundige verhandeling vande fermentatie*, Middelburg and Amsterdam octavo 1676: relief, tailpiece, fruit and mermaids, no border; 31 × 46 millimetres
Goeree 4. *Nieuwe en geneeskundige verhandeling vande fermentatie*, Middelburg and Amsterdam octavo 1676: relief, open shadowed initial 'I', inverted, stem and leaf background, no border; 18 × 16 millimetres

Goeree 5. *Nieuwe en geneeskundige verhandeling vande fermentatie*, Middelburg and Amsterdam octavo 1676: relief, headpiece, stems, leaves, rose and crown, no border; 17 × 45 millimetres

Goeree 6. *Nieuwe en geneeskundige verhandeling vande fermentatie*, Middelburg and Amsterdam octavo 1676: relief, open shadowed initial 'B', stem and flower background, no border; 23 × 21 millimetres

Goeree 7. *Nieuwe en geneeskundige verhandeling vande fermentatie*, Middelburg and Amsterdam octavo 1676: relief, open shadowed initial 'B', stem and leaf background, no border; 18 × 19 millimetres

Goeree 8. *Nieuwe en geneeskundige verhandeling vande fermentatie*, Middelburg and Amsterdam octavo 1676: relief, tailpiece, hanging inverted triangular garland, leaves, stem, fruit and flowers, no border; 33 × 43 millimetres

Goeree 9. *Genees-middelen in s'menschen lichaam*, Middelburg and Amsterdam octavo 1677: relief, tailpiece, human face with floral collar, no border; 12 × 18 millimetres

Goeree 10. *Genees-middelen in s'menschen lichaam*, Middelburg and Amsterdam octavo 1677: relief, open shadowed initial 'H', stem and leaf background, no border; 20 × 19 millimetres

Goeree 11. *Genees-middelen in s'menschen lichaam*, Middelburg and Amsterdam octavo 1677: relief, open shadowed initial 'D', stem and leaf background, no border; 19 × 19 millimetres

Goeree 12. *Genees-middelen in s'menschen lichaam*, Middelburg and Amsterdam octavo 1677: relief, tailpiece, bear holding stems and leaves, no border; 35 × 53 millimetres (see: Figure 42)

Goeree 13. *Genees-middelen ontrent de deelen en sieketen des menschen lichaams*, Amsterdam octavo 1681: relief, open shadowed initial 'N', stem and leaf background, no border; 25 × 24 millimetres

Goeree 14. *Genees-middelen ontrent de deelen en sieketen des menschen lichaams*, Amsterdam octavo 1681: relief, tailpiece, arabesque, no border; 24 × 25 millimetres.

Goeree 15. *Genees-middelen ontrent de deelen en sieketen des menschen lichaams*, Amsterdam octavo 1681: relief, open shadowed initial 'S', stem and leaf background, no border; 15 × 15 millimetres

Goeree 16. *Genees-middelen ontrent de deelen en sieketen des menschen lichaams*, Amsterdam octavo 1681: relief, open shadowed initial 'I', Adam and Eve, naked gender neutral, single border; 21 × 21 millimetres.

Hoorn:

Hoorn 1. *Diatribæ duæ medico-philosophicæ*, Amsterdam octavo 1681: relief, open shadowed initial 'H', stem and leaf background, no border; 15 × 14 millimetres

Hoorn 2. *Diatribæ duæ medico-philosophicæ*, Amsterdam octavo 1681: relief, open shadowed initial 'W', leaf background, no border; 18 × 18 millimetres.

Huguetan:

Huguetan 1. *Opera omnia*, Lyon quarto 1676: engraving, printer's device, armillary sphere and cherubs, lettered VNIVERSITAS RERUM VT PVLVIS IN MANVTE HOVAE [The whole of things is as dust in the hand of Jehovah] on a scroll, cloud background, no border; 43 × 78 millimetres (plate marks 56 × 80 millimetres)

Huguetan 2. *Opera omnia*, Lyon quarto 1676: relief, headpiece, stems, leaves, rabbits, satyrs, and fleur-de-lys, no border; 30 × 120 millimetres (see: Figure 21)
Huguetan 3. *Opera omnia*, Lyon quarto 1676: relief, open shadowed initial 'S', stem, leaf, and flower, animal background, no border; 44 × 44 millimetres
Huguetan 4 *Opera omnia*, Lyon quarto 1676: relief, headpiece, stems, leaves, buds, bird, and squirrels, human face with moustache and pointed beard wearing glasses, no border; 22 × 130 millimetres (see: Figure 22)
Huguetan 5. *Opera omnia*, Lyon quarto 1676: relief, open shadowed initial 'I', stem, leaf and flowers background, no border; 25 × 24 millimetres
Huguetan 6. *Opera omnia*, Lyon quarto 1676: fleuron, spray; 5 × 5 millimetres
Huguetan 7. *Opera omnia*, Lyon quarto 1676: relief, open shadowed initial 'A', stem, leaf and flower background, no border; 24 × 24 millimetres
Huguetan 8. *Opera omnia*, Lyon quarto 1676: relief, tailpiece, floral basket, no border; 65 × 85 millimetres (see: Figure 43)
Huguetan 9. *Opera omnia*, Lyon quarto 1676: fleuron, spray; 6 × 5 millimetres
Huguetan 10. *Opera omnia*, Lyon quarto 1676: fleuron, scroll; 5 × 2 millimetres
Huguetan 11. *Opera omnia*, Lyon quarto 1676: relief, open initial 'F', leaf background, no border; 16 × 18 millimetres
Huguetan 12. *Opera omnia*, Lyon quarto 1676: fleuron, fleur-de-lys; 5 × 4 millimetres
Huguetan 13. *Opera omnia*, Lyon quarto 1676: relief, bordered and solid initial 'F', leaf and flower background, white on black, single serrated border; 16 × 16 millimetres
Huguetan 14. *Opera omnia*, Lyon quarto 1676: relief, open initial 'V[U]', leaf background, no border; 10 × 13 millimetres
Huguetan 15. *Opera omnia*, Lyon quarto 1676: relief, bordered and solid initial 'C', leaf and flower background, white on black, single serrated border; 16 × 16 millimetres
Huguetan 16. *Opera omnia*, Lyon quarto 1676: relief, closed initial 'V', stem and leaf background, white on black, single serrated border; 16 × 16 millimetres (see: Figure 68)
Huguetan 17. *Opera omnia*, Lyon quarto 1676: relief, closed initial 'Q', leaf background, white on black, in 8 panels, inner serrated and outer lined border; 16 × 16 millimetres
Huguetan 18. *Opera omnia*, Lyon quarto 1676: relief, closed initial 'I' factotum, with 4 flowers, nine borders (from inside: dashed, ruled, dashed, lined, serrated, dashed, serrated [2], lined); 16 × 16 millimetres
Huguetan 19. *Opera omnia*, Lyon quarto 1676: relief, closed initial 'O', flower background, white on black, inner dashed circular, outer serrated borders; 16 × 16 millimetres
Huguetan 20. *Opera omnia*, Lyon quarto 1676: relief, open initial 'I', leaf background, no border; 14 × 14 millimetres
Huguetan 21. *Opera omnia*, Lyon quarto 1676: relief, open shadowed initial 'A', stem and leaf background, no border; 14 × 14 millimetres
Huguetan 22. *Opera omnia*, Lyon quarto 1676: relief, tailpiece, floral basket, no border; 42 × 51 millimetres
Huguetan 23. *Opera omnia*, Lyon 1676: relief, open shadowed initial 'P', stem and leaf background, no border; 13 × 13 millimetres
Huguetan 24. *Opera omnia*, Lyon quarto 1676: relief, open initial 'D', stem and leaf background, no border; 22 × 24 millimetres
Huguetan 25. *Opera omnia*, Lyon quarto 1676: relief, tailpiece, floral basket, no border; 33 × 39 millimetres

Huguetan 26. *Opera omnia*, Lyon quarto 1676: relief, open shadowed initial 'I', stem and leaf, animal and locusts background, no border; 22 × 22 millimetres (see: Figure 69)
Huguetan 27. *Opera omnia*, Lyon quarto 1676: fleuron, stem, and flowers; 3 × 9 millimetres
Huguetan 28. *Opera omnia*, Lyon quarto 1676: relief, open shadowed initial 'D', stem, leaf, and flowers; no border; 24 × 24 millimetres
Huguetan 29. *Opera omnia*, Lyon quarto 1676: relief, tailpiece, floral basket, initialled P G (probably the cutter), no border; 81 × 93 millimetres (see: Figure 44)
Huguetan 30. *Opera omnia*, Lyon quarto 1676: relief, open initial 'E', stem, leaf and bird, no border; 23 × 22 millimetres
Huguetan 31. *Opera omnia*, Lyon quarto 1676: relief, open initial 'A', stem and leaf, no border; 21 × 23 millimetres
Huguetan 32. *Opera omnia*, Lyon quarto 1676: relief, open initial 'N', stem, leaf and owl's face background, no border; 22 × 23 millimetres
Huguetan 33. *Opera omnia*, Lyon quarto 1676: relief, open initial 'Q', stem, leaf and hart background, no border; 22 × 23 millimetres (see: Figure 70)
Huguetan 34. *Opera omnia*, Lyon quarto 1676: relief, bordered and solid initial 'R', eight flowers background, white on black, outer serrated border; 16 × 16 millimetres
Huguetan 35. *Opera omnia*, Lyon quarto 1676: relief, open shadowed initial 'A', stem and leaf background, no border; 10 × 12 millimetres
Huguetan 36. *Opera omnia*, Lyon quarto 1676: relief, open initial 'Q', leaf, buds, eagle pecking at a snail background, no border; 20 × 20 millimetres (see: Figure 71)
Huguetan 37. *Opera omnia*, Lyon quarto 1676: relief, bordered and closed initial 'E' with eight surrounding panels, two alternating designs, one with four leaf and floral, the other with three leaf components, white on black, single serrated border; 16 × 16 millimetres
Huguetan 38. *Opera omnia*, Lyon quarto 1676: fleuron, scrolls; 6 × 5 millimetres
Huguetan 39. *Opera omnia*, Lyon quarto 1676: relief, open shadowed initial 'A', leaf and flower background, no border; 8 × 9 millimetres
Huguetan 40. *Opera omnia*, Lyon quarto 1676: relief, solid initial 'C', leaf and flower background, no border; 10 × 10 millimetres
Huguetan 41. *Opera omnia*, Lyon quarto 1676: relief, headpiece, stem, leaf, flower, scroll, snail, unclothed males riding a bull and a goat, garlanded African female, one eye closed, no border; 28 × 120 millimetres (see: Figure 23)
Huguetan 42. *Opera omnia*, Lyon quarto 1676: relief, open shadowed initial 'Q', scrolls and face of sun background, no border; 25 × 25 millimetres
Huguetan 43. *Opera omnia*, Lyon quarto 1676: relief, headpiece, stem, leaf, flower and bird, no border; 20 × 113 millimetres
Huguetan 44. *Opera omnia*, Lyon quarto 1676: relief, open initial 'I', historiated with king and humble subject, double-lined border; 21 × 21 millimetres (see: Figure 72)
Huguetan 45. *Opera omnia*, Lyon quarto 1676: relief, tailpiece, floral basket, no border: 59 × 82 millimetres (see: Figure 45)
Huguetan 46. *Opera omnia*, Lyon quarto 1676: relief, tailpiece, floral basket, no border: 35 × 40 millimetres
Huguetan 47. *Opera omnia*, Lyon quarto 1676: relief, open initial 'M', leaf background, no border; 20 × 20 millimetres
Huguetan 48. *Opera omnia*, Lyon quarto 1676: relief, open shadowed initial 'A', stem, flower and seahorses, no border; 22 × 22 millimetres (see: Figure 73)

Huguetan 49. *Opera omnia*, Lyon quarto 1676: relief, tailpiece, floral basket, no border; 41 × 47 millimetres

Huguetan 50. *Opera omnia*, Lyon quarto 1676: relief, open shadowed initial 'A', stem and leaf design, no border; 16 × 17 millimetres

Huguetan 51. *Opera omnia*, Lyon quarto 1676: relief, tailpiece, floral basket, no border; 23 × 38 millimetres

Huguetan 52. *Opera omnia*, Lyon quarto 1676: relief, open shadowed initial 'I', stem, flower, goats and serpent background, no border; 20 × 20 millimetres (see: Figure 74)

Huguetan 53. *Opera omnia*, Lyon quarto 1676: relief, open shadowed initial 'H', stem, leaf and flower background, no border; 12 × 13 millimetres

Huguetan 54. *Opera omnia*, Lyon quarto 1676: relief, open shadowed initial 'A', stem, leaf, and flower background, no border; 12 × 13 millimetres

Huguetan 55. *Opera omnia*, Lyon quarto 1681: relief, headpiece, leaves, griffins, people as insects, three central fleur-de-lys, no border; 31 × 112 millimetres

Huguetan 56. *Opera omnia*, Lyon quarto 1681: relief, open initial 'A', leaf design, cross-hatching, white on black background, double-lined border; 20 × 20 millimetres

Huguetan 57. *Opera omnia*, Lyon quarto 1681: relief, tailpiece, stem, leaf and interlaced arabesque, no border; 60 × 75 millimetres (see: Figure 46)

Huguetan 58. *Opera omnia*, Lyon quarto 1681: fleuron, crossed leaf design; 8 × 9 millimetres

Huguetan 59. *Opera omnia*, Lyon quarto 1681: fleuron, scrolls; 5 × 5 millimetres

Huguetan 60. *Opera omnia*, Lyon quarto 1681: relief, open shadowed initial 'F', stem and leaf design, no border; 18 × 18 millimetres

Huguetan 61. *Opera omnia*, Lyon quarto 1681: relief, closed initial 'F', stem and leaf design, on white, no border; 8 × 8 millimetres

Huguetan 62. *Opera omnia*, Lyon quarto 1681: relief, closed initial 'V', stem and leaf design, on white, no border; 8 × 8 millimetres

Huguetan 63. *Opera omnia*, Lyon quarto 1681: relief, open initial 'Q', bird in flight design, white on black background, double-lined border; 11 × 11 millimetres

Huguetan 64. *Opera omnia*, Lyon quarto 1681: relief, open initial 'I', stem design, white on black background, double-lined border; 13 × 13 millimetres

Huguetan 65. *Opera omnia*, Lyon quarto 1681: relief, open initial 'O', stem and flower design, white on black background, double-lined border; 10 × 10 millimetres

Huguetan 66. *Opera omnia*, Lyon quarto 1681: relief, closed initial 'I', stem and leaf design, no border; 8 × 8 millimetres

Huguetan 67. *Opera omnia*, Lyon quarto 1681: relief, closed initial 'A', stem and leaf design, no border; 8 × 8 millimetres

Huguetan 68. *Opera omnia*, Lyon quarto 1681: relief, closed initial 'D', stem, flower and bird design, single border; 16 × 17 millimetres

Huguetan 69. *Opera omnia*, Lyon quarto 1681: relief, open initial 'I', naked bald male figure with stem and leaf design, double border; 24 × 23 millimetres

Huguetan 70. *Opera omnia*, Lyon quarto 1681: relief, open shadowed initial 'E', stem and leaf design, no border; 23 × 23 millimetres

Huguetan 71. *Opera omnia*, Lyon quarto 1681: relief, open shadowed initial 'N', stem and leaf with central partial mask design, no border; 20 × 19 millimetres

Huguetan 72. *Opera omnia*, Lyon quarto 1681: relief, open shadowed initial 'D', stem and leaf with central mask design, no border; 20 × 20 millimetres

Huguetan 73. *Opera omnia*, Lyon quarto 1681: relief, open initial 'I', two naked children dancing, double border; 17 × 18 millimetres

Huguetan 74. *Opera omnia*, Lyon quarto 1681: relief, closed initial 'R', stem and leaf design, no border; 8 × 8 millimetres

Huguetan 75. *Opera omnia*, Lyon quarto 1681: relief, open initial 'C', squirrel with leaf and stem design, no border; 20 × 20 millimetres

Huguetan 76. *Opera omnia*, Lyon quarto 1681: relief, closed initial 'A', stem and leaf design, no border; 8 × 8 millimetres

Huguetan 77. *Opera omnia*, Lyon quarto 1681: relief, open initial 'Q', human face with flower and stem design, no border; 29 × 29 millimetres

Huguetan 78. *Opera omnia*, Lyon quarto 1681: relief, open initial 'I', locusts with leaf and stem design, no border; 22 × 22 millimetres

Huguetan 79. *Opera omnia*, Lyon quarto 1681: relief, closed initial 'E', factotum with four flowers, four leaf designs, nine borders (from inside: dashed, ruled, dashed, lined, serrated, dashed, serrated [2], lined); 16 × 16 millimetres

Huguetan 80. *Opera omnia*, Lyon quarto 1681: fleuron, fleur-de-lys; 5 × 5 millimetres

Huguetan 81. *Opera omnia*, Lyon quarto 1681: relief, tailpiece, flower basket, no border; 38 × 51 millimetres

Huguetan 82. *Opera omnia*, Lyon quarto 1681: relief, headpiece, Egyptian woman with flower baskets, two mythical figures and scrolls, no border; 23 × 93 millimetres

Huguetan 83. *Opera omnia*, Lyon quarto 1681: relief, headpiece, stem and floral design, no border; 34 × 12 millimetres

Huguetan 84. *Opera omnia* Lyon quarto 1681: relief, open shadowed initial 'M', stem and leaf with human head design, no border; 20 × 20 millimetres

Huguetan 85. *Opera omnia* Lyon quarto 1681: relief, open shadowed initial 'A', stem and leaf with human figure, and swans with human faces design, no border; 30 × 30 millimetres

Huguetan 86. *Opera omnia* Lyon quarto 1681: relief, open shadowed initial 'A', leaf and stem design, no border; 19 × 19 millimetres

Huguetan 87. *Opera omnia* Lyon quarto 1681: relief, closed initial 'H', stem and leaf design, no border; 8 × 8 millimetres.

Leers:

Leers 1. *Pharmaceutice rationalis* (part 1), The Hague duodecimo 1674: relief, tailpiece, hanging inverted triangular garland, leaves and buds, no border; 16 × 23 millimetres

Leers 2. *Pharmaceutice rationalis* (part 1), The Hague duodecimo 1674: relief, open shadowed initial 'Q', stem and leaf background, no border; 15 × 15 millimetres

Leers 3. *Pharmaceutice rationalis* (part 1), The Hague duodecimo 1674: relief, open shadowed initial 'A', stem and leaf background, no border; 13 × 13 millimetres

Leers 4. *Pharmaceutice rationalis* (part 1), The Hague duodecimo 1675: relief, tailpiece, flowers, interlaced stems and leaves, no border; 24 × 29 millimetres

Leers 5 *Pharmaceutice rationalis* (part 1), The Hague duodecimo 1675: relief, open shadowed initial 'Q', stem, leaf, and flower background, no border; 19 × 19 millimetres

Leers 6. *Pharmaceutice rationalis* (part 1), The Hague duodecimo 1675: relief, tailpiece, interlaced stems and leaves, no border; 26 × 31 millimetres

Leers 7. *Pharmaceutice rationalis* (part 1), The Hague duodecimo 1675: relief, open shadowed initial 'A', stem and flower background, no border; 19 × 19 millimetres

Leers 8. *Pharmaceutice rationalis* (part 2), The Hague duodecimo 1677: relief, open shadowed initial ‘A’, stem and flower background, no border; 15 × 15 millimetres

Leers 9. *Pharmaceutice rationalis* (part 2), The Hague duodecimo 1677: relief, open shadowed initial ‘D’, stem and leaf background, no border; 15 × 14 millimetres

Leers 10. *Pharmaceutice rationalis* (part 2), The Hague duodecimo 1677: relief, tailpiece, inverted triangular garland, leaves, stem and flowers, no border; 21 × 28 millimetres

Leers 11. *Pharmaceutice rationalis* (part 2), The Hague duodecimo 1677: relief, headpiece, leaves, stem, flower, bird and basket (cut down from a larger ornament and inverted), no border; 19 × 56 millimetres (see: Figure 24)

Leers 12. *Pharmaceutice rationalis* (part 2), The Hague duodecimo 1677: relief, tailpiece, leaves, stem, buds and squirrel design, no border; 28 × 36 millimetres (see: Figure 47)

Leers 13. *Pharmaceutice rationalis* (part 2), The Hague duodecimo 1677: relief, open shadowed initial ‘I’, stem and leaf background, no border; 19 × 15 millimetres.

Lucas:

Lucas 1. *Cerebri anatome*, Amsterdam duodecimo 1676: relief, tailpiece, rosette, stems and buds, no border; 20 × 27 millimetres

Lucas 2. *Cerebri anatome*, Amsterdam duodecimo 1676: relief, tailpiece, stems and buds, no border; 27 × 33 millimetres.

Malachin:

Malachin 1. *Opera omnia*, Venice folio 1720: engraving, printer’s device, cartouche with crowns, arabesque with leaves, lettered M G D A, single-lined border; 79 × 115 millimetres

Malachin 2. *Opera omnia*, Venice folio 1720: relief, open shadowed initial ‘N’, stem and leaf design, double-lined border; 36 × 40 millimetres

Malachin 3. *Opera omnia*, Venice folio 1720: relief, tailpiece, inverted triangle, stem, leaves worked into central human face, no border; 50 × 77 millimetres (see: Figure 48)

Malachin 4. *Opera omnia*, Venice folio 1720: relief, headpiece, urn, flowers, leaves, two semi-recumbent figures each supported on stems by one arm, no border; 44 × 73 millimetres (see: Figure 25)

Malachin 5. *Opera omnia*, Venice folio 1720: relief, open shadowed initial ‘I’, stem and leaf design, male and female figures, no border; 35 × 35 millimetres

Malachin 6. *Opera omnia*, Venice folio 1720: relief, tailpiece, basket, flower, stems and leaf background, no border; 44 × 65 millimetres

Malachin 7. *Opera omnia*, Venice folio 1720: relief, open shadowed initial ‘A’, stem and leaf design, double-lined border; 35 × 35 millimetres

Malachin 8. *Opera omnia*, Venice folio 1720: relief, open shadowed initial ‘Q’, stem and leaf, fleur-de-lys design, double-lined border; 32 × 32 millimetres

Malachin 9. *Opera omnia*, Venice folio 1720: relief, open shadowed initial ‘E’, stem and leaf, peacock, diagonally lined design, double-lined border; 33 × 33 millimetres (see: Figure 75)

Malachin 10. *Opera omnia*, Venice folio 1720: relief, open shadowed initial ‘D’, stem and leaf, human figure design, no border; 32 × 32 millimetres.[49]

[49] As discussed in chapter 12, the same ‘D’ (Malachin 10) is found on the cancelled sheet (†8v, page [16]) in one copy of *Opera omnia* published by Ruinetti and Storti (1708: 8H.c3). It is not clear when this cancellans was printed

Roycroft:

Roycroft 1. *Diatribæ duæ medico-philosophicæ*, London octavo 1659: fleuron, urn; 6 × 6 millimetres
Roycroft 2. *Diatribæ duæ medico-philosophicæ*, London octavo 1659: fleuron, heraldic badge, and coronet; 9 × 6 millimetres
Roycroft 3. *Diatribæ duæ medico-philosophicæ*, London octavo 1659: fleuron, heraldic badge, and coronet; 9 × 5 millimetres
Roycroft 4. *Diatribæ duæ medico-philosophicæ*, London octavo 1659: fleuron, heraldic badge, and coronet; 9 × 6 millimetres
Roycroft 5. *Diatribæ duæ medico-philosophicæ*, London octavo 1659: fleuron, heraldic badge, and coronet; 9 × 6 millimetres
Roycroft 6. *Diatribæ duæ medico-philosophicæ*, London octavo 1659: fleuron, heraldic badge, and coronet; 9 × 5 millimetres
Roycroft 7. *Diatribæ duæ medico-philosophicæ*, London octavo 1659: fleuron, spray; 8 × 5 millimetres
Roycroft 8. *Diatribæ duæ medico-philosophicæ*, London octavo 1659: fleuron, fleur-de-lys; 3 × 2 millimetres.
Roycroft 9. *Diatribæ duæ medico-philosophicæ*, London octavo 1659: relief, open initial 'I' on leaves, no border; 18 × 17 millimetres
Roycroft 10. *Diatribæ duæ medico-philosophicæ*, London octavo 1659: fleuron, heraldic badge, and coronet; 9 × 4 millimetres
Roycroft 11. *Diatribæ duæ medico-philosophicæ*, London duodecimo 1660: fleuron, spray; 6 × 5 millimetres
Roycroft 12. *Diatribæ duæ medico-philosophicæ*, London duodecimo 1660: fleuron, scroll; 4 × 8 millimetres
Roycroft 13. *Diatribæ duæ medico-philosophicæ*, London duodecimo 1660: fleuron, spray; 5 × 4 millimetres
Roycroft 14. *Diatribæ duæ medico-philosophicæ*, London duodecimo 1660: fleuron, fleur-de-lys; 6 × 4 millimetres
Roycroft 15. *Diatribæ duæ medico-philosophicæ*, London duodecimo 1660: fleuron, fleur-de-lys; 6 × 4 millimetres
Roycroft 16. *Diatribæ duæ medico-philosophicæ*, London duodecimo 1660: fleuron, urn; 6 × 4 millimetres
Roycroft 17. *Diatribæ duæ medico-philosophicæ*, London duodecimo 1660: fleuron, rosette; 5 × 5 millimetres
Roycroft 18. *Diatribæ duæ medico-philosophicæ*, London duodecimo 1660: fleuron, coiled rosettes; 5 × 10 millimetres
Roycroft 19. *Diatribæ duæ medico-philosophicæ*, London duodecimo 1660: relief, open shadowed initial 'D' on flowers and leaves, no border; 22 × 20 millimetres
Roycroft 20. *Diatribæ duæ medico-philosophicæ*, London duodecimo 1660: fleuron, acorn; 6 × 2 millimetres
Roycroft 21. *Diatribæ duæ medico-philosophicæ*, London duodecimo 1662: relief, head-piece, leaves, stems, rose, thistle, and fleur-de-lys, no border; 16 × 56 millimetres (see: Figure 26)

and, although the decorated initial 'D' may first have been in the possession of Ruinetti, it has been classified as one of Malachin's ornaments.

Roycroft 22. *Diatribæ duæ medico-philosophicæ*, London duodecimo 1662: relief, open shadowed initial 'S' on leaves, no border; 25 × 25 millimetres

Roycroft 23. *Diatribæ duæ medico-philosophicæ*, London duodecimo 1662: relief, open shadowed initial 'D' on leaves, no border; 17 × 17 millimetres

Roycroft 24. *Diatribæ duæ medico-philosophicæ*, London duodecimo 1662: relief, open shadowed initial 'I' on leaves, no border; 19 × 20 millimetres

Roycroft 25. *Diatribæ duæ medico-philosophicæ*, London duodecimo 1662: relief, headpiece, deconstructed caduceus with strapwork, lined border; 8 × 55 millimetres (see: Figure 27)

Roycroft 26. *Diatribæ duæ medico-philosophicæ*, London duodecimo 1677: relief, open shaded initial 'S' on stems, double-lined border; 16 × 16 millimetres

Roycroft 27. *Diatribæ duæ medico-philosophicæ*, London duodecimo 1677 relief (inverted), headpiece, deconstructed caduceus, or mythical coiled animals, lined border; 9 × 55 millimetres

Roycroft 28. *Cerebri anatome*, London octavo 1664: fleuron, thistle; 5 × 4 millimetres

Roycroft 29. *Cerebri anatome*, London octavo 1664: relief, open shadowed initial 'N' on corn stooks and leaves, no border; 20 × 20 millimetres

Roycroft 30. *Pathologiæ cerebri* London quarto 1667: relief, open shadowed initial 'I', angels blowing pipes, with cockerels, strapwork, double-lined border; 36 × 36 millimetres (see: Figure 76)

Roycroft 31. *Pathologiæ cerebri* Oxford and London quarto 1667: fleuron, spray; 5 × 4 millimetres

Roycroft 32. *Pathologiæ cerebri* Oxford and London quarto 1667: fleuron, spray; 5 × 4 millimetres

Roycroft 33. *Pathologiæ cerebri* Oxford and London quarto 1667: fleuron, spray; 5 × 4 millimetres

Roycroft 34. *Pathologiæ cerebri* Oxford and London quarto 1667: fleuron, spray; 5 × 4 millimetres

Roycroft 35. *Pathologiæ cerebri* Oxford and London quarto 1667: fleuron, spray; 5 × 4 millimetres

Roycroft 36. *Pathologiæ cerebri* Oxford and London quarto 1667: fleuron, spray; 7 × 5 millimetres

Roycroft 37. *Pathologiæ cerebri*, London duodecimo 1678: relief, headpiece, corn stook, ravens, stems, and leaves, no border; 23 × 62 millimetres (see: Figure 28)

Roycroft 38. *Pathologiæ cerebri*, London duodecimo 1678: relief, open shadowed initial 'Q' on leaves, no border; 21 × 20 millimetres

Roycroft 39. *Pathologiæ cerebri*, London duodecimo 1678: relief, headpiece, cherubs riding seahorses, crowned head, leaves and stems, cartouche border; 24 × 50 millimetres (see: Figure 29)

Roycroft 40. *Pathologiæ cerebri*, London duodecimo 1678: relief, open shadowed initial 'I' on leaves, border; 13 × 14 millimetres

Roycroft 41. *Affectionum quæ dicuntur hystericæ et hypochondriac*, London duodecimo 1678: relief, open shadowed initial 'R' on leaves, no border; 13 × 14 millimetres.

Ruinetti:

Ruinetti 1. *Opera omnia*, Venice folio 1708: relief, open shadowed initial 'C', stems and leaves design, no border; 41 × 41 millimetres

Ruinetti 2. *Opera omnia*, Venice folio 1708: relief, open shadowed initial 'S', stems and leaves design, no border; 33 × 32 millimetres

Ruinetti 3. *Opera omnia*, Venice folio 1708: relief, tailpiece, inverted triangle, lion's head with mane of stems, leaves and flowers, no border; 49 × 58 millimetres (see: Figure 49)

Ruinetti 4. *Opera omnia*, Venice folio 1708: relief, headpiece, urns, seated figures in a landscape with distant roofed building, leaping harts, single-lined border; 32 × 161 millimetres

Ruinetti 5. *Opera omnia*, Venice folio 1708: relief, open initial 'T', male figure apparently about to strike a figure lying in bed with a raised dagger being restrained by a third, female, figure background, double-lined border; 34 × 35 millimetres (see: Figure 77)

Ruinetti 6. *Opera omnia*, Venice folio 1708: tailpiece, urn with stems and flowers, no border; 59 × 70 millimetres

Ruinetti 7. *Opera omnia*, Venice folio 1708: tailpiece, oval framed face with stems, leaves and flowers, no border; 29 × 63 millimetres

Ruinetti 8. *Opera omnia*, Venice folio 1708: tailpiece, spray of leaves, no border; 30 × 46 millimetres

Ruinetti 9. *Opera omnia*, Venice folio 1708: relief, open shadowed initial 'D', leaf design, double-lined border; 30 × 29 millimetres

Ruinetti 10. *Opera omnia*, Venice folio 1708: tailpiece, spray of stems, leaves and flower, no border; 37 × 42 millimetres (see: Figure 50)

Ruinetti 11. *Opera omnia*, Venice folio 1708: relief, headpiece, figure with basket of flowers, birds, stem and leaf background, no border; 33 × 172 millimetres (see: Figure 30)

Ruinetti 12. *Opera omnia*, Venice folio 1708: relief, open shadowed initial 'I', stem and leaf design, double-lined border; 32 × 32 millimetres

Ruinetti 13. *Opera omnia*, Venice folio 1708: relief, open initial 'D' two figures in a landscape, one standing with staff, the other kneeling and gazing at an angel in the cloud, scroll lettered NVNTIO VOCAV(I) [I inform, I have called]; double-lined border; 30 × 29 millimetres (see: Figure 78)

Ruinetti 14. *Opera omnia*, Venice folio 1708: relief, tailpiece, sphere with flames (perhaps a bomb or firework), no border; 87 × 90 millimetres (see: Figure 51)

Ruinetti 15. *Opera omnia*, Venice folio 1708: relief, open shadowed initial 'O', angel with headdress, leaf design, double-lined border; 35 × 35 millimetres (see: Figure 79)

Ruinetti 16. *Opera omnia*, Venice folio 1708: relief, open shadowed initial 'A', stem and leaf design, double-lined border; 34 × 34 millimetres

Ruinetti 17. *Opera omnia*, Venice folio 1708: tailpiece, basket of fruit, flowers with stem and leaves, no border; 22 × 90 millimetres

Ruinetti 18. *Opera omnia*, Venice folio 1708: tailpiece, winged angel with stems, leaves and flowers, no border; 51 × 119 millimetres (see: Figure 52)

Ruinetti 19. *Opera omnia*, Venice folio 1708: relief, open shadowed initial 'D', stem and leaf background, no border; 26 × 26 millimetres

Ruinetti 20. *Opera omnia*, Venice folio 1708: relief, open shadowed initial 'Q', stem and leaf design, double-lined border; 36 × 36 millimetres

Ruinetti 21. *Opera omnia*, Venice folio 1708: relief, open shadowed initial 'Q', stem and leaf design, double-lined border; 38 × 38 millimetres

Ruinetti 22. *Opera omnia*, Venice folio 1708: relief, open shadowed initial 'R', stem and leaf design, no border; 24 × 24 millimetres

Ruinetti 23. *Opera omnia*, Venice folio 1708: relief, open shadowed initial 'I', stem, leaf and flower design, double-lined border; 25 × 25 millimetres

Ruinetti 24. *Opera omnia*, Venice folio 1708: relief, tailpiece, twin angels aloft holding a crown and sprays, no border; 29 × 57 millimetres (see: Figure 53)
Ruinetti 25. *Opera omnia*, Venice folio 1708: relief, open initial 'C', figure blowing a horn, leaf design, no border; 27 × 28 millimetres
Ruinetti 26. *Opera omnia*, Venice folio 1708: relief, open shadowed initial 'E', stem and leaf design, double-lined border; 32 × 32 millimetres
Ruinetti 27. *Opera omnia*, Venice folio 1708: relief, open shadowed initial 'Q', stem and leaf design, no border; 21 × 21 millimetres
Ruinetti 28. *Opera omnia*, Venice folio 1708: relief, tailpiece, oval framed reindeer, square cartouche, single-lined border; 104 × 88 millimetres (see: Figure 54)
Ruinetti 29. *Opera omnia*, Venice folio 1708: relief, open initial 'Q', stem and leaf design, single-lined border; 22 × 22 millimetres
Ruinetti 30. *Opera omnia*, Venice folio 1708: relief, open initial 'A', stem and leaf design, no border; 25 × 24 millimetres
Ruinetti 31. *Opera omnia*, Venice folio 1708: relief, tailpiece, flower and leaves, no border; 30 × 38 millimetres
Ruinetti 32. *Opera omnia*, Venice folio 1708: relief, open shadowed initial 'A', flowers, stem and leaf design, double-lined border; 34 × 33 millimetres
Ruinetti 33. *Opera omnia*, Venice folio 1708: relief, open shadowed initial 'I', stem and leaf design, double-lined border; 23 × 23 millimetres
Ruinetti 34. *Opera omnia*, Venice folio 1708: relief, tailpiece, inverted triangle, angel with leaves, no border; 44 × 51 millimetres.

Schagen:

Schagen 1. *Diatribæ duæ medico-philosophicæ*, Amsterdam duodecimo 1663: fleuron, spray; 3 × 3 millimetres (see: Figure 31)
Schagen 2. *Diatribæ duæ medico-philosophicæ*, Amsterdam duodecimo 1663: fleuron, rosette; 4 × 4 millimetres (see: Figure 31)
Schagen 3. *Diatribæ duæ medico-philosophicæ*, Amsterdam duodecimo 1663: relief, open shadowed initial 'D', stem and leaf background, no border; 17 × 17 millimetres
Schagen 4. *Diatribæ duæ medico-philosophicæ*, Amsterdam duodecimo 1663: relief, open shadowed initial 'D', stem and leaf background, no border; 12 × 12 millimetres
Schagen 5. *Diatribæ duæ medico-philosophicæ*, Amsterdam duodecimo 1663: relief, open shadowed initial 'I', dentelle background, no border; 13 × 13 millimetres
Schagen 6. *Diatribæ duæ medico-philosophicæ*, Amsterdam duodecimo 1663: relief, tailpiece, inverted triangle, stem, leaves, and tulips, no border; 32 × 38 millimetres
Schagen 7. *Diatribæ duæ medico-philosophicæ*, Amsterdam duodecimo 1663: relief, headpiece, stem, flower, scroll and beaked animals, no border; 5 × 50 millimetres
Schagen 8. *Diatribæ duæ medico-philosophicæ*, Amsterdam duodecimo 1663: relief, open shadowed initial 'E', leaf background, no border; 12 × 11 millimetres
Schagen 9. *Diatribæ duæ medico-philosophicæ*, Amsterdam duodecimo 1663: relief, headpiece, interlaced stems, leaves, coiled serpents and birds, central X / ∇, no border; 10 × 49 millimetres (see: Figure 32)
Schagen 10. *Diatribæ duæ medico-philosophicæ*, Amsterdam duodecimo 1663: relief, open shadowed initial 'C', stem and leaf background, no border; 16 × 16 millimetres (see: Figure 80)

Schagen 11. *Diatribæ duæ medico-philosophicæ*, Amsterdam duodecimo 1663: relief, tailpiece, inverted triangular arabesque, no border; 25 × 38 millimetres
Schagen 12. *Diatribæ duæ medico-philosophicæ*, Amsterdam duodecimo 1669: relief, headpiece, hounds, stems, leaves, and flowers, no border; 4 × 49 millimetres
Schagen 13. *Diatribæ duæ medico-philosophicæ*, Amsterdam duodecimo 1669: relief, open shadowed initial 'C', spiral stem and leaf background, no border; 16 × 16 millimetres
Schagen 14. *Cerebri anatome*, Amsterdam duodecimo 1664: relief, open shadowed initial 'A', dentelle background, no border; 13 × 13 millimetres
Schagen 15. *Cerebri anatome*, Amsterdam duodecimo 1664: relief, open shadowed initial 'N' (inverted), dentelle background, no border; 13 × 13 millimetres
Schagen 16. *Cerebri anatome*, Amsterdam octavo 1666: relief, tailpiece, hanging inverted triangular garland, leaves and buds, pendants, no border; 18 × 24 millimetres (see: Figure 55)
Schagen 17. *Cerebri anatome*, Amsterdam octavo 1666: relief, open shadowed initial 'A', spiral stem and leaf background, no border; 17 × 17 millimetres
Schagen 18. *Cerebri anatome*, Amsterdam octavo 1666: relief, open shadowed initial 'N', spiral stem and leaf background, no border; 17 × 17 millimetres
Schagen 19. *Cerebri anatome*, Amsterdam octavo 1666: relief, tailpiece, hanging inverted triangular garland, fruit, leaves and buds, leaf pendants, no border; 37 × 51 millimetres (see: Figure 56)
Schagen 20. *Cerebri anatome*, Amsterdam octavo 1666: relief, open shadowed initial 'P', spiral stem and leaf background, no border; 17 × 17 millimetres
Schagen 21. *Cerebri anatome*, Amsterdam octavo 1666: relief, open shadowed initial 'D', spiral stem and leaf background, no border; 17 × 18 millimetres
Schagen 22. [*De ratione motus musculorum*]. Amsterdam octavo 1667: fleuron, arabesque; 9 × 13 millimetres.

Someren:

Someren 1. *De anima brutorum*, Amsterdam duodecimo 1674: fleuron, stems and flower; 4 × 9 millimetres
Someren 2. *De anima brutorum*, Amsterdam duodecimo 1674: relief, open shadowed initial 'Q', stem and leaf background, no border; 15 × 15 millimetres
Someren 3. *De anima brutorum*, Amsterdam duodecimo 1674: relief, open shadowed initial 'E', stem and flower background, no border; 16 × 16 millimetres
Someren 4. *De anima brutorum*, Amsterdam duodecimo 1674: relief, tailpiece, hanging inverted triangular garland, leaves and buds, pendants, no border; 20 × 27 millimetres
Someren 5. *De anima brutorum*, Amsterdam duodecimo 1674: relief, open shadowed initial 'A', stem and flower background, no border; 15 × 15 millimetres.

Storti:

Storti 1. *Opera omnia*, Coloniæ folio 1694: engraving, printer's device, two unclothed angels linking arms through lion's head and holding a scroll lettered FORTITVDO OMNIA VINCIT [Strength conquers all], Minerva with lance and shield in a landscape with buildings, oval panel with monogram, cartouche garland of flowers; 112 × 151 millimetres (plate marks, 117 × 154 millimetres; see: Figure 15)
Storti 2. *Opera omnia*, Coloniæ folio 1694: relief, open initial 'C', urn with leaves, horned heads with human faces background, double-lined border; 43 × 42 millimetres

Storti 3. *Opera omnia*, Coloniæ folio 1694: relief, open shadowed initial 'S', stems and leaves design, no border; 33 × 32 millimetres

Storti 4. *Opera omnia*, Coloniæ folio 1694: relief, tailpiece, stems, leaves and rose background, no border; 33 × 47 millimetres

Storti 5. *Opera omnia*, Coloniæ folio 1694: relief, open shadowed initial 'T', stems and leaves design, no border; 35 × 34 millimetres

Storti 6. *Opera omnia*, Coloniæ folio 1694: relief, tailpiece, basket of flowers, stems and leaf background, no border; 25 × 62 millimetres

Storti 7. *Opera omnia*, Coloniæ folio 1694: relief, tailpiece, human face with headdress of stems, leaves, and flowers, no border; 37 × 54 millimetres

Storti 8. *Opera omnia* Coloniæ folio 1694: relief, open initial 'C' stems and leaves design, single-lined border; 28 × 28 millimetres

Storti 9. *Opera omnia*, Coloniæ folio 1694: relief, tailpiece, intertwined stems, leaves and flowers, no border; 38 × 44 millimetres

Storti 10. *Opera omnia*, Coloniæ folio 1694: relief, open initial 'D' stems and leaves, human figure in flight design, double-lined border; 34 × 34 millimetres

Storti 11. *Opera omnia*, Coloniæ folio 1694: relief, tailpiece, Gemini, stems, leaves and flowers, no border; 43 × 59 millimetres (see: Figure 57)

Storti 12. *Opera omnia*, Coloniæ folio 1694: relief, headpiece, angels playing viols, scroll-work, angel's head, no border; 32 × 147 millimetres (see: Figure 33)

Storti 13. *Opera omnia*, Coloniæ folio 1694: relief, open shadowed initial 'I', stems and leaves design, no border; 32 × 33 millimetres

Storti 14. *Opera omnia*, Coloniæ folio 1694: relief, tailpiece, inverted triangle, human head with open mouth, stems, leaves and flowers, two doves eating fruit, no border; 103 × 129 millimetres

Storti 15. *Opera omnia*, Coloniæ folio 1694: relief, open shadowed initial 'O', stems and leaves design, no border; 34 × 33 millimetres

Storti 16. *Opera omnia*, Coloniæ folio 1694: relief, open shadowed initial 'A', stems and leaves design, no border; 33 × 33 millimetres

Storti 17. *Opera omnia*, Coloniæ folio 1694: relief, tailpiece, inverted triangle, human head with open mouth, stems, leaves and flowers, two doves eating buds, no border; 66 × 91 millimetres (see: Figure 58)

Storti 18. *Opera omnia*, Coloniæ folio 1694: relief, open initial 'D' lion's face with mane of stems and leaves design, no border; 33 × 33 millimetres

Storti 19. *Opera omnia*, Coloniæ folio 1694: relief, open shadowed initial 'Q', stems and leaves design, no border; 33 × 33 millimetres

Storti 20. *Opera omnia*, Coloniæ folio 1694: relief, fleuron scroll; 7 × 7 millimetres

Storti 21. *Opera omnia*, Coloniæ folio 1694: relief, open shadowed initial 'I', stems and leaves, no border; 25 × 25 millimetres

Storti 22. *Opera omnia*, Coloniæ folio 1694: relief, open shadowed initial 'R', stems and leaves design, no border; 24 × 24 millimetres

Storti 23. *Opera omnia*, Coloniæ folio 1694: relief, open shadowed initial 'C', stems and leaves design, no border; 25 × 24 millimetres

Storti 24. *Opera omnia*, Coloniæ folio 1694: relief, tailpiece, winged angels with stems, leaves and flowers, no border; 62 × 89 millimetres (see: Figure 59)

Storti 25. *Opera omnia*, Coloniæ folio 1694: relief, headpiece, female face with stems, leaves and fruit, no border; 36 × 170 millimetres (see: Figure 34)

Storti 26. *Opera omnia* Coloniæ folio 1694: relief, open initial 'E' stems and leaves, no border; 32 × 33 millimetres

Storti 27. *Opera omnia*, Coloniæ folio 1694: relief, open shadowed initial 'Q', stems and leaves, no border; 33 × 33 millimetres

Storti 28. *Opera omnia*, Coloniæ folio 1694: relief, open shadowed initial 'A', stems and leaves design, no border; 24 × 24 millimetres.

Tournes:

Tournes 1. *Opera omnia*, Geneva quarto 1676: relief, printer's device, two female figures, one 'Justice' in profile blindfolded with sword and scales, the other 'Prudence' (partly robed) with serpent and cup, central armorial design with cartouche, monograms in double-lined circular borders, lettered (upper) SADT and (lower) motif incorporating I A S, central inscription 'QVOD TIBI FIERI NON VIS, ALTERI NEFECERIS' [Do unto others as you would have them do unto you],[50] no border; 48 × 76 millimetres

Tournes 2. *Opera omnia*, Geneva quarto 1676: relief, headpiece, leaf, stem, flower, mermaids, squirrels eating nuts, and lion's head, no border; 28 × 114 millimetres (see: Figure 35)

Tournes 3. *Opera omnia*, Geneva quarto 1676: relief, criblé, open initial 'E', intertwined stems and leaf, white on black background, single-lined border; 42 × 42 millimetres

Tournes 4. *Opera omnia*, Geneva quarto 1676: relief, headpiece, cherub's face and wings, hanging garland of stems and fruit background, no border; 25 × 110 millimetres (see: Figure 36)

Tournes 5. *Opera omnia*, Geneva quarto 1676: relief, criblé, open initial 'S', intertwined stems and leaf, white on black background, single-lined border; 42 × 42 millimetres

Tournes 6. *Opera omnia*, Geneva quarto 1676: relief, open initial 'D', three male figures, two unclothed, each with staff, white on black background, single-lined border; 27 × 27 millimetres (see: Figure 81)

Tournes 7. *Opera omnia*, Geneva quarto 1676: fleuron, spray; 5 × 4 millimetres

Tournes 8. *Opera omnia*, Geneva quarto 1676: fleuron, strapwork; 4 × 8 millimetres

Tournes 9. *Opera omnia*, Geneva quarto 1676: relief, criblé, open initial 'D', stems and leaf, white on black background, single-lined border; 28 × 28 millimetres

Tournes 10. *Opera omnia*, Geneva quarto 1676: relief, tailpiece, basket of flowers and fruit, no border; 39 × 59 millimetres

Tournes 11. *Opera omnia*, Geneva quarto 1676: fleuron, acorn (rotated); 4 × 2 millimetres

Tournes 12. *Opera omnia*, Geneva quarto 1676: fleuron, spray; 6 × 9 millimetres

Tournes 13. *Opera omnia*, Geneva quarto 1676: relief, open initial 'F', capped and cloaked male figure, crouching and walking through a wood, white on black background, single-lined border; 21 × 21 millimetres

Tournes 14. *Opera omnia*, Geneva quarto 1676: relief, open initial 'V', hooded and smocked figure killing a boar with his dagger, white on black background, single-lined border; 21 × 20 millimetres (see: Figure 82)

Tournes 15. *Opera omnia*, Geneva quarto 1676: relief, criblé, open initial 'I', stems, leaves and dragon, white on black background, single-lined border; 28 × 28 millimetres

[50] See: The Gospel according to Matthew, chapter 7, verse 12, which is part of the Sermon on the Mount.

Tournes 16. *Opera omnia*, Geneva quarto 1676: relief, open initial 'E', naked hatted male figure blowing an Alpine horn, white on black background, single-lined border; 27 × 27 millimetres (see: Figure 83)

Tournes 17. *Opera omnia*, Geneva quarto 1676: relief, tailpiece, floral basket, no border; 49 × 56 millimetres

Tournes 18. *Opera omnia*, Geneva quarto 1676: fleuron, strapwork; 3 × 9 millimetres

Tournes 19. *Opera omnia*, Geneva quarto 1676: fleuron, spray; 4 × 2 millimetres

Tournes 20. *Opera omnia*, Geneva quarto 1676: relief, criblé, open initial 'V', stems, leaves and angel, white on black background, single-lined border; 27 × 27 millimetres

Tournes 21. *Opera omnia*, Geneva quarto 1676: relief, open initial 'C', hooded and smocked figure by a river bank gaffing a fish, white on black background, single-lined border; 27 × 27 millimetres (see: Figure 84)

Tournes 22. *Opera omnia*, Geneva quarto 1676: relief, tailpiece, basket of fruit, no border; 38 × 52 millimetres

Tournes 23. *Opera omnia*, Geneva quarto 1676: relief, open initial 'A', two head-garlanded figures hauling a fishing net, white on black background, single-lined border; 27 × 27 millimetres (see: Figure 85)

Tournes 24. *Opera omnia*, Geneva quarto 1676: relief, open initial 'C', two satyrs, one blowing an Alpine horn, white on black background, single-lined border; 20 × 20 millimetres

Tournes 25. *Opera omnia*, Geneva quarto 1676: relief, criblé, open initial 'I', leaves and dragon, white on black background, single-lined border; 28 × 28 millimetres

Tournes 26. *Opera omnia*, Geneva quarto 1676: relief, headpiece, four females with dogs on leashes, chariot with reindeer, no border; 21 × 105 millimetres (see: Figure 37)

Tournes 27. *Opera omnia*, Geneva quarto 1676: relief, open initial 'N', leaves with seated satyr speaking, white on black background, single-lined border; 26 × 27 millimetres (see: Figure 86)

Tournes 28. *Opera omnia*, Geneva quarto 1676: relief, open initial 'T', leaves with two clothed seated male figures conversing, white on black background, single-lined border; 21 × 21 millimetres

Tournes 29. *Opera omnia*, Geneva quarto 1676: relief, criblé, open initial 'D', leaves with one fashioned as human face, white on black background, single-lined border; 27 × 27 millimetres

Tournes 30. *Opera omnia*, Geneva quarto 1676: relief, criblé, open initial 'I', intertwined stems and leaves, white on black background, single-lined border; 42 × 42 millimetres

Tournes 31. *Opera omnia*, Geneva quarto 1676: fleuron, spray (rotated); 4 × 3 millimetres

Tournes 32. *Opera omnia*, Geneva quarto 1676: relief, criblé, open initial 'Q', leaves and dragon, white on black background, single-lined border; 27 × 26 millimetres

Tournes 33. *Opera omnia*, Geneva quarto 1676: relief, open initial 'Q', leaves and child climbing a tree with a bird on the branch, white on black background, single-lined border; 21 × 21 millimetres

Tournes 34. *Opera omnia*, Geneva quarto 1676: relief, open initial 'I', flowers and coiled serpents, white on black background, single-lined border; 21 × 21 millimetres

Tournes 35. *Opera omnia*, Geneva quarto 1676: relief, headpiece, stems, flowers, fruit and angels with viol and lute, no border; 20 × 102 millimetres (see: Figure 38)

Tournes 36. *Opera omnia*, Geneva quarto 1676: relief, criblé, open initial 'I', stems, leaves and satyr, white on black background, single-lined border; 27 × 27 millimetres

Tournes 37. *Opera omnia*, Geneva quarto 1676: relief, open initial 'I', naked male with bow, arrow, and quiver shooting past a hart, white on black background, single-lined border; 28 × 28 millimetres (see: Figure 87)

Tournes 38. *Opera omnia*, Geneva quarto 1676: relief, open initial 'Q', kneeling male figure with plumed hat and banner, white on black background, single-lined border; 27 × 27 millimetres

Tournes 39. *Opera omnia*, Geneva quarto 1676: relief, headpiece, intertwined stems, leaves, flowers, fruit, horse, snail, birds, serpents, lion, central unclothed female figure with each arm around a lion and stag, no border; 27 × 119 millimetres (see: Figure 39)

Tournes 40. *Opera omnia*, Geneva quarto 1676: relief, open initial 'R', stems, leaves, bird and griffin background, no border; 28 × 29 millimetres

Tournes 41. *Opera omnia*, Geneva quarto 1676: relief, open initial 'I', stem, leaf and flower background, no border; 28 × 29 millimetres

Tournes 42. *Opera omnia*, Geneva quarto 1676: fleuron, strapwork; 3 × 2 millimetres

Tournes 43. *Opera omnia*, Geneva quarto 1676: relief, open initial 'C', stem, leaf, flower, and unclothed winged angel background, no border; 28 × 28 millimetres

Tournes 44. *Opera omnia*, Geneva quarto 1676: relief, criblé, open initial 'A', stems, leaves and face, white on black background, single-lined border; 26 × 26 millimetres

Tournes 45. *Opera omnia*, Geneva quarto 1676: relief, open initial 'A', two serpents with human hatted heads, white on black background, single-lined border; 21 × 21 millimetres (see: Figure 88)

Tournes 46. *Opera omnia*, Geneva quarto 1676: relief, open initial 'M', leaves, winged angel and basket, white on black background; single-lined border; 21 × 21 millimetres

Tournes 47. *Opera omnia*, Geneva quarto 1676: relief, open shadowed initial 'A', stems scrolled into human faces in profile and floral headdress background, no border; 27 × 27 millimetres

Tournes 48. *Opera omnia*, Geneva quarto 1676: relief, open initial 'A', Neptune attacking lamb with a trident, distant mountains and cloudy sky, white on black background, four lined borders with additional scrolls (upper and left); 42 × 42 millimetres

Tournes 49. *Opera omnia*, Geneva quarto 1676: relief, open initial 'O', three human head and torsos in profile, dagger and shield, white on black background, single-lined border; 20 × 20 millimetres

Tournes 50. *Opera omnia*, Geneva quarto 1676: relief, open initial 'A', leaves with human figure crouching, white on black background, single-lined border; 21 × 21 millimetres

Tournes 51. *Opera omnia*, Geneva quarto 1680: relief, new version of the Tournes printer's device (Tournes 1) but with the upper monogram reworked, undecipherable but presumably a version of SADT, no border; 48 × 76 millimetres

Tournes 52. *Opera omnia*, Geneva quarto 1680: relief, open initial 'L', two children, one seated and unclothed, the other walking, each with a staff, in a wood, white on black background, single-lined border; 27 × 27 millimetres

Tournes 53. *Opera omnia*, Geneva quarto 1680: relief, fleuron, rosette; 3 × 2 millimetres

Tournes 54. *Opera omnia*, Geneva quarto 1680: relief, open initial 'V', hooded and smocked figure killing a boar with his dagger, white on black background, single-lined border; 21 × 21 millimetres

Tournes 55. *Opera omnia*, Geneva quarto 1680: relief, criblé, open initial 'E', stem, leaves one shaped as male human figure with beard, white on black background, single-lined border; 28 × 28 millimetres

Tournes 56. *Opera omnia*, Geneva quarto 1680: relief, criblé, open initial 'C', stems, leaves one shaped as female human figure, white on black background, single-lined border; 27 × 27 millimetres

Tournes 57. *Opera omnia*, Geneva quarto 1680: relief, open initial 'T', leaves with two clothed seated male figures conversing, white on black background, single-lined border; 21 × 21 millimetres

Tournes 58. *Opera omnia*, Geneva quarto 1680: relief, open initial 'R', seated child playing amongst trees and flowers, white on black background, single-lined border; 27 × 27 millimetres

Tournes 59. *Opera omnia*, Geneva quarto 1695: relief, fleuron, spray; 4 × 3 millimetres

Tournes 60. *Opera omnia*, Geneva quarto 1695: relief, open initial 'T', child with staff riding a swan, white on black background, single-lined border; 27 × 27 millimetres (see: Figure 89)

Tournes 61. *Opera omnia*, Geneva quarto 1695: relief, fleuron, rosette; 4 × 4 millimetres

Tournes 62. *Opera omnia*, Geneva quarto 1695: relief, fleuron, strapwork; 3 × 5 millimetres

Tournes 63. *Opera omnia*, Geneva quarto 1695: relief, open initial 'D', child with stem and leaves, white on black background, single-lined border; 21 × 20 millimetres

Tournes 64. *Opera omnia*, Geneva quarto 1695: relief, fleuron, scroll; 6 × 6 millimetres

Tournes 65. *Opera omnia*, Geneva quarto 1695: relief, open initial 'D', female figure with stem and leaves, white on black background, single-lined border; 21 × 21 millimetres

Tournes 66. *Opera omnia*, Geneva quarto 1695: relief, solid initial 'F', intertwined stems and leaves, black on white, double-lined border; 20 × 20 millimetres

Tournes 67. *Opera omnia*, Geneva quarto 1695: relief, criblé, open initial 'E', stems, leaves and flower, white on black background, single-lined border; 28 × 28 millimetres

Tournes 68. *Opera omnia*, Geneva quarto 1695: relief, open shadowed initial 'V', stems and leaf, white on black background, single-lined border; 27 × 27 millimetres

Tournes 69. *Opera omnia*, Geneva quarto 1695: relief, fleuron, scroll; 4 × 3 millimetres

Tournes 70. *Opera omnia*, Geneva quarto 1695: relief, criblé, open initial 'C', stem, leaves one shaped as male human figure with crown and beard, white on black background, single-lined border; 28 × 28 millimetres (see: Figure 90)

Tournes 71. *Opera omnia*, Geneva quarto 1695: relief, tailpiece, basket of leaves with female face as bas, garland of stems and leaf, pendants, background, no border; 50 × 75 millimetres (see: Figure 60)

Tournes 72. *Opera omnia*, Geneva quarto 1695: relief, fleuron, scroll; 4 × 8 millimetres

Tournes 73. *Opera omnia*, Geneva quarto 1695: relief, fleuron, scroll; 5 × 11 millimetres

Tournes 74. *Opera omnia*, Geneva quarto 1695: relief, fleuron, scroll; 4 × 6 millimetres.

Vlacq:

Vlacq 1. *Diatribæ duæ medico-philosophicæ*, The Hague duodecimo 1662: relief, headpiece, intertwined stems and leaves, rose and thistle, crossed maces, no border; 26 × 56 millimetres

Vlacq 2. *Diatribæ duæ medico-philosophicæ*, The Hague duodecimo 1662: fleuron, acorn; 5 × 2 millimetres

Vlacq 3. *Diatribæ duæ medico-philosophicæ*, The Hague duodecimo 1662: fleuron, stems, and flower; 3 × 9 millimetres.

Wetstein:

Wetstein 1. *Opera omnia*, Amsterdam quarto 1682: relief, printer's device, globe, classical figure on plinth, caduceus, seated scholastic with beard and book, foot placed on seated animal with human head, pile of six books, lighted lamp, pyramid, star of David, scroll inscribed CONSULTORIBUS ISTIS [With them as advisers], no border; 47 × 48 millimetres

Wetstein 2. *Opera omnia*, Amsterdam quarto 1682: relief, open shadowed initial 'S', stem, leaf and flower background, no border; 25 × 25 millimetres

Wetstein 3. *Opera omnia*, Amsterdam quarto 1682: relief, headpiece, stems, leaves, fruit, urn, no border; 25 × 132 millimetres

Wetstein 4. *Opera omnia*, Amsterdam quarto 1682: relief, open shadowed initial 'T', stem, leaf and flower background, no border; 25 × 25 millimetres

Wetstein 5. *Opera omnia*, Amsterdam quarto 1682: relief, tailpiece, stems, leaves, fruit, urn, no border; 48 × 60 millimetres

Wetstein 6. *Opera omnia*, Amsterdam quarto 1682: relief, open shadowed initial 'D', stem and leaf background, no border; 26 × 26 millimetres

Wetstein 7. *Opera omnia*, Amsterdam quarto 1682: relief, open shadowed initial 'I', stem and leaf background, no border; 26 × 26 millimetres

Wetstein 8. *Opera omnia*, Amsterdam quarto 1682: relief, open shadowed initial 'E', stem and leaf background, no border; 27 × 27 millimetres

Wetstein 9. *Opera omnia*, Amsterdam quarto 1682: relief, open shadowed initial 'C', stem and leaf background, no border; 27 × 27 millimetres

Wetstein 10. *Opera omnia*, Amsterdam quarto 1682: relief, tailpiece, seated bear with sprays in each paw, serpents; 42 × 80 millimetres (see: Figure 61)

Wetstein 11. *Opera omnia*, Amsterdam quarto 1682: relief, open shadowed initial 'A', stem and leaf background, no border; 26 × 26 millimetres

Wetstein 12. *Opera omnia*, Amsterdam quarto 1682: relief, open shadowed initial 'Q', stem and leaf background, no border; 27 × 27 millimetres

Wetstein 13. *Opera omnia*, Amsterdam quarto 1682: tailpiece, basket of leaves and flower, no border; 51 × 66 millimetres

Wetstein 14. *Opera omnia*, Amsterdam quarto 1682: relief, open shadowed initial 'A', stem and leaf background, no border; 19 × 19 millimetres

Wetstein 15. *Opera omnia*, Amsterdam quarto 1682: relief, open shadowed initial 'R', stem and leaf background, no border; 26 × 26 millimetres

Wetstein 16. *Opera omnia*, Amsterdam quarto 1682: relief, tailpiece, stems, leaves, flowers, urn, snail and insects, no border; 69 × 77 millimetres

Wetstein 17. *Opera omnia*, Amsterdam quarto 1682: relief, open shadowed initial 'Q', stem and leaf background, no border; 19 × 19 millimetres; 9 × 10 millimetres

Wetstein 18. *Opera omnia*, Amsterdam quarto 1682: relief, headpiece, stems, flowers, hares, goats, male figures with bow and arrow, Bacchus seated supporting peacocks, no border; 35 × 140 millimetres

Wetstein 19. *Opera omnia*, Amsterdam quarto 1682: relief, tailpiece, intertwined stems, leaves, lances, central urn with X / ∇ and lettered I D I, design, no border; 32 × 43 millimetres (see: Figure 62)

Wetstein 20. *Opera omnia*, Amsterdam quarto 1682: relief, open shadowed initial 'A', leaf background, no border; 30 × 30 millimetres

Wetstein 21. *Cerebri anatome*, Amsterdam duodecimo 1683: relief, printer's device, winged angel blowing two horns astride armillary sphere balanced on one foot, two clothed figures, one using an optical cross-staff, the other a spade, scroll inscribed VIVITUR INGENIO [Lives on by his genius], no border;[51] 29 × 29 millimetres

Wetstein 22. *Cerebri anatome*, Amsterdam duodecimo 1683: relief, open shadowed initial 'A', leaf background, no border; 12 × 12 millimetres

Wetstein 23. *Cerebri anatome*, Amsterdam duodecimo 1683: relief, open shadowed initial 'I', leaf background, no border; 11 × 11 millimetres

Wetstein 24. *Cerebri anatome*, Amsterdam duodecimo 1683: relief, open shadowed initial 'N', leaf background, no border; 12 × 12 millimetres.

Zyll:

Zyll 1. *De urinis*, Utrecht octavo 1670: relief, tailpiece, swag of fruit and flowers draped through two rings, no border; 34 × 57 millimetres (see: Figure 63).

Engraved plates and the printed works of Thomas Willis

The seventeenth and eighteenth century issues of Thomas Willis's books are well known for the engraved plates that illustrate the scientific content of four works. There is no direct evidence that Willis drew sketches from the dissections. Rather, he is explicit that these were the work of others. Varying considerably in their artistry and detail, the main interest lies in anatomical depictions of the brain and nerves in animals and man contained in *Cerebri anatome* and *Nervorum descriptio et usus*, and in *De anima brutorum*. The often-stated view is that these illustrations are by Christopher Wren but it does not take much of an eye to see that more than one artist is at work. Furthermore, in understanding the overall coherence of Willis's writings, the plates in *De motu musculori* and the two parts of *Pharmaceutice rationalis* are no less illuminating.

On leaving Westminster School in London, aged 15 years, Wren moved to his father's house outside Oxford where he made contact with Charles Scarburgh (1615–1694) who acted as his physician and cured Wren 'from recent sickness as from the hand of God'. Later, anticipating the work of William Croone (1633–1684) and Thomas Willis, and building on ideas propagated by William Harvey (1578–1657) and others, Wren wrote a 'treatise on the motion of muscles, explaining the whole anatomy by models form'd in pasteboards'. He presented these to Scarburgh.[52] Wren's mentor in Oxford was John Wilkins (1614–1672),

[51] The full quote is: 'Vivitur ingenio, cæteris mortis erunt [He lives by his genius and all else is mortal]'. This is a line attributed to Publius Vergilius Maro (70–19 BC) allegedly lamenting the death of his patron Gaius Maecenas (68–8 BC). But, as has been pointed out, Virgil pre-deceased his patron so this attribution needs qualification. The words are inscribed on the pedestal supporting the skeleton in early printings of plate 22 from Andreas Vesalius, *De humani corporis fabrica libri septem*, (1543): page 164. They are present in the editions from 1555: page 204; 1568: page 124; and 1725 (volume I, between pages 140–1); but missing from *Bruxellensis icones anatomicæ* (1934) in which plates were printed from the original blocks. Singer and Rabin, *A prelude to modern science* (1946) reproduce the image without the inscription (page xi), describing this as 'From the Fabrica' but without offering a date; Saunders and O'Malley, *The illustrations from the works of Andreas Vesalius of Brussels* (1950): page 87 also show the plate without its inscription and write: 'in the original version of the plate, the motto *Vivitur ingenio, cætera mortis erunt*—"Genius lives on, all else is mortal"—was inserted on the side of the tomb'. It seems that the woodblock lacked any lettering and, in early issues, was run twice through the press in order to print image and text on one leaf.

[52] See: William Carleton Gibson, 'The biomedical pursuits of Christopher Wren. The Monkton Copeman lecture of the Worshipful Society of Apothecaries read at the Wellcome Institute of the History of Medicine on 4 March 1970', *Medical History* 1970: 14; 331–41, citing Christopher Wren (1645–1747), *Parentalia: or, memoirs of the family*

warden of Wadham College which Wren attended: 'that prodigious young scholar Mr Christopher Wren presented me with a piece of marble which he has stain'd with a lively red very deepe, as beautiful as if it had been natural'. Wren moved to All Souls where John Evelyn (1620–1706), visiting the College, remarked: 'after dinner I visited that miracle of a youth Mr Christopher Wren, a nephew of the Bishop of Ely'; and soon after Evelyn was at Wadham where he saw the various working models that Wren had created.[53] Having met Thomas Willis and other members of the Oxford Experimental Philosophical Club through Wilkins, Wren acted as one of Willis's technical assistants and may have used this opportunity to pay his way through Oxford. The evidence for his involvement in Willis's work comes from the author himself and several other contemporary sources. Willis confirms that Wren was frequently present at anatomical dissections 'to confer and reason about the parts' and 'was pleased out of his singular humanity, wherewith he abounds, to delineate with his own most skilful hands many Figures of the brain and Skull, whereby the work might be more exact'.[54]

Only one original drawing of an anatomical preparation attributable both to Wren and Willis survives. This depicts an haemorrhagic ulcer affecting a section of small intestine. It is in watercolour and lettered in ink by an unidentified hand with the names of Thomas Willis (upper left) and Christopher Wren (lower right); that of Wren is similar to his signature on a letter from 1682.[55] With the original watercolour is a note in manuscript, possibly written by William Gibson (1913–2009):[56]

> The drawings illustrate a portion of small intestine. On the left, haemorrhagic ulceration is seen through the thickness of the wall. On the right the intestine has been opened to expose the mucosa. In this lies a haemorrhagic ulcer. In Willis's *Pharmaceutice rationalis* (1678 [*sic*]), in the section on putrid fevers, Willis writes: "A dysentery is a distemper frequent in continual feavers ... The cause of it is wont to be ... a certain infection impressed on the blood and so intimately confused with it ... that it cannot be pulled away from the blood; wherefore the thrusting forwards towards the intestines unlocks the little mouths of the arteries and makes there little ulcers and exudations and flowings forth of the blood ...". Willis describes cases of such fever (possibly typhoid) in 1656–1658, whilst he was working with Christopher Wren. This drawing is probably from such a case.

Wren was technically innovative. Combining his knowledge of engineering with Harvey's work on the circulation, and focusing on the hollow nature of vessels and nerves, Wren instituted intravenous injections using sharpened quills, and used these to investigate the

of the Wrens ... chiefly of Sir Christopher Wren ... Compiled, by his son Christopher, now published by his grandson, Stephen Wren, Esq., with the care of Joseph Ames, London (1750). The models were lost in the Fire of London.

[53] See: Gibson (1970): page 334.

[54] See: 'The preface to the reader', *The anatomy of the brain* (1681): page [54].

[55] See: Kerry Downes, 'Sir Christopher Wren. An exhibition selected by Kerry Downes at the Whitechapel Art Gallery 9 July–26 September 1982', London (1982): #6, pages 46 (II.6)–47; #13, pages 56–7 (III.13); and Gibson (1970): plate I at page 332, and page 336 attributing the discovery of the provenance to Dr Noël Poynter (1908–1979).

[56] A letter to the Wellcome Institute from Alasdair Coles, Pembroke College, Oxford, dated 3 October 1986, reports the opinion of a pathologist at Glasgow University, that the drawing: 'almost certainly represents typhoid fever of the lower ileum. It would have been common at the time and is typically described as showing shallow longitudinal ulcers which in fact lie over the Peyer's patches. I think I can see 3 such ulcers in [the] two segments. Page 631 of Muir's *Textbook of pathology* shows this well; I think I can see the swollen lymphoid follicles, illustrated in Fig. 19.57, on [the] right hand specimen, in the brown segment at the top. There are two well circumscribed nodules just adjacent to the ulcer. In my opinion, you can be confident that this picture does illustrate typhoid lesions in the small intestine.'

circulation, slaying many animals in the process.[57] This expertise was used to inject the vessels of the brain with India ink and a preservative: 'let a dyed liquor, and contained in a large squirt or pipe, be injected upwards in the trunk [of an artery] of one side: after once or twice injecting, you shall see the tincture or dyed liquor to descend from the other side by the trunk of the opposite artery'. In Oxford, Wren invented a perspectograph that allowed a draughtsman to trace the lines of any object or landscape. This was used in delineating the topography of the brain but more as an artistic device than as an attempt at realist representation. Wren's contributions to *Cerebri anatome* were drafted in the spring of 1663. One informant is Richard Lower. In a letter to Robert Boyle (4 June 1663), Lower confirms that:[58]

> Dr Wren hath drawn most excellent schemes of the brain, and the several parts of it, according to the doctor's design, and the next week he will have finished the scheme of the eighth pair of nerves, and then all the work is at an end.

This is confirmed by Hooke who comments favourably in a letter to Boyle on the careful and detailed drawings made by Wren for the group of 'neurologists'. Hooke writes:[59]

> Mr Lower was to have waited upon you, and was sorry to miss you here in town. He had Dr. Willis's services to have presented to you, whose book he tells me is within a little while to come forth, and he added, that Dr Wren had drawn the pictures very curiously for it; and I am glad to hear it will afford such considerable discoveries, which I doubt not but you know.

According to an unattributed annotation in the British Museum copy, the plates in *Cerebri anatome* (1664: **2A**) were engraved by David Loggan. Horace Walpole (1717–1797) quotes the opinion of Vertue that Loggan was the engraver.[60] The illustrations are described as schematic and linear with details suppressed in order to emphasize conceptual rather than realistic spatial arrangements, and the artistic style conditioned by geometry and the rules of mathematics. This is certainly true of the later examples showing the nerves, which are strictly diagrammatic in contrast to images of the brain viewed from the base or cut in coronal and sagittal planes. John Fulton (1899–1960) considered that the engravings show a better understanding of the anatomy of the brain than Willis's explanations.[61] Perhaps influenced by Wren, Thomas Willis did himself adopt an architectural metaphor for his work on the brain: 'There remains not only the outward Courts and Porches of this Fabrick, as it were of a certain Kingly Palace, but also its intimate Recesses and private Chambers'.[62]

That Wren was involved is certain but not so clear is which of the original drawings can be attributed to him, which to Richard Lower, and which to someone else. Opinions differ.

[57] According to his son, Wren was offered a servant of the French ambassador on whom to experiment but was prevented from injecting an emetic by the prolonged fainting attack of the subject: see Wren (1750): page 64, cited by Allister Neher, 'Christopher Wren, Thomas Willis and the depiction of the brain and nerves', *Journal of Medical Humanities* 2009: 30; 191–200, at page 195.

[58] See: William Feindel, 'The life of Thomas Willis'. In: *The anatomy of the brain and nerves*, Montreal (1965, volume 1): pages 20–1 for full text of this letter.

[59] See: Feindel (1965): page 22. In referring to this correspondence, Gibson (1970): page 337 may have allowed himself some etymological freedom since whether Hooke really used the collective term 'neurologists' in his correspondence from that time is unclear.

[60] See: Horace Walpole, *Anecdotes of painting*, volume 3, London (1762–1771): page 91; cited by HR [Harold] Denham, 'A bibliographic survey of Cerebri anatome'. In: Feindel (1965): page 71.

[61] Cited in Gibson (1970): page 336.

[62] See: 'The conclusion', *The anatomy of the brain* (1681): page 192.

At one extreme is the view that Wren drew and engraved all the plates in *Cerebi anatome* (1664).[63] HJR Wing considers that Figures I–III (Pl.1–Pl.3) and V–VIII (Pl.5, Pl.6, Pl.8 and Pl.9) of *Cerebri anatome* are by Wren, and the remainder by Richard Lower.[64] William Gibson is more vague: 'during the spring of 1663, Wren drew the illustrations for much of Willis's great book Cerebri anatome... while Wren was designing the Sheldonian Theatre in Oxford he was doubling as Willis's trusted dissector'.[65] Trevor Hughes shows Figure I from *Cerebri anatome* (Pl.1) as 'Christopher Wren's drawing' and, without citing his authority, illustrates Tabula IX (Pl.13) as 'Richard Lower's drawing of the autonomic nervous system'.[66] William Feindel argues that the thirteenth table (Pl.15) and, with similarities to images of the cerebral sinuses in Lower's *Tractatus de corde* (1669: Tab.5, Fig. 4), the two unnumbered plates depicting the cerebral vessels and the third, fourth, fifth and sixth cranial nerves (Pl.7 and Pl.10) are each by Lower.[67] He goes further and suggests that Lower's figure showing the cerebral venous sinuses may originally have been intended for Chapter VI of *Cerebri anatome* where Willis describes injected ink passing from arteries into veins and then into the sinuses. Since Willis's figures and tables are numbered I–XIII yet *Cerebri anatome* contains fifteen plates, it seems self-evident that the two unnumbered illustrations (Pl.7, Pl.10) were added as an afterthought. This is further supported by the fact that, as Feindel points out, the description of Pl.7 is on an interleaf in the quarto and an otherwise blank page in the octavo issues, indicating that these plates and their explanations were added after the main text had been set and the available plates numbered.[68]

Any ambiguity as to the provenance of the figures and tables in *Cerebri anatome* is resolved by a clear statement from Willis in the preface that, in addition to Wren, Lower was responsible for images depicting the nerves (Tabulæ IX–XIII):[69]

> For having prosecuted, with a most exact search all the divarications, wandring on every side of the Nerve, how minute or small soever, and immersed, and variously unfolded within other Bodies, and so turning over the Labyrinths of the Branches, and shoots of every pair ... he [Lower] drew out with his own hand the Schemes, Images or Draughts of them, also of many passages of the Blood, as they appear in this Tract; which indeed that they might be faithfully shewn, without any falsity or errour, he causes that no Table might contain scarce any line or the most light passage, whose conformation and exact habitude he had not found proved by the marks or inspection of many Animals for that purpose killed.

One interpretation of what happened requires consideration of the plates in *Cerebri anatome* alongside those published in *De anima brutorum* (1672). These were also engraved by David Loggan. As a starting point, the manuscript annotation in a copy of *De anima brutorum* at The Queen's College, Oxford, by Theophilus Metcalfe (fl.1635) reads:[70]

63 See: Neher (2009): page 193.

64 See: HJR (John) Wing, *A bibliography of Dr. Thomas Willis (1621–1675)* submitted as part requirement for the University of London Diploma in Librarianship (1962): page 11.

65 See: Gibson (1970): page 336.

66 See: J Trevor Hughes *Thomas Willis 1621–1675*, London (1991): page 71.

67 Unusually, Feindel (1965): page 37 gets his details wrong in referring to the four small figures of the plate 'facing page 86': it is at page 106 in the quarto and page 56 in the octavo edition.

68 See chapter 6 for more detailed discussion.

69 See: *The anatomy of the brain* (1681): pages 53–4.

70 See: Philip Oldfield *A bibliography of Thomas Willis's* De anima brutorum (typescript, 1991): footnote 3 page 5; also mentioned is a catalogue issued by Dawson's of Pall Mall, 'The Royal Society of London for the promotion of natural knowledge 1660–1960: a tercentenary tribute London' (1961): #1801 in which it is claimed that Wren engraved the plates for *De anima brutorum*. Oldfield points out that, unlike the acknowledgement to Wren

> Figuras in hoc Libro contentas (quae mea quidem sententia paene aequiparent Cowperianas) ipse manu sua designavit Dno. Christ. Wren Eques; & postea exsculp. curavit: ubi etiam eas, quas in tractatu Loweriano de Corde invenias.
>
> [The figures contained in this book (which at least in my opinion are almost as good as Cowper´s) Mr. Christopher Wren Esq. drew by hand and later engraved: he also provided those that one can find in Lower's tract on the heart].

This statement fails to acknowledge that Tabula I is not original to *De anima brutorum* but copied from Marcello Malpighi's (1628–1694) treatise on the silkworm.[71] A further point to be considered is why, when *Cerebri anatome* and *De anima brutorum* each contain engraved plates, none are present in *Pathologiæ cerebri* which also lends itself to illustration. At the risk of censure in the absence of evidence, the following sequence of events that takes into account the dates of these publications and, more especially, the inclusion of images can be proposed.

In the early 1660s, Willis and Wren were working together in Oxford and, with demonstrable skills as a draughtsman, Wren agreed to record their dissections as images that Loggan would engrave. Lower, inferior as an artist but close to the work and engaged with Willis in medical practice, was party to this arrangement. As the need to complete the work and have the plates ready for binding with the printed sheets became increasingly urgent, and Wren still had not completed the task, Lower stepped in and drew several images for *Cerebri anatome* allowing the book to be published in 1664. Willis and Wren may have had in mind providing illustrations for *Pathologiæ cerebri* (1667) but these were either lost at the time of the fire of London, or (more probably) Wren was then busy with architectural matters relating to damaged buildings and hence distracted from producing anatomical drawings. Wren's son considered that his father regretted moving on from scientific work to become an architect: 'King Charles II had done him a disservice in taking him from the pursuit of those studies, and obliging him to spend all his time in rubbish'.[72] But after 1667 Wren was able to complete the four drawings illustrating comparative anatomy of the brain and nerves in various animal species and these duly appeared in *De anima brutorum* (1672). The somewhat risky suggestion, much influenced by artistry of the fifteen plates in *Cerebri anatome*, the eight in *De anima brutorum* and the seven in *Tractatus de corde*, is that Christopher Wren drew Figures I, II, III, IV, V, VI, VII, and VIII of *Cerebri anatome* (1664); and was responsible for Tabulæ V, VI, VII, and VIII of *De anima brutorum* (1672). The other eleven plates, Tabulæ IX, X, XI, XII, and XIII and the two unnumbered plates from *Cerebri anatome*, and Tabulæ I, II, III, and IV from *De anima brutorum*, are the work of Richard Lower. In support of the position that Wren was involved with the illustrations of both works is the very close similarity between Figura VII (Pl.8) in *Cerebri anatome* and Tabula V in *De anima brutorum* (Pl.23). The dissection is the same but the plane in which the tissue is cut differs as does the outline, especially in the upper part.[73] Against this analysis is the evidence from

in *Cerebri anatome*, there is no such mention in *De anima brutorum* nor in the account of his life written by Wren's son and published by his grandson (1750). Oldfield anticipates the suggestion that four of the plates are held over from *Cerebri anatome* and are by Wren.

[71] See: Marcelli Malpighi, *De bombyce*, London (1669).

[72] British Museum MSS Add 25071, folio 38v: cited by Neher (2009): footnote 5, page 192.

[73] In *The anatomy of the brain* (1681), the legend at page 94 reads: '*The Seventh Figure*, SHews the Brain of a Sheep bent back and cut a little open in the places where they stick together near the streaked bodies, that its

Lower, cited earlier, relating to Wren's responsibility for images of the eighth pair of nerves (wandring nerve, or vagus in modern terminology); and some similarity between images of the human brain and the four depicting the nervous system of the silkworm, oyster, lobster, and earthworm.

There is no preface to *De motu musculari* (1670) and nothing to identify the person who drew and engraved the four figures of muscle. These do show some similarity in design to the six images included by Lower in *Tractatus de corde* (1669: Tab. 3, Figs 1–6), making it possible that Lower was responsible for the illustrations in these two books published a year apart. By comparison with *Cerebri anatome* and *De anima brutorum*, the fourteen plates in *Pharmaceutice rationalis* (parts 1 and 2) are relatively crude and uninformative. Christopher Wren can have had nothing to do with their production. The first are diagrams of the stomach and intestines with various coats stripped away to show the blood vessels and nerve network. The later ones depict the lungs and trachea to show blood vessels, lymphatics, and nerves. Although Willis writes in his preface to the reader of help from John Masters (fl.1672–1680)[74] and Edmund King (*c.*1630–1709) in 'illustrating the pharmaceutical Doctrin', this may imply elucidating the concepts rather than illustrating the work.

Enumerating illustrations in the printed works

Whilst it may seem straightforward to count the number of plate leaves that should be present in the original and collected editions, this exercise is not so simple. Even the most diligent and experienced bibliographers have made mistakes. Many a distinguished bookseller has offered items that appear to be complete but are not; parted with copies that are declared incomplete but are not; or given up in exasperation at trying to work out what should be present.

The numbers apart, it is often stated that the plates for one edition were later reused for another issue or edition. Whilst is it true that the features shown and the lettering are consistent, not infrequently lines were added or cross-hatching altered and page numbers scratched out or edited, making for different states of a particular plate. For example, page numbers appropriate for the quarto issue of *Cerebri anatome* (1664: **2A**) are found on plate leaves in some copies of the octavo issue (**2B1**), whereas these are corrected in what can be assumed to be second states (**2B2**). Some plates were obviously reengraved by copying an existing version but differ in size from their predecessors. More than one plate might be arranged on the press, rotated, or otherwise moved around in order to accommodate everything on a single printed sheet. When the same plates were used to print illustrations for more than one issue, sometimes separated by several years and with other imprints intervening for which better preserved engravings were used, systematic degeneration with cracking and loss of detail are apparent. Eventually the printer tired of these imperfect versions and the plate was reengraved. The sheet on which several figures from a single engraving had been printed was sometimes cut and the individual parts separately bound. Conversely, several

interior substance may be turned the inside out, and unfolded on a plain.' In *De anima brutorum* etc (1683), the legend at page 27 reads: 'The Fifth Table, Shews the Figure of the Brain of a Sheep roled forth, and derased, and as it were made bare of the Flesh, in many places, that the Marrowy tracts may be seen'.

[74] See: William Munk, *The roll of the Royal College of Physicians of London*, 1518–1700, volume I, London (1861): page 410 for discussion of John Masters and his engagement with Willis in preparation of *De anima brutorum* (1672) and *Pharmaceutice rationalis* (1674, 1675).

that were normally distributed may be found as one composite engraving printed on a single large folding sheet. In the last two editions of *Opera omnia*, the figures are printed within the main text.

It follows that the only reliable method for enumerating accurately the illustrations and collating any one copy is to start with the images, proceed to list the number of engravers' plates (numbered and unnumbered), and then count the number of leaves or folding sheets. For the original Latin issues printed in England, the numbers are:

Cerebri anatome (1664: **2A**), twenty-three images on fifteen plates usually bound as fifteen leaves.
De motu musculorum (1670: **4A**), four images on two plates usually bound as two leaves.
De anima brutorum (1672: **5A**), sixteen images on eight plates usually bound as eight leaves.
Pharmaceutice rationalis (part 1, 1674: **6A**), twelve images on six plates usually bound as six leaves.[75]
Pharmaceutice rationalis (part 2, 1675: **6E**), twenty-five images on eight plates usually bound as eight leaves (Pl.34 has two components but these are part of the same anatomical structure and so should be counted as one, image 59).
Together, there are eighty images on thirty-nine plates usually bound as thirty-nine leaves.

Assessing the correct number of illustrations becomes more complicated when considering the editions of *Cerebri anatome* published in Amsterdam by Schagen (1664: **2C1**; 1666: **2D**), and those published by Commelin (1664: **2C2**; 1667: **2E1**). One problem relates to the inclusion of *De ratione motus musculorum* and its plate leaf.[76] Schagen and Commelin both had access to the text of *De ratione motus musculorum*. Each used his own title page and made slight differences to the preliminaries. Both had the fifteen engravings for *Cerebri anatome* but only Commelin included the plate to Croone's treatise. Therefore the correct number of images and engravings for this edition of *Cerebri anatome* is twenty-three and fifteen for any imprint by Schagen but twenty-five and sixteen for Commelin's editions. Any copy of Schagen's *Cerebri anatome* with the Croone plate has been made up with Commelin's issue of *De ratione motus musculorum*. But there are two further confusions in assessing the correct number of illustrations, plates, and sheets for each edition. First, if the engraved title page used in his 1666 edition (**2D**) and available only to Schagen (F.2a1) is counted (incorrectly since it is a frontispiece and does not directly illustrate the main text), the count for Schagen is twenty-four images and sixteen engravings. Much more problematic is that, from the outset, the Dutch publishers printed illustrations on one sheet from several engraved on a single large plate. This applies both to *Cerebri anatome* and the third edition of *De anima bruutorum* published by Someren (1674: **5C**). Comparing the incomplete plate marks on one or more sides with lines printed on the remaining edges, or evidence that a larger sheet had been torn or cut before binding, does not make it possible to count how many plates were

[75] One minor confusion is that, numbered Tabulæ 1–VI in part 1 and 1–VIII in part 2, all of which lack page placements, the plates in *Pharmaceutice rationalis* are almost invariably confused in the first complete issue (1679: **6I**) and found in the wrong part of the book.

[76] See chapter 6 for details of arrangements between Gerbrandt Schagen (b.1633) and Caspar Commelin (1636–1693) and their dealings with the engraver Salomon Savry (1594–1683).

placed on the rolling press in order to print these illustrations. All that can be counted is the number of separate areas that were engraved and intended as independent illustrations.[77]

These issues carry over to the Latin collected editions published in continental Europe.[78] Some editions of the *Opera omnia* include both Croone's *De ratione motus musculorum* and Willis's *De motu musculari*, each with their respective illustrations. Only Wetstein's *Opera omnia* (**8E**) omits Croone's treatise and hence its plate. He also cut down several larger engravings into individual plates. Therefore Wetstein's edition should have eighty images printed from thirty-nine plates bound as thirty-eight sheets. With the decision to include images on the printed page in the first folio edition of the *Opera omnia* (1694: **8F**), many illustrations were reengraved on independent plates. Others were combined. This changes the totals for the folio editions to eighty-two images on thirty-two plates printed on thirty separate pages or plate leaves.

No less confusing are the collected works in English published originally as three independent volumes (1679: **9A**, 1681: **9B**, and 1683: **9D**) but brought together in varying arrangements that constitute three separate collected editions (1681: **9C**, 1684 [1]: **9E**, and 1684 [2]: **9F**). The two dated 1684 each advertise forty copper plates on the title page, a number that reflects the sum of those from the original Latin treatises. But this is not correct, as the difficulties experienced by one distinguished bibliographer indicate. When Harold Denham tackled the task of enumerating illustrations in the English translations, his initial summary of what had to be reconciled made the following points:[79]

The remaining medical works (1681) and *Pharmaceutice rationalis* (1679) were planned as a single edition in two volumes even though the second was published first.

The *Term Catalogue* for February 1681 advertised: 'Dr. Willis's practice of *Physick*: being all the medical Works of that renowned and famous Physician; containing these ten several Treatises . . . With thirty-two Copper plates'.

Although this equates to eighteen advertised on the title page of *The remaining medical works*, and fourteen in *Pharmaceutice rationalis*, 'there are actually only sixteen' in the first named volume.

The advertisement placed two years later at the end of *Concerning the soul of brutes* changed: 'Doctor Willis's Practice of Physick, being all the Medical Works of that Renowned and Famous Physician, Containing these ten treatises . . . With Thirty Copper Plates'.[80]

The title *Dr Willis's practice of physick* was used for the collected edition of 1684 advertised 'With forty copper plates' and there is 'no other known edition of Willis to which it can refer'.

This volume included 'new versions of the 1679–1681 edition' together with *Concerning the soul of brutes*, some plates from 1679 and 1681 having been reengraved.

[77] Even after allowing for this distinction, HJR Wing and HR Denham each make a mistake in their listing of 'plates' for the Dutch editions of 1664–1667. HJR Wing 10 (Schagen 1664: **2C1**) excludes Croone's essay and therefore correctly calls for 15 engraved plates. HJR Wing 11 (Commelin 1664: **2C2**) includes Croone's treatise and lists that plate. Although the copy HJR Wing examined lacked all the plates for *Cerebri anatome*, we can assume that number to be 15 making the correct total of 16 for this issue. HJR Wing 12 and 13 are the 1666 issues (**2D**) and correctly he calls for 15 plates, omitting that for *De ratione motus musculorum*. However, HJR Wing 14 (Commelin 1667: **2E1**) is described as having the same number of plates as HJR Wing 10, i.e. fifteen, whereas a complete copy has 16. Denham 3 is equivalent to HJR Wing 10 (**2C1**) and calls for fifteen plates; and Denham 4 is equivalent to HJR Wing 11 (**2C2.c1**) and calls for 16 plates. Both are correct. However, Denham 5 and 6 (Schagen 1666: **2D**) are equivalent to HJR Wing 12 and 13 but Denham calls for 16 plates, and also the engraved title page. This is incorrect since HJR Wing 12 and 13 do not have the Croone plate. Denham 7 is equivalent to HJR Wing 14 (**2E1**) and correctly calls for 16 plates.

[78] Tournes's 1695 edition (**8G**) includes a Latin translation of *A plain and easie method* which does not affect the number of illustrations.

[79] See: Denham (1965): pages 80–3.

[80] See: Thomas Willis, *Two discourses concerning the soul of brutes*, London (1683): at Kk1v page [8].

From this it would follow that Denham's calculation of the number of 'plates' in *Dr Willis's practice of physick* (1684: **9F**) is 14 + 16 (18–2) + 8 = 38 rather than the forty specified on the title page. But Denham assumed that all references to numbers of plates were anticipating the final edition from 1684 (**9F**). He had not identified the 1681 issue of *Dr Willis's practice of physick* (**9C**) or the first issue of the collected works from 1684 (**9E**) which included some of its sheets. Two changes had been made in reengraving plates for the only edition he identified (1684: **9F**): the two plates for *Cerebri anatome* Figuræ I and II (Pl.1 and Pl.2) were printed from one engraving on a single leaf, as were the four images for *Of muscular motion* (Pl.17 and Pl.18).

Denham returned to the problem in correspondence with Mrs Strachan who had purchased a copy of *Dr Willis's practice of physick* (1684: now **9F**) and was writing, on the recommendation of Edwin Clarke (1919–1996), to seek guidance on whether or not her copy was complete.[81] Admitting that it was now some time since he had conducted his research and referring to notes made whilst working on a bibliography of Thomas Willis which, to the detriment of posterity, was never completed, rather than relying on the printed advertisements, he sent back his assessment based on examination of copies which he considered correct for a perfect copy. Mrs Strachan was reassured that:

> On the plates I have no doubt that you have the correct number in your copy. The figure should be 38 but, as you have noted, irregularities arise because plates are sometimes combined on a single sheet. No other plates (except portraits) were made for Willis's works as shown by the following enumeration of all the plates which occur in separate or collected editions:
>
> Of Musculary Motion: 1 plate with 4 figures
>
> Anatomy of the Brain: 13 numbered plates plus 2 unnumbered (usually between VI and VII and between VIII and IX)
>
> Pharmaceutice Rationalis 1: 6 plates
>
> Pharmaceutice Rationalis 2: 8 plates
>
> Soul of Brutes: 8 plates
>
> Making a total of 38
>
> However, there is an additional plate in some Latin editions of *Cerebri anatome* and in most of the Latin Collected editions which belongs to an appended work by another author, William Croone* (*Entitled 'De ratione motus musculorum'); this was omitted from the English editions. Also in some of the Opera Omnia, the plate to Musculary Motion is printed in two separate halves so that these editions could be regarded as possessing 40 plates in all. This suggests a possible explanation for the erroneous number of plates given on the title page of the 1684 edition.
>
> It seems more than coincidental that a similar mistake was made in the earlier English edition of Thomas Willis's treatises. The first part of this was published in 1681 two years after the second part (Pharmaceutice Rationalis). It was entitled 'The Remaining Medical Works' and corresponds to (1) and (2) in my description of the 1684 edition or Vol. 1 of

[81] Details of this correspondent are described in a letter to the author from Harold Denham on another topic dated 16 June 1998 in which he mentions that Mrs Strachan had made contact soon after Denham retired in 1982: 'I think from New Zealand and I have the impression that she (and her husband) were not collectors but acquired the book at random'. The copy was sold by a Cambridge-based dealer in antiquarian medical books with the binding already restored by Bernard Middleton in 1984. Therefore Mrs Strachan must have been keen to realize a profit from her purchase without much delay, having been reassured by Harold Denham that it was complete.

> the Latin collected editions (except for the omission of the work by Croone), which would probably have contained the two extra plates mentioned above.
>
> The title page of this 1681 edition gives 18 plates (the number in the Latin edition) instead of the correct 16. Perhaps whoever drafted this title page did not have access to the plates at the time and therefore used the Latin edition to count the plates, overlooking the fact that this included an additional work with an extra plate and that the plate to Muscular Motion had been split into two halves.
>
> The editor of the 1684 volume may have perpetuated the error by taking the figure from the 1681 title page and simply adding the number of plates in Pharmaceutice Rationalis (1679) and Soul of Brutes (1683).
>
> If so, he had not studied the advertisement in Soul of Brutes for the two previous volumes (here called Practice of Physick), which mentions a total of 30 plates, the correct figure.

Poor Mrs Strachan simply wanted to know whether her copy was complete and worth reselling. Denham failed to distinguish plates from leaves. He did not explain that Tabula VI (Pl.24) and VII (Pl.25) in *Concerning the soul of brutes*, which is present in both 1684 editions of *Dr Willis's practice of physick* (**9E** and **9F**), are printed from individual plates on a single leaf. Nor did he point out that, in the only edition he was considering (**9F**), Figuræ I and II (Pl.1 and Pl.2) from *The anatomy of the brain*, and Tabulæ VII and VIII in *Pharmaceutice rationalis* part 2 (Pl.39 and Pl.40), are each printed from single plates. Therefore, *Dr Willis's practice of physick* (1684[1]: **9E**) collates as:

> *Of musculory motion*; four images on two plates printed on one sheet
> *The anatomy of the brain*, twenty-three figures on fifteen plates printed on fifteen sheets
> *Pharmaceutice rationalis* (part 1) twelve images on six plates printed on six sheets
> *Pharmaceutice rationalis* (part 2) twenty-five images on seven plates printed on six sheets (Tabs VII and VIII on a single sheet)
> *Concerning the soul of brutes*, sixteen images on eight plates printed on seven sheets (Tabs VI and VII on a single sheet)
> The total is eighty images on thirty-eight plates printed on thirty-five sheets.

And *Dr Willis's practice of physick* (1684[2]: **9F**) collates as:

> *Of musculory motion*; four images on one plate printed on one sheet
> *The anatomy of the brain*, twenty-three figures on fourteen plates printed on fourteen sheets
> *Pharmaceutice rationalis* (part 1) twelve images on six plates printed on six sheets
> *Pharmaceutice rationalis* (part 2) twenty-five images on seven plates printed on six sheets (Tabs VII and VIII on a single sheet)
> *Concerning the soul of brutes*, sixteen images on eight plates printed on seven sheets (Tabs VI and VII on a single sheet)
> The total is eighty images on thirty-six plates printed on thirty-four sheets.

Against this background, Table 1 shows the collation for each of Willis's works containing an engraved frontispiece, portrait, or anatomical illustrations. Table 2 shows the state for each image in those books which contain one or other of these illustrations. The legends in Latin are reproduced in the bibliographical descriptions for each illustrated book. English translations appear as the legends to figures 97–112, 120–1, 123–30, 131–6, and 138–45.

Table 1 A summary of the number of images, printers' plates, and plate leaves in the works of Thomas Willis

Title	Engraved title page	Portrait	Individual images	Printers' plates	Plate leaves
Diatribæ duæ medico-philosophiæ (1659)	–	–	–	–	–
Cerebri anatome (1664)	–	–	23 (images 1–23)	15 (plates 1–15)	15
Pathologiæ cerebri (1667)	–	Pt.1a1	–	–	–
De motu musculori (1670)	–	[Pt.1a1]	4 (images 26–29)	2 (plates 17–18)	2
De anima brutorum (1672)	–	–	16 (images 30–45)	8 (plates 19–26)	8
Pharmaceutice rationalis (1674: part1)	Fell 3	–	12 (images 46–57)	6 (plates 27–32)	6
Pharmaceutice rationalis (1675: part 2)	Fell 9	–	25 (images 58–82)	8 (plates 33–40)	8
The London practice of physick (1685)	–	Pt.1f1	–	–	–
A plain and easie method (1691)	–	Pt.1f1	–	–	–
[*De ratione motus musculorum*] (1664)	–	–	[2] (images 24–25)	[1] (plate 16)	[1]
Total in original editions	2	2	80 [82]	39 [40]	39 [40]
Dr Willis's practice of physick (1681: as for 1684 [1])	–	Pt.1a1	80 (images 1–23, 26–82)	38 (plates 1–15, 19–39/40)	35
Dr Willis's practice of physick (1684 [1])	–	Pt.1a1	80 (images 1–23, 26–82)	38 (plates 1–15, 19–39/40)	35
Of musculary motion	–	–	4 (images 26–29)	2 (plates 17–18)	1
The anatomy of the brain	–	–	23 (images 1–23)	15 (plates 1–15)	15
Pharmaceutice rationalis (part 1)	–	–	12 (images 46–57)	6 (plates 27–32)	6
Pharmaceutice rationalis (part 2)	–	–	25 (images 58–82)	7 (plates 33–39/40)	6
Concerning the soul of brutes	–	–	16 (images 30–45)	8 (plates 19–26)	7
Dr Willis's practice of physick (1684 [2])	–	–	80 (images 1–23, 26–82)	36 (plates 1/2, 3–15, 19–39/40)	34
Of musculary motion	–	–	4 (images 26–29)	1 (plates 17/18)	1
The anatomy of the brain	–	–	23 (images 1–23)	14 (plates 1/2, 3–15)	14
Pharmaceutice Rationalis (part 1)	–	–	12 (images 46–57)	6 (plates 27–32)	6
Pharmaceutice Rationalis (part 2)	–	–	25 (images 58–82)	7 (plates 33–39/40)	6
Concerning the soul of brutes	–	–	16 (images 30–45)	8 (plates 19–26)	7

Table 2 The different states of engraved frontispieces, portraits, and plates in the works of Thomas Willis

Number	Short title	Place of publication and format	Year	Frontispiece	Portrait 1	Plate 1	Plate 2	Plate 3	Plate 4	Plate 5	Plate 6	Plate 7	Plate 8	Plate 9	Plate 10	Plate 11	Plate 12	Plate 13	Plate 14	Plate 15	Plate 16
1B	*Diatribæ duæ*	London duodecimo	1660	F.1a1	–	–	–	–	–	–	–	–	–	–	–	–	–	–	–	–	–
1C	*Diatribæ duæ*	London duodecimo	1662	F.1a1	–	–	–	–	–	–	–	–	–	–	–	–	–	–	–	–	–
1D1	*Diatribæ duæ*	The Hague duodecimo	1662	F.1b1	–	–	–	–	–	–	–	–	–	–	–	–	–	–	–	–	–
1D2	*Diatribæ duæ*	London duodecimo	1662	F.1b1	–	–	–	–	–	–	–	–	–	–	–	–	–	–	–	–	–
1E	*Diatribæ duæ*	Amsterdam duodecimo	1663	F.1c1	–	–	–	–	–	–	–	–	–	–	–	–	–	–	–	–	–
1F	*Diatribæ duæ*	Amsterdam duodecimo	1669	F.1c2	–	–	–	–	–	–	–	–	–	–	–	–	–	–	–	–	–
1I	*Diatribæ duæ*	London duodecimo	1677	F.1a1	–	–	–	–	–	–	–	–	–	–	–	–	–	–	–	–	–
2A	*Cerebri anatome*	London quarto	1664	–	–	Pl.1a1	Pl.2a1	Pl.3a1	Pl.4a1	Pl.5a1	Pl.6a1	Pl.7a1	Pl.8a1	Pl.9a1	Pl.10a1	Pl.11a1	Pl.12a1	Pl.13a1	Pl.14a1	Pl.15a1	–
2B1	*Cerebri anatome*	London octavo	1664	–	–	Pl.1a1	Pl.2a1	Pl.3a1	Pl.4a1	Pl.5a1	Pl.6a1	Pl.7a2	Pl.8a1	Pl.9a1	Pl.10a1	Pl.11a1	Pl.12a1	Pl.13a1	Pl.14a1	Pl.15a1	–
2B2	*Cerebri anatome*	London octavo	1664	–	–	Pl.1a2	Pl.2a2	Pl.3a2	Pl.4a2	Pl.5a2	Pl.6a2	Pl.7a2	Pl.8a2	Pl.9a2	Pl.10a2	Pl.11a2	Pl.12a2	Pl.13a2	Pl.14a2	Pl.15a2	–
2C1.c1	*Cerebri anatome*	Amsterdam duodecimo	1664	–	–	Pl.1b1	Pl.2b1	Pl.3b1	Pl.4.b1	Pl.5b1	Pl.6b1	Pl.7b1	Pl.8b1	Pl.9b1	Pl.10b1	Pl.11b1	Pl.12b1	Pl.13b1	Pl.14b1	Pl.15b1	–
2C1.c2	*Cerebri anatome*	Amsterdam duodecimo	1664	–	–	Pl.1b1	Pl.2b1	Pl.3b1	Pl.4.b1	Pl.5b1	Pl.6b1	Pl.7b1	Pl.8b1	Pl.9b1	Pl.10b1	Pl.11b1	Pl.12b1	Pl.13b1	Pl.14b1	Pl.15b1	Pl.16a1
2C2.c1	*Cerebri anatome*	Amsterdam duodecimo	1664	–	–	Pl.1c1	Pl.2c1	Pl.3c1	Pl.4.c1	Pl.5c1	Pl.6c1	Pl.7c1	Pl.8c1	Pl.9c1	Pl.10c1	Pl.11c1	Pl.12c1	Pl.13c1	Pl.14c1	Pl.15c1	Pl.16a1
2C2.c2	*Cerebri anatome*	Amsterdam duodecimo	1664	–	–	Pl.1c1	Pl.2c1	Pl.3c1	Pl.4.c1	Pl.5c1	Pl.6c1	Pl.7c1	Pl.8c1	Pl.9c1	Pl.10c1	Pl.11c1	Pl.12c1	Pl.13c1	Pl.14c1	Pl.15c1	Pl.16a1
2D1	*Cerebri anatome*	Amsterdam octavo	1666	F.2a1	–	Pl.1b2	Pl.2b2	Pl.3b2	Pl.4b2	Pl.5b2	Pl.6b2	Pl.7b2	Pl.8b2	Pl.9b2	Pl.10b2	Pl.11b1	Pl.12b1	Pl.13b1	Pl.14b2	Pl.15b1	–
2D2	*Cerebri anatome*	Amsterdam octavo	1666	F.2a1	–	Pl.1b2	Pl.2b2	Pl.3b2	Pl.4b2	Pl.5b2	Pl.6b2	Pl.7b2	Pl.8b2	Pl.9b2	Pl.10b2	Pl.11b1	Pl.12b1	Pl.13b1	Pl.14b2	Pl.15b1	–
2E 1	*Cerebri anatome*	Amsterdam duodecimo	1667	–	–	Pl.1c1	Pl.2c1	Pl.3c1	Pl.4.c1	Pl.5c1	Pl.6c1	Pl.7c1	Pl.8c1	Pl.9c1	Pl.10c1	Pl.11c1	Pl.12c1	Pl.13c1	Pl.14c1	Pl.15c1	Pl.16a1
2E 2	*Cerebri anatome*	Amsterdam duodecimo	1676	–	–	Pl.1c1	Pl.2c1	Pl.3c1	Pl.4.c1	Pl.5c1	Pl.6c1	Pl.7c1	Pl.8c1	Pl.9c1	Pl.10c1	Pl.11c1	Pl.12c1	Pl.13c1	Pl.14c1	Pl.15c1	–
2F	*Cerebri anatome*	Amsterdam duodecimo	1683	–	–	Pl.1b3	Pl.2b3	Pl.3b3	Pl.4.b3	Pl.5b3	Pl.6b3	Pl.7b3	Pl.8b3	Pl.9b3	Pl.10b3	Pl.11b1	Pl.12b1	Pl.13b1	Pl.14b2	Pl.15b1	–
3A	*Pathologiæ cerebri*	London quarto	1667	–	Pt.1a1	–	–	–	–	–	–	–	–	–	–	–	–	–	–	–	–
3B1	*Pathologiæ cerebri*	Amsterdam duodecimo	1668	–	Pt.1b1	–	–	–	–	–	–	–	–	–	–	–	–	–	–	–	–
3B2	*Pathologiæ cerebri*	London duodecimo	1668	–	Pt.1b1	–	–	–	–	–	–	–	–	–	–	–	–	–	–	–	–
3B3.c1	*Pathologiæ cerebri*	Amsterdam duodecimo	1670	–	Pt.1b1	–	–	–	–	–	–	–	–	–	–	–	–	–	–	–	–
3B3.c2	*Pathologiæ cerebri*	Amsterdam duodecimo	1670	–	Pt.1b1	–	–	–	–	–	–	–	–	–	–	–	–	–	–	–	–
4A	*Affectionum quæ dicuntur* etc.	Oxford & London quarto	1670	–	Pt.1a1	–	–	–	–	–	–	–	–	–	–	–	–	–	–	–	–
4B1	*Affectionum quæ dicuntur* etc.	Leyden duodecimo	1671	–	–	–	–	–	–	–	–	–	–	–	–	–	–	–	–	–	–
4B2	*Affectionum quæ dicuntur* etc.	Leyden duodecimo	1671	–	–	–	–	–	–	–	–	–	–	–	–	–	–	–	–	–	–
4C	*Affectionum quæ dicuntur* etc.	London duodecimo	1678	–	–	–	–	–	–	–	–	–	–	–	–	–	–	–	–	–	–
5A1	*De anima brutorum*	Oxford quarto	1672	–	–	–	–	–	–	–	–	–	–	–	–	–	–	–	–	–	–
5A2	*De anima brutorum*	Oxford quarto	1672	–	–	–	–	–	–	–	–	–	–	–	–	–	–	–	–	–	–
5A3	*De anima brutorum*	Oxford quarto	1672	–	–	–	–	–	–	–	–	–	–	–	–	–	–	–	–	–	–
5A4	*De anima brutorum*	London quarto	1672	–	–	–	–	–	–	–	–	–	–	–	–	–	–	–	–	–	–
5A5	*De anima brutorum*	London quarto	1672	–	–	–	–	–	–	–	–	–	–	–	–	–	–	–	–	–	–
5B1	*De anima brutorum*	London octavo	1672	–	–	–	–	–	–	–	–	–	–	–	–	–	–	–	–	–	–

Plate 17	Plate 18	Plate 19	Plate 20	Plate 21	Plate 22	Plate 23	Plate 24	Plate 25	Plate 26	Plate 27	Plate 28	Plate 29	Plate 30	Plate 31	Plate 32	Plate 33	Plate 34	Plate 35	Plate 36	Plate 37	Plate 38	Plate 39	Plate 40
–	–	–	–	–	–	–	–	–	–	–	–	–	–	–	–	–	–	–	–	–	–	–	–
–	–	–	–	–	–	–	–	–	–	–	–	–	–	–	–	–	–	–	–	–	–	–	–
–	–	–	–	–	–	–	–	–	–	–	–	–	–	–	–	–	–	–	–	–	–	–	–
–	–	–	–	–	–	–	–	–	–	–	–	–	–	–	–	–	–	–	–	–	–	–	–
–	–	–	–	–	–	–	–	–	–	–	–	–	–	–	–	–	–	–	–	–	–	–	–
–	–	–	–	–	–	–	–	–	–	–	–	–	–	–	–	–	–	–	–	–	–	–	–
–	–	–	–	–	–	–	–	–	–	–	–	–	–	–	–	–	–	–	–	–	–	–	–
–	–	–	–	–	–	–	–	–	–	–	–	–	–	–	–	–	–	–	–	–	–	–	–
–	–	–	–	–	–	–	–	–	–	–	–	–	–	–	–	–	–	–	–	–	–	–	–
–	–	–	–	–	–	–	–	–	–	–	–	–	–	–	–	–	–	–	–	–	–	–	–
–	–	–	–	–	–	–	–	–	–	–	–	–	–	–	–	–	–	–	–	–	–	–	–
–	–	–	–	–	–	–	–	–	–	–	–	–	–	–	–	–	–	–	–	–	–	–	–
–	–	–	–	–	–	–	–	–	–	–	–	–	–	–	–	–	–	–	–	–	–	–	–
–	–	–	–	–	–	–	–	–	–	–	–	–	–	–	–	–	–	–	–	–	–	–	–
–	–	–	–	–	–	–	–	–	–	–	–	–	–	–	–	–	–	–	–	–	–	–	–
–	–	–	–	–	–	–	–	–	–	–	–	–	–	–	–	–	–	–	–	–	–	–	–
–	–	–	–	–	–	–	–	–	–	–	–	–	–	–	–	–	–	–	–	–	–	–	–
–	–	–	–	–	–	–	–	–	–	–	–	–	–	–	–	–	–	–	–	–	–	–	–
–	–	–	–	–	–	–	–	–	–	–	–	–	–	–	–	–	–	–	–	–	–	–	–
–	–	–	–	–	–	–	–	–	–	–	–	–	–	–	–	–	–	–	–	–	–	–	–
–	–	–	–	–	–	–	–	–	–	–	–	–	–	–	–	–	–	–	–	–	–	–	–
–	–	–	–	–	–	–	–	–	–	–	–	–	–	–	–	–	–	–	–	–	–	–	–
–	–	–	–	–	–	–	–	–	–	–	–	–	–	–	–	–	–	–	–	–	–	–	–
–	–	–	–	–	–	–	–	–	–	–	–	–	–	–	–	–	–	–	–	–	–	–	–
Pl.17a1	Pl.18a1	–	–	–	–	–	–	–	–	–	–	–	–	–	–	–	–	–	–	–	–	–	–
Pl.17b1	Pl.18b1	–	–	–	–	–	–	–	–	–	–	–	–	–	–	–	–	–	–	–	–	–	–
Pl.17b1	Pl.18b1	–	–	–	–	–	–	–	–	–	–	–	–	–	–	–	–	–	–	–	–	–	–
Pl.17a1	Pl.18a1																						
–	–	Pl.19a1	Pl.20a1	Pl.21a1	Pl.22a1	Pl.23a1	Pl.24a1	Pl.25a1	Pl.26a1	–	–	–	–	–	–	–	–	–	–	–	–	–	–
–	–	Pl.19a1	Pl.20a1	Pl.21a1	Pl.22a1	Pl.23a1	Pl.24a1	Pl.25a1	Pl.26a1	–	–	–	–	–	–	–	–	–	–	–	–	–	–
–	–	Pl.19a1	Pl.20a1	Pl.21a1	Pl.22a1	Pl.23a1	Pl.24a1	Pl.25a1	Pl.26a1	–	–	–	–	–	–	–	–	–	–	–	–	–	–
–	–	Pl.19a1	Pl.20a1	Pl.21a1	Pl.22a1	Pl.23a1	Pl.24a1	Pl.25a1	Pl.26a1	–	–	–	–	–	–	–	–	–	–	–	–	–	–
–	–	Pl.19a1	Pl.20a1	Pl.21a1	Pl.22a1	Pl.23a1	Pl.24a1	Pl.25a1	Pl.26a1	–	–	–	–	–	–	–	–	–	–	–	–	–	–
–	–	Pl.19a2	Pl.20a2	Pl.21a2	Pl.22a2	Pl.23a2	Pl.24a2	Pl.25a2	Pl.26a2	–	–	–	–	–	–	–	–	–	–	–	–	–	–

(continued)

Table 2 Continued

Number	Short title	Place of publication and format	Year	Frontispiece	Portrait 1	Plate 1	Plate 2	Plate 3	Plate 4	Plate 5	Plate 6	Plate 7	Plate 8	Plate 9	Plate 10	Plate 11	Plate 12	Plate 13	Plate 14	Plate 15	Plate 16
5B2.c1	*De anima brutorum*	London octavo	1672	–	–	–	–	–	–	–	–	–	–	–	–	–	–	–	–	–	–
5B2.c2	*De anima brutorum*	London octavo	1672	–	–	–	–	–	–	–	–	–	–	–	–	–	–	–	–	–	–
5B3	*De anima brutorum*	Amsterdam octavo	1672	–	–	–	–	–	–	–	–	–	–	–	–	–	–	–	–	–	–
5C	*De anima brutorum*	Amsterdam octavo	1674	–	–	–	–	–	–	–	–	–	–	–	–	–	–	–	–	–	–
6A1	*Pharmaceutice rationalis* (part I)	Oxford quarto	1674	–	–	–	–	–	–	–	–	–	–	–	–	–	–	–	–	–	–
6A2	*Pharmaceutice rationalis* (part I)	Oxford quarto	1674	–	–	–	–	–	–	–	–	–	–	–	–	–	–	–	–	–	–
6B1	*Pharmaceutice rationalis* (part I)	Oxford duodecimo	1674	–	–	–	–	–	–	–	–	–	–	–	–	–	–	–	–	–	–
6B2	*Pharmaceutice rationalis* (part I)	Oxford & London duodecimo	1674	–	–	–	–	–	–	–	–	–	–	–	–	–	–	–	–	–	–
6C	*Pharmaceutice rationalis* (part I)	The Hague duodecimo	1674	F.3a1	–	–	–	–	–	–	–	–	–	–	–	–	–	–	–	–	–
6D	*Pharmaceutice rationalis* (part I)	The Hague duodecimo	1675	F.3a1	–	–	–	–	–	–	–	–	–	–	–	–	–	–	–	–	–
6E	*Pharmaceutice rationalis* (part II)	Oxford quarto	1675	–	–	–	–	–	–	–	–	–	–	–	–	–	–	–	–	–	–
6F	*Pharmaceutice rationalis* (part II)	Oxford duodecimo	1675	–	–	–	–	–	–	–	–	–	–	–	–	–	–	–	–	–	–
6G	*Pharmaceutice rationalis* (part II)	The Hague duodecimo	1677	–	–	–	–	–	–	–	–	–	–	–	–	–	–	–	–	–	–
6H	*Pharmaceutice rationalis* (part I)	Middelburg octavo	1677			–	–	–	–	–	–	–	–	–	–	–	–	–	–	–	–
6I	*Pharmaceutice rationalis* (parts I & II)	Oxford octavo	1679	–	–	–	–	–	–	–	–	–	–	–	–	–	–	–	–	–	–
6J	*Pharmaceutice rationalis* (part II)	Amsterdam octavo	1681			–	–	–	–	–	–	–	–	–	–	–	–	–	–	–	–
7A1	*A plain and easie method*	London octavo	1691	–	Pt.1f1	–	–	–	–	–	–	–	–	–	–	–	–	–	–	–	–
7A2	*A plain and easie method*	London octavo	1691	–	Pt.1f1	–	–	–	–	–	–	–	–	–	–	–	–	–	–	–	–
8A.c1	*Opera medica & physica*	Lyons quarto	1676	–	Pt.1c1	Pl.1e1	Pl.2e1	Pl.3e1	Pl.4e1	Pl.5e1	Pl.6e1	Pl.7e1	Pl.8e1	Pl.9e1	Pl.10e1	Pl.11e1	Pl.12e1	Pl.13e1	Pl.14e1	Pl.15e1	Pl.16b1
8A.c2	*Opera medica & physica*	Lyons quarto	1676	–	Pt.1c1	Pl.1e1	Pl.2e1	Pl.3e1	Pl.4e1	Pl.5e1	Pl.6e1	Pl.7e1	Pl.8e1	Pl.9e1	Pl.10e1	Pl.11e1	Pl.12e1	Pl.13e1	Pl.14e1	Pl.15e1	Pl.16b1
8B1	*Opera omnia*	Geneva quarto	1676	–	Pt.1d1	Pl.1f1	Pl.2f1	Pl.3f1	Pl.4f1	Pl.5f1	Pl.6f1	Pl.7f1	Pl.8f1	Pl.9f1	Pl.10f1	Pl.11f1	Pl.12f1	Pl.13f1	Pl.14f1	Pl.15f1	Pl.16c1
8B2	*Opera omnia*	Coloniæ Allobrogum quarto	1676	–	Pt.1d1	Pl.1f1	Pl.2f1	Pl.3f1	Pl.4f1	Pl.5f1	Pl.6f1	Pl.7f1	Pl.8f1	Pl.9f1	Pl.10f1	Pl.11f1	Pl.12f1	Pl.13f1	Pl.14f1	Pl.15f1	Pl.16c1
8B3	*Opera omnia*	Coloniæ Allobrogum quarto	1676	–	Pt.1d1	Pl.1f1	Pl.2f1	Pl.3f1	Pl.4f1	Pl.5f1	Pl.6f1	Pl.7f1	Pl.8f1	Pl.9f1	Pl.10f1	Pl.11f1	Pl.12f1	Pl.13f1	Pl.14f1	Pl.15f1	Pl.16c1
8C1	*Opera omnia*	Geneva quarto	1680	–	Pt.1d2	Pl.1f1	Pl.2f1	Pl.3f1	Pl.4f1	Pl.5f1	Pl.6f1	Pl.7f1	Pl.8f1	Pl.9f1	Pl.10f1	Pl.11f1	Pl.12f1	Pl.13f1	Pl.14f1	Pl.15f1	Pl.16c1
8C2	*Opera omnia*	Coloniæ Allobrogum quarto	1680	–	Pt.1d2	Pl.1f1	Pl.2f1	Pl.3f1	Pl.4f1	Pl.5f1	Pl.6f1	Pl.7f1	Pl.8f1	Pl.9f1	Pl.10f1	Pl.11f1	Pl.12f1	Pl.13f1	Pl.14f1	Pl.15f1	Pl.16c1
8D	*Opera omnia*	Lyons quarto (2 volumes)	1681	–	Pt.1c1	Pl.1e1	Pl.2e1	Pl.3e1	Pl.4e1	Pl.5e1	Pl.6e1	Pl.7e1	Pl.8e1	Pl.9e1	Pl.10e1	Pl.11e1	Pl.12e1	Pl.13e1	Pl.14e1	Pl.15e1	Pl.16b1
8E	*Opera omnia*	Amsterdam quarto	1682	F.4a1	Pt.1e1	Pl.1c2	Pl.2c2	Pl.3c2	Pl.4c2	Pl.5c2	Pl.6c2	Pl.7c2	Pl.8c2	Pl.9c2	Pl.10c2	Pl.11c2	Pl.12c2	Pl.13c2	Pl.14c2	Pl.15c2	–
8F	*Opera omnia*	Coloniæ Allobrogum folio	1694	–	Pt.1g1	Pl.1g1	Pl.2g1	Pl.3g1	Pl.4g1	Pl.5g1	Pl.6g1	Pl.7g1	Pl.8g1	Pl.9g1	Pl.10g1	Pl.11g1	Pl.12g1	Pl.13g1	Pl.14g1	Pl.15g1	Pl.16d1
8G	*Opera omnia*	Coloniæ Allobrogum quarto	1695	–	Pt.1d2	Pl.1f1	Pl.2f1	Pl.3f1	Pl.4f1	Pl.5f1	Pl.6f1	Pl.7f1	Pl.8f1	Pl.9f1	Pl.10f1	Pl.11f1	Pl.12f1	Pl.13f1	Pl.14f1	Pl.15f1	Pl.16c1
8H.c1	*Opera omnia*	Venice folio	1708	–	Pt.1g1	Pl.1g1	Pl.2g1	Pl.3g1	Pl.4g1	Pl.5g1	Pl.6g1	Pl.7g1	Pl.8g1	Pl.9g1	Pl.10g1	Pl.11g1	Pl.12g1	Pl.13g1	Pl.14g1	Pl.15g1	Pl.16d1
8H.c2	*Opera omnia*	Venice folio	1708	–	Pt.1g1	Pl.1g1	Pl.2g1	Pl.3g1	Pl.4g1	Pl.5g1	Pl.6g1	Pl.7g1	Pl.8g1	Pl.9g1	Pl.10g1	Pl.11g1	Pl.12g1	Pl.13g1	Pl.14g1	Pl.15g1	Pl.16d1
8H.c3	*Opera omnia*	Venice folio	1708	–	Pt.1g1	Pl.1g1	Pl.2g1	Pl.3g1	Pl.4g1	Pl.5g1	Pl.6g1	Pl.7g1	Pl.8g1	Pl.9g1	Pl.10g1	Pl.11g1	Pl.12g1	Pl.13g1	Pl.14g1	Pl.15g1	Pl.16d1
8I	*Opera omnia*	Venice folio	1720	–	Pt.1g1	Pl.1g2	Pl.2g2	Pl.3g2	Pl.4g2	Pl.5g2	Pl.6g2	Pl.7g2	Pl.8g2	Pl.9g2	Pl.10g2	Pl.11g2	Pl.12g2	Pl.13g2	Pl.14g2	Pl.15g2	Pl.16d2

Plate 17	Plate 18	Plate 19	Plate 20	Plate 21	Plate 22	Plate 23	Plate 24	Plate 25	Plate 26	Plate 27	Plate 28	Plate 29	Plate 30	Plate 31	Plate 32	Plate 33	Plate 34	Plate 35	Plate 36	Plate 37	Plate 38	Plate 39	Plate 40
–	–	Pl.19a2	Pl.20a2	Pl.21a2	Pl.22a2	Pl.23a2	Pl.24a2	Pl.25a2	Pl.26a2	–	–	–	–	–	–	–	–	–	–	–	–	–	–
–	–	Pl.19a2	Pl.20a2	Pl.21a2	Pl.22a2	Pl.23a2	Pl.24a2	Pl.25a2	Pl.26a2	–	–	–	–	–	–	–	–	–	–	–	–	–	–
–	–	Pl.19a2	Pl.20a2	Pl.21a2	Pl.22a2	Pl.23a2	Pl.24a2	Pl.25a2	Pl.26a2	–	–	–	–	–	–	–	–	–	–	–	–	–	–
–	–	Pl.19b1	Pl.20b1	Pl.21b1	Pl.22b1	Pl.23b1	Pl.24b1	Pl.25b1	Pl.26b1	–	–	–	–	–	–	–	–	–	–	–	–	–	–
–	–	–	–	–	–	–	–	–	–	Pl.27a1	Pl.28a1	Pl.29a1	Pl.30a1	Pl.31a1	Pl.32a1	–	–	–	–	–	–	–	–
–	–	–	–	–	–	–	–	–	–	Pl.27a1	Pl.28a1	Pl.29a1	Pl.30a1	Pl.31a1	Pl.32a1	–	–	–	–	–	–	–	–
–	–	–	–	–	–	–	–	–	–	Pl.27a2	Pl.28a2	Pl.29a2	Pl.30a2	Pl.31a2	Pl.32a2	–	–	–	–	–	–	–	–
–	–	–	–	–	–	–	–	–	–	Pl.27a2	Pl.28a2	Pl.29a2	Pl.30a2	Pl.31a2	Pl.32a2	–	–	–	–	–	–	–	–
–	–	–	–	–	–	–	–	–	–	Pl.27b1	Pl.28b1	Pl.29b1	Pl.30b1	Pl.31b1	Pl.32b1	–	–	–	–	–	–	–	–
–	–	–	–	–	–	–	–	–	–	Pl.27b2	Pl.28b2	Pl.29b2	Pl.30b2	Pl.31b2	Pl.32b2	–	–	–	–	–	–	–	–
–	–	–	–	–	–	–	–	–	–	–	–	–	–	–	–	Pl.33a1	Pl.34a1	Pl.35a1	Pl.36a1	Pl.37a1	Pl.38a1	Pl.39a1	Pl.40a1
–	–	–	–	–	–	–	–	–	–	–	–	–	–	–	–	Pl.33a1	Pl.34a1	Pl.35a1	Pl.36a1	Pl.37a1	Pl.38a1	Pl.39a1	Pl.40a1
–	–	–	–	–	–	–	–	–	–	–	–	–	–	–	–	Pl.33b1	Pl.34b1	Pl.35b1	Pl.36b1	Pl.37b1	Pl.38b1	Pl.39b1	Pl.40b1
–	–	–	–	–	–	–	–	–	–	Pl.27b2	Pl.28b2	Pl.29b2	Pl.30b2	Pl.31b2	Pl.32b2	–	–	–	–	–	–	–	–
–	–	–	–	–	–	–	–	–	–	Pl.27a3	Pl.28a3	Pl.29a3	Pl.30a3	Pl.31a3	Pl.32a3	Pl.33a2	Pl.34a2	Pl.35a2	Pl.36a2	Pl.37a2	Pl.38a2	Pl.39a2	Pl.40a2
–	–									–	–	–	–	–	–	Pl.33c1	Pl.34c1	Pl.35c1	Pl.36c1	Pl.37c1	Pl.38c1	Pl.39c1	Pl.40c1
–	–	–	–	–	–	–	–	–	–	–	–	–	–	–	–	–	–	–	–	–	–	–	–
–	–	–	–	–	–	–	–	–	–	–	–	–	–	–	–	–	–	–	–	–	–	–	–
Pl.17d1	Pl.18d1	Pl.19d1	Pl.20d1	Pl.21d1	Pl.22d1	Pl.23d1	Pl.24d1	Pl.25d1	Pl.26d1	Pl.27e1	Pl.28e1	Pl.29e1	Pl.30e1	Pl.31e1	Pl.32e1	Pl.33e1	Pl.34e1	Pl.35e1	Pl.36e1	Pl.37e1	Pl.38e1	Pl.39e1	Pl.40e1
Pl.17d1	Pl.18d1	Pl.19d1	Pl.20d1	Pl.21d1	Pl.22d1	Pl.23d1	Pl.24d1	Pl.25d1	Pl.26d1	Pl.27e1	Pl.28e1	Pl.29e1	Pl.30e1	Pl.31e1	Pl.32e1	Pl.33e1	Pl.34e1	Pl.35e1	Pl.36e1	Pl.37e1	Pl.38e1	Pl.39e1	Pl.40e1
Pl.17e1	Pl.18e1	Pl.19e1	Pl.20e1	Pl.21e1	Pl.22e1	Pl.23e1	Pl.24e1	Pl.25e1	Pl.26e1	Pl.27f1	Pl.28f1	Pl.29f1	Pl.30f1	Pl.31f1	Pl.32f1	Pl.33f1	Pl.34f1	Pl.35f1	Pl.36f1	Pl.37f1	Pl.38f1	Pl.39f1	Pl.40f1
Pl.17e1	Pl.18e1	Pl.19e1	Pl.20e1	Pl.21e1	Pl.22e1	Pl.23e1	Pl.24e1	Pl.25e1	Pl.26e1	Pl.27f1	Pl.28f1	Pl.29f1	Pl.30f1	Pl.31f1	Pl.32f1	Pl.33f1	Pl.34f1	Pl.35f1	Pl.36f1	Pl.37f1	Pl.38f1	Pl.39f1	Pl.40f1
Pl.17e1	Pl.18e1	Pl.19e1	Pl.20e1	Pl.21e1	Pl.22e1	Pl.23e1	Pl.24e1	Pl.25e1	Pl.26e1	Pl.27f1	Pl.28f1	Pl.29f1	Pl.30f1	Pl.31f1	Pl.32f1	Pl.33f1	Pl.34f1	Pl.35f1	Pl.36f1	Pl.37f1	Pl.38f1	Pl.39f1	Pl.40f1
Pl.17e1	Pl.18e1	Pl.19e1	Pl.20e1	Pl.21e1	Pl.22e1	Pl.23e1	Pl.24e1	Pl.25e1	Pl.26e1	Pl.27f1	Pl.28f1	Pl.29f1	Pl.30f1	Pl.31f1	Pl.32f1	Pl.33f1	Pl.34f1	Pl.35f1	Pl.36f1	Pl.37f1	Pl.38f1	Pl.39f1	Pl.40f1
Pl.17e1	Pl.18e1	Pl.19e1	Pl.20e1	Pl.21e1	Pl.22e1	Pl.23e1	Pl.24e1	Pl.25e1	Pl.26e1	Pl.27f1	Pl.28f1	Pl.29f1	Pl.30f1	Pl.31f1	Pl.32f1	Pl.33f1	Pl.34f1	Pl.35f1	Pl.36f1	Pl.37f1	Pl.38f1	Pl.39f1	Pl.40f1
Pl.17d1	Pl.18d1	Pl.19d1	Pl.20d1	Pl.21d1	Pl.22d1	Pl.23d1	Pl.24d1	Pl.25d1	Pl.26d1	Pl.27e1	Pl.28e1	Pl.29e1	Pl.30e1	Pl.31e1	Pl.32e1	Pl.33e1	Pl.34e1	Pl.35e1	Pl.36e1	Pl.37e1	Pl.38e1	Pl.39e1	Pl.40e1
Pl.17f1	Pl.18f1	Pl.19b2	Pl.20b2	Pl.21b2	Pl.22b2	Pl.23b2	Pl.24b2	Pl.25b2	Pl.26b2	Pl.27b3	Pl.28b3	Pl.29b3	Pl.30b3	Pl.31b3	Pl.32b3	Pl.33b2	Pl.34b2	Pl.35b2	Pl.36b2	Pl.37b2	Pl.38b2	Pl.39b2	Pl.40b2
Pl.17g1	Pl.18g1	Pl.19f1	Pl.20f1	Pl.21f1	Pl.22f1	Pl.23f1	Pl.24f1	Pl.25f1	Pl.26f1	Pl.27g1	Pl.28g1	Pl.29g1	Pl.30g1	Pl.31g1	Pl.32g1	Pl.33g1	Pl.34g1	Pl.35g1	Pl.36g1	Pl.37g1	Pl.38g1	Pl.39g1	Pl.40g1
Pl.17e1	Pl.18e1	Pl.19e1	Pl.20e1	Pl.21e1	Pl.22e1	Pl.23e1	Pl.24e1	Pl.25e1	Pl.26e1	Pl.27f1	Pl.28f1	Pl.29f1	Pl.30f1	Pl.31f1	Pl.32f1	Pl.33f1	Pl.34f1	Pl.35f1	Pl.36f1	Pl.37f1	Pl.38f1	Pl.39f1	Pl.40f1
Pl.17g1	Pl.18g1	Pl.19f1	Pl.20f1	Pl.21f1	Pl.22f1	Pl.23f1	Pl.24f1	Pl.25f1	Pl.26f1	Pl.27g1	Pl.28g1	Pl.29g1	Pl.30g1	Pl.31g1	Pl.32g1	Pl.33g1	Pl.34g1	Pl.35g1	Pl.36g1	Pl.37g1	Pl.38g1	Pl.39g1	Pl.40g1
Pl.17g1	Pl.18g1	Pl.19f1	Pl.20f1	Pl.21f1	Pl.22f1	Pl.23f1	Pl.24f1	Pl.25f1	Pl.26f1	Pl.27g1	Pl.28g1	Pl.29g1	Pl.30g1	Pl.31g1	Pl.32g1	Pl.33g1	Pl.34g1	Pl.35g1	Pl.36g1	Pl.37g1	Pl.38g1	Pl.39g1	Pl.40g1
Pl.17g1	Pl.18g1	Pl.19f1	Pl.20f1	Pl.21f1	Pl.22f1	Pl.23f1	Pl.24f1	Pl.25f1	Pl.26f1	Pl.27g1	Pl.28g1	Pl.29g1	Pl.30g1	Pl.31g1	Pl.32g1	Pl.33g1	Pl.34g1	Pl.35g1	Pl.36g1	Pl.37g1	Pl.38g1	Pl.39g1	Pl.40g1
Pl.17g2	Pl.18g2	Pl.19f2	Pl.20f2	Pl.21f2	Pl.22f2	Pl.23f2	Pl.24f2	Pl.25f2	Pl.26f2	Pl.27g1	Pl.28g1	Pl.29g2	Pl.30g2	Pl.31g1	Pl.32g1	Pl.33g1	Pl.34g1	Pl.35g2	Pl.36g2	Pl.37g1	Pl.38g1	Pl.39g1	Pl.40g1

(continued)

Table 2 Continued

Number	Short title	Place of publication and format	Year	Frontispiece	Portrait 1	Plate 1	Plate 2	Plate 3	Plate 4	Plate 5	Plate 6	Plate 7	Plate 8	Plate 9	Plate 10	Plate 11	Plate 12	Plate 13	Plate 14	Plate 15	Plate 16
9A1	*Pharmaceutice rationalis* (English)	London folio	1679	–	–	–	–	–	–	–	–	–	–	–	–	–	–	–	–	–	–
9A2.c1	*Pharmaceutice rationalis* (English)	London folio	1679	–	–	–	–	–	–	–	–	–	–	–	–	–	–	–	–	–	–
9A2.c2	*Pharmaceutice rationalis* (English)	London folio	1679	–	–	–	–	–	–	–	–	–	–	–	–	–	–	–	–	–	–
9B1.c1	*The remaining medical works*	London folio	1681	–	Pt.1a1	Pl.1a3	Pl.2a3	Pl.3a3	Pl.4a3	Pl.5a3	Pl.6a3	Pl.7a3	Pl.8a3	Pl.9a3	Pl.10a3	Pl.11a3	Pl.12a3	Pl.13d1	Pl.14d1	Pl.15a3	–
9B1.c2	*The remaining medical works*	London folio	1681	–	Pt.1a1	Pl.1a3	Pl.2a3	Pl.3a3	Pl.4a3	Pl.5a3	Pl.6a3	Pl.7a4	Pl.8a3	Pl.9a3	Pl.10a3	Pl.11a3	Pl.12a3	Pl.13d1	Pl.14d1	Pl.15a3	–
9B2	*The remaining medical works*	London folio	1681	–	Pt.1a1	Pl.1a3	Pl.2a3	Pl.3a3	Pl.4a3	Pl.5a3	Pl.6a3	Pl.7a4	Pl.8a3	Pl.9a3	Pl.10a3	Pl.11a3	Pl.12a3	Pl.13d1	Pl.14d1	Pl.15a3	–
9C	*Dr Willis's practice of physick*	London folio	1681	–	Pt.1a1	Pl.1a3	Pl.2a3	Pl.3a3	Pl.4a3	Pl.5a3	Pl.6a3	Pl.7a3	Pl.8a3	Pl.9a3	Pl.10a3	Pl.11a3	Pl.12a3	Pl.13d1	Pl.14d1	Pl.15a3	–
9D	*Two discourses concerning the soul of brutes*	London folio	1683	–	–	–	–	–	–	–	–	–	–	–	–	–	–	–	–	–	–
9E.c1	*Dr Willis's practice of physick*	London folio	1684	–	Pt.1a1	Pl.1a3	Pl.2a3	Pl.3a3	Pl.4a3	Pl.5a3	Pl.6a3	Pl.7a4	Pl.8a3	Pl.9a3	Pl.10a3	Pl.11a3	Pl.12a3	Pl.13d1	Pl.14d1	Pl.15a3	–
9E.c2	*Dr Willis's practice of physick*	London folio	1684	–	Pt.1a1	Pl.1a3	Pl.2a3	Pl.3a3	Pl.4a3	Pl.5a3	Pl.6a3	Pl.7a4	Pl.8a3	Pl.9a3	Pl.10a3	Pl.11a3	Pl.12a3	Pl.13d1	Pl.14d1	Pl.15a3	–
9F	*Dr Willis's practice of physick*	London folio	1684	–	–	Pl.1d1	Pl.2d1	Pl.3d1	Pl.4d1	Pl.5d1	Pl.6d1	Pl.7d1	Pl.8d1	Pl.9d1	Pl.10d1	Pl.11d1	Pl.12d1	Pl.13d2	Pl.14d2	Pl.15d1	–
10A1.c1	*London practice of physick*	London octavo	1685	–	Pt.1f1	–	–	–	–	–	–	–	–	–	–	–	–	–	–	–	–
10A1.c2	*London practice of physick*	London octavo	1685	–	Pt.1f1	–	–	–	–	–	–	–	–	–	–	–	–	–	–	–	–
10A1.c3	*London practice of physick*	London octavo	1685	–	Pt.1f1	–	–	–	–	–	–	–	–	–	–	–	–	–	–	–	–
10A2.c1	*London practice of physick*	London octavo	1689	–	Pt.1f1	–	–	–	–	–	–	–	–	–	–	–	–	–	–	–	–
10A2.c2	*London practice of physick*	London octavo	1689	–	Pt.1f1	–	–	–	–	–	–	–	–	–	–	–	–	–	–	–	–
10A2.c3	*London practice of physick*	London octavo	1689	–	Pt.1f1	–	–	–	–	–	–	–	–	–	–	–	–	–	–	–	–
10A3.c1	*London practice of physick*	London octavo	1692	–	Pt.1f1	–	–	–	–	–	–	–	–	–	–	–	–	–	–	–	–
10A3.c2	*London practice of physick*	London octavo	1692	–	Pt.1f1	–	–	–	–	–	–	–	–	–	–	–	–	–	–	–	–
10A4	*London practice of physick*	London octavo	1695	–	Pt.1f1	–	–	–	–	–	–	–	–	–	–	–	–	–	–	–	–

Plate 17	Plate 18	Plate 19	Plate 20	Plate 21	Plate 22	Plate 23	Plate 24	Plate 25	Plate 26	Plate 27	Plate 28	Plate 29	Plate 30	Plate 31	Plate 32	Plate 33	Plate 34	Plate 35	Plate 36	Plate 37	Plate 38	Plate 39	Plate 40
–	–	–	–	–	–	–	–	–	–	Pl.27a4	Pl.28a4	Pl.29a4	Pl.30a4	Pl.31a4	Pl.32a4	Pl.33a3	Pl.34a3	Pl.35a3	Pl.36a3	Pl.37a3	Pl.38a3	Pl.39a3	Pl.40a3
–	–	–	–	–	–	–	–	–	–	Pl.27a5	Pl.28a4	Pl.29a4	Pl.30a4	Pl.31a4	Pl.32a4	Pl.33a3	Pl.34a3	Pl.35a3	Pl.36a3	Pl.37a3	Pl.38a3	Pl.39a3	Pl.40a3
–	–	–	–	–	–	–	–	–	–	Pl.27a5	Pl.28a4	Pl.29a4	Pl.30a4	Pl.31a4	Pl.32a4	Pl.33a3	Pl.34a3	Pl.35a3	Pl.36a3	Pl.37a3	Pl.38a3	Pl.39a3	Pl.40a3
Pl.17a2	Pl.18a2	–	–	–	–	–	–	–	–	–	–	–	–	–	–	–	–	–	–	–	–	–	–
Pl.17a2	Pl.18a2	–	–	–	–	–	–	–	–	–	–	–	–	–	–	–	–	–	–	–	–	–	–
Pl.17a2	Pl.18a2	–	–	–	–	–	–	–	–	–	–	–	–	–	–	–	–	–	–	–	–	–	–
Pl.17a2	Pl.18a2	–	–	–	–	–	–	–	–	Pl.27a5	Pl.28a4	Pl.29a4	Pl.30a4	Pl.31a4	Pl.32a4	Pl.33a3	Pl.34a3	Pl.35a3	Pl.36a3	Pl.37a3	Pl.38a3	Pl.39a3	Pl.40a3
–	–	Pl.19c1	Pl.20c1	Pl.21c1	Pl.22c1	Pl.23c1	Pl.24c1	Pl.25c1	Pl.26c1														
Pl.17a2	Pl.18a2	Pl.19c1	Pl.20c1	Pl.21c1	Pl.22c1	Pl.23c1	Pl.24c1	Pl.25c1	Pl.26c1	Pl.27c1	Pl.28c1	Pl.29c1	Pl.30c1	Pl.31c1	Pl.32c1	Pl.33d1	Pl.34d1	Pl.35d1	Pl.36d1	Pl.37d1	Pl.38d1	Pl.39d1	Pl.40d1
Pl.17a2	Pl.18a2	Pl.19c1	Pl.20c1	Pl.21c1	Pl.22c1	Pl.23c1	Pl.24c1	Pl.25c1	Pl.26c1	Pl.27c1	Pl.28c1	Pl.29c1	Pl.30c1	Pl.31c1	Pl.32c1	Pl.33d1	Pl.34d1	Pl.35d1	Pl.36d1	Pl.37d1	Pl.38d1	Pl.39d1	Pl.40d1
Pl.17c1	Pl.18c1	Pl.19c1	Pl.20c1	Pl.21c1	Pl.22c1	Pl.23c1	Pl.24c1	Pl.25c1	Pl.26c1	Pl.27c1	Pl.28c1	Pl.29c1	Pl.30c1	Pl.31c1	Pl.32c1	Pl.33d1	Pl.34d1	Pl.35d1	Pl.36d1	Pl.37d1	Pl.38d1	Pl.39d1	Pl.40d1
–	–	–	–	–	–	–	–	–	–	–	–	–	–	–	–	–	–	–	–	–	–	–	–
–	–	–	–	–	–	–	–	–	–	–	–	–	–	–	–	–	–	–	–	–	–	–	–
–	–	–	–	–	–	–	–	–	–	–	–	–	–	–	–	–	–	–	–	–	–	–	–
–	–	–	–	–	–	–	–	–	–	–	–	–	–	–	–	–	–	–	–	–	–	–	–
–	–	–	–	–	–	–	–	–	–	–	–	–	–	–	–	–	–	–	–	–	–	–	–
–	–	–	–	–	–	–	–	–	–	–	–	–	–	–	–	–	–	–	–	–	–	–	–
–	–	–	–	–	–	–	–	–	–	–	–	–	–	–	–	–	–	–	–	–	–	–	–
–	–	–	–	–	–	–	–	–	–	–	–	–	–	–	–	–	–	–	–	–	–	–	–
–	–	–	–	–	–	–	–	–	–	–	–	–	–	–	–	–	–	–	–	–	–	–	–

The further use of Willis's illustrations

As acknowledged in the legend and text of chapter 3, the four figures of Tabula 1 in *De anima brutorum* are copied from Marcello Malpighi's *De Bombyce* (1669) published by John Martyn (1618–1678) and James Allestry, printers to the Royal Society. Willis's Figure I is Malpighi's Tabula IV, Fig. II; Willis's Figura II is Malpighi's Tabula III, Figure 1; Willis's Figura III is Malpighi's Tabula III, Fig. III; and Willis's Figura IIII is one image from the two that make up Malpighi's Tabula III, Fig. IIII. With this exception, and discounting the illustrations for Croone's essay, the remaining 80 images on 39 plates used in the printed works of Thomas Willis were original, even if individual details were already known and the presentational arrangements familiar.

After Andreas Vesalius (1514–1564) published *De humani corporis fabrica libri septem* (1543) and Bartolomew Eustachius (1500–1574) had produced his plates (1552: but lost until first published in 1714), depictions of the brain were often used to illustrate anatomical works. Andreas Laurentius (1558–1609) included twenty images that were copied, more or less faithfully, from Vesalius.[82] Johan Vesling (1598–1649) used thirteen images in three plates, which also mimicked Vesalius in style, but added sections of the cerebellum; dissection of the spinal cord, nerve roots and brachial and lumbar plexuses; and an improved view of the base of the brain including the blood vessels.[83] Nathanael Highmore (1613–1685), known to Willis, included an original view of the sagittal sinus orientated as in dissections of Vesalius, and an image of the skull base with various structures wholly or partially removed.[84] Thomas Bartholin (1616–1680) published an adaptation of his father's (Caspar Bartholin: 1585–1629) anatomical work with seven folding sheets and a large number of engravings included within the text or occupying the entire recto or verso of plate leaves.[85] Liber III deals with the head and has nine plates engraved by S Voort-Scamp (nd) but taken from Vesalius and other earlier anatomists. Libellus III on the nerves has six plates which are equally derivative. These were the images with which Willis, Lower, and Wren would have been familiar.

The most significant set of plates depicting the nervous system, from the same period as Willis but published after his death, was that of Raymond Vieussens (*c.*1635–1715).[86] Liber I deals with the brain and contain XVII plates. Liber II describes the spinal cord and contains Tabulæ XVIII–XXI, which are superior to Willis. Liber III is on the nerves and brachial and lumbar plexuses and includes Tabulæ XXII–XXX, several of which are on folding sheets and remarkable for being lifesize representations of the dissected human arm and leg. By any analysis, Vieussens advanced anatomy of the human nervous system

[82] See: Andreas Laurentius, *Historia anatomica humani corporis et singularum eius partim multis controversus & observationibus nouis illustrata*, Frankfurt (1600): pages 207 and 209 with legends at pages 206, 208, and 210.

[83] See: Johan Vesling, *Syntagma anatomicum, locis plurimis auctum, emendatum, novisque iconibus diligenter exornatum*, Padua (1647): Tabulæ I, II, and III, Cap. XIV, pages 185, 189, and 195 with legends at pages 181–3, 187–8, and 191–4.

[84] See: Nathanael Highmore, *Corporis humani disquisitio anatomica; in qua sanguinis cirrculationem in quavis corporis particula plurimis typis novis, ac ænygmatum medicorum succincta dilucidatione ornatam profequutus est*, The Hague (1651): Tab XV, page 211 with legend at pages 212–13.

[85] See: Thomas Bartholin, *Institutiones anatomicæ, novis recentiorum opinionibus & observationibus, quarum innumere hactenus edite non sunt figuris que aucte*, Lugduni Batavorum [Leiden] (1641): liber III, pages 240–307.

[86] Vieussens work was printed in several issues and editions starting with: Raymindi Vieussens, *Neurographia universalis hoc est omnium corporis humani nervorum, simul & cerebri, medulæque spinalis. Descriptio anatomica; eaque integra et accurata, variis iconibus fideliter & ad vivum delineatis, aréque incisis illustrata: cum ipsorum actione et usu, physico discursu explicatis*, Lugduni [Lyon] (1684). This was reprinted as 'Editio nova' (1685); *Editio in Germania prima, ob causas in nova præsatione allegatas adornata, & adjecto rerum indice aucta*, Frankfurt (1690); *Editio novissima*, Lugduni (1716); *Nova editio*, Tolosæ [Toulouse] (1775); and perhaps others.

beyond Willis, in terms of complexity of dissection and details of the brain and peripheral nerves. That said, the image of the base of the brain with the vessels, Tabula IV pasted onto Eijv at page 36, is much inferior to Figura I from *Cerebri anatome* (1664: Pl.1). Also in France, Vincent Droüin (1660–1722) included nine plates containing 24 images.[87] The second figure shows the base of the brain but without any blood vessels. Although in no sense copies, other perhaps than in the orientation of some dissections, the seven images on five plates included in Humphry Ridley's (1653–1708) monograph on the human brain, the first written in English, are inferior to Willis. Figure I showing the base of the brain without a completed circle does include the arterial supply of the spinal cord originating from the right vertebral artery.[88]

Vieussens, Droüin, and Ridley may have benefited from Willis's descriptions but their images were original. Others were less restrained and, with no very strict rules on copyright, it did not take long for the illustrations—especially those of the brain—to be copied, with or without attribution.[89] Gerard Blasius (1625–1682) anticipated his edition of the *Opera omnia* (1682: **8E**) by including in two earlier publications plates copied from Willis. In his short treatise, *Anatome medullæ spinalis et nervorum* (1666), Blasius refers extensively to Willis in the text between pages 24 and 38. He reproduces Tabula XIII using an original unaltered plate (Pl.15c1) from Commelin's 1664 edition of *Cerebri anatome* and *Nervorum descriptio et usus* (**2C2**) as one of three folding sheets, together with Willis's legend.[90] Blasius includes an additional Figura VI, not taken from Willis but relating to his work, on one of the two other folding sheets. His legend reads:

> Arteriæ ſpinalis circa medullæ ſpinalis ſuperficiem poſticam quæ vertebrarû ſpinas reſpicit, ſeſe exhibentis diviſiones & ramificationes proponit, prout in corpore equino ſeſe nobis manifeſtavit, & delineandem ex poſuit; ubi [Represents the posterior surface of the spinal artery around the spinal marrow, which faces the processes of the vertebrae and shows its divisions and ramifications, in so far as it presented itself to us and exposed itself for drawing]
>
> A.A.A. Corpus medullæ ſpinalis [The body of the spinal medulla]
> B.B Arteria ſpinalis [spinal artery]
> C.C.C. Eius rami, laterales, aut ex mente Dn. Willis lateralia principia. [Its lateral branches, or, according to Mr. Willis, its lateral beginnings]
> D. Vertebrales arteriæ. [Vertebral arteries]
> B [E]. Bifurcatio arteriæ dictae, ubi alia annotatur cum axillaribus unio quam in figurâ additâ Dni. Willis [the bifurcation of the said artery, where the other (bifurcation) is designated together with the axillary arteries in the same way as in the added figure of Mr. Willis]
> F.F Spinalis medullæ principium intra cranium. [The beginning of the spinal medulla within the skull]

[87] See: [Vincent Denis] Mr Droüin, *Description du cerveau, des principales distributions de ses dix paires de nerfs, & des organes des sens. Avec les figures*, Paris (1691).

[88] See: Humphry Ridley, *The anatomy of the brain containing its mechanism and physiology; together with some new discoveries and corrections of ancient and modern authors upon that subject. To which is annex'd a particular account of animal functions and muscular motion*, London (1695).

[89] The details that follow are intended to be illustrative not comprehensive. The selected works are taken in the order of publication, whether or not the illustrations are copied from Willis or original to those authors but important in the context of Willis's works.

[90] See: Gerardi Blasii, *Anatome medullæ spinalis et nervorum inde provenientium*, Amsterdam (1666).

Blasius also included four plates from Willis in *Anatome animalium* (1681): Figuræ II (Pl.2, image 2)[91] and VIII (Pl.9, image 12) from *Cerebri anatome*; and Tabulæ V (Pl.23, image 42) and VI (Pl.24, image 43) from *De anima brutorum*.[92] There are no illustrations from Willis in any other of Blasius's works from this period.[93]

In 1682, Thomas Gibson (1647–1722) published a work in English on human anatomy. This was anonymous but the author is identified in 'the second edition, corrected and inlarged both in the discourse and figures'.[94] Gibson makes clear that 'its ornaments are in a great measure borrow'd, but it fears not to be unplum'd and laught at ... seeing it struts not in them as its own, but has everywhere the ingenuity to confess the true Owners'. The authorities include 'Dr. Willis *de Cerebro, de sanguinis Incalescentia sive Accensione Exercitatio Medico-Physica,* and *de primis viis, & de respirationis organis, in the first and second part of his Pharmaceutice Rationalis*'.[95] Gibson includes four plates taken from Willis's works.

Tabula II has five images from *Pharmaceutice rationalis* part 1: '*representeth the several Coats of the Stomach with their fibres*': these are Tabulæ II (Pl.28, image 47), III (Pl.29, image 48), and IV (Pl.30, images 49–51).

Tabula XIII has four images from *Pharmaceutice rationalis* part 2: '*Representeth one Lobe of the Lungs, with its Lobules, Membranous interstices,* &c'; these are Tabulæ I (rotated: Pl.33, image 58), III (Pl.35, images 60–61), and IV (Pl.36, image 62 only).

Tabula XIV has two figures, the upper from *Cerebri anatome*: 'Representeth the outer or upper superficies of the Brain taken out of the Skull; where the *Limbus* of the Brain being loosed from its coherence with other parts by Membranes, is lifted up and bent forwards, that the *Crura* of the *Medulla oblongata*, the *Fornix, Nates* and *Testes* with the *Glandula pinealis*, and other processes may be clearly seen': this is Figura III (Pl.3, image 3). The figure depicting a transverse section of the eye is from another source [William Briggs (1642–1704) *Ophthamographia, sive oculi eiusque partium descriptio anatomica* (1676)].

Tabula XV has five images, the first from *Cerebri anatome*: 'Representeth the basis of an humane Brain taken out of the Skull, with the roots of the Vessels cut off short': this is Figura I (Pl.1, image 1). The other figures are from Joseph Guichard Duvernoy [1648–1730: *Traité de l'organe de l'ouïe* [A treatise of the organ of hearing, (1683), not listed by Gibson in his introduction].

In 1685, Martin Lister (1639–1712), physician, arachnologist, and conchologist, published privately a collection of plates with descriptions on shells in which he reproduced the two

[91] Because the entirety of each engraving was not always copied, plate and image numbers are given.

[92] See: Gerardi Blasii, *Anatome animalium, terrestrium variorum, volatilium, aquatilium, serpentum, insectorum, ovorumque, structuram naturalem ex veterum, recentiorum, propriisque observationibus proponens figuris variis illustrata*, Amsterdam (1681).

[93] See: Gerardi Blasii, *Medicina universa*, Amsterdam (1665); Gerardi Blasii, *Anatome contracta in gratiam discipulorum conscripta, & editia*, Amsterdam (1666): Gerardi Blasii, *Miscellanea anatomica hominis*, Amsterdam (1673): Gerardi Blasii *Observata anatomica*, Lyon (1674): and Gerardi Blasii *Observationes medicæ rariores*, Amsterdam (1677).

[94] See: Thomas Gibson, *The anatomy of human bodies epitomized wherein all parts of man's body, with their actions and uses, are succinctly described, according to the newest doctrine of the most accurate and learned modern anatomists*, London (1684). Gibson's work proved popular and was issued eight times between 1682 and 1721.

[95] Gibson also draws upon Richard Lower's *Tractatus de corde*, London (1669); John Mayow's *Tractatus quinque; medico-physici, &c.*, Oxford (1674); Walter Needham's *disquisitio anatomica de formato fœtu*, London (1667); William Croone's *De ratione motus musculorum*, London (1664); and Nicolas Steno's *de Glandulis Oris, & novis earundem vasis observationes anatomicæ*, Copenhagen (1661) and *De musculis & glandulis observationum specimen*, Copenhagen (1664).

figures from *De anima brutorum* (Tabula II: Pl.20, images 34–35) depicting the oyster. These are reengraved with the legends reordered but faithfully transcribed. The two plates were re-used in a second publication, retaining the original numbering and identical other than the addition of *Tab. 5* and *Tab. 6* to the engravings from Willis, in the sequence of nine leaf size or folding illustrations to the work.[96]

Also in 1685 appeared the most extensive contemporary reproduction of text and illustrations from the works of Thomas Willis, by Daniel Le Clerc (1652–1728) and Jean-Jacques Manget (1652–1742).[97] It is a magnificent work. The purpose of *Bibliotheca anatomica* (1685) was to reprint attributed selections from the most important treatises relating to anatomy published since the mid-sixteenth century. The two volumes are organized topographically. There is a spectacular engraved title page showing a human dissection with several figures surrounding the anatomical table, similar in design to that in the Amsterdam edition of *Cerebri anatome* (1666: F.2a1) but more elaborate and allegorical. The book has six entries for Thomas Willis and a large number of illustrations from his treatises. These are reengraved and regrouped using templates taken from Jean-Antoine Huguetan:[98]

Tomus primus: *Primarum viarum descriptio*; pages 101–10. The text corresponds to *Pharmaceutice rationalis*, part 1, section I, caput II, page 6, paragraph 2 through to the end of the chapter at page 32. Tabula I, figures IV–VII; and Tabula II, figures I–VIII correspond to Pl.27 (image 46), Pl.28 (image 47), Pl.30 (images 49–50); Pl.29 (image 48), Pl.30 (image 51), Pl.31 (image 52) and Pl.32 (images 53–57). The legends are fully transcribed.

Tomus secundus: *De respirationis organis et usu dissertatio*: pages 134–47 (but paginated as 172–81, 144–7). The text corresponds to *Pharmaceutice rationalis*, part 2, section I, caput I, page 2, paragraph 2 through to the end of that chapter at page 33. One figure within this sequence of text, at page 175, is from Frederik Ruysch (1638–1731). Tabula XLII (the first five figures are from Malpighi), figures VI–IX; Tabula XLIII, figures I–VI; and Tabula XLIV, figures 1–15 correspond to Pl.34 (image 59) and Pl.35 (images 60–61), reversed; Pl.33 (image 58), rotated; Pl.36 (images 62–64) and Pl.37 (images 65–67), reversed; Pl.38 (images 68–75) and Pl.39 (images 76–79), reversed; and Pl.40 (images 80–82), reorientated. The legends are fully transcribed.

De cerebro tractatus: pages 241–94. The text corresponds to the entirety of *Cerebri anatome*, starting at page 1, paragraph 1 through to the end of Caput XX. Tabula XLVII, figures I–II; Tabula XLVIII, figures I–II; Tabula XLIX, figures I–II; and Tabula XL, figures I–VI correspond to Pl.1 (image 1); Pl.2 (image 2); Pl.3 (image 3); Pl.4 (image 4);

[96] See: Martini Lister, *Historiæ sive synopsos methodicæ conchyliorum quorum omnium pictura, ad vivum delinatæ, exhibutur*, volume I, London (1685): plates 195 and 196; and Martini Lister, *Conchyliorum bivalvium utrisque aquæ exercitatio anatomica tertia, huic accessit medicinalis de calculo humano*, Symptibus authoris impressa, London (1696). See also Henry Oldenburg's letter to Lorenzo Magalotti (1637–1712) of 13 June 1672, extolling the virtue of these plates: Royal Society Library. MS. O 2, no. 87; and *The correspondence of Henry Oldenburg*, volume IX (1672–1673). Eds. A. Rupert Hall and Marie Boas Hall, Madison (1973): pages 106–8.

[97] See: Daniel Le Clerc and Jean-Jacques Manget, *Bibliotheca anatomica sive recens in anatomia inventorum. thesaurus locupletissimus, in quo integra atque absolutissima totius corporis humani descriptio euisdémque oeconomia è præstantissimorum quorúmque anatomicorum tractatibus singularibus, tum hactenus in lucem editis, tum etiam ineditis, concinnata exhibetur. Adiecta est partum omnium administratio anatomica, cum variis earundem præparationibus curiosissimis. Digesserunt, tractatus suppleverunt argumenta, notulas, & observationes anatomico-practitas addiderunt. Daniel Le Clerc & I. Iacobus Mangetus, M.M. D.D. cum indicibus necessariis, figurísque* æneis, 2 volumes, Genevæ (1685). Volume I has 37 plates with other figures printed within the text. Volume 2 has the remaining plates, 38–85 with one extra inserted between LXVI and LXVII.

[98] See: chapter 12, *Opera medica & physica* Lyons (1676: **8A**).

Pl.5 (image 5); Pl.6 (image 6); Pl.7 (unnumbered 1: images 7–10); Pl.8 (image 11); and Pl.9 (image 12). The legends are fully transcribed. The editors include an extensive footnote on pages 248–9, marked at 'de *Cerebro* * in *glandulam pituitariam* ...' which relates to '*... *Diemerbrœckius Corporis humani Anatomes lib* 3 *p. n.* 530. 531'. There is a further footnote on page 285, column 2, marked at 'de quibus postea, cum * νευρολ ογίαν integram institutemus ...' which reads '**Illa videbitur suo loco scilicet in quarta huius Bibliothecæ parte*' [This will be seen in its (proper) place, that is, in the fourth part of this Bibliotheca];[99] and others at pages 247, 289, 290, and 293.

Exercitatio medico-physica. De motu musculari: pages 552–63. The text is fully reproduced. Tabula LXVI, figures I–IV correspond to Pl.17 (images 26–27) and Pl.18 (images 28–29). The legends are fully transcribed.

Nervorum descriptio et usus: pages 598–632. The text is fully reproduced but the chapters are renumbered I–IX in Le Clerc and Manget whereas they are sequential with *Cerebri anatome*, i.e. XXI–XXIX in the original edition. Pl.10 (images 13–14) is printed within the text at page 604. Tabulæ LXVII; LXVIII; LXIX, figures I and II; and LXX, figures I–V correspond to Pl.11 (image 15); Pl.12 (image 16); Pl.13 (image 17); Pl.14 (image 18); and Pl.15 (images 19–23). The legends are fully transcribed. There is an extensive footnote on pages 610–11 marked at 'cum vero his * fibræ pro motu locali requisitæ defunt ...', which relates to the work of Malpighi.[100]

Arteriæ descriptio anatomica: pages 633–4. The text starts at page 279, paragraph 2 through to page 283, paragraph 3 omitting the final eleven lines of the chapter. There are no illustrations.

The second reproduction of text by Manget is the section on 'Stupiditas' in his monumental *Bibliotheca medico-practica* (1695–1698). This corresponds to *De anima brutorum*, page 504, caput XIII, paragraph 1 through to the end of the chapter at page 516. It is signed '*Thom. Willis. De morbis ad animum corpoream*'. There are no illustrations.

Changes were made when Le Clerc and Manget published a second edition of *Bibliotheca anatomica* (1699) with much new material added.[101] There are now 120 numbered plates with five extras: two are inserted between LXXIV and LXXV; one between LXXV and LXXVI, and one between LXXVIII and LXXIX. At least one of these is from Ridley (1695: and marked 'see pages 406 and 407') but placed in a section of text relating to Theodor Kerckring (1638–1693). The fifth is attributed to Clopton Havers (1657–1702), or possibly Henrici Eysonii (nd), and inserted between LXXXV and LXXXVI, marked 'see page 482'. There are no changes to the entries for Thomas Willis or the illustrations to his works from 1685 other than altered indicators on the engravings for page placements corresponding to:

Tomus prima: Primarum viarum descriptio: pages 100–9; De respirationis organis et usu dissertatio: pages 970–[9]82.

99 These comments correspond to *Cerebri anatome* (1664): pages 39 and 229, respectively. See chapter 18 for further mention of Isbrand van Diemerbroeck (1609–1674).

100 This corresponds to *Nervorum descriptio et usus* (1664): page 333.

101 See: Jo. Jac. Manget, *Bibliotheca medico-practica sive rerum medicarum thesaurus cumulatissimus quo omnes prorsus humani corporis morbosæ affectiones tum artem medicam in genere, tum chirurgicam in specie, spectantes ordine alphabetico explicantur. Et per curationes, consilia, observationes, ac cadaverum anatomicas inspectiones, tam hinc inde proprias, quàm à variis, iisque præstantissimis authoribus, veteribus & recentioribus, petitas, abundè, imò & curiosè, tractantur*, two volumes, Genevæ (1699).

Tomus secundus: De cerebro tractatus: pages 3–56: Exercitatio medico-physica. De motu musculorum: pages 543–53; Nervorum descriptio et usus: pages 586–620:[102] and Arteriæ descriptio anatomica: pages 666–7.

Later, Le Clerc and Manget's compendium of anatomical texts was translated into English.[103] Willis's importance is much reduced. The translator does not reproduce blocks of text, as before, but contributions of the various authors are rewritten into his own narrative. Presented in the first person, '*The Learned Willis's* Exercitatio Medico Physica *concerning the Motion of the Muscles*' page 251–65 corresponds (roughly) to *Of musculary motion* (1681), page 34, paragraph 1 to page 46, paragraph 1, omitting the remaining nine paragraphs. Neither '*A general description of the membranes, nerves, fibres, veins and arteries: taken from* St Hilaire, Le Clerk, Glisson, Willis, Vieussens, Diemerbroeck, &c.' pages 393–404; nor '*Of the diseases of the* head *and their cures, from* Michaelis, Willis, St Hilaire, Cole, &c.' pages 660–674, contain original text. However Tabulæ VI, figure III; and IX, figures II, IV, and V, at page 652 are taken from Willis. These correspond to *Pharmaceutice rationalis* part 2, Pl.37 (image 67, the left half only); and *Cerebri anatome* Pl.15, figures 1, 2 (with part of figure 4 added) and 3 (images 19–22).

The most comprehensive borrowing of plates from Willis, disconnected from the accompanying text, is found in the appendix forming a third section of James Drake's (1667–1707) *Anthropologia nova*.[104] Issued with the 1707 and 1717 editions but omitted in 1727 (and a later issue, 1750), the appendix was published separately in 1728. Drake's use of images depended on plagiarism by Steven Blankaart (or Blancard: 1650–1702).[105] These works can conveniently be considered together, by reference to Drake. Although his preface to the main work sets out Drake's methods and many of his sources, there is no mention of Willis.[106]

> I had ... engag'd to the *Booksellers* who print this, to draw up a short System upon the Figures of *Blancard*, which they, without my Advice had purchas'd, in expectation of having that done by the late Ingenious Dr. *Havers*, (according to a Contract they had made with him) which now is fall'n to my Share; which Figures were procur'd at his Instance,

[102] These leaves are mispaginated in some copies as: 578–612.

[103] Daniel Le Clerc, *Bibliotheca anatomica, medica, chirurgica, &c. Containing a description of the several parts of the body: each done by some one or more eminent physician or chirurgeon; with their diseases and cures. Wherein are not only all the tracts of use that are in the second edition of the bibliotheca anatomica, lately publish'd by Daniel Clericus and Jacob Mangetus, in two volumes in folio, but an addition also of near double the number of other curious tracts, which were either omitted in the said bibliotheca, or have been publish'd since, some of them translated, others faithfully abridg'd; very few of which were ever before in English. Illustrated with several added figures, done by the best artists, and from the truest designs; as will appear from the name to each figure*, London (1711–1714).

[104] See: James Drake, *Anthropologia nova: or a new system of anatomy. Describing the animal oeconomy and a short rationale of many distempers incident to human bodies. In which are inserted divers anatomical discoveries, and medicinal observations, with the history of the parts. Illustrated with above four score figures drawn after the life. And to every chapter a syllabus of the parts describ'd, for the instruction of young anatomists*, two volumes, London (1707); with *The appendix to Dr. Drake's Anthropologia nova; or new system of anatomy. With fifty-one copper plates*, London (1728).

[105] See: Steph. Blancardi, *Anatomia reformata, sive concinna corporis humani. Dissectio, ad neotericorum mentem adornata, plurimisque tabulis chalcographicis illustrata. Accedit eiusdem authoris de Balsamatione, nova methodus, nemine antehac hoc modo descripta*, Lugduni Batavorum (1688). See: KF Russell, *British anatomy 1525–1800. A bibliography*, Melbourne (1963): pages 102–3 for details of the fifty-one plates forming the appendix which are taken from Blankaart with the original copper plates reused and page placements originally engraved outside the single-lined border at the top right partially erased: 'Drake explains why he uses these plates in the preface to his book. His printer purchased the plates for use in a book by Clopton Havers who died before the text was written'. Plates in Drake's 1728 issue of the appendix are faithfully reengraved but with differences of detail and there is no mention of the original source in the preface to the second edition.

[106] Blankaart does mention in his own preface: '*Bartholinus* uterque, *Willis, Malpighus, Graaf, Harvæus, Louwerus, Steno, Wharton, Needham, Glissonius, Ruisch, Vernay, Kerkingius, Bodloo, Leeuwenhoek* &c', although as Drake points out, these sources are not given in the individual legends.

> and make the Appendix to this work ... The Figures in the *Appendix* (annex'd to the first Volume) were of the first Edition of Dr. *Stephen Blancard*'s *Anatomia Reformata*, and are Borrow'd from other Books of *Anatomy*; from which, and Autopsy, the Explications here annex'd are written; and not from that Collector's Account of them; which is full of Gross Mistakes, tho he did no more than Transcribe the Explications of their Original Authors.

However, unlike Blankaart, in his appendix Drake does attribute images to the authors from whose works they are taken.[107] He draws, in part, on each of Willis's books that contain illustrations. In the text that follows, it may be confusing that Drake and Willis each refer to Tabs. and Figs. Drake uses Roman notations in his narratives (i.e. IV) and Arabic on the engraved plates (i.e. 4). This anomaly is maintained but the reference to illustrations reproduced by Drake in the appendix to *Anthropologia nova* and their source in the works of Willis should be clear.

Drake, Tab III (opposite page 5), Figures IV and V are from *Pharmaceutice rationalis* part 2. Figure 4 (unlabelled) is crudely adapted from Tabula VI (Pl.38, images 68–75); Figure 5 is Plate VII, Figure 4 (Pl.39, image 79).

Drake Tab IV (opposite page 7), Figures I, II, and III are from *Cerebri anatome*. Figure 1 is unnumbered plate 1, Fig IIII (Pl.7, image 10); Figure 3 is Fig I (rotated) from the same plate (Pl.7, image 7); Figure 2 is from Tab XIII, Fig 2 (Pl.15, image 20).

Drake Tab VIII (opposite page 11), Figures IV, V, VI, and VIII are from *Pharmaceutice rationalis* part 2. Figures 4, 5, and 6 are imperfectly copied from Tab IV figures 1, 2, and 3 (Pl.36, images 62–64); Figure 8 is plate VIII, Figure 1 (Pl.40, image 80); and Figure 9 (not attributed by Drake) is Figure 2 from the same plate (Pl.40, image 81).

Drake Tab IX (opposite page 12), Figures I and II are from *Pharmaceutice rationalis* part 2. Figure 1 (rotated) is Tab 1 (Pl.33, image 58); Figure 2 depicts both juxtaposed parts of the image at Tab II (Pl.34, image 59).

Drake Tab X (opposite page 14), Figures I and III are from *Pharmaceutice rationalis* part 2. These are Tabula III, Figures 1 and 2 (Pl.35, images 60–61).

Drake Tab XI (opposite page 15), Figure 2 is from *Cerebri anatome*. It is Figura I (Pl.1, image 1).

Drake Tab XII (opposite page 16), Figures I and II are from *Cerebri anatome*. Figure 1 is Figura III (Pl.3, image 3); and Figure 2 is Figura V (Pl.5, image 5).

Drake Tab XIII (opposite page 18), Figure 1 is from *De anima brutorum*. It is Tab V (Pl.23, image 42).[108]

Drake Tab XIV (opposite page 20), Figures I and II are from *De anima brutorum*. Figure 1 is Tab VI (Pl.24, image 43); and Figure 2 is Tab VIII (Pl.25, image 44).

Drake Tab XV (opposite page 21), Figures II, IV, V, and VI are from *Cerebri anatome*. Figure 2 is Tabula XII (Pl.14, image 18); Figure 4 is Tabula XIII Fig 1 (Pl.15, image 19); and Figures 5 and 6 are from unnumbered 2, Figures 1 and 2 (Pl.10, images 13–14).

Drake Tab XVI (opposite page 24), Figures I and II are from *Cerebri anatome* and Figure III is from *Pharmaceutice rationalis* part 2. Figure 1 is an adaptation of Tabula IX (Pl.11, image 15) and Tab XI (Pl.13, image 17); Figure 2 is Tabula XIII, Figure 3 (Pl.15, image 21); and Figure 3 is Tabula V, Figure 2 (Pl.37, image 66). As Drake explains: 'From

[107] This differs from Drake's two main volumes: volume II, Tab XV at page 276 showing the base of the brain and vascular supply of the upper cord is from Ridley (1695), Figure I, but unattributed; and Tabula XVI is Ridley's Figures VI and VII, also unattributed. Ridley is not mentioned in Drake's preface.

[108] As noted elsewhere, the dissection and its representation are almost the same as *Cerebri anatome* Figura VII (**Pl.8**, image 11) but subtly different in some details.

Dr Willis, but very ill copy'd wherefore the Original Figure is here referr'd to; see the Doctor's ninth and eleventh Tables of his Anatomy of the Brain.'

Drake Tab XXVI (opposite page 53), Figures I, II, and IV are from *Pharmaceutice rationalis* part 1. Figure 1 is Tab 1 (Pl.27, image 46, but elaborated to show the duodenum attached to the pylorus); Figure 2 is Tab V (Pl.31, image 52); and Figure 4 is based upon Tabula IV, Figures 1, 2, and 3 (Pl.30, images 49–51). As Drake explains: 'This is patch'd together from Dr Willis, but so very ill composed, that no Explication can afford and tolerable idea of what it pretends to represent, wherefore it shall be passed by.'

Drake Tab XXVII (opposite page 54), Figures I and II are crudely adapted from *Pharmaceutice rationalis* part 1. They are based on the five components of Tab VI (Pl.32, images 53–57) but markedly different from the originals.

Drake Tab XXXVIII (opposite page 73), Figures III, IV, V, and VI are from *De motu musculari*. These are Figuræ 1 and II (Pl.17, images 26–27); and Figura III and IV (Pl.18, images 28–29).

Much superior to French texts incorporating the work of other anatomists, including Willis, is that of Petro Tarin (*c.*1725–*c.*1761). As with Le Clerc and Manget's *Bibliotheca anatomica*, this little-known work is important in gathering examples of images relating to the brain from the most significant anatomists working up to the end of the seventeenth century.[109] The three parts are: 'De genuinâ cavitatum cerebri cerebelli descriptione'; 'De cavitatum cerebri & cerebelli variorum iconum relatione'; and 'De variis, autorum, cavitatum cerebri & cerebelli descriptionibus'. The eighteen plates comprise fifteen separate configurations: three—Tabulæ I, II, and III—are reproduced both in black and white and in colour 'imprimé par Richomme l'Aine'. This is Jacques-Nicolas Richomme (1724–1783), whose firm flourished between 1750 and 1818. The plates combine 14 (apparently) original engravings and 106 copied from other works, accompanied by detailed legends explaining the anatomical features and with commentaries on the original contributions. The images (in colour and black and white) in Tabula I (figures 1–6), Tabula II (figures 1–6) and Tabula III (figures 1 and 2) appear to be original to Tarin. Four of Willis's plates from *Cerebri anatome* are reproduced. The rest come from many different sources:[110]

Tabula X, Figure 1 is from Ridley. Figures 2 and 3 are from Bartholin. Figures 4 and 5 are from Willis (*Cerebri anatome*: Pl.8, image 11; and Pl.9, image 12). Tarin refers to

[109] See: Petro Tarin, *Adversaria anatomica, de omnibus corporis humani partium, tum descriptionibus, cum picturis*, Paris (1750).

[110] Although not cited by Tarin, most of the books from which the images are taken can be identified. Some but not all are already cited and omitted from this footnote. Tabula IV reproduces thirteen images from Magnus Hundt (1449–1515: Tarin's figures 1 and 4), Berengario da Carpa (*c.*1460–1530: figures 2 and 3), Johann Dryander (1500–1560: figures 5, 6, and 7), Charles Estienne (1504–1564: figures 8, 9, 10, and 11) and Vesalius (figures 12 and 13). Table V has thirteen images taken from Vesalius (1543: figures 1–12) and Eustachius (figure 13). Tabula VI has nine images from Eustachius (figures 1–3), Costanzo Varolio (1543–1575: figures 4 and 5) and Giovanni Battista Cortesi (1554–1636: figures 6–9). Tabula VIII (misnumbered VII) has nine images all from Giulio Casserii (*c.*1561–1616) in the commentary by Daniel Bucretius (i.e. Daniel Rindfleisch: 1562–1621). Tabula VIII has nine images taken from the same work (figures 1–3), another by Casserius (figure 4) and Vesling (figures 5–9). Tabula IX has nine images from Vesling (figures 1 and 3), Highmore (figures 2 and 4) and Steno (figures 5, listed as 4, and 6–9). Tabula XI has three images from Govert Bidloo (1649–1713: figure 1, somewhat plagiarized by William Cowper, 1666–1709), Hubero (not identified: figure 2) and Eustachius (figure 3). Tabula XIII has eight images taken from Lorenz Heister (1683–1758: figures 1 and 2), René-Jacques Croissant de Garengeot (1688–1759: figure 3), Carl August von A Bergen (1704–1759: figure 4, labelled 3), Joseph Lieutaud (1703–1780: figure 5, labelled 7, and 6 and 7) and Johann Georg Duvernoy (1691–1759: figure 8). Tabula XIV has six images taken from Ridley (figure 1) and Jean Baptiste Bonhomme (nd: figures 2–6). Tabula XV has nine images taken from Morandi Morando (1693–1756: figures 1 and 2) and Bonhommio (nd: figures 3–9).

Willis is his notes for this legend alongside Vesling and Bartholin. Figures 6–8 are from Verheyeno (i.e. Philip Verheyen: 1648–1711).[111]

Tabula XII, Figures 1 and 2, are from *Cerebri anatome*: Figura III: Pl.3, image 3; and IV: Pl.4, image 4. Figures 3–10 are from Vieussens but the legend for Figure 8 is omitted.

Finally, it is worth mentioning a detail in William Hogarth's (1697–1764) reworking of an unpublished satirical engraving, 'Enthusiasm Delineated', as 'Credulity, Superstition and Fanaticism' (1762). The iconography is a hectic mix of religious and secular scenes that does not flatter either the preacher in his pulpit nor the members of his congregation engaged in various unsavoury activities. In the foreground is Mary Toft (1701–1763) who pretended to have given birth to rabbits, a hoax that evidently took in some of the doctors who attended her. Down the right hand side are two scales that measure the levels of credulity, superstition, and fanaticism of the congregation. The depiction of ghosts on the capital of the lower meter was probably inspired by the infamous hoax of the Cock Lane Ghost in 1762. Below the image, an inscription on a separate plate reads under the title: 'Believe not every Spirit, but try the Spirits whether they are of God: because many false Prophets are gone out into the World'.[112] Standing on copies of John Wesley's (1703–1791) sermons and John Glanvill's (1636–1680) book on witchcraft is the religious thermometer that measures emotional states from a central reading of lukewarm. Upward movement indicates the heat of love towards lust, ecstasy, madness, and raving; downward movement represents the coolness of low spirits to sorrow, agony, settled grief, despair, madness, and suicide. At the base of the instrument is a depiction of the base of the brain with an auricle stuck onto the temporo-parietal cortex. It is crude and might have been taken from various sources but some structures are apparent including certain vessels and cranial nerves, which are reminiscent of Willis and Wren's much famed and often reproduced depiction (Pl.1).

[111] See: Philippo Verheyen, *Corporis humani anatomia in qua omnia tam veterum, quam recentiorum anatomicorum inventa. Methodo novâ, & intellectu facillimâ describuntur, ac tabulis æneis repræsentantur*, Lovani [Leuven] (1676).

[112] See: 'The first epistle general of John', chapter IV, verse 6.

4

'The mystery and school house of nature'

Bibliography and the works of Thomas Willis

There is no readily available bibliography of the printed works of Thomas Willis. In August 1962, HJR (John) Wing wrote '*A bibliography of Dr. Thomas Willis (1621–1675)*' submitted in part requirement for the University of London Diploma in Librarianship.[1] This was never published but three manuscript copies exist: one in the possession of Mr HJR Wing; the second sold by him at auction in 2009 and in the author's collection; and the third held by the University of London Library from where it can be borrowed. Over the years, Mr Wing has generously made available his copy to those writing on Thomas Willis, some of whom prepared brief short title lists of the main editions and issues of the books. As part of the tercentenary edition, *The anatomy of the brain and nerves*, William Feindel (1918–2014) produced an introductory volume that included as Part V, 'A bibliographic survey of *Cerebri anatome*' by Harold Denham (1917–1999).[2] This leans heavily on HJR Wing's list but has some differences (see: Figure 91). Philip Oldfield, former rare books librarian at the University of Toronto, has written 'A bibliography of Thomas Willis's *De anima brutorum*' (typescript, *c.*1991) but this was never published. Mr Oldfield has been generous in making available copies of his bibliography which has many scholarly footnotes and is additionally valuable for having a copy-by-copy comparison of the variant settings of twenty-five examples of the ordinary Oxford quarto 1672 issue (**5A2**), ten others of the large paper issue (**5A1**), and differences in the cancelled title page on three copies of the 'third' London quarto issue (1672: **5A4**) which otherwise uses the original sheets of the ordinary Oxford issue. He also compared between one and twenty-seven copies of each of the subsequent issues and editions of *De anima brutorum* (**5B–5C**).

Many libraries and individual collectors list copies of the printed works of Thomas Willis. No attempt has been made to document their holdings in this bibliography. Presumably Willis kept copies of some or all of the books published in his lifetime but, if so, their fate is unknown and no example of a book with his ownership inscription has

[1] In a letter dated 5 March 2010, John Wing wrote that once he became aware that a bibliography was required for part 2 of the diploma in librarianship, he asked for advice from his former employer, WG Hiscock (nd), deputy librarian at Christ Church, who suggested Thomas Willis. Not until Wing visited the Wellcome Library did he discover that Harold Denham was working on the same subject. In the preface, John F Fulton, *A bibliography of two Oxford physiologists. Richard Lower 1631–1691, John Mayow 1643–1679*, (1935), reprinted from *The Oxford Bibliographical Society Proceedings and Papers*, volume IV, part I, Oxford (1935): pages 1–62, writes: 'I hope in the future to take up Thomas Willis, Robert Hooke, and several others who played a prominent part in Oxford during the Restoration'. But this bibliography of Willis also never materialized.

[2] See: Thomas Willis, *The anatomy of the brain and nerves*, Ed. William Feindel, Montreal (1965): pages 67–104. Harold Denham was chief cataloguer in the Wellcome Library from 1951 to 1982 and was instrumental in compiling the *Catalogue of printed books* (1962–2006). He had worked in Watford Public Library before the Second World War, for much of which he was a prisoner in Singapore, and at the Royal College of Physicians before joining the Wellcome Trust. The first volume of the Wellcome catalogue, compiled from cards and typed slips, was ready by 1962, the third with his name on the title page by 1976, and the fourth after his retirement in 1995. His plans for a bibliography of Thomas Willis for Fellowship of the Library Association were thwarted by the Association's bureaucracy but his notes were used for the 1965 tercentenary volumes. See John Symons, 'Harold Richard Denham 1917–1999', *Medical History* 1999: 43; 514.

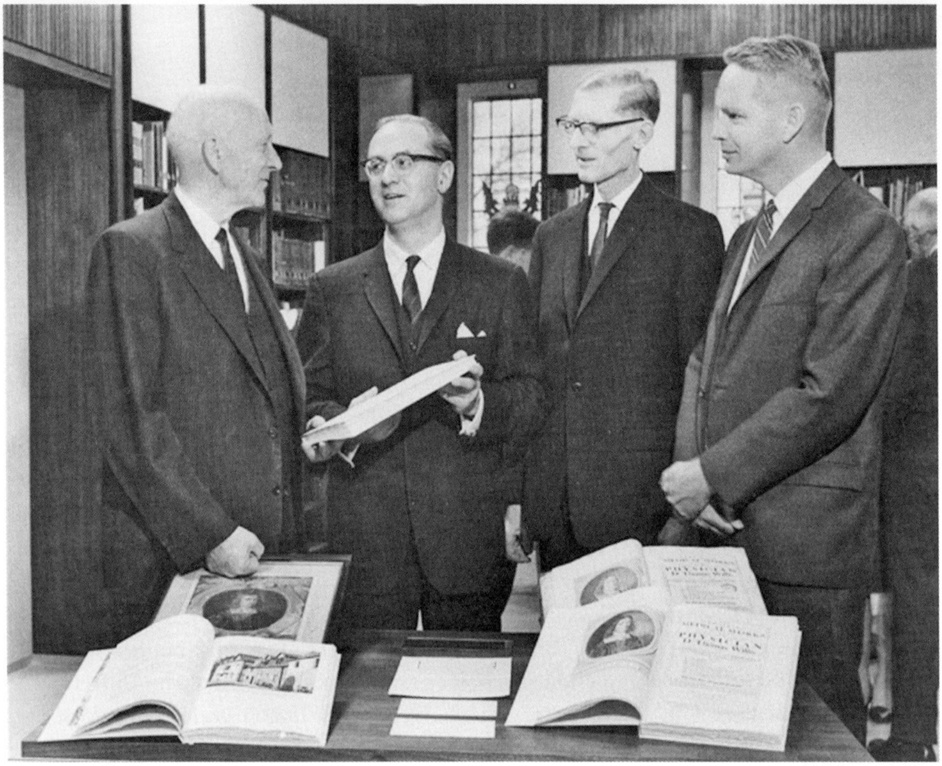

Figure 91 Wilder Penfield, William Feindel, Harold. Denham, and Robin Farr (McGill University Press) celebrating publication of the Tercentenary edition of 'Dr. Thomas Willis' "The anatomy of the brain and nerves"' in the Wellcome Camera of the Osler Library. Collection of William Feindel, originally printed in the McGill University Bulletin for November 1965–1966.

been identified. It is nevertheless instructive to get a sense of which copies were known to, and presumably read by, Willis's contemporaries. John Locke (1632–1704) had copies of: *Diatribæ duæ medico-philosophicæ* 1660 (**1B**);[3] *Cerebri anatome* 1664 (either the quarto or octavo edition: **2A** or **2B**); *Pathologiæ cerebri* 1667 (**3A**); and *Opera omnia* Amsterdam 1682 (**8E**).[4] Browne Willis (1682–1760) listed his grandfather's books in the *General dictionary* (1741).[5] Apart from some additional comments and details, this was copied from Anthony Wood (1632–1695) and retains all the existing errors:[6]

[3] Numbers refer to chapters 5–14 in this catalogue, as explained next.

[4] See: J Harrison and P Laslett, *The library of John Locke Oxford Bibliographical Society*, Oxford (1965).

[5] See: [Browne Willis], 'Willis (Thomas)'. In: [John Bernard, Thomas Birch, John Locke, and other hands] *A general dictionary, historical and critical: in which a new and accurate translation of that celebrated Mr. Bayle with the corrections and observations printed in the late edition at Paris, is included; and interspersed with several thousand lives never before published. The whole containing the history of the most illustrious persons of all ages and nations, particularly those of Great Britain and Ireland, distinguished by their rank, actions, learning and other accomplishments*, volume X, London (1741): pages 171–5; and chapter 1 for further details.

[6] See: [Anthony Wood] *Athenæ Oxoniensis. An exact history of all the writers and bishops who have had their education in the most ancient and famous University of Oxford, from the fifteenth year of King Henry the Seventh, Dom. 1500, to the end of the year 1690. Representing the birth, fortune, preferment, and death of all those authors and prelates, the great accidents of their lives, and the fate and character of their writings. To which are added, the Fasti*

Diatribæ duæ medico-philosophicæ, The Hague octavo 1659 (**1A3**); with *Dissertatio epistolica de urinis* listed separately as part of that work
Diatribæ duæ medico-philosophicæ, London duodecimo 1660 (**1B**)
Diatribæ duæ medico-philosophicæ, London duodecimo 1662 (**1C**), added in parentheses to 1817 edition
Diatribæ duæ medico-philosophicæ, London duodecimo '1665' (**1D**).[7]

Wood notes that this title was: 'Answer'd by Edm. De Meara a Doctor of Physic at Bristol, and Fellow of the College of Physicians. See more in Rich. Lower, an 1690'. The 1817 edition also draws attention in a footnote to Coxly Cosin's *Willisius malevindicatus sive Medicus Oxoniensis mendacitatis et inscitiæ detectus* (1667).[8]

Cerebri anatome, London quarto 1664 (**2A**), added as a footnote to the 1817 edition
Cerebri anatome, London octavo 1664 (**2B**)
Cerebri anatome, Amsterdam duodecimo 1667 with *De ratione motus musculorum* (**2E1**)

Wood adds here his much quoted remark: 'Whatsoever is anatomical in that Book, the Glory thereof belongs to the said Dr. Lower, whose indefatigable Industry at Oxon produced that elaborate Piece'.

Pathologiæ cerebri, Oxford quarto 1667 (**3A**)
Pathologiæ cerebri, Amsterdam duodecimo '1669' (**3B1**)[9]
Pathologiæ cerebri, London duodecimo 1668 (**3B2**)

Wood adds: 'An account of which is in the *Philosophical Transactions*, num 31'.

Affectionum quæ dicuntur hystericæ et hypochondriacæ, London quarto 1670 with *De sanguinis* and *De motu musculari* (**4A**)
Affectionum quæ dicuntur hystericæ et hypochondriacæ, Leyden duodecimo 1671 (**4B1** or **4B2**)

Referring to the *Exercitationes medico-physicæ duæ*, Wood adds: 'An account of both of them are in *Phil. Transact*. Num 57'.

De anima brutorum, London quarto 1672 (**5A4** or **5A5**)
De anima brutorum, London octavo 1672 (**5B1** or **5B2**)
De anima brutorum, Amsterdam duodecimo 1674 (**5C**)

or Annals, of the said University, for the same time, volume 1, London (1690): pages 402–3, entries 364–5; *Athenæ Oxoniensis*, volume 2, London (1721): pages 549–52, entry 408; and *Athenæ Oxoniensis*, volume 3, London, and Oxford (1817): pages 1048–53, entry 550. See chapter 1 for further details of these books.

[7] In *Athenæ Oxoniensis* (1690), Wood writes 'Lond. 1660. 65 &c.'. In the 1817 edition this is altered to: "Lond. 1660 [1662, Bodl. Crynes 213] 65, &c'. Browne Willis has this as: 'London 1660, 1665 &c'. Whatever editions each had in mind, there is no 1665 printing of *Diatribæ duæ*.
[8] See: Walter Harris (1686–1761), *The whole works of Sir James Ware concerning Ireland*: volume III, Containing, the writers of Ireland, Dublin (1739–1746): pages 169, 190 in which Ware mentions that 'Coxly Cosin M.D. wrote a defence (as it is there said) of Dr Willis'. See chapter 15 for discussion of Edmund de Meara's commentaries on Thomas Willis and responses from Richard Lower.
[9] This may refer either to Amsterdam 1668 or 1670.

Wood adds: 'And also of this [i.e. *Philosophical Transactions*], num 83. All which books, except *Affectionum quæ dicuntur*, &c. and that *De anima brutorum* were translated into English by S.P, esq; ---- Lond. 1681. Fol.'

Pharmaceutice rationalis (Part 1), Oxford quarto 1674 (**6A1**)
Pharmaceutice rationalis (Part 1), Oxford duodecimo 1674 (**6B1**), omitted by Wood (1691 and 1817) but added by Browne Willis
Pharmaceutice rationalis (Part 2), Oxford quarto 1675 (**6E**)
Pharmaceutice rationalis (Part 2), Oxford duodecimo 1674 (**6F**), omitted by Wood (1691 and 1817) but listed by Browne Willis
Pharmaceutice rationalis (Parts 1 and 2), Oxford octavo 1679 added as a footnote to the 1817 volume (**6I**)

Wood writes: 'Published by Dr Jo. Fell, who in a Postscript added to the Author's Preface, gives some running Account of the said Author, but false as to his Parent.' Wood then explains that *Pharmaceutice rationalis* was translated into English by 'Anon. Lond. 1679. fol. but being not well done it was corrected by S.P esq.'

A plain and easie method, London octavo 1690, date of publication corrected to 1691 in a footnote to the 1817 volume (**7A1**)
A plain and easie method, London octavo '1722', added in a footnote to the 1817 volume (**7B**)[10]
Opera omnia, Geneva quarto 1676 (**8B**)
Opera omnia, Amsterdam quarto 1682 (**8E**)
Pharmaceutice rationalis, London folio 1679 (**9A**)
The remaining medical works, London folio 1681 (**9B**)
The London practice of physic, London octavo 1685 (**10A1**)

Referring to *The London practice of physick*, Wood adds: 'This Translation is said to be different from that containing the same Pieces contained in his former translation of all his Works in fol.'

Neither Wood nor Browne Willis necessarily owned these books. Browne Willis's possessions were distributed after his death in 1760. Three books were acquired in 1939 for St Martin's Church, Fenny Stratford, founded by Browne Willis in memory of his grandfather. They came from Aspley House, built about 1690 for William Norcliffe (d.1717). Aspley House is 5.8 miles from Fenny Stratford and 7.3 miles from the site of Browne Willis's manor house at Water Eaton. It was in the possession of Charles Downes (d.1909), a great-great-grandson of Browne Willis's daughter Mary Hervey (née Willis). The contents were auctioned after the death of Downes's widow. The books were Lot 846. These are kept in the church.[11] One is a copy of *Two discourses concerning the soul of brutes* (1683: **9D**).[12] It is in a nineteenth-century binding and unsigned apart from some insignificant annotations. Browne Willis usually inscribed his books and the earlier provenance of this copy is unknown.

[10] The correct date is 1721.
[11] See: http://bedsarchives.bedford.gov.uk/CommunityArchives/AspleyGuise/AspleyHouse.aspx.
[12] Access to the three books was kindly made by Canon Father Victor Bullock of St Martin's Church. The two others are: Browne Willis, *A survey of cathedrals*, three volumes, London (1752); and Browne Willis, *The history and antiquities of the town, hundred, and deanry of Buckingham*, London (1755).

More direct evidence comes from the Willis Fleming Historical Trust.[13] In the nineteenth century, the library of the family seat at Stoneham Park, Hampshire, had some copies of Thomas Willis's books. It is not certain when these were all acquired. Some were definitely in the possession of Browne Willis; others are on the aforementioned list but not necessarily his copies. The items from Stoneham Park are: *Diatribæ duæ* (1660: **1B**, listed earlier); *Cerebri anatome* (1666: **2D**, not listed earlier); *Pathologæ cerebri* (1667: **3A**, listed earlier); *Affectionum quæ dicuntur hysteriæ et hypochondriacæ* (1670: **4A**, listed earlier) with a manuscript note by Browne Willis relating to two portraits at Whaddon Hall, Buckinghamshire; *De anima brutorum* (1672: **5A**, listed earlier); *Pharmaceutice rationalis* parts 1 and 2 (1674–1675: **6A** and **6E**, listed earlier) with a manuscript note by Browne Willis referring to John Fell's postscript and the copy of an epigram written by Caspar Needham (1622–1679) on hearing the news of Willis's death, dated Oxford 1674 or 1675);[14] *Opera Omnia* (1676: **8B**, listed earlier); *Opera omnia* (1682: **8E**, listed earlier); and *The remaining medical works* (1681: **9B**, listed earlier) with inscription and annotations by Browne Willis. The library was dispersed in the nineteenth century and the present whereabouts of these books are unknown.

Printing in the seventeenth century

By the time that Thomas Willis published his first book in 1659, printing with movable type had been in use in the West for approximately 200 years and without much alteration in how books were made. Economic in its architecture, aesthetically pleasing, and easy to handle, the well-constructed book had already achieved its status as one of the great engineering feats of mankind. Beyond the hands-on account by Joseph Moxon (1627–1691) of printing in the seventeenth century,[15] descriptions of how books were made in that period lean heavily on the standard works by Ronald McKerrow (1872–1940);[16] Fredson Bowers (1905–1991),[17] and Philip Gaskell (1925–2001)[18] who, from different perspectives, describe the principles of formulae and collation, and practical aspects of presswork, handling of sheets, printing, binding, and selling of books.

Publishing a book in the seventeenth century involved several trades. Frequented by scholars, the printer's workshop was a busy place providing space for cultural and intellectual activity. The printer supervised translation, copy-editing, indexing, illustration, engraving, composition, imposition, and correction. He bought ready-made type and paper which represented about 50% of the cost of producing a printed book. Binding was usually carried out elsewhere. The punchcutter carved and filed each letter or symbol in reverse on the end of a steel rod. This was driven into a block of copper which became the matrix fitted into a typecaster's mould into which a molten mixture of lead, tin and antimony was poured

[13] Details kindly provided by Harry Willis Fleming, personal communication 21 June 2020.

[14] This is unrecorded but may possibly be confused with Nathanael Williams, *A pindarique elegie on the most learned and famous physitian Dr* Willis, Oxford (1675) with a further edition, with a new title, Oxford (1676). Different copies of each part of *Pharmaceutice rationalis* (1674; 1675) in the library of St John's College, Oxford, have the inscription 'Liber Coll. S. Joan: Bapt: Oxon: Ex Dono Brown Willis Armigeri', presumably in the hand of the librarian, and may have been given to the College with other items from Browne Willis in 1738.

[15] See: Joseph Moxon, *Mechanick exercises: or, the doctrine of handy-works. Applied to the art of printing. The second volume* (1683–1684). Eds. Herbert Davis and Harry Carter, London (1958).

[16] See: Ronald B McKerrow, *An introduction to bibliography for literary students*, Oxford (1927)

[17] See: Fredson Bowers, *Principles of bibliographical description*, Princeton (1949, new edition 1986).

[18] See: Philip Gaskell, *A new introduction to bibliography*, Oxford (1972).

to produce individual characters, once more in reverse.[19] Stored according to the frequency with which each letter and symbol was used, the compositor selected items from the upper or lower case, and added spaces so that the line was justified to the right. Sometimes a word was split and hyphenated, contracted, or deliberately misspelt in order to justify the line.[20]

Paper was made from linen rags or vegetable extracts mixed with water. A wire covered wooden frame was dipped into the pulp, the paper turned out, and pressed, sized, and allowed to dry, traces of the mould being seen as chain lines. A device, the watermark, was added to indicate the place of manufacture and size of the sheet (see: Figure 92).[21] From 1670, a second 'counter-mark', usually the maker's initials, also appeared on the sheet. The folding of that sheet determined the format. A standard ream consisted of 480 identically marked sheets of which around 430 were likely to be usable. Most paper used prior to 1670 came from France. Later white paper was made in eastern England, especially Lincoln and Norwich.

Each sheet was signed at the foot of the first few leaves allowing the printer to organize material and guide the binder in ensuring that the folded leaves were gathered and sewn in the correct order.[22] Most books were produced in folio, quarto, octavo, and duodecimo and using roman type with some italic and greek letters.[23] Catchwords linking the continuity of text across page breaks served much the same purpose, but these were mainly used by the printer to ensure that the impositions were correct and text not omitted in moving around the formes (see: Figure 93). It is remarkable that more major type setting mistakes were not made. The only example detected in this bibliography is in the Amsterdam issue of *Diatribæ duæ medico-philosophicæ* (1669: **1F**) in which the compositor seems to have picked up in the manuscript at the wrong place and left an awkwardly typeset leaf.[24] Pagination provided another method of achieving accuracy in the sequence of leaves but was the least reliable of the three systems. Marginal notes and other additions might be added to help the reader

[19] See: Gaskell (1972): pages 12, 23; and 9, Fig 1a and b for depiction of the punch and features of individual letters. Some were cast as diphthong, ligatures, and tied letters (æ and œ; ct and st), the ampersand (& or &), amphora (@), or pilcrow (¶).

A set of roman alphabet consisted of around 150 typefaces, as did italic, mainly through the use of swash and non-swash italic capitals. A skilled worker could produce 4000 pieces of type per day, but there would be many imperfections and variations. In the seventeenth century most type was bought from foundries in Antwerp, Frankfurt, and Paris. The University presses in Oxford and Cambridge obtained their type from the Low Countries.

[20] For these and many other practical details, see: McKerrow (1927): pages 9, 56; and Gaskell (1972): page 45.

[21] See: Gaskell (1972): pages 57–77; and McKerrow (1927): page 172. Gaskell illustrates typical watermarks and corresponding sheet sizes at pages 68–75. In a folio edition, the watermark is central and the chain lines vertical; in quarto, the watermark is on its side and the chain lines horizontal; in octavo the watermark is vertical in the central fold with chain lines vertical; and, with some variation, duodecimo has horizontal chain lines and a watermark at the foreedge of the leaf. In the common duodecimo format the lower portion of the sheet is cut away and, folded twice, sewn into the centre of the upper section folded as 'octavo' to form 12 pages; another arrangement is to fold the intact sheet horizontally in a 'Z' shape—the top forward and the bottom backwards—and the whole then twice folded vertically, the distinction detected by different placement of the watermark and orientation of the chain lines.

[22] See: McKerrow (1927): pages 155–63. Signatures use the 23 letter Latin alphabet with I or J and U or V and omitting W. $1–2 in quarto, $1–4 in octavo, and $1–5 in duodecimo are usually signed. Each alphabetical sequence in quarto should include 92 leaves and 184 pages, and 184 leaves and 368 pages in octavo. Omission of signatures or gaps in pagination may have occurred when composition was distributed to different workers each of whom was given an estimate, which might prove inaccurate, of the number of leaves that person was required to set. This is the best explanation for the omission of sheet 'O' in all copies of *Two discourses concerning the soul of brutes* (1683: **9D**) with matching errors of pagination, since the text and catchwords are continuous across the gap.

[23] See: Cristina Dondi, 'The European printing revolution'. In: Eds. Michael F Suarez and HR Woudhuysen, *The Oxford companion to the book*, volume I, Oxford (2010): pages 53–61 for details of the relative frequency of printing in each format.

[24] See chapter 5 for details.

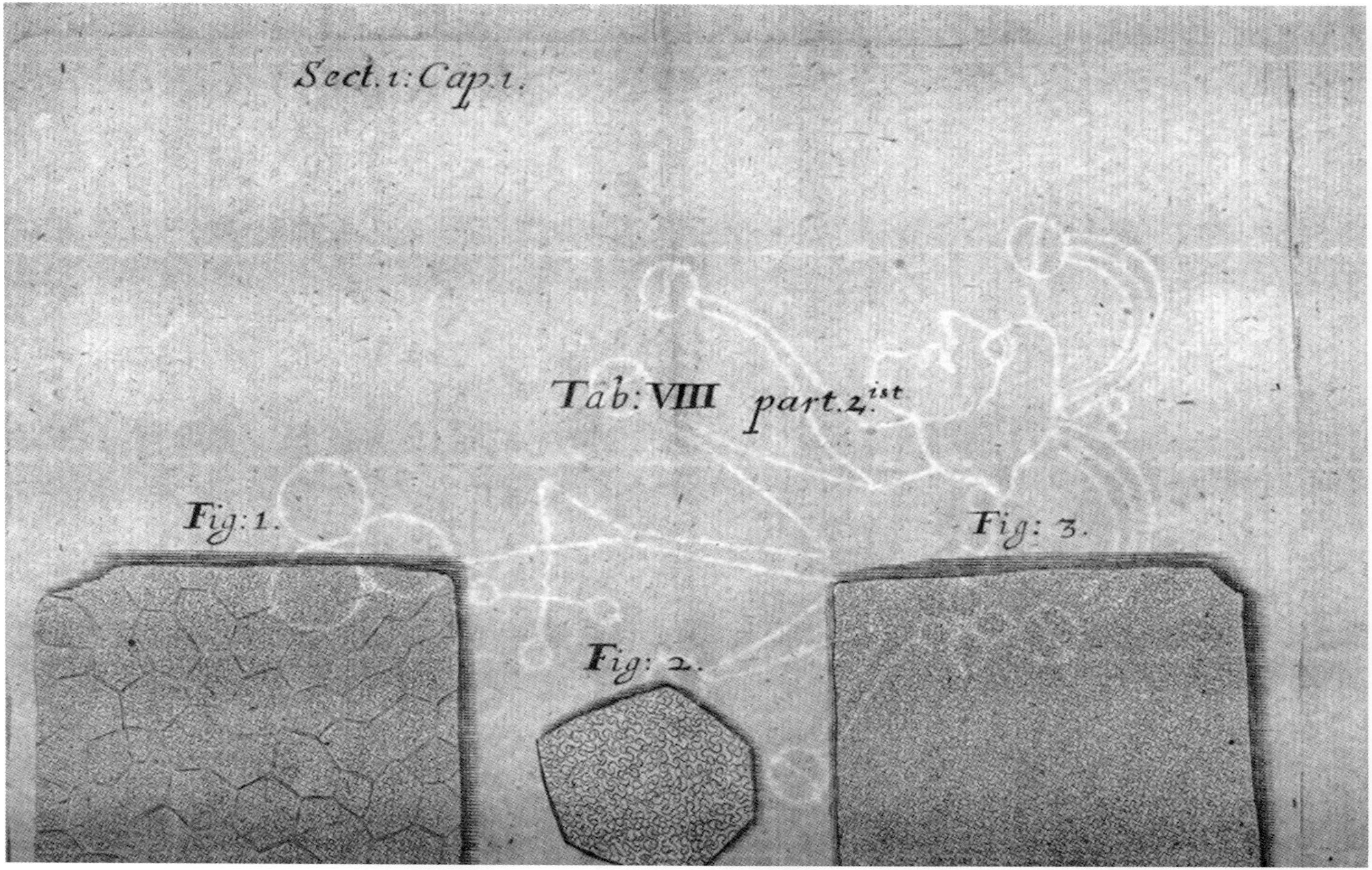

Figure 92 Chain lines and watermark showing the 'fool's cap' on the sheet used for Tabula VIII in *Pharmaceutice rationalis* part 2, London 1679.

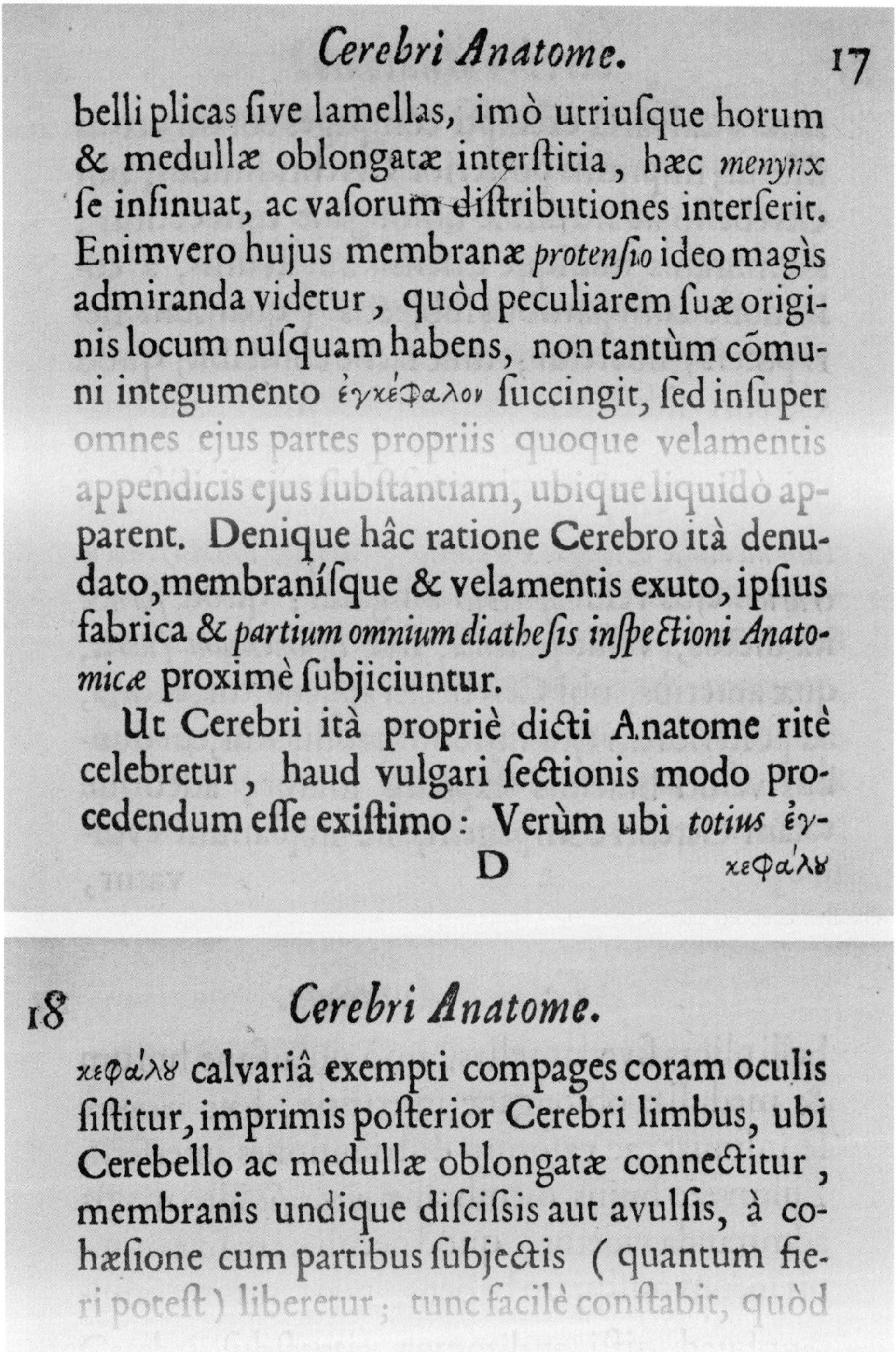

Cerebri Anatome. 17

belli plicas ſive lamellas, imò utriuſque horum & medullæ oblongatæ interſtitia, hæc *menynx* ſe inſinuat, ac vaſorum diſtributiones interſerit. Enimvero hujus membranæ *protenſio* ideo magìs admiranda videtur, quòd peculiarem ſuæ originis locum nuſquam habens, non tantùm cõmuni integumento ἐγκέφαλον ſuccingit, ſed inſuper omnes ejus partes propriis quoque velamentis appendicis ejus ſubſtantiam, ubique liquidò apparent. Denique hâc ratione Cerebro ità denudato, membraníſque & velamentis exuto, ipſius fabrica & *partium omnium diatheſis inſpectioni Anatomicæ* proximè ſubjiciuntur.

Ut Cerebri ità propriè dicti Anatome ritè celebretur, haud vulgari ſectionis modo procedendum eſſe exiſtimo: Verùm ubi *totius* ἐγ-

D κεφάλȣ

18 *Cerebri Anatome.*

κεφάλȣ calvariâ exempti compages coram oculis ſiſtitur, imprimis poſterior Cerebri limbus, ubi Cerebello ac medullæ oblongatæ connectitur, membranis undique diſciſsis aut avulſis, à cohæſione cum partibus ſubjectis (quantum fieri poteſt) liberetur; tunc facilè conſtabit, quòd

Figure 93 Leaves from *Cerebri anatome*, London 1664 showing roman, greek, and italic type; headline, signature, and catchwords.

access key passages. Errors of signatures, catchwords, and pagination are frequently present in Willis's books.[25]

The compositor worked from the author's manuscript but the printer might make edits in order to confine the text to a defined number of sheets. Punctuation remained the responsibility of the printer, not the author, and styles varied. Most compositors set type from the beginning of the main text, later adding preliminaries and title pages.[26] Therefore the roman signatures, A–Z, generally start after the preliminaries which are either signed using upper or lower case roman letters (A, B: these then being repeated at the first sheet of main text starting with A; or less ambiguously as: a, b, c) and other indicators such as *, **, π, ¶, ã, ẽ, ĩ, õ, or ũ. Since several of Thomas Willis's books include a detailed 'elenchus rerum' (contents list) and some also have an alphabetical index allowing relevant sections to be searched, the preliminaries are often extensive, requiring the use of many such symbols, especially for the *Opera omnia* printed in Lyon and Geneva (1676–1681: **8A–8D**).

Correctly organized impositions on each forme were surrounded by a 'chase', the edges filled with 'furniture' to create the margins, everything 'locked' with 'wedges' or 'quoins', and proud letters hammered down [27] Once the first side of the sheet was printed, the batch was turned over and the second forme used within two or three days, at most, to impress the reverse pages before the paper had dried and the two sides disproportionately shrunk.[28] A pin hole and the use of standard furniture helped to align the placement of type on each side of the sheet. A dry run produced a proof often using second quality paper kept for that purpose and not intended for publication, ensuring that everything was ready for the definitive impression. Seventeenth-century ink consisted of varnish made from boiled linseed or nut oil mixed with resin to stop it spreading on the wet paper, coloured with lampblack made from the smoke of burning resin and calcified to preserve the colour. Red (vermilion) ink was made from mercuric sulphide.

Stop press corrections were made during the run for a whole impression which might involve printing up to 1250 sheets in a single day. Errors tended to cluster on pages printed from a single forme. Philip Oldfield has analysed with great care the variations according to inner and outer formes in the settings of *De anima brutorum* (1672: **5A**).[29] The proof was then checked against the original manuscript although this might already have been amended in order to accommodate everything within a defined number of sheets. Taken as a whole, the process was imperfect for many understandable reasons. Although printing was a craft, the workforce of journeymen was casual and standards generally rather poor in seventeenth-century England, at least by comparison with continental Europe. No copy of the printed works of Thomas Willis is free from textual and typographical errors. Although some text was left 'standing' for reuse at a later date, in practice the printer rarely possessed enough type to set an entire book, let alone leave the entirety untouched in case another impression was needed. Formes already printed in sufficient numbers for an impression were therefore soon redistributed.[30] The evidence from the printed works of Thomas Willis

[25] The two most egregious examples in Thomas Willis's books are *De anima brutorum* (1672: **5A**) and *The London practice of physick* (1685: **10A**).

[26] See: Gaskell (1972): pages 40–3 who assesses the work-rate of skilled compositors at up to 60,000 ens (each being half a line or c30 letters) per week. Errors were common due to weariness, good and bad days, and other distractions due to broken tools, disagreements amongst the men, drunkenness, and other practical problems.

[27] See Gaskell (1972): pages 118–34 for a detailed description of the construction of fixed and moving parts, and the workings of the wooden hand-press. Depending on the format 2, 4, 8, 12, 16, 18, or 24 pages would be imposed on each forme.

[28] See: Gaskell (1972): page 132.

[29] See: Oldfield (typescript, 1991): pages 12–14.

[30] The amount varied but Gaskell (1972): page 38 points out that, late in the sixteenth century, the Cambridge University printer Thomas Thomas (1553–1588) had *c.*1400 kg of type of which 40% was worn and waiting to be

suggests that when a new edition was needed, the compositor took up an existing copy and slavishly reproduced its type setting so that many of the initial errors and quirks were reinserted, and some new ones introduced. Also apparent is that attention to detail varied between these skilled workers, or they grew tired, since errors of headlines and signatures, for example, tend to cluster.

Once all the sheets were ready (and in their various states after stop press amendments), and the preliminaries and title page printed, everything was offered for sale and that issue of the book deemed to be complete. The printer determined the print run based on assessment of how well the book might sell. He needed to cover his costs and pay wages for the amount of composition and presswork done by each employee, and maintain the work force by ensuring regular activity of the presses.[31] Syndicates were formed to share risks and this left journeymen free to move from one shop to another when business was slack. Editions were limited by the Stationers' Company to 1500 copies but this restriction was not necessarily followed. For all these reasons a print run of under 1000 made good sense for a learned or technical work.

Unbound sheets were distributed to the bookseller. The customer might buy a ready bound copy over the counter but more often ordered a bespoke binding leaving the bookseller to make the arrangements, or took a bundle of folded sections to the bindery. Buying a book therefore involved two prices, one for the sheets and another for the binding. Different copies of the same book were rarely uniform. But by the 1660s it became increasingly easy to purchase smaller format books ready bound, whereas larger volumes were still more usually sold as folded sheets. Most of Willis's books published in England first appeared in quarto format, soon followed by editions in octavo and duodecimo. A stitch piercing the folded sheets horizontally was considered cumbersome leading to sewing through the back fold with individual gatherings secured by cords placed across the spine to create the textblock. Sewing two or more folded sheets as one to form a single gather was common and necessary in order to avoid too bulky a back to the book, especially with folio printing. Once folded and sewn, gatherings were held in the desired order with threads and the outermost front and back leaves protected, either with blanks forming part of the first and last signature or temporary paper covers.[32] Later, leather was used to cover the upper and lower boards, the threads secured and endpapers added to disguise the hinged joint. Many leathers were used, the commonest being tanned calfskin, pigskin, vellum (calf or sheepskin), and goatskin (turkey or morocco). The boards were often decorated in blind-stamp or gilt using hot metal tools.

The book could not be read until bolts connecting individual leaves on the top and fore-edge had been opened with a knife, leaving rough or deckled margins which the binder

melted down, 22% was standing in pages, 22% standing in formes, and 16% ready for new use. About 50 kg type was required for the two formes used to print each sheet. When text was reset for further formes of the same book, the letters were washed with alkali, or stipped, but the furniture, quoins, and headlines might be set aside as a skeleton for reuse with newly composed text of the next forme.

[31] Gaskell (1972): pages 164–72 estimates that most investment was in type with the purchase of presses representing 5–15%, and the rest on stocks of paper, ink, and other materials. For a detailed analysis of the work and productivity of individual workshops, especially in the year 1668, see: DF McKenzie, 'Printing and publishing 1557–1700: constraints on the London book trades'. In: Eds. John Barnard and DFM McKenzie, *The Cambridge history of the book in Britain*, volume IV 1557–1695, Cambridge (2002): pages 553–67.

[32] The blank might start or complete the signature, or be within and folded out. Marbled paper covers, unusual in the seventeenth century, are occasionally found as covers of Willis's works (see, as examples, **2D2**; and part 2 of **8C1** in original printer's marbled paper covers, as issued).

sometimes trimmed. The even surface might then be gilded or decorated (see **8C1**). Partially unopened examples of Willis's books are rarely found but uncut copies with deckled edges do survive. Self-evidently, the latter tend to have slightly larger leaf sizes (see **2D2**). The availability of books was advertised through lists printed independently or as part of the press work using end material in a book already in production. Best known amongst Thomas Willis's writings is the list of books sold by Richard Davis (1618–*c.*1693) appended to the final gathering of *De anima brutorum* (1672: **5A1–5A3**), which has been the cause of much bibliographic confusion. Davis took 'over the cost and risk of marketing books which the university delegates were glad to print but lacked the organisation to distribute'.[33]

Authors of books in the seventeenth century rarely benefited from sales or commissions. Royalties were not paid to the author, who wrote for reputation, not profit. Publication often depended on a patron, duly acknowledged in the preliminary leaves in most of Willis's books whilst he earned his living as a physician. What the patron had to provide for the printer to proceed with production of the book is unclear.[34] Books sold for around 1*d* per 3 sheets until 1550 rising by around 40% thereafter but with notable exceptions. In general the total cost was around 8s–16s per copy but some of Willis's books were more expensive. The advertisement for *Dr Willis's practice of physick* (1684: **9E** and **9F**) appearing in *Concerning the soul of brutes* (1683: **9D**) and the Hilary *Term Catalogue* for 1680 and 1681 printed in February 1681, listed the price at thirty shillings.[35]

The principles of bibliography

Bibliography concerns the architecture of books as material objects. The unit is the perfected sheet as printed on a given occasion. A further run of the press might incorporate minor changes whilst leaving the imposition largely unchanged. How the available printed sheets were eventually gathered and assembled by the binder is a subsidiary matter. Bibliography describes what the printer intended, albeit with inferences made on information that is missing or ambiguous. It also acknowledges the process whereby some sheets were altered and therefore in different states before being offered for sale. Bibliographies usually provide details of a series of publications, linked by author or subject matter, sufficient to bring an ideal copy of each item to mind. This descriptive information may then serve as the basis for subsequent textual analysis. Within the general structure, some variation of method is allowable. No one system suits all tastes. Bibliography is based on discrete categories: impression, state, issue, and edition. The experts do not always agree on their boundaries.

Sheets printed in one batch comprise an impression of that book. Reuse of formes containing unaltered type in order to make available further copies at a later date constitutes a new impression. It may not always be easy to distinguish one impression from another and, as explained next, for some experts the interval between passing sheets through the press may be such as to constitute a new issue. However the economics of printing made retention

[33] See: John Barnard and Maureen Bell, 'The English provinces'. In: Barnard and McKenzie (2002): page 671.

[34] A degree of organization occurred in England when the trades of text-writer, limner, or illuminator, binder, bookseller, and printer were regulated through a guild (dating from 1403) that eventually became the Stationers' Company. It exerted influence and distributed resources, had privileges, and arbitrated disputes in the various trades concerned with production and selling of written material. The company received its Royal Charter, endorsing its monopoly on printing and effectively confining activities to London, in 1557.

[35] See: Edward Arber, *The Term Catalogues, 1668–1709 A.D. A contemporary bibliography of English literature in the reigns of Charles II, William and Mary, and Anne*, catalogue IV number 2, London (1903–1906): page I 431.

of standing type impractical in the seventeenth century and new impressions do not affect the bibliography of Thomas Willis.

Stop press alterations were made when an error was detected, the type loosened, an individual letter slipped, or as a result of some other mechanical accident. Depending on the details, these changes represent new states of individual leaves. Therefore it is difficult to make decisions about state based on examination of a single copy.

An issue is the entirety of copies intended to be sold in one batch produced from one or more impressions that retains existing typesetting but may include altered states. Variations made outside that period constitute a new issue. Bowers' position on this is pragmatic and not strictly mechanical.[36] The definition of issue is therefore more an administrative matter than typographical arrangement. Unlike state, issue refers to the whole book not its individual parts. Alterations might be required leading to a new issue because an existing printer had lost interest or died, new material had come to light, the rights had been transferred, or time had passed so that a new date was required. Alterations to textual details and headlines, pagination, and ornaments may be found. A new issue can also reasonably be described for large paper copies containing extra decorative or dedicatory content, or when preliminary leaves are changed.[37] For practical purposes, the bibliographer is usually alerted to a new issue by a change to the title page.[38] Particular difficulties arise with respect to illustrations since these are produced independently of the printed text. Bowers considers that decisions on state and issue based on differences in plates should be applied to the book as a whole, even if the printed text is unaltered.[39]

Allowing for minor alterations, as mentioned, an edition is all the copies of a book printed from the same setting of type. Any substantial resetting of type, even in the same format, amounts to a new edition.[40] In a collected work, each individual part should be considered as existing issues which happen to have been brought together if the original typesetting, signatures, and independent title pages are preserved. Any other alterations are likely to constitute a new edition, as does the inclusion of a collective title page for works originally printed in several parts.

The ideal copy is that which is considered most faithful to the original intentions of the author and printer with respect to the text and contents. It is not necessarily the first (or the last) printing and may have cancelled leaves or alterations. Where variations exist, much forensic work may be needed to identify the ideal copy. A blank interrupting continuous text is likely to have been intended for cancellation but preserved without that amendment. A blank between

[36] Bowers (1986) in particular accommodates variations within state which other experts would consider a new issue. See pages 79, 80, and 103 for discussion of 'separate' and 'reissues', and his acceptance that others may classify these as new editions.

[37] The large paper copy, more luxurious and sometimes with extra embellishments, is not necessarily the first printed. Press work generally settled down during the impression making it convenient to print the more luxurious large copy version later.

[38] McKerrow (1927): page 176, and Bowers (1986): page 78 differ in their emphasis on the title page. Bowers argues that a change of date (perhaps to enlarge the impression and add to sales, and occasionally to correct an error or typographical irregularity) or to the name(s) of the printer(s) and bookseller(s), are variations of state and not a new issue. The same applies to the addition of extra leaves (errata, advertisements, dedications, and other material in the preliminaries, and secondary titles without cancellation of the first), all geared towards producing the ideal copy.

[39] See: Bowers (1986): page 77.

[40] The edition is considered new even if resetting incorporates some standing type held back in anticipation of reuse at a later date. More generally, it is unfortunate for the amateur that different experts vary in their position on just how much alteration and reimposition of formes is tolerated within a single issue, albeit with leaves in different states. The situation is not helped by the fact that publishers may claim 'new edition' for printings that bibliographers would classify as 'issues' or 'states'.

sections of a collected work is more likely to belong in the ideal copy but may have been excised in some copies by the binder. The same applies particularly to first or last blank leaves. Alterations to headlines, pagination, and catchwords do not necessarily discard one state in favour of the next in determining the ideal copy. Nor are aberrations of ordering the preliminaries reasons for choosing an example closest to the ideal copy, since these may merely reflect the binder's handling of the sheets irrespective of what the printer intended.[41]

Most of these bibliographical problems arise with respect to the printed works of Thomas Willis. To anticipate a few examples: there are large paper copies which incorporate the coat of arms of Gilbert Sheldon as an extra head piece (*De anima brutorum* 1672: **5A1**); correction of typographical errors on title pages (*Cerebri anatome* 1664: **2C2.c1** and **2C2.c2**); the same text published with different preliminaries (*Cerebri anatome* duodecimo, 1664: **2C1** and **2C2**) or title pages (**8B1, 8B2,** and **8B3**); headers and pagination corrected and new errors introduced (*The London practice of physick* 1685–1692: different copies of **10A1**, **10A2**, and **10A3**); plates included that have different states (*Cerebri anatome* 1664: **2B1** and **2B2**); title pages cancelled listing different printers and publishers (*Pharmaceutice rationalis* 1679: **9A1** and **9A2**; *The remaining medical works* 1681: **9B1** and **9B2**); extra leaves added to otherwise complete signatures (*Cerebri anatome* 1664: **2A** and **2B**); cancelled pages printed and either or both the cancellandum and cancellans bound in (*De anima brutorum* 1672: **5A**; *Pathologiæ cerebri* 1667: **3A**; *Opera omnia* 1708: **8H.c3**); and leaves or sheets that were intended by the printer routinely omitted before sale (*A Plain and easie method* 1691: **7A2**). An example of the binder guided by the order of erroneous signatures rather than flow of the text, is provided by the 1667 Amsterdam printing of *De ratione motus musculorum*, published as part of *Cerebri anatome* (**2E1**). B3 is missigned B4, and vice versa. They are bound as 'B3' followed by 'B4'. This creates confusion with the pagination which, after B2v, page 28, runs: 31–2, 29–30, 33–4 with corresponding discontinuity of catchwords and text. Everything would have been restored for the reader by simply binding 'B4' before 'B3'. With the benefit of hindsight, it is clear that many of Thomas Willis's books never achieved their ideal status. Modern bibliography seeks to move away from the concept of the ideal copy and emphasise information available from binding, annotation, and provenance as indicators of the subsequent use of a particular copy.

A system of bibliography for the printed works of Thomas Willis

This bibliographical catalogue describes 103 copies of books, considered as ten separate publications but carrying fifteen different titles, containing various combinations of the fourteen treatises of Thomas Willis printed in Latin, English, or Dutch across the period of interest

[41] Selecting the ideal copy and deciding on its authenticity may be problematic. Bowers (1986) and Gaskell (1972) suggest clues that help distinguish copies that are as first printed, reprinted, incomplete, or made-up. Errors of signature and pagination may or may not be corrected for a new impression of an existing text. A complete change in signatures clearly indicate a new setting of the text. Early editions may end in the middle of a sheet whereas reprints are adjusted so as to avoid this awkwardness by varying page size and spacing. Pages may be missing and that copy improved by insertion of leaves from the same or another edition. Conversely, it is possible that these leaves were never intended to be present and making-up spuriously creates a non-existent edition. Apart from chain lines and watermarks, the continuity of damp-staining and other blemishes is a useful guide. Feathered in patches may be especially deceptive. Most cancellation consists of single leaves. This may be detected by a stub of the original leaf, an incorrect signature, text that does not align with neighbouring pages, the wrong number of text lines or chain lines, and a watermark that differs from the rest of the book.

(1659–1721).[42] Other copies that differ from those described are certain to be exist. The entries in this bibliography are:

- *Diatribæ duæ medico-philosophicæ* (1659–1687: treatises 1–3), sixteen entries
- *Cerebri anatome* (1664–1683: treatises 4–5), thirteen entries
- *Pathologiæ cerebri* (1667–1678: treatises 6–7), seven entries
- *Affectionum quæ dicuntur hystericæ et hypochondriacæ* (1670–1678: treatises 8–10), four entries
- *De anima brutorum.* (1672–1674: treatise 11), ten entries
- *Pharmaceutice rationalis* (1674–1679: treatises 12–13), twelve entries
- *A plain and easie method* (1691–1721: treatise 14), five entries
- *Opera omnia* or *Opera medica et physica* (1676–1720: treatises 1–13, variously including William Croone's treatise *De ratione motus musculorum*, and with treatise 14 in one edition), fifteen entries
- *Pharmaceutice rationalis* (1679: treatises 12–13, 7), three entries
- *The remaining medical works* (1681: treatises 1–6, 9–10), three entries
- *Dr Willis's practice of physick* (1681: treatises 1–7, 9–10, 12–13), one entry
- *Two discourses concerning the soul of brutes* (1683: treatise 11), one entry
- *Dr Willis's practice of physick* (1684: treatises 1–7, 9–13), three entries
- *The London practice of physick* (1685–1695: extracts from treatises 2, 6–7, 11–13), nine entries
- *Dr Willis's receipts for the cure of all distempers* (1701: not specified but also extracted from treatises 2, 6–7, 11–13), one entry.

The system adopted for bibliographic description is based upon principles advocated by experts, especially Bowers (1986), in terms of categories of information that are included and level of detail but is nonetheless slightly idiosyncratic.

[1]. *Classification.* The short title, format, place, and year of publication are given for each entry numbered by order of publication for each main work within ten categories. The two parts of *Pharmaceutice rationalis* (1674 and 1675) are combined in one section, as are all of the English translations (1679–1684) as another, separate from the two extracts in English (1685–1701). Entries are classified alphabetically by year of printing within each category and further subclassified, where appropriate, for each new issue or state of a particular copy. For example, **2C1.c2** is the second title, the third edition, its first issue, but a second copy with one or more leaves in a different state.

[2a]. *Title page.* A quasi-facsimile transcription of the title page is given. Borders are described, as is underlining of the text. Line breaks are indicated by |. Roman, italic, and Old English type are preserved. Spelling, use of upper and lower case, punctuation and hyphens are as printed, including VV for W, V for U, j for i, and roman ſ for s and italic *ſ* for *s* in lower case. Ligatures and diphthongs (æ / Æ and œ / Œ; ct; st) and accents are as printed. Differences in type size are not described. Mottoes are transcribed and, where

[42] These numbers may seem awkward but are based on analysis of the publication history and contents of each publication or 'book'. The two parts of *De anima brutorum* are treated as one book and one title since they always appear as a single publication. *Pharmaceutice rationalis* was originally published in two parts, but here considered as one book and one title. The same collective title was used for the English translation which is treated as an independent book with a single title combining the two parts. *Opera omnia* or *Opera medica et physica*, are considered as one title and book. *Dr Willis's practice of physick* is considered as one book containing three components each with its own title. Extracts from the treatises included in *The London practice of physick* and *Dr Willis's receipts* are considered as one book but two titles.

necessary, given as translations in []. Titles are condensed only when these are identical to a preceding entry.

[2b]. *Subsidiary subtitle*(s). These are treated as for the main title.

[3]. *Collation*. The format is indicated.[43] Signatures are specified within the 23-letter Latin alphabet (specifying I / J and U / V) with an indication of which leaves are signed, listing errors and anomalies for that particular book. Title pages, half titles, imprimatur leaves and statements of dedication are unsigned; and the number of leaves signed is usually less on half than whole sheets in the same book. These normal variations, which usually relate to preliminaries and endpages, are not listed.[44] Recto and verso (r and v) are used to describe individual pages. Text printed in two columns is specified as 1 and 2 to indicate left and right. Completion of each 23 letter sequence is indicated, ie A–Z^4, a–z^4 rather than straddling more than one alphabetical sequence, i.e. A–z^4. Signatures with letters that repeat are printed as such: A, Aa, Aaa. Identical signatures within a single section are indicated by superscript: A, ^{2}A, ^{3}A. Separate sections that repeat the same signature are indicated: A, 2A, 3A, etc. but only at the start of each subheading. π is used to denote extra unsigned preliminaries. χ is used to indicate extra leaves inserted after the first signed text leaf, usually A1. The placement of these leaves within a given signature is indicated. Any identified cancelled leaves are indicated: e.g. C^4 (C2.3 cancelled). The total number of leaves including blanks is given. Pagination is specified as: unnumbered preliminaries [], followed by text as printed indicating breaks or errors of sequence. A final unnumbered blank verso is indicated as: 1–295 [296]. Endpages not forming part of the text are numbered as []. A summary of the correct number of pages is given allowing for errors in sequence and reconciled with the format. Individual errors of pagination not affecting the overall sequence are identified.

[4]. *Type*. The usual number of lines on a full page without paragraph breaks, excluding headlines and direction lines is given.[45] The height of twenty lines and the width of one typical line, with and without marginal notes, are given in millimetres. Specification of the type is not given, nor are details of the paper, chain lines, and watermarks described.[46]

[5]. *Contents*. All significant headings of preliminary and text leaves are transcribed with lettering and punctuation as printed in roman, italic, or Old English type retaining VV for W, V for U, j for i, roman f for s, and italic *ſ* for *s* but without line breaks. Signature and page limits for these entries are given. Decisions on binding in a particular copy may appear to make page numbers out of sequence with signatures. References to erroneous signatures are indicated, i.e. [Aa4]r. Page numbers are as printed, i.e. '234'. Printing errors and variations affecting the main text are not described although even a superficial reading shows many in every copy examined.

[6]. *Headlines*. These are not faithfully reproduced since they often alter page by page or between chapters but variations within a particular sequence that reflect type setting rather than the mechanics of printing are noted.[47]

[43] See: Gaskell (1972) pages 84–7 for a guide to assessing format using dimensions, chain lines, watermarks, and number of leaves in each gathering; and Figures 46–63, pages 88–105, for the organization of pages on the outer and inner formes.

[44] In the Dutch translations, signatures are above, and in others below, footnotes. Press figures, placed at the foot of a page and identifying one pressman's work, do not feature regularly in seventeenth century books: any that may be present are not noted.

[45] This does occasionally vary within sections of a single copy.

[46] See: Gaskell (1972): table 1 page 15 and table 2 page 16 for classification of typefaces; and pages 17–39 for description and illustration of various typefaces in use during the seventeenth and later centuries.

[47] The headline is all the material printed across the top of the page, including the pagination; and the direction line at the foot of the page includes the signature, catchword, and any other running instructions. Occasionally it

[7]. *Catchwords.* Where a catchword is called for but omitted or incorrect, the error is identified. Errors in the separate catchwords for the text and footnote in Dutch translations with running footnotes are noted. Partial abbreviations are not noted. The majority of errors relate not to the catchword but setting of the word on the consecutive page, it being easier for the typesetter to see from the manuscript what comes next as he reaches the foot of a page but sometimes forgetting when he moves, perhaps after an interval, to the other forme and has to refer back. There is also a tendency for errors to cluster indicating more or less diligence amongst individuals in typesetting catchwords.[48] There is much variation in the use of catchwords across blank pages, on selected preliminary leaves particularly dedications, and where a catchword might straddle 'FINIS' onto the first page of an index. The lists of errors reflect the style adopted for a particular book and therefore may appear inconsistent across entries.

Both for headlines and running instructions, no mention is made where a letter has not fully imprinted, tilted, or slipped; nor are occasional extra marks at the edge of individual characters.

[8]. *Frontispiece and engraved title pages.* These are numbered, e.g. F.1a1, with text and lettering transcribed retaining VV for W, V for U, j for i, roman f for s, and italic *ſ* for *s* but without line breaks. The engraver is identified if shown or otherwise known. Sheet, plate, and figure sizes are given as height × width in millimetres.

[9]. *Portraits.* These are numbered, e.g. Pt.1a1, with text and lettering transcribed retaining VV for W, V for U, j for i, roman f for s, and italic *ſ* for *s*. The engraver is identified if shown or otherwise known. Sheet, plate, and figure sizes are given as height × width in millimetres.

The absence of engraved frontispieces, portrait, printers' ornaments, decorated initials, and illustrations is noted for books that do not call for one or other of these features.

[10]. *Printers' ornaments.* Printers' devices, head, and tailpieces and fleurons are listed for each publisher in numerical order of appearance, with their classification, e.g. {**Roycroft 1**}, and locations by signature and page number, for each title in sequence through to completion of that printer's publications of Willis's works. The plural is used even when one individual is identified on the title page on the basis that many others were actively involved in printing the book. Earlier use of the same ornament or cross-referencing to another printer already listed are noted. These ornaments are separately listed and described in chapter 3.

[11]. *Decorated initials.* Each decorated capital letter is listed separately from the ornaments using the same descriptive method.

[12]. *Engraved plates.* Plates are numbered, Pl.1 (image 1)—Pl.40 (images 80–82), to indicate the order of appearance of the forty anatomical plates and the order in sequence of the separate images that appear on each (sometimes ≤ eight): a–g refer to reengravings of the original illustration; 1, 2, and 3 refer to further minor alterations of state, usually indicating revised page placements. For example Pl.4b2 is Figura IIII (image 4) from *Cerebri anatome* (1666: **2D**) with the figure reengraved and alteration to the page placement from the earlier use of that plate (1664: **2C**). 'Folding' describes sheets that unfold and may be smaller or larger than 'leaf size'. 'Cropped' usually indicates peculiarities of a particular copy although some sheets, such as Pl.5, lack the upper margin of the cranium in most copies examined,

is not easy to decide on the intended setting: for example where the chapter changes on a printed page, some headlines refer to the preceding chapter, some to the new chapter, and some to both.

[48] Headings and signatures are part of the skeleton forme, page numbers, and signature letters being changed during imposition and therefore accounting for their many errors, whereas catchwords would be set with the text.

perhaps reflecting a defect on the engraved plate. Sizes of the figures, plate and sheet are given with height × width in millimetres. Reference is made to an earlier entry when an original engraving has been reused, but since this is a copy-specific bibliography the individual sheet sizes are given.[49] The title of the illustration is transcribed as printed in roman or italic: e.g. Figura, *Tabula*, Fig., *Tab.*, etc. The figure legends in Latin or English at first appearance are as printed but not repeated for each issue and edition. Placement by the binder with respect to signatures and pagination is noted. This is not repeated with minor variation in the ordering of a group of plates, or their insertion before or after the relevant text page or printed legend. However, marked inconsistencies between the printed page placement and location of the bound leaf are identified when these suggest confusion between author, printer, and binder that informs the bibliography of that entry.

[13]. *Copy*. Location of the preferred copy (and accession or shelf number where relevant) is given with details of any apparent defects.[50] DASC (#1 of 3) indicates that the author has used his copy and that this is one of three in the collection. The numbers assigned by HJR Wing, Harold Denham, and Philip Oldfield (where appropriate) are given but other bibliographic entries are not listed.[51] Although not described in detail, the binding and its lettering, repairs or current state, endpapers, and dimensions of the leaves, height × width in millimetres, and boards excluding curvature of the spine, height × width (to the hinge, resulting in the stated width of the binding sometimes being less than that of the leaves) × depth in millimetres, are given. Ownership inscriptions ('undeciphered' where illegible and 'unidentified' when not traced) and bookplates are noted but no attempt has been made to transcribe the many and varied annotations relating to the texts. Shelf marks are transcribed since these may help experts in tracing further the provenance of individual copies.

Short title listing of the printed works of Thomas Willis

Book 1. 1659 containing treatises: 1. *De fermentatione*; 2. *De febribus*; and 3. *De urinis*

- **1A1.c1.** *Diatribæ duæ medico-philosophicæ* London octavo 1659
- **1A1.c2.** *Diatribæ duæ medico-philosophicæ* London octavo 1659
- **1A2.** *De motu naturali inorganico* [*Diatribæ duæ medico-philosophicæ*] London octavo 1659
- **1A3.** *Diatribæ duæ medico-philosophicæ* The Hague octavo 1659
- **1B.** *Diatribæ duæ medico-philosophicæ* London duodecimo 1660
- **1C.** *Diatribæ duæ medico-philosophicæ* London duodecimo 1662
- **1D1.** *Diatribæ duæ medico-philosophicæ* The Hague duodecimo 1662
- **1D2.** *Diatribæ duæ medico-philosophicæ* London duodecimo 1662
- **1E.** *Diatribæ duæ medico-philosophicæ* Amsterdam duodecimo 1663
- **1F.** *Diatribæ duæ medico-philosophicæ* Amsterdam duodecimo 1669
- **1G.** [*Diatribæ duæ medico-philosophicæ*] *De urinis* Trajecti ad Rhenum octavo 1670

[49] Images printed from the same plate may differ in size due to variation in paper shrinkage during drying which is estimated to allow differences of ≤ 3 millimetres.

[50] With almost no exceptions, the copy is one chosen because it has the fewest obvious defects.

[51] Readers may be irritated not to find the English Short Title Catalogue entry number. This is easily located but the many qualifications needed to align some entries and explain apparent discrepancies were considered unhelpful.

- 1H. [*Diatribæ duæ medico-philosophicæ*: *De fermentatione*] *Nieuwe en Geneeskundige verhandeling vande fermentatie ofte rising* Middelburg and Amsterdam octavo 1676
- 1I. *Diatribæ duæ medico-philosophicæ* London duodecimo 1677
- 1J. [*Diatribæ duæ medico-philosophicæ*: *De febribus, De urinis*] *Nieuwe Verhandeling van de koorsen* Amsterdam octavo 1681
- 1K1. [*Diatribæ duæ medico-philosophicæ*: *De urinis*] *Dissertation sur les urines* Paris duodecimo 1683
- 1K2. [*Diatribæ duæ medico-philosophicæ*: *De urinis*] *Dissertation sur les urines* Paris duodecimo 1687

Book 2. 1664 containing treatises: 4. *Cerebri anatome*; and 5. *Nervorum descriptio et usus*

- 2A. *Cerebri anatome* London quarto 1664
- 2B1. *Cerebri anatome* London octavo 1664
- 2B2. *Cerebri anatome* London octavo 1664
- 2C1.c1. *Cerebri anatome* Amsterdam duodecimo 1664
- 2C1.c2. *Cerebri anatome* Amsterdam duodecimo 1664
- 2C2.c1. *Cerebri anatome* Amsterdam duodecimo 1664
- 2C2.c2. *Cerebri anatome* Amsterdam duodecimo 1664
- 2D1. *Cerebri anatome* Amsterdam octavo 1666
- 2D2. *Cerebri anatome* Amsterdam octavo 1666
- 2E1. *Cerebri anatome* Amsterdam duodecimo 1667
- 2E2. *Cerebri anatome* Amsterdam duodecimo 1676
- 2F. *Cerebri anatome* Amsterdam duodecimo 1683
- 2G. [*De ratione motus musculorum*] Amsterdam octavo 1667

Book 3. 1667 containing treatises: 6. *De morbis convulsivis*; and 7. *De scorbuto*

- 3A. *Pathologiæ cerebri* Oxford and London quarto 1667
- 3B1. *Pathologiæ cerebri* Amsterdam duodecimo 1668
- 3B2. *Pathologiæ cerebri* London duodecimo 1668
- 3B3.c1. *Pathologiæ cerebri* Amsterdam duodecimo 1670
- 3B3.c2. *Pathologiæ cerebri* Amsterdam duodecimo 1670
- 3C. *Pathologiæ cerebri* [Scurvey] Middelburg octavo 1676 (same as 1H)
- 3D. *Pathologiæ cerebri* London duodecimo 1678

Book 4. 1670 containing treatises: 8. *Affectionum quæ dicuntur hystericæ et hypochondriacæ*; 9. *De sanguinis accensione*; and 10. *De motu musculari*

- 4A. *Affectionum quæ dicuntur hystericæ et hypochondriacæ* London quarto 1670
- 4B1. *Affectionum quæ dicuntur hystericæ et hypochondriacæ* Leyden duodecimo 1671
- 4B2. *Affectionum quæ dicuntur hystericæ et hypochondriacæ* Leyden duodecimo 1671
- 4C. *Affectionum quæ dicuntur hystericæ et hypochondriacæ* London duodecimo 1678

Book 5. 1672 containing treatise: 11. *De anima brutorum*

- 5A1. *De anima brutorum* Oxford quarto 1672
- 5A2. *De anima brutorum* Oxford quarto 1672

- **5A3.** *De anima brutorum* Oxford quarto 1672
- **5A4.** *De anima brutorum* London quarto 1672
- **5A5.** *De anima brutorum* London quarto 1672
- **5B1.** *De anima brutorum* London octavo 1672
- **5B2.c1** *De anima brutorum* London octavo 1672
- **5B2.c2.** *De anima brutorum* London octavo 1672
- **5B3.** *De anima brutorum* Amsterdam octavo 1672
- **5C.** *De anima brutorum* Amsterdam duodecimo 1674

Book 6a. 1674 containing treatise: 12. *Pharmaceutice rationalis* (part 1); with
Book 6b. 1675 containing treatise: 13. *Pharmaceutice rationalis* (part 2)

- **6A1.** *Pharmaceutice rationalis* (Part 1) Oxford quarto 1674
- **6A2.** *Pharmaceutice rationalis* (Part 1) Oxford and London quarto 1674
- **6B1.** *Pharmaceutice rationalis* (Part 1) Oxford duodecimo 1674
- **6B2.** *Pharmaceutice rationalis* (Part 1) Oxford and London duodecimo 1674
- **6C.** *Pharmaceutice rationalis* (Part 1) The Hague duodecimo 1674
- **6D.** *Pharmaceutice rationalis* (Part 1) The Hague duodecimo 1675
- **6E.** *Pharmaceutice rationalis* (Part 2) Oxford quarto 1675
- **6F.** *Pharmaceutice rationalis* (Part 2) Oxford duodecimo 1675
- **6G.** *Pharmaceutice rationalis* (Part 2) The Hague duodecimo 1677
- **6H.** [*Pharmaceutice rationalis* (Part 1)] *D'algemeene en bysondere wercking der genees-middelen in s'menschen lichaam* Middelburg and Amsterdam octavo 1677
- **6I.** *Pharmaceutice rationalis* (Parts 1 and 2) Oxford octavo 1679
- **6J.** [*Pharmaceutice rationalis* (Part 2)] *Vervolg of tweede deel der redenkundige verhandeling van de kragt en werking der genees-middelen* Amsterdam octavo 1681

Book 7. 1691 containing treatise: 14. *A plain and easie method for preserving those that are well from the infection of the plague.*

- **7A1.** *A plain and easie method* London octavo 1691
- **7A2.** *A plain and easie method* London octavo 1691
- **7A3.** *A plain and easie method* London octavo 1691 [1692]
- **7A4.** *A plain and easie method* London octavo 1695
- **7B.** *A plain and easie method* London octavo 1721

Book 8. 1676 *Opera omnia* or *Opera medica et physica* containing treatises: 1–13 (14)[52]

- **8A.c1** *Opera medica & physica* Lyons quarto 1676
- **8A.c2** *Opera medica & physica* Lyons quarto 1676
- **8B1.** *Opera omnia* Geneva quarto 1676
- **8B2.** *Opera omnia* Coloniæ Allobrogum quarto 1676
- **8B3.** *Opera omnia* Coloniæ Allobrogum quarto 1676
- **8C1.** *Opera omnia* Geneva quarto 1680
- **8C2.** *Opera omnia* Coloniæ Allobrogum quarto 1680

[52] The Latin translation of *A plain and easie method* is only present in **8G**, with a title-page dated 1694.

- **8D.** *Opera omnia* Lyons quarto 1681
- **8E.** *Opera omnia* Amsterdam quarto 1682
- **8F.** *Opera omnia* Coloniæ folio 1694
- **8G.** *Opera omnia* Coloniæ Allobrogum quarto 1695
- **8H.c1.** *Opera omnia* Venice folio 1708
- **8H.c2.** *Opera omnia* Venice folio 1708
- **8H.c3.** *Opera omnia* Venice folio 1708
- **8I.** *Opera omnia* Venice folio 1720

Book 9. English translations: containing treatises 12–13, 7 (**9A**); 1–6, 9–10 (**9B**); 1–7, 9–10, 12–13 (**9C**); 11 (**9D**); 1–7, 9–13 (**9E, 9F**)

- **9A1.** *Pharmaceutice rationalis* London folio 1679
- **9A2.c1.** *Pharmaceutice rationalis* London folio 1679
- **9A2.c2.** *Pharmaceutice rationalis* London folio 1679
- **9B1.c1.** *The remaining medical works* London folio 1681
- **9B1.c2.** *The remaining medical works* London folio 1681
- **9B2.** *The remaining medical works* London folio 1681
- **9C.** *Dr Willis's practice of physick* London folio 1681
- **9D.** *Two discourses concerning the soul of brutes* London folio 1683
- **9E.c1.** *Dr Willis's practice of physick* London folio 1684
- **9E.c2.** *Dr Willis's practice of physick* London folio 1684
- **9F.** *Dr Willis's practice of physick* London folio 1684

Book 10. Extractions in English from treatises: 2, 6, 7, 11–13 (**10A, 10B**)

- **10A1.c1.** *The London practice of physick* London octavo 1685
- **10A1.c2.** *The London practice of physick* London octavo 1685
- **10A1.c3.** *The London practice of physick* London octavo 1685
- **10A2.c1.** *The London practice of physick* London octavo 1689
- **10A2.c2.** *The London practice of physick* London octavo 1689
- **10A2.c3.** *The London practice of physick* London octavo 1689
- **10A3.c1.** *The London practice of physick* London octavo 1692
- **10A3.c2.** *The London practice of physick* London octavo 1692
- **10A4.** *The London practice of physick* London octavo 1695
- **10B.** *Dr Willis's receipts for the cure of all distempers* London duodecimo 1701.

5

'Those first forgotten particles'

Diatribæ duæ medico-philosophicæ (1659–1687)

Diatribæ duæ medico-philosophicæ (1659), in fact containing three treatises (*De fermentatione, De febribus,* and *De urinis*), was published when Thomas Willis was aged 38. Unusually for works printed in his lifetime, the first issues were in octavo, not quarto, format (**1A1–1A3**). Willis turned to a printer and booksellers based in London for the publication of his first book. Furthermore, in the year of publication, sheets were available in the Netherlands under the imprint of Adriaan Vlacq (1600–1667) who was already well known in London and Oxford (**1A3**).[1] Thereafter duodecimo editions appeared in London, The Hague, and Amsterdam (1660–1677: **1B–1F** and **1I**). Together with the work on scurvy (first published in 1667: **3A**) these three treatises were translated into Dutch between 1676 and 1681 (**1H** and **1J**). As with his Dutch translations of *Pharmaceutice rationalis* (parts 1 and 2: **6H**, **6J**), Dr (Antonius) de Heide (1646–*c*.1702) added a large number of footnotes as commentary on Willis's works.[2] *De urinis* was also published from Utrecht, in Latin, as part of a collected work on urines by various authors (**1G**). Unlike any other of Willis's writings, this treatise was also translated into French (1683, 1687; **1K1**, **1K2**).

The 1659 octavo edition

De fermentatione was completed by June 1656. Samuel Hartlib (1600–1662) noted that Willis 'hath written a treatise De Fermentatione'; and Robert Wood (1622–1685) wrote to Hartlib suggesting that:[3]

> If the Booke you write of de Fermentatione be Mr Willis his of Oxford, I am confident it is an excellent peece, having formerely seen some sheets of his upon ye subject, when we met a Club, at Oxford.

There are three issues of the 1659 octavo edition, with one (at least) having leaves in more than one state. There is an additional sheet signed H* containing preliminary material for *De febribus* which may initially have been overlooked, or not available, when the manuscript was first typeset. Sheet Z has an added bifolium and therefore comprises 10 leaves. These

[1] See chapter 2 for details of Vlacq's time as a bookseller in England from 1632 to 1642.

[2] It is clear that work is needed on the content and significance of these footnotes by an authority on Dutch medicine in the seventeenth century.

[3] See: Robert Frank, 'Thomas Willis and his circle: brain and mind in seventeenth-century medicine'. In: Ed. GS Rousseau, *The languages of psyche*, Berkeley (1990): page 116, footnote 33.

features are common to all three issues. Where they differ is in the text of the title pages. The variations of state arise from the signing of sheet H*.

Priority remains a matter of speculation. A case can be made for the copy in the Bodleian Library (**1A1.c1**), which was bought by John Aubrey (1626–1697) from James Allestry (d.1670) in 1658 for 3s 6d. This has the inscription 'T. Willis A^{e}de Chr^{ti}' in red pencil and with other annotations in Aubrey's hand on the endpapers and within the text.[4] John Fulton (1899–1960) states that this is the first issue and a very rare book (he owned a copy bought at Christie's on 15 June 1925).[5]

There are several bibliographical points relating to sheet H*. The text of *De fermentatione* (but with the incorrect headline *De febribus*) ends at H1r, page 97, with H1v, page [98] blank. There is no catchword to H2r, page 1, which starts the text of *De Febribus*. The preface to *De febribus*, the Elenchus rerum, and the Errata are printed on the extra sheet, signed H*, bound between H1v, page [98], and H2r, page 1. Bibliographic description would be relatively straightforward were it not for two other anomalies. The first leaf of sheet H* is signed H2*; and although the flow of text and catchwords for the preface, elenchus rerum, and errata leaf are all in sequence and correct, H* is inconsistently signed. Assuming that the John Aubrey copy has priority, signatures on the eight leaves follow the sequence: H2*, H3*, H4*, 5 unsigned leaves.[6]

An alternative interpretation is that the copy at St John's College Library, which has the same signatures for sheet H* but a different title page, has priority (**1A2**). *De motu naturali inorganico* is the heading of the first chapter of 'De fermentatione' and it could be argued that this was taken as the initial collective title before the more general suggestion of *Diatribæ duæ medico-philosophicæ* was adopted (see: Figure 94). Self-evidently, neither description is strictly correct since the 'Diatribæ duæ [two discourses]', are followed, '*His acceſſit* [after comes]', by the treatise 'Of urines'. The note in the Bodleian Library catalogue referring to this holding at St John's College describes *De motu naturali inorganico* as a 'reissue with the title page reset'. Whenever it was first issued, this is also an extremely rare book.[7]

Different states for the signing of some leaves of sheet H* are found in a second Bodleian Library copy inscribed by Richard Frewin (1681–1761) in 1703 whilst he was a student at Christ Church (**1A1.c2**). This was subsequently acquired for the Radcliffe Library with the rest of Frewin's books. H* follows the sequence H2*, H3* signed H2*, H4*, H5* signed H4*, 4 unsigned leaves. Little is gained by speculating which states of sheet H* came first off the press, although it could be argued that incorrect signing of H3* and H5* indicates an earlier state than found in the Aubrey copy (**1A1.c1**) and Dutch issue of *Diatribæ duæ* (**1A3**) in which the signatures on these two pages are in sequence. Presumably both states of sheet H* were in the print shop and randomly allocated to different copies.

[4] See: John Aubrey, *Brief lives with an apparatus for the lives of our English mathematical writers*, volume 2. Ed. Kate Bennett, Oxford (2015): page 1478.

[5] See: John Fulton, *A Bibliography of two Oxford physiologists: Richard Lower 1631–1691, John Mayow 1643–1679*, Oxford (1935): page 13. Fulton describes the claim by TS Patterson in *Isis* 1931; 15: page 66 describing Vlacq, The Hague, as the first issue as an error.

[6] With H1* signed H2*, the sheet is referred to in this bibliography as H2*–H9* rather than H1*–H8*+1.

[7] One early reference to this title is in Francis Bernard (1627–1698). *A catalogue of the library of the late learned D Francis Bernard*, London (1698): page 169, #1739. Bernard also had a copy of the issue entitled *Diatribæ duæ medico-philosophicæ* listed on page 131, #411. Most of Bernard's books went to John Trotter (1667–1718) and remained with that family in Scotland until 1947 but the fate of Willis's books is not known.

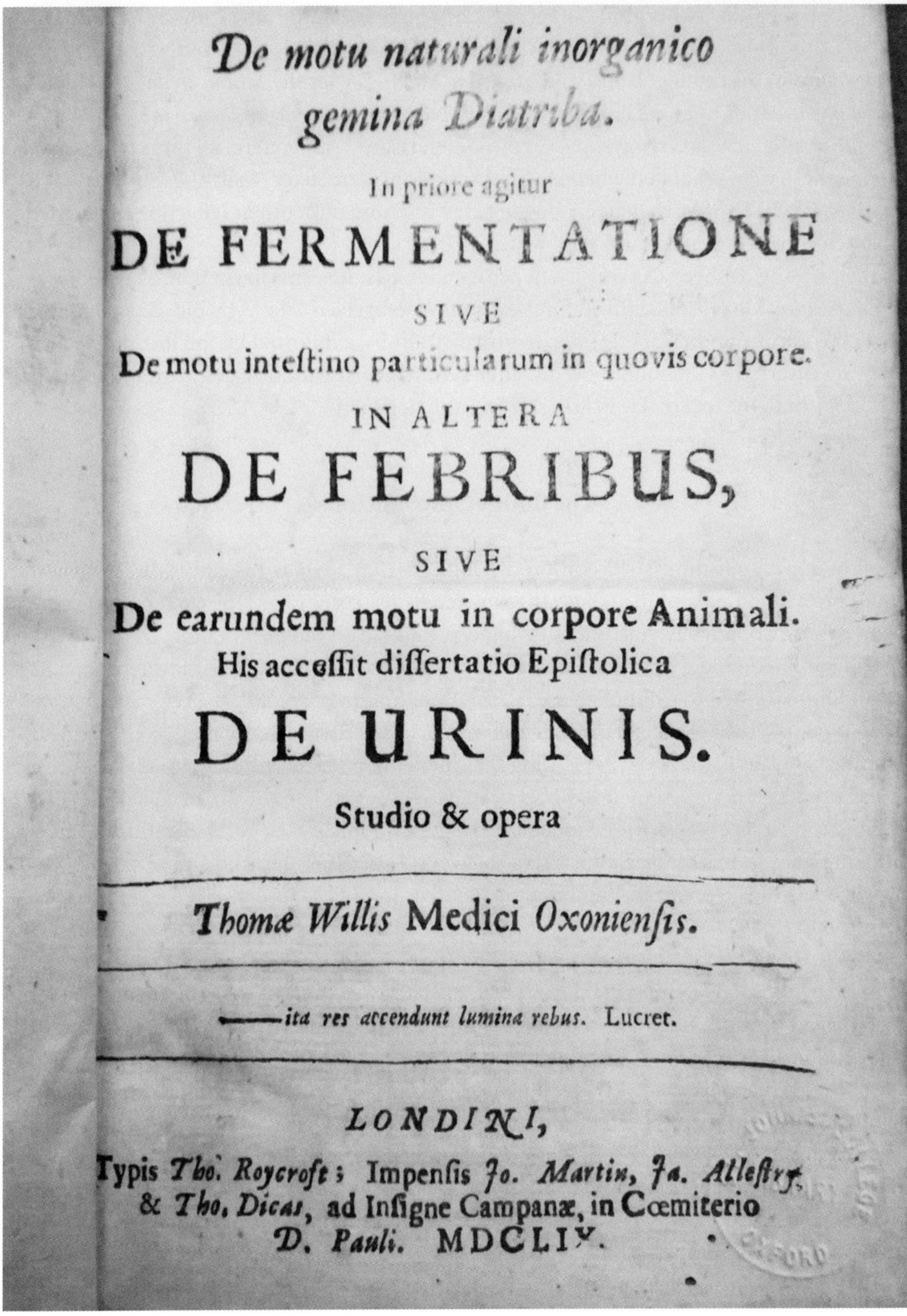
De motu naturali inorganico gemina Diatriba.

In priore agitur

DE FERMENTATIONE

SIVE

De motu inteſtino particularum in quovis corpore.

IN ALTERA

DE FEBRIBUS,

SIVE

De earundem motu in corpore Animali.

His acceſſit diſſertatio Epiſtolica

DE URINIS.

Studio & opera

Thomæ Willis Medici *Oxonienſis.*

—*ita res accendunt lumina rebus.* Lucret.

LONDINI,

Typis *Tho.* *Roycroft*; Impenſis *Jo. Martin*, *Ja. Alleſtry*, & *Tho. Dicas*, ad Inſigne Campanæ, in Cœmiterio *D. Pauli.* MDCLIV.

Figure 94 Variant title page from Thomas Willis's first publication. No other copy identified. *By* permission of the President and the Fellows of St John's College, Oxford.

It has to be assumed that the Dutch issue follows copies already available in England late in 1658. It is unlikely that, whatever favours may have been granted to Adriaan Vlacq, he would have been in a position to sell his issue before John Aubrey obtained a copy from the printer, James Allestry. Only the Dutch issue is mentioned by Browne Willis (1682–1760) in the listing of books by his grandfather, which is largely taken from Anthony Wood (1632–1695).[8] This is also the issue cited by Albrecht von Haller (1708–1777) but without mention of *De urinis* in his catalogue entry: 'Ej *diatribæ duæ*, 1. *de fermentatione, ſ. de motu inteſtino particularum in quocunque corpore. 2. de febribus, ſ de motu earundem in ſanguine animali* Haag 1659'. The few surviving copies of the Dutch issue (**1A3**) contain all three treatises even though these were separated when Dutch translations were made. In listing only the first two treatises, it is likely that Haller's catalogue entry is wrong rather than reflecting the existence of Dutch copies, as printed and sold, which lack *De urinis*.[9]

The printing of sheet Z is consistent across all issues. It seems likely that, as with the preliminaries for *De febribus*, those for *De urinis* also arrived late. Z4* and Z5* contain the 'Elenchus rerum' and errata leaf for that treatise, and are followed by the text of 'De urinis'. They are inserted as a bifolium bound after Z3v, page [4] with its catchword linking across the bifolium to the text of 'De urinis' starting at Z4r, page 1.

The duodecimo editions

The London duodecimo 1660 edition of *Diatribæ duæ* (**1B**) is the only work by Thomas Willis printed in England to include an engraved frontispiece (F.1a1). The scene is allegorical and depicts two females, one unclothed and presumed to represent nature, illuminated by rays of the sun directed by instruments held by the second female figure, clothed and in front a building, assumed to symbolize medicine. As set out in chapter 3, the engraving quotes a line from Lucretius (99–55 BC), which also appears on the title page of the 1659 edition (**1A**). The adjacent leaf has a poem explaining that medicine uses her torch to understand nature and the two sisters spread their light between each other and on the earth.

The frontispiece was reused, unaltered for the London 1662 and 1667 editions (**1C** and **1I**), but in new states in the Netherlands 1662, 1663 (**1C, 1D1, 1E**) and 1669 (**1F**).[10] In resetting the text of the poem for the London 1662 edition (**1C**), accents were added to several words: *hâc*, line 2; *porrectâ*, line 3; *indè*, line 4; '*tribuêre*' (line 5); and '*tribuëre*' (line 6). The change to '*tribuêre*', but the not the other alterations in accent, was made in both lines 5 and 6 for the Dutch 1662 edition (**1D1**) and its London issue (**1D2**). A further change was made to '*tribuëre*' (in both lines 5 and 6) for the London 1677 edition (**1I**). The use of 'tribuêre' indicates that the 'e' is long, and the form should be read as 'tribuerunt', third person plural; the accent in 'tribuëre' makes the 'e' short, indicating that the infinitive, 'to contribute', is intended. The poem was omitted from the Dutch issues for 1663 and 1669 (**1E, 1F**).

As noted by HJR Wing, the final 'ta' in 'Auctario locupletata' on the title page of the London duodecimo edition 1660 (**1B**) is always added in pen and ink but corrected in print thereafter.[11] He adds that 'in the majority of copies the engraved plate and the leaf on which

[8] See: [Browne Willis], 'Willis (Thomas)'. In: [John Bernard, Thomas Birch, John Locke, and other hands] *A general dictionary, historical and critical*, volume X (1741): pages 171–5; and chapter 4.

[9] See: Albrecht von Haller, *Bibliotheca medicinæ practicæ qua scripta ad partem medicinæ practicam facientia a rerum initiis ad A. MDCCLXXV recensentur*: Tomus III *Ab Anno* 1648 *Ad. A.* 1685; page 73. Haller lists later editions of *Diatribæ duæ* (1660–1669) and gives an abbreviated account of the contents of all three treatises in the text that follows.

[10] Johann-Friedrich Gmelin, *Geschichte der chemie seit dem widderaufleben der wissenschaften*, Volume 1 Göttingen (1797): page 673 lists an Amsterdam edition for 1665 but without further details. Although mentioned in various recently published accounts of seventeenth-century medicine, this edition has not been identified. It is not listed in the online Short Title Catalogue for the Netherlands. Copies of the 1663 edition are sometimes bound with works by other authors dated 1665; there may also be confusion with Lower's *Diatribæ Thomæ Willisii* which was published in 1665 in London and 1667 in Amsterdam.

[11] See: HJR Wing, *A bibliography of Dr. Thomas Willis (1621–1675)*, typescript (1962): page 5.

the poem is printed precede the title page but it is evident from the BM copy that they were printed as R11 and R12'. Both copies examined for this bibliography have these leaves bound as printed at R11 and R12.[12]

The point that printers rarely had sufficient material to retain standing type for books that were already published is well made by the fact that Thomas Roycroft (d.1677) reset type from 1660 for the 1662 edition (**1C**). In this case there was an additional need to make changes. Mention is made on the 1662 title page of Willis's appointment in 1660 as Sedleian professor in Oxford and it was appropriate therefore to include the dedication to Gilbert Sheldon (1598–1677), Bishop of London, and later Archbishop of Canterbury. This is printed on A4r–A5v, pages [7–10]. The engraved frontispiece and its poem are brought forward and printed as A1v, page [2], and A2r, page [3]. R9 and R12 are left blank and R10 and R11 are used for an advertisement of books for sale by John Martin (1618–1678), James Allestry, and Thomas Dicas (fl.1660–1669). The distribution of text for *De fermentatione* differs from the 1660 edition at B1r–B2r, pages 1–3, *De febribus* at F1r–F4v, pages 97–104, and *De urinis* at P11r–P12r, pages 333–5. Although everything is reset and some text added, thereafter the same content is accommodated on all other leaves, albeit occasionally with different line breaks. The opportunity was taken to correct several errors of catchword and a few others were introduced.

But there was another problem. It seems that, presumably copying from the octavo edition, once more the printer forgot to set the preface to *De febribus*. His solution was to print this on the four unused leaves of a^{12}. But because they relate to the second treatise, these leaves were signed f^{*4} and intended as preliminaries to the text of *De febribus* starting at F1r, page 97. Of the two copies examined for this bibliography, one has f^{*4} placed between E12v–F1r, pages 96–7, where these leaves naturally belong. The other has f^{*4} bound in the middle of the Elenchus rerum after a4 which, in terms of textual continuity, is inappropriate. In other copies it is found after a8 preceding the text of 'De fermentatione'. Both arrangements are understandable in terms of the printed sheet but still out of place in terms of the text. The catchwords make clear that these four leaves were an after-thought. There is no position where a catchword links to f*1r. However 'DE' at E12v, page 96, does link to F1r, page 97; and f*4v has the same catchword 'DE' indicating that, once his omission had been noticed but without bothering to alter E12, this is where the printer intended f^{*4} to be bound. Wherever f4 happens to be bound, the London duodecimo 1662 edition (**1C**) therefore has six extra leaves (a7 and a8, and f*1–4) compared to the 1660 edition (**1B**).

Adriaan Vlacq's duodecimo edition printed in The Hague (1662: **1D1**) is not conspicuous for its accuracy. All copies have *Actuario* for *Auctario* on the title page and *accesſit* replaces the more usual *acceſſit* or *acceſsit*. The same sheets with the reengraved frontispiece, repunctuated poem, and reset text and printers' ornaments are used in (at least) one copy with a London title page printed by Thomas Roycroft, John Martin, James Allestry, and Thomas Dicas (**1D2**).[13] In reproducing the errors introduced by Vlacq, this is likely to be a reissue of the Dutch imprint (**1D1**) rather than an independent London edition. That **1D2** is not just a made up copy of **1D1** with a London title page borrowed from **1C** is excluded by the fact that the settings of **1C** and **1D2** differ throughout even though both were printed by Roycroft for Martin, Allestry, and Dicas in 1662. Taken together, the duodecimo 1662 editions and issues provide further evidence for close cooperation between Adriaan Vlacq and his former colleagues in England.

[12] An ideal copy, bound as intended, would collate: π^2 (= R12, R11), A^{12}, a^6, B–Q^{12}, R^{10} (-R11, -R12 = π1, π2).

[13] The copy in the British Library (RB.23.a.11685) was acquired from the library of Hugh Sinclair (1910–1990), Oxford physician and nutritionist, and is used as the description for 1D2, next.

In his duodecimo 1663 and 1669 editions (**1E** and **1F**), Gerbrandt Schagen (b.1633) designates himself 'GERBRANDUS SCHAGHEN'. He omits the dedication to Sheldon and crowds some of the other text reducing his preliminaries from Vlacq's twenty-two (A^{12} Aa^{10}) to sixteen (A^{12} a^4). The engraved frontispiece is a mirror image of the duodecimo London 1660 (**1B**), 1662, (**1C**), and The Hague 1662 (**1D1**) and London 1662 (**1D2**) editions and issues. In its third state, Schagen adds his name and place of publication to the frontispiece for his Amsterdam 1663 edition (**1E**). Later he further amends the engraving to include the new date, 1669, in blank space underneath his name (**1F**).

Schagen resets the text for the 1669 edition with fewer and narrower lines per page (**1F**). This contains an error, apparently unique in Thomas Willis's works. In the middle of chapter VII of *De fermentatione*, B12r, page [47], is blank whereas B12v, page 48, has printed text. Although the pagination remains in sequence across this leaf, something is clearly wrong. The catchword at B11v, page 46, (fer-) links to C1r, page 49, (fermentefcibilis);[14] and the text is also continuous without involving B12. Nothing is missing despite the blank page. What has happened is that the thirty-eight lines of text at B12v, page 48, reappear where they belong as the last thirty-five lines of C2v, page 52 (starting in the middle of a line) and the first five lines of C3r, page 53. The book is in common duodecimo with the watermark at the foreedges of leaves 11 and 12 on most sheets, but this mark is not visible on either B11 or B12. The best explanation for the incomplete and inappropriate printing of B12 is that the typesetter working on the outer forme took up the wrong part of the manuscript when he reached B12v, page 48. Later he realized the error and therefore did not bother to set the inner forme at B12r, page 47. He decided not to discard the sheet with its erroneous page of text since that would have involved extensive reworking of the whole outer forme of sheet B. Rather, leaving in place the redundant B12, he picked up the correct place in the manuscript and carried on setting text at C1r, page 49, reaching and resetting the redundant text on B12v, page 48, at C2v–C3r, pages 52–3. HJR Wing who examined two copies makes no mention of this but does refer to leaf B12, page 47, as 'cancelled' in one example (Royal Society of Medicine) so presumably the error was resolved in some copies of this issue.[15]

The three treatises included in *Diatribæ duæ* were translated into Dutch, as was *De scorbuto* (1670, see **3C**). Although there is a subsidiary title page dated 1676 for the treatise on scurvy, this work is listed on the collective 1676 title page indicating that 'Of fermentation' and 'Of scurvy' were published as one work (**1H**). 'Of fevers' and 'Of urines' appeared later in Dutch, but printed together, in 1681 (**1J**). The 1676 and 1681 volumes each have explanatory footnotes. Where these extend across two pages, there are independent catchwords both for the main text and the footnotes.

Although the text is reset for the London duodecimo 1677 edition (**1I**), printing of the preface to 'De febribus' and the signing of f*4 remain unchanged, with erratic placement of those leaves in different copies as in the London duodecimo 1662 edition (**1C**). This is the only edition of *Diatribæ duæ* advertised in the *Term Catalogue*, at a price of 3s:

> Trinity 1677 July 5th, III, Numb 12, I 285, column 1, *Books reprinted.*
>
> Diatribæ Duæ Medico-Philosophicæ. Quarum Prior agit *De Fermentatione, sive de Motu Intestino particularum in quovis Corpore.* Altera, *De Febribus, sive de motu earundem*

[14] Misprinted in both copes as 'fermentefcibills'.

[15] Due to the circumstances of 2020 and 2021, this copy could not be directly examined, and therefore the variant state is not included in the present bibliography.

in sanguine Animalium. His accessit Dissertatio Epistolica *De Urinis*. Studio Tho. Willis. Editio Quarta ab auctore recognita, atque ab eodem multiplici auctuario locupletata. In Twelves. Price, bound, 3s. Printed for Sam. Carr in St. *Paul's* Churchyard.

The French translation of 'Of urines' published in duodecimo by Laurent d'Houry (1644–1725) in 1683 (**1K1**) has a full sheet (8 leaves) alternating with a half sheet (4 leaves) and catchwords only at the interval between each signature. Unless standing type was retained and reprinted, sheets of the original impression must still have been available when this was reissued in 1687 (**1K2**), now with d'Houry's address altered from 'ruë S. Jacques au S. Efprit pres les Mathurins' to 'ruë S. Jacques, devant la Fontaine S. Severin au Saint Efprit'. In place of the headpiece with leaves and buds that decorated his title page in 1683, d'Houry used a simple arrangement of three fleurons made up of two fleur-de-lys placed on their sides above a single shield with crossed lances.

1A1.c1. DIATRIBÆ DUÆ MEDICO-PHILOSOPHICÆ, London octavo 1659

The first issue of the first edition of Willis's first book [HJR Wing 1].

Title page: *Diatribæ duæ Medico-philofophicæ* | *quarum prior agit* | DE FERMENTATIONE | SIVE | *De motu inteftino particularum in quovis corpore.* | ALTERA | DE FEBRIBUS, | SIVE | De motu earundem in fanguine Animalium | Differtatio Epiftolica | DE URINIS. | [rule] | STUDIO | *Thomæ Willis* Medici *Oxonienfis.* | [rule] | *—ita res accendunt lumina rebus.* Lucret. 1. I. | [rule] | *LONDINI,* | Typis *Tho. Roycroft*; Impenfis *Jo. Martin*, *Ja. Alleftry*, | & *Tho. Dicas*, ad Infigne Campanæ, in Cœmiterio | *D. Pauli.* MDCLIX.

Collation: octavo; 23 letter roman alphabet using I and V: A^8, B–G^8, H^8 + H^{*8} [these 16 leaves signed: H, H2*, H3*, H4*, 5 unsigned, H2, H3, H4, 4 unsigned], I–Y^8, Z^{10} [signed: Z, Z2, Z3, Z4*, unsigned, Z4, 4 unsigned], Aa–Cc^8; $1–4 signed apart from: N2 signed L2, P2 signed p2.

218 leaves: paginated as [16], 1–97 [98], [16], 1–239 [240], [8], 1–52, [6].

Type: 35 lines: height (20 lines) 80 millimetres, width 81 millimetres.

Contents: **A1r–v**, page [1–2], blank; **A2r** title, page [3]; **A2v**, page [4], blank; **A3r–A4r**, page [5–7], Amico Lectori Præfatio. [De Fermentatione]; **A4v–A5v**, page [8–10], AUTHORI *In illius diatribas Medico-philofophicas Carmen gratulatorium* … [signed] *Phillipus Fell, Med. Stud. Oxon.*; **A6r–A8r**, page [11–15], Elenchus rerum [De Fermentatione]; **A8v**, page [16], Errata [De Fermentatione] Typothetarum παραράματα saltem illa, quæ Lectori minus attento molestiam factura videntur; (alia enim datâ opera præterimus) ita corrigi poterunt. [Of the printers' errors only those which seem a possible cause of trouble to a less attentive Reader; (indeed, the others I passed over, given the trouble) so they can be corrected], 9 lines listing 28 errors.

Blr–Hlr, pages 1–97, [text] DE FERMENTATIONE, five De *motu* corporum naturalium *inorganico*.; **H1v**, page [98], blank.

H2*r–H5*v, pages [1–8], *Amico Lectori PRÆFATIO.* [De Febribus]; **H6*r–H9*r**, pages [9–15], Elenchus rerum [De Febribus]; **H9*v**, page [16], Errata [De Febribus], 18 lines listing 68 errors.

H2r–Zlr, pages 1–239, [text] DE FEBRIBUS; **Z1v**, page [240], blank.

Z2r–Z3v, page [1–4], *De Urinis.* Diſſertatio Epiſtolica AD virum Doctiſſimum, mihique AMICISSIMUM, D. RADULPHUM BATHURST, Med Doct. & Collegii S. Sanctæ Trinitatis Oxon. ſocium; **Z4*r–Z5*r**, page [5–7], Elenchus rerum [De Urinis]; **Z5*v**, page [8], Errata [De Urinis], 4 lines listing 10 errors.

Z4r–Cc5v, page 1–52, [text] DE URINIS.

Cc6r–Cc7r, pages [1–3], Theſe Books following, are to be ſold by John Martin, James Alleſtre, and Thomas Dicas, at the Bell in St Pauls Churchyard; **Cc7v**, page [4], blank; **Cc8r–v**, pages [5–6], blank.

Headlines and *Catchwords*: '31' left not right at **E4r**, page 31; '74' right not left at **L1v**, page 74, [corrected in manuscript]; *Febrmentatione.* for *Fermentatione.* at **H1r**, page 97; *De Febribus.* for *De Urinis.* at **Aa1r**, page 11.

fermenteſcit for menteſcit at **C7v** / **C8r**, pages 30 / 31; ciunt. for unt, at **D5r** / **v**, pages 41 / 42; radicalis for dicalis at **E1v** / **E2r**, pages 50 / 51; ribus for vaporibus at **G7r** / **v**, pages 93 / 94; CAp for CAP at **H8*r** / **v**, pages [13] / [14]; moris for humoris at **H3r** / **v**, pages 3 / 4; 2.Quod for II. Quod at **H4v** / **H5r**, pages 6 / 7; tis for rentis at **I3r** / **v**, pages 19 / 20; rapidor for pidior at **M4v** / **M5r**, pages 70 / 71; xtione for mixtione at **M6v** / **M7r**, pages 74 / 75; Cum for I. Cum at **M7v** / **M8r**, pages 76 / 77; Ob for XII. Ob at **O1r** / **v**, pages 95 / 96; Pulsu for pulsu at **O3v** / **O4r**, pages 100 / 101; tionem for mitionem at **P5v** / **P6r**, pages 118 / 119; eo (letters vertically displaced) for dem at **R2r** / **v**, page 145 / 146; periclofum for periculoſum at **S5r** / **v**, pages 167 / 168; eius for præcipue [but ('quos malum illus' evidently missing and added in pen and ink] at **S7r** / **v**, pages 171 / 172; pore for torpor at **Y8v** / **Z1r**, pages 238 / 239; no catchword at **Z5*r** / **v**, pages [7–8]; and rimum for mum at **Z4r** / **v**, pages 1 / 2.

Frontispiece: none.

Portrait: none.

Printers' ornaments: single row of 12 fleurons at ***A3r***, page [5] {**Roycroft 1**}; single row of 13 fleurons, ##1, 3, 9, and 12 {**Roycroft 2**}; ##2 and 5 {**Roycroft 3**}; #4 {**Roycroft 4**}; ##6, 10, and 11 {**Roycroft 5**}; #7 {**Roycroft 6**}; ##8 and 13 {**Roycroft 7**} at ***A4v***, page [8]; single row of 29 fleurons at ***A6r***, page [11]; **H6*r,** page [9] {**Roycroft 8**}; single row of 14 fleurons, ##1, 5, and 7 {**Roycroft 10**}; ##2, 6, and 12 {**Roycroft 5**}; ##3, 8, 10, and 14 {**Roycroft 7**}; #4 {**Roycroft 2**}; ##9 and 11 {**Roycroft 3**}; and #13 {**Roycroft 6**} at **H2*r**, page [1]; single row of 13 fleurons, ##1, 3, 9, and 12 {**Roycroft 2**}; ##2 and 5 {**Roycroft 3**}; #4 {**Roycroft 4**}; ##6, 10, and 11 {**Roycroft 5**}; #7 {**Roycroft 6**}; ##8 and 13 {**Roycroft 7**} at **Z4*r**, page [5].

Decorated I at **B1r**, page 1 {**Roycroft 9**}.

Illustrations: none.

Copy: Bodleian Library (Ashm. D 65). Early calf boards with double lines off-centre and at edges, spine (detached) with nine double lined panels, paper label D. 65, original endpapers. Leaves 167 × 108 millimetres, boards 172 × 112 × 34 millimetres. Inscribed: (1) T. Willis A^{e}de Ch^{ti}; (2) John Aubrey. 1658. é Societ Medy Templi; (3) others (unidentified).[16]

1A1.c2. DIATRIBÆ DUÆ MEDICO-PHILOSOPHICÆ, London octavo 1659

The first issue of the first edition of Willis's first book, with altered signing of sheet H* [not distinguished from HJR Wing 1].

As in **1A1.c1** apart from:

Collation: octavo; 23 letter roman alphabet using I and V: A^8, B–G^8, H^8 + $H*^8$ [these 16 leaves signed: H, H2*, H3* signed H2*, H4*, H5* signed H4*, 4 unsigned, H2, H3, H4, 4 unsigned], I–Y^8, Z^{10} [signed: Z, Z2, Z3, Z4*, unsigned, Z4, 4 unsigned], Aa–Cc^8; $1–4 signed apart from: N2 signed L2, P2 signed p2.

Copy: Bodleian Library (RR.z.210). Early calf boards with double lines off-centre and at edges, spine (rebacked) with seven double lined panels and red gilt edged label WILLIS | DE | FERMENT | & DE | FEBR:, original endpapers. Leaves 166 × 105 millimetres, boards 170 × 110 × 33 millimetres. Inscribed: R. Frewin 1703. Bookplate E. BIBL. RADCL.[17]

1A2. DIATRIBÆ DUÆ MEDICO-PHILOSOPHICÆ, London octavo 1659

The second issue of the first edition of Willis's first book, retitled and with the reference to Lucretius abbreviated, and sheet H* as originally signed [not distinguished from HJR Wing 1].

Title page: *De motu naturali inorganico* | *gemina Diatriba.* | In priore agitur | DE FERMENTATIONE | SIVE | De motu inteſtino particularum in quovis corpore. | IN ALTERA | DE FEBRIBUS, | SIVE | De earundem motu in corpore Animali. | His acceſſit

[16] See: Bennett [Aubrey] (2015): page 1478 for mention of the annotations. The manuscript entries in this copy deserve detailed study. They appear on the free and paste-down endpapers (front and back), title page, preface, and final blank. There are also occasional annotations in the text. The book was bought by John Aubrey for 3s 6d from James Allestry in 1658. His name is inscribed twice but not in the same hand and using a different notation for the sum involved. The signature 'T. Willis', is in Aubrey's hand. A third annotation indicates that the book passed from Aubrey to the 'Mus. Ashmol' sometime after 1683. The annotations at the back are in several different scripts, including the one that inscribed 'T. Willis' in red pencil, and relate to various remedies and how best they are made.

[17] Richard Frewin owned this copy whilst studying medicine at Christ Church. He was a renowned physician but also described as professor of chemistry (1708) in Oxford and elected Camden professor of ancient history (1727) upon which he spent one hundred pounds on books, the better to discharge the duties of his office. Frewin bequeathed his house in Oxford, now Frewin Hall, for use of the regius professor of medicine, and 2300 books to the Radcliffe Library.

diſſertatio Epiſtolica | DE URINIS. | [rule] | Studio & opera | [rule] | *Thomæ Willis* Medici *Oxonienſis.* | [rule] | *—ita res accendunt lumina rebus.* Lucret. | [rule] | *LONDINI,* | Typis *Tho. Roycroft*; Impenſis *Jo. Martin, Ja. Alleſtry,* | & *Tho. Dicas*, ad Inſigne Campanæ, in Cœmiterio | *D. Pauli.* MDCLIX.

Then as in **1A1.c1**.

Copy: St John's College Library, Oxford (HB4 / 4.b.4.21). Original calf with triple-lined edges, spine with ten triple-lined bands, paper label TA2, original free endpapers and binder's stubs. Leaves 168 × 105 millimetres, boards 172 × 108 × 35 millimetres. Inserted: bookplate of St John's College, Oxford.

1A3. DIATRIBÆ DUÆ MEDICO-PHILOSOPHICÆ, The Hague octavo 1659

The third issue of the first edition of Willis's first book, with resetting of the title page and H* as originally signed [not distinguished from HJR Wing 1].

Title page: DIATRIBÆ DUÆ | MEDICO- | PHILOSOPHICÆ | Quarum Prior agit de | FERMENTATIONE | Sive | *De motu inteſtino particularum in quovis corpore.* | Altera de | FEBRIBVS, | Sive | *De motu earundem in ſanguine Animalium* | His acceſſit Diſſertatio Epiſtolica de | VRINIS. | Studio THOMÆ WILLIS Medici Oxonienſis. | *—ita res accendunt lumina rebus.* Lucret. 1. I. | HAGÆ-COMITIS, | [short rule] | Apud ADRIANUM VLACQ | M. DC. LIX.

Then as in **1A1.c1** apart from:

Contents: **Z4*r–Z5*r**, pages [5–7] bound before **Z2r–Z3v**, pages [1–4].

Copy: Leiden University Library (620 G 10), lacking *A*1 (blank). Original vellum, spine with small paper labels G20 (×2), not lettered, original endpapers. Leaves 171 × 108 millimetres, boards 176 × 105 × 35 millimetres. Stamped: (1) Ex Legato VERRIJST. ACAD. LVGD. (on title page below the printer's name); and (2) ACAD. LVGD (on upper and lower edges).[18]

1B. DIATRIBÆ DUÆ MEDICO-PHILOSOPHICÆ, London duodecimo 1660

The second edition of Willis's first book, with the allegorical engraved frontispiece in its first state (see: Figure 95) [HJR Wing 2].

[18] The book was evidently part of a legacy to the University of Leiden from A. Verrijst (nd) about whom little is known other than that, in 1784, he published a paper on the 'Usefulness of "cortex perneranus" in the treatment of malignant autumnal fevers', perhaps explaining his interest in Willis's treatise on fevers. He is mentioned in AJ van der Aa, *Biographisch Woordenboek der Nederlanden* [Biographical Dictionary of the Netherlands] volume 19 [letter V] (1876): page 190.

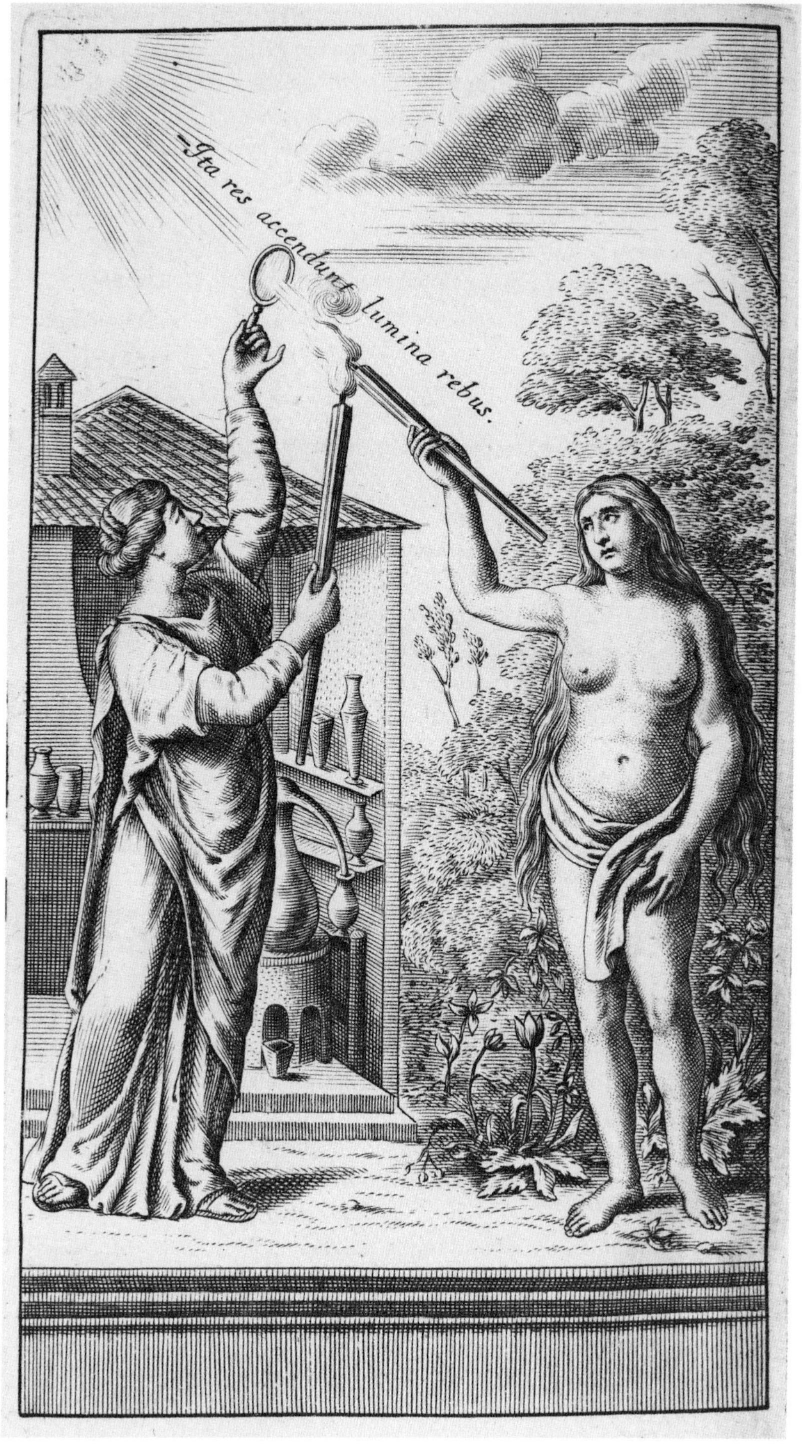

Figure 95 Engraved allegorical frontispiece: *Diatribæ duæ medico-philosophicæ*, London, 1660 (F.1a1).

Title page: *Diatribæ duæ Medico-philoſophicæ,* | *Quarum prior agit* | DE | FERMENTATIONE | SIVE | *De motu inteſtino particularum in quovis corpore.* | ALTERA | DE FEBRIBUS, | SIVE | De moto earundem in ſanguine Animalium. | *His acceſsit* | Diſſertatio Epiſtolica | DE URINIS. | [rule] | STUDIO | *Thomæ Willis Medici Oxonienſis.* | [rule] | Editio Secunda, | *Ab Authore recognita, atque ab eodem* | *multiplici Auctario locupletata* | [rule] | *LONDINI,* | Typis *Tho. Roycroft*; Impenſis *Jo. Martin, Ja.* | *Alleſtry,* & *Tho. Dicas,* ad Inſigne Campanæ, in | Cœmiterio *D. Pauli.* MDCLX.

Collation: duodecimo; 23 letter roman alphabet using I: A^{12}, a^{6}, B–R^{12}; $1–5 signed apart from: A2 signed *A*2, a2 signed *a*2, a3 signed *a*3.

210 leaves: paginated as [36], 1–376, [8]. Mispaginated: 175 for 178, 149 for 249.

Type: 42 lines; height (20 lines) 52 millimetres, width 61 millimetres.

Contents: **Alr**, page [1], title; **A1v**, page [2] blank; **A2r–A3v**, pages [3–6], Amico Lectori Præfatio. [De Fermentatione]; **A4r–v**, pages [7–8], AUTHORI *In illius diatribas Medico-philoſophicas, Carmen gratulatorium* ... [signed] *Philippus Fell. Med. Stud. Oxon.*; **A5r–A8r**, pages [9–15], Elenchus rerum, IN TRACTATU DE FERMENTATIONE.; **A8v–A12v**, pages [16–24], Elenchus rerum IN TRACTATU DE *FEBRIBUS.*; **A12v–alv**, pages [24–26], Elenchus Rerum *in diſſertatione* DE URINIS.; **a2r–a5v**, pages [27–34], Amico Lectori PRÆFATIO. [De Febribus]; **a6r**, page [35], blank; **a6v**, page [36], Errata, 34 lines listing 98 errors.

Blr–El2v, page 1–96, [text] DE FERMENTATIONE, ſive De *motu* corporum naturalium *inorganico.*; **Flr–P8v**, pages 97–328, [text] DE FEBRIBUS.; **P9r–P10v**, pages 329–32, DE URINIS. *Diſſertatio Epiſtolica* AD Virum Doctiſſimum mihique AMICISSIMUM, D. RADULPHUM BATHURST, Med Doct. & Collegii S. Sanctæ Trinitatis Oxon. ſocium.; **Pllr–R8v**, pages 333–76, [text] DE URINIS.

R9r–R10v, pages [1–4], A Catalogue of Books Printed for *John Martin, James Alleſtry*, and *Thomas Dicas*: And are to be ſold at the *Bell* in St *Pauls Church-yard*; **R11r**, page [5], blank, **R11v**, page [6], Engraved allegorical frontispiece; **R12r**, page [7], [poem] ARtis *ope ætherios* Natura *exſuſcitat ignes,* | *Et cœlo attonitos, hac famulante vocat.* | *Huic mox acceptas porrecta lampade flammas* | *Reddit, & inde novum creſcit utrique jubar.* | Sic lucem *unanimes* terris *tribuere* ſorores, | *Et* lucem *unanimes ſic tribuere* ſibi.; **R12v**, page [8], blank.

Headlines and *Catchwords*: '64' placed right not left at **D8v**, page 64; FEBIRBUS. for FEBRIBUS. at **H8r**, page 159; **I8r**, page 183, **K8r**, page 207; **L8r**, page 231, **M6r**, page 251; **O1v**, page 290.

ſepe for ſæpe at **B6r / v**, pages 11 / 12; hæc for hęc at **C11r / v**, pages 45 / 46; anæ for anę at **G12r / v**, pages 143 / 144; ſœpius for ſæpius at **I7r / v**, pages 181 / 182; Propter for propter at **O8v / O9r**, pages 304 / 305; quoris for liquoris at **Q8r / v**, pages 351 / 352.

Frontispiece: **F.1a1.** Engraved allegorical frontispiece with oblique text: *–Ita res accendunt lumina rebus* [diagonal, top left to bottom right]. 145 × 80 millimetres (sheet), 122 × 68 millimetres (plate marks), 118 × 65 millimetres (image).

Portrait: none.

Printers' ornaments: double row of 11 fleurons {**Roycroft 11**} over 7 fleurons, #6 inverted, separated between ##3 / 4, 6 / 7 by : {**Roycroft 12**} at *A2r*, page [3]; single row of 13 fleurons separated between ##5 / 6, 8 / 9 by : {**Roycroft 13**} at **A4r**, page [7]; single row of 13 fleurons ##1, 2, 4, 6, and 11 {**Roycroft 14**}; ## 3, 5, 7, 8, 9, 10, 12, and 13 separated between ##4 / 5, 9 / 10 by : {**Roycroft 15**} at A5r, page [9]; single row of 11 fleurons {**Roycroft 16**} and 2 adjacent fleurons {**Roycroft 17**} with a rule below at **A8v**, page [16]; single row of 22 fleurons separated between ##11 / 12 by : {**Roycroft 8**} at A12v, page [24]; double row of 11 fleurons separated between ##6 / 7 by • {**Roycroft 11**} , over 6 fleurons {**Roycroft 18**} at **a2r**, page [27]; double row of 22 above 22 similar (inverted) fleurons {**Roycroft 20**} at **B1r**, page 1; **R9r**, page [1]; single row of 14 fleurons ##1, 5, 6, 8, 10, and 12 {**Roycroft 14**}; ##2, 3, 4, 7, 9, 11, 13, and 14 {**Roycroft 15**} at **F1r**, page 97; double row of 14 fleurons ##1, 5, 6, 8, 10, and 12 {**Roycroft 14**}; ##2, 3, 4, 7, 9, 11, 13, and 14 {**Roycroft 15**}over 6 fleurons {**Roycroft 18**} at **P11r**, page 333.

Decorated D at **a2r**, page [27] {**Roycroft 19**}; I at **B1r**, page 1 {**Roycroft 9**}.

Illustrations: none.

Copy: DASC (#1 of 2). Early full sprinkled calf, spine (relaid) with four raised bands and four gilt decorated panels, lettered DE | FERMEN, original endpapers. Leaves 145 × 80 millimetres, boards 152 × 83 × 22 millimetres. Inserted: bookplate, Hopetoun. Inscribed: William Feindel, Montréal. Early shelf mark K 3 14.[19]

1C. DIATRIBÆ DUÆ MEDICO-PHILOSOPHICÆ, London duodecimo 1662

The third edition of Willis's first book, with the allegorical engraved frontispiece in its first state [HJR Wing 3].

Title page: *Diatribæ duæ Medico-Philoſophicæ*: | *Quarum prior agit* | DE | FERMENTATIONE, | SIVE | *De motu inteſtino particularum in quovis corpore*; | ALTERA | DE FEBRIBUS, | SIVE | De motu earundem in ſanguine Animalium. | *His acceſsit* | Diſſertatio Epiſtolica | DE URINIS. | [rule] | STUDIO | THOMÆ WILLIS, *ex Æde* Chriſti | OXON. M. D. & in iſta Celeberrima Academia | Naturalis Philoſophiæ Profeſſoris *Sidleiani*. | [rule] | Editio Tertia, | *Ab Authore recognita, atque ab eodem multiplici Auctario* | *locupletata* [not centred] | [rule] | *LONDINI*, | Typis *Tho. Roycroft*; Impenſis *Jo. Martin, Ja.* | *Alleſtry*, & *Tho. Dicas*, ad Inſigne Campanæ, | in Cœmeterio *D. Pauli*, MDCLXII.

[19] The bookplate, with the mottoes 'Tria juncta in uno' and 'At spes non fracta', is from Hopetoun, the ancestral home in South Queensferry, near Edinburgh, of the Earl of Hopetoun, now also the Marquess of Linlithgow. The bookplate and shelf marks appear to match those used *c.*1750 during the lifetime of the second Earl, John Hope (1704–1781), whose son, James Hope-Johnstone (1741–1816) was elected FRSE. No one of the Earls appears to have had an interest in medicine. William Feindel (1918–2014) was a Canadian neurosurgeon and head of the Montreal Neurological Institute. He developed a lifelong interest in Thomas Willis whilst working in Oxford as a Rhodes Scholar during the 1940s when he started to acquire copies of the printed works, a number of which subsequently came into the present collection.

Collation: duodecimo; 23 letter roman alphabet using I: A[12], a[8], B–E[12], f*[4], F–R[12]; $1–5 signed apart from: -D3.

216 leaves: paginated as [40], 1–96, [8], 97–376, [8]. Mispaginated: 26 for 29.

Type: 42 lines; height (20 lines) 57 millimetres, width 61 millimetres.

Contents: **A1r**, page [1], blank; **A1v**, page [2], [poem] ARtis *ope ætherios* Natura *exſuſcitat ignes, / Et cœlo attonitos, hâc ſamulante, vocat. / Huic mox acceptas porrectâ lampade flammas / Reddit, & indè novum creſcit utrique jubar. /* Sic lucem *unanimes* terris *tribuêre* ſorores, / *Et* lucem *unanimes ſic tribuëre* ſibi.; **A2r**, page [3], engraved allegorical frontispiece; **A2v**, page [4], blank; **A3r**, page [5], title; **A3v**, page [6], blank; **A4r–A5v**, pages [7–10], Reverendiſſimo in *CHRISTO* Patri, ac Domino, D[no.] GILBERTO Epiſcopo LONDINENSI, & Sacelli Regii Decano. … [signed] *Humillimus, & æternùm Addictiſſimus* THO. WILLIS.; **A6r–A8r**, pages [11–15], Amico Lectori Præfatio [De Fermentatione]; **A8v**, page [16], blank; **A9r–A9v**, pages [17–18], AUTHORI, *In illius Diatribas Medico-Philoſophicas, Carmen gratulatorium.* … [signed] *Philippus Fell, Med. Stud. Oxon.*; **A10r–a1r**, pages [19–25], Elenchus rerum IN TRACTATU DE FERMENTATIONE.; **a1v–a5v**, pages [26–34], Elenchus Rerum IN TRACTATU DE *FEBRIBUS*.; **a6r–a7r,** pages [35–7], Elenchus Rerum *in Diſſertatione* DE URINIS.; **a7v**, page [38], blank; **a8r**, page [39], Errata, 22 lines listing 61 errors; **a8v**, page [40], blank.

Blr–E12v, pages 1–96, [text] DE FERMENTATIONE, ſive De *motu* corporum naturalium *inorganico.*

f1*r–f4*v, pages [1–8], Amico Lectori PRÆFATIO. [De Febribus].

Flr–P8v, pages 97–328, [text] DE FEBRIBUS.; **P9r–P10v**, pages 329–32, DE URINIS *Diſſertatio Epiſtolica* AD Virum Doctiſſimum mihíque AMICISSIMUM, D. RADULPHUM BATHURST, Med. Doct. & Collegii S. Sanctæ Trinitatis Oxon. Socium.; **Pllr–R8v**, pages 333–76, [text] DE URINIS.; **R9r–v**, pages [1–2], blank.

R10r–R11v, pages [3–6], CATALOGUS *Librorum, qui proſtant venales apud* Joannem Martin, Jacobum Alleſtry, & Thomam Dicas, *ad Inſigne* Campanæ *in Cœmeterio* Paulino.; **R12r–v**, pages [7–8], blank.

Headlines and *Catchwords*: Elenchus for Elenchus at **a2r**, page 27; FEBRIIBUS for FEBRIBUS at **K5v**, page 202.

No catchword at **A5v / A6r**, pages [10] / [11]; **A9v / A10r**, pages [18] / [19]; non for miscibile at **F7v / F8r**, pages 110 / 111; optimè for optime at **F8r / v**, pages 111 / 112; culum for triculum at **K7v / K8r**, pages 206 / 207; propter for Propter at **O8v / O9r**, pages 304 / 305; phuræ for Sulphureȩ at **S9r / v**, pages 353 / 354; isve for iſve at **R1r / v**, pages 361 / 362.

Frontispiece: **F.1a1.** Engraved allegorical frontispiece with oblique text: *Ita res accendunt lumina rebus* [diagonal, top left to bottom right]; 145 × 80 millimetres (sheet), 122 × 68 millimetres (plate marks), 118 × 65 millimetres (image).

Portrait: none.

Printers' ornaments: headpiece at **A4r**, page [7]; **B1r**, page 1; **P11r**, page 333; **R10r**, page [3] (inverted) {**Roycroft 21**}; single line of 12 fleurons separated between ##6 / 7 by : and ##7 / 8 by • at **A6r**, page [11]; single line of 12 fleurons separated between ##6 / 7 by : at **a1v**, page [26] {**Roycroft 14**}; single line of 20 fleurons separated by | between ##5 / 6, 11 / 12, 16 / 17 at **A9r**, page [17]; single line of 20 fleurons separated by : between ##7 / 8, 14 / 15 at **a6r**, page [35] {**Roycroft 8**}; single line of 10 fleurons separated by | between ##6 / 7 at **A10r**, page [19]; single line of 10 fleurons separated by : between ##5 / 6 at **f*1r**, page [1] {**Roycroft 11**}; headpiece at **F1r**, page 97 {**Roycroft 25**}; single line of 21 fleurons at **P9r**, page 329 {**Roycroft 8**}.

Decorated S at **A4r**, page [7] {**Roycroft 22**}; D at **A6r**, page [11] {**Roycroft 23**}; D at **f*1r**, page [1] {**Roycroft 19**}; I at **B1r**, page 1 {**Roycroft 24**}.

Illustrations: none.

Copy: DASC (#1 of 2), lacking R12 (blank). Later full sprinkled calf, spine with four raised bands, label WILLIS | DE FERMEN | DE FEBRIB | DE URINIS, new endpapers. Leaves 150 × 80 millimetres, boards 152 × 83 × 30 millimetres. Inscribed: Wm Feindel. Shelf mark: T126 / W67 / 662.

1D1. DIATRIBÆ DUÆ MEDICO-PHILOSOPHICÆ, The Hague duodecimo 1662

The first issue of the fourth edition of Willis's first book, described as the third edition, with the allegorical frontispiece in its second state [HJR Wing 4].

Title page: *Diatribæ duæ Medico-Philoſophicæ:* | *Quarum prior agit* | *DE* | FERMENTATIONE | *SIVE* | *De Motu inteſtino particularum in* | *quovis corpore*; | *ALTERA* | DE FEBRIBUS, | SIVE | De motu earundem in ſanguine | Animalium. | *His acceſſit* | Diſſertatio Epiſtolica | DE URINIS. | [rule] | STUDIO | THOMÆ WILLIS, *ex Aede* Chriſti | OXON. M.D. & in iſta celeberrima Academia | Naturalis Philoſophiæ Profeſſoris *Sidleiani.* | [short rule] | Editio Tertia, | *Ab Authore recognita, atque ab eodem multiplici* | *Actuario locupletata.* | [short rule] | HAGÆ-COMITIS, | Ex Typographia ADRIANI VLACQ. | M. DC. LXII.

Collation: duodecimo; 23 letter roman alphabet using I: $A^{12,}$ Aa^{10}, B–Q^{12}, R^{8}; \$1–5 signed apart from: A5 for A4, -A5, Aa2 for Aa3, Aa3 for Aa4, Aa4 for Aa5, +Aa5 for Aa6, +Aa6 for Aa7, +C6, +R6, +R7, +R9 for R8.

210 leaves: paginated as [44], 1–376. Mispaginated: 24 for 22, 146 for 170, 214 for 222, 332 for 342.

Type: 42 lines; height (20 lines) 57 millimetres, width 61 millimetres.

Contents: **A1r**, page [1], engraved allegorical frontispiece; **A1v**, page [2], [rule] [poem] ARtis *ope ætherios* Natura *exſuſcitat ignes, / Et cœlo attonitos, hac ſamulante, vocat. / Huic mox acceptas porrecta lampade flammas / Reddit, & inde novum creſcit utrique jubar.* / Sic lucem *unanimes* terris *tribuêre* ſorores, / *Et* lucem *unanimes ſic tribuere* ſibi. [rule]; **A2r**, page [3], title; **A2v**, page [4], blank; **A3r**–[**A4**]**v**, pages [5–8], Reverendiſſimo in *CHRISTO* Patri, ac Domino,

D^{no} GILBERTO Epiſcopo LONDINENSI, & Sacelli Regii Decano. … [signed] *Humillimus, & æternùm addictiſſimus THO. WILLS.*; **A5r–A7r**, pages [9–13], Amico Lectori PRÆFATIO [De Fermentatione]; **A7v**, page [14], blank; **A8r–A8v**, pages [15–16], AUTHORI, *In illius Diatribas Medico-Philoſophicas, Carmen gratulatorium.* … [signed] *Philippus Fell, Med. Stud. Oxon.*; **A9r–A12r**, pages [17–23], Elenchus rerum IN TRACTATU DE FERMENTATIONE.; **A12v–[Aa4]v**, pages [24–32], Elenchus Rerum IN TRACTATU DE *FEBRIBUS*.; **[Aa5]r–[Aa6]r**, pages [33–5], ELENCHUS RERUM *In Diſſertatione* DE URINIS.; **[Aa6]v**, page [36], blank; **[Aa7]r–Aa10v**, pages [37–44], Amico Lectori. PRÆFATIO. [De Febribus].

Blr–El2v, pages 1–96, [text] DE FERMENTATIONE, SIVE De *motu* corporum naturalium *inorganico*.; **Flr–P8v**, pages 97–328, [text] DE FEBRIBUS.; **P9r–P10v**, pages 329–32, DE URINIS *Diſſertatio Epiſtolica* AD Virum Doctiſſimum mihique AMICISSIMUM, D. RADULPHUM BATHURST, Med Doct. & Collegii S. Sanctæ Trinitatis Oxon. Socium.; **Pllr–R8v**, pages 333–76, [text] DE URINIS.

Headlines and *Catchwords*: headlines correct [switch from De FERMENTATIONE to DE FERMENTATIONE at **C1r–E12v**, pages 25–96].

No catchword at **[A4]v / A5r**, page [8] / [9]; **A8v / A9r**, page [16] / [17]; **[Aa6]r** / v, pages 35 / 36; **[Aa7]r** / v, pages 37 / 38; quenti for insuper at **B2r / v**, pages 3 / 4; Quia for Quin at **C3r / v**, pages 29 / 30; nimè for nime at **D3r / v**, pages 53 / 54; nitor for gnitur at **D6r / v**, pages 59 / 60; ducunt for cunt at **F9v / F10r**, pages 114 / 115; stinum for num at **H11r / v**, pages 165 / 166; propter for Propter at **O8v / O9r**, pages 304 / 305; phuræ for Sulphureæ at **S9r / v**, pages 353 / 354.

Frontispiece: **F.1b1.** Engraved allegorical frontispiece with oblique text: *Ita res accendunt lumina rebus* [diagonal, top left to bottom right]; 150 × 80 millimetres (sheet), 125 × 70 millimetres (plate marks), 116 × 65 millimetres (image).

Portrait: none.

Printers' ornaments: headpiece at **A3r**, page [5]; **P11r**, page 333 {**Vlacq 1**}; single line of 17 fleurons at **A5r**, page [9]; **A8r**, page [15]; **A9r**, page [17]; **A12v**, page [24]; **[Aa5]r**, page [33]; single line of 17 fleurons separated by ٦ between ##5 / 6 with rule over single line of 17 (inverted) fleurons separated by ٦ between ##8 / 9 at **B1r**, page 1; single line of 17 fleurons with rule under at **F1r**, page 97 {**Vlacq 2**}; line of 17 fleurons {**Vlacq 2**} over line of 6 fleurons {**Vlacq 3**} at [Aa7]**r**, page [37]; single line of 6 fleurons {**Vlacq 3**} at **P9r**, page 329.

No decorated initials.

Illustrations: none.

Copy: DASC (#1 of 3), of which one copy lacks the printed frontispiece at A1r, despite having the poem intact at A1v, illustrating an error liable to occur in moving the printed sheet from the hand press for addition of the engraving using the rolling press. Early full vellum, spine lettered 234 | WILLIS | IS 1E 8ZA | AGA | 1667, original endpapers. Leaves 150 × 78 millimetres, boards 157 × 85 × 25 millimetres. Inserted: bookplate EX LIBRIS FRANZ SONDHEIMER.[20]

[20] Franz Sondheimer (1926–1981) moved from Germany to England in 1937 and studied chemistry. After working in Israel (1956–1964) he was Royal Society research professor first in Cambridge and then at University

1D2. DIATRIBÆ DUÆ MEDICO-PHILOSOPHICÆ, London duodecimo 1662

The second issue of the fourth edition of Willis's first book, described as the third edition, with the title page reset and the allegorical frontispiece in its second state [not distinguished from HJR Wing 4].

Title page: *Diatribœ duœ Medico-Philoſophicœ:* | *Quarum prior agit* | *DE* | FERMENTATIONE | *SIVE* | *De Motu inteſtino particularum in* | *quovis corpore*; | *ALTERA* | DE FEBRIBUS, | SIVE | De motu earundem in ſanguine | Animalium. | *His accesſit* | Diſſertatio Epiſtolica | DE URINIS. | [rule] | STUDIO | THOMÆ WILLIS, *ex Aede* Chriſti | OXON. M.D & in iſta celeberrima Academia | Naturalis Philoſophiæ Profeſſoris *Sidleiani.* | [short rule] | Editio Tertia, | *Ab Authore recognita, atque ab eodem multiplici* | *Actuario locupletata.* | [rule] | *LONDINI,* | Typis *Tho. Roycroft*; Impenſis *Jo. Martin, Ja.* | *Alleſtry,* & *Tho. Dicas,* ad inſigne Campanæ, | in Cœmeterio *D. Pauli,* MDCLXII.

Then as in **1D1**.

Copy: British Library (RB.23.a.11685). Original vellum, gilt blind coat of arms on upper and lower boards, spine with labelled WILLIS | Medicina, original endpapers. Leaves 148 × 81 millimetres, boards 158 × 83 × 30 millimetres. Bookplate of HUGH MACDONALD SINCLAIR. Inscribed: (1) Præſse et Prodeſse; (2) Præſse et Prodeſse Morrÿ B.M.V [Beatae Mariae Virginis]. Sac: Ord. Cist: ad S. Crucem Catalogo jnſsority [??] N.j. Shelf marks: (1) 3. XX.k; (2) VI Ek. M12; (3) RB.23.a.11685.[21]

1E. DIATRIBÆ DUÆ MEDICO-PHILOSOPHICÆ, Amsterdam duodecimo 1663

The fifth edition of Willis's first book, with the allegorical frontispiece reversed and in its third state (see: Figure 96) [HJR Wing 5].

Title page: *Diatribœ duœ Medico-Philoſophicœ:* | Quarum prior agit de | FERMENTATIONE, | *SIVE* | De motu inteſtino particularum | in quovis corpore; | *ALTERA* | DE FEBRIBUS, | *SIVE* | De motu earundem in ſangui- | ne Animalium. | *His acceſſit Diſſertatio Epiſtolicœ* | DE URINIS. | STUDIO | THOMÆ WILLIS, *ex Æde* Chriſti | Oxon. M.D. & in iſta Celeberrima Academia | Naturalis Philoſophiæ Profeſſoris *Sidleiani.* | EDITIO | *Poſtrema prioribus longè emendatior at-* | *que auctior.* | [ornament] | AMSTELODAMI, | [short rule] | Apud GERBRANDUS SCHAGHEN | M DC LXIII.

College London. He was elected FRS for his work on synthesis of hormones and other natural products. This copy was subsequently owned by William Feindel.

[21] Hugh Macdonald Sinclair was a physician interested in nutrition who emphasized the role of 'bad fats' in human disease. He claimed descent from Woldonius, Viking monarch of Finland, and the St Clair cousins of William the Conqueror. His academic career was in Oxford and, later, Reading. Sinclair intended to found an International Institute of Human Nutrition at his home, Lady Place, including a library to house his collection of *c.*300 000 reprints and books. At his death, the University of Reading established the Hugh Sinclair professorship and Unit of Human Nutrition.

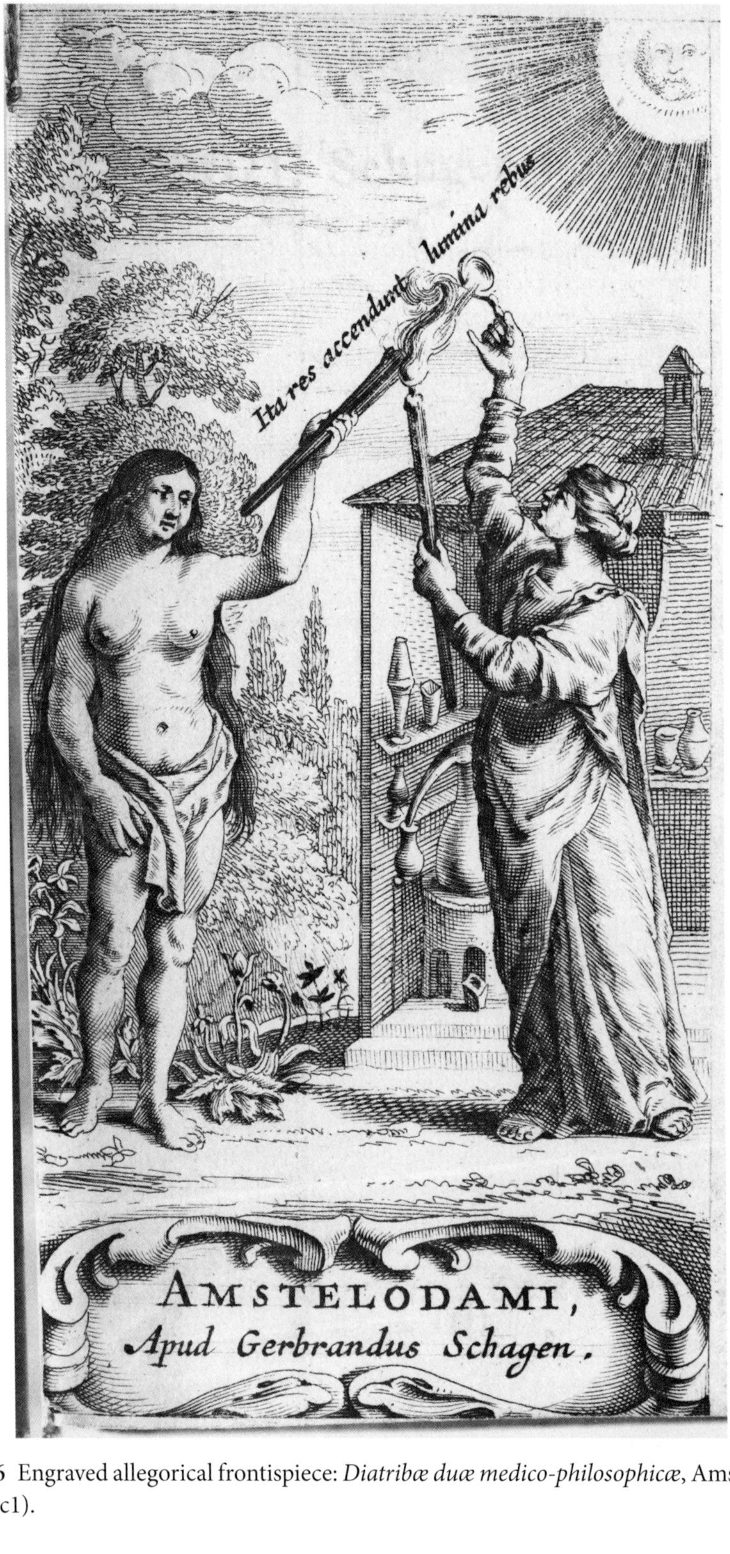

Figure 96 Engraved allegorical frontispiece: *Diatribæ duæ medico-philosophicæ*, Amsterdam, 1663 (F.1c1).

Collation: duodecimo; 23 letter roman alphabet using I: A^{12}, a^{4}, B–Q^{12}, R^{8}; $1–6 signed apart from: F5 signed F, G4 signed G2, +I7, +L7, +M7, +O7, +P7, +Q7.

204 leaves: paginated as [32], 1–376.

Type: 42 lines; height (20 lines) 54 millimetres, width 59 millimetres.

Contents: **A1r**, page [1], engraved allegorical frontispiece; **A1v**, page [2], blank; **A2r**, page [3], title; **A2v**, page [4], blank; **A3r–A4r**, pages [5–7], Amico Lectori PRÆFATIO. [De Fermentatione]; **A4v–A5r**, pages [8–9], *AUTHORI*, In illius Diatribas Medico-Philoſophicas, *Carmen gratulatorium*. ... [signed] PHILIPPUS FELL, *Med. Stud. Oxon.*; **A5v–A8v**, pages [10–16], ELENCHUS RERUM *In Tractatu* DE FERMENTATIONE.; **A9r–a1r**, pages [17–25], ELENCHUS RERUM *In Tractatu* DE FEBRIBUS.; **a1v–a2v**, pages [26–28], ELENCHUS RERUM *In Diſſertatione* DE URINIS.; **a2v–a4v**, pages [28–32], Amico Lectori. PRÆFATIO. [De Febribus].

Blr–El2v, pages 1–96, [text] DE FERMENTATIONE, *SIVE* De *motu* corporum naturalium *inorganico*.; **F1r–P8v**, pages 97–328, [text] DE FEBRIBUS.; **P9r–P10v**, pages 329–32, DE URINIS Diſſertatio Epiſtolica A D *Virum Doctiſſimum mihique* AMICISSIMUM, D. RADULPHUM BATHURST, Med. Doct. & Collegii S. Sanctæ Trinitatis Oxon. Socium.; **Pllr–R8v**, pages 333–76, [text] DE URINIS.

Headlines and *Catchwords*: no ⁚ after header at **D9v**, page 66; **E1v**, page 74; **N7v**, page 278; **N8v**, page 280; **O9v**, page 306; and **O10v**, page 308.

gitat for agitat at **B5v** / **B6r**, pages 10 / 11; ina for in at **D4r** / **v**, pages 55 / 56; phurea for phureo at **E2r** / **v**, pages 75 / 76; turbatur for turpatur at **P6r** / **v**, pages 323 / 324.

Frontispiece: **F.1c1.** Engraved allegorical frontispiece with oblique text: *Ita res accendunt lumina rebus* [diagonal, bottom left to top right] AMSTELODAMI, *Apud Gerbrandus Schagen.*; 131 × 70 millimetres (sheet), 130 × 67 millimetres (plate marks), 126 × 65 millimetres (image).

Portrait: none.

Printers' ornaments: design of four fleurons, one rotated to the left and one to the right above two inverted {**Schagen 1**}, the upper pair separated by one fleuron {**Schagen 2**}, on the title page at **A2r**, page [3]; two rows each made up of 14 fleurons, the lower inverted, with 2 others (rotated) at the left and right margins {**Schagen 1**}, separated by a central row of 12 fleurons {**Schagen 2**} at **B1r**, page 1; tailpiece at **E12v**, page 96 {**Schagen 6**}; headpiece at **F1r**, page 97 {**Schagen 7**}; headpiece at **P11r**, page 333 {**Schagen 9**}; and tailpiece at **R8v**, page 376 {**Schagen 11**}.

Decorated D at **A3r**, page [5] {**Schagen 3**}; D at **a2v**, page [28] {**Schagen 4**}; I at **B1r**, page 1 {**Schagen 5**}; E at **F1r**, page 97 {**Schagen 8**}; C at **P11r**, page 333 {**Schagen 10**}.

Illustrations: none.

Copy: DASC (#1 of 2). Early full vellum with faded signature on front cover, faded shelf mark on spine, original endpapers. Leaves 132 × 70 millimetres, boards 140 × 72 × 23 millimetres. Inscribed on title page (unidentified).

1F. DIATRIBÆ DUÆ MEDICO-PHILOSOPHICÆ, Amsterdam duodecimo 1669

The sixth edition of Willis's first book, with the allegorical frontispiece reversed and in its fourth state [HJR Wing 6].

Title page: *Diatribæ duæ Medico-Philoſophicæ*: | Quarum prior agit de | FERMENTATIONE, | *SIVE* | De motu inteſtino particularum | in quovis corpore; | *ALTERA* | DE FEBRIBUS, | *SIVE* | De motu earundem in ſangui- | ne Animalium. | *His acceſsit Diſſertatio Epiſtolica* | DE URINIS. | STUDIO | THOMÆ WILLIS, *ex Æde* Chriſti | Oxon M.D. & in iſta Celeberrima Academia | Naturalis Philoſophiæ Profeſſoris *Sidleiani.* | EDITIO | *Poſtrema prioribus longè emendatior* | *atque auctior.* | [ornament] | AMSTELODAMI, | [short rule] | Apud GERBRANDUS SCHAGHEN. | M DC LXIX.

Collation: duodecimo; 23 letter roman alphabet using I: $*^{12}$, $**^{6}$, A–R^{12}; \$1–6 signed (all leaves 5 and 6 in italics).

222 leaves: paginated as [36], [Fol] 1–408. Mispaginated: page 47 blank and unnumbered, 156 for 159, 278 for 178, 295 for 195, 196 for 198, 197 for 199, 226 for 229, and 226 for 326.

Type: 41 lines; height (20 lines) 53 millimetres, width 58 millimetres.

Contents: ***1r**, page [1], engraved frontispiece, ***1v**, page [2], blank; ***2r**, page [3], title; ***2v**, page [4], blank; ***3r**–***4r**, pages [5–7], Amico Lectori. PRÆFATIO. [De Fermentatione]; ***4v**–***5r**, pages [8–9], *AUTHORI*, In illius Diatribas Medico-Philoſophicas. *Carmen gratulatorium. …* [signed] PHILIPPUS FELL, *Med. Stud. Oxon.*; ***5v**–***9r**, pages [10–17], ELENCHUS RERUM *In Tractatu* DE FERMENTATIONE.; ***9v**–****2v**, pages [18–28], ELENCHUS RERUM *In Tractatu* DE FEBRIBUS.; ****2v**–****4r**, pages [28–31], ELENCHUS RERUM *In Diſſertatione* DE URINIS.; ****4v**–****6v**, pages [32–6], Amico Lectori. PRÆFATIO. [De Febribus].

A1r–E5r, pages 1–105, [text] DE FERMENTATIONE, *SIVE* De *Motu* corporum naturalium *inorganico.*; **E5r–P11v**, pages 105–358, [text] DE FEBRIBUS

P12r–Q1v, pages 359–62, DE URINIS Diſſertatio Epiſtolica A D *Virum Doctiſſimum mihique* AMICISSIMUM, D. RADULPHUM BATHURST, Med. Doct. & Collegii S. Sanctæ Trinitatis Oxon. Socium.

Q2r–R12v, pages 363–408, [text] DE URINIS.

Headlines and *Catchwords*: ELENCVS for ELENCHUS at ****1r**–****4r**, pages [25]–[31]; ':' for '.' after header at **A2r**, page 3; **A10r**, page 19; **A10v**, page 20; **C6v**, page 60; **C7r**, page 61; **D1r**, page 73; **D2v**, page 76; **D9v**, page 90; text blank and no page number at **B12r**, page 47; FERMENTATIONEj for FERMENTATIONE. at **D7r**, page 85; FERBRIBUS. for FEBRIBUS. at **E7v**, page 110.

ELEN for In at ***9r** / **v**, pages [17] / [18]; pif- for Pifcium at **E2r** / **v**, pages 99 / 100; quæ) for que) at **G1v** / **G2r**, pages 146 / 147; primum for Primum at **L8v** / **L9r**, pages 256 / 257; Quoad for Quod at **L12r** / **v**, pages 263 / 264.

Frontispiece: **F.1c2.** Engraved allegorical frontispiece with oblique text: *Ita res accendunt lumina rebus* [diagonal, bottom left to top right] AMSTELODAMI, *Apud Gerbrandus Schagen. Anno 1669.*; 133 × 72 millimetres (sheet), 131 × 70 millimetres (plate marks), 126 × 65 millimetres (image).

Portrait: none.

Printers' ornaments: design of four fleurons, one rotated to the left and one to the right above two inverted {**Schagen 1**}, the upper pair separated by one fleuron {**Schagen 2**}, on the title page at ***2r**, page [3]; tailpiece at ****6v**, page [36] {**Schagen 6**}; headpiece at **A1r**, page 1{**Schagen 12**}; tailpiece at **P11v**, page 358 {**Schagen 11**}.

Decorated D at ***3r**, page [5] {**Schagen 3**}; I at **A1r**, page 1 {**Schagen 5**}; C at **Q2r**, page 363 {**Schagen 13**}.

Illustrations: none.

Copy: DASC (#1 of 2). Early full vellum with stubs of ties (missing), spine with shelf mark 126, original endpapers. Leaves 127 × 71 millimetres, boards 133 × 72 × 40 millimetres.

IG. [DIATRIBÆ DUÆ MEDICO-PHILOSOPHICÆ] DE URINIS, Trajecti ad Rhenum (Utrecht) octavo 1670

The seventh issue of the treatise on urines from Willis's first book, printed within a collected work on urines [HJR Wing 66].

In: ACTUARII | JOHANNIS ZACHARIÆ | FILII, | *Græciæ Medici principis*, | DE | URINIS | LIBRI VII. | Accedunt huic editioni aliorum medi- | corum differtationes de Urinis, | *Quorum nomina verfa pagina indicat.* | [printers' ornament] | TRAJECTI Ad RHENUM | Ex Officinà GISBERTI à ZYLL, Bibliopolæ | Anno cIↃ IↃ c LXX. [22]

[22] The collective title is slightly confusing. Depending on how the count is made, the volume either consists of eight or eleven separate items. It is made up of four works by Actuarius, together comprising seven libri, and four by other authors: [1] Actuarius, *De differentiis omnibus urinarum*; [2 and 3] Actuarius, *De judiciis urinarum*; [4 and 5] Actuarius, *De caufis urinarum*; and [6 and 7] Actuarius, *De prævidentiis ex urinis*. This is followed by [8] Jodoci Willichii, *De probationibus urinarum, cum scholis medicis Hyeronimi Reusneri M. D. & Remedia plurima ex urina defumpta*; [9] Thomas Willis's *Differtatio de urinis*; [10] Guielmi Straneni, *Difputationes medicæ tres, de erroribus popularibus prima, de fallaci urinarum judico*; and [11] Aristotelis Stagiritæ & Antonii Tilefii, *Liber de coloribus*. The book collates as *8, A^8–V^2, *A^6*, *B^8–Z^8*, Aa^8–Gg^8. 400 leaves: paginated as [16], 1–320, 1–224, 227–[461], [3]. The Wellcome copy (EPB/B10244) lacks the half-title, π1, whereas the British Library copy (540.d.22) is complete and has this leaf bound following the final work, after Gg6v, page [3].

Collation: octavo; 23 letter roman alphabet using I: [Willis's treatise, the ninth of eleven] π1, *V*6r–*Bb*4v: $1–5 signed.

39 leaves: paginated as 301–78.

Type: 30 lines; height (20 lines) 82 millimetres, width 65 millimetres.

Contents: [9]. **π1r**, page [1], half-title, THOMÆ WILLIS *Diſſertationes* DE URINIS., **π1v**, blank (bound in the preliminaries before *1); ***V*6r–V7r**, pages 301–3, THOMÆ WILLIS ELENCHUS RERUM *In diſſertatione* DE URINIS.; **V7v–X1v**, pages 304–8, DE URINIS DISSERTATIO EPISTOLICA A D *Virum Doctiſſimum mihique* AMICISSIMUM, D. RADULPHUM BATHURST, Med. Doct. & Collegii S. Sanctæ Trinitatis Oxon. Socium.

X2r–Bb4v, pages 309–78, [text] DE URINIS.

Headlines and *Catchwords*: no '.' after header at **X2v**, page 310; **Y2r–v**, pages 325–6; **Z7v–Z8v**, pages 352–4; **Aa3v–Aa4r**, pages 360–1; **Aa6v**, page 366; **Bb3r**, page 375; *359* for 359 at **Aa3r**, page 359.

nem for eorumque at **Y8v / Z1r**, pages 338 / 339.

Frontispiece: none.

Portrait: none.

Printers' ornament: tailpiece at **Bb4v**, page 378 {**Zyll 1**}.

No decorated initials.

Illustrations: none.

Copy: DASC, lacking X^8. Original paper boards, spine with shelf mark No jj and red paper label O 192, red bordered white paper label *Willis Thomas Dissertation. de urinis*, original endpapers. Leaves 150 × 100 millimetres, boards 157 × 100 × 45 × millimetres. Shelf mark: O- I|3 e192. Stamped: Ad Bibliothecam FT Minor Suazen Sidet (unidentified).

1H. [DIATRIBÆ DUÆ MEDICO-PHILOSOPHICÆ] DE FERMENTATIONE, Middelburg and Amsterdam octavo 1676

A Dutch translation of the treatises on fermentation and on scurvy from Willis's first and third books, respectively [Wing 67].

Title page: [1]. TH. WILLIS. | *Nieuwe en Geneeſkundige verhandeling vande* | FERMENTATIE | ofte RYSING, | Hoedanig ons die inde beſchouwing aller | MINERALEN, PLANTEN, DIEREN, | En andere lichamen, ten aanſien harer voort-teeling, aangroejing, | verwiſſeling, ſterven en ontdoeninge, als in der ſelver | CHYMISCHE Behandeling | Voorkomt. | *Leerende uit d' Algemeene Grond-veſt der Stof-* | *ſcheyding, op een ligt verſtanelijke manier de ware kenniſſe der Natuur-* | *kundige beginſelen tot alle Genees-kundige waar-nemingen, en* | *ARTZENY* Bereidingen | *Over-brengen.* | Benneffens een Tractaat van des | SCHEURBUIKS OORSPRONG, | Soorten, toevallen en konſtige Geneſing, volgens de Nieu- | we *Chymiſche Gronden* van den ſelven Autheur. | *Beide nu eerſt tot dienſt der Heel-meeſters en Apotekers* | *uyt het Latÿn vertaalt en door-gaans met Aan-* | *teykeningen en Blat-wÿſer verrÿkt.* | [ornament] | Tot MIDDELBURGH, | [short rule] | By *Wilhelmus Goeree*, Book-verkooper in *Cicero*. En ſijn mede te be- | komen, tot *Amſterdam*, by *Ioh. Ianſonius van Waaſberge*. 1676.[23]

[2]. (as in **3C**) DES | SCHEUR—BUIKS | Oorſprong, ſoorten, toe-vallen | en konſtige Geneſing, volgens | de nieuwe Chijmiſche Gronden, | *Van den Vermaarden Heer* | THOMAS WILLIS, | *Hoog-Leeraar tot Oxfordt*; *Nauw-* | *keuriger als oyt verhandelt.* | Nu eerſt uit het Latijn Vertaalt, en met | Genees-kundige Aan-teykeningen en Blad- | wijſer Verrijkt. | [printers' ornament] | Tot MIDDELBURGH, | [short rule] | By *Wilhelmus Goeree*, Book-verkooper | in Cicero. 1676.[24]

Collation: octavo; 23 letter roman alphabet using I and V: $*^6$, A–K^8, L^2, M–Z^8, Aa^8; \$1–5 signed apart from: *4 signed *5, B3 signed B5, -G5, -I2, Aa1 signed A2.

192 leaves: paginated as [12], [Fol] 1–344, [28].

Type: 35 lines; height (20 lines) 68 millimetres, width 61 millimetres (77 with marginal notes).

Contents: ***1r**, page [1], title; ***1v**, page [2], blank; ***2r**–***3v**, pages [3–6], Voor-reden van *Thomas Willis*, Aanden Weet-gierigen LESER.; [***4r**]–***6v**, pages [7–12], Den Oversetter *Tot den LESER*.[25]

A1r–**L2v**, pages 1–164, [text] Van de Fermentatie, of natuurlijke beweging, die ſonder Werktuig in de lichamen verwerkt werd.[26]

M1r, page [165], [second title page]; **M1v**, page 166, blank; **M2r**–**M4v**, pages 167–72, Den Overſetter *Tot den LESER*.; **M5r**–**Z2v**, pages 173–344, [text] Verhandeling Van het SCHEUR—BUIK.[27]

[23] Underlined text originally printed in red. 'TH. WILLIS. *New and Medical treatise on* FERMENTATION or ACCENSION, How this appears to us in the consideration of all MINERALS, PLANTS, ANIMALS And other bodies, with respect to their procreation, growth, transmutation, demise and dissolution, as well as in their CHEMICAL Treatment *Teaching from the General Foundation of separation of Matter, to pass on in an easily understandable manner the true knowledge of the Physical principles of all Medical observations, and* PHARMACEUTICAL Recipes. In addition a Treatise on the ORIGIN of SCURVY, Categories, complications, and artful Curation, according to the new *Chemical Foundations* of the same Author. *Both only now for the benefit of Surgeons and Apothecaries Translated from Latin and throughout enriched by Comments and Index.* In MIDDELBURGH, At *Wilhelmus Goeree*, Bookseller in *Cicero*. And they are also available in *Amsterdam*, at *Joh. Jansonius van Waasberge*. 1676'.

[24] 'ABOUT SCURVY Origin, categories, complications and artful Curation, according to The new Chemical Foundations, *Of the Famous Gentleman* THOMAS WILLIS, Professor in Oxford, explained more precisely than before. Only now Translated from Latin, and enriched with Medical Comments and Index In MIDDELBURGH, At *Wilhelmus Goeree*, Bookseller in Cicero. 1676'.

[25] 'Preface of *Thomas Willis*, To the curious READER'; and 'The Translator *To the READER*'.

[26] 'About the Fermentation, or natural movement, which took place in the bodies without Instrument'.

[27] 'The Translator *to the READER*' and 'Treatise On SCURVY'.

Z3r–Aa6r, pages [1–23], Blad- Wijſer [Index]; **Aa6v–Aa8v** [24–8], blank.

Headlines and *Catchwords*: inconsistent use of 'van' on versos throughout: Van de for vande at **E5v–F3v**, pages 74–86; **G3v**, page 102; van de for vande on versos only at **F4v–F6v**, pages 88–92, **G2v**, page 100, **G5v–G6v**, pages 106–8; Van't for van't at **G8v**, page 112; **H1v**, page 114; **H5v**, page 122; **H6v**, page 124; **I1v**, page 130; **I2v**, page 132; **I4v**, page 136; **K1v**, page 146; **K5v**, page 154; **K6v**, page 156; **L1v**, page 162; **L2v**, page 164; Vande for Van de at **R4v**, page 252, **S5v**, 270, and **T1v**, page 278; *Bloed* for *Zenu-sap* at **Q1r**, page 229; *uit 't Zenu-sap ontſtaande* for *uit het Bloed enZen. Enz.* at **R2r**, page 247.

No catchword at ***6v / A1r**, page [12] / 1; uit- for (*o*) uit at **A2r / v**, pages 3 / 4; aan for (*a*) aan at **A3r / v**, pages 5 / 6; de geeſt for geeſt at **A4v / A5r**, pages 8 / 9; Wat for wat at **D1v / D2r**, pages 50 / 51; (*d*) pijpjes for *d* pijpjes at **E1r / E1v**, pages 65 / 66; onder for dericheide at **K5r / v**, pages 153 / 154; verbrand for brand at **N6r / v**, pages 191 / 192; op-sie for opsie at **Q3r / Q3v**, pages 233 / 234; *Her* for *ſenen* at **Q5r / v**, pages 237 / 238 (footnote); ſterk for ſterck at **R5v / R6r**, pages 254 / 255.

Frontispiece: none.

Portrait: none.

Printers' ornaments: tailpiece at ***6v**, page [12] {**Goeree 3**}; headpiece at **M1r**, page 165 {**Goeree 5**}; tailpiece **Aa6r**, page [23] {**Goeree 8**}.

Decorated A at ***2r**, page [3] {**Goeree 1**}; W at [*4]r, page [7] {**Goeree 2**}; I at **A1r**, page 1{**Goeree 4**}; B at **M2r**, page 167 {**Goeree 6**}; B at **M5r**, page 173 {**Goeree 7**}.

Illustrations: none.

Copy: DASC. Original full vellum, spine with faded lettering in manuscript, original end-papers. Leaves 155 × 95 millimetres, boards 165 × 97 × 30 millimetres.

11. DIATRIBÆ DUÆ MEDICO-PHILOSOPHICÆ, London duodecimo 1677

The seventh edition of Willis's first book, with the engraved frontispiece in its first state [HJR Wing 7].

Title page: *Diatribæ duæ Medico-Philoſophicæ*: | Quarum Prior agit | DE | FERMENTATIONE, | SIVE, DE | MOTU inteſtino particularum in quovis corpore; | ALTERA, DE | FEBRIBUS, | SIVE, DE | MOTU earundem in Sanguine Animalium. | His acceſſit | Diſſertatio Epiſtolica de | URINIS. | [rule] | STUDIO | THOMÆ WILLIS, ex *Æde Chriſti* Oxon. | M.D. & in iſta celeberrima Academia Na- | turalis Philoſophiæ Profeſſoris *Sidleiani.* | [rule] | Editio Quarta, | Ab AUTHORE recognita, atque ab eodem | multiplici Auctario locupletata. | [rule] | *LONDINI.* | Typis *T.R.* Impenſis *J. Martyn,* proſtant apud *Sa-* | *muelem Carr,* Bibliopolam. MDCLXXVII.

Collation: duodecimo; 23 letter roman alphabet using I: A^{12}, a^{8}, f^{*4}, B–Q^{12}, R^{8}, S^{4}; $1–5 signed apart from: -D3, E2 signed F2, M3 signed N3, -R5.

216 leaves: paginated as [48], 1–376, [8]. Mispaginated: 142 for 143.

Type: 42 lines; height (20 lines) 57 millimetres, width 59 millimetres.

Contents: **A1r**, page [1], blank; **A1v**, page [2], [poem] ARtis *ope ætherios* Natura *exſuſcitat ignes, / Et cœlo attonitos, hâc ſamulante, vocat. / Huic mox acceptas porrectâ lampade flammas / Reddit, & indè novum creſcit utrique jubar. /* Sic lucem *unanimes* terris *tribuëre* ſorores, / *Et* lucem *unanimes ſic tribuëre* ſibi.; **A2r**, page [3], engraved allegorical frontispiece; **A2v**, page [4], blank; **A3r**, page [5], title; **A3v**, page [6], blank; **A4r–A6r**, pages [7–11], Reverendiſſimo in *CHRISTO* Patri, Honoratiſſimoque Domino D^no.^ GILBERTO Divinâ Providentiâ Archiepiſcopo *Cantuarienſi, Totius ANGLIÆ Primati & Metropolitano, & Sereniſſimæ REGIÆ Majeſtati à Conſiliis Sanctoribus.* ... [signed] *Clementiæ veſtræ Humillimus, & æternùm Addictiſſimus THO. WILLIS.*; **A6v**, page [12], blank; **A7r–A9v**, pages [13–18], Amico Lectori PRÆFATIO. [De Fermentatione]; **A10r–A10v**, page [19–20], AUTHORI *In illius Diatribas Medico-Philoſophicas* CARMEN GRATULATORIUM ... [signed] *Philippus Fell. Med. Stud. Oxon.*; **A11r–a2r**, pages [21–7], Elenchus RERUM IN TRACTATU DE FERMENTATIONE.; **a2v–a6v**, pages [28–36] Elenchus RERUM IN TRACTATU DE FEBRIBUS.; **a7r–a8r**, pages [37–9], Elenchus RERUM in Diſſertatione De URINIS.; **a8v**, page [40], blank; **f*1r–f*4v**, pages [41–8] *AMICO LECTORI* PRÆFATIO. [De Febribus].

B1r–E12v, pages 1–96, [text] DE FERMENTATIONE, sive De *motu* corporum naturalium *inorganico.*; **F1r–P10v**, pages 97–328, [text] DE FEBRIBUS.

P9r–P11r, pages 329–33, DE URINIS *Diſſertatio epiſtolica* AD Virum Doctiſſimum mihique AMICISSIMUM, D. RADULPHUM BATHURST, Med. Doct. & Collegii S. Sanctae Trinitatis Oxon. Socium.

P11r–R12v, pages 333–76, [text] DE URINIS.

S1r–S4v, pages [1–8], Catalogus librorum qui proſtant venales apud *Joannem Martyn* ad Inſigne *Campanæ* in Cœmeterio *Paulino*.

Headlines and *Catchwords*: no ⁚ after header at **a1r**, page [25]; **B12r**, page 23; EE FEBRIBUS for DE FEBRIBUS at **F2v**, page 100; DEFEBRIBUS for DE FEBRIBUS at **H7r–H8r**, pages 157–159; DB FEBRIBUS for DE FEBRIBUS at **H9r**, page 161.

No catchword at **A10v / A11r**, pages [20]–[21]; particulæ for ticulæ at **A12r / v**, pages [23] / [24]; cipuè for cipue at **F3r / v**, pages 101 / 102; optimè for optime at **F8r / v**, pages 111 / 112; cebat for ſcebat at **I4r / v**, pages 175 / 176; par for ticulis at **K1r / v**, pages 193 / 194; inanita for nanita at **K10v / K11r**, pages 212 / 213; factam for fectem at **K12v / M1r**, pages 240 / 241; Alexiphar for alixiphar at **M2r / v**, pages 243 / 244; φωνία for ἀφωνία at **N7v / N8r**, pages 278 / 279; propter for Propter at **O8v / O9r**, pages 304 / 305; phureæ for Sulphureæ at **Q9r / v**, pages 355 / 356.

Frontispiece: **F.1a1**. Engraved allegorical frontispiece with oblique text (diagonal, top left to bottom right): –*Ita res accendunt lumina rebus*: 150 × 89 millimetres (sheet), 122 × 69 millimetres (plate marks), 118 × 66 millimetres (image).

Portrait: none.

Printers' ornaments: headpiece at **A4r**, page [7]; **B1r**, page 1; **P11r**, page 333 {**Roycroft 21**}; row of 20 fleurons with : between ##11 / 12 at **A10r**, page [19]; and : between ##10 / 11 with #20 rotated at **a7r**, page [37]; and with #20 upright at **P9r**, page 329 {**Roycroft 8**}; row of 3 fleurons {**Roycroft 11**} and 7 fleurons {**Roycroft 17**} at **A11r**, page [21]; and with : between ##5 / 6 at **a2v**, page [28]; headpiece {**Roycroft 27**} at **F1r**, page 97.

Decorated S at **A4r**, page [7] {**Roycroft 26**}; D at **A7r**, page [13] {**Roycroft 23**}; D at **f*1**, page [41] {**Roycroft 19**}; I at **B1r**, page 1 {**Roycroft 24**}.

Illustrations: none.

Copy: Wellcome (EPB/A/53351). Original calf boards (detached), spine with three raised bands and red label WILLIS | DIATRIBAE | 1677 (later pen and ink), lacking endpapers. Leaves 150 × 89 millimetres, boards 157 × 90 × 27 millimetres. Inserted: bookplate CE BAGGE MD. Shelf marks: (1) A.xxx.w; (2) 53351 / A; (3) 13 A; (4) 31141. Inscribed: Wm Goulis [?] Coll. Wadh (unidentified).[28]

1J. [DIATRIBÆ DUÆ MEDICO-PHILOSOPHICÆ] DE FEBRIBUS, DE URINIS, Amsterdam octavo 1681

Dutch translation of the treatises on fevers and on urines from Willis's first book [not listed by HJR Wing].

Title page: T. WILLIS | Nieuwe Verhandeling van de | KOORSEN, | Of | *Der zelver beweging in 't bloed* | *der Dieren,* | Als ook een befchryving der | MENSCHELYKE | WATEREN. | *Tot dienft en gemeene nut van alle Lief-hebbers.* | Uit het Latyn vertaalt, en met noodige aan- | teikeningen verrykt, | DOOR S. B. *Med. Doct.* | [ornament] | t'AMSTERDAM.[*] | [rule] | By JOHANNES ten HOORN, Boekverkooper | tegen over 't Oude Heere Logement. 1681.[29]

Collation: octavo; 23 letter roman alphabet using I and V: $*^4$, A–Z^8; Aa–Hh^8, Ii^4; \$1–5 signed apart from: Dd3 signed Dd5.

[28] Charles Elsdon Bagge (d.1799) studied medicine (MB 1774, MD 1779) and was subsequently a fellow of Caius College, Cambridge. He practised briefly in London (MRCP 1779, FRCP 1780) and at Lynn Regis (King's Lynn) and finally East Dereham where he died (*c.*1798). Several surviving items with his bookplate are recorded.

[29] 'T. WILLIS New Treatise of the FEVERS, Or, *Their movement in the Blood of Animals,* As well as a description of the HUMAN WATERS. *To The benefit and general utility of all Interested persons.* Translated from Latin, and enriched with necessary notes, By S.B. *Physician* In AMSTERDAM. At JOHANNES ten HOORN, Bookseller across the Old Hotel for Gentlemen. 1681.'

[*] Underlined text originally printed in red.

256 leaves: paginated as [8], 1–416, [6], 417–490, [8]. Mispaginated: as [8], 1–257, 238–353, 254, 355–357, 360–375, 276, 377–397 [398]; [6], 399–423, 414, 425–465, 468–473 [474], [8].

Type: 34 lines; height (20 lines) 69 millimetres, width 61 millimetres (76 millimetres with marginal notes).

Contents: ***1r** title, page [1]; ***1v** blank, page [2]; ***2r–*3v**, pages [3–6], OPDRACHT en VOORREDEN. *Aan den Voordeſtigen Heer, de Heer* JOHAN VAN DUEREN *S. Theol. C. Med. & Philoſ. Doctor, out Schepen &c. tot Gorkum. . . .* [signed] Amſterdam MDCLXXXI, den 12 Junii. *Ootmoedige Dienaar en Vriend* S BLANKAART *Med. Doct.*;[30] ***4r–v**, pages [7–8], KORTE INHOUD. *Van de Hooſt-ſlukken* des BOEKS, Handelende van de Koorsen.; ***4v**, page [8], KORTE INHOUD. *Van de Hooſt-flukken* des BOEKS, Handelende van de Pis.

A1r–Cc8r, pages 1–'397', [text] THOMAS WILLIS Verhandeling der KOORSEN.; **Cc8v**, page ['398'], blank.

Dd1r, page [1], [half-title] T. WILLIS Beſchryving der MENSCHELYKE WATEREN.; **Dd1v**, page [2]; blank; **Dd2r–[Dd3]v**, pages [3–6], Briefs gewyſe Beſchryving der Menſchelyke Wateren, *Aan den zeer geleerden, en mynen zeer beminden Heer* RADOLPH BATHURST, *Genees-kundige, en Makker van 't geſelſchap der Dry-eenigheid tot Oxford.*[31]

Dd4r–Hh8r, pages '399'–'473', [text] T. WILLIS. Verhandeling van de MENSCHELYKE WATEREN.; **Hh8v**, page '474', blank.

Ii1r–Ii4v, pages [1–8], AANWYSER, *Der voornaamſte ſaken, die in de verhandeling der* KOORSEN *En Pisbegrepen zyn.*

Headlines and *Catchwords*: *d'Ontleding* for *d'Ontlediging* at **A1v**, page 2; *dagelykze* for *dagelykse* at **F4v**, page 88; *derdendaagſe* for *derden-daagſe* at **F5v**, page 90; *koors* for *Koors* at **G2r**, page 99; **G4r**, page 103; **H3r**, page 117, *koorſen* for *Koorſen* at **G7r**, page 109; *Peſt-en quaadaardige* for *peſt-en quaadaardige* at **S1v**, page 254; **S3v**, page '258'; *Kinder-pokjes* for *kinder-pokjes* at **S5v**, page '262'; *Maſelen* for *maſelen* at **S6r**, page '263'; **T4r**, page '283'; *kraam-kooſen* for *Kraam-kooſen* at **X3r**, page '305'; **Z2r**, page '335'; **Z3r**, page '337'; *algemeene Korſen* for *algemeene korſen* at **Z6v**, page '344'; *Van de veelte en koleur* for *in de pis der ziekeni* at **Ff1r**, page '425'.

No catchword at ***3v** / ***4r**, pages [6] / [7]; ſtof- for (*o*) Stoffcheiders at **A2v** / **A3r**, pages 4 / 5; koor for Koorſen at **K7v** / **K8r**, pages 158 / 159; de for welke at **T8v** / **V1r**, page '284' / '285'; Eens for Eenſ at **Z2v** / **Z3e**, pages '336' / '337'; lym- for ymagtig[32] at **Ee2v** / **Ee3r**, pages '412' / '413'; Re- for AAN at **Hh8r–Ii1r**, pages '473'–[1].

[30] 'DEDICATION and PREFACE. *To the Highly Respectable Gentleman, Mr.* JOHAN VAN DUEREN *S. Theol. Med. & Philos. Doctor, former Alderman in Gorkum . . . Humble Servant and Friend* S. BLANKAART *Med. Doct.* Amsterdam MDCLXXXI, on June 12th. / BRIEF TABLE OF CONTENTS. The chapters of the BOOK, with a Treatise on the Fevers. / BRIEF TABLE OF CONTENTS. The chapters of the BOOK, with a Treatise on the Urine.'

[31] 'THOMAS WILLIS Description of the HUMAN WATERS / Description in the form of Letters on the Human Waters, *To the highly learned and to me very dear Gentleman* RADOLPH BATHURST, *Physician, and Fellow of Trinity College in Oxford.*'

[32] DASC (#2) has '*gylis' added as a catchword in pen and ink but the asterisk relates to '*en 't voe-' earlier in the text, not type that follows onto the next page.

Frontispiece: none.

Portrait: none.

Printers' ornaments: tailpiece on title page at ***1r**, page [1] {**Schagen 16**}; **Hh8r**, page 473 {**Schagen 19**}.

Decorated D at ***4r**, page [7] {**Leers 9**}; H at **Dd2r**, page [3] {**Hoorn 1**}; W at **Dd4r**, page '399' {**Hoorn 2**}.

Illustrations: none.

Copy: DASC (#1 of 2). Original full calf; spine (relaid with small upper part missing) with four raised bands, gilt tooling, and label WILLIS | VAN DE | COORSEN, original endpapers. Leaves 147 × 88 millimetres, boards 154 × 94 × 37 millimetres. Inscribed: Wm Feindel Montréal. Stamped: S DOBBELEERS-VERSIENE VELDSTRAAT, 62 BORGERHOUT-ANTWERPEN (presumed bookseller, unidentified).

1K1. [DIATRIBÆ DUÆ MEDICO-PHILOSOPHICÆ] DISSERTATION SUR LES URINES, Paris duodecimo 1683

First issue of the French translation of the treatise on urines from Willis's first book [HJR Wing 65].

Title page: DISSERTATION | SUR | LES URINES. | Tirée des Ouvrages de | WILLIS tres— celebre | Medecin d'Angleterre. | *Nouvellement miſe en François,* | *Par **** | [ornament] | A PARIS, | Chez LAURENT D'HOURY, | ruë S. Jacques au S. Eſprit | prés les Mathurins. | [rule] | M. DC. LXXXIII. | *Avec Approbation & Permiſſion.*

Collation: duodecimo; 23 letter roman alphabet using I: ã^{8} (-a8), A^{8} B^{4}–L^{8} M^{4}, N^{8}, O1 (= a8); $i–iiij and i–ii signed, apart from:–ãiiij.

88 leaves: paginated as [14], 1–162. Mispaginated: 13 for 133.

Type: 24 lines; height (20 lines) 94 millimetres, width 59 millimetres.

Contents: (converting signatures to Arabic numbers) **ã1r**, page [1], title; **ã1v**, page [2], blank; **ã2r–ã6v**, pages [3–12], EPISTRE EN FORME de diſſertation à Monſieur Rodolphe Bathhurſt Docteur en Medecine, & mon Collegue dans le College de la Sainte Trinité d'Oxford.; **ã7r**, page [13], TABLE des Chapitres.; **ã7v**, page [18], *APPROBATION.* LA Faculté aprés avoir vû la traduction d'un Traité des Urines tiré des Ouvrages de WILLIS, conſent ſon Edition. Ce troiſième Juillet 1682. Lienard *Doyen. VEu l'Approbation, permis d'imprimer. Fait ce ſeptième Aouſt* 1682. DE LA REYNIE.

A1r–O1v, pages 1–162, [text] DISSERTATION SUR LES URINES.

Headlines and *Catchwords*: no ⁚ after header at **ã5r**, page [9]; *Vrines* for *Urines* at **H2r**, page 91; **H3r**, page 93; **I8r**, page 111; **K3r**, page 117; **K4r**, page 119; **L1r**, page 121; **L6r**, page 131; **M4r**, page 143; **N4r**, page 151; **N5r**, page 153.

Present only at interval between signatures, i.e. **A8v** / **B1r**, pages 16 / 17, apart from: no catchword at **L8v** / **M1r**, pages 136 / 137.

Frontispiece: none.

Portrait: none.

Printers' ornaments: headpiece at title page **ã1r**, page [1] {**D'Houry 1**}; headpiece at **ã2r**, page [3]; **A1r**, page 1 {**D'Houry 2**}; tailpiece at **ã6v**, page [12] {**D'Houry 4**}; row of 12 fleurons ##1–3, 5, 7, and 10 {**D'Houry 5**} and ##4, 6, 8, 9, 11, and 12 {**D'Houry 6**} with : between ##5 / 6, 8 / 9 at **ã7r**, page [13]; row of 12 fleurons ##1–5, 7, 9–11 {**D'Houry 5**}, ##6, 8, and 12 {**D'Houry 6**} with *:* between ##9 / 10 at **ã7v**, page [14]; two rows of fleurons (three upper and two lower) at **C2r**, page 27; **G8v**, page 88 {**D'Houry 8**}; tailpiece at **O1v**, page 162 {**D'Houry 9**}.

Decorated M at **ã2r**, page [3] {**D'Houry 3**}; Q at **A1r**, page 1{**D'Houry 7**}.

Illustrations: none.

Copy: Wellcome (14328214). Original full sprinkled calf, spine with five raised bands, gilt tooling, and label TRAI | DES | URIN, original endpapers. Leaves 153 × 85 millimetres, boards 158 × 89 × 18 millimetres. Ex libris R Deschamps Anno 1741 (unidentified). Shelf marks: (1) E xii f; (2) 53359 / A; (3) I^{II}; (4) 42550.

1K2. [DIATRIBÆ DUÆ MEDICO-PHILOSOPHICÆ] DISSERTATION SUR LES URINES, Paris duodecimo 1687

Second issue of the French translation of the treatise on urines from Willis's first book, with the title page reset [not distinguished from HJR Wing 65].

Title page: DISSERTATION | SUR | LES URINES. | Tirée des Ouvrages de | VVILLIS tres—celebre | Medecin d'Angleterre. | *Nouvellement mif en François,* | *Par* *** [not centred] | SECONDE EDITION. | [printers' ornaments] | A PARIS, | Chez LAURENT D'HOURY, | ruë S. Jacques, devant la Fontaine | S. Severin au Saint Efprit | [rule] | M. DC. LXXXVII. | *Avec Approbation & Permiffion.*

Then as in **1K1** apart from:

Collation: Mispaginated: 13 for 133, altered to 135 for 133.

Printers' ornaments: headpiece replaced by inverted triangle of three fleurons, two upper {**D'Houry 10**} and one lower {**D'Houry 11**}, on title page at **ã1r**, page [1].

Illustrations: none.

Copy: DASC. Original full sprinkled calf, spine with five raised bands, gilt tooling, and label DISSER | LES | URINE, original endpapers. Leaves 153 × 85 millimetres, boards 159 × 90 × 17 millimetres. Inserted: bookplate (1) e Bibliotheca Andreae Comitis Renard; (2) Ex libris hans joachim reuter. Inscribed: Buichen (unidentified).[33]

[33] Several books have appeared on the market since the 1990s containing the crested bookplate of Andreae Comitis Renard (nd), engraved in 1769 by CF Holtmann (nd), and that of Hans by Hans Joachim Reuter (1923–2003), who served in the Second World War on the Eastern Front but returned to Germany when injured in 1942 and studied medicine in Tübingen and Heidelberg. After qualification in 1950 he trained in urology and worked in Stuttgart publishing a renowned endoscopic atlas in two volumes (1963–1980).

6

'Addicted to the opening of heads'

Cerebri anatome (1664–1683)

Cerebri anatome cui accessit nervorum deſcriptio et usus, containing his fourth and fifth treatises, is Thomas Willis's second book and the first to be illustrated.[1] It was completed at Beam Hall, which Willis leased from Corpus Christi College, in 1662. The imprimatur is dated 20 January 1663.[2] Quarto and octavo editions with the title page dated 1664 were printed and sold in London. Two duodecimo editions were published from Amsterdam in the same year.[3] There were four further editions from 1666 to 1683, the first octavo and the others in duodecimo format. Harold Denham (1917–1999) provides a useful narrative of the early publication history.[4]

The London issues

It is reasonable to conclude that although production of the London quarto (**2A**) and octavo (**2B**) editions may have overlapped, the quarto appeared first.[5] There was a degree of co-operation between James Flesher (d.1670) and Thomas Roycroft (d.1677)—who printed the quarto and octavo editions, respectively—and the booksellers for each, John Martyn (1618–1680) and James Allestry (d.1670). Both editions ran into difficulties. The most obvious problem relates to the fifteen plate leaves. These are headed Figuræ I–VIII and Tabulæ IX–XIII, with two unnumbered. As explained in chapter 3, the plates are designated Pl.1–Pl.15 in this bibliography, in the order in which they are usually bound: Figuræ I–VI, unnumbered 1, Figuræ VII–VIII, unnumbered 2, and Tabulæ IX–XIII.

Allowing for some speculation, it seems likely that the two unnumbered plates (Pl.7, Pl.10) did not become available until production of the quarto issue was already well advanced.

[1] See chapter 3 for discussion of provenance for the artwork; and chapter 16 for an account of the anatomical information depicted in the illustrations.

[2] It is sometimes argued that the imprimatur may not be called for in the earliest issue. For example a bookseller's entry for *c.*2016 reads: 'This copy was bound without the imprimatur leaf, which may not have been added to the first copies issued. A copy sold at Sotheby's in 1967 (16–17 October, lot 359), uncut in the original boards, lacked the imprimatur leaf. It is also lacking from several copies in institutional collections (e.g. one of the two Wellcome copies).' This defence seems improbable given that the imprimatur was needed to authorize publication. It is dated 20 January 1663 and printed as part of the first sheet at A1 and not as an added leaf. It is best to regard copies without the imprimatur as incomplete.

[3] A copy inscribed by Thomas Willis to Stephen Wentworth esq. is dated 23 January 1664: see Hans Sallander, *Bibliotheca Walleriana. A catalogue of the Erik Waller collection*, Stockholm (1955): page 453, #10315.

[4] See: Harold Denham, In: Ed. William Feindel; *Thomas Willis, The anatomy of the brain and nerves*. Tercentenary edition, volume I, Montreal (1965): pages 67–104.

[5] See: HJR Wing, *A bibliography of Dr Thomas Willis (1621–1675)*, typescript (1962): pages 10–12; and Denham (1965); pages 70 and 85, each of whom gives priority to the quarto. Waller prefers the octavo but without giving reasons: see Sallander (1955): page 453, #10314. Denham (1965): page 72 states that the octavo issue was being prepared before the quarto was published and makes the further point that the printer worked independently from Willis's original manuscript.

The other thirteen were already engraved and numbered. The lack of indicative page placements on the plates beyond Figura VIII (Pl.10) suggests that the printer and engraver were working simultaneously. Because the text had not been set, instructions on where to bind Tabulæ IX–XIII (Pl.11–Pl.15) could not yet be provided. Why the designation changed from Figura to Tabula is not clear but since this is consistent between the plates and their explanatory text, the engraver was presumably following the printer's example. Typesetting of the text had reached somewhere between sheets Q and Qq when the two unnumbered illustrations arrived. The text relevant to the first (Pl.7) was already printed and the type may even have been redistributed. Therefore the explanatory legend had to be printed on an extra leaf signed * with instructions to insert this between P1 and P2, pages 106 and 107 ('interpag. 106 & 107'), which an informed reader, presumably Willis, considered most appropriate. With the second late arrival, unnumbered 2 (Pl.10), there was time to engrave an indicative placement, '*Pag: 302*', and set the legend at Qq2r–Qq3v, pages 299–302, in continuity with typesetting and pagination of the main text.

A different solution was adopted by Thomas Roycroft for the London octavo edition (**2B**). The leaf containing explanatory text for the first unnumbered plate (Pl.7) was again signed * but with an indication to place this at 'Pag. *56*'. Rather than adding an interleaf, it was printed on a8 which would otherwise have been blank since all the preliminaries were accommodated on the 30 pages of A^8, a1–a7. The legend for Pl.7 is usually bound after E4v, page 56, where, contextually, it belongs. The decision was taken not to alter pagination of the adjacent text, which is continuous across E4v, page 56, and E5r, page 57. However in some copies, this leaf is found after a7, page [30], where it was printed. Therefore, wherever * is placed, the octavo issue has page E4v and a second leaf (*) sharing the same pagination, one as '56' and the other as 'Pag. *56*'.[6]

The London octavo has a list of errata, and most of the mistakes listed in the quarto are not present. This does not necessarily establish priority for one or other edition, if the typesetters were working independently from different copies of the manuscript. But the most parsimonious explanation is that it was possible to correct the printed mistakes, widely distributed throughout the quarto, when completing the octavo edition without constantly stopping the press.

It is generally stated that the same plates were used to print illustrations for the quarto (**2A**) and octavo (**2B**) editions. This is correct in principle but requires qualification. In what must be the earliest copies to be distributed (**2B1**), Figuræ I–VIII (Pl.1–6, Pl.8–9), are in the same state as the quarto edition but with the page indicators scored through in pen and ink. In one instance, the new page placement is added, also in manuscript (second unnumbered, Pl.10).[7] However, the first unnumbered plate (Pl.7) is in a new state with '*Pag 56*' now engraved on blank space in the top right corner. Tabulæ IX–XIII (Pl. 11–15) remain unnumbered and are therefore in the same state as the quarto issue. These minor amendments to the illustrations provide further evidence that the octavo followed the quarto edition.

[6] HJR Wing (1962): page 12 also states that the legend for Figure VII (Pl.7) is printed on a cancelled leaf at F3. Only the cancellans is present in all copies examined. The text of this legend is identical to that in the quarto issue, correcting any error that may have required a cancelled leaf.

[7] The probability that sheets and illustrations for the quarto and octavo editions were being gathered and distributed almost certainly from the same workshop and at much the same time is made clear by one copy of the quarto (formerly in the collection of James Tait Goodrich [1946–2020] and now 2A, copy #3) in which Pl.10, the second unnumbered, is present with the placement '*Pag. 302*' printed in the top right corner and bound correctly at page 302, as expected, but with a duplicate on which '*302*' is scored through and 158 added in manuscript and the plate leaf bound at page 158, as in copies of **2B1**.

However a further complication is revealed from copies of the London octavo edition (**2B2**), which must have been put together at a later date. Here the engraved plates have been extensively reworked. The page placements at top right, previously scored through in manuscript, are now erased on the plate (leaving some residual traces) and replaced by details engraved in blank space at the top left corner (apart from Figura VIII, Pl.9 where the new page placement overlies the original fully erased engraving). Details have also been added to Tabulæ IX–XIII (Pl.11–PL.15). With two exceptions, these page numbers are correct for sheets of the London octavo edition. The second unnumbered plate (Pl.10) is marked 'p: 69' and bound at F3r, page 69, within the text of *Cerebri anatome*. Its legend is at L7v–L8v, pages 158–160, in the text of *Nervorum descriptio et usus* where the plate belongs. Tabula XII (Pl.14) is marked 'p: 231' and therefore bound at Q4r, page 231. This has the legend for Tabula XI (Pl.13) which is also marked 'p 231' and correctly placed. Conversely, the legend for Tabula XII (Pl.14) is at Q6r, page 235. Not unreasonably, the second unnumbered plate (Pl.10) and Tabula XII (Pl.14) are found at pages 69 and 231, as instructed, respectively. The errors are in the engraving, not the binding.

But the changes did not stop there. Because the plate and text leaves were printed independently, the availability of each did not necessarily match. The stock of illustrations had periodically to be replenished in order to supplement text sheets and make up copies for sale. The plates had been stored badly or the copper damaged by earlier inking and wiping. This led to two problems. Over time, cracks started to appear, especially affecting Figuræ IIII (Pl.4), unnumbered 1 (Pl.7), and VII (Pl.8), and Tabulæ IX, XI and XII (Pl.11, Pl.13, and Pl.14). Furthermore, Tabulæ IX and XI (Pl.11, Pl.13) had each lost a corner and lower part. Even more problematic was that details of the engraving had been partly erased. Rather than going to the expense of commissioning new engravings, the decision was taken to persist with these damaged plates by extensive reworking of lines, contours, and cross-hatching. Superficially these features appear very different to those in the quarto edition (**2A**) and earlier octavo (**2B1**) copies but closer scrutiny shows evidence for the original work of the burin over which new details have been scored. At what point the damaged engravings were first put back into use, so as to make good sheets of the London octavo, is unclear. The provenance of the copy used in this bibliography which shows these features (**2B2**) puts this at before 1672.[8] And, as explained in chapter 13, those to whom ownership of the engravings passed continued to use many in their increasingly damaged state when printing copies of *The remaining medical works* in 1681 (**9B**).

The Amsterdam issues: printing

Apart from resetting the type for duodecimo format, changes were made to the edition printed when *Cerebri anatome* went to Amsterdam in 1664. The imprimatur, dedication to Gilbert Sheldon (1598–1677), and verse by Philip Fell (*c.*1632–1682) were omitted. Because the errata were corrected, the assumption is that the London octavo edition was used for typesetting. The problematic legend for the first unnumbered illustration (Pl.7) was now integrated into the text. Copies using the same printed sheets were sold by two

[8] See chapter 2 for details of unsold copies of *Cerebri anatome* (1664), the quarto and octavo not distinguished, which were assigned by Thomas Roycroft's widow to Robert Scott (1632–1710) as late as 1683.

different booksellers, Gerbrandt Schagen (b.1633) and Caspar Commelin (1636–1693).[9] Although they worked independently, albeit with a degree of collaboration, the evidence suggests an uneasy relationship. As a result, their issues of *Cerebri anatome* show several differences other than variant title pages. HJR Wing and Harold Denham give priority to Schagen's issue, and this seems correct.[10] Denham notes that Commelin's title page shows evidence of hasty preparation since there are three literal errors. Of the two copies examined for this bibliography, **2C2.c1** has all three typographical errors: '*iu*' (corrected to '*in*' in **2C2.c2**); 'Cereberrima' corrected in pen and ink to 'Celeberimma' in both; and 'Seidleiani' not corrected to 'Sidleiani' in either. Copies sold by each bookseller have some individual leaves in different states. The main bibliographic issues relate to the preliminaries and inclusion, or not, of *De ratione motus musculorum* (1664) and its illustration published anonymously by William Croone (1633–1684) earlier that year.

Schagen's 1664 issue has twelve preliminary leaves ($*^{12}$), of which $*1$ is blank. He appears not, at that stage, to have had access to Croone's treatise. HJR Wing and Denham were able to examine a single copy of Schagen's issue containing only *Cerebri anatome* which, although still catalogued by the Wellcome Library, is now 'missing'. The two copies used for this bibliography each have Croone's treatise bound at the back. However, Commelin is identified as the publisher and these copies merely reflect the decision to bind the two works together. It seems safe to assume that Croone's essay was not intended as part of Schagen's 1664 duodecimo issue (**2C1.c1**).

What happened next is that Commelin published *Cerebri anatome* with *De ratione motus musculorum* and listed both on the collective title page. That Commelin chose not to name the correct author, or perhaps did not know Croone's identity, has led to much confusion.[11] His title page was printed as part of an added bifolium for which the conjugate sheet is the Benevolo lectori, which mentions the treatise on muscular motion. The printer's statement indicates that this work came to hand when the main text of *Cerebri anatome* was already in the press and that Willis had not been consulted about its inclusion. In justifying the decision to publish Croone's essay with *Cerebri anatome*, Commelin refers to 'the great affinity between the two works so that they seem in many ways to complement one another'. Presumably, including Croone's treatise placed Commelin at a commercial advantage.

Various arrangements for accommodating the extra bifolium in the preliminary leaves are found in examples of Commelin's issue. Denham collates the copy he studied as $*^{12}$, and his description of the contents makes clear that the blank at $*1$ and Schagen's title page ($*2$) are removed and replaced by Commelin's bifolium, making twelve leaves: $*^{12}$ ($-*1$, $-*2$) $+\pi 2$. HJR Wing examined a copy (in the Wren Library, Trinity College, Cambridge) in which the blank at $*1$ is removed, Commelin's bifolium inserted, but Schagen's title page still retained. His

[9] HJR Wing was unable to make direct comparison of the typesetting and printer's errors of the main text and wrote in correspondence dated 15 September 2003: 'I would like to know if ... they are identical ... In other words did Commelin acquire Schagen's unsold stock and reissue it with his own title page?' The sheets are identical.

[10] In correspondence dated 27 October 2003, HJR Wing writes: 'I had always assumed that Schagen was the first 1664 Amsterdam edition of the *Cerebri anatome* and that Commelin was later in the same year but I cannot prove it. When I compiled my bibliography the only copy of the latter was at Trinity College, Cambridge. I assume that Commelin thought that the best way to publish the anonymous work *De ratione motus musculorum* was to add it to another medical work of an author already established on the continent but again I have no proof'. Denham (1965): page 73 goes further in referring to the contract with Savry: 'Apart from the evidence as to the date of Schagen's issue, the document is of interest for the light it throws on Commelin's role. Whereas it might otherwise have been thought that he had merely taken over the completed sheets from Schagen and used them for his own purposes, it is now apparent that he played an active part in the preparation of the original edition, although his name does not occur in the imprint.'

[11] See: Denham (1965): page 74, footnote: 'Typographus; presumably refers to Commelin, as the person who had the work printed, even if he did not print it on his own press. Another printer commissioned by Commelin would be unlikely to have so much influence on publishing policy'.

collation is therefore *12 (–*1) +π2, making thirteen leaves. Of the two copies examined for this bibliography one conforms to Denham's collation. The other offers a third variation: *12 (–*2 [Schagen's title page]) +π2, also thirteen preliminary leaves (**2C2.c1**).[12]

There are independent signatures and pagination for the Amsterdam 1664 duodecimo issue of Croone's treatise. Its subsidiary title page includes a quote from Aristotle's (384–322 BC) *De partibus animalium* (*c.*350 BC): *Ἐν πᾶσι τοῖς φυσικοῖς ἐνεστί τι θαυμαστόν.* [There is something admirable in all physical matters]. Neither title page identifies the author. But one copy of Schagen's issue shows the manoeuvres adopted in order to sell books. Schagen's name is on the title page, which lists *De ratione motus musculorum*, and his preliminaries and text sheets are bound before Commelin's printing of Croone's essay (**2C1.c2**). At a casual glance, this appears to confound the conclusion that, at least in 1664, Schagen did not have access to Croone's treatise. But closer scrutiny shows that the top half of Commelin's title page has been cut and glued over Schagen's title page;[13] and the conjugate leaf of the Commelin bifolium has been discarded. It is hard to imagine this manipulation being done by a binder or the owner, Francisci [?], who, in 1666, inscribed the lower half of Schagen's title page. Neither would have had access to the two title pages, and the assumption must be that Schagen or someone close to him was the perpetrator of this seventeenth century cut-and-paste. At the very least, the evidence indicates that sheets of Schagen's and Commelin's duodecimo issues of *Cerebri anatome*, and Commelin's printing of Croone's essay, were available simultaneously to Amsterdam booksellers in 1664.

Several changes were made by Schagen for his 1666 edition (**2D**). This is especially important for the image that forms the engraved title page (F.2a1: dated 1665). Schagen reset the type for octavo format and did now have access to the text of *De ratione motus musculorum*. The signatures and pagination are continuous with *Cerebri anatome*. Croone's treatise remains anonymous. Schagen's intention was to replace the Elenchus rerum with a list of chapter headings and a final Index alphabeticus. But delays seem to have occurred so that the first issue (**2D1**) has only the relatively uninformative list of chapters, and neither the Elenchus rerum nor the more detailed index. Once the Index alphabeticus was ready, Schagen reissued *Cerebri anatome* with a new sheet, *8, bound after Croone's treatise (**2D2**). HJR Wing describes a final gathering of *6 and Denham, more accurately, indicates *7. But both are wrong. The copy described in this bibliography also has *8r–v, blank, followed by a ¾ binder's stub before the final gathering of folding sheets containing the illustrations printed as composites (see next). As with Schagen's 1664 edition, the illustration to Croone's treatise (Pl.16) is not present in either issue of **2D**.[14]

The last three Amsterdam issues are described as 'Editio ultima priori emendatior'. The first, published by Commelin in 1667 (**2E1**), uses many text sheets set identically to his 1664 issue, but there are differences. Notwithstanding his earlier publication, there is no mention of *De ratione motus musculorum* on the collective title page. Although it seems somewhat late to have developed scruples, Denham argues that Commelin may have omitted this detail

[12] The recto of the blank leaf, *1, shows offsetting of type from a full page of text from *Cerebri anatome*, too faint to identify but clearly indicating that this leaf left the print shop and is not a binder's endpaper.

[13] The pirated upper half of Commelin's title page in **2C1.c2** has '*in*', 'Ce<u>r</u>eberrima' uncorrected (providing further evidence that this leaf was obtained from the printshop) in addition to 'Se<u>i</u>dleiani'.

[14] HJR Wing (1962): #12, page 14 describes the engraved title and fifteen plates whereas Denham (1965): #5, page 89 calls for sixteen, 'as in No. 4 [i.e. Commelin 1664]'; and he also mentions the engraved title page. If Denham considers that Pl.16 is called for, his description is incorrect. Denham (1965): page 89 also misprints Typograph*icus* for typographus in his description of the contents at Z5r–v, pages [3–4]. Waller (1955): #10317, page 453 calls for 17 plates *and* the engraved title, which presumably means that the sections of Tabula XIII were cut and bound separately in each of his two copies and counted individually.

through uncertainty as to whether Croone would consent to the inclusion of his treatise in association with a work by Willis. In the event permission was obtained (see next). The leaf from the bifolium conjugate with the 1664 Commelin title page with Willis's letter to the printer (Benevolo Lectori Sal. D Typographus) is omitted, thereby restoring the collation to $*^{12}$ with *1 blank, *2r Commelin's 1667 title page, followed by the Amico lectori præfatio at *3r. In describing this edition, Denham refers to two conjugate stubs in the National Library of Medicine copy, as indicated to him by Mr RJ Durling (1932–1999): 'apparently of cancelled leaves, following the title page. He suggests that the existing title page is a cancellans. However, I have no further evidence of this at present. The stubs are not in the Wellcome Library copy'. Nor are they present in the copy examined for this bibliography. Because the Elenchus rerum is retained, Denham speculates that the relationship with Schagen had deteriorated to the extent that the Index alphabeticus was not made available to him, just as the illustration to Croone's treatise was evidently withheld from Schagen. Although the text largely follows the setting from 1664, this changes after L12, page 264. Whereas the Schagen and Commelin 1664 duodecimo issues (**2C1** and **2C2**) each have six leaves in the final signature (ending M5r, page 273; M5v, blank; M6r–v, blank), the text is reset by Commelin in 1667 from M3v, page 270, so that everything beyond the legend for Figura XIII is accommodated on three printed pages (M3v, M4r–v, pages 270–2).[15]

De ratione motus musculorum, separately signed and paginated, is also reset and printed on A1r–B5v, pages [1]–34, compared to A1r–B4v, pages [1]–32, in 1664. By incorrectly signing B3 as B4, and vice versa, which were duly bound in numerical sequence, discontinuities of pagination, catchword, and flow of the narrative were introduced. Had the error been noticed, confusion would have been solved by binding these leaves in reverse order. For the first time since his treatise was printed (either in London or Amsterdam), Croone is identified as the author on the title page. A2r–v, pages [3–4], contain correspondence from Croone to Commelin. In translation:[16]

> We commit this treatise to a second edition and lest the censors, dear Reader, think that we have ornamented it with a certain fictitious name we have printed a letter of the author himself which he wrote in reply to a letter of ours in which the work in question was desired to be corrected and enlarged.
>
> Caspar Commelin
> The Very Famous Printer
> Amsterdam
>
> Although your letter came to me directly my dear Commelin I would certainly have answered it more fittingly and so would have acted according to your wish, except that,

[15] HJR Wing (1962): #14, page 15 describes a copy of Commelin's imprint from 1667 without *De ratione motus musculorum* and considers this 'another issue of No. 10', i.e. Schagen 1664, despite the fact that, as he mentions, the final signature is limited to M^4 and the pagination ends at 272.

[16] The translation is from LG Wilson, 'William Croone's theory of muscular contraction', *Notes and Records of the Royal Society of London* 1961: 16; page 177, endnote 38. Wilson transcribes 'Caspar' as 'Gaspar'. At pages 167–8, Wilson suggests that Croone may have delayed allowing his name to be identified or revising his treatise because of criticism from Nicolas Steno (1638–1686) of Croone's belief, shared with Willis, that muscle does not expand during contraction and the need therefore to revise his position. Croone did eventually refine his ideas on muscular contraction in a lecture delivered at the Surgeons's Theatre in 1675 published as 'An hypothesis of the structure of a muscle' in Robert Hooke's (1635–1703) *Philosophical Collections* (1675), number 11; pages 22–5, which filled a gap in production of *Philosophical Transactions of the Royal Society* when publication lapsed due to lack of funds. See JF Fulton, *Selected readings in the history of physiology*, Springfield (1930): page 186.

almost at the same time, I also received a letter from Paris by which it was made known to me that a Treatise on Muscles of that distinguished gentleman my very good friend Dr. Steno is now in press there. One or two years ago there took place a considerable intercourse between that gentleman and I at Montpellier and we talked much together on this question. I wished to know fully what he, who is remarkable for the highest ingenuity, and diligence, had contributed to this very matter from his store. For I do not have such faith in my opinion that I would not wish to test it first by the judgment of others (which was my strongest reason for writing) before I shall bring into the light to those things which themselves (it seems to me) the mind must ponder further to confirm. You see dear Sir that I do not have any improper reason for publishing this Edition; meanwhile I am very unwell, my affairs are such that I am compelled to deny you that which, if it were of any value or moment, I would think it glorious to be struck with your imprint, the Commelin Press and to be ornamented with your type.

Yours most devotedly,
William Croone
M.D. and Fellow of the Royal College
of Physicians and of the Royal Society.

For if you are certain to print this treatise again, lest your edition seem to the ordinary reader to be a very faulty one of Willis (also a Fellow of the same Society), you may if you like add this letter in place of a preface.

Schagen was clearly not party to the arrangement with Croone and earlier in the same year published his Dutch translation of William Croone's *De ratione motus musculorum* wrongly attributed to Thomas Willis (**2G**), without the plate, and with an additional section providing a register of human muscles by Joannes Baptiste van Lamzweerde (fl.1657–*c.*1700).

Jean Maximilian Lucas (1647–1697) reset the title page but used the available sheets (or standing type) of Commelin's edition (1667) in his reissue of *Cerebri anatome* (1676; **2E2**). Lucas also published William Croone's *De ratione motus musculorum* (1676), replacing his name as bookseller on the title page but using Commelin's sheets (retaining the awkward signatures and binding of B3 and B4). Although this was an independent publication, it seems likely that in having access to Commelin's material, Lucas's intention was exactly to reproduce the complete 1667 edition.[17] Copies of Lucas's issue are complete without *De ratione motus musculorum*, but both texts are sometimes bound as one volume. Henry Wetstein (1649–1726) reset the text for his edition (1683; **2F**) closely following Commelin's format and retaining a few errors to headlines and catchwords, correcting others, and introducing a few new mistakes. Copies of Wetstein's 1683 duodecimo edition do not include Croone's essay.

HJR Wing mentions that 'Manget *Bibliotheca scriptorum medicorum* Tomus II (1731) lists another edition [of *Cerebri anatome*] published at London (1670) and another at Amsterdam (1674). No examples were found in the libraries visited nor in the *Index Catalogue of the library of the Surgeon General's Office* nor the London edition in the *Term Catalogues* or [Donald] *Wing* so they have not been included in the general bibliography'.[18] There is no reason to think that these editions of *Cerebri anatome* were ever published.

[17] *Cerebri anatome* (1676) and *De ratione motus musculorum* (1676), published by Lucas are listed as independent publications in the Short Title Catalogue for the Netherlands (#4 and #5, respectively).
[18] See: HJR Wing (1962): pages 10–11.

The Amsterdam duodecimo issues: illustrations

It will already be clear that there were differences in how Schagen and Commelin dealt with the illustrations for *Cerebri anatome.*[19] Denham makes the point that 'Schagen and Commelin shared possession of the original plates, as Salomon Savry (1594–1683) testified that he had received one from each of the publishers. The plates referred to are clearly those of the English edition as the text reads "een ... copere plaet uyt Willis de Cerebri Anatomie".'[20]

This quote is slightly ambiguous in that it leaves open whether Schagen and Commelin shared the same set of engraved plates. Examination of their various issues and editions makes clear that they did not. The figure sizes used by Schagen and Commelin are not identical, and the engravings differ in detail and lettering.[21] But there are enough similarities to indicate that the same workshop was used or that the engraver working for Commelin copied the material available to Schagen, or vice versa. Both Schagen and Commelin economized by placing several illustrations on one large engraved plate which was printed on a single sheet. The intention was to cut these along horizontal and vertical lines indicated by the engraver and bind the parts individually, as found in many copies. Two, at least, survive in copies of Schagen's 1666 octavo edition (**2D**) with the large sheet uncut and bound as printed. In order to arrange everything neatly in a rectangle, one illustration on each is rotated (see next). In fact, the plate marks visible on one or more (but never all four) sides and the lines showing where cuts should be made, indicate that all of the illustrations, both for Schagen and Commelin, were printed as composites on large sheets. Most were then cut and bound individually at an appropriate place in the text.

Denham states that, on 29 June 1664 together with Commelin's business partner, Michael de Groot (nd), Schagen and Commelin signed an agreement with Savry to engrave 'two plates' for *Cerebri anatome*, one contract coming from each publisher, to be delivered within 8 days for a fee of 15 guilders. What remains unclear is exactly how many engravings were involved in these contracts. One interpretation is that there were two plates, as stated: one possibly the unique engraved title page, eventually used by Schagen in 1666 (F.2a1), and the other the illustration for William Croone's treatise, *De ratione motus musculorum*, which remained only in the possession of Commelin. Two plates might also refer to two of the large engravings on which several images were grouped (see next). A different interpretation is that Savry produced two versions of all the engravings since it is clear that two complete sets were in circulation. Because the individual illustrations are all cut from much larger printed sheets, the number of engraver's plates needed to illustrate *Cerebri anatome cui accessit nervorum deſcriptio et usus* was probably reduced by one-half compared with the London editions. The buying power of 15 guilders in the middle of the seventeenth century was equivalent to €150 in 2021.

The evidence from copies of Schagen's 1664 duodecimo (**2C1**) and 1666 octavo (**2D**) editions indicates that most images were engraved vertically, but three were rotated and placed horizontally for printing:

> Tabula XII (Pl.14) is horizontal above Figura III (Pl.3, left) and Figura I (Pl.1, right), both vertical. All three may be found on a sheet with vertical chain lines (it follows that when cut and bound individually, Tabula XII has horizontal chain lines)

[19] See also chapter 3 for further details.

[20] See: Denham (1965): page 73 and footnotes.

[21] Where diagonal lines are engraved as cross-hatching, Commelin's are usually top left to bottom right and Schagen's top right to bottom left. These are the natural strokes of right and left handed engravers moving the plate against the burin. One of Schagen's plates (Tabula IX, Pl.9b1) has faint lines in the top right corner close to the more deeply engraved markings suggesting that these were copied from an original version as part of a rough draft. Commelin's (Tabula IX, Pl.9c1) lacks this feature, but which was engraved first remains unclear.

Tabula XI (Pl.13) is horizontal above Tabula XIII (Pl.15), which is vertical, on a sheet with horizontal chain lines (it follows that when cut and bound individually, Tabula XI has vertical chain lines)

Figura II (Pl.2), Figura IIII (Pl.4), Figura V (Pl.5) come from the lower left corner of sheets with horizontal chain lines

Figura VI (Pl.6), unnumbered 1 (Pl.7) and Figura VIII (Pl.9) come from the lower right corner of sheets with horizontal chain lines

Figura VII (Pl.8) comes from the upper right corner of a sheet with horizontal chain lines

Unnumbered 2 (Pl.10) comes from the upper left of a sheet with horizontal chain lines

Tabula IX (Pl.11) comes from the lower left of a sheet with vertical chain lines

Tabula X (Pl.12) comes from the lower right of a sheet with vertical chain lines.

The attempt at reconstructing rectangles from all these illustrations in order to determine the exact number of large engravings provided for Schagen proves frustrating since, with plate marks and lines removed by cropping, the jigsaw puzzle cannot be completed.

The same exercise can be carried out for Commelin's engravings, using copies of the 1664 and 1667 duodecimo editions (**2C2**, **2E1**), and Lucas's 1676 (**2E2**) duodecimo edition which used the same plates in altered states. In Lucas's edition:

Tabula XII (Pl.14) is horizontal above Figura III (Pl.3, left) and Figura I (Pl.1, right), both vertical. All three may be found on a sheet with vertical chain lines (it follows that when cut and bound individually, Tabula XII has horizontal chain lines)

Tabula IX (Pl.11) is printed to the left of Tabula X (Pl.12) on a sheet with vertical chain lines (but, as bound in the copy used for this bibliography, the sheet is inverted)[22]

Tabula XI (Pl.13) is horizontal above Tabula XIII (Pl.15), which is vertical, on a sheet with horizontal chain lines (it follows that when cut and bound individually, Tabula XI has vertical chain lines).

Thereafter, the illustrations are individual, as are all fifteen in copies of Commelin's editions examined for this bibliography:

Figura 2 (Pl.2) and unnumbered 1 (Pl.7) come from the lower left corner of a sheet with horizontal chain lines

Figura V (Pl.5) comes from the lower left of a sheet with horizontal chain lines, printed with Figura 6 (Pl.6) at the right corner; the tear is awkward and, in **2E1**, a section of Pl.6 is still attached to the corresponding edge of Figura V

Figura IIII (Pl.4) and Figura VIII (Pl.9) come from the lower right corner of a sheet with horizontal chain lines

Unnumbered 2 (Pl.10) comes from the upper left corner of a sheet with horizontal chain lines. This is a different arrangement from Schagen's engraving

Figura VII (Pl.8) comes from the upper right corner of a sheet with horizontal chain lines. This is a different arrangement from Schagen's engraving.

[22] It follows that the same arrangement was originally in place for Tabula IX and X in Schagen's set.

There is one further complexity relating to the Dutch duodecimo editions. It seems that Schagen and Commelin had lost interest in *Cerebri anatome* by the late 1660s, and both sets of engravings came into the possession of Hendrik Wetstein. He used the Commelin plates in his 1682 quarto edition of the *Opera omnia* (**8E**) but cut these down so that plate marks surround all sides of Figuræ II (Pl.2), III (Pl.3), V (Pl.5), VI (Pl.6), unnumbered 1 (Pl.7), VII (Pl.8), VIII (Pl.9), unnumbered 2 (Pl.10), Tabulæ XI (Pl.13) and XIII (Pl.15); whereas only Figuræ 1 (Pl.1) and III (Pl.3) and Tabulæ IX (Pl.11) and XII (Pl.14) are incomplete and might have been cut from larger printed sheets. But after manipulating the plates in 1682, these may have no longer been usable. For this, or some other reason, Wetstein switched to Schagen's set when he published his Amsterdam 1683 duodecimo edition of *Cerebri anatome*, cutting each illustration from the large printed sheets.[23]

William Croone and *De ratione motus musculorum*: a summary

De ratione motus musculorum was first published anonymously in 1664 and printed in London by 'F Hayes. For sale by S. Thompson, at the sign of the Bishop in St Paul's Cemetry'. It may be useful to summarize its subsequent history in the context of the printed works of Thomas Willis.

The treatise was first reprinted, separately signed, and paginated, and bound with Commelin's edition of *Cerebri anatome* (1664: **2C2**) together with the illustration (Pl.16). This was not a misunderstanding on authorship but reflected the perceived complementarity of the two works. Commelin's text sheets were either acquired by Schagen in 1664 or purchased independently and bound together at the request of individual owners. The treatise is next seen, with a separate title page dated 1665 but, again without an author, in Schagen's edition of *Cerebri anatome* (1666: **2D1** and **2D2**), neither issue of which included the two images engraved on a single plate (Pl.16). Commelin issued a further edition in 1667 (**2E1**) in which he identified Croone as the author: *Studio Guglielmi Croone MD e Coll Med Lond ac Societatis Regalis Socii*. This was presumably a few months after Schagen had published his Dutch translation of *De ratione motus musculorum* attributed to Thomas Willis, again without the plate (**2G**).

The matter was not finally settled by Commelin's declaration of William Croone as the author of *De ratione motus musculorum* in 1667. The confusion persisted because Willis himself wrote a treatise on muscle entitlted *De motu musculari* (1670: **4A**). In the collected editions of Willis's works published by Jean-Antoine Huguetan (1647–*c*.1750: 1676, 1681; **8A**, **8D**) both treatises are included with *De ratione motus musculorum* correctly attributed to Croone and *De motu musculari* to Willis. But the Samuel de Tournes (1628–1695) editions (1676, 1680, 1695, **8B**, **8C**, **8G**) have *De ratione motus musculorum* as anonymous, and *De motu musculari* correctly attributed to Willis. De Tournes explains his position:

> BENEVOLIS LECTORIBVS TYPOGRAPHVS S. TRACTATUM De Ratione Motus Mufculorum (*etfi Authoris Anonymi*) Anatomiæ Cerebri, Nervorumque Defcriptioni *ab* Excellentifs. Viro D. THOMA WILLIS M.D. Celeberrimo *inftitutæ, fubnectere non*

[23] Since only one copy has been examined for this bibliography, it is possible that Wetstein kept both sets in use and therefore that copies of the 1683 duodecimo edition of *Cerebri anatome* will be found with Commelin's plates in altered states.

incongruum duxi; vel eâ potiſſimum ratione (ut alias, tum à Materiæ affinitate, tum ab Operis præſtentiâ petitas, miſſas faciam,) quòd in prioribus Editionibus magno cum Doctorum applauſu, & sine ullâ, quod ſciam, Clariſſimi D. *WILLIS querelâ, appoſitus reperiatur.* Valete.

[THE PRINTER GREETS THE BENEVOLENT READERS. I thought it not unsuitable to attach A TREATISE on The Manner of the Movement of Muscles (*though from an Anonymous Author*) to the Anatomy of the Brain and the Description of Nerves, written by the most excellent Man, the very Famous Mr. THOMAS WILLIS M.D.; *primarily for the reason (which makes that I must overlook other* [works] *in demand because of affinity to the Subject as well as of availabilty of the Work) that it is found added to earlier Editions, with great acclaim of Doctors and, as far as I know, without any complaint of the very Famous Mr. WILLIS.* Farewell.]

Lucas reissued William Croone's *De ratione motus musculorum* using Commelin's sheets but with his own title page (1676: **2E2**). However, Wetstein appears not to have had, or chose not to include, these sheets in his edition (1683: **2F**); or perhaps, by then, the Commelin stock was exhausted. Wetstein later endorsed his position by omitting *De ratione motus musculorum* but including Willis's *De motu musculari* in his edition of *Opera omnia* (1682: **8E**). However, *De ratione motus musculorum*, correctly attributed to Croone, returns in the Gasparas Storti (nd) *Opera omnia* (1708: **8H**) and the Joannes Malachinum (nd: 1720: **8I**) folio editions. The English translations are correct in that Samuel Pordage's *The remaining medical works* (1681: **9B**) omits 'On the Reason for the movement of the muscles'; nor is it included in *Dr Willis's practice of physick* (1684[1], 1684[2]; **9E**, **9F**).

2A. CEREBRI ANATOME, London quarto 1664

The first edition of Willis's second book, and the first of his works to include illustrations [HJR Wing 8, Denham 1].

Title page: CEREBRI | ANATOME: | CUI ACCESSIT | *NERVORUM DESCRIPTIO* | ET USUS. | STUDIO | THOMÆ WILLIS, ex *Æde Chriſti* | *Oxon.* M. D. & in iſta Celeberrima | Academia Naturalis Philoſophiæ Pro- | feſſoris *Sidleiani.* | [rule] | *LONDINI,* | Typis *Ja. Fleſher,* Impenſis *Jo. Martyn* & *Ja. Alleſtry* | apud inſigne Campanæ in Cœmeterio | *D. Pauli.* [rule over date] M DC LXIV.

Collation: quarto; 23 letter roman alphabet using I and V: A^4, a–d^4, B–I^4, K–O^4, P^4 (P1+*1), Q–T^4, V^4, X–Z^4, Aa–Ii^4, Kk–Tt^4, Vv^4, Xx–Zz^4, Aaa–Iii^4, Kkk–Mmm^4; $1–3 signed apart from: *a*1 signed a1, *Iii–Mmm*^{4} signed in italic apart from Kkk3 and Lll3.

249 leaves: paginated as [40], 106, [2: 'inter pag. 106 & 107' signed *], 107–456.

Type: 27 lines; height (20 lines) 115 millimetres, width 97 millimetres.

Contents: **A1r**, page [1], blank; **A1v**, page [2], Imprimatur, Jan. 20. 1663. THO. GRIGG R. in Chriſto Pat. Ac. D^{no} D. *Humfr.* Epiſc. *Lon.* À ſac. Domeſticis.; **A2r**, page [3], title; **A2v**, page [4], blank; **A3r–a1r**, pages [5–9], REVERENDISSIMO In Chriſto Patri, & Domino,

Domino GILBERTO, Providentia Divina, Archiepiſcopo *Cantuarienſi,* totius *Angliæ* Primati & Metropolitano; & Auguſtiſſimo Principi CAROLO II. M. *Britanniæ, Franciæ,* & *Hiberniæ* Regi, à Secretioribus Conſiliis ... [signed] *Clementiæ veſtræ Clientem humillimum & aſtrictiſsimum,* THO. WILLIS.; **a1v–a3v**, pages [10–14], Amico Lectori Præfatio.; **a4r–v**, pages [15–16], AUTHORI In Cerebri Anatomen carmen ... [signed] Philippus Fell, *A.M. & Collegii Omnium Animarum in Acad.* Oxon, *Socius.*; **b1r–c3v**, pages [17–30], *Elenchus rerum.* [Cerebri anatome]; **c4r–d4r**, pages [31–9], Elenchus rerum. *Nervorum deſcriptio & uſus.*; **d4v**, page [40], Errata, 14 lines listing 22 corrections.

B1r–Nn1r, pages 1–273 plus inserted leaf between pages 106 and 107, [text] *CEREBRI ANATOME.*; **Nn1v–Mmm4v**, pages 274–456, [text] Nervorum deſcriptio & uſus.

Headlines and *Catchwords*: *Elenchus rerum* for Elenchus rerum at **b1r**, page 17.

No catchword at **a3v / a4r**, pages [14] / [15]; **d4r / v**, pages [39] / [40]; **d4v / B1r**, page [40] / 1; **Zz4v / Aaa1r**, pages 360 / 361.

Frontispiece: none.

Portrait: none.

Printers' ornaments: two rows each of 12 fleurons, lower inverted, at **B1r**, page 1 {**Allestry 1**}.

No decorated initials.

Illustrations: **Pl.1a1**. Plate 1 (image 1): *Figura I.^a* (headline, centre),[24] *pag: 25* (headline, right), *de medio T vid pag: 414* (footer, right); lettering to depict structures (in multiples of ≤ 4) A–I, K–T, V–Y, a. Folding, 238 × 207 millimetres (sheet); 212 × 184 millimetres (plate marks);[25] 194 × 175 millimetres (figure). Legend: *Figura prima* Cerebri humani Cranio exempti baſin cum Vaſorum abſciſſorum radicibus oſtendit. Plate inserted before legend at **E1r–v**, pages 25–6 (see: Figure 97 and dust wrapper).

Pl.2a1. Plate 2 (image 2): *Figura II.^da.* (headline, centre), *pag: 27* (headline, right), *de medio S vid pag; 414* (footer, right); lettering to depict structures (in multiples of ≤ 4) A–I, K–T, V–X. Leaf size, 187 × 144 millimetres (sheet); 157 × 116 millimetres (plate marks); 135 × 103 millimetres (figure). Legend: *Figura Secunda* Cerebri Ovini cranio exempti baſin & vaſorum abſciſſorum radices oſtendit, ubi arteriæ omnes ab atramento uni carotidum injecto, atratæ & conſpectiores redduntur. Plate inserted before legend at **E2r–v**, pages 27–8 (see: Figure 98).

Pl.3a1. Plate 3 (image 3): *Fig: III.* (headline, centre), *pag: 49.* (headline, right); lettering to depict structures (in multiples of ≤ 2) A–P. Folding, 229 × 204 millimetres (sheet); 213 × 183 millimetres (plate marks); 196 × 180 millimetres (figure). Legend: *Figura Tertia* Cerebri humani cranio exempti ſuperficiem extimam ſive ſuperiorem exhibet, ubi Cerebri Limbus à

[24] As printed, most abbreviations in superscript have ⁚ placed under the lettering but this is here displaced to precede the roman numeral. Others are reproduced as printed.

[25] With the descriptions that follow printers' plate sizes have been estimated when these are not visible based on any available copy.

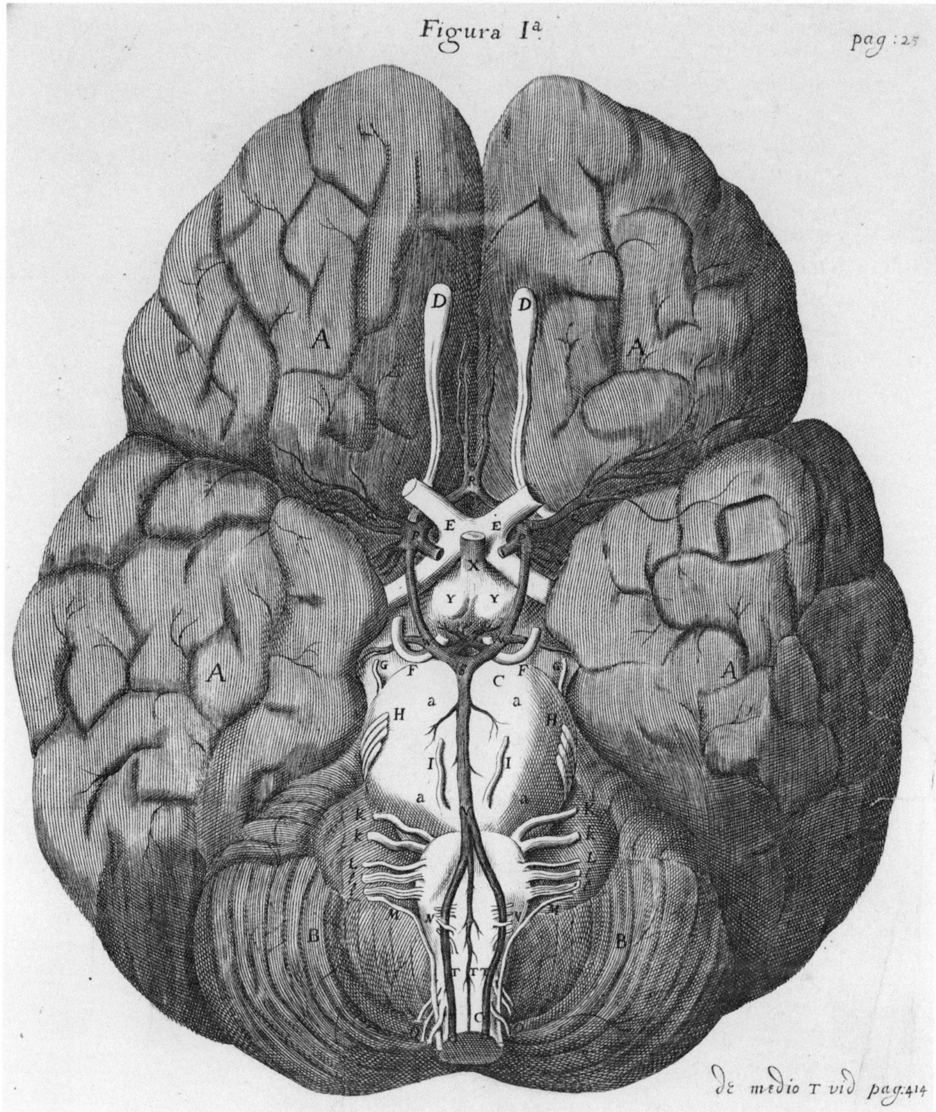

Figure 97 Plate 1 (image 1). The Firſt Figure SHews the Baſis of an humane Brain taken out of the Skull, with the Roots of the Veſſels cut off. Image from *Cerebri anatome* 1664; legend from *The remaining medical works* 1681.

nexu cum aliis partibus, per membranas facto, ſolutus, elevator & anteriùs flectitur, ut Crura medullæ oblongatæ, Fornix, Nates & Teſtes cum glandula pineali, aliíque proceſſus clarè & diſtinctè conſpiciantur. Plate inserted before legend at **H1r–H2r**, pages 49–51 (see: Figure 99).

Pl.4a1. Plate 4 (image 4): *Fig: IIII.* (headline, centre), *pag: 51* (headline, right); lettering to depict structures (in multiples of ≤ 2) A–N, O. Ruled border. Leaf size, 187 × 144 millimetres (sheet); 147 × 111 millimetres (plate marks); 116 × 94 millimetres (figure). Legend: *Figura Quarta.* Effigies Cerebri humani, quod cujuſdam Adoleſcentis, ab ipſa nativitate Fatui, & ex eorum numero qui vulgò Lemurum ſubdititii perhibentur, fuerat; Cujus Cerebri moles, cùm

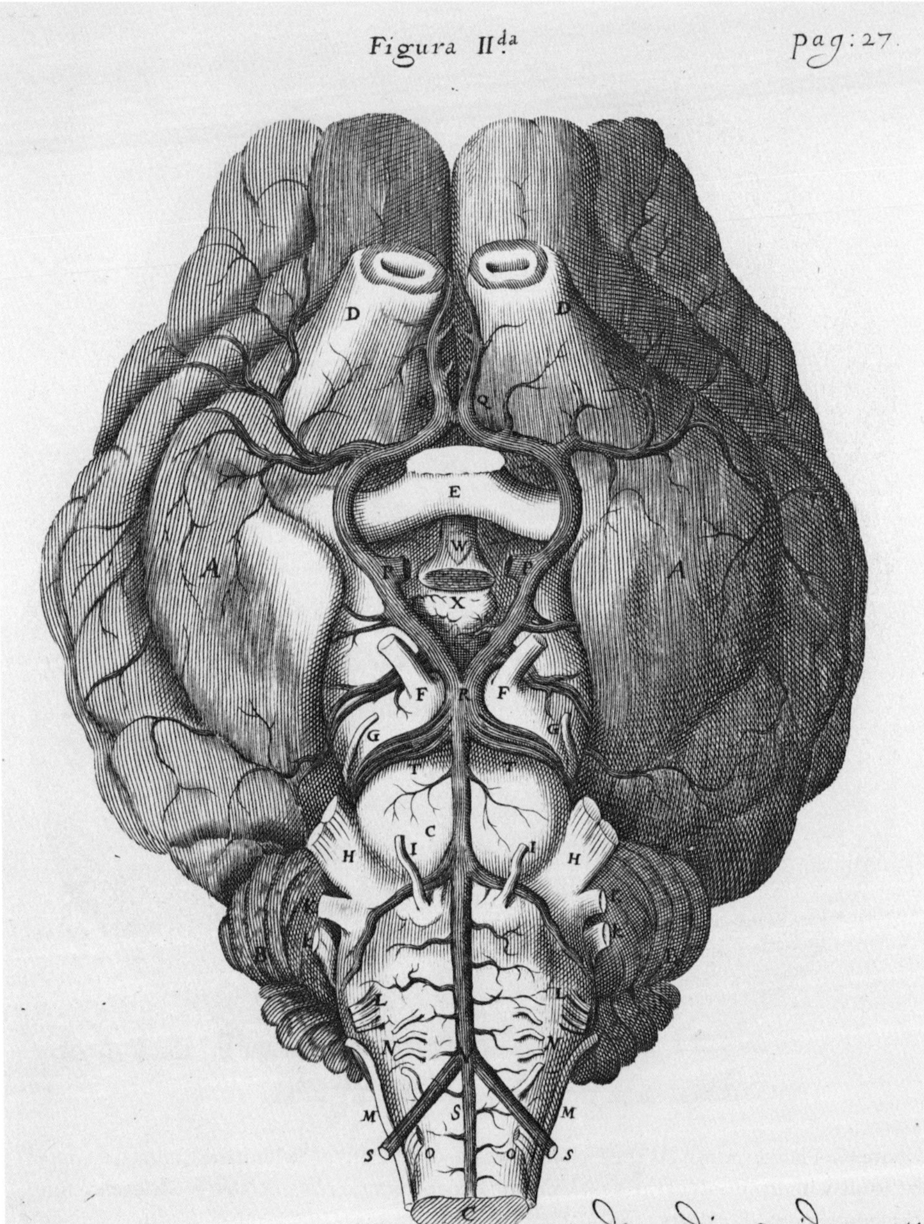

Figure 98 Plate 2 (image 2). The Second Figure Shews the Bafis of a Sheeps Brain taken out of the Skull, and the Roots of the Veffels cut off, where all the Arteries, by Ink being injected into one of the Carotides, are made black and more conspicuous. Image from *Cerebri anatome* 1664; legend from *The remaining medical works* 1681.

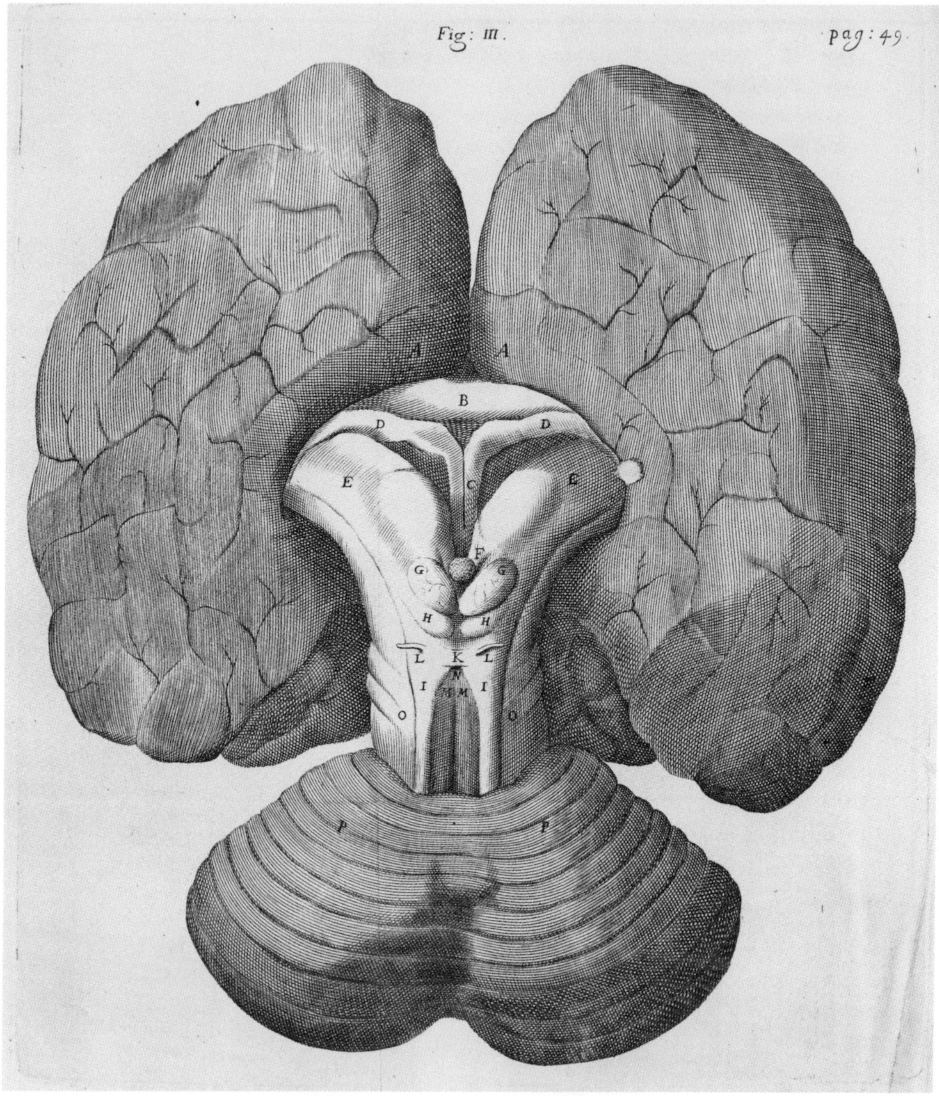

Figure 99 Plate 3 (image 3). The Third Figure SHews the outmoſt or ſuperior Superficies of the humane Brain taken out of the Skull; where the border of the Brain being looſned from the knitting of the other Parts, made by the membranes, is elevated and turned outward, that the ſhanks of the oblong Marrow, the Fornix or arched Vault, the Nates and Teſtes, with the pineal Kernel, and other Proceſſes, may be clearly and diſtinctly beheld. Image from *Cerebri anatome* 1664; legend from *The remaining medical works* 1681.

tenuior ac ſolito minor fuit, limbus ejus ulteriùs elevari & reflecti potuit, ut interiora quævis penitiùs conſpicerentur. Plate inserted before legend at **H2r–v**, pages 51–2 (see: Figure 100).

Pl.5a1. Plate 5 (image 5): *Figura V.* (headline, centre), *pag: 63* (headline, right); lettering to depict structures (in multiples of ≤ 2) A–Q. Folding, 234 × 190 millimetres (sheet); 210 × 145 millimetres (plate marks); 182 × 133 millimetres (figure). Legend: *Figura Quinta* Exhibet Cranii humani baſin interiorem; ubi oſtenditur quo ritu Vaſa cujuſque generis, Cerebro

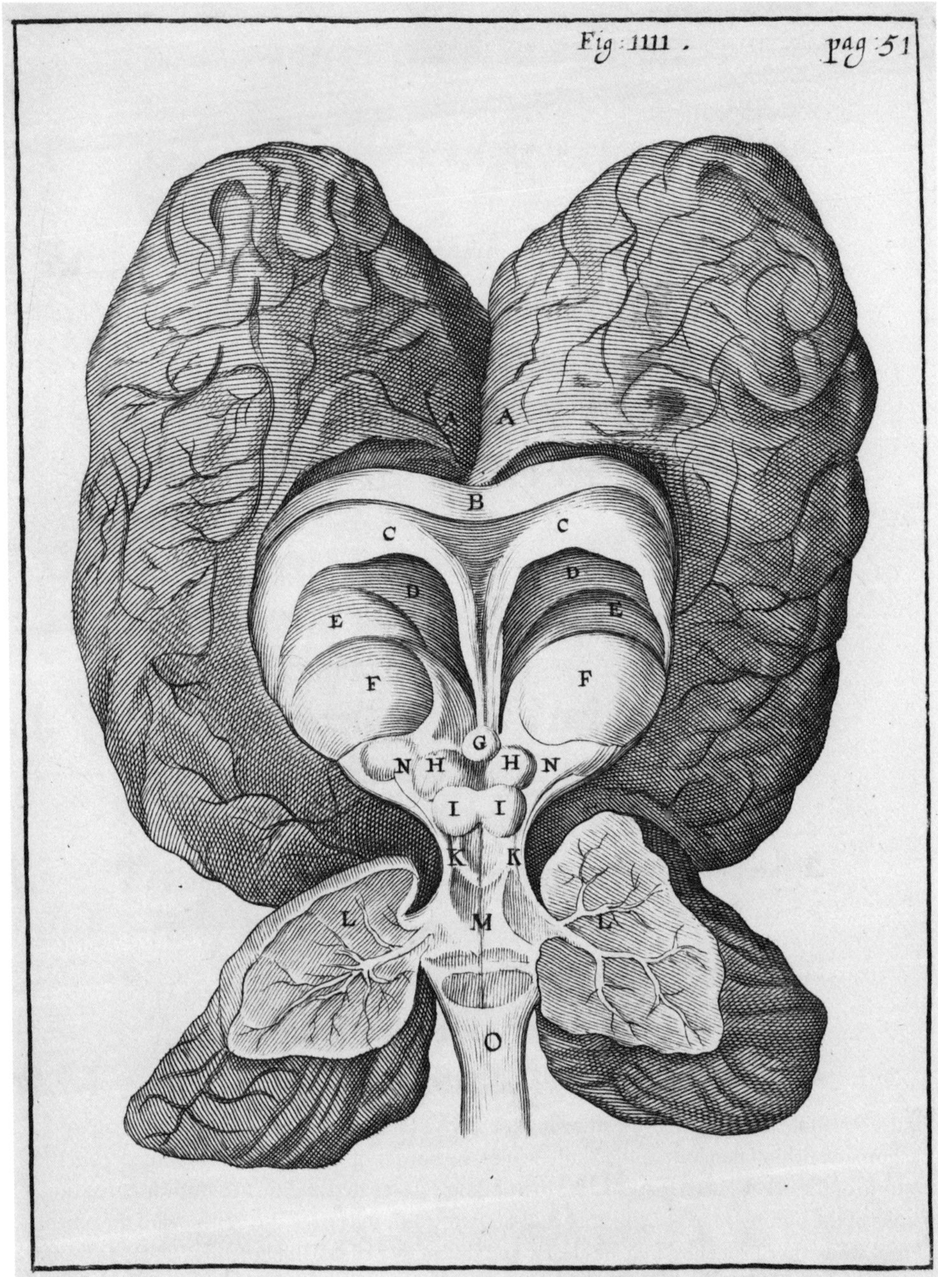

Figure 100 Plate 4 (image 4). The Fourth Figure. The Effigies of an humane Brain of a certain Youth that was fooliſh from his birth, and of that ſort which are commonly termed Changelings; the bulk of whoſe brain, as it was thinner and leſſer than is uſual, its border could be farther lifted up and turned back, that all the more interior parts might be more deeply held together. Image from *Cerebri anatome* 1664; legend from *The remaining medical works* 1681.

abſciſſa, & Cranio egreſſura, ſub Dura matre reconduntur. Plate inserted before legend at **I4r–v**, pages 63–4 (see: Figure 101).

Pl.6a1. Plate 6 (image 6): *Fig: VI.*[a] (headline, centre), *pag: 64* (headline, right); lettering to depict structures (in multiples of ≤ 2) A–N. Folding, 231 × 144 millimetres (sheet); 212 × 140 millimetres (plate marks); 197 × 130 millimetres (figure). Legend: *Figura Sexta* Exhibet Calvariæ Vitulinæ baſin; ubi oſtenditur quo ritu vaſa Cerebro abſciſſa & cranio egreſſura ſub dura matre demerguntur. Plate inserted within legend at **I4v–K1r**, pages 64–5 (see: Figure 102).

Pl.7a1. Plate 7 (images 7–10): [Unnumbered 1] *Fig: I*; *Fig: II*; *Fig: III* (header, centre above each image), *Fig: 1111* (left of image); lettering on each figure to depict structures (in multiples of ≤ 4) A–D; A–D, d, E–F; A, a, B–C; and A–D. Leaf size, 188 × 144 millimetres (sheet); 198 × >142 millimetres (plate marks, cropped); 28 × 98 millimetres, 82 × 94 millimetres, 38 × 26 millimetres, 76 × 26 millimetres (figures). Legend: *Figura Prima* Exhibet Arteriæ Carotidis aſcenſum, & ſitum intra Cranium Humanum, priuſquam verſùs Cerebrum effertur; *Figura Secunda* Arteriarum Carotidum aſcenſum, & ſitum intra Cranium Equinum exhibet; *Figura Tertia* Exhibet Rete mirabile, cum glandula pituitaria in Cranio vitulino; *Figura Quarta* Oſtendit quo ritu ſinus lateralis in venam jugularem cum diverticulo appenſo cedit. Plate inserted after legend at **P1 +*1r–v**, page Inter pag. 106 & 107–[-] (see: Figure 103).

Pl.8a1. Plate 8 (image 11): *Fig: VII.*[a] (headline, centre), *pag: 131* (headline, right); lettering to depict structures (in multiples of ≤ 2) A–I, K–T, V–X. Folding, 238 × 144 millimetres (sheet); 225 × 129 millimetres (plate marks); 194 × 105 millimetres (figure). Legend: *Figura Septima* Exhibet Cerebrum ovinum reclinatum, & in cohæſionum locis, juxta corpora ſtriata, aliquatenus diſciſſum, ut interior ejus compages evolvi, ac in planum explicari queat. Plate inserted before legend at **S2r–S3r**, pages 131–3 (see: Figure 104).

Pl.9a1. Plate 9 (image 12): *Fig: VIII.*[a], *pag: 167* (headline, centre and right); lettering to depict structures (in multiples of ≤ 2) A–I, K–T, V–X. Leaf size, 187 × 144 millimetres (sheet); 135 × 100 millimetres (plate marks); 111 × 96 millimetres (figure). Legend: *Figura Octava* Medullam oblongatam Capite Ovino exemptam, cum Cerebro abſciſſo & amoto, cúmque Cerebello, & corpore uno ſtriato, per medium diſſectis, aliáque præcipuè ad Caudicem medullarem pertinentia repræſentat. Plate inserted before legend at **Y4r–v**, pages 167–8 (see: Figure 105).

Pl.10a1. Plate 10 (images 13–14): [Unnumbered 2] *Fig: I.* (headline, centre), *Pag: 302* (headline, right), *Fig: II* (lower, centre); lettering to depict structures (in multiples of ≤ 2) A–H, a–r; and A–K, a–i. Folding, 226 × 144 millimetres (sheet); 200 × >138 millimetres (plate marks, cropped); 126 × 115 millimetres, 50 × 114 millimetres (figures). Legend: Hæc Figura Nervorum Paris Quinti & Sexti Ramificationes exhibet; Figura Secunda exhibet nervos omnes, qui ſcilicet à nervi tertii, quarti, quinti, & ſexti Paris profecti, oculi muſculis aliiſque partibus impenduntur. Plate inserted after legend at **Qq2r–Qq3v**, pages 299–302 (see: Figure 106).

Pl.11a1. Plate 11 (image 15): *Tabula IX.*[a] (headline, right); lettering to depict structures (in multiples of ≤ 4, with repetition for different structures, admixture of upper and lower case and erratic ordering) A–I, K–M, *H*, a–c, f–i, l–q, s–t, v–x, α–ω, 1–5, *, □, Δ and ·.

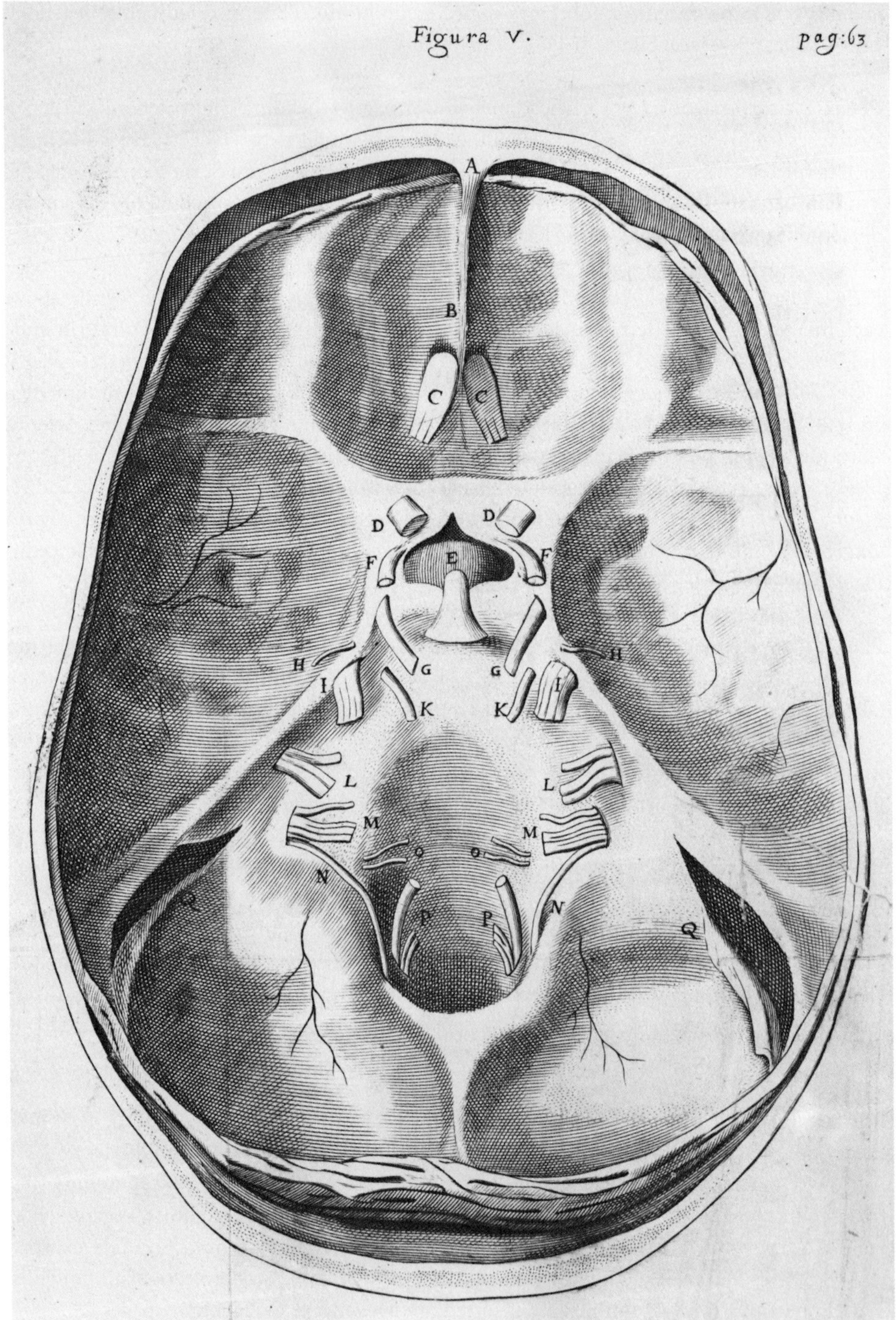

Figure 101 Plate 5 (image 5). The Fifth Figure. SHews the interior Baſis of an humane Skull; where is ſhewn after what manner the Veſſels of every kind cut off from the Brain, and about to go out of the Skull, are hid or laid up under the dura Mater. Image from *Cerebri anatome* 1664; legend from *The remaining medical works* 1681.

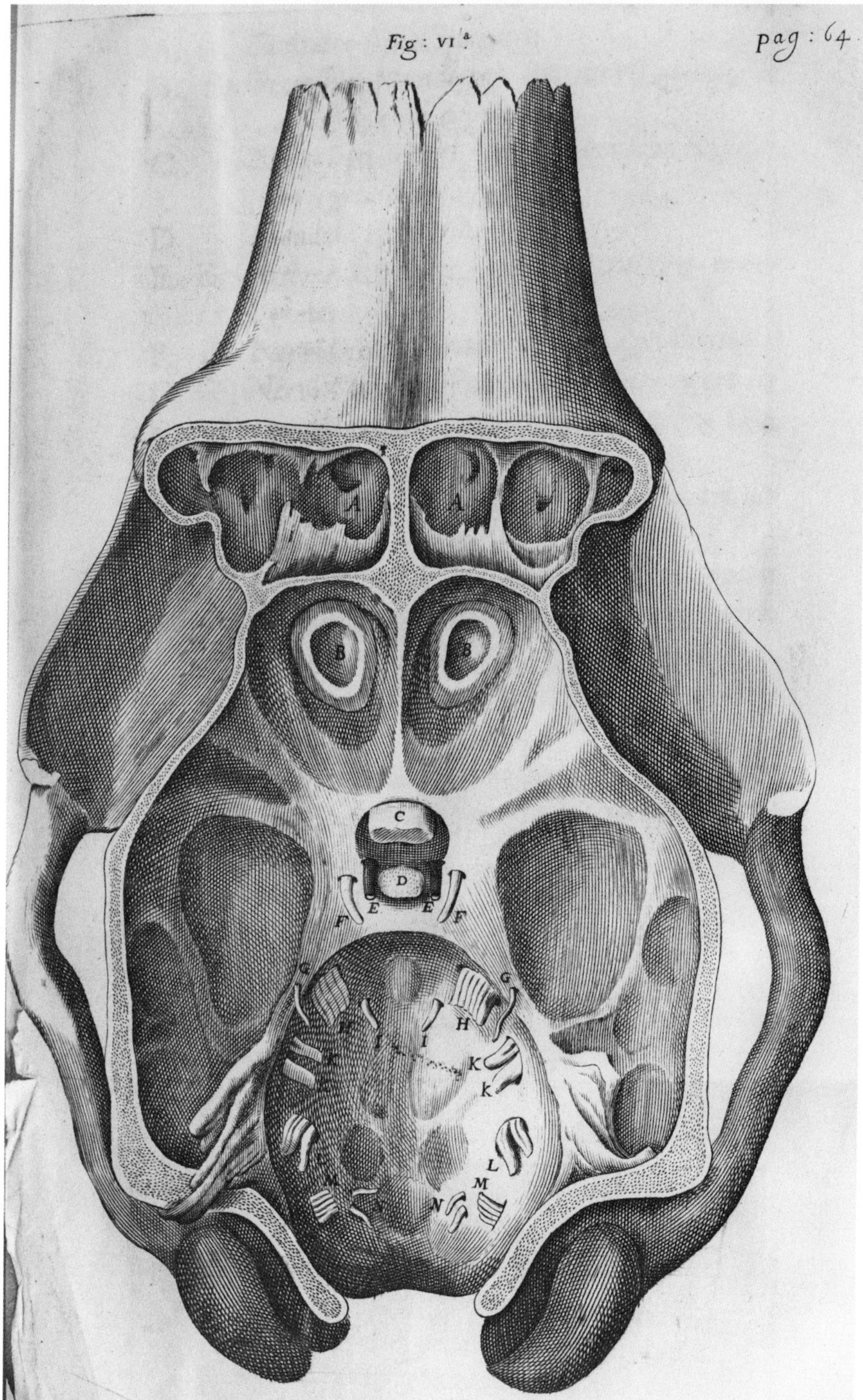

Figure 102 Plate 6 (image 6). The Sixth Figure. SHews the Bafis of a Calfs Skull; where is fhewn after what manner the Veffels cut off from the Brain, and about to go out from the Skull, are drowned under the dura Mater. Image from *Cerebri anatome* 1664; legend from *The remaining medical works* 1681.

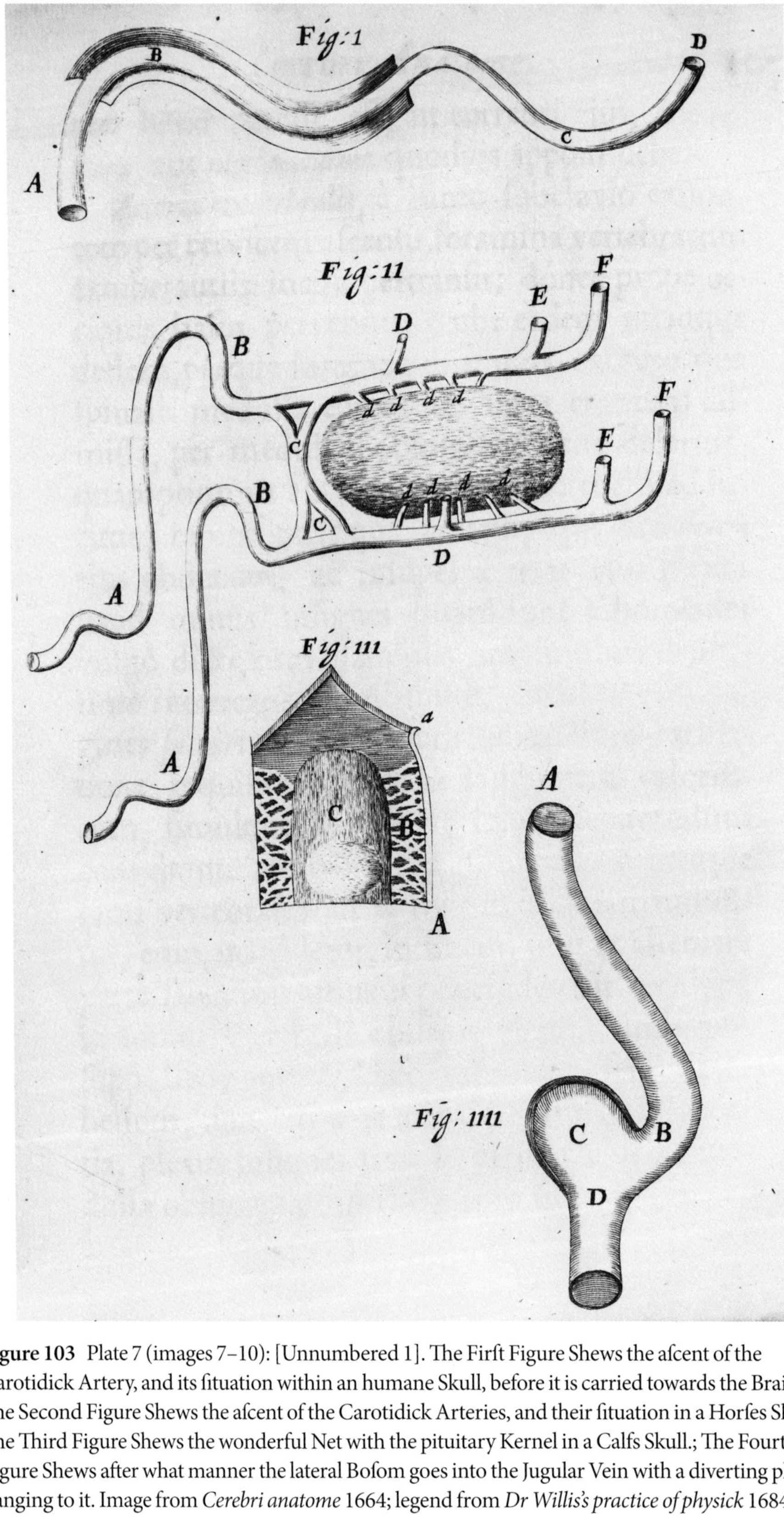

Figure 103 Plate 7 (images 7–10): [Unnumbered 1]. The Firſt Figure Shews the aſcent of the Carotidick Artery, and its ſituation within an humane Skull, before it is carried towards the Brain.; The Second Figure Shews the aſcent of the Carotidick Arteries, and their ſituation in a Horſes Skull.; The Third Figure Shews the wonderful Net with the pituitary Kernel in a Calfs Skull.; The Fourth Figure Shews after what manner the lateral Boſom goes into the Jugular Vein with a diverting place hanging to it. Image from *Cerebri anatome* 1664; legend from *Dr Willis's practice of physick* 1684.

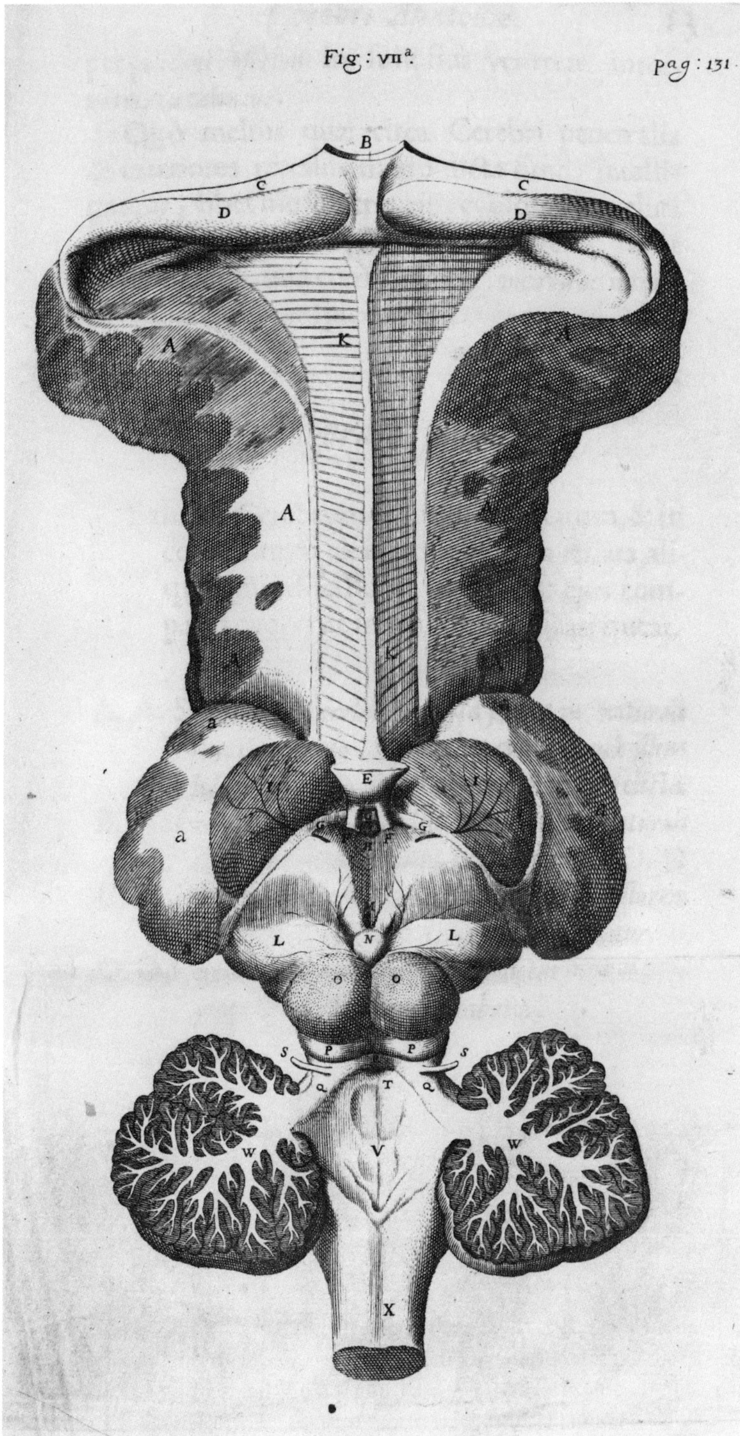

Figure 104 Plate 8 (image 11). *The Seventh Figure* SHews the Brain of a Sheep bent back and cut a little open in the places where they ſtick together near the ſtreaked bodies, that its interior ſubſtance may be turned the inſide out, and unfolded on a plain. Image from *Cerebri anatome* 1664; legend from *The remaining medical works* 1681.

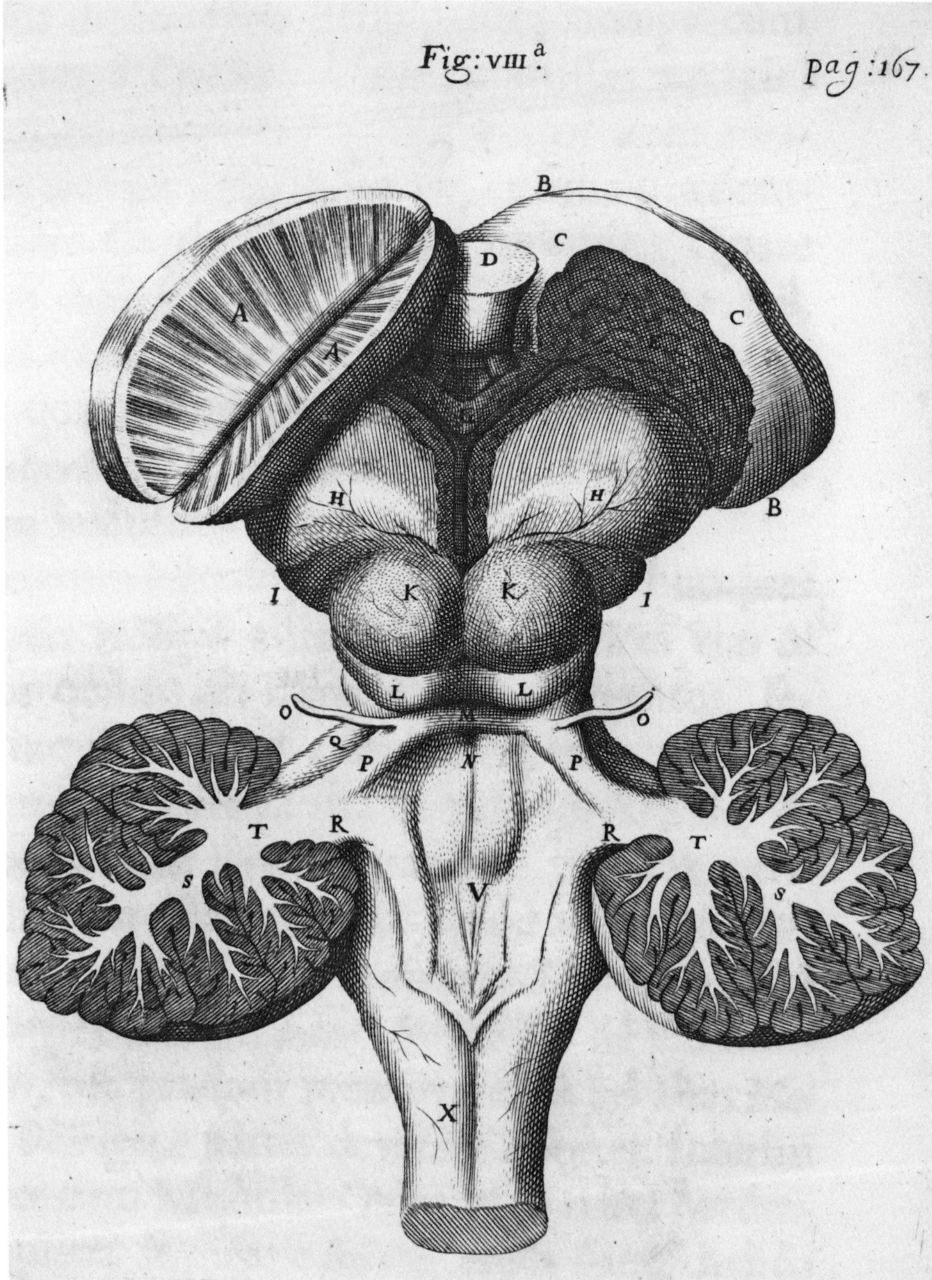

Figure 105 Plate 9 (image 12). The Eighth Figure. REprefents the oblong Marrow taken out of the Head of a Sheep with the Brain cut off and removed, and with the Cerebel and one ftreaked Body cut in two in the middle, and the other things chiefly belonging to the medullar Trunk. Image from *Cerebri anatome* 1664; legend from *Dr Willis's practice of physick* 1684.

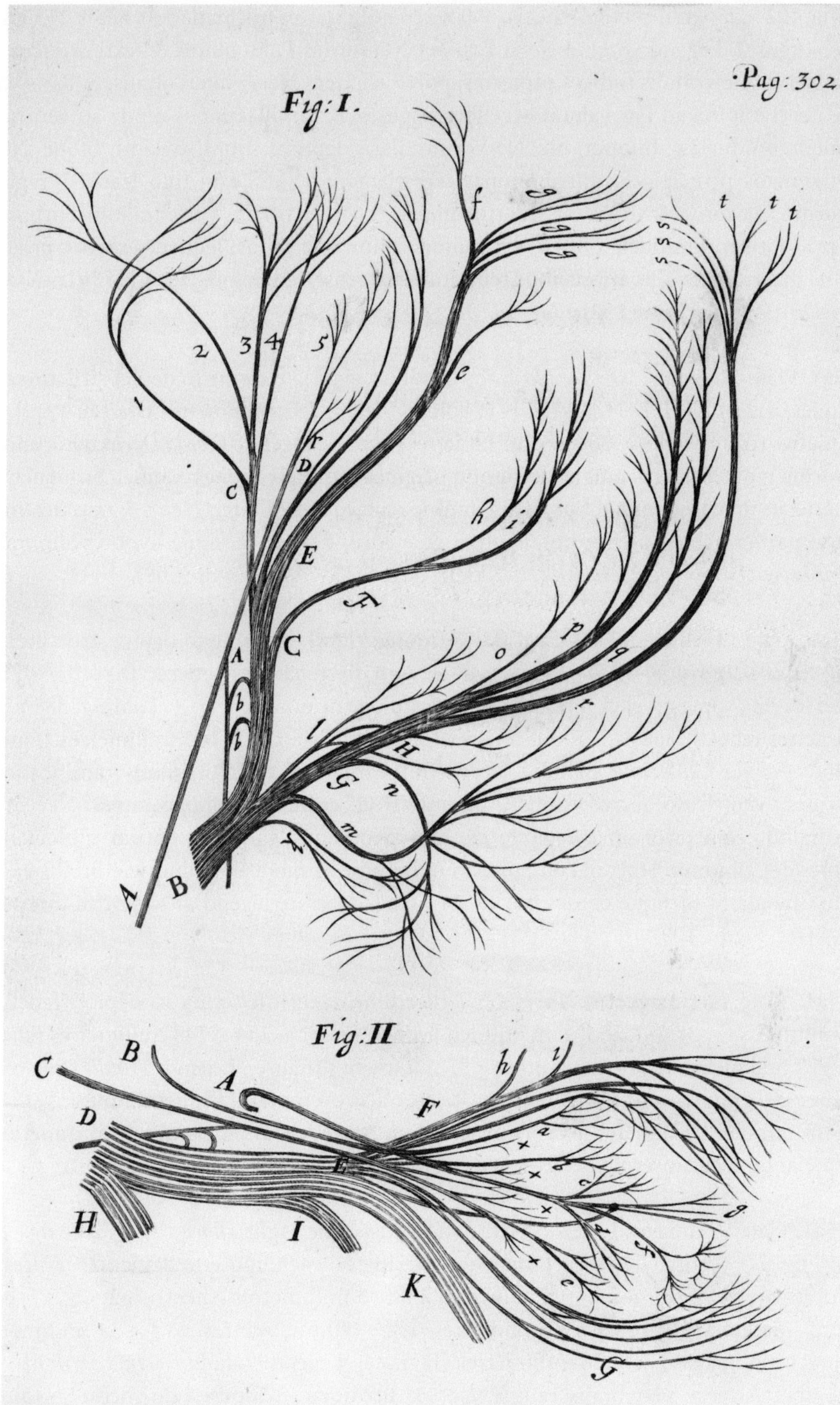

Figure 106 Plate 10 (images 13 and 14): [Unnumbered 2]. This figure ſhews the Branchings of the fifth and ſixth pair of Nerves. The Second Figure ſhews all the Nerves, which being carried from the Nerves of the third, fourth, fifth and ſixth Pair, are beſtowed upon the Muſcles and other parts of the Eye. Image from *Cerebri anatome* 1664; legend from *The remaining medical works* 1681.

Folding, 402 × 250 millimetres (sheet); 390 × 223 millimetres (plate marks); 383 × 215 millimetres (figure). Legend: *Tabula Nona* Exhibet Nervorum Paris quinti & ſexti origines, ab iiſque Nervi intercoſtalis radices proſectas; porrò eiuſdem Nervi intercoſtalis, & Paris vagi, atque nervi è ſpina ad Par vagum acceſſori origines, & ramificationes uſque ad ventriculi regionem productas: Inſuper hîc Nervorum Paris ſeptimi, noni, decimi, atque Nervi diaphragmatis principia & diſtributiones repræſentantur; atque in toto tractu è regione Nervorum præcordis & viſceribus inſertorum, origines Nervorum Vertebralium, eorúmque cum prioribus communicationes deſcribuntur. Totum hoc Tabula ſequens exhibet, prout in homine diverſum ab aliis animalibus reperitur. Plate inserted before legend at ***Iii*1r–*Kkk*1v**, pages 425–34 (see: Figure 107).

Pl.12a1. Plate 12 (Image 16): *Tabula X.*^{ma} (headline, right); lettering to depict structures (in multiples of ≤ 4) A–H, L–N, i–k, n, 1–3. Folding, 398 × 282 millimetres (sheet); 393 × 265 millimetres (plate marks); 378 × 257 millimetres (figure). Legend: *Tabula Decima* Eorundem Nervorum qui in priori Tabula deſcribuntur origines & ramificationes exhibet, prout illarum aliquæ ſecùs in Brutis animalibus ac in Homine reperiunter / Cæteri Nervi & ramificationes illorum pariter habent ac in priori Figura, quæ eorundem in Homine hypotypoſin refert. Plate inserted before legend at ***Kkk*2r–Kkk3r**, pages 435–7 (see: Figure 108).

Pl.13a1. Plate 13 (Image 17): *Tabula X1.*^{ma} (footer, right); lettering to depict structures (in multiples of ≤ 9) A–I, K–L, a–i, k–t, v, x, α–ψ (with discrepancies between the lettering and legend leaving some greek symbols missing from one or other), ʘ, ♀, ♂. Folding, 385 × 202 millimetres (sheet); 368 × 178 millimetres (plate marks); 358 × 164 millimetres (figure). Legend: *Tabula Undecima* Exhibet Nervorum Paris vagi & Intercoſtalis ramificationes inferiores, ventriculo ſc. & totius Abdominis viſceribus diſtributas; item Nervorum vertebralium, qui priorum è regione conſiſtunt, cúmque aliquibus eorum inoſculantur, origines deſcribuntur. Horum configuratio in homine ac quadrupedibus ferè ſimilis exiſtit, ut hæc Tabula ſit utriſque communis. Plate inserted before legend at **Kkk4r–Lll3r**, pages 439–5 (see: Figure 109).

Pl.14a1. Plate 14 (Image 18): *Tabula XII* (headline, right); lettering to depict structures (in multiples of ≤ 3) A–I, K, f, g, h, i. Ruled border. Folding, 254 × 144 millimetres (sheet); 226 × 77 millimetres (plate marks); 220 × 37 millimetres (figure). Legend: *Tabula Duodecima* Exhibet integram medullam Spinalem, ſpecu oſſeo exemptam, & membranâ inveſtiente diſſectâ ſemiexemptam, ut nervorum omnium vertebralium origines & productiones conſpiciantur. Plate inserted before legend at **Lll4r–v**, pages 447–8 (see: Figure 110).

Pl.15a1. Plate 15 (Images 19–23): *TABVL. XIII* (headline, right), *fig: 1.*^{ma}, *fig. 2*$^{da..}$, *fig. 3.*$^{tia..}$, *fig 4*^{ta}, *fig: 5.*$^{ta.}$ (centre above each image); lettering on each figure to depict structures (in multiples of ≤ 4) A–H, a–i, k–n. Folding, 372 × 233 millimetres (sheet); 362 × >217 millimetres (plate marks); 168 × 79 millimetres, 174 × 70 millimetres, 294 × 34 millimetres, 275 × 41 millimetres, 76 × 26 millimetres (Figures). Legend: *Tabula Decima tertia. Figura I.* Exhibet Arteriæ vertebralis ramificationes, utrinque in ſuperiorem medullæ ſpinalis partem, ínque poſteriorem medullæ oblongatæ, exporrectas; *Figure II.* Exhibet venas vertebrales, quæ arteriis ſupradictis pares ſunt; item ſinûs vertebralis portionem ſuperiorem, ac utriuſque inter ſe ac ſinus laterales capitis, & inter venas jugulares, communicationes; *Figure III.* Exhibet Arteriam Spinalem, quæ intra ſpecum oſſeum, juxta interiorem medullæ ſuperficiem, ab occipite ad os Sacrum, ad formam Inſtitæ reticularis, producitur; *Figure*

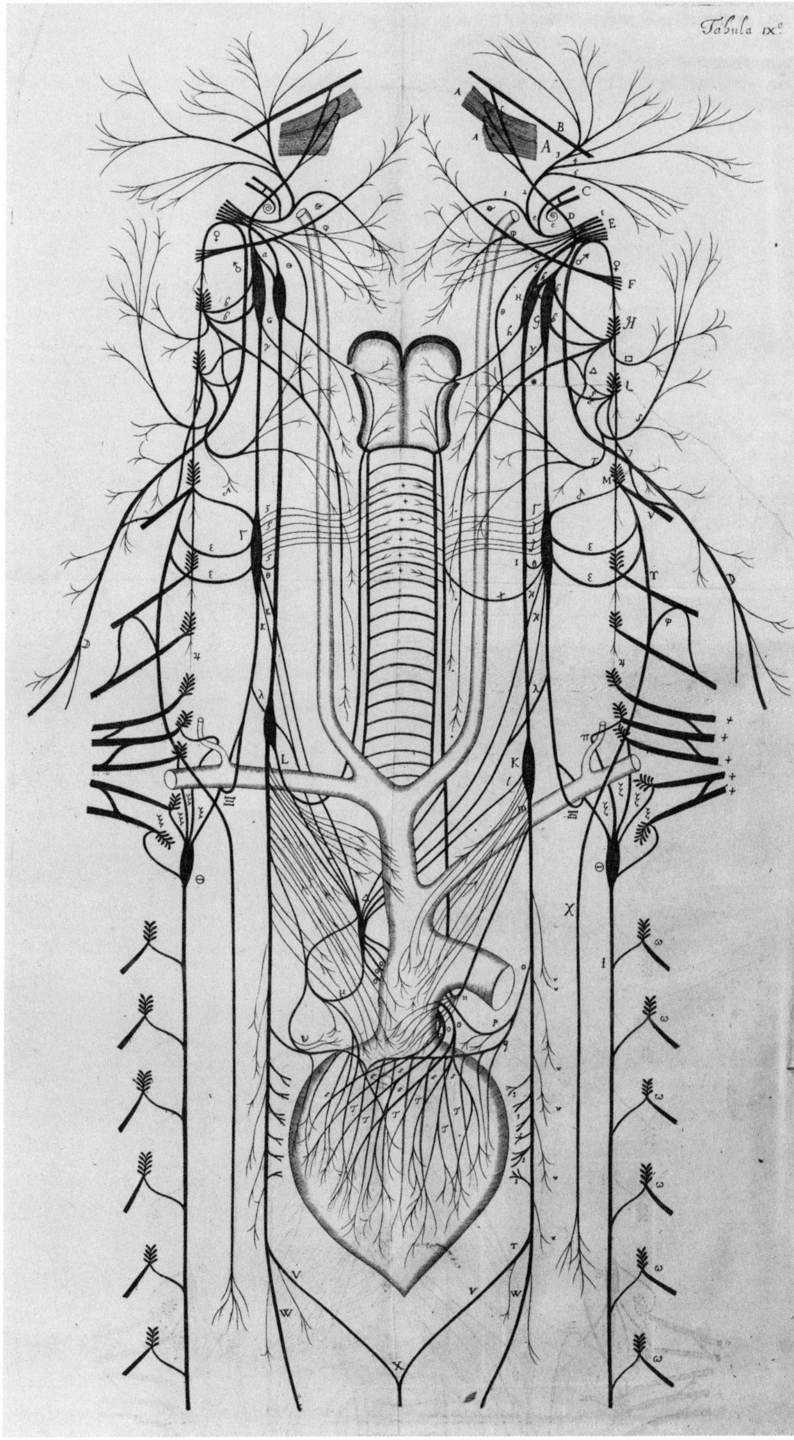

Figure 107 Plate 11 (image 15). *The Ninth Table* Shews the beginnings of the fifth and ſixth pair of Nerves, and the Roots of the Intercoſtal Nerve proceeding from them; moreover, the Origines and Branchings out of the ſame Intercoſtal nerve and the wandring Pair, and of the acceſsory Nerve produced out of the Spine to the wandering Pair carried to the Region of the Ventricle. Beſides, here are repreſented the beginnings and diſtributions of the ſeventh, ninth, tenth Pair of Nerves, and of the Nerve of the Diaphragma; alſo the beginnings of the Vertebral Nerves in their whole Tract from the Region of the Nerves inſerted in the *Præcordia* and *Viſcera* are deſcribed, and their Communications with the former. All this whole following Table ſhews how it is found in Man different from other living Creatures. Image from *Cerebri anatome* 1664; legend from *The remaining medical works* 1681.

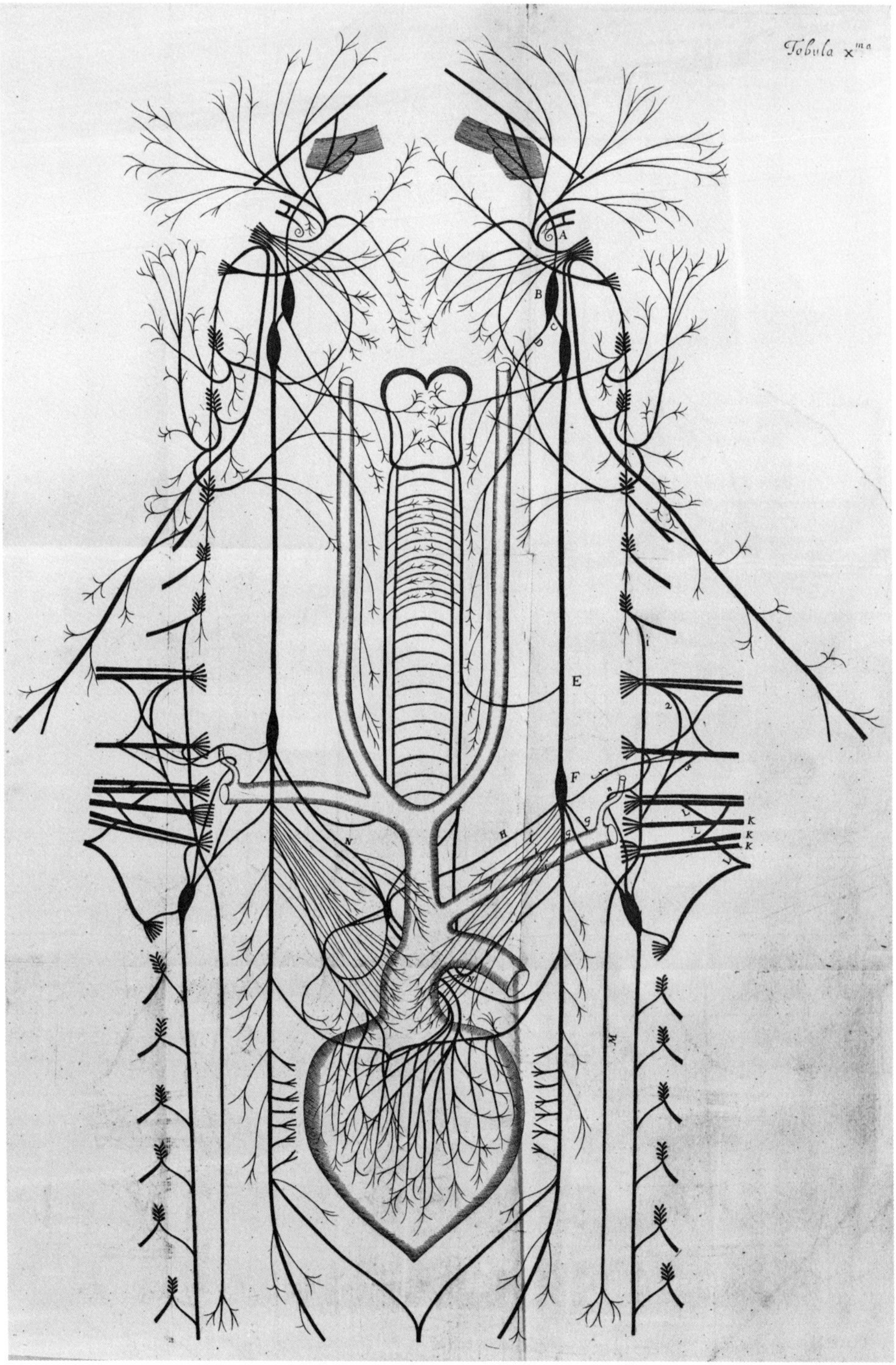

Figure 108 Plate 12 (image 16). *The Tenth Table* Shews the beginnings and Branchings out of the ſame Nerves which were deſcribed in the former Table, as ſome of them are found in brute Beaſts otherwiſe than in Man / The other Nerves and their Branchings out are as in the other Figure, which ſhews the pattern of them in Man. Image from *Cerebri anatome* 1664; legend from *The remaining medical works* 1681.

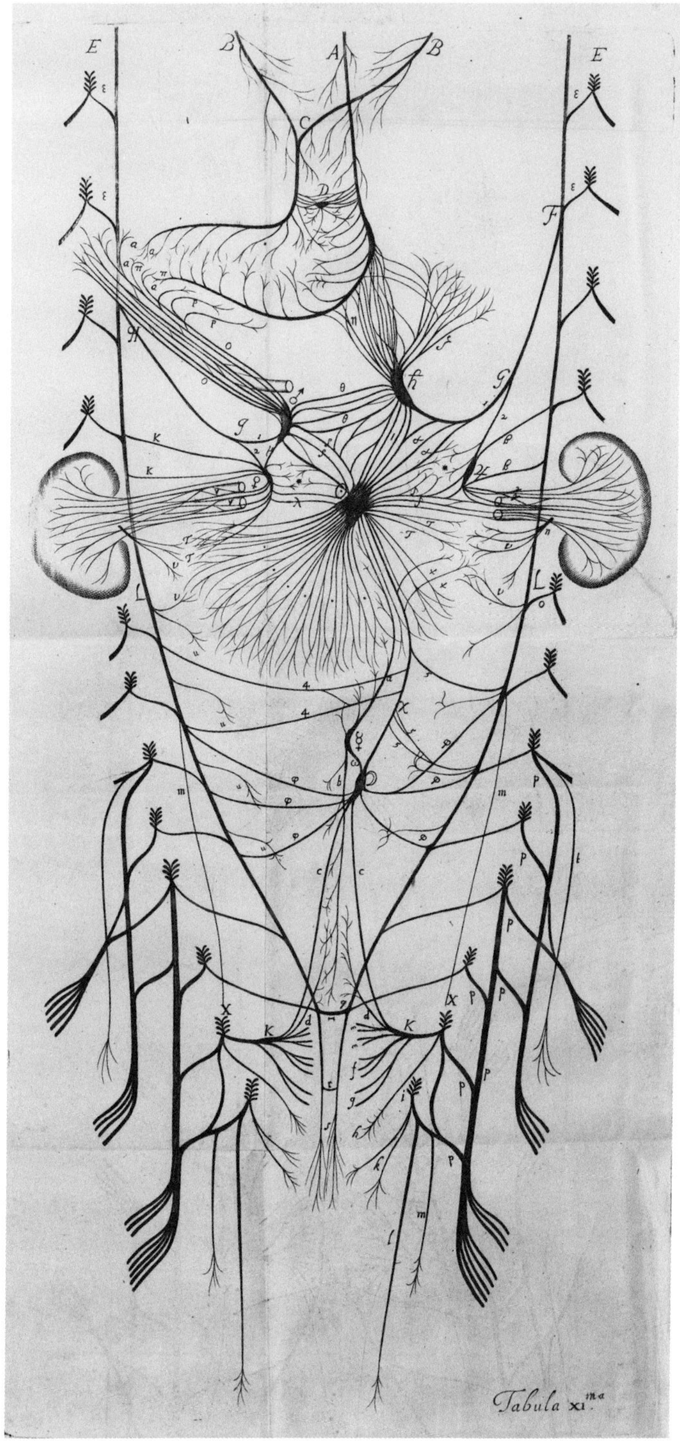

Figure 109 Plate 13 (image 17). *The Eleventh Table* Shews the lower Branchings out of the wandring and the Intercoſtal Pair diſtributed to the Ventricle and the *Viſcera* of the Abdomen; alſo the beginnings of the Vertebral Nerves, which are placed over againſt the former, and are ingraffed into ſome of them. The figure of theſe in Man and in the four-footed Beaſts is almoſt alike, ſo that this Table may be common for both. Image from *Cerebri anatome* 1664; legend from *The remaining medical works* 1681.

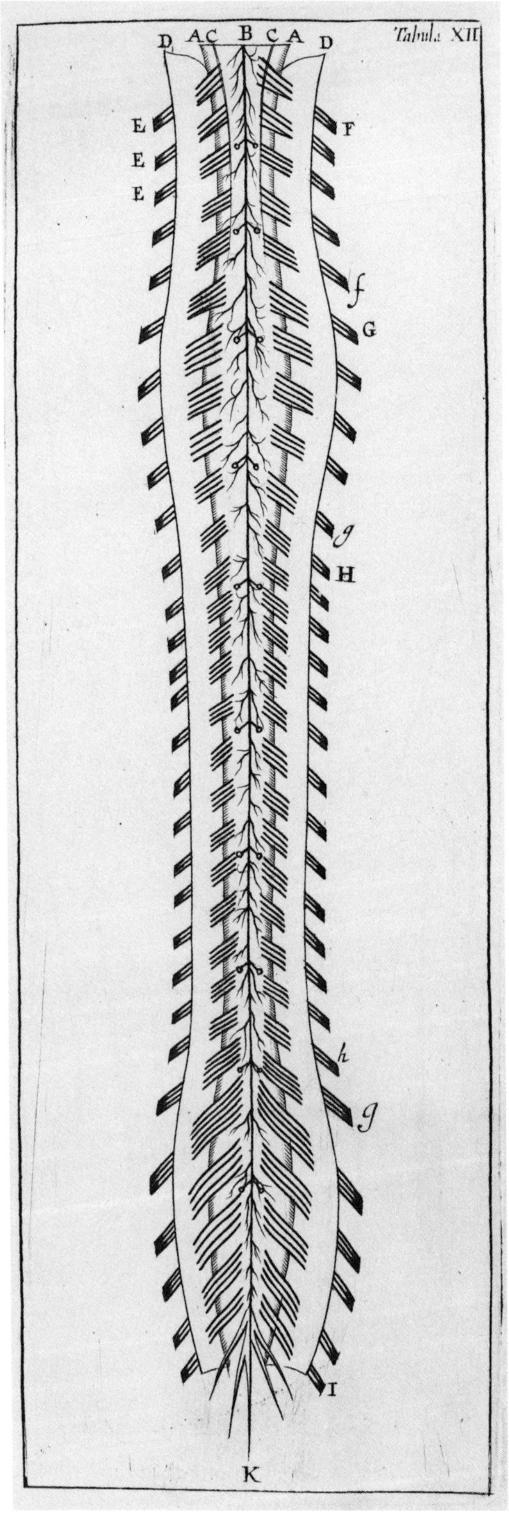

Figure 110 Plate 14 (image 18). *The Twelfth Table* Shews the Spinal Marrow whole taken out of its bony Den, and half taken from the Membrane cloathing it, being diffected, that the beginnings and productions of all the Vertebral Nerves might be feen together. Image from *Cerebri anatome* 1664; legend from *The remaining medical works* 1681.

IIII. Sinûs ſpinalis divaricationes in toto ductu ejus exhibet; *Figura V*. Exhibet ſinûs ſpinalis Iconem in cane, qui non utì in vitulo, ove, porco, & pleriſque aliis, commiſſuras in toto ductu habet, ſed tantùm in parte inſima & ſuprema, ubi per tres aut quatuor proceſſus tranſverſos inter ſe communicat. Plate inserted before legend at ***Mmm*1r–*Mmm3*v**, pages 449–54 (see: Figure 111).

Copy: DASC (#1 of 3): early full calf with gilt tooled device on upper and lower boards (winged crusader with sword aloft standing astride supine horned figure: unidentified), spine with five raised bands and six gilt decorated panels, unlettered, restored with new front endpapers. Leaves 185 × 143 millimetres, boards 198 × 147 × 45 millimetres.

2B1. CEREBRI ANATOME, London octavo 1664

The second edition of Willis's second book, with illustrations from the quarto edition in their first state altered in pen and ink [HJR Wing 9, Denham 2].

Title page: CEREBRI | ANATOME: | CUI ACCESSIT | *Nervorum Deſcriptio* | ET USUS. | [rule] | STUDIO | THOMÆ WILLIS, | Ex *Æde Chriſti Oxon.* M D. & in | iſta Celebrerrima Academia Naturalis | Philoſophiæ Profeſſoris *Sidleiani.* | [rule] | *LONDINI,* | Typis *Tho. Roycroft*, Impenſis *Jo. Martyn* | & *Ja. Alleſtry* apud inſigne Campanæ in | Cœmeterio *D. Pauli.* [rule over date] M.DC.LXIV.

Collation: octavo; 23 letter roman alphabet using I: A^8, a^8 (-a8), B–D^8, E^8 (E4 + *1 = a8), F–Q^8; \$1–4 signed apart from: -B4, a8 signed *; F3 is a cancelled leaf.[26]

136 leaves: paginated as [30] 1–56, [2: recto numbered Pag. 56, verso unnumbered], 57–240.

Type: height (20 lines) 57 millimetres, width 69 millimetres.

Contents: **A1r**, page [1], blank; **A1v**, page [2], Imprimatur, Jan. 20. 1663. THO. GRIGG R in Chriſto Pat. ac. D^no^ D. *Humfr.* Epiſc. *Lon.* à ſac. Domeſticis.; **A2r**, page [3], title; **A2v**, page [4], blank; **A3r–A5r**, pages [5–9], REVERENDISSIMO *In Chriſto Patri, & Domino, Domino* GILBERTO, *Providentia Divina, Archiepiſcopo* Cantuarienſi, *totius* Angliæ *Primati & Metropolitano; & Auguſtiſsimo Principi* CAROLO II. *M.* Britanniæ, Franciæ, & Hiberniæ *Regi, à Secretioribus Conſiliis.* ... [signed] *Clementiæ veſtræ Clientem humillimum & aſtrictiſſimum,* THO. WILLIS.; **A5v–a1r**, pages [10–17], Amico Lectori Præfatio.; **a1v–a2r**, pages [18–19], AUTHORI In Cerebri Anatomen carmen. ... [signed] *Philippus Fell*, A.M. & Collegii Omnium Animarum in Acad. *Oxon.* Socius.; **a2v–a5v**, pages [20–6], *Elenchus rerum.* [Cerebri anatome]; **a6r–a7v**, pages [27–30], *Nervorum deſcriptio & uſus.*

B1r–K8r, pages 1–143, plus inserted leaf *1r–v, 'Pag. 56'-[-], between pages 56–7, [text] CEREBRI ANATOME.; **K8v**, page 144, blank; **L1r–Q8v**, pages 145–240, [text] *NERVORUM* Deſcriptio & Uſus.

[26] This is pointed out by HJR Wing (1962): page 12, and consistent with difference in the paper and the presence of a stub onto which the cancellans is pasted.

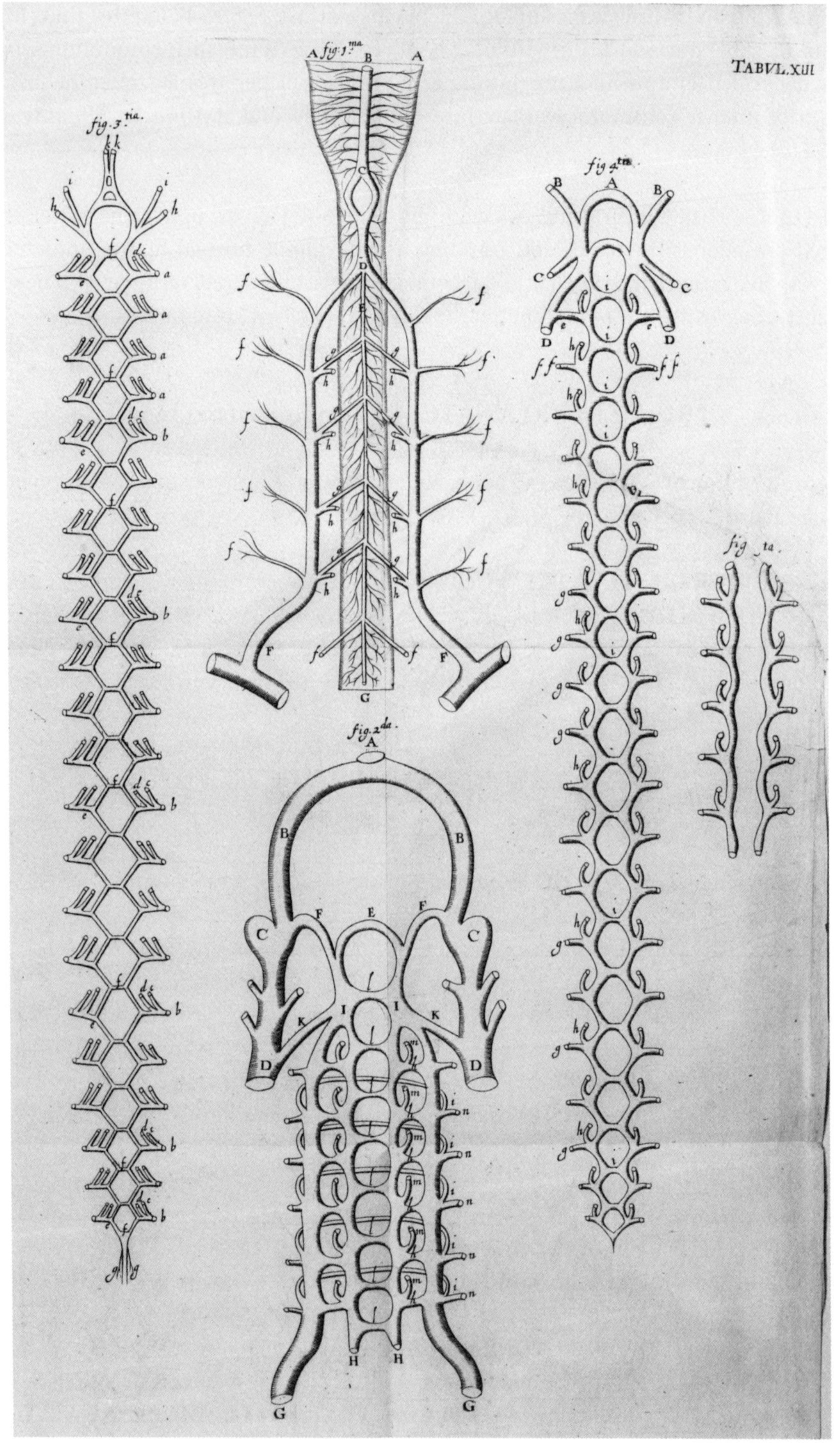

Figure 111 Plate 15 (images 19–23). *The Thirteenth Table*. FIGURE I. Shews the branchings forth of the Vertebral artery reaching out, on both ſides into the ſuperiour part of the Spinal Marrow, and into the hinder Region of the oblong Marrow.; FIGURE II. Shews the Vertebral Veins which are Companions to the aboveſaid Arteries; alſo the upper portion of the Vertebral

Headlines and *Catchwords*: ufus: for ufus. at **Q8r**, page 239.

No catchword at **A5r / v**, pages [9] / [10].

Frontispiece: none.

Portrait: none.

Printers' ornaments: row of 14 fleurons {**Roycroft 15**} and two rows each of 12 fleurons, the lower inverted, separated between ##6 / 7 by : {**Roycroft 17**} at **A3r**, page [5]; row of 11 fleurons {**Roycroft 11**} above two rows each of 15 fleurons, the lower inverted {**Roycroft 28**} at **A5v**, page [10]; row of 14 fleurons {**Roycroft 15**} above single row of 12 fleurons separated by : between ##6 / 7 {**Roycroft 17**} at **a1v**, page [18]; row of 14 fleurons {**Roycroft 15**} separated by | between ##5 and 6, 9 and 10, at **B1r**, page 1; two rows of 14 fleurons separated by | between ##6 / 7, 9 / 10 (upper), and 14 fleurons (inverted) separated by | between ##5 / 6, 9 / 10 (lower) {**Roycroft 15**}, with middle row of 12 fleurons separated by : between ##4 / 5, 7 / 8 {**Roycroft 17**} at **L1r**, page 145.

Decorated I {**Roycroft 9**} at **B1r**, page 1; N {**Roycroft 29**} at **L1r**, page 145.

Illustrations: As in **2A** apart from:

Pl.1a1. Plate 1 (image 1): *page 25* (headline, right) scored through, pag: 414 (footer, right) scored through and altered in pen and ink to 217. Folding, 222 × 195 millimetres (sheet). Inserted before legend at **B7r–v**, pages 13–14.

Pl.2a1. Plate 2 (image 2): *pag: 27* (headline, right) scored through. Folding, 162 × 133 millimetres (sheet). Inserted within legend at **B7v–B8r**, pages 14–15.

Pl.3a1. Plate 3 (image 3): *pag: 49* (headline, right) scored through. Folding, 242 × 188 millimetres (sheet). Inserted within legend at **C5v–C6r**, pages 26–7.

Pl.4a1. Plate 4 (image 4): *pag: 51* (headline, right) scored through. Folding, 150 × 115 millimetres (sheet). Inserted before legend at **C6r–C6v**, pages 27–8.

Pl.5a1. Plate 5 (image 5): *pag: 63* (headline, right) scored through. Folding, 206 × 150 millimetres (sheet). Inserted after legend at **D1v**, page 34.

Bofom and the communications of either among themfelves and lateral Bofoms of the Head, and between the Jugular Veins.; FIGURE III. Shews the Spinal Artery which is produced within the bony Den nigh the more inward Superficies of the Marrow, from the hinder part of the Head to the *Os Sacrum*, in the fhape of a Net-work purl.; FIGURE IV. Shews the Branchings out of the Spinal Bofom in its whole paffage.; FIGURE V. Shews the Image of the Spinal Bofom in a Dog, which hath not joynings together in its whole paffage, as it is in a Calf, Sheep, Hog, and many others, but only in the loweft and uppermoft part, where it communicates with it felf by three or four crofs Proceffes. Image from *Cerebri anatome* 1664; legend from *The remaining medical works* 1681.

Pl.6a1. Plate 6 (image 6): *pag: 64* (headline, right) scored through. Folding, 220 × 147 millimetres (sheet). Inserted before legend at **D2r**, page 35.

Pl.7a2. Plate 7 (images 7–10): *pag: 56* (headline, right). Folding, 202 × 143 millimetres (sheet). Inserted after legend at **E4 + *1r–v**, 'Pag. 56' / -.

Pl.8a1. Plate 8 (image 11): *pag: 131* (headline, right) scored through. Folding, 222 × 125 millimetres (sheet, cropped). Inserted before legend at **F3r–v**, pages 69–70.

Pl.9a1. Plate 9 (image 12): *pag: 167* (headline, right) scored through. Leaf size, 150 × 92 millimetres (sheet, cropped). Inserted within legend at **G4v–G5r**, pages 88–9.

Pl.10a1. Plate 10 (images 13–14): [*pag:*] *302* scored through and 158 added in pen and ink (headline, right). Folding (bound horizontally), 203 × 150 millimetres (sheet). Inserted within legend at **L7v–L8v**, pages 158–60.

Pl.11a1. Plate 11 (image 15): Folding, 385 × 238 millimetres (sheet, cropped). Inserted before legend at **P8r–Q2v**, pages 223–38.

Pl.12a1. Plate 12 (image 16): Folding, 385 × 275 millimetres (sheet, cropped). Inserted before legend at **Q3r–v**, pages 229–30.

Pl.13a1. Plate 13 (image 17): Folding, 377 × 179 millimetres (sheet, cropped). Inserted before legend at **Q4r–Q5v**, pages 231–4.

Pl.14a1. Plate 14 (image 18): Folding, 241 × 94 millimetres (sheet). Inserted before legend at **Q6r**, page 235.

Pl.15a1. Plate 15 (images 19–23): Folding, 374 × 217 millimetres (sheet). Inserted within legend at **Q7r–Q8r**, pages 237–9.

Copy: DASC. Early full roan with gilt edges, spine with five raised bands and five gilt decorated panels, label CEREB | ANATO with gilt border, restored, original endpapers. Leaves 150 × 95 millimetres, boards 155 × 100 × 30 millimetres. Bookplate: Docteur François Moutier.[27]

2B2. CEREBRI ANATOME, London octavo 1664

A later issue of the second edition of Willis's second book, with illustrations from the quarto edition extensively reworked and in their second state [not distinguished from HJR Wing 9, Denham 2].

[27] François Moutier (1881–1961) was a physician and poet based in Paris who contributed to neurology and gastroenterology. He had trained with Édouard Brissaud (1852–1909) and Pierre Marie (1853–1940) and wrote his thesis on Broca's aphasia (1907: pages 774). Moutier was a well-published poet whose verse reflected his experience in the First World War and echoed a plea for Christianity and humanity.

As in **2B1** apart from:

Collation: *1 = a8 bound, as printed, after a7.

136 leaves: paginated as [32] 1–240.

Illustrations: plates with page placements revised, extensively worn, and reworked, several cracked and with corners missing [marked †]:

Pl.1a2. Plate 1 (image 1): *pag: 25* (headline, right) partly erased and *p. 13* added (headline, left). Folding, 222 × 189 millimetres (sheet).

Pl.2a2. Plate 2 (image 2): *pag: 27* erased and *p. 14* added (headline, left). Folding, 167 × 125 millimetres (sheet).

Pl.3a2. Plate 3 (image 3): *pag: 49* erased and *p 26* added (headline, left). Folding, 230 × 186 millimetres (sheet).

Pl.4a2. Plate 4 (image 4): *pag: 51* erased and *p: 27:* added (headline, left). Folding, 158 × 113 millimetres (sheet).

Pl.5a2. Plate 5 (image 5): *pag: 63* erased and *p: 35:* added (headline, left). Folding, 215 × 145 millimetres (sheet).

Pl.6a2. Plate 6 (image 6): *pag: 64* erased and *p: 35.* added (headline, left). Folding, 222 × 146 millimetres (sheet).

Pl.7a2†. Plate 7 (images 7–10): Folding, 208 × 153 millimetres (sheet). Inserted after **E4v**, page 56; legend after **a7v**, page [30].

Pl.8a2†. Plate 8 (image 11): *pag: 131* partly erased and *p: 69:* added (headline, left). Folding, 235 × 138 millimetres (sheet).

Pl.9a2. Plate 9 (image 12): *pag: 167* erased and p: *88* overprinted (headline, right). Folding, 147 × 106 millimetres (sheet).

Pl.10a2. Plate 10 (images 13–14): *pag: 302* partly erased and *p: 69*: added (headline, left). Folding, 210 × 150 millimetres (sheet, folding). Inserted before legend for Figura VII at **F3r–v**, pages 69–70.

Pl.11a2†. Plate 11 (image 15): *p: 223* added (headline, left). Folding, 396 × 236 millimetres (sheet).

Pl.12a2. Plate 12 (image 16): *p: 229* added (headline, left). Folding, 402 × 269 millimetres (sheet).

Pl.13a2†. Plate 13 (image 17): *p: 231* added (headline, left). Folding, 350 × 188 millimetres (sheet).

Pl.14a2†. Plate 14 (image 18): *Tabula XII* erased (and with the upper right corner lost), and *p 231* added (headline, left). Folding, 240 × 92 millimetres (sheet). Inserted before **Q4r**, page 231, legend at **Q6r**, page 235.

Pl.15a2. Plate 15 (images 19–23): *p. 236* added (headline, left). Folding, 369 × 222 millimetres (sheet).

Copy: DASC. Early full calf, spine with five raised bands and five gilt decorated panels, lettered WILLIS | ANATOME with gilt border, new front endpaper, original pastedown, and rear endpapers. Leaves millimetres, boards 159 × 97 × 32 millimetres. Inscribed: Ex libris [writing inked over] 1672.

2C1.c1. CEREBRI ANATOME, Amsterdam duodecimo 1664

The first issue of the third edition of Willis's second book, with reengraved illustrations in their first state [HJR Wing 10, Denham 3].

Title page: CEREBRI | ANATOME: | *Cui acceſſit* | NERVORUM | Deſcriptio & Uſus. | STUDIO | THOMÆ WILLIS, | *Ex Æ*de Chriſti Oxon. *M. D. & in iſta* | *Celeberrima Academia Naturalis Philoſo-* | *phiæ Profeſſoris* Sidleiani. | [ornament] | AMSTELODAMI, | [short rule] | Apud GERBRANDUM SCHAGEN. | M. DC. LXIV.

Collation: duodecimo; 23 letter roman alphabet using I: $*^{12}$, A–I^{12}, K–L^{12}, M^{6}; $1–6 signed apart from: *6 signed L6.

150 leaves: paginated as [24], 1–273 [274], [2]. Mispaginated: 144 for 134, 246 for 264.

Type: 41 lines; height (20 lines) 53 millimetres, width 56 millimetres.

Contents: ***1r–v**, pages [1–2], blank; ***2r**, page [3], title; ***2v**, page [4], blank; ***3r–*5v**, pages [5–10], AMICO LECTORI PRÆFATIO.; ***6r–*10r**, page [11–19], Elenchus rerum. [Cerebri anatome]; ***10v–*12v**, pages [20–24], [Elenchus rerum] Nervorum deſcriptio & uſus.

A1r–G10v, pages 1–164, [text] CEREBRI ANATOME.; **G11r–M5r**, page 165–273, [text] NERVORUM Deſcriptio & Uſus.; **M5v**, page 274, blank; **M6r–v**, pages [1–2], blank.

Headlines and *Catchwords*: headlines correct.

quibus for Glandulam at **B5r** / v, page 33 / 34; ultoro for ultro at **D12v** / **E1r**, pages 96 / 97.

Frontispiece: none.

Portrait: none.

Printers' ornament: tailpiece at ***2r**, page [3] {**Schagen 11**}.

Decorated 'A' at ***3r**, page [5] {**Schagen 14**}; 'I' at **A1**, page 1 {**Schagen 5**}; 'N' at **G10r**, page 165 {**Schagen 15**}.

Illustrations: reengraved, lettering and legends as in **2A**:

Pl.1b1. Plate 1 (image 1): Figura 1[a] (headline centre), *Pag. 15* (headline, right), *de medio T vid pag. 248* (footer, right). Folding, 225 × 180 millimetres (sheet); printed from a plate measuring 296 × 376 millimetres (plate mark at lower border, no lines); 186 × 166 millimetres (figure). Inserted before legend at **A8r–v**, pages 15–16.

Pl.2b1. Plate 2 (image 2): Fig. II.[da] (headline, centre), *pag. 16.* (headline, right), *de medio S vid pag. 248* (footer, right). Folding, 163 × 122 millimetres (sheet); printed from a larger plate, lines 137 × 101 millimetres (plate marks at left and lower borders; lines on all four edges, continuing upwards and to the right); 130 × 100 millimetres (figure). Inserted within legend at **A8v–A9r**, pages 16–17.

Pl.3b1. Plate 3 (image 3): Fig. III. (headline, centre), *Pag. 29* (headline, right). Folding, 222 × 190 millimetres (sheet); printed from a plate measuring 296 × 376 millimetres (no plate marks or lines); 190 × 173 millimetres (figure). Inserted after legend at **B3v**, page 30.

Pl.4b1. Plate 4 (image 4): Fig. IIII. (headline, centre), *pag. 30.* (headline, left). Folding, 171 × 110 millimetres (sheet); printed from a larger plate, lines 147 × *c.*105 millimetres (plate mark at left and lower borders; line at upper edge); 113 × 93 millimetres (figure). Inserted within legend at **B3v–B4r**, pages 30–1.

Pl.5b1. Plate 5 (image 5): *Fig. V.* (headline, left), *p: 38* (headline, right). Folding, 216 × 163 millimetres (sheet); printed from a larger plate, lines 192 × 152 millimetres (plate mark at left and lower borders; lines at upper and right edges); 179 × 133 millimetres (figure). Inserted following legend at **B7v**, page 38.

Pl.6b1. Plate 6 (image 6): *Fig. VI* (headline, left), *p. 39* (headline, right). Folding, 202 × 163 millimetres (sheet, cropped); printed from a larger plate, lines 182 × 143 millimetres (plate marks at right and lower borders; lines at upper and left edges); 172 × 127 millimetres (figure). Inserted before legend at **B8r**, page 39.

Pl.7b1. Plate 7 (images 7–10) [Unnumbered 1]: Fig. I; Fig. II; Fig. III (headlines, above each figure); Fig. IIII. (right of figure), *pag. 65.* (headline, right). Folding, 177 × 128 millimetres (sheet, cropped); printed from a larger plate, lines 145 × 100 millimetres (plate marks at right and lower borders; lines at upper and left edges, continuing upwards and to the left); 26 × 94 millimetres, 71 × 93 millimetres, 35 × 27 millimetres, 72 × 25 millimetres (figures). Inserted within legend at **C8v–C9v**, pages 64–66.

Pl.8b1. Plate 8 (image 11): *Fig VII* (headline left), *p. 80* (headline, right). Folding, 204 × 158 millimetres (sheet); printed from a larger plate, lines 197 × 145 millimetres (plate marks at upper and right borders; lines at left and lower edges); 192 × 105 millimetres (figure). Inserted within legend at **D4r–D5r**, pages 79–81.

Pl.9b1. Plate 9 (image 12): Fig. VIII (headline, centre), *pag. 101.* (headline, right). Folding, 173 × 118 millimetres (sheet); printed from a larger plate, lines 138 × 97 millimetres (plate marks at right and lower borders; lines on all four edges, continuing upwards and to the left); 108 × 95 millimetres (figure). Inserted before legend at **E3r–v**, pages 101–102.

Pl.10b1. Plate 10 (images 13–14) [Unnumbered 2]: *Fig: I.*; *Fig: II.* (above each figure), *p. 180* (headline, right). Folding, 194 × 150 millimetres (sheet); printed from a larger plate, lines 190 × 149 millimetres (plate marks at upper and left borders; lines at right and lower edges); 125 × 112 millimetres, 55 × 114 millimetres (figures). Inserted within legend at **H6r–H7v**, pages 179–82.

Pl.11b1. Plate 11 (image 15): *Tabula.* IX.^{a} (headline, right). Folding, 298 × 183 millimetres (sheet); printed from a larger plate (plate marks at left and lower borders; no lines); 273 × 153 millimetres (figure). Inserted within legends for Tabulæ IX–XIII at **L7v–M6r**, pages 254–73.

Pl.12b1. Plate 12 (image 16): *Tabula* X.^{ma} (headline, right). Folding, 300 × 212 millimetres (sheet); printed from a larger plate (plate marks at right and lower borders; no lines); 267 × 182 millimetres (figure). Inserted within legends for Tabulæ IX–XIII at **L7v–M6r**, pages 254–73.

Pl.13b1. Plate 13 (image 17) *Tabula* XI.^{ma} (footer, right). Folding, 305 × 135 millimetres (sheet); printed from a plate measuring 298 × 382 millimetres (plate marks at upper, left, and lower borders; line at right edge); 276 × 125 millimetres (figure). Inserted within legends for Tabulæ IX–XIII at **L7v–M6r**, pages 254–73.

Pl.14b1. Plate 14 (image 18): *Tabula* XII (headline, right), no ruled border to inner margin of plate. Folding, 231 × 72 millimetres (sheet); printed from a plate measuring 296 × 376 millimetres (plate marks at upper, right, and lower borders); 213 × 37 millimetres (figure). Inserted within legends for Tabulæ IX–XIII at **L7v–M6r**, pages 254–73.

Pl.15b1. Plate 15 (images 19–23) distributed as four separate leaves: Tab. XIII (headline, right above Figure 2), *Fig. 1.*^{ma} (header, centre), *Fig. 2.*^{da} (header within figure), *Fig. 3.*^{tia} (header, straddling upper part of figure), *Fig. 4.*^{ta} (header, centre) and *Fig. 5.*^{ta} (header, centre). Folding, 176 × 115 millimetres, 174 × 108 millimetres, 303 × 75 millimetres, 130 × 66 millimetres (sheets); printed from a plate measuring 298 × 382 millimetres (plate marks at left, right, and lower borders, lines above figures 1, 2, and 5, and figures 3 and 4); 162 × 77 millimetres, 168 × 68 millimetres, 284 × 30 millimetres, 267 × 33 millimetres, 72 × 25 millimetres (figures). Inserted within legends for Tabulæ IX–XIII at **L7v–M6r**, pages 254–73.

Copy: DASC, lacking *1, A8, and C9. Early full vellum, spine lettered in manuscript Tho Willis | Anatome | Cerebr | 1 *B*, original endpapers. Leaves 132 × 75 millimetres, boards 142 × 76 × 30 millimetres. Inscribed (inked over) *599 Path* [obscured].

2C1.c2. CEREBRI ANATOME, Amsterdam duodecimo 1664

The first issue of the third edition of Willis's second book, with reengraved illustrations in their first state, the upper half of the title page from **2C2** pasted over **2C1.c1** to reflect inclusion in the bound volume of *De ratione motus musculorum* [not distinguished from HJR Wing 9, Denham 3].[28]

[28] See introductory notes for justification of including this made-up copy.

Title page: [1]. CEREBRI | ANATOME, | NERVORUMQUE | Deſcriptio & Uſus, | STUDIO | THOMÆ WILLIS, | *Ex Æde Chriſti Oxon. M. D. & in iſtâ | Cereberrima Academia Naturalis Philoſo— | phia Profeſſoris* Seidleiani. | Acceſſit | *Viri cujuſdam Clariſsimi* | De Ratione Motûs | MUSCULORUM | Tractatus ſingularis. | . . . (pasted over lower part of title page for 2C1.c1) [printers' device] | AMSTELODAMI, | [short rule] | Apud GERBRANDUM SCHAGEN. | M. DC. LXIV.

[2]. DE | RATIONE | MOTUS | MUSCULORUM. | *Ἐν πᾶσι τοῖς φυσικοῖς ἐνεστί τι θαυμαστόν.* | Ariſt. de Part. Animal. | [printers' device] | AMSTELODAMI, | [rule] | Apud CASPARUM COMMELINUM. | M. DC. LXIV.

Then as in [1]. **2C1c1** and [2]. **2C2** (next) apart from:

Illustrations: variation in sheet sizes and occasional binding positions.

Copy: DASC, lacking *6 signed L6, *7, and Figuræ V and VI. Early full calf with double lined border, spine with five raised bands and five gilt decorated panels, lettered CEREB | ANATO, original endpapers. Leaves 133 × 72 millimetres, boards 137 × 75 × 25 millimetres. Inscribed on lower part of title (Schagen) Ex libris Francisci (surname obscured) 1666.

2C2.c1. CEREBRI ANATOME, Amsterdam duodecimo 1664

The second issue of the third edition of Willis's second book, with reset title page in its first state, *iu* for *in*, 'Cereberrima' corrected in pen and ink to 'Celeberrima', and Seidleiani, with the text and illustration of *De ratione motus musculorum* [HJR Wing 11, Denham 4].

Title page: [1]. CEREBRI | ANATOME, | NERVORUMQUE | Deſcriptio & Uſus, | STUDIO | THOMÆ WILLIS, | *Ex Æde* Chriſti Oxon. *M. D. & iu iſtâ* | *Cer*[l]*eberrima Academia Naturalis Philoſo— | phia Profeſſoris* Seidleiani. | Acceſſit | *Viri cujuſdam Clariſsimi* | De Ratione Motûs | MUSCULORUM | Tractatus ſingularis. | [printers' device] | AMSTELODAMI, | [short rule] | Apud CASPARUM COMMELINUM. | M. DC. LXIV.

[2]. DE | RATIONE | MOTUS | MUSCULORUM. | *Ἐν πᾶσι τοῖς φυσικοῖς ἐνεστί τι θαυμαστόν.* | Ariſt. de Part. Animal: | [printers' device] | AMSTELODAMI, | [rule] | Apud CASPARUM COMMELINUM. | M. DC. LXIV.[29]

Collation: duodecimo; 23 letter roman alphabet using I: $*^{12}$ (-*2), π^2, A–I^{12}, K–L^{12}, M^6, $^2A^{12}$, $^2B^4$; \$1–6 signed apart from: *6 signed L6.

167 leaves: paginated as [26], 1–273 [274], [2], 1–32. Mispaginated: 144 for 134, 246 for 264.

[29] The quote from Aristotle reads: 'There is something admirable in all physical matters.'

Then as in **2C1.c1** apart from:

Contents: [1]. ***1r–v**, pages [1–2], blank; **π1r**, page [3], title; **π1v**, page [4], blank; **π2r–v**, pages [5–6], BENEVOLO LECTORI Sal. D. TYPOGRAPHUS., until

[2]. **A1r**, page [1], title; **A1v**, page [2], blank; **A2r–B4v**, pages 3–32, [text] DE RATIONE MOTUS MUSCULORUM. [William Croone].

Headlines and *Catchwords*: [1]. Headlines correct.

Catchwords correct.

[2]. Headlines correct.

4. Re for 3. Re at **A2r / v**, pages [Fol.] 3 / 4.

Frontispiece: none.

Portrait: none.

Printers' ornament: printers' device: [1]. **π1r**, page [1], title page {**Commelin 1**}.

Decorated P at ***2r**, page [5] {**Commelin 2**}.

[2]. **A1r**, page [1], title page {**Commelin 1**}.

Decorated D at **A2r**, [Fol.] 3 {**Commelin 3**}.

Illustrations: lettering and legends as in **2A**:

Pl.1c1. Plate 1 (image 1). Figura 1.[a] (headline centre), *pag. 15.* (headline, right), *de medio T vid pag. 248* (footer, right). Folding, 229 × 200 millimetres (sheet); printed from a larger plate, lines 217 × 179 millimetres (plate marks at right and lower borders, lines on all four edges); 188 × 168 millimetres (figure). Inserted before legend at **A8r–v**, pages 15–16.

Pl.2c1. Plate 2 (image 2). Fig. II.*[da]*. (headline, centre), *pag. 16* (headline, right), *de medio S vid pag 248.* (footer, right). Folding, 161 × 140 millimetres (sheet); printed from a larger plate, lines 144 × 117 millimetres (plate marks at left and lower borders; lines on all four edges, continuing upwards and to the right); 133 × 102 millimetres (figure). Inserted before legend at **A8v–A9r**, pages 16–17.

Pl.3c1. Plate 3 (image 3). Fig. III. (headline, centre), *pag 29.* (headline, right). Folding, 224 × 205 millimetres (sheet); printed from a larger plate (plate marks at left and lower borders; lines at left and lower edges); 193 × 174 millimetres (figure). Inserted before legend at **B3r–v**, pages 29–30.

Pl.4c1. Plate 4 (image 4). Fig. IIII. (headline, centre), *pag. 30* (headline, right). Folding, 151 × 128 millimetres (sheet); printed from a larger plate, lines 144 × 117 millimetres (plate marks at right and lower borders; lines on upper and left edges, continuing upwards and left); 115 × 93 millimetres (figure). Inserted within legend at **B3v–B4r**, pages 30–1.

Pl.5c1. Plate 5 (image 5). Fig. V. (headline; left), *pag. 38.* (headline, right). Folding, 190 × 150 millimetres (sheet, cropped); printed from a larger plate *c.*185 × 148 millimetres (plate mark at left and lower borders; line on right edge); 179 × 131 millimetres (figure, cropped at upper margin). Inserted following legend at **B7v**, page 38.

Pl.6c1. Plate 6 (image 6). Fig. VI. (headline, left), *pag. 39.* (headline, right). Folding, 182 × 145 millimetres (sheet, cropped); printed from a larger plate, lines 178 × 146 millimetres (plate marks at right and lower borders; line on upper and left edges); 172 × 128 millimetres (figure). Inserted before legend at **B8r**, page 39.

Pl.7c1. Plate 7 (images 7–10) [Unnumbered 1]: Fig. I.; Fig. II; Fig. III (headlines, above figures); Fig. IIII (right, of figure), *pag. 65* (headline, right). Folding, 165 × 147 millimetres (sheet, cropped); printed from a larger plate, lines 143 × 120 millimetres (plate marks at left and lower borders; lines on upper and right edges); 26 × 95 millimetres, 76 × 93 millimetres, 36 × 28 millimetres, 73 × 25 millimetres (figures). Inserted within legend at **C8v–C9v**, pages 64–6.

Pl.8c1. Plate 8 (image 11). Fig VII[a] (headline left), *pag. 80.* (headline, right). Folding, 204 × 147 millimetres (sheet, cropped); printed from a larger plate, lines 196 × 143 millimetres (plate marks at upper and right borders; lines on left and lower edges); 191 × 103 millimetres (figure). Inserted before legend at **D4r–D5r**, pages 79–81.

Pl.9c1. Plate 9 (image 12). Fig. VIII (headline, centre), *pag. 101* (headline, right). Folding, 159 × 147 millimetres (sheet); printed from a larger plate, lines 144 × 117 millimetres (plate marks at right and lower borders; lines on all four edges, continuing at upper and lower to the left); 112 × 95 millimetres (figure). Inserted before legend at **E3r–v**, pages 101–2.

Pl.10c1. Plate 10 (images 13–14) [Unnumbered 2]: Fig. I.; Fig. II. (above each figure), *pag. 180.* (headline, right). Folding, 193 × 147 millimetres (sheet, cropped); printed from a larger plate, lines 188 × 147 millimetres (plate marks at upper and left borders; lines on right and lower edges); 125 × 113 millimetres, 48 × 112 millimetres (figures). Inserted within legend at **H6r–H7v**, pages 179–82.

Pl.11c1. Plate 11 (image 15). *Tabula IX [a].* (headline, right). Folding, 304 × 184 millimetres (sheet); printed from a larger plate, lines 293 × 168 millimetres (plate marks at upper, left, and lower borders; lines on all four edges); 277 × 153 millimetres (figure). Inserted within legends for Tabulæ IX–XIII at **L7v–M6r**, pages 254–73.

Pl.12c1. Plate 12 (image 16). *Tabula X [ma]* (headline, right). Folding, 307 × 215 millimetres (sheet); printed from a larger plate, lines 296 × 203 millimetres (plate marks at upper, right, and lower borders; line on left edge); 272 × 184 millimetres (figure). Inserted within legends for Tabulæ IX–XIII at **L7v–M6r**, pages 254–73.

Pl.13c1. Plate 13 (image 17). *Tabula XI.[ma]* (footer, right). Folding, 305 × 149 millimetres (sheet); printed from a larger plate, lines 292 × 135 millimetres (plate marks at upper, left, and lower borders; lines on all four edges); 278 × 126 millimetres (figure). Inserted within legends for Tabulæ IX–XIII at **L7v–M6r**, pages 254–73.

Pl.14c1. Plate 14 (image 18). *Tabula XII* (headline, right, no ruled border to inner margin of plate). Folding, 240 × 78 millimetres (sheet); printed from a larger plate (plate mark at right border, line on right edge); 218 × 38 millimetres (figure). Inserted within legends for Tabulæ IX–XIII at **L7v–M6r**, pages 254–73.

Pl.15c1. Plate 15 (images 19–23). *Tab. XIII* (headline, right above Figure 2), *Fig. 1.*^{ma} (header, centre), *Fig. 2.*^{da} (header within figure), *Fig. 3.*^{tia} (header, straddling upper part of figure), *Fig. 4.*^{ta} (header, centre) and *Fig. 5.*^{ta} (header, centre). Folding, 241 × 296 millimetres (sheet); printed from a larger plate, lines >240 × 296 millimetres (plate marks at right and lower borders, line at left edge and above figures 3 and 4); 163 × 77 millimetres, 168 × 69 millimetres, 285 × 31 millimetres (placed horizontally), 272 × 35 millimetres (placed horizontally), 73 × 25 millimetres (Figures). Inserted within legends for Tabulæ IX–XIII at **L7v–M6r**, pages 254–73.

Pl.16a1. Plate 16 (images 24 and 25). *Fig. 1.* (headline, left), *Fig. 2.* (headline, right), lettered A–V, Z, k, l, n, m, q, y, 1, 3, 4, and 8. Ruled border. Folding, 175 × 150 millimetres (sheet); 168 × 139 millimetres (plate marks); 132 × 57 millimetres, 115 × 66 millimetres (figures). Inserted between **2B2v–B3r**, pages 28–9. No legend but text at ¶35 describes the figures, 'Hæc autem ægrè ab iis affenſum impetrabunt …… eò forſan minus à veritate aliena quæ diximus exiſtimabit' (see: Figure 112).[30]

Copy: DASC. Early full calf, spine with five raised bands and five gilt decorated panels; lettered CEREBR | ANATO, original endpapers. Leaves 130 × 70 millimetres, boards 137 × 75 × 30 millimetres. Inscribed Rouhier p[undeciphered] No 499.

2C2.c2. CEREBRI ANATOME, Amsterdam duodecimo 1664

The second issue of the third edition of Willis's second book, with reset title page in its second state, 'Cereberrima' corrected in pen and ink to 'Celeberrima', '*iu*' corrected to '*in*', Seidleiani uncorrected, with text and illustration of *De ratione motus musculorum* [not distinguished from HJR Wing 11, Denham 4].

Title page: [1]. CEREBRI | ANATOME, | NERVORUMQUE | Deſcriptio & Uſus, | STUDIO | THOMÆ WILLIS, | *Ex Æde* Chriſti Oxon. *M. D. & in iſtâ* | *Cer*[l]*eberrima Academia Naturalis Philoſo— | phia Profeſſoris* Seidleiani. | Acceſſit | *Viri cujuſdam Clariſsimi* | De Ratione Motûs | MUSCULORUM | Tractatus ſingularis. | [printers' device] | AMSTELODAMI, | [short rule] | Apud CASPARUM COMMELINUM. | M. DC. LXIV.

[2]. DE | RATIONE | MOTUS | MUSCULORUM. | *Ἐν πᾶσι τοῖς φυσικοῖς ἐνεστί τι θαυμαστόν.* | Ariſt. de Part. Animal: | [printers' device] | AMSTELODAMI, | [rule] | Apud CASPARUM COMMELINUM. | M. DC. LXIV.

[30] See chapter 3 for full transcription and translation.

Then as in **2C2.c1** apart from:

Illustrations: variation in sheet sizes and occasional binding positions.

Copy: DASC, lacking *1, page [1], blank. Early vellum; lettered anatome | Willis, original endpapers. Leaves 133 × 76 millimetres; boards 137 × 76 × 27 millimetres. Recent crude architectural drawing with annotations in French on endpapers.

2D1. CEREBRI ANATOME, Amsterdam octavo 1666

The first issue of the fourth edition of Willis's second book, with the engraved title page depicting Thomas Willis and others, and without the Index alphabeticus [HJR Wing 12, Denham 5].

Title page: [1]. CEREBRI | ANATOME: | CUI ACCESSIT. | Nervorum Deſcriptio | ET USUS. | STUDIO | THOMÆ WILLIS, | Ex Æde Chriſti Oxon. M. D. & in | iſta Celeberrima Academia Naturalis Phi- | loſophiæ Profeſſoris Sidleiani. | *Acceſſit viri cujuſdam Clariſſimi de Ratione* | *Motus Muſculorum tractatus Singularis.* | [ornament] | AMSTELODAMI, | Apud GERBRANDUM SCHAGEN, | M. DC. LXVI.

[2]. DE | RATIONE | MOTUS | MUSCULORUM. | *Ἐν πᾶσι τοῖς φυσικοῖς ἐνεστί τι θαυμαστόν.* | Ariſt. de Part. Animal. | [ornament] | AMSTELODAMI, | [rule] | Apud GERBRANDUM SCHAGEN, | M. DC. LXV.

Collation: octavo; 23 letter roman alphabet using I and V: A–I ^{8}, K–T^{8}, V^{8}, X–Z^{8}, Aa–Bb^{8}; $1–5 signed apart from: -B1, B2 signed 2B, -B3, -B4, -B5, -C3, -C4, -C5, -D2, -D3, -D4, -D5, -O4, -R5, -Z4, -Z5, and -Bb3.

200 leaves: paginated as [16], 1–342, [4], 1–37 [38]. Mispaginated: 25 for 21, 232 for 242, 278 for 288; 5 for 10, 32 for 33.

Type: 34 lines; height (20 lines) 69 millimetres, width 70 millimetres.

Contents: **A1r**, page [1], engraved title page; **A1v**, page [2], blank; **A2r**, page [3], title; **A2v**, page [4], blank; **A3r–A6v**, pages [5–12], *Amico Lectori Præfatio.*; **A7r–A8r**, page [13–15], INDEX.; **A8v**, page [16], blank.

B1r–O6r, pages 1–203, [text] CEREBRI ANATOME.; **O6v–Z3v**, pages 204–342, [text] NERVORUM Deſcriptio & Uſus.

Z4r, page [1], title; **Z4v**, page [2], blank; **Z5r–v**, pages [3–4], BENEVOLO LECTORI Sal. D. TYPOGRAPHUS.

Z6r–Bb8r, [Fol.] pages 1–37, [text] DE RATIONE MOTUS MUSCULORUM. [William Croone]; **Bb8v**, page [38], blank.

Headlines and *Catchwords*: no ⁚ after headline at **B1v**, page 2; **B2r**, page 3; **B4v**, page 8; **B8v**, page 16; **C2r**, page 19; **C2v**, page 20; **C3v**, page 22; **C5r**, page 25; **D7r**, page 45 and **D8v**,

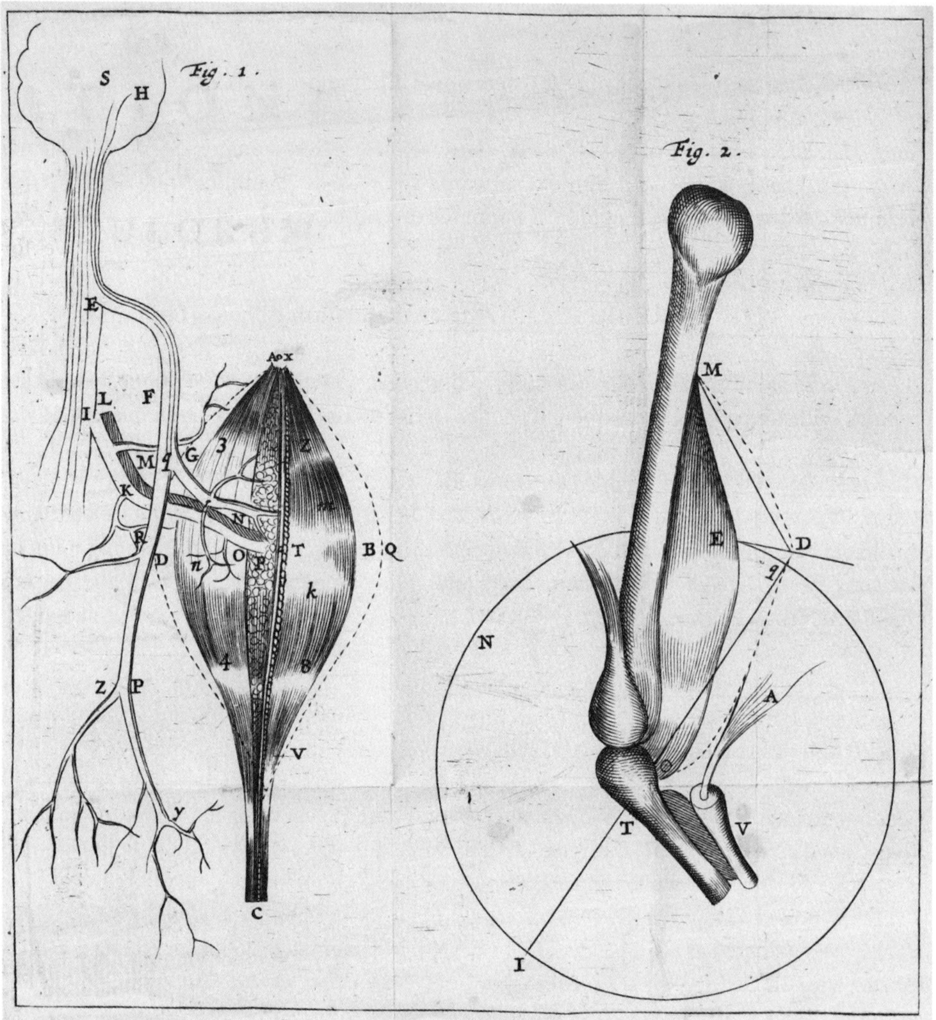

Figure 112 Plate 16 (images 24–25): [William Croone] 1664. No legend but the text at ¶35 describes the figures. In translation: 'But these explanations will scarcely gain access to those whose minds are occupied by that opinion concerning inflation on account of the spirit, since they will hardly believe that these very quick agitations of the limbs, which we observe, and the extremely rapid alternations of tensions and relaxations in antagonistic muscles, can result from them. But I say that all these things are carried out by these causes even in an instant. Indeed, at the same time that these fibrils of the nerve HEG, extended to the brain, are struck, these droplets of liquor exude continuously from all its branchlets, just as liquor spurts out at once when the piston of a syringe is pushed in very lightly. For it must be understood that the whole body is filled completely with spirituous and vital juices. Like water added to oil of vitriol, so this liquor instantly rouses an effervescence in the blood. In the same instant blood flows through the artery IKO like water from an opened pipe. No sooner does the muscle begin to swell at its boundary than the fibres are also contracted, and so everything occurs at once as if in the twinkling of an eye. However that effervescence which I have mentioned ceases very rapidly and the very active spirits are dissipated through the membranes of the muscle almost in an instant and, unless a new impulse arrives at once, the muscle is immediately pulled back and made flaccid when the imbalance of the circulation of the blood ceases due to the contraction of the fibres of the antagonist. And the blood immediately flows out in greater quantity through the vein LMN. Hence, also, excessively violent

page 48; ⁏ for ⁖ after headline at **B5r**, page 9; **B5v**, page 10; **C4v**, page 24; **C8r**, page 31; **C8v**, page 32; **D5r**, page 41; **E1r**, page 49; **O3r**, page 197; **O3v**, page 198.

habuit for exciſtit at **B2r** / v, pages 3 / 4; no catchword at **B2v** / **B3r**, pages 4 / 5; **B5r** / v, pages 9 / 10; **B7v** / **B8r**, pages 14 / 15; **B8v** / **C1r**, pages 16 / 17; **C6v** / **C7r**, pages 28 / 29; **C8r** / v, pages 31 / 32; **D1v** / **D2r**, pages 34 / 35; **D4v** / **D5r**, pages 42 / 43; **D5r** / v, pages 43 / 44; **D6r** / v, pages 45 / 46; af- for eendunt at **D3r** / v, pages 37 / 38; in for aliis at **D4r** / v, pages 41 / 42; partes for hæ at **G8r** / v, pages 95 / 96; ganglio for glioforme at **Q3r** / v, pages 229 / 230; Ve- for necne at **Q8r** / v, pages 239 / 240; Enim for Euim at **R2r** / v, pages 243 / 244; eoque for eoq; at **R6r** / v, pages 251 / 252; Quæ for in at **R8v** / **S1r**, pages 256 / 257; *bello* for *lari* at **S2v** / **S3r**, pages 260 / 261; di for hi at **T7r** / v, pages 285 / 286; *Plures* for ζζ *Plures* at **Y1v** / **Y2r**, pages 322 / 323; *Pro-* for ςς *Pro-* at **Y2r** / v, pages 323 / 324; *Ner-* for ζ *Ner* at **Y6v** / **Y7r**, pages 330 / 331; Ω *Plexus* for ω *Proceſſus* at **Y6v** / **Y7r**, pages 332 / 333; Qnin for Quin at **Aa4r** / v, pages 13 / 14; ren- for decurrent at **Bb4v** / **Bb5r**, pages 30 / 31.

Frontispiece: engraved title page, **F.2a1**: CEREBRI ANATOME *Cui acceſſit* NERVORUM Deſcriptio & Uſus STUDIO THOMÆ WILLIS. AMSTELODAMI Apud GERBRANDUM SCHAGEN. M. DC. LXV. 150 × 92 millimetres (sheet); 125 × 80 millimetres (plate marks); 113 × 75 millimetres (figure). Inserted before title page at **A1r**, page [1] (see: Figures 113–114).

Portrait: none.

Printers' ornaments: tailpiece at **A2r**, page [1] {**Schagen 16**}; **Z4r**, page [1] {**Schagen 19**}.

Decorated A at **A3r**, page [5] {**Schagen 17**}, N at **O6v**, page 204 {**Schagen 18**}, P at **Z5r**, page [3] {**Schagen 20**}; D at **Z6r**, page 1{**Schagen 21**}.

Illustrations: as in **2C1.c1** apart from:

Pl.14b2, **Pl.3b2** and **Pl.1b2** on a single sheet. Plate 14 (image 18): *Tabula XII* (headline, centre; vertical); Plate 3 (image 3): Fig: III. (headline, centre), *Pag. 37* (headline, right); Plate

---

activity exhausts the spirits and makes them break out through sweats. This is also the reason why the limbs are very painful and weak after more violent movements of the body (especially in those who are not accustomed to them). The sudden erection of the penis resulting from sexual thoughts and its flaccidity after emission of semen, the sudden flushing of the whole face from shame, the instantaneous recession of the blood from every part of the body to the inside in fear, all show how rapidly the blood flows in and flows out again. Moreover the smaller the ratio of the sustained weight to the moving force, the more rapidly the distances ED and qD are travelled. Hence heavy weights attached to a bladder are fairly quickly raised by inflating the bladder with air or with water. Then, one must think that, while part of the arm which is close to the joint or to the centre of rotation travels this smaller distance qD, the other extremity traverses a much longer distance in the same time. Finally, if one considers carefully that those spirits about which people make so much noise are found nowhere in the body outside the blood and the nervous fluid, and are in fact liquids, he would judge that what we have said is perhaps the less inconsistent with the truth.' Image from *Cerebri anatome* (Amsterdam) 1664.

See: William Croone, 'On the reason of the movement of the muscles', translated by Paul Maquet, *Transactions of the American Philosophical Society* 2000; 90: 1–130 at pages 123 / 125.

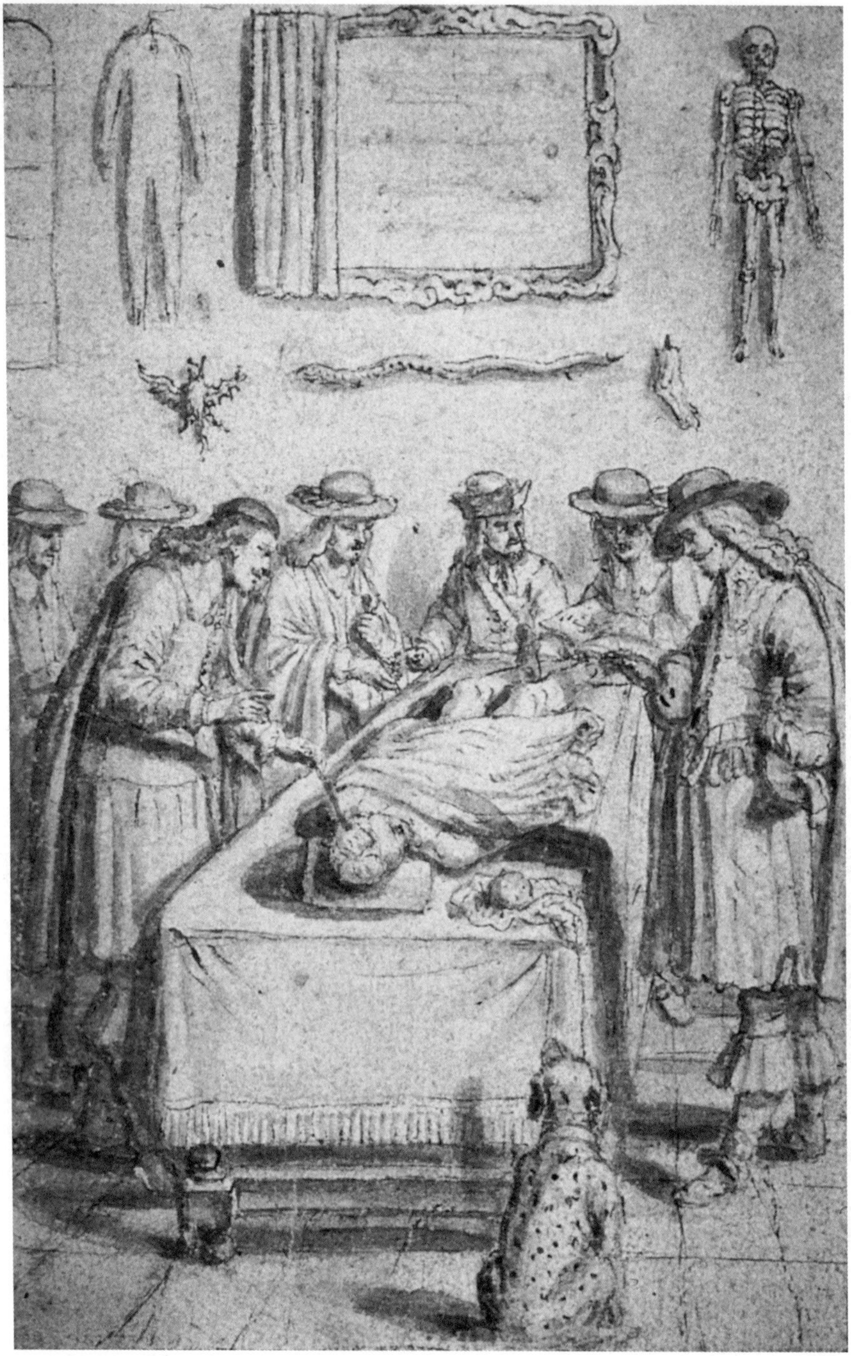

Figure 113 Early draft of the engraved title page for *Cerebri anatome* 1666.
Reproduced courtesy of the US National Library of Medicine.

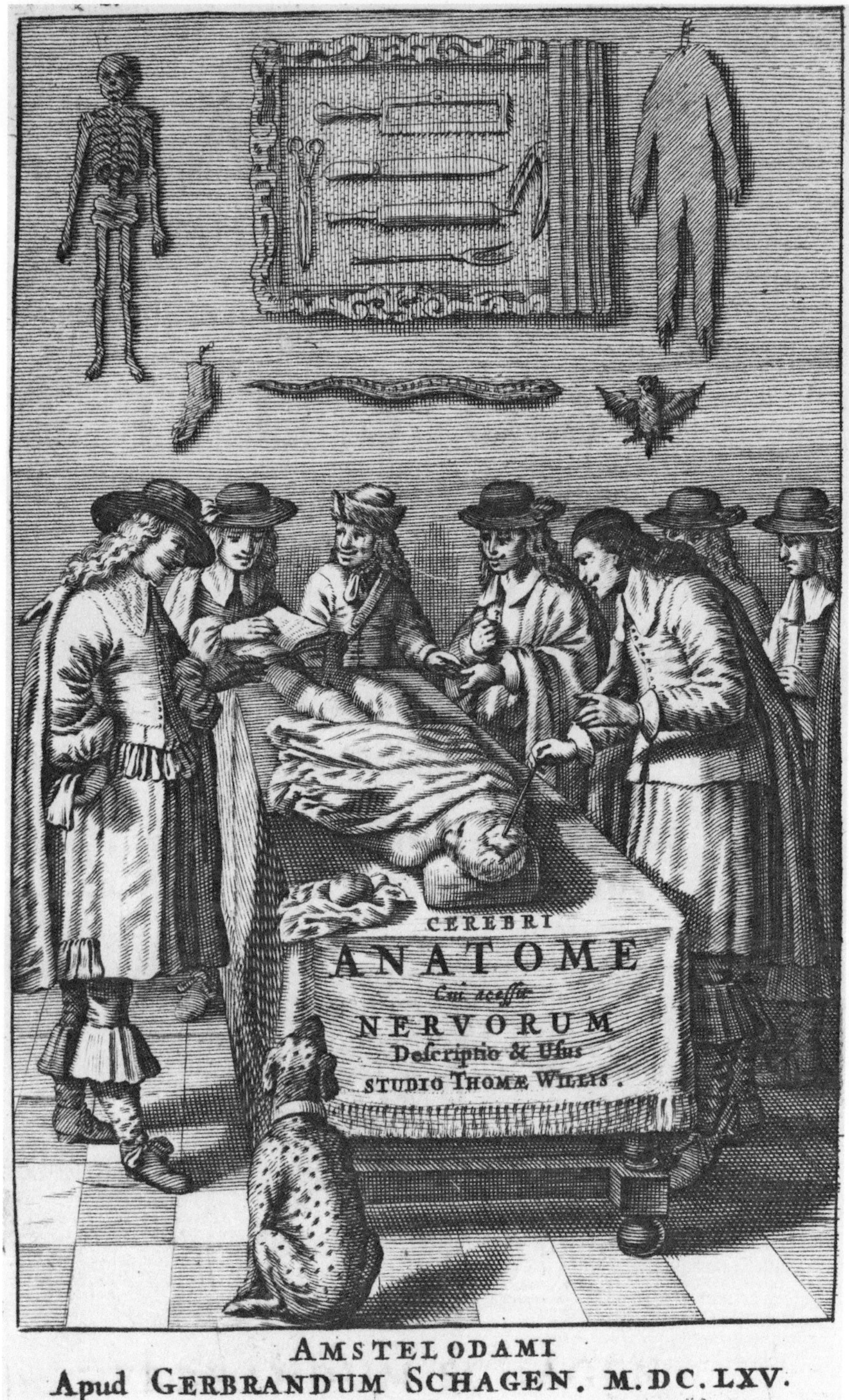

Figure 114 Engraved title page thought to depict Thomas Willis, Richard Lower, John Hemming. Christopher Wren, Thomas Millington, Edmund King, John Locke, and Robert Hooke: *Cerebri anatome* 1666 (F.2a1).

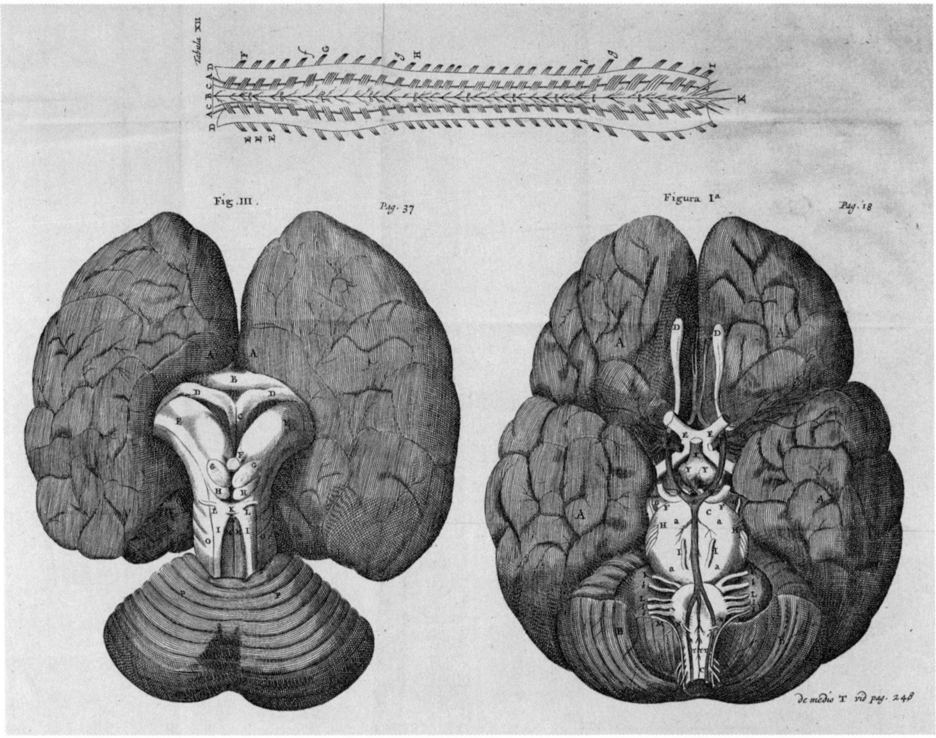

Figure 115 Printed sheet from a large engraving of engraving of Tabula XII, Pl.14d1. Plate 14 (image 18); Figura III, Pl.3a3. Plate 3 (image 3); and Figura I, Pl.1a3. Plate 1 (image 1). Image from *Cerebri anatome* 1666.

1 (image 1): Figura 1^{a} (headline centre), *Pag. 18.* (headline, right), *de medio T vid pag. 248* (footer, right). Folding, 278 × 372 millimetres (sheet). Inserted within legend for *Figura prima* at **C1v–C2r**, pages 18–19 (see: Figure 115).[31]

Pl.2b2. Plate 2 (image 2). Fig. II.^{da} (headline, centre), *pag. 20* (headline, right), *de medio S vid pag. 248* (footer, right). Folding, 154 × 110 millimetres (sheet). Inserted before legend at **C2v–C3r**, pages 20–1.

Pl.4b2. Plate 4 (image 4). *pag. 38* (headline, left), Fig. IIII. (headline, centre). Folding, 154 × 110 millimetres (sheet). Inserted within legend at **D3v–D4r**, pages 38–9.

Pl.5b2. Plate 5 (image 5). *Fig. V* (headline; left), *p. 47.* (headline, right). Folding, 190 × 146 millimetres (sheet). Inserted before legend at **D8r–v**, pages 47–8.

Pl.6b2. Plate 6 (image 6). *Fig. VI* (headline, left), *pag. 49* (headline, right). Folding, 180 × 145 millimetres (sheet). Inserted before legend at **E1r**, page 49.

[31] See also: legends for *Figura Tertia* at D3r–v, pages 37–8; and *Tabula Duodecima* at Y4r–v, pages 327–8 where, although the text is correct, *Tabula Duodecima* is incorrectly listed as *Tabula Decima*.

Pl.7b2. Plate 7 (images 7–10) [Unnumbered 1]: Fig. I; Fig. II; Fig. III (headers, above each image); Fig. IIII (headline, right, of figure), *pag. 81* (header, right). Folding, 154 × 110 millimetres (sheet). Inserted before **G1r–v**, pages 81–2.

Pl.8b2. Plate 8 (image 11). *Fig. VII* (headline, left), *p. 99* (headline, right). Folding, 204 × 143 millimetres (sheet). Inserted before legend at **H2r–v**, pages 99–100.

Pl.9b2. Plate 9 (image 12). Fig. VIII (headline, centre), *pag. 125* (headline, right). Folding, 154 × 108 millimetres (sheet). Inserted before legend at **I7r–v**, pages 125–6.

Pl.10b2. Plate 10 (images 13–14) [Unnumbered 2]: *Fig: I.*; *Fig: II* (above each figure), *p. 222* (headline, right). Folding, 193 × 145 millimetres (sheet). Inserted within legend at **P7r–P8v**, pages 222–4.

Pl.11b1. Plate 11 (image 15): *Tabula IX.*^{a} (headline, right). Folding, 290 × 167 millimetres (sheet). Inserted within legend at **X7r–Y3v**, pages 318–26.

Pl.12b1. Plate 12 (image 16): *Tabula X.*^{ma} (headline, right). Folding, 292 × 200 millimetres (sheet). Inserted before legend for Tabula X incorrectly headed '*Tabula Duodecima*' at **Y3r**, page 327.

Pl.13b1. Plate 13 (image 17): *Tabula XI.*^{ma} (footer, right). Folding, 300 × 140 millimetres (sheet). Inserted before legend at **Y5r–Y7v**, pages 329–34.

Pl.15b1. Plate 15 (images 19–23): Figures 1, 2, and 5 and separated by a ruled line above Figures 3 and 4 printed horizontally; *Fig. I.*^{ma} (header, left), *Fig. 5*^{ta} (header, centre), *Fig. 2.*^{da}, *Tab. XIII.* (headline, right), *Fig. 3.*^{tia} (header, lower left: vertical), *Fig.4.*^{ta} (header, lower right: vertical). Folding, 266 × 303 millimetres (sheet). Inserted before legend for Tabula X at **Y8r**, page 335.

Copy: DASC. Recent limp vellum with new endpapers. Leaves 154 × 93 millimetres, boards 157 × 95 × 26 millimetres. Inscribed: Dr Brian Gough 5|11|51, £5.10.0.[32]

2D2. CEREBRI ANATOME, Amsterdam octavo 1666

The second issue of the fourth edition of Willis's second book, with the engraved title page depicting Thomas Willis and others, and an additional sheet containing the Index alphabeticus [HJR Wing 13, Denham 6].

32 [Wilfred] Brian Gough (1909–1999) qualified in medicine from Birmingham Medical School where he worked in the city as a general practitioner, and anaesthetist to the Solihull Hospital and the Birmingham and Midlands Hospital for Women. He was president of the Birmingham Medical Institute. An archive of personal and professional correspondence, including material about local institutions with which he was involved, and on his interests in medical history, was passed to the Birmingham University Archives and is now in the Wellcome Library. Gough's medical and scientific library was sold at auction by Phillips, London, on 5 November 1999.

As in **2D1** apart from:

Collation: A–I ^{8}, K–T^8, V^8, X–Z^8, Aa–Bb^8, *^{8}; $1–5 signed.

208 leaves: paginated as [16], 1–342, [4], 1–37 [38], [16].

Contents: after **Bb8v**, page [38], ***1–*7**, pages [1–14], INDEX ALPHABETICUS RERUM POTISSIMARUM, *In* CL. WILLISII *Anatomia Cerebri occurrentium.*; ***8r–v**, pages [15–16], blank.

Headlines and *Catchwords*: [*^{8}] correct.

[*^{8}] correct.

Then as in **2D1** apart from:

Illustrations: **Pl.13b1**. Plate 13 (image 17) printed with **Pl.15b1**. Plate 15 (images 19–23): Folding, 388 × 308 millimetres (sheet). Inserted after ***8 + 1v**, page [18] (see: Figure 116).

Copy: DASC (#1 of 2). Twentieth-century morocco with gilt lined borders to central motif depicting the circle of Willis, spine with the same motif and gilt lines, lettered WILLIS | [short rule] | CEREBRI | ANATOME | [motif depicting the circle of Willis, different from the upper cover] | 1666, gilt to upper edges, leather continued onto inner upper and lower boards with corner floral ornaments, marbled endpapers, and original paper wrapper bound at the end. Leaves 155 × 104 millimetres (uncut with deckled edges), boards 165 × 108 × 33 millimetres. Inscribed: 'This book bound in morocco by Mr John Grabau in 1947. (October). The back strip ornament is a copy of the circle of Willis, Figura 1^a—The front cover ornament is from Dandy, "Intracranial arterial aneurysms", Comstock. Ithaca NY, 1944. P. 77 issue. This page is one of the original paper covers.' Loosely inserted invoice from John F. Grabau, 429 Parkdale Ave, Buffalo, N.Y dated Oct. 15, 1947 to Dr W.B. Hamby for the binding, $75.00 PD. BY CK. # 4199 $75.00, 10-18-47.[33]

2E1. CEREBRI ANATOME, Amsterdam duodecimo 1667

The fifth edition of Willis's second book, based on **2C2** but reset with changes to the preliminaries, some other leaves, and sheets M^4, ^{2}A^{12}, and ^{2}B^6 [HJR Wing 14, Denham 7].

[33] John F Grabau (1878–1948), considered one of the most artistic bookbinders in the United States, never duplicated his creative designs. He was apprenticed in the printing shops of Gies & Co. and the bookbindery of Peter Paul, A.T. Brown's Printing House, and the Roycrofters in East Aurora, all in New York State. He worked independently in Buffalo from 1905 and was renowned for his lettering, tooling and use of Levant morocco leather. Even in the early years, his bindings cost up to $200. This volume, invoiced on 15 October 1947, typifies these features and must have been one of his last decorative bindings. Wallace B Hamby (1903–1999) established neurosurgery at Buffalo in 1933 and became known for his work on the treatment of cerebral aneurysms and arteriovenous malformations on which he wrote a monograph (*Intracranial aneurysms* 1952). He returned as professor of neurosurgery at the Cleveland Clinic (1960–1969), where he had previously trained in surgery and neuropathology (1929–1934), before retiring to Florida maintaining his interest in medical history and publishing books on the case reports and autopsy records, and influence on surgery, of Ambrose Paré (1510–1590). In commissioning the decorative binding on his copy of *Cerebri anatome* from John Grabau, it was appropriate that the upper cover included an image from Walter Dandy's (1886–1946) *Intracranial arterial aneurysms* (1944): figure 30, page 77 which, in the original, is signed HAGER '40. Dorcas Hager Padget (1906–1973) had been introduced to Dandy in 1926 by Max Brödel (1870–1941) and continued to illustrate his works until Dandy's death in 1946. Figure 30 also has an acknowledgement to the neuro-opthalmologist Dr Frank Walsh (1895–1978).

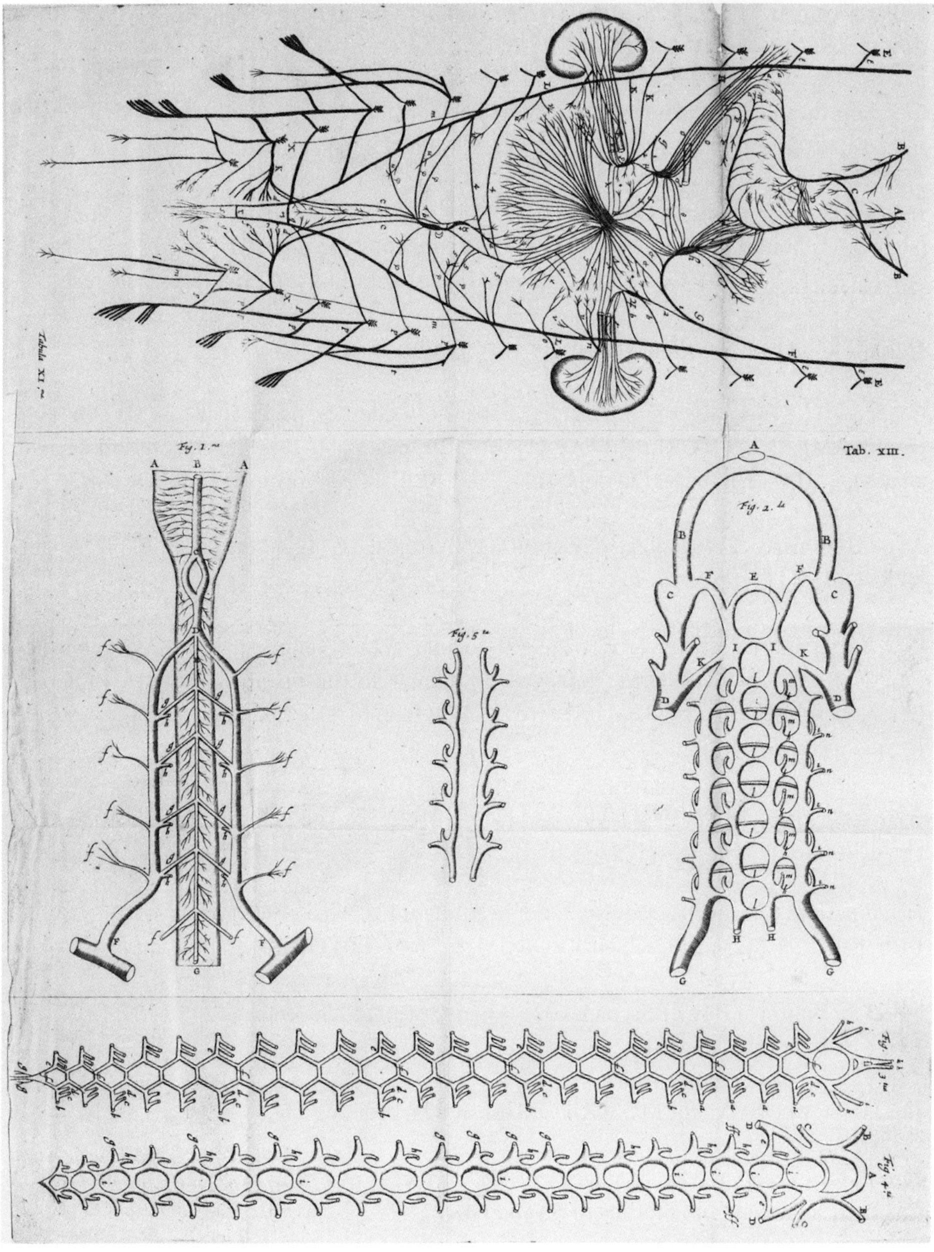

Figure 116 Printed sheet from a large engraving of Tabula XI, Pl.13b1. Plate 13 (image 17); and Tabula XIII, Pl.15b1. Plate 15 (images 19–23). Image from *Cerebri anatome* 1666.

Title page: [1]. CEREBRI | ANATOME, | *Cui acceffit* | NERVORUM | Defcriptio & Ufus. | STUDIO | THOMÆ WILLIS, | *Ex Æ*de Chrifti Oxon. *M. D. & in ifta* | *Celeberrima Academia Naturalis Philofo-* | *phiæ Profefforis* Sidleiani. | Editio ultima priori emendatior. | [printers' device] AMSTELODAMI, | Apud CASPARUM COMMELINUM. | M. DC. LXVII.

[2]. DE | RATIONE | MOTUS | MUSCULORUM. | *Studio* | GULIELMI CROONE, | *M. D. è Coll. Med. Lond. ac Societatis* | *Regalis Socii.* | *'Εν πᾶσι τοῖς φυσικοῖς ἐνεστί τι θαυμαστόν.* | Arift.

de Part. Animal. | *Editio ſecunda priori Emendatior.* | [printers' device] | AMSTELODAMI, | Apud CASPARUM COMMELINUM. | M. DC. LXVII.

Collation: duodecimo; 23 letter roman alphabet using I: $*^{12}$, A–I^{12}, K–L^{12}, M^4, $^2A^{12}$, $^2B^6$; $1–6 signed apart from: [1] *6 signed L6; [2] -A2, B3 signed B4, B4 signed B3.

166 leaves: paginated as [1–24], 1–272, [1]–34, [2]. Mispaginated: [1] 56 for 76; [2] B3 (signed B4) bound before B4 (signed B3) so that pagination after **B2v**, page 28, follows the sequence: 31–2, 29–30, 33–4 with corresponding discontinuity of catchwords and text.

Type: 41 lines: height (20 lines) 52 millimetres, width 56 millimetres.

Contents: [1]. ***1r–v**, pages [1–2], blank; ***2r**, page [3], title; ***2v**, page [4], blank; ***3r–*5v**, pages [5–10], AMICO LECTORI PRÆFATIO.; ***6r–*10r**, pages [11–19], Elenchus rerum. [Cerebri anatome], ***10v–*12v**, pages [20–4], ELENCHUS RERUM Nervorum deſcriptio & uſus.

A1r–G10v, pages 1–164, [text] CEREBRI ANATOME.; **G11r–M4v**, pages 165–272, [text] NERVORUM Deſcriptio & Uſus.

[2]. **A1r**, page [1], title; **A1v**, page [2], blank; **A2r–v**, pages [3–4], *Lectori benevolo* TYPOGRAPHUS SALUTEM., followed by a letter to the printer … [signed] è Colleg. Gresham. Jul. 25. St. V. 1667. GULIELMUS CROONE, M. D. *è Coll. Med. Lond. ac Societatis Regalis Socius.*

A3r–B5v, pages 5–34, [text] DE RATIONE MOTUS MUSCULORUM.; **B6r–v**, pages [1–2], blank.

Headlines and *Catchwords*: [1]. No ⁚ after headline at **I3r**, page 197; & for ET at **L1r**, page 241; **L10r**, page 259; **M2r** page 267; NERVORUM, &c. for NERVORUM at **L4v**, page 248.

bulu3 for bulum at **B4v** / **B5r**, pages 32 / 33; m for (uti at **L5r** / **v**, page 249 / 250; L. D. L. for L. L. L. at **L11r** / **v**, pages 261 / 262.

[2]. MUSCVLORUM. for MUSCULORUM. at **B2r**, page 27.

cerebri for Cerebri at **A8r** / **v**, pages 15 / 16; [correct at **B2v–B5r**, pages 28–33, allowing for incorrect signatures and binding of B3 and B4].

Frontispiece: none.

Portrait: none.

Printers' ornaments: printers' device at ***1r**, page [3]; **2A1r**, page 1 {**Commelin 1**}.

Decorated A at ***3r**, page [5] {**Commelin 4**}; I at **A1r**, page 1 {**Commelin 5**}; and N (inverted) at **G10r**, page 165 {**Schagen 15**}.

Illustrations: as in **2C2.c1** apart from variation in sheet sizes and occasional binding positions.

Copy: DASC, lacking *1, blank. Original calf with blind stamped fleur de lys corners and lined borders, later spine with five panels each having a gilt acorn ornament with double ruled lines, label WILLIS | CEREBRI | ANATOME, original front endpapers, rear free endpaper lacking. Leaves 130 × 75 millimetres, boards 133 × 74 × 33 millimetres. Inscribed: (1) (undeciphered); (2) Yelloly. Coll. of Edinburgh (×2). Stamped and with book label: Norfolk and Norwich United Medical Book Society.[34]

2E2. CEREBRI ANATOME, Amsterdam duodecimo 1676

A reissue of the fifth edition of Willis's second book, with the title page and subsidiary title page reset and at least one page in an altered state [HJR Wing 15, Denham 8].

Title page: [1]. CEREBRI | ANATOME, | *Cui accefsit* | NERVORUM | Defcriptio & Ufus. | STUDIO | THOMÆ WILLIS, | *Ex Æ*de Chrifti Oxon. *M.D. & in ifta Celeber* | *rima Academia Naturalis Philofophiæ* | *Profefforis* Sidleiani. | Editio ultima priori emendatior. | [ornament] | AMSTELODAMI, | [rule] | Apud JOANNEM MAXIMILIANUM | LUCAS. M. DC. LXXVI.

[2]. DE | RATIONE | MOTUS | MUSCULORUM. | *Studio* | GULIELMI CROONE, | *M. D. è Coll. Med. Lond. Ac Societatis* | *Regalis Socii.* | *'Εν πᾶσι τοῖς φυσικοῖς ἐνεστί τι θαυμαστόν.* | Arift. de Part. Animal. | *Editio fecunda priori Emendatior.* | [ornament] | AMSTELODAMI, | Apud JOANNEM MAXIMILIANUM | LUCAS. M. DC. LXXVI.

Then as in **2E1** apart from:

Catchwords: [1]. bulu3 for bulum at **B4v** / **B5r**, pages 32 / 33; L. D. L. for L. L. L. at **L11r** / **v**, pages 261 / 262 [m for (uti at **L5r** / **v**, pages 249 / 250, corrected].

Printers' ornament: [1]. Tailpiece at [1] ***2r**, page [3], title page {**Lucas 1**}.

[2]. Tailpiece at **A1r**, page [1], title page {**Lucas 2**}.

Illustrations: **Pl.14c1**, **Pl.3c1**, and **Pl.1c1**. (images 18, 3, and 1) combined on a single leaf. Folding, 283 × 360 millimetres (sheet). Bound upside-down and inserted before legend for Figura I at **A8r–v**, pages 15–16.

Pl.11c1 (image 15) and **Pl.12c1** (image 16) combined on a single sheet. Folding, 374 × 293 millimetres (sheet). Bound upside-down and inserted before legend for unnumbered 2 at **H6r**, page 179.

[34] John Yelloly (1774–1842) of Alnwick, Northumberland, graduated from the University of Edinburgh (1799) and was appointed physician to the London Hospital (1807–1818). With Alexander John Gaspard Marcet (1870–1822), he founded the Royal Medical and Chirurgical Society (1805), and was responsible for development of the library. He was elected FRS on 5 May 1814. After moving to Norfolk, Yelloly was appointed to the Norfolk and Norwich Hospital (1820–1832). In 1840, he was thrown onto his head from a phaeton and became paralysed on the right side. Later he developed a left hemiparesis from apoplexy from which he died three days later. The Norwich Philosophical Society (founded 1812) whose members included poets, painters, and philosophers as well as scientists, chemists and doctors became the Norwich and Norfolk United Medical Book Society in *c.*1827. It merged with the Norwich Pathological Society in 1848 to become the Norwich Medical Society and, in 1867, was renamed the Norwich Medico-Chirurgical Society.

Pl.13c1 (image 17) and **Pl.15c1** (images 19–23) combined on a single sheet. Folding, 377 × 296 millimetres (sheet). Inserted before legend for Tabula IX at **L7v**, page 254.

Copy: DASC. The description of images combined on one sheet relates to the copy held at Wadham College, Oxford. The author's copy has these images cut and bound individually. Original calf, spine (restored) with five raised bands, gilt decorated panels, lettered CEREB | ANATO, original endpapers. Leaves 130 × 71 millimetres, boards 137 × 74 × 33 millimetres. Inscribed: Ex libris andros denesde (?) doct. med.[35]

2F. CEREBRI ANATOME, Amsterdam duodecimo 1683

The sixth edition of Willis's second book, reset following the format of Commelin's 1667 edition (2E1) but with Schagen's engraved plates in their third states [HJR Wing 16, Denham 9].[36]

Title page: CEREBRI | ANATOME, | *Cui acceſſit* | NERVORUM | Deſcriptio & Uſus. | STUDIO | THOMÆ WILLIS, | *Ex* Æde Chriſti Oxon. *M. D. & in iſta Celeberrima* | *Academia Naturalis Philoſophiæ* | *Profeſſoris* Sidleiani. | Editio ultima priori emendatior. | [printers' device] | *AMSTELÆDAMI,* | Sumtibus HENRICI WETSTENII, | CIↃ IↃC LXXXIII.

Collation: duodecimo; 23 letter roman alphabet using I: *12, A–I^{12}, K–L^{12}, M^{4}; $1–6 signed apart from: +*7, G3 signed G2.

148 leaves: paginated as [24], 1–272. Mispaginated: 83 for 85, 288 for 188, 296 for 196, 130 for 230.

Type: 41 lines; height (20 lines) 52 millimetres, width 58 millimetres.

Contents: ***1r–v**, pages [1–2], blank; ***2r**, page [3], title; ***2v**, page [4], blank; ***3r–*5v**, pages [5–10], AMICO LECTORI PRÆFATIO; ***6r–*10r**, pages [11–19], Elenchus rerum [Cerebri anatome]; ***10v–*12v**, pages [20–4], ELENCHUS RERUM Nervorum deſcriptio & uſus.

A1r–G10v, pages 1–164, [text] CEREBRI ANATOME; **G11r–M4v**, pages 165–272, [text] NERVORUM Deſcriptio & Uſus.

Headlines and *Catchwords*: no ⁚ after headline at ***4r**, page [7]; **B6v**, page 36, **B8v**, page 40, **C5v**, page 58, **C10v**, page 68, **D9r**, page 89; **K3r**, page 221; & for ET at **I5r**, page 201, **L1r**, page 241; NERVORUM, &tc for NERVORUM. at **L4v**, page 248; ⁚ added after headline at **L7v**, page 254.

[35] This may be André Denesde (nd) who was active as a physician in the faculty of medicine and pharmacy at the University of Poitiers between 1710 and 1734. In the description of Yates Thompson 45, the British Library catalogue refers, as part of the provenance of this Book of Hours, to inscriptions of dates and names for several members of the Denesde family active in the seventeenth and eighteenth centuries, including André Denesde.

[36] In considering the duodecimo publications of Commelin (1667: **2E1**), Lucas (1676: **2E2**) and Wetstein (1683: **2F**), HJR Wing refers to Commelin (1667, #14) as 'another edition of no. 10 [i.e. Schagen 1664: **2C1**]'; Lucas 1676 as 'another issue of no. 14 [i.e. Commelin 1667]' and Wetstein 1683 'as in no. 14' [i.e. Commelin 1667]'; see Wing (1962): pages 15–16. Denham has these three books as Commelin 1667 'a new edition', Lucas 1676, 'a reissue of no. 7 [i.e. Commelin 1667]'; and Wetstein 1683 'a reprint of no. 8 [i.e. Lucas 1676 and, hence, Commelin 1667]'; see Denham (1965): pages 91–3. Neither set of statements is strictly correct.

diffic- for diffectione at **D8r / v**, pages 39 / 40; rranf for tranf at **I12v / K1r**, pages 216 / 217; *tfinctu-* (initial *t* inverted) for *ftinctus* at **L3r / v**, pages 245 / 246; L. D. L. for L. L. L. at **L11r / v**, pages 261 / 262.

Frontispiece: none.

Portrait: none.

Printers' ornament: printers' device on title page at ***2r**, page [3] {**Wetstein 21**}.

Decorated A at ***3r**, page [5] {**Wetstein 22**}; I at **A1r**, page 1 {**Wetstein 23**}; N at **G11r**, page 165 {**Wetstein 24**}.

Illustrations: as in **2C1** apart from:

Pl.1b3. Plate 1 (image 1) Figura 1[a] (headline centre), *Pag. 15.* (headline, right), *de medio T vid pag. 248.* (footer, right). Folding, 225 × 180 millimetres (sheet). Inserted before legend for Figura I at **A8r–v**, pages 15–16.

Pl.2b3. Plate 2 (image 2) Fig. II.*[da]* (headline, centre), *pag. 16* (headline, right), *de medio S vid pag. 248.* (footer, right). Folding, 163 × 122 millimetres (sheet). Inserted within legend for Figura II at **A8v–A9r**, pages 16–17.

Pl.3b3. Plate 3 (image 3) Fig. III. (headline, centre), *Pag. 29.* (headline, right). Folding, 222 × 190 millimetres (sheet). Inserted after legend for Figura III at **A8v–A9r**, pages 16–17.

Pl.4b3. Plate 4 (image 4) Fig. IIII. (headline, centre), *pag. 31.* (headline, left). Folding, 171 × 110 millimetres (sheet). Inserted within text of CAPUT IV between **B4v–B5r**, pages 32–33.

Pl.5b3. Plate 5 (image 5) *Fig. V* (headline; left), *p 38* (headline, right). Folding, 216 × 163 millimetres (sheet). Inserted following legend for Figura V at **B7v**, page 38.

Pl.6b3. Plate 6 (image 6) *Fig. VI* (headline, left), *p. 39* (headline, right). Folding, 202 × 163 millimetres (sheet). Inserted before legend for Figura VI at **B8r**, page 39.

Pl.7b3. Plate 7 (images 7–10) [Unnumbered 1]: Fig. I; Fig. II; Fig. III (headers, above each image); Fig. IIII (header, right, of figure), *pag. 65.* (header, right). Folding, 177 × 127 millimetres (sheet). Inserted within legend for unnumbered figure 1 at **C8v–C9v**, pages 64–6.

Pl.8b3. Plate 8 (image 11) *Fig. VII* (headline left), *p. 80.* (headline, right). Folding, 204 × 157 millimetres (sheet). Inserted within legend for Figura VII at **D4r–D5r**, pages 79–81.

Pl.9b3. Plate 9 (image 12) Fig. VIII (headline, centre), *pag. 101.* (headline, right). Folding, 173 × 118 millimetres (sheet). Inserted before legend for Figura VIII at **E3r–v**, pages 101–2.

Pl.10b3. Plate 10 (images 13 and 14) [Unnumbered 2]: *Fig: I.*; *Fig: II.* (above each figure), *p. 180.* (headline, right). Folding, 194 × 143 millimetres (sheet). Inserted within legend for unnumbered figure 2 at **H6r–H7v**, pages 179–82.

Pl.11b1. Plate 11 (image 15) *Tabula IX.*[a] (headline, right). Folding, 299 × 180 millimetres (sheet). Inserted within legends for Tabulæ IX–XIII at **L7v–M4v**, pages 254–272.

Pl.12b1. Plate 12 (image 16) *Tabula X.*[ma] (headline, right). Folding, 300 × 212 millimetres (sheet). Inserted within legends for Tabulæ IX–XIII at **L7v–M4v**, pages 254–72.

Pl.13b1. Plate 13 (image 17) *Tabula XI.*[ma] (footer, right). Folding, 305 × 132 millimetres (sheet). Inserted within legends for Tabulæ IX–XIII at **L7v–M4v**, pages 254–72.

Pl.14b2. Plate 14 (image 18) *Tabula XII* (headline, right). Folding, 231 × 67 millimetres (sheet). Inserted within legends for Tabulæ IX–XIII at **L7v–M4v**, pages 254–72.

Pl.15b1. Plate 15 (images 19–23) Tab. XIII. (headline, right), *Fig. 1.*[ma] (header, centre), *Fig. 2.*[da] (header within figure), *Fig. 3.*[tia] (header, straddling upper part of figure), *Fig. 4.*[ta] (header, centre) and *Fig. 5* [ta] (header, centre). Folding (1) figures 1, 5, and 2, 171 × 284 millimetres; (2) figures 3 and 4, 290 × 75 millimetres (sheets). Inserted within legends for Tabulæ IX–XIII at **L7v–M4v**, pages 254–72.

Copy: British Library (7421 a 23). Original vellum (block loose), spine lettered Willis, original endpapers. Leaves 130 × 75 millimetres, boards 138 × 77 × 28 millimetres. Inscribed: [1] (name undeciphered) Dr Heberden in his Introd. to the Study of Physick recommends Willis *Cerebri anatome* amongst others, but adds 'I think a Man may pass over the Uses, and be content with only what He says of the nerves and Brain: and no one can be too exact in his knowledge of the course of the intercostal nerve and of the eight pairs of nerves', see [p]. 19; (2) Inst. *Willis* show'd spontaneous actions here / and why involuntary motions there / & how the spirits by mechanic laws / in wild careers tumultuous riots cause. Garth C[anto]. 6; (3) J Hacket (unidentified). Stamped: BRITISH MUSEUM I 5 NO 86.[37]

2G. [DE RATIONE MOTUS MUSCULORUM], Amsterdam octavo 1667

Dutch translation of William Croone's *De ratione motus musculorum* attributed to Thomas Willis [not previously recorded].

[37] The reference in an eighteenth-century hand to William Heberden's (1710–1801) 'Introd. To the Study of Physick' raises a bibliographic issue that puts into doubt a later 'find'. In 1929, Hoeber, New York, published 'An introduction to the study of physic by William Heberden', reprinted, with additions and corrections from *Annals of Medical History* 1928: 10: 226–41 and 349–67 with a prefatory essay by LeRoy Crummer (1871–1934). It is stated elsewhere that 'this unpublished original manuscript of Heberden was a lucky find by Dr. Crummer in a little second-hand book shop in the south of London. Picked up as a medical manuscript in Wales the week before by the bookseller, the volume handed to Dr. Crummer had written on the title page "An Introduction to the Study of Physic" and beneath this the signature "William Heberden".' Crummer was a cardiologist and bibliophile who scoured Europe for books. He became professor of the history of medicine, and was associate editor of *Annals of Medical History*. See also chapter 16 and Samuel Garth (1661–1719), *The dispensary. A poem in six cantos*. London (1699): page 91, Canto VI, ll 7–10. The printed text reads 'Then, *Willis*, why spontaneous Actions here, / And whence involuntary Motions there: / And how the Spirits by mechanick Laws, / in wild Careers, tumultuous Riots cause.

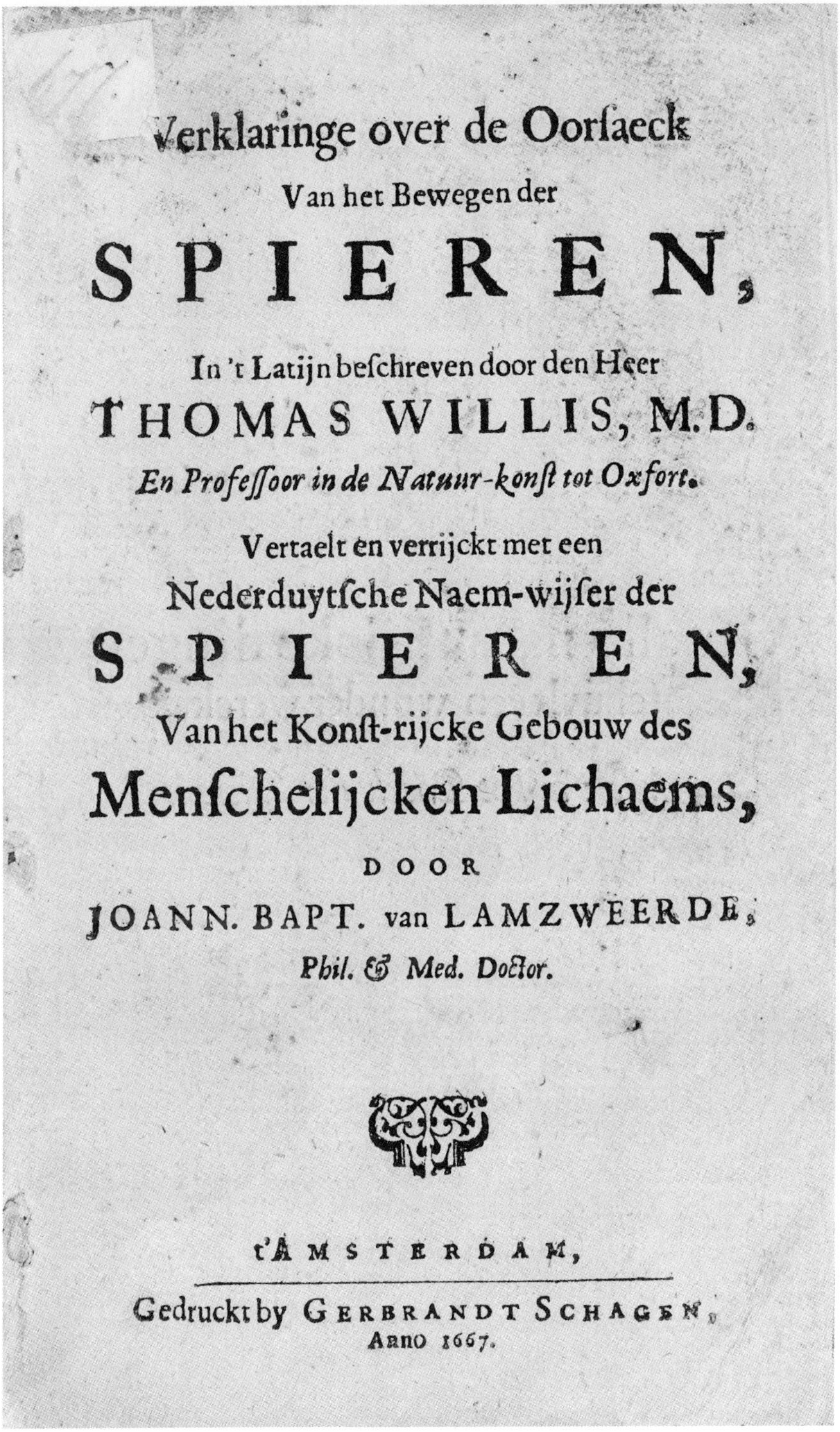

Verklaringe over de Oorſaeck
Van het Bewegen der
SPIEREN,
In 't Latijn beſchreven door den Heer
THOMAS WILLIS, M.D.
En Profeſſoor in de Natuur-konſt tot Oxfort.
Vertaelt en verrijckt met een
Nederduytſche Naem-wijſer der
SPIEREN,
Van het Konſt-rijcke Gebouw des
Menſchelijcken Lichaems,
DOOR
JOANN. BAPT. van LAMZWEERDE,
Phil. & Med. Doctor.

t'AMSTERDAM,
Gedruckt by GERBRANDT SCHAGEN,
Anno 1667.

Figure 117 Title page of William Croone's *De ratione motus musculorum* translated into Dutch and attributed to Thomas Willis. The only known copy.

Title page: Verklaringe over de Oorſaeck | Van het Bewegen der | SPIEREN, | In 't Latijn beſchreven door den Heer | THOMAS WILLIS, M.D. | *En Profeſſoor in de Natuur-konſt tot Oxfort.* | Vertaelt en verrijickt met een | Nederduytſche Naem-wijſer der | SPIEREN, | Van het Konſt-rijcke Gebouw des | Menſchelijcken Lichaems, | DOOR | JOANN. BAPT. van LAMZWEERDE, | *Phil. & Med. Doktor.* | [ornament] | t'AMSTERDAM, | [short rule] | Gedruckt by GERBRANDT SCHAGEN. | Anno 1667.[38]

Collation: octavo; 23 letter roman alphabet: A–D^8, E^4; \$1–5 signed.

36 leaves: paginated as [8] 9–66, 63–4, [2], 67–[68].

Type: 37 lines; height (20 lines) 69 millimetres, width 74 millimetres.

Contents: **A1r**, page [1], title; **A1v**, page [2], In alle natuurlijcke dingen ſchuylt een wonder werck. *Ariſt: in het Boeck der Dieren.*; **A2r–A3v,** pages [3–6], *Den wel-geleerde, en ſeer behendige Sny-Konſtenaer, en Heere* Dr. FREDERICUS RUYSCH, *En de ſeer ervaren Meeſters,* JAN COENDERDING, DANIEL FLORIANUS, NICOLAUS FRUYT, AUGUSTUS MEYERT, ABRAHAM HONDECOETER, MARTEN KRIECK, Voorzitter, en Opper-Vooghden van de Kamer der Hant-Artzenye Tot AMSTERDAM ... signed JOH. BAPT. van LAMZWEERDE.; **A4r–v**, pages [7–8], Konſt-lievende LEESER.

A5r–C7r, pages 9–45, [text] VERKLARINGE *Over de Oorzaeck van de beweginge der* SPIEREN.; **C7v** page [46], blank; **C8r–E2v**, pages 47–66, '63–64', [text] NAEM-WYSER DER SPIEREN.; **E3 r–v**, pages [1–2], blank.

E4r, page 67, [concluding text] NAEM-WYSER DER SPIEREN.; **E4v**, page 68, Op den Naam-wijſer der spieren, Door den voornamen Genees-Heer JOAN. BAPT. van LAMZWEERDE in 't licht gebracht ... [signed] Meditando JOAN BLASIUS, Adv^{t}.[39]

Headlines and *Catchwords*: headlines correct.

Rirsum for Sursum at **D2r / v**, pages 51 / 52.

Printers' ornament: fleuron at **A1r**, page [1] {**Schagen 22**}.

Frontispiece: none.

[38] Treatise on the cause of the movement of muscles, written in Latin by Mr THOMAS WILLIS, Doctor of Medicine and Professor of Physick in Oxford. Translated and extended with a Dutch register of muscles, in the miraculous structure of the human body, BY JOANN[ES] BAPT[IST]. VAN LAMZWEERDE, Doctor of Philosophy and Medicine in Amsterdam. Printed by GERBRANDT SCHAGEN, in the year 1667.

[39] A1v, page [2], In all things of nature a miraculous work is hidden. *Aristotle in The Book of* Animals; A2r–A3v, pages [3–6], *To the very learned and very able Anatomist Mr.* Dr. FREDERICUS RUYSCH, *and to the very experienced Masters* JAN COENDERDING, DANIEL FLORINS, NICHOLAS FRUYT, AUGUSTUS MEYERT, ABRAHAM HONDECOETER, MARTEN KRIECK, President and *chief Guardians* of the Chamber of Medicine in AMSTERDAM ... [signed] your Humble Servant JOH. BAPT. Van LAMZWEERDE; A4r–v, pages [7–8], Art loving READER, A5r–C7r, pages 9–45, [text] EXPLANATION *about the cause of the movement of* MUSCLES; C7v, page [46], blank; C8r–E2r, pages [1–2], blank; E4r, page 67, [concluding text] REGISTER OF THE NAMES OF MUSCLES, E4v, page 68, On the Register of the names of muscles, brought to light by the respected Physician JOAN. BAPT. Van LAMZWEERDE ... For contemplation added by JOAN BLASIUS.

Portrait: none.

Illustrations: none.

Copy: DASC. Original limp vellum with stitching, no endpapers. Leaves 158 × 93 millimetres, limp covers 155 × 93 × 6 millimetres. Inscribed: Daernandris Jeyth Den 8 januarisis (unidentfied). Inserted: small label marked 677.

7

'A certain physiologie and pathology of the brain and nervous stock'

Pathologiæ cerebri (1667–1678)

Thomas Willis's sixth and seventh treatises—*De morbis convulsivis* under the general title of *Cerebri pathologiæ*, and *De Scorbuto*—were first published as his third book in a quarto edition from Oxford and London (1667: **3A**). This was followed by duodecimo issues from Amsterdam and London (1668, 1670, and 1678: **3B** and **3D**). A Dutch translation of *De scorbuto* with *De fermentatione* was published from Middelburg in octavo (1676: **3C**; see also **1H**).

The Oxford and London quarto edition

It seems likely that James Allestry (d.1670) either lost the quarto sheets of *Pathologiæ cerebri* in the Great Fire of London or was unable to continue his plans to publish these treatises. The book also has the stamp of Thomas Roycroft (1637–1677) in that many of the printers' ornaments are those he had used for printing *Diatribæ duæ* in 1660 and 1662 (**1B**, **1C**). An arrangement was evidently made with William Hall (fl.1656–1672) in Oxford who had a close association with the University press.[1] Eventually the book was printed, 'excudebat', from Oxford, and sold, 'apud Insigne', from Duck Lane in London (1667: **3A**). The Oxford association is evident from the fact that the book has the imprimatur of John Fell (1625–1686), vice-chancellor, and is the first to include the engraved portrait of Willis by David Loggan (1634–1692), who was based in Oxford. Attention has not previously been drawn to the cancelled leaf in *De scorbuto* at Rr1. In the copy considered for this bibliography the cancellandum and the cancellans are both present, making a volume with 171 leaves (compared with 170 as described by HJR Wing).[2] The texts start to differ in the last three lines at Rr1r, page 313 extending to line 3 at Rr1v, page 314. The cancellandum reads:

> … in victu; quippe vir Inſigniſſimus poſt negotia, & ſtudia ſeveriora ad μεσονύκτιον ſæpe protracta, tunc temporis cænare, & ſtatim à Lienis, alio- [catchword, rumque] / rumque forsan viſcerum, fermenta morbida ſanguini ſuppeditantium, diatheſi valetudinariâ …

[1] See: Harry Carter *A history of the Oxford University press*, Oxford (1975): pages 194–7 for details of the Oxford firm of Hall family printers which survived into the 1960s. In the 1660s, John Hall (former printer to the University press) had six apprentices; and a seventh worker was added when William Hall took over and was required to provide 'meate, drinke, washing and lodging, shoes and stockings'. William's son (also William) served John Fell for seven years from 1672 to learn the art of letter founding:

[2] The cancellans is present in one of the copies in the Bodleian Library inscribed R. Frewin (1701): the cancellandum is present in the other Bodleian copy, and that in St John's College Library. No one of these copies has both.

> [Of course this excellent man, after his work and rather serious study, often past midnight, was wont to have his meal only then, and suddenly, by a feeble disposition of the internal organs of the spleen or others, mixing morbid fermentations in great quantity with the blood . . .].

The cancellans reads:

> . . . in victu; quippe vir Inſigniſſimus poſt negotia, & ſtudia ſeveriora ad μεσονύκτιον ſæpe protracta, tunc temporis cænare, & ſtatim Lecto commiſſus obdor- [catchword, mire] / mire ſolebat: Porro hic morbus partium oriebatur, à Lienis, aliorumque forſan viſcerum, fermenta morbida ſanguini ſuppeditantium, diatheſi valetudinariâ: . . .
>
> [Of course this excellent man, after his work and rather serious study, often past midnight, was wont to have his meal only then, and to drop off to sleep immediately on having conveyed himself to bed: subsequently this disease of his [body] parts may have originated, by a feeble disposition of the internal organs of the spleen or others, mixing morbid fermentations in great quantity with the blood . . .].

After Rr1v, page 314, line 3 the texts are identical but the line breaks remain different to the foot of page 314 ending 'in appendice nervoſa, at- [catchword, que] / que circa . . .'. The cancellans makes the point that going to bed on a full stomach risks disordered fermentation. This correction is present in all subsequent Latin printings of *De scorbuto* (**3B**, **3D**) and (presumably) in the Dutch translation (**3C**).

The London and Amsterdam duodecimo editions

Issues of the 1668 duodecimo edition were printed and distributed in Amsterdam and London (**3B1** and **3B2**). These differ only on the title pages. Unusually for a book of that period, James Allestry prints the date in Arabic numerals. He decorates that leaf with a tail-piece, whereas Daniel Elsevier uses his printer's device. The Amsterdam 1670 issue retains the original sheets (**3B3**). However these three issues also have leaves in different states making for further variation between copies. As with other of Willis's publications where sheets remained available over time, these alterations do not represent systematic correction. Most examples of the 1668 Amsterdam and London issues (**3B1**, **3B2**) have O2 signed N2;[3] mispagination of 203 for 103, 253 for 153, and 147 for 247; and catchword errors at H11r / v, pages 189 / 190, and K2v / K3r, pages 220 / 221. When sheets were gathered for sale in 1670, some of these errors were retained, others amended, and one newly introduced. In the two copies from 1670 examined for this bibliography, O2 is correctly signed and A5 and E5 are reset as A5 and E5; and page 153 is correctly numbered. Mispagination of 147 for 247 remains in one copy (**3B3.c1**) but is corrected in the other, as is the catchword error at K2v / K3r, pages 220 / 221 (**3B3.c2**). A new error, 379 for 279, is newly introduced and present in both copies. It is likely that many other combinations of leaves in altered states exist, randomly allocated to examples of the 1668 or 1670 issues.

[3] The error is present in all copies used for this bibliography, but (as HJR Wing indicates) O2 is signed correctly in the Wellcome Library copy (EPB/A/53352).

The Amsterdam duodecimo issue from 1668 has priority over the London imprint. HJR Wing takes as his authority the analysis of Charles Pieters (nd).[4] But, in a somewhat convoluted account, Pieters merely explains (correctly) that there are two duodecimo 1668 issues, each with the same imprimatur from John Fell and each with O2 signed N2. He explains that the Amsterdam duodecimo 1670 issue retains the imprimatur but now has O2 correctly signed (as detailed earlier). HJR Wing concludes that Elsevier printed copies bearing the Allestry imprint but 'whether Allestry commissioned Elsevier to print some copies for him or whether Elsevier printed them without his knowledge must remain, for the moment, unanswered'. Because Allestry's premises had been destroyed in the Great Fire of 1666, leaving him almost ruined, HJR Wing clearly supports the view that Elsevier was printing books for the London market as a favour to Allestry, much as William Hall had done in Oxford at a time when Allestry, in 1667, had not yet managed to reestablish his London business,[5] rather than pirating an existing publication for sale in Amsterdam. Negotiations may have been through James's brother, Richard Allestry (1619–1681), who was often in Holland as a secret agent on behalf of Charles II (1630–1685). Allestry carried back orders to bishops in England instructing them to maintain the Anglican tradition, resulting in his arrest on a charge of treason and imprisonment in Lambeth Palace until the restoration.

The assumption that Elsevier provided printed sheets to Allestry is supported, indirectly, by consideration of the printers' ornaments. In general, although fleurons and decorated initials are occasionally found, head and tailpieces were not much used in the issues of Willis's works published in England at that time. Allestry's duodecimo London issue has a tailpiece on the title page comprising an inverted floral design with a human face worked into the foliage, typical of several used by continental printers, and a headpiece at A1r, page 1, with the chi-delta design first used by Gerbrandt Schagen in 1663 (Schagen 9: **1E**). Another unusual feature of the 1668 issues is the use of an otherwise blank page, here *6v, page [12], on which to print the portrait (Pt.1b1) rather than this being bound in as a separate leaf. The engraver copied the Loggan portrait from the 1667 issue directly onto the copperplate resulting in reversal of the printed image.

The Dutch translation

HJR Wing suggests that the Dutch translation (1676: **3C** and **1H**) is probably by Steven Blankaart (1650–1702).[6] Although the treatise on scurvy has its own title page, it seems unlikely that this was printed independently from the translation of *De fermentatione* since the volume has a collective title page, also dated 1676, which refers to 'Beneffens een Tractaat van des Scheurbuiks … Aanteykeningen en Blat-wÿſer verrÿkt'[7]:

[4] See: Charles Pieters *Annales de l'imprimerie des Elsevier: ou histoire de leur famille et de leurs editions*, Gand [Ghent] (1858): pages 300–1.

[5] See: HJR Wing, *Christ Church Newsletter* (2011–2012): page 19 for comment that Allestry's premises in St Paul's Churchyard were unusable and not surveyed for damage until 10 July 1668.

[6] Wing takes his entry from *The catalogue of the library of the surgeon general's office*, second series, volume 21, Authors and subjects, Waterworth-Zysman, Catalogue, Washington (1916): page 141, and refers to this as a translation of Willis's *De fermentatione* without mentioning the second treatise. Incorrectly, the Surgeon General and HJR Wing each transcribe the publisher's name as W. Goetree. Steven Blankaart was a Dutch physician, iatrochemist, and entomologist, who proved the existence of a capillary system without fully realizing the significance of his findings. His approach to science was deductive and Cartesian. Blankaart was in favour of prohibition on the use of alcohol.

[7] See chapter 5 for transcription of the Dutch text in full.

In addition a Treatise on the ORIGIN of SCURVY, Categories, complications, and artful Curation, according to the new *Chemical Foundations* of the same Author. *Both only now for the benefit of Surgeons and Apothecaries. Translated from Latin and throughout enriched by Comments and Index.*

The Dutch octavo issue is typographically unusual in that, when a footnote straddles two pages, the first has its own catchword independent of that relating to the main text.

The 'fourth' London edition

The final duodecimo edition of *Pathologiæ cerebri* (1678: **3D**) was printed by Samuel Roycroft (1657–1717) for John Martyn (1618–1680). This is reset and contains more printers' ornaments and decorated initials than Thomas Willis's other books printed in England. The type setting of the endpages is sloppy: 'ELENCHUS RERUM IN TRACTATU DE MOR*BB*IS CONVULSIVIS.' at O8r, page [327]; 'ELENCHUS RERUM IN TRACTATU *EE* SCORBUTO.' at P2v, page [340]. The pagination is chaotic. The 1678 duodecimo is described as the fourth edition. This is understandable since others had appeared in 1667 (**3A**), 1668 (**3B1** and **3B2**), and 1670 (**3B3**) but, correctly, HJR Wing draws attention to the fact that there is no trace of a third London edition. This final edition was advertised in the *Term Catalogue* and the price, 3 shillings, duly noted:

> Easter 1678 May 14th, III Numb 15, I 315, column 1, *Books reprinted.*
>
> *Pathologiæ Cerebri et nervosi generis Specimen.* In quo agitur *De morbus Convulsivis et de Scorbuto.* Studio Tho. Willis, M.D. In Twelves. Price, bound, 3s. Printed for J. Martyn at the Bell in St. *Paul's* Churchyard.

3A. PATHOLOGIÆ CEREBRI, Oxford and London quarto 1667

The first edition of Willis's third book, with first appearance of the engraved portrait of Thomas Willis by David Loggan [HJR Wing 17].

Title page: PATHOLOGIÆ | CEREBRI, | ET | NERVOSI GENERIS | SPECIMEN. | In quo agitur De | MORBIS CONVULSIVIS, | ET DE | SCORBUTO. | STUDIO | THOMÆ WILLIS, Ex *Æde Chrifti Oxon.* M. D. | & in ifta Celeberrimâ Academiâ Naturalis Philo- | fophiæ Profefforis Sidleiani, nec non Inclyti | Medic. Coll. Londin. & Societatis | Regiæ ibidem, Socii. | [rule] | *OXONII,* | Excudebat *Guil. Hall,* Impenfis *Ja. Alleftry,* apud Infigne | Rofæ Coronatæ in Vico Vulgo dicto *Duck-lane,* MDCLXVII.

Collation: quarto; 23 letter roman alphabet using I and U: A^4, a–c^4, B–Z^4, Aa–Qq^4, Rr^2 (Rr1 + 1); $1–2 signed apart from: C[1] for *c*[1], +*c*3, +Z3.

171 leaves: paginated as [32], 1–202, [2], 203–78, 289–314, 313–14, 315–16 (i.e. 1–310). Mispaginated: 230 for 130.

Type: 35 lines; height (20 lines) 92 millimetres, width 102 millimetres (120 with marginal notes).

Contents: **A1r**, page [1], title; **A2v**, page [2], Imprimatur, Septemb. 25. 1667. JOHANNES FELL. VICE-CANCELLARIUS OXON:; **A2r–A3v**, pages [3–6] REVERENDISSIMO In Chriſto Patri, & Domino, Domino GILBERTO, Providentia Divina, Archiepiſcopo *Cantuarienſi*, totius *Angliæ* Primati & Metropolitano; & Auguſtiſſimo Principi CAROLO II. M. *Britanniæ*, *Franciæ*, & *Hiberniæ* Regi, à Secretioribus Conſiliis. … [signed] *Quod animitus precatur Clementiæ veſtræ Humillimus cultor, Cliens addictiſſimus* THO: WILLIS.; **A4r–a1v**, pages [7–10], Amico Lectori Præfatio.; **a2r–b4r**, pages [11–23], ELENCHUS RERUM IN TRACTATU DE MORBIS CONVULSIVIS.; **b4v–c4r**, pages [24–31], ELENCHUS RERUM IN TRACTATU DE SCORBUTO.; **c4v**, page [32], *ERRATA*, 15 lines listing 46 corrections.

B1r–Dd1v, pages 1–202, [text] [De morbis convulsivis]; **Dd2r**, page [1], [half title] [rule] Tractatus Secundus DE SCORBVTO. [rule]; **Dd2v**, page [2], blank; **Dd3r–Rr** (Rr +1)–**Rr2v**, pages 203–'316' (i.e. 310), [text] TRACTATUS SECUNDUS DE SCORBUTO.

Headlines and *Catchwords*: no '.' after headline at ***a*3r**, page [13]; ***b*3r–v**, pages [21–2], ***c*2v–*c*3r**, pages [28–9]; ***c*4r**, page [31]; *SCORBUTO* for *SCORBVTO* at **Rr1 + 1r–v**, pages [313–14].

CAP. for Febris at ***b*2r / v**, page [17] / [18]; a for à at **C3v / C4r**, page 14 / 15; Epilepſie for 2. Epilepſie at **D4v / E1r**, page 24 / 25; tam: for tam; at **E1v / E2r**, page 26 / 27; tius for tiùs at **E4r / v**, page 31 / 32; In for Methodus at **F4v / G1r**, page 40 / 41; pone for ponè at **H3v / H4r**, page 54 / 55; quemvis for vis at **N4r / v**, page 95 / 96; nerant; for nerant: at **S2v / S3r**, page 132 / 133; facile for facilè at **Z4r / v**, page 175 / 176; guine for sanguine at **Z4v / Aa1r**, page 176 / 177; *con* for *om*: at **Mm4v / Nn1r**, page 270 / 271.

Frontispiece: none.

Portrait: **Pt.1a1**: [Engraved portrait of Thomas Willis] *D: Loggan: delin: et ſculpt*: *ÆTATIS SUÆ, 45*. 195 × 150 millimetres (sheet), 187 × 139 millimetres (plate marks), 184 × 135 millimetres (image; see: Figure 118).

Printers' ornaments: single row of 23 fleurons {**Roycroft 15**} separated by a single fleuron {**Roycroft 8**} between ##11 / 12 at **B1r**, page 1; two rows each of 28 fleurons, upper ##1–5, 9, 10, 13–16, 18, 20, 22–26, 28 {**Roycroft 31**}; ##6–8, 11, 12, 21, 27 {**Roycroft 32**}; #17 {**Roycroft 33**}; #19 {**Roycroft 34**} separated by *ſ* between #14 / 15; and lower ##1, 4, 6, 10, 16–18, 21, 22, 25, 26 {**Roycroft 34**}; ##2, 3, 5, 8, 12, 13, 15, 19, 20, 23, 24 {**Roycroft 31**}; ##7, 27, 28 {**Roycroft 33**}; ##9, 11 {**Roycroft 32**}; #14 {**Roycroft 35**} separated by : between ##6 / 7, 20 / 21, at **Dd1v**, page 202; single row of 19 fleurons {**Roycroft 36**} at **Dd3**, page 203.

Decorated I at **B1r**, page 1 {**Roycroft 30**}.

Illustrations: none.

Copy: DASC. Original full calf with blind tooling, spine (rebacked) with four raised bands and five gilt decorated panels, label WILLIS | CEREBRI, new endpapers. Leaves 195 × 150

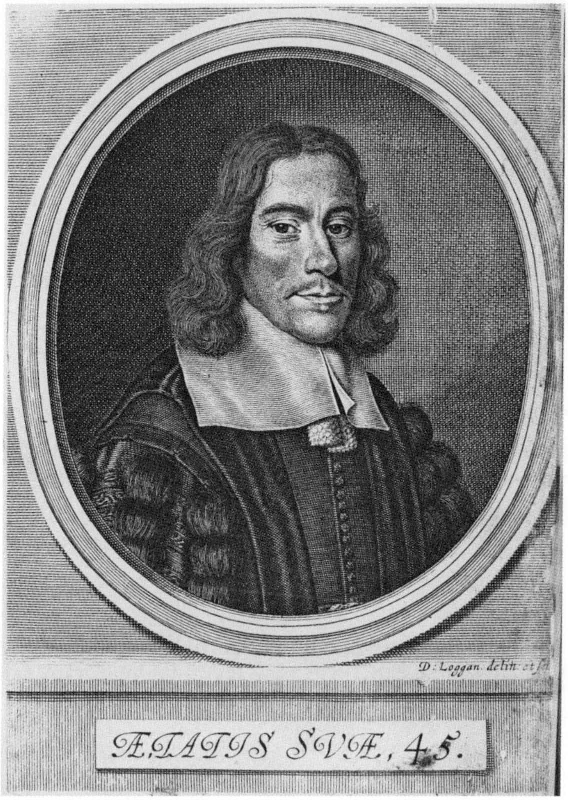

Figure 118 Portrait of Thomas Willis engraved by David Loggan: *Pathologiæ* cerebri 1667 (Pt.1a1).

millimetres, boards 200 × 160 × 32 millimetres. Bookplate F.M.R. WALSHE MD FRS. Inscribed: (at one time on original front free endpaper, now lost) Wm Feindel Montréal.[8]

3B1. PATHOLOGIÆ CEREBRI, Amsterdam duodecimo 1668

The first issue of the second edition of Willis's third book, with the portrait reengraved and printed as part of the first preliminary sheet [HJR Wing 18].

Title page: PATHOLOGIÆ | CEREBRI, | ET | NERVOSI GENERIS | SPECIMEN. | *In quo agitur de* | MORBIS CONVULSIVIS, | ET DE | SCORBUTO. | Studio | THOMÆ WILLIS, *ex Æde Chrifti Oxon. M. D. &* | *in ifta celeberrima Academia Naturalis Philofophiæ* | *Profefforis*

[8] Sir Francis Walshe FRS (1885–1973) was a neurologist appointed to the consultant staff of the National Hospital, Queen Square, and University College Hospital. He was not an experimentalist but contributed to human neurophysiology through observation and interpretation of disease. Unlike William Feindel (1918–2014) from whom this copy was obtained, Walshe was an avid reader but not a noted bibliophile. Although there are occasional annotations in Latin and Greek script, the earlier provenance of the copy is unknown.

Sidleiani, nec non inclyti Med. Coll. | *Londini, & Societatis Regiæ ibidem Socii.* | [printers' device] | *AMSTELODAMI,* | Apud DANIELEM ELZEVIRIUM, | CIↃ IↃC LXVIII.

Collation: duodecimo; 23 letter roman alphabet using I: $*^6$, A–0^{12}, P–Q^6; $1–7 signed apart from -K5, O2 signed N2, -P5, -P6, -Q5, -Q6.

186 leaves: paginated as [12], 1–338, [22]. Mispaginated: 203 for 103, 253 for 153, 147 for 247.

Type: 40 lines; height (20 lines) 52 millimetres, width 50 millimetres (60 with marginal notes).

Contents: ***1r**, page [1], title; ***1v**, page [2], Imprimatur, Septemb. 25. 1667. JOHANNES FELL. *Vice-Cancellarius Oxon.*; ***2r**–***3v**, pages [3–6], *Reverendiſſimo in Chriſto Patri, & Domino*, D. GILBERTO, Providentia Divina, Archiepiſcopo Cantuarienſi, totius Angliæ Primati & Metropolitano; & Auguſtiſſimo Principi CAROLO II. M. Britanniæ, Franciæ & Hiberniæ Regi, à ſecretioribus Conſiliis. ... [signed] *Clementiæ veſtræ humillimus cultor, Cliens addictiſſimus* THOM. WILLIS.; ***4r**–***6r**, page [7–11], Amico Lectori Præfatio.; ***6v**, page [12], engraved portrait.

A1r–**K4v**, pages 1–224, [text] TRACTATUS PRIMUS DE MORBIS CONVULSIVIS.; **K5r**, page [225], [half title] TRACTATUS SECUNDUS DE SCORBUTO.; **K5v**, page [226], blank; **K6r**–**P1v**, pages 227–338, [text] TRACTATUS SECUNDUS DE SCORBUTO.

P2r–**Q1v**, pages [1–12] ELENCHUS RERUM IN TRACTATU DE MORBIS CONVULSIVIS.; **Q2r**–**Q5r**, pages [13–19], ELENCHUS RERUM IN TRACTATU DE SCORBUTO.; **Q5v**–**Q6v**, pages [20–22], blank.

Headlines and *Catchwords*: headlines correct.

vulgo for valde at **H11r** / **v**, pages 189 / 190; *lapii* for *julapii* at **K2v** / **K3r**, pages 220 / 221.

Frontispiece: none.

Portrait: **Pt.1b1**: at *6v, page [12], *ÆTATIS SUÆ, 45.* 130 × 75 millimetres (sheet), 109 × 65 millimetres (plate marks), 107 × 64 millimetres (image; see: Figure 119).

Printers' ornaments: printers' device at *1r, page [1] {**Elsevier 1**}; headpiece at **A1r**, page 1; **K6r**, page 227 {**Schagen 9**}; tailpiece at **K4v**, page 224; **P1v**, page 338; **Q1v**, page [12] {**Elsevier 4**}.

Decorated I at *2r, page [3] {**Elsevier 2**}; Q at *4r, page [7] {**Elsevier 3**}; I at **A1r**, page 1; **K6r**, page 227 {**Elsevier 5**}.

Illustrations: none.

Copy: DASC (#1 of 2). Original full calf; spine with five raised bands and five gilt decorated panels and edges, labelled WILLIS | PATHOL, original endpapers. Leaves 130 × 75

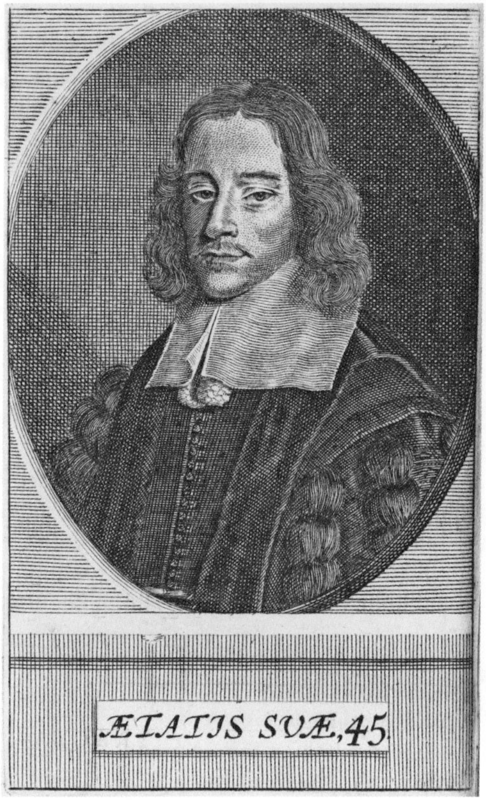

Figure 119 Portrait of Thomas Willis: *Pathologiæ cerebri* 1668 (Pt.1b1).

millimetres, boards 137 × 85 × 25 millimetres. Inscribed: (1) ex Libris [Raymond] ?Rubrio (unidentified); (2) ?De Sesse medicin.[9]

3B2. PATHOLOGIÆ CEREBRI, London duodecimo 1668

The second issue of the second edition of Willis's third book, with the title page reset, the date in Arabic numerals [HJR Wing 19].

Title page: PATHOLOGIÆ | CEREBRI, | ET | NERVOSI GENERIS | SPECIMEN. | *In quo agitur de* | MORBIS CONVULSIVIS, | ET DE | SCORBUTO. | Studio | THOMÆ WILLIS, *ex Æde Chriſti Oxon. M. D. &* | *in iſta celeberrima Academia Naturalis Philoſophiæ* | *Profeſſoris Sidleiani, nec non inclyti Med. Coll.* | *Londini, & Societatis Regiæ ibidem Socii.* | [ornament] | *LONDINI,* | Apud JACOBUM ALLESTRY, Regalis | Societatis Typographum. 1668.

Then as in **3B1** apart from:

Printers' ornament: tailpiece at ***1r**, page [1] {**Elsevier 4**}.

[9] This may be Martín Sessé [y Lacasta] (1751–1808) who was a military physician from 1779 but better known as a botanist expert on the flora of Mexico.

Copy: DASC. Later full calf with blind tooling, spine with six gilt lines and blind tooling in three panels, labels PATHOLOGIÆ | CEREBRI | – |THOMÆ | WILLIS / LOND. 1668, original endpapers. Leaves 127 × 75 millimetres, boards 133 × 82 × 24 millimetres. Shelfmark: S: ff: 4.[10]

3B3.c1. PATHOLOGIÆ CEREBRI, Amsterdam duodecimo 1670

The third issue of the second edition of Willis's third book, with the title page reset and variant states of some leaves [HJR Wing 20].

Title page: PATHOLOGIÆ | CEREBRI, | ET | NERVOSI GENERIS | SPECIMEN. | *In quo agitur de* | MORBIS CONVULSIVIS, | ET DE | SCORBUTO. | Studio | THOMÆ WILLIS, *ex Æde Chrifti Oxon. M. D. &* | *in ifta celeberrima Academia Naturalis Philofophiæ* | *Profefforis Sidleiani, nec non inclyti Med. Coll.* | *Londini, & Societatis Regiæ ibidem Socii.* | [printers' device] | *AMSTELODAMI,* | Apud DANIELEM ELZEVIRIUM, | CIↃ IↃC LXX.

Then as in **3B1** apart from:

Collation: A5 signed A5; E5 signed E5, (O2 correctly signed).

Mispaginated: 203 for 103, (253 for 153 corrected), 147 for 247, and 379 for 279.

Copy: DASC. Early full calf, spine with four raised bands and gilt edges (restored), original endpapers. Leaves 130 × 72 millimetres, boards 135 × 75 × 23 millimetres.

3B3.c2. PATHOLOGIÆ CEREBRI, Amsterdam duodecimo 1670

The third issue of the second edition of Willis's third book, with further variant states of some leaves [not distinguished from HJR Wing 20].

As in **3B3.c1** apart from:

Collation: Mispaginated: 203 for 103 (253 for 153 and 147 for 247 corrected), 379 for 279.

Catchwords: lapii for julapii at **K2v / K3r**, pages 220 / 221 corrected.

Copy: DASC. Early full calf, spine with five raised bands and five gilt panels with gilt fleuron and edges, label PATHOL | CEREB, original endpapers (no free end papers). Leaves 132 × 72 millimetres, boards 138 × 80 × 24 millimetres. Inscribed: in French (undeciphered) but appearing to make the point that these two works were first published in London and that they relate to Glisson and others.

[10] This copy has three leaves of printers' waste from Simon Patrick (1626–1707) *A continuation of the Friendly debate by the same author*, London (1669): pages 93 / 94, 63 / 64, and a stub with type on the recto and verso, bound after Q6. See chapter 1 for further mention of Bishop Patrick.

3C. (see 1H) [ON SCURVY], Middelburg octavo 1676

The Dutch translation of the treatise on scurvy from Willis's third book [HJR Wing 67].

Title page: DES | SCHEUR—BUIKS | Oorſprong, ſoorten, toe-vallen | en konſtige Geneſing, volgens | de nieuwe Chijmiſche Gronden, | *Van den Vermaarden Heer* | THOMAS WILLIS, | *Hoog-Leeraar tot Oxfordt; Nauw- | keuriger als oyt verhandelt.* | Nu eerſt uit het Latijn Vertaalt, en met | Genees-kundige Aan-teykeningen en Blad- | wijſer Verrijkt. | [ornament] | Tot MIDDELBURGH, | [short rule] | By *Wilhelmus Goeree*, Book-verkooper | in Cicero. 1676.[11]

Collation: octavo; 23 letter roman alphabet using V: M–Z^8, Aa^8; $1–5 signed.

104 leaves, [Fol.] pages [165]–344, [28].

Type: 35 lines; height (20 lines) 68 millimetres, width 62 millimetres (76 with marginal notes).

Contents: **M1r**, page [165], title page; **M1v**, page 166, blank; **M2r–M4v**, pages 167–72, Den Overſetter *Tot den LESER.*[12]

M5r–Z2v, pages 173–344, [text] Verhandeling Van het SCHEUR-BUIK.

Z3r–Aa6r, pages [1–23], Blad–Wijſer; **Aa6v–Aa8v**, pages [24–8], blank.

Headlines and *Catchwords*:*'t Bloed* for*'t Zenu-sap* at **Q1r**, page 229;*'t Zenu-sap ontſtaande.* for *het Bloed enZen. Enz.* at **R2r**, page 247; *Vande* for *Van de* at **R4v**, page 252; **S5v**, page 270; **T1v**, page 278.

verbrand for brand at **N6r / v**, pages 191 / 192; walgren for Walgren at **P6v / P7r**, pages 222 / 223; op-sie for opsie at **Q3r / Q3v**, pages 233 / 234; ſterk for ſterck at **R5v / R6r**, pages 254 / 255; ß *pont* for ß pont at **V8r / v**, pages 307 / 308 (footnote).

Frontispiece: none.

Portrait: none.

Printers' ornaments: headpiece at **M1r**, page 165 {**<u>Goeree 5</u>**}; tailpiece at **Aa6r**, page [23] {**<u>Goeree 8</u>**}.

Decorated B at **M2r**, page 167 {**<u>Goeree 6</u>**}; B at **M5r**, page 173 {**<u>Goeree 7</u>**}.

Illustrations: none.

[11] ABOUT SCURVY Origin, categories, complications and artful Curation, according to The new Chemical Foundations, *Of the Famous Gentleman* THOMAS WILLIS, Professor in Oxford, explained more precisely than before. Only now translated from Latin, and enriched with Medical Comments and Index At MIDDELBURGH, For *Wilhelmus Goeree*, Bookseller in Cicero. 1676.

[12] The Translator *to the READER* / Treatise On SCURVY / Index.

Copy: DASC. Original full vellum, spine with faded lettering in manuscript, original endpapers. Leaves 155 × 95 millimetres, binding 165 × 103 × 35 millimetres.

3D. PATHOLOGIÆ CEREBRI, London duodecimo 1678

The third edition of Willis's third book, but described as the fourth presumably on the basis that one or other of the London (1668) and Amsterdam (1668 or 1670) issues of the second edition constituted a third 'edition' [HJR Wing 21].

Title page: PATHOLOGIÆ | CEREBRI, | ET | NERVOSI GENERIS | SPECIMEN. | *In quo agitur de* | MORBIS CONVULSIVIS, | ET DE | SCORBUTO. | [rule] | STUDIO | THOMÆ WILLIS, ex *Æde Chriſti* OXON. | M. D. & in iſta celeberrima Academia Na- | turalis Philoſophiæ Profeſſoris *Sidleiani.* | [rule] | Editio Quarta, | Ab AUTHORE recognita, atque ab eodem | multiplici Auctario locupletata. | [rule] | *LONDINI,* | Typis S. *Roycroft*; Impenſis *Jo. Martyn*, ad Inſig- | ne Campanæ, in Cœmeterio D. *Pauli*, MDCLXXVIII.

Collation: duodecimo; 23 letter roman alphabet using I: a^6, $A–0^{12}$, P^6; $1–5 signed apart from: B4 signed B3, C4 signed C5, -D4, -G5, -H4, -I5, K5 signed K3, -O5, -P5.

180 leaves: paginated as [12], 1–[346], [2]. Mispaginated: 351 for 135, 666 for 266, -327, -330, -331, -334, -335, 536 for 336, -337–46.

Type: 42 lines; height (20 lines) 57 millimetres, width 50 millimetres (67 with marginal notes).

Contents: **a1r–v**, pages [1–2], blank; **a2r**, page [3], title; **a2v**, page [4], blank; **a3r–a4v**, pages [5–8] *Reverendiſſimo in Chriſto Patri, & Domino*, D. GILBERTO, Providentia Divina, Archipiſcopo Cantuarienſi, totius Angliæ Primati & Metropolitano; & Augustiſſimo Principi CAROLO II. M. Britanniæ, Franciæ & Hiberniæ Regi, à ſecretioribus Conciliis … [signed] *Clementiæ veſtræ cultor, Cliens addictiſſimus* THO. WILLIS.; **a5r–a6v**, pages [9–12], Amico Lectori Præfatio.

A1r–I12v, pages 1–216, [text] TRACTATUS PRIMUS DE MORBIS CONVULSIVIS.; **K1r**, page [217], [half title] TRACTATUS SECUNDUS DE SCORBUTO.; **K1v**, page [218], blank; **K2r–07v**, pages 219–326, [text] TRACTATUS SECUNDUS DE SCORBUTO.

O8r–P2r, pages [327]–[339], ELENCHUS RERUM. IN TRACTATU DE MORBBIS CONVULSIVIS.; **P2v–P5v**, pages [340–6], ELENCHUS RERUM. IN TRACTATU EE SCORBUTO.; **P6r**–v, pages [1–2], blank.

Headlines and *Catchwords*: DE MORBIS for CONVULSIVIS. at **B2r**, page 27; **B3r**, page 29; **[B4]r**, page 31; CONVULSIVIS. for DE MORBIS at **B3v**, page 30; ⁚ after headline at **B7v**, page 38; **B11v**, page 46; **B12v**, page 48; **C2v**, page 52; **C3v**, page 54; **C[4]v**, page 56; **C5v**, page 58; **C10v**, page 68; **C11v**, page 70; **D3v**, page 78; **D5v**, page 82; **D12v**, page 96; **E2v**, page 100; **E3v**, page 102; **E4v**, page 104; **E6v**, page 108; **F4v**, page 128; **F9v**, page 138; **G8v**, page 160; **H5v**, page 178; **I3v**, page 198; **I8v**, page 208; CONVILSIVI. for CONVULSIVIS. at **C[4]r**, page 55; ⁏ for ⁚ after headline at **H3r**, page 173; **I9r**, page 209; no ⁚ after headline at **H6r**, page 179; **H8r**, page 183; **I7r**, page 205; **K8r**, page 231; **N9v**, page 258; **M1v**, page [266]; **M5r**, page 273; **N2r**, page 291; **N9v**, page 306; ELENCAUS RERUM. for ELENCHUS RERUM. at **O11v**, page 334.

No catchword at **D7r / v**, pages 85 / 86; nem for mnem at **D12v / E1r**, pages 96 / 97; metu for tu at **H9r / v**, pages 185 / 186; grui for fuſceptionem at **K8r / v**, pages 231 / 232; 4. A for 5. Aqua at **M9r / v**, pages 281 / 282; De for *De* at **N4v / N5r**, pages 296 / 297; **N7v / N8r**, pages 302 / 303.

Frontispiece: none.

Portrait: none.

Printers' ornaments: headpiece at **a3r**, page [5] {**Roycroft 37**}; K2r, page 219 {**Roycroft 39**}.

Decorated I at **a3r**, page [5]; **A1r**, page 1 (inverted) {**Roycroft 9**}; Q at **a5r**, page [9] {**Roycroft 38**}; I at **K2r**, page 219 {**Roycroft 40**}.

Illustrations: none.

Copy: DASC. Original full calf with blind tooling, spine three raised bands with gilt lines (rebacked), label WILLIS | PATHOLOGIÆ | CEREBRI | SPECIMEN | 1678. Inserted: book label (front pastedown) and stamped (title page) Norfolk and Norwich United Medical Book Society. Inscribed: (1) Wm Feindel Montréal (upside down); (2) Jno Stubbing Hanc librum jure tenet ['my book']. Ex libris Johannes Stubbingi (unidentified); (3) Jno Stubbing (title page). Shelfmarks: (1) g–y x pic; (2) W735p 1678 10546.[13]

[13] See chapter 6, **2E1**, for details of the Norwich and Norfolk United Book Society.

8

'An Iliad of evils in the head'

Affectionum quæ dicuntur hystericæ et hypochondriacæ (1670–1678)

Affectionum quæ dicuntur hystericæ et hypochondriacæ, *De sanguinis accensione*, and *De motu musculari*, Willis's eighth, ninth, and tenth treatises, were first published as his fourth book in 1670. The account of hysteria and hypochondria is a rapidly written response to a publication in the same year by Nathanael Highmore (1613–1685),[1] provoked by Willis's comments in *Pathologiæ cerebri* (1667: **3A**) criticising Highmore's earlier work on this topic from 1660.[2] Quarrelling with one of his contemporaries was nothing new for Thomas Willis. The second of these three treatises, *De sanguinis accensione*, is Willis's final statement on fermentation. After the confusion of including William Croone's *De ratione motus musculorum* (1664) and its plate in the Amsterdam editions of *Cerebri anatome*, not fully resolved until 1667 (**2E1**), the third treatise published in 1670 is *De motu musculari*, Willis's account of muscular motion, with four figures engraved on two plates (Pl.17 and Pl.18).

The publication history followed the usual sequence: an initial quarto edition, published in London now that Willis had moved from Oxford (1670: **4A**); two issues of a duodecimo edition printed in Leiden by arrangement or piracy (1671: **4B1** and **4B2**); and a further duodecimo edition from London (1678: **4C**). The quarto is relatively unadorned. There are no printer's ornaments or decorated initials although use is made of several large capital letters, each occupying several lines of text.[3] The portrait is printed at A1v, page 2, as part of the first sheet. The book ends with a brief list of four errata and the somewhat weary suggestion, Rogandus eſt lectòr ut cætera corrigat, 'The reader is asked to correct the rest'.

Willis presented a copy to the Royal Society on 17 March 1670. It was reviewed in the *Philosophical Transactions*.[4] Priced at 2s 6d, the book was noted (with two almost identical entries) in the *Term Catalogue*:

> Easter 1670 May 17th, I Numb. 7, I 29, column 2, *Physick*.
>
> *AFFECTIONUM quæ dicuntur Hystericæ et Hypochondriacæ pathologia spasmodica vindicata*, Contra Responsionem epistolarem N*athaniel Highmori*, M.D. Cui accesserunt Exercitationes Medico-Physicæ duæ. 1. *De sanguine accensione*. 2. *De motu Musculari*.

[1] See: *De hysterica & hypochondriaca passione responsio epistolaris ad Doctorem Willis*, London (1670).

[2] See: *Exercitationes duae. Quarum prior de paſſione hyſterica: altera de affectione hypochondriaca*, Oxford (1660).

[3] These are: Q, 24 × 20 millimetres, at A3r, page [5]; R, 20 × 21 millimetres, at B1r, page (1); J, 20 × 9 millimetres, at G4r, page 47; C, 20 × 19 millimetres, at K4r, page '69', i.e. 71; and O, 11 × 11 millimetres, at P2v, page 108.

[4] See: [Anon], III. *Affectionum quæ dicuntur hysterica & hypochondriacæ pathalogia spasmodica vindicata, contra responsion. epistol. Nathanaelis Highmori M. D. cui accessere exercitat. Medico-physicæ duæ, I. De Sanguinis Accension. 2. De Motu Musculari*, Auth. Tho. Willis M. D. Nat. Philos. Prof. Oxon, nec non med. Coll. Londini & Soc. Regiæ Sodalis. Londini apud Jac. Allestry In 4°, *Philosophical Transactions of the Royal Society*, December 1670, Vol V, number 57, page 1178; and see chapter 17 for discussion.

Studio T. Willis, M.D. Coll. *Londini*, et Societatis Regii, socii. In Quarto. Price, stitcht, 2s. 6d. Printed for J. Allestry at the Rose [and Crown] in St. *Paul's* Churchyard.

Easter 1670 May, II Numb. 1, I 35/6, column 2/1, *Libri Latini.*

AFFECTIONUM quæ dicuntur Hystericæ et Hypochondriacæ pathologia spasmodica vindicata, Contra Responsionem epistolarem N*athanael Highmori*, M.D. Cui accesserunt Exercitationes Medico-Physicæ duæ: 1. *De sanguinis accensione.* 2. *De motu Musculari.* Studio T. Willis, M.D. Coll. *Londini.*, et Societatis Regii, socii. In Quarto. Price, stitcht, 2s. 6d. Printed for J. Allestry at the Rose [and Crown] in St. *Paul's* Churchyard.

There is nothing of note bibliographically relating to the 1671 Leiden duodecimo edition. This appeared in two issues which differ only in order of names for the two booksellers on the title pages. The fact that the publishers did not have access to the original plates and therefore had the illustrations reengraved suggests that, by comparison with Daniel Elsevier and the duodecimo Amsterdam edition of *Pathologiæ cerebri* (**3B1**),[5] there was no cooperation between James Allestry (d.1670) and the Dutch booksellers. But quite what local rivalries required Felicem Lopez (fl.1664–1693) and Cornelius Driehuysen (fl.1663–1671) to reverse the order of their names on the title page of some copies is unclear.

With the London duodecimo edition of 1678, publication of *Affectionum quæ dicuntur hystericæ et hypochondriacæ* was complete and no further editions in Latin appeared. The plates used by James Allestry were still available and reused, although the plate sizes were slightly reduced perhaps in order to fit a different forme. Publication was again noted in the *Term Catalogue* at a price now reduced to 1s 6d:

Trinity 1678 June 22nd, III numb 16, I 322/3, column 2/1, *Books reprinted. Affectionum quæ dicuntur Hystericæ et Hypochondriacæ Pathologia Spasmodica vindicata, contra refponfionem Epistolarem* Nath. Highmori *M. D.* Cui accesserunt Exercitationes Medico-Physicæ duæ. 1. *De sanguinis accenssione.* 2. *De Motu musculari.* Studio T. Willis, ex æde *Chriſti Oxon*, M.D. Editio Tertia, ab authore recognita, atque ab eodem multiplici auctuario locupletata. In Twelves. Price, bound, 1s 6d. Printed for J. Martyn at the Bell in S. *Paul's* Churchyard.

Affectionum quæ dicuntur hystericæ et hypochondriacæ is included in the Latin collected editions of Willis's works (**8A–8I**), but not in either *The remaining medical works* (1681: **9B**) or *Dr Willis's practice of physick* (1694: **9E**, **9F**). It is the only treatise of Thomas Willis that remains to be translated into English.

4A. AFFECTIONUM QUÆ DICUNTUR HYSTERICÆ ET HYPOCHONDRIACÆ, London quarto 1670

The first edition of Willis's fourth book [HJR Wing 22].

Title page: AFFECTIONUM | Quæ dicuntur | *HYSTERICÆ* & *HYPOCHONDRIACÆ* | Pathologia Spaſmodica vindicata, | Contra | RESPONSIONEM EPISTOLAREM |

[5] See chapter 7 for details.

NATHANAEL. HIGHMORI, M. D. | Cui acceſſerunt | Exercitationes Medico-Phyſicæ Duæ. | 1. *De Sanguinis Accenſione.* | 2. *De Motu Muſculari.* | [rule] | Studio | *THO. WILLIS* M. D. Natur. Philoſo- | phiæ Profeſſoris. *Oxon.* necnon Inclyti Me- | dic. Coll. *Londin.* & Societat. Reg. Socii. | [rule] | [ornament] | [double rule] | *LONDINI,* | Apud *Jacobum Alleſtry*, Societatatis Regiæ Typographum, | in Cœmeterio *D. Pauli.* M DC LXX.

Collation: quarto; 23 letter alphabet using I: [A]^4, B–P^4; \$1–2 signed.

60 leaves: paginated as [8], 1–112 each enclosed in (). Mispaginated: 69 for 71.

Type: 35 lines; height (20 lines) 92 millimetres, width 97 millimetres.

Contents: **A1r**, page [1], blank; **A1v**, page [2], portrait; **A2r**, page [3], title; **A2v**, page [4], blank; **A3r–A4r**, pages [5–7], AMICO LECTORI PRÆFATIO.; **A4v**, page [8], blank.

B1r–G3r, pages 1–45 [Text] AD Virum Doctiſsimum *NATHANAEL. HIGHMORUM*, M. D.; **G3v**, page 46, blank; **G4r–K3r**, pages 47–69, [Text] DE SANGUINIS INCALESCENTIA SIVE ACCENSIONE Exercitatio Medico-phyſica.; **K3v**, page 70, blank; **K4r–P2r**, page ['69']–107, [Text] DE MOTU MUSCULARI Exercitatio Medico-phyſica.

P2v–P3r, pages 108–9, *Elenchus Materiæ.* De Affectibus Hyſtericis, & Hypochondriacis.; **P3r–P3v**, pages 109–10, Elenchus Materiæ Excertationis de Accenſione Sanguinis.; **P3v–P4v**, pages 110–12, Elenchus Materiæ Excertationis de Motu Muſculari.; **P4v**, page 112, Errata, 3 lines listing 4 errors. Rogandus eſt lector ut cætera corrigat.

Headlines and *Catchwords*: preliminaries, correct; no headlines included in the main text.

ubiq; for ubique at **B2r / v**, pages 3 / 4; Quod for Quòd at **F4v / G1r**, pages 40 / 41; ſiùs for ſius at **I2r / v**, pages 59 / 60; perma for Perma at **O3r** / v, pages 101 / 102.

Frontispiece: none.

Portrait: **Pt.1a1.** *D: Loggan: delin: et ſculp: ÆTATIS SUÆ, 45.* 193 × 143 millimetres (sheet); 187 × 139 millimetres (plate, cropped); 184 × 138 millimetres (image, cropped).

Printers' ornaments: row of 3 fleurons {**Roycroft 14**} on title page at **A2r**, page [3]: headpiece at **A3r**, page [5] {**Allestry 2**}; row of 16 fleurons at **B1r**, page (1); **G4r**, page (47); **K4r**, page '(69)' i.e. (71) {**Allestry 3**}.

No decorated initials.

Illustrations: **Pl.17a1.** Plate 17 (images 26–27): *Fig. I.* (headline, centre, upper), *Fig. II.* (headline, centre, lower); lettering to depict structures A–E. Folding, 168 × 336 millimetres (sheet); 127 × 171 millimetres (plate marks); 28 × 143 millimetres, 50 × 158 millimetres (figures). Legend: FIGURA I. Exhibet muſculum simplicem regulatem, juxta Φάσιν naturalem, deſcriptum, in cujus ventre, fibræ carneæ apertæ ab invicem deducuntur, ut fibrillæ membranaceæ meliùs conſpiciantur. FIGURA II. Exhibet muſculum ſimplicem, poſt Tendinem diſciſſum, eiúſq; portiones divulſas, in medio fiſſum, ut interior fibrarum

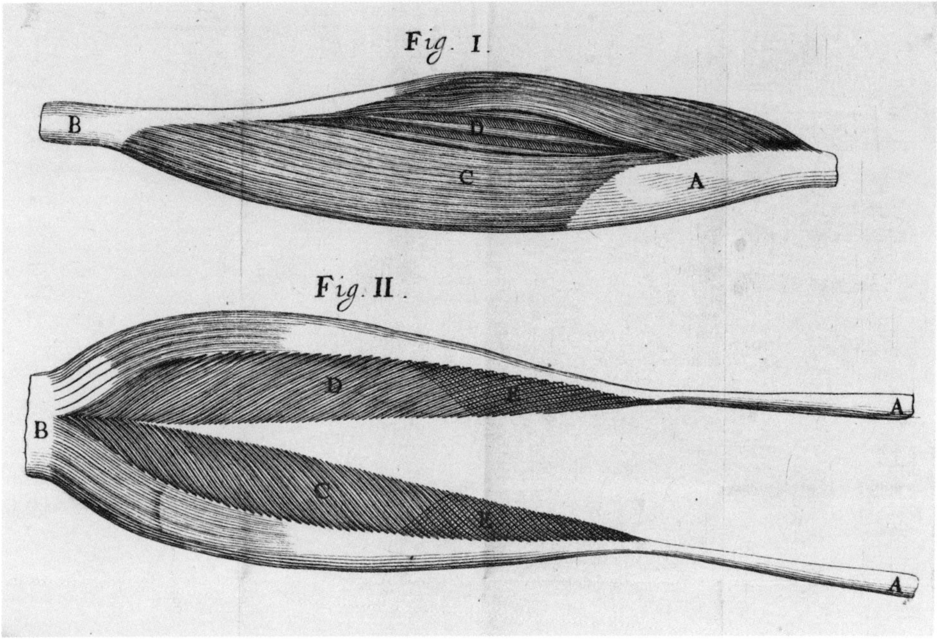

Figure 120 Plate 17 (images 26–27). The Firſt Figure *SHews a simple regular muſcle, deſcribed according to its natural appearance, in the Belly of which the Fleſhy fibres being opened, are diduced one from another, that the membranaceous Fibrils may be the better beheld.*; The Second Figure *Shews a simple Muſcle cleft in the middle, after the Tendon being cut off, and portions of it pulled away, that the interiour ſeries of the fleſſhy Fibres, or their commixtures or mingling with the Tendons, may appear*. Image from *De motu musculari* 1670; legend from *The remaining medical works* 1681.

carnearum ſeries, earumq; cum Tendinibus commiſſuræ appareant. Inserted after errata at **P4v**, page 112 (see: Figure 120).

Pl.18a1. Plate 18 (images 28–29): *Fig. III.* (headline, centre, upper), *Fig. IV.* (headline, centre, lower); lettering to depict structures A–G. Folding, 168 × 336 millimetres (sheet); 129 × 172 millimetres (plate marks); 30 × 155 millimetres, 42 × 164 millimetres (figures). Legend: FIGURA III. Exhibet muſculum quendam minùs compoſitum, cujus binis ventribus carneis, etiam bini Tendines compoſiti, (quatuor ſimplicibus æquales) deſtinantur. FIGURA IV. Exhibet muſculum regularem compoſitum in medio diviſum, & apertum, ità ut utriuſq; ventris facies interior appareat. Inserted after errata at **P4v**, page 112 (see: Figure 121).

Copy: Wellcome (EPB/B/63465). Modern full morocco, spine and corners black, boards maroon, spine lettered (vertical) WILLIS. T.—AFFECTIONES HYSTERICÆ 1670, new endpapers. Leaves 193 × 143 millimetres, boards 197 × 146 × 13 millimetres. Bookplate: The Library of the Wellcome Institute for the History of Medicine MEDICAL SOCIETY OF LONDON DEPOSIT Accession Number Press Mark WILLIS T. Inscribed: (1) XVI_3 (twice); (2) 63465 / B. Stamped: (1) Medical Society of London; (2) BRITISH MUSEUM SALE DUPLICATE 1787.

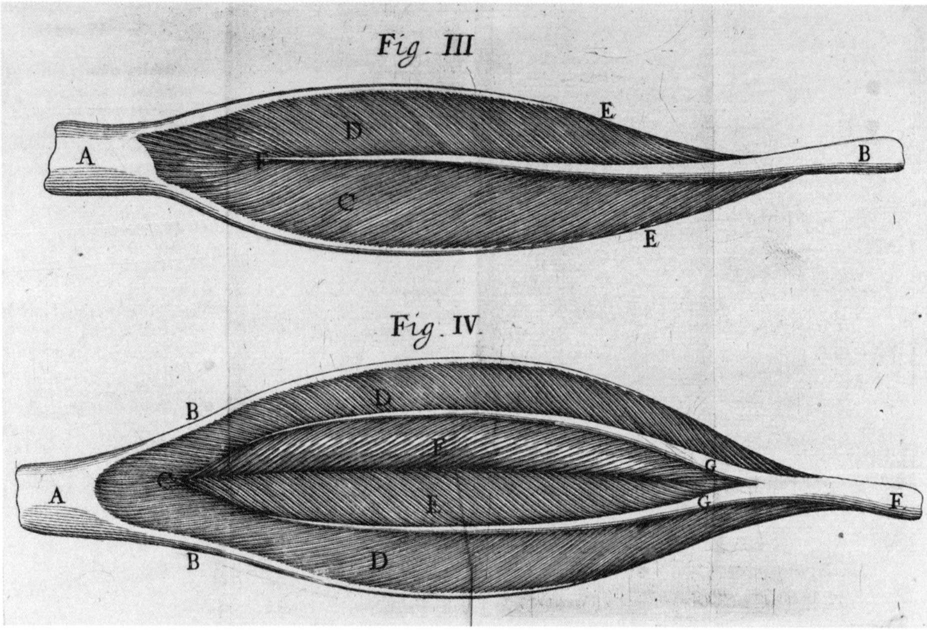

Figure 121 Plate 18 (images 28–29). The Third Figure *Exhibits a certain Mufcle lefs compounded, to whofe two flefhy Bellies two compounded Tendons alfo (equal to four fimple ones) are deftinated.*; The Fourth Figure *Shews a regular compounded Mufcle, divided and opened in the middle, fo that the interiour face of either Belly may appear.* Image from *De motu musculari* 1670; legend from *The remaining medical works* 1681.

4B1. AFFECTIONUM QUÆ DICUNTUR HYSTERICÆ ET HYPOCHONDRIACÆ, Leyden duodecimo 1671

The first issue of the second edition of Willis's fourth book, listing the bookseller Cornelius Driehuysen before Felix Lopez [HJR Wing 23].

Title page: AFFECTIONUM | Quæ dicuntur | HYSTERICÆ | *ET* | HYPOCHONDRIACÆ | Pathologia Spafmodica vindicata, | Contra | *Refponfionem Epiftolarem* | NATHANAEL. HIGHMORI, M. D. | *Cui accefferunt* | Exercitationes Medico- | Phyficæ Duæ. | 1. *De Sanguinis Accenfione.* | 2. *De Motu Mufculari.* | Studio *THO. WILLIS* M. D. Na- | tur. Philofophiæ Profeffor. *Oxon.* nec | non Inclyti Medic. Coll. *Londin.* & | Societat. Reg. Socii. | [ornament] | *LUGD. BATAV.* | *Apud* {CORNEL. DRIEHUYSEN, | {FELICEM LOPEZ, | {CIƆ IƆ C LXXI.

Collation: duodecimo; 23 letter roman alphabet: A–G^{12}, H^{6}; $1–6 signed apart from: -B5, D3 signed D4, +D7, +F7, +G7.

90 leaves; paginated as [6], 1–172, [2].

Type: 30 lines; height (20 lines) 68 millimetres, width 49 millimetres.

Contents: **A1r**, page [1], title; **A1v**, page [2], blank; **A2r–A3v**, pages [3–6], AMICO LECTORI *PRÆFATIO.*

A4r–D1v, pages 1–68, [Text] AD Virum Doctiffimum NATHANAEL. HIGHMORUM, M. D.; **D2r–E7r**, pages 69–103, [Text] DE Sanguinis Incalefcentia *SIVE* ACCENSIONE *Exercitatio Medico-phyfica.*; **E7v–G12v**, pages 104–62, [Text] DE MOTU MUSCULARI *Exercitatio Medico-phyfica.*

H1r–H2r, pages 163–5, *Elenchus Materiæ.* De Affectibus Hyftericis, & Hypochondriacis.; **H2v–H3v**, pages 166–8, *Elenchus Materiæ* Excertationis de Accenfione Sanguinis; **H4r–H5v**, pages 169–72, *Elenchus Materiæ* Excertationis de Motu Mufculari.; **H6r–v**, pages [1–2], blank.

Headlines and *Catchwords*: page numbers contained as () apart from [] at **B5r**, page 27; **B11r**, page 39; **B12v**, page 42; **C11r–C12v**, pages 63–6; **D2v–D6r**, pages 70–7; **D10r–D11r**, pages 85–7; **E4v–E5v**, pages 98–100; **F12r–G2v**, page 137–42; **G6v–G9r**, pages 150–5; (109) | for (109) at **E10r**, page 109.

ptoma- for tomate at **A8v** / **A9r**, pages 10 / 11; rum for um at **D5r** / **v**, pages 75 / 76.

Frontispiece: none.

Portrait: none.

Printers' ornament: headpiece at **A1r**, page [1] {**Driehuysen 1**}.

Decorated R at **A4r**, page 1{**Driehuysen 2**}; I at **D2r**, page 69 {**Driehuysen 3**}.

Illustrations: lettering and legends as in **4A**:

Pl.17b1. Plate 17 (images 26–27): *Fig. I.* (headline, centre, upper), *Fig. II.* (headline, centre, lower). Folding, 134 × 177 millimetres (sheet); 113 × 165 millimetres (plate marks); 28 × 138 millimetres, 44 × 157 millimetres (figures). Inserted before legends for Figuræ I and II at **G11r–v**, pages 159–60.

Pl.18b1. Plate 18 (images 28–29): *Fig. III.* (headline, centre, upper), *Fig. IV.* (headline, centre, lower). Folding, 134 × 177 millimetres (sheet); 113 × 165 millimetres (plate marks); 30 × 151 millimetres, 42 × 160 millimetres (figures). Inserted within legends for Figuræ III and IV at **G11v–G12v**, pages 160–2.

Copy: DASC, lacking H6 (blank). Recent full calf with blind double lines and fleurons at corners, spine with four raised bands, labelled WILLIS | HYSTER, new endpapers. Leaves 127 × 73 millimetres, boards 132 × 75 × 15 millimetres. Bookplate of Jan van Gijn.[6]

[6] See acknowledgements for details.

4B2. AFFECTIONUM QUÆ DICUNTUR HYSTERICÆ ET HYPOCHONDRIACÆ, Leyden duodecimo 1671

The second issue of the second edition of Willis's fourth book, listing the bookseller Felix Lopez before Cornelius Driehuysen [HJR Wing 24].

Title page: AFFECTIONUM | Quæ dicuntur | HYSTERICÆ | *ET* | HYPOCHONDRIACÆ | Pathologia Spaſmodica vindicata, | Contra | *Reſponſionem Epiſtolarem* | NATHANAEL. HIGHMORI, M. D. | *Cui acceſſerunt* | Exercitationes Medico- | Phyſicæ Duæ. | 1. *De Sanguinis Accenſione.* | 2. *De Motu Muſculari.* | Studio *THO. WILLIS* M. D. Na- | tur. Philoſophiæ Profeſſor. *Oxon.* nec | non Inclyti Medic. Coll. *Londin.* & | Societat. Reg. Socii. | [ornament] | *LUGD. BATAV.* | *Apud* {FELICEM LOPEZ, | {CORNELIUM DRIEHUYSEN, | {CIↃ IↃ C LXXI.

Then as in **4B1**.[7]

Copy: DASC (#1 of 2). Original full calf, spine with five raised bands and gilt decorated panels, label WILLI | MEDI, original endpapers. Leaves 130 × 70 millimetres, boards 138 × 78 × 18 millimetres. Shelf marks: N42 and 16.806.

4C. AFFECTIONUM QUÆ DICUNTUR HYSTERICÆ ET HYPOCHONDRIACÆ, London duodecimo 1678

The third edition of Willis's fourth book, reusing the two plates from the London quarto edition (1670) [HJR Wing 25].

Title page: AFFECTIONUM | Quæ dicuntur | HYSTERICÆ | ET | HYPOCHONDRIACÆ | Pathologia Spaſmodica vindicata, | Contra | Reſponſionem Epiſtolarem | NATHANAEL HIGHMORI. M D | Cui acceſſerunt | Exercitationes Medico- | Phyſicæ Duæ, | 1. *De ſanguinis Accenſione.* | 2. *De Motu Muſculari.* | [rule] | STUDIO | THOMÆ WILLIS, *ex Æde Chriſti* OXON. | M. D. & in iſta celeberrima Academia Natu- | ralis Philoſophiæ Profeſſoris *Sidleiani.* | [rule] | Editio Tertia, | Ab AUTHORE recognita, atque ab eodem | multiplici Auctario locupletata. | [rule] | *LONDINI,* | Typis *S. Roycroft*, Impenſis *J. Martyn*, ad Inſig- | ne Campanæ Cœmeterio D. *Pauli*, MDCLXXVIII.

Collation: duodecimo; 23 letter roman alphabet: A–E^{12}; \$1–5 signed apart from A4 signed B4.

60 leaves; paginated as [6], 1–105, [9]. All page numbers within ().

Type: 42 lines; height (20 lines) 58 millimetres, width 52 millimetres.

Contents: **A1r**, page [1], title; **A1v**, page [2], blank; **A2r**–**A3r**, pages [3–5], AMICO LECTORI *PRÆFATIO.*; **A3v**, page [6], blank.

[7] Unlike **4B1**, the catchword is ugi- for fugi- at C9r / v, pages 59 / 60. Whilst this can be explained by failure of 'f' to imprint, there is no impression on the paper. Although this may be a second state for C9, it does not resolve the decision to order **4B1** ahead of **4B2**.

A[B]4r–C1v, pages 1–44, AD Virum Doctiffimum NATHANAEL HIGHMORIUM, M.D. [text] Affectionum quæ dicuntur hyftericæ & hypochondriacæ; **C2r–D1r**, pages 45–67, [text] DE Sanguinis Incalefcentia *SIVE* ACCENSIONE, *Exercitatio Medico-phyfica.*; **D1v–E8r**, pages 68–105, [text] DE MOTU MUSCULARI *Exercitatio Medico-phyfica.*

E8v–E9v, pages [1–3], *Elenchus Materiæ.* De Affectibus Hyftericis & Hypochondriacis.; **E9v–E10v**, pages [3–5], *Elenchus Materiæ.* Exercitationis de Accenfione Sanguinis.; **E10v–E12r**, pages [5–8], *Elenchus Materiæ.* Exercitationis de Motu Mufculari.; **E12v**, page [9], blank.

Headlines and *Catchwords*: no headlines.

quam for ficubi at **A7v / A8r**, pages 8 / 9; tius for tiùs at **B3r / B3v**, pages 23 / 24; no catchword at **C1v / C2r**, pages 44 / 45; **D1r / D1v**, pages 67 / 68.; cupavreit for cupaverit at **C11v / C12r**, pages 64 / 65; dinosas for tendinosis at **D11v / D12r**, pages 88 / 89.

Frontispiece: none.

Portrait: none.

Printers' ornament: headpiece at **A2r**, page [3] {**Roycroft 21**}.

Decorated R at **A[B]4r**, page 1 {**Roycroft 41**}; I at **C2r**, page 45 {**Roycroft 24**}.

Illustrations: as in **4A** apart from:

Pl.17a1. Plate 17 (images 26–27): Folding, 128 × 183 millimetres (sheet). Inserted within legends for Figuræ I–IV at **E6v–E8r**, pages 102–5.

Pl.18a1. Plate 18 (images 28–29): Folding, 128 × 188 millimetres (sheet). Inserted within legends for Figuræ I–IV at **E6v–E8r**, pages 102–5.

Copy: Cambridge University Library (Keynes.U.8.31). Original full calf with blind central double-lined panel and fleurons at each corner, boards with gilt edges, spine with four raised bands, no lettering, original endpapers. Leaves 147 × 84 millimetres, boards 152 × 87 × 15 millimetres. Inscribed: (1) Geoffrey Keynes; (2) Ex libris Sam. De la Rose (unidentified); (3) Robert Kelsatt / Kelsall. kk. (unidentified); (4) 'Bok. 050' (cropped, possibly a bookseller's code for price 5s).[8]

[8] Sir Geoffrey Keynes (1887–1982) was a physician and surgeon who made important contributions to blood transfusion, and the management of breast cancer and myasthenia gravis. He was also a scholar of English literature and medical history. During a long career, Keynes published around fifty books including bibliographies of Thomas Browne (1924), William Harvey (1928), Robert Hooke (1960), Timothy Bright (1962), and William Petty (1971). His autobiography, *The gates of memory*, Oxford (1981), describing the many prominent friends and relatives with whom he interacted during the twentieth century was published when he was aged 94. Keynes's working papers and many items from his large collection of books are in the Cambridge University Library. See chapter 17 for discussion of Geoffrey Keynes on the history of myasthenia gravis.

9

'To understand all things but itself'

De anima brutorum (1672–1674)

Willis's fifth book, *De anima brutorum*, containing the two parts of his eleventh treatise, and the third to include illustrations, appeared in quarto, octavo, and duodecimo editions published in Oxford, London, and Amsterdam between 1672 and 1674. It is already the subject of an excellent but unpublished bibliography by Philip Oldfield.[1]

The Oxford and London quarto edition

The quarto edition was printed for the University press and sold in Oxford by Richard Davis (1646–1688). Distribution in London was entrusted to the press's principal agents, William Wells (fl.1641–73) and Robert Scott (fl.1661–1691).[2] There are differences between the Oxford and London issues apart from changes to the title page. Some copies from Oxford are on large paper, and many of these have variant settings compared to those on ordinary paper and the London issue. The advertisement for books sold by Richard Davis was mainly pertinent to Oxford and eventually discarded, although sometimes found as part of the London issue. The imprimatur leaf, of most significance for Oxford, was used for another purpose in the London issue. Even though the overall design and appearance are attractive, accuracy of the typesetting was far from satisfactory. Errors of signature, pagination, headings, and catchwords are present throughout. Many went unnoticed or were left unchanged. Others were corrected and some new ones introduced on variant states of individual leaves.[3] The main problem relates to the final signature. The various inconsistencies were largely resolved for the three issues of the octavo and single duodecimo editions.

De anima brutorum was one of eight titles planned by John Fell (1625–1686) when he set up the reorganized University press in November 1671. The imprimatur was received from the vice-chancellor, Peter Mews (1619–1706), on 12 December 1671. Oldfield explains that Thomas Yate (fl.1660–1681), principal of Brasenose College and a member of Fell's four man partnership, informed Leoline Jenkins (1625–1685) on 2 January 1672 that the printing would soon be completed. However the problem that arose with the index (see next) held up publication to the third week of April.[4] On 24 April, Henry Oldenburg (1619–1677) reported

[1] See: Philip M Oldfield, *A bibliography of Thomas Willis's De anima brutorum*, unpublished typescript (1991): pages 1–50.

[2] HJR Wing considers the London quarto issue to be much the rarer and he was only able to describe a single copy, unseen, from the library of Sir Geoffrey Keynes (1887–1982). Philip Oldfield (1991) located copies in the libraries of the Universities of Cambridge, Edinburgh, and British Columbia. Several copies have been offered for sale in recent years.

[3] At least six states of the quarto edition can be identified, and others must exist.

[4] See: Oldfield (1991): page 3, footnote 3, citing All Souls MS.239, folio 641; and Falconer Madan, 'The Oxford Press, 1650–1675: the Struggle for a Place in the Sun', *The Library*, 4th series, volume 6 (1925): page. 138.

to the Royal Society that Willis's book was published. The author gave a copy to the Society on 1 May and it was reviewed in *Philosophical Transactions* on 30 May.[5] A presentation copy from Willis to John Wilkins (1614–1672), bishop of Chester, is dated 26 April 1672.[6] The first announcements of publication appeared in the *Term Catalogue* for 13 May 1672 and the *London Gazette*, number 677, on Thursday 16 May 1672. Neither indicated that the price of a bound small paper copy was 10 shillings.[7]

Easter 1672 May 13th, II Numb. 9, I 105, column 1/2, *Libri Latini.*

De Anima Brutorum quæ Hominis Vitalis ac Sensitiva est, Exercitationes Duæ. Prior *Physiologica, ejusdem Naturam, Partes, Potentias et Affectiones, tradit.* Altera *Pathologica Morbos qui ipsam, et sedem ejus primariam, nempe cerebrum et nervosum genus afficiunt, explicat, eorumque Therapeias instituit.* Studio Thomæ Willis, M.D. Philosophiæ Natural. Profess. *Sidleian Oxon*, necon incliti med. Coll. *Lond.*, et Societ. Reg. Socii. Printed for Richard Davis in *Oxford.* In Quarto.

The problem of the final signature

De anima brutorum is notorious for the difficulty in resolving what happened with the final sheet, Zzz^4. Different interpretations have been offered. The most parsimonious is the analysis of HJR Wing supplemented by that of Philip Oldfield, although a few further points can be made.[8] Three complications arose, the first of which was resolved before any sheets were distributed.

Zzz1r–v, pages 561–2, are followed by the final printing of the text at Zzz2r which is (appropriately) unsigned but wrongly paginated '565'. There follows a catalogue of books to be sold by Richard Davis, ordered by folio, quarto, octavo, and duodecimo, starting at Zzz2v and ending at Zzz4v to complete that quarto sheet. Two changes were then made, but probably not at the same time.

First, the printer realized that he had omitted the index. His solution was to add one full and one half sheet, collating as Zzz Aaaa^4, pages [1–8], and Bbbb^2, pages [9–12]. He reprinted the final page of text as a cancellans at Zzz Aaaa1r leaving the erroneous pagination as '565'. This gave him space to print the index as eleven (unnumbered) pages from

[5] See: *Philosophical Transactions of the Royal Society*, volume 7 (1672): pages 4071–3; and chapter 17 for details.

[6] Let us hope that he had time to read it before his death on 19 November 1672. Oldfield (1991): page 8, footnote 2, notes that the copy was subsequently owned by Robert Hooke (1635–1703) and is now in the Wellcome Library. It is inscribed on the title page: 'Given me by ye Reuerend Dr John Tillotson Dean of Canterbury for a remembrance of John L^d B^p of Chester. R Hooke Oct 8 1673'.

[7] See: Oldfield (1991): page 8, footnote 4, who points out that the price is given in Robert Clavell's *A catalogue of all the books printed in England since the dreadful fire of London, in 1666. to the end of Michaelmas Term, 1672*, London (1673): page 29.

[8] See: HJR Wing, *A bibliography of Dr. Thomas Willis (1621–1675)* (1962): pages 28–9. Wing has as his starting point the analysis made by Falconer Madan, *Oxford Books* volume III (1651–1680), Oxford (1931): pages 273–4: 'All went well to the end of p.562 (=Zzzl) with the catchword "morbi-". Then was printed the second leaf of Zzz with (on the recto) the remaining part of the text with "Finis" and (on the verso) "Errata". But the publisher had forgotten the Index, which took eleven pages and was bound to precede the Errata: and he also wanted to add his own Catalogue of published books (five pages). So the printer (1) tore off Zzz2, (2) printed a new Zzz2 bearing on the recto the end of the text as before, and on the verso, the first page of the Index, paging the new leaf on the recto 565 (for 563), with sign. "Zzzz Aaaa", (3) the rest of the index—which has no paging or signatures'. Most would agree with Wing's conclusion: 'this is Madan's view on the complicated structure at the end of this book but I think he is mistaken'.

Zzz Aaaa1v–Bbbb2v. The cancellans appears in two states: one is signed Zzz Aaaa and the other (incorrectly) Zzzz Aaaa.[9] Both are found in the five copies examined for this bibliography: Zzz Aaaa (**5A3**, Oxford; and **5A5**, London) and Zzzz Aaaa (**5A1**, **5A2**, Oxford; and **5A4**, London). This indicates that the Oxford and London issues used the same batch of randomly allocated printed sheets.

Having made good his omission of the index, the printer was then faced with the dilemma of what to do with the original page 565 on Zzz2r, now a cancellandum, and the advertisements for Richard Davis's books printed on Zzz2v–Zzz4v. In the event the decision was taken to retain these leaves but cross through page '565' in pen and ink to indicate that this was cancelled. The binder was advised to place Zzz2–Zzz4 with Davis's advertisements after the newly printed sheets, Zzz(z) Aaaa^4 and Bbbb^2, so that the index followed the main text now ending on the cancellans Zzz Aaaa1r, page '565'. Collation of the earliest issue therefore ends: ... Zzz1v, page 562; Zzz Aaaa1r, page '565' (i.e. 563), cancellans; Zzz Aaaa1v–Bbbb2v, pages [11], Index alphabeticus; Zzz2r, page '565' (i.e. 563), cancellandum (scored through in pen and ink); Zzz2v–4v, catalogue of Richard Davis's books.

The problem of the errata

The second problem requiring adjustment after the first sheets had been printed and distributed, but probably before any reached London, was the recognition of various errors (and failure to notice many others).[10] Therefore an errata sheet was printed. HJR Wing and Oldfield consider Falconer Madan (1851–1935) to be mistaken in suggesting that Zzz2v was used and the leaf simply reversed and inserted after the index. Madan seems wrong for three reasons: no such copy has been seen; Zzz2 never appears without the rest of that sheet; and the first page of Richard Davis's catalogue is invariably printed on Zzz2v. Rather, the printer typeset a separate errata slip on spare paper and pasted it over the cancellandum, Zzz Aaaa1r, page '565'. HJR Wing finds that interpretation consistent with the different watermarks found in some copies.[11] Not unreasonably, Oldfield, who also notes this arrangement, describes the errata slip as Cccc1r; and he considers Cccc1v, invisible when pasted in, to be blank.[12]

A different solution was used for copies of the London issue which did not involve pasting Cccc1r over the cancelled Zzz2r, or binding this as an extra leaf. In resetting the preliminaries naming the London booksellers, the imprimatur, printed at π1 (r or v: with the corresponding face blank), was no longer needed and this was used for the errata leaf. Copies of the London quarto appear with the errata (now printed on π1r and separated from its conjugate leaf π2) either placed within the preliminaries after A4, or following the catalogue of books to be sold by Richard Davis in Oxford, still not discarded, after Bbbb2v.

[9] This was noted by Oldfield (1991) but only in copies of the ordinary issues from Oxford.

[10] See: chapter 3 for speculation that the consignment of sheets for two books sent in 1671 to Robert Scott by John Fell in the 'Flying coach' included those for *De anima brutorum*.

[11] That the errata appeared after the dilemma of the index had been resolved is indicated by its absence from any of the three Oxford copies examined for this bibliography, even though it may be present in copies that were bound and sold in Oxford after the initial batch of sheets had been distributed.

[12] Where it is present, the errata leaf in copies of the Oxford imprint is unsigned, whether or not it is pasted onto the cancelled Zzz2r or bound as a separate leaf. Oldfield (1991) found the errata leaf in fourteen of twenty-eight copies examined, in eight of which it was pasted over the cancelled Zzz2v. Of the remainder, Zzz2v is marked in pen and ink for cancellation in seven (of fourteen).

The problem of the variant settings

Pagination of the quarto edition of *De anima brutorum* is chaotic.[13] The interval of sixteen numbered pages from 16 to 33 corresponds to one complete quarto sheet but the signatures, catchwords, and text are continuous from B4v, page 16, to C1r, page 33, and nothing is missing. Presumably this error of pagination reflects the work of different compositors whose estimates of the number of pages needed to accommodate their allocation of the text proved inaccurate. With one exception, this interval and the many other individual pagination errors were never corrected.[14] However, other settings were altered and Philip Oldfield has carried out page-by-page comparison of twenty-eight copies, with diligence that is beyond the scope of this bibliography. His guidance has been used to check variations in the five copies that have been considered. Following Oldfield, all large paper copies but only a few of those on ordinary paper have Gilbert Sheldon's (1598–1677) coat of arms on the dedicatory epistle at A1r, page [5].[15] This is an engraving, not a relief, and was printed by putting the sheet twice through the press (see: Figure 122). The setting of descriptive titles for the two dedicatory epistles varies:

> *REVERENDISSIMO* | In Chrifto Patri & Domino Domino | GILBERTO | Providentia Divina Archiepifcopo *Cantua-* | *rienfi*, totius *Angliæ* Primati & Metropolitano, & Au- | guftiffimo Principi CAROLO II. M. *Britanniæ*, | *Franciæ* & *Hiberniæ* Regi à Secretioribus Confiliis. (Oldfield A)

This is usually linked to variant setting of the second epistle:

> ERUDITISSIMIS | *ET* | VENERABILIBUS VIRIS | Mihique æternum colendis | D. VICE-CANCELLARIO | DOCTORIBUS & MAGISTRIS | Qui in Celeberrimâ Univerfitate Oxonienfi | BONAS LITERAS | Diligentifsime Excolunt, | Egregie Ornant, | Feliciffime Promovent. | *Salutem.* (Oldfield A).

The other settings usually found together are:

> REVERENDISSIMO | In Chrifto Patri & Domino | Domino | GILBERTO | Providentia Divina Archiepifcopo *Can* | *tuarienfi*, totius *Angliæ* Primati & | Metropolitano, & Auguftiffimo Prin- | cipi CAROLO II. M. *Britanniæ Fran-* | *ciæ* & *Hiberniæ* Regi, à Secretiori- | bus Confiliis. (Oldfield B)

> ERUDITISSIMIS | *ET* | VENERABILIBUS VIRIS | Mihique aeternum colendis | D.VICE-CANCELLARIO | DOCTORIBUS ET MAGISTRIS | Qui in Celeberrimâ Univerfitate Oxonienfi | BONASLITERAS | *DILIGENTISSIME EXCOLUNT* | Egregie ornant | FELICISSIME PROMOVENT. | *Salutem.* (Oldfield B).

[13] The pages are made up as: [56] preliminaries; 547 text (as 16, 33–562, '565' cancellans); [17] catalogue, '565' cancellandum, index = 310 leaves. Copies with the errata sheet as a bound in leaf rather than pasted over the cancellandum have 311 leaves.

[14] Oldfield (1991) points out that the mispagination 358 for 360 is corrected in two of 28 copies examined. Of the five considered for this bibliography, only **5A5** is correct.

[15] For reasons that are not given, HJR Wing (1962): page 28 considers that the sheet on which the dedication appears without the coat-of-arms is probably the earlier.

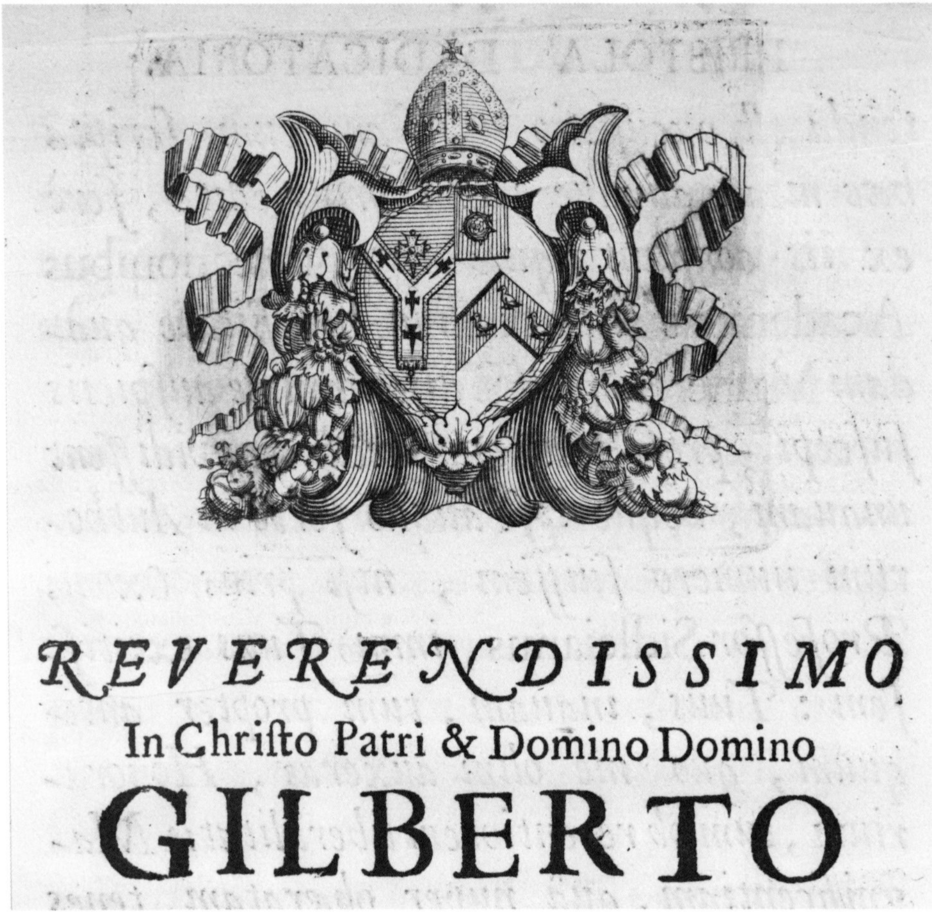

Figure 122 Gilbert Sheldon's coat of arms: *De anima brutorum* 1672 (Fell 1).

Oldfield also draws attention to the two settings of PARS SECUNDA at Hh2r, page 259, with one measuring 82 millimetres and the second (less common) 77 millimetres. He lists a large number of variant states in the headlines and links these either to the outer or inner forme. Oldfield notes:

> With the exception of sheet K, variations in running titles occur on one side of the forme only in any given gathering. Of thirteen copies that show variations in K, six have them in the outer forme only, the remaining seven in both inner and outer formes. 'B' variants occur almost exclusively in copies of the ordinary trade issue. Only two large paper copies had any of the 'B' variants, both in the outer forme of gathering K. Variations in gatherings K, Ii, and Ss are quite common, in Mm less so, and quite scarce in Cc and Gg.

Clearly the different compositors to whom formes were assigned varied in their attention to detail. Of the five copies of the Oxford or London issues examined for this bibliography, apart from the narrower PARS SECUNDA at page 259 and the change at Gg2v, page 252, CAP. XVI *vs* CAP. XVI, each of these alternate settings is present. But there is uneven distribution of 'A' or 'B' within the same copy and no two are identical. It follows that these changes were made whilst proofreading the first side of the printed sheet, which might have been the outer or inner forme, so that errors present on the reverse side were retained when that sheet was perfected. Binders and booksellers received a random allocation of sheets resulting in an almost infinite number of possible page-by-page comparisons, although variants 'A' are more usually seen than 'B'. Oldfield having drawn attention to these variations, one further point can be made. Of the five copies examined for this bibliography, two (Oxford, 5A2; London 5A5) have *U* (swash) for *V* in *Visu* at Cc3v, page 222 and Cc4r, page '233'; and all five have *U* (swash) for *V* at Bb3v, page 214; Bb4r, page 215; Bb4v, page 216; Dd1r, page 225; and Dd1v, page 226.[16] The descriptions of individual copies that follows assign either 'A' or 'B' affecting individual leaves within the nine relevant signatures (one each for the outer and inner formes of signature K), as follows:

K signature
- Page 89: (A) CAP. V. present; '&' of '& Habitus' above space between 'interim' and 'à' in line 1 at K1r, *versus* (B) CAP. V. absent; '&' of '& Habitus' above 'im' of 'interim'
- Page 90: (A) CAP. V. present; 'A' of 'Animæ' above 'qu' of 'Vnicuique' in line 1 at K1v, *versus* (B) CAP. V. absent; 'A' of 'Animæ' above 'a' of 'animali'
- Page 91: (A) CAP. V. present at K2r, *versus* (B) CAP. V. absent
- Page 92: (A) CAP. V. present; 'A' of 'Animæ' above 'a' of 'animalibus' in line 1 at K2v, *versus* (B) CAP. V. absent; 'A' of 'Animæ' above 'm' of 'animalibus'
- Page 94: (A) CAP. V. at K3v, *versus* (B) CAP. IV
- Page 96: (A) CAP. V. at K4v, *versus* (B) CAP. VI

Bb signature
- Page 214: (A) *U* (swash) for *V* in *Visu* at Bb3v, *versus* (B) *V* in *Visu*
- Page 215: (A) *U* (swash) for *V* in *Visu* at Bb4r, *versus* (B) *V* in *Visu*
- Page 216: (A) *U* (swash) for *V* in *Visu* at Bb4v, *versus* (B) *V* in *Visu*

Cc signature
- Page 218: (A) italic *V* in *Viſu* at Cc1v, *versus* (B) roman V in V*iſu*
- Page 219: (A) italic *V* in *Viſu* at Cc2r, *versus* (B) roman V in V*iſu*
- Page 222: (A) non-swash *V* in *Viſu* at Cc3v, *versus* (B) *U* (swash) in *Viſu*
- Page '233' (223): (A) non-swash *V* in *Viſu* at Cc4r, *versus* (B) *U* (swash) in *Viſu*

Dd signature
- Page 225: (A) *U* (swash) for *V* in *Visu* at Dd1r, *versus* (B) *V* in *Visu*
- Page 226: (A) *U* (swash) for *V* in *Visu* at Dd1v, *versus* (B) *V* in *Visu*

Gg signature
- Page 252: (A) CAP. XVI at Gg2v, *versus* (B) CAP. XVI.

Ii signature
- Page 272: (A) italic *C* in *Cephalalgia* at Ii4v, versus (B) roman C in C*ephalalgia*

Mm signature
- Page 290: (A) italic *C* in *Cephalalgiæ* and *Curatio* at Mm1v, *versus* (B) roman C in C*ephalalgiæ* and C*uratio*
- Page 291: (A) italic *C* in *Curatio* at Mm2r, versus (B) roman C in C*uratio*
- Page 294: (A) italic *C* in *Cephalalgiæ* and *Curatio* at Mm3v, versus (B) roman C in C*ephalalgiæ* and C*uratio*
- Page 295: (A) italic *C* in *Cephalalgiæ* at Mm4r, *versus* (B) roman C in C*ephalalgiæ*

[16] Since those newly listed for signatures Bb and Dd affect the recto and verso of individual leaves, these must involve the outer and inner formes. However, no examples of the B variant are present in any of the five copies examined for this bibliography and the *U* (swash) for *V* in *Visu* may therefore invariably be present.

Ss signature

- Page 340: (A) italic *P* in *Pervigilio* at Ss2v, *versus* (B) roman P in P*ervigilio*
- Page 341: (A) italic *P* in *Pervigilio* at Ss3r, *versus* (B) roman P in P*ervigilio*.

The title pages

De anima brutorum is unusual in that the printer included a vertical half title (g2v). The purpose of vertical half titles in books of this period, mainly from Oxford, was either to mark unsold stock in the printer's shop or to identify the book with the foreedge outermost on the owner's shelves.[17] Details on the title page changed for the quarto London issue from Ric Davis to William Wells and Robert Scott but (as pointed out by Philip Oldfield) it was also reset. This affects the Æ of DUÆ which is under 'ti' of 'Sensitiva' (Oxford) and 'a' of 'Sensitiva' (London); the 'P' of 'PHYSIOLOGICA' which is above the 'N' of 'Naturum' (Oxford) and the 'tu' of 'Naturam' (London); 'tradit' which is followed by '⁚' (Oxford) and ':' (London); the 'N' of 'NEMPE' which is above the 'er' of 'Nervorum' (Oxford) and 'N' of 'Nervorum' (London); and 'eorumque' (Oxford) and 'eorúmque' (London). In addition there is variable use of swash and non-swash capital italics (swash 'Æ' of 'DUÆ', Oxford; swash 'U' of 'DUÆ', London).

Priority

Against this background, it may not be especially useful to order the appearance of quarto copies with leaves in different states. It is logical to assume that copies were available in Oxford before the London issue. The large paper copy may have been issued first. If so, what can reasonably be considered to be one of the earliest available examples, the large paper copy presented by Willis to the Royal Society one week after publication, has the cancellans with index (partly unopened) bound before the cancellandum with ink crossing out, Richard Davis's advertisements, no errata leaf, Oldfield settings A with 'Diligentiſsime Excolunt.', and the wider (and more usual) PARS SECUNDA at Hh2r, page 259, measuring 82 millimetres.

The illustrations

As acknowledged by Willis, the four figures of Tabula 1 in all issues and editions of *De anima brutorum* are copied from Marcello Malpighi's (1628–1694) treatise on the silkworm.[18] Illustrations in the Oxford and London quarto issues are printed from the same plates and in the same states. Apart from variation in inking, there is no sign of wear. Although more than one impression may have been made, the illustrations are indistinguishable. But there is one detail that may previously have escaped attention and is made clear by the binder who handled sheets for the London issue (**5A5**).

[17] The fact that one copy examined for this bibliography of *Dr Willis's practice of physick* (1684: **9E**) has a vertical half title in manuscript which is bound at a place convenient for covering the foreedge suggests that the latter interpretation is correct. The vertical half title is found in the Oxford and London imprints; and although it is possible that this was eventually excluded from the London issue, any copy lacking g2 is best considered incomplete.

[18] See: Marcelli Malpighi, *De bombyce*, London (1669); and chapter 3 for further details.

In this copy, Tabula I (Pl.19) is bound at Xx4v, page 368. Although casual inspection suggests that this is simply misplaced from G2v, page 68, where Tabula II (Pl.20), Tabula III (Pl.21), and Tabula IIII (Pl.22) are found, closer scrutiny shows that an attempt has been made to erase the number '3' before '68' on the page placements for Tabula I (Pl.19), Tabula II (Pl.20), and Tabula III (Pl.21). Conversely Tabula IIII (Pl.22) is correctly marked, 'page 68' and both the spacing and appearance show that this has not been amended. That the placements were all intended to be at page 68 is clear from the text at G2v which deals with comparative anatomy in the lobster and invertebrates, and where the legends for Pl.19–Pl.22 are printed in sequence at F2r–G2v, pages 59–68. Conversely the text at Xx4v, page 368, concerns 'vertigine' in man. It follows that, in one instance, a diligent but scientifically uninformed binder receiving the illustration with less than complete alteration of the page placement made an understandable mistake and misplaced Tabula I (Pl.19). The error is with the engraving of Tabulæ I, II, and III and a valiant attempt at correction before the sheets were printed. It would be instructive if a copy was to be identified in which the indicative placement 'page 368' has not been amended and all three illustrations (Pl.19–Pl.21) are bound at Xx4v, page 368.

The engraved plates used to print the eight illustrations were made available to other booksellers during 1672, and remained in reasonably good condition despite being reprinted in slightly different states for the octavo copies sold in London and Amsterdam. The illustrations were newly engraved for the duodecimo edition printed in Amsterdam (1674).

The octavo issues

Apart from the format, other changes were made when the octavo edition was printed (**5B**). It is found in three issues, one with the title page in two different states. Clearly these were all planned from the start, and the differences merely reflect distribution arrangements for the entire edition. There is a new imprimatur, granted by Samuel Parker (1640–1688), chaplain to archbishop Sheldon of Canterbury. Philip Oldfield points out that, according to the register of the Stationers' Company (Liber F), permission to print this edition was granted on 5 January 1672 before the quarto edition was first available in April 1672.[19] He explains that entry in the register provided a record of permission to print the work and staked a claim to copyright. Why registration was needed for a book already authorized may have been due to the fact that ownership of the octavo edition of *De anima brutorum* was held by Walter Kettilby (fl.1669–1711), a London bookseller not previously connected with Willis's books who needed to document that he had acquired the copyright. The *Term Catalogue* advertisement for this edition did not appear until 21 November 1672. The price was 5 shillings bound:

> Michaelmas 1672 November 21st, II Number 11, I 123, column 2, *Books reprinted.*
>
> *De Anima Brutorum quæ hominis vitalis ac sensitiva est, Exercitationes Duæ. Prior Physiologica, ejusdem naturam, partes, potentias et affectiones, tradit. Altera Pathologica morbos qui ipsam, et sedem ejus primariam, nempe cerebrum et nervosum genus afficiunt, explicat, eorumque Therapeias instituit.* Cum Figuris Æneis. Studio Thomæ Willis, M.D. In Octavo. Price, bound, 5s.

[19] See: Oldfield (1991): page 17.

Priority cannot be established for the three octavo issues but Oldfield favours that printed by 'EF' and sold by Richard Davis (**5B1**).[20] Oldfield has noticed a variant state of the title page for the issue sold by Wells and Scott, each of which is represented by the copies examined for this bibliography: the differences are 'partes' (**5B2.c1**) in place of 'Partes' (**5B2.c2**) at line 8; and 'Affectiones' (**5B2.c1**) in place of 'affectiones' (**5B2.c2**) at line 9, each with different spacing. HJR Wing and Philip Oldfield are agreed that the Amsterdam issue (**5B3**) was printed in London. Oldfield argues that distribution was hampered by the war between Britain and the Netherlands, which broke out on 19 February 1672 and lasted until February 1674. In altering the page placements on engravings used for the octavo edition, the ambiguity of 'page 368' for Tabulæ I–III (**Pl.19–Pl.21**) was resolved.

The Amsterdam duodecimo edition

The text was reset for duodecimo format in 1674 and the illustrations all reengraved. The only variant noticed by Oldfield is that, as in the copy used for this bibliography, P3 is unsigned in three of seven copies examined. There is one slight anomaly. Looked at casually, although in fact correct, the page placement for Tabula VIII (Pl.26) might be read as 'page. 209'; and this plate leaf is incorrectly bound before I9r, page 209, rather than at E7r, page 109, where it belongs. Unlike the London and Amsterdam quarto and octavo editions, but as with the Dutch issues of *Cerebri anatome*, more than one illustration was engraved on the same plate. Some edges are visible as are lines to indicate where cuts should be made, but no one illustration is surrounded on all sides by plate marks. It is not possible to match up the eight illustrations into coherent patterns from which to estimate the number that were engraved. Tabula I (Pl.19) and Tabula VIII (Pl.26) each have an upper and left side plate mark. Tabula II (Pl.20) has a plate mark at the right and lower border. Tabula III (Pl.21) has a plate mark at the left border and an engraved line at the right edge. Tabula IIII (Pl.22) has a plate mark at the lower and right edges and an engraved line at the upper edge. Tabula V (Pl.23) has a plate mark at the right border and an engraved line at the upper edge. Tabula VI (Pl.24) has an engraved line at the right edge. Tabula VII (Pl.25) has neither print marks nor engraved lines.

5A1. DE ANIMA BRUTORUM, Oxford quarto 1672

The first issue of the first edition of Willis's fifth book, on large paper with the Oxford imprint, imprimatur, first setting of the dedication to Gilbert Sheldon, Oldfield settings AAAAAAAAA for variant headlines, cancellans (signed Zzzz Aaaa) and cancellandum after Zzz1, Ric Davis' catalogue and the index but without the errata [HJR Wing 26, Oldfield A1].

Title page: DE | ANIMA BRUTORUM | Quæ Hominis Vitalis ac Senſitiva eſt, | *EXERCITATIONES DUÆ.* | Prior | PHYSIOLOGICA | Ejuſdem Naturam, Partes, Potentias & Affectiones tradit. | Altera | PATHOLOGICA | Morbos qui ipſam, & ſedem ejus Primariam, | NEMPE | Cerebrum & Nervoſum Genus afficiunt, | *explicat, eorumque Therapeias inſtituit.* | Studio *THOMÆ WILLIS* M.D. | Philoſophiæ Natural. Profeſſ. Sidleian. *Oxon.* | Nec Non |

[20] See chapter 3 for details of Elizabeth Fletcher and the books of Thomas Willis with which she was associated.

Inclyti Med. Coll. Lond. & Societ. Reg. Socii. | *OXONII.* | E THEATRO SHELDONIANO. | Impenſis RIC. DAVIS. | [rule] | Anno Dom. M. DC. LXXII.

Collation: quarto, 23 letter roman alphabet using I and V, Vu and Vuu: π^2, A^4, b–f^4, g^2, $^2A^4$, B–Z^4, Aa–Zz^4, Aaa–Zzz^4, Zzzz $Aaaa^4$, $Bbbb^2$. $1–2 signed, apart from: -A2, -b2, -f2, -B2, +E3, +I3, +K3, +L3, +M3, +Q3, +T3, +X3, +Y3, +Z3, +Dd3, +Ee3, +Kkk3, -Zzz2, Aaaa1 signed Zzzz Aaaa, -Bbbb2.

310 leaves: paginated as [56], 1–16, 33–255, [256–8], 259–'565' (i.e. = 547), [17]. Mispagination 97 for 67, 193 for 191, 194 for 192, 233 for 223, 343 for 243, 292 for 262, 293 for 263, 311–18 for 321–8, 331 for 330, 330 for 331, 324 for 332, 325 for 333, 358 for 360, 311 for 411, 334 for 434, 412 for 512, 336 for 536, and 565 for 563 (cancellans and cancellandum).

Type: 34 lines; height (20 lines) 93 millimetres, width 100 millimetres (120 millimetres with marginal notes).

Contents: [Oldfield setting A in dedication and epistle] **π1r**, page [1]; blank; **π1v**, page [2], Imprimatur. Decemb. 12. 1671. *PET. MEWS Vice-Cancellarius.*; **π2r**, page [3], title; **π2v**, page [4], blank; **A1r–A2v**, pages [5–8], *REVERENDISSIMO* In Chriſto Patri & Domino Domino GILBERTO Providentia Divina Archiepiſcopo *Cantuarienſi*, totius *Angliæ* Primati & Metropolitano, & Auguſtiſſimo Principi CAROLO II. M. *Britanniæ*, *Franciæ* & *Hiberniæ* Regi à Secretioribus Conſiliis … [signed] Clementiæ veſtræ Cultorem humillimum, ſervum devotiſſimum THO. WILLIS.; **A3r–A4r**, pages [9–11], ERUDITISSIMIS *ET* VENERABILIBUS VIRIS Mihique æternum colendis D. VICE-CANCELLARIO DOCTORIBUS & MAGISTRIS Qui in Celeberrimâ Univerſitate Oxonienſi BONAS LITERAS Diligentiſsime Excolunt, Egregie Ornant, Feliciſſime Promovent. *Salutem.*… [signed] *Clariſsimi Domini Veſtrum omnium Cultori addictiſſimo* THO. WILLIS.; **A4v**, page [12], blank; **b1r–c1r**, pages [13–21], PRÆFATIO Ad Lectorem.; **c1v**, page [22], blank; **c2r–d4v**, pages [23–36], ELENCHUS RERUM In Tractatu DE ANIMA BRUTORUM, Sive parte primâ.; **e1r–f4r**, pages [37–51], ELENCHUS RERUM. PARS II. PATHOLOGICA; **f4v**, page [52], blank; **g2r**, page [53] blank; **g2v**, page [54] WILLIS DE Anima Brutorum. [vertical half title]; **g1r**, page [55]; DE ANIMA BRUTORUM *QUÆ HOMINIS VITALIS AC SENSITIVA EST*, Pars Prima PHYSIOLOGICA Ejuſdem Naturam, partes, Potentias & affectiones tradens. [half title]; **g1v**, [page 56], blank

2A1r–Gg4r, pages 1–'255', [text] DE ANIMA BRUTORUM [pars prima]; **Gg4v**, page ['256'], blank.

Hh1r, page ['257'], PARS SECUNDA PATHOLOGICA SIVE De Morbis Quæ ad Animum Corpoream, ejuſque ſubjecta, ſcilicet Cerebrum, & Genus Nervoſum ſpectant. [half title]; **Hh1v**, page ['258'], blank; **Hh2r–Zzz1v**, pages '259–562'; **Zzzz Aaaa** 1r, page '565', i.e. 563 (cancellans), [text] PARS SECUNDA.

Zzzz Aaaa1v–Bbbb2v, pages [1–11], INDEX ALPHABETICVS Rerum & Verborum.; **Zzz2r**, page [12], cancellandum (crossed through in pen and ink); **Zzz2v–Zzz4v**, pages [13–17], A CATALOGUE *of ſome Books Printed for, and to be ſold by* Richard Davis *in Oxford.*

[**Cccc1r–v**, Errata, 12 lines correcting 21 errors in the text, not present].

Headlines and *Catchwords*: Oldfield settings: K outer forme, A; K inner forme, A; Bb signature, A; Cc signature, A; Dd signature, A; Gg signature, A; Ii signature, A; Mm signature, A; Ss signature, A. ELENCHUS RRERUM. for ELENCHUS RERUM. at **c4v**, page [28]; **e2r**, page [39]; no '.' after headline at **d2v**, page [32]; **f2v**, page [48]; **K4v**, page '96'; **P2r**, page '131'; **R4r**, page '151'; **Ff2r**, page '343'; **Pp1v**, page '314'; **Rr3r**, page '325'; **Ll3r**, page '469'; no ',' after headline at **C1v**, page '34'; no 'CAP' headline at **A1r**, page 1; **G3r**, page '69'; **I4r**, page '87'; **K4r**, page '95'; **M3v**, page '110'; **Hh2r**, page '259'; **Yy2v**, page '372'; **Aaa4v**, page '392'; **Ggg1r**, page '433'; **Iii3v**, page '454'; **Nnn3r**, page '485'; **Ppp4v**, page '504'; **Rrr3r**, page '517'; **Vuu3r**, page '543'; CAP. XIII. for CAP. XII. at **Y1r**, page '185'; *De Cephalalgia.* for *Cephalalgiæ Curatio.* at **Kk4r–v**, pages '279–80'; CAP. IV. for CAP. VI. at **Rr4r**, page '335'; CAP. XI. for CAP. IX. at **Kkk2v**, page '460'; **Kkk4v**, page '464'; CAP. XIV. for CAP. XV. at **Zzzz Aaaa1**, page '565'; **Zzz2r**, page '565'.

No catchword at: **A2v** / **A3r**, pages [8] / [9]; *CAP*. for CAP. at **d3v** / **d4r**, pages [34] / [35]; ceptu for ptu at **B1r** / **v**, pages 9 / 10; *Tabula* for Tabula at **F2v** / **F3r**, pages '60 / 61'; flammam for flamam at **Y4r** / **v**, pages '193 / 194'; quod for quot at **Ee2v** / **Ee3r**, pages '236 / 237'; butus for imbutus at **Kk4v** / **Ii1r**, pages '264 / 265'; *Tabul* for *f. Tabul* at **Ll4v** / **Mm1r**, pages '288 / 289'; *bus* for *ribus* at **Nn1r** / **v**, pages '297 / 298'; no catchword at **Ccc2v** / **Ccc3r**, pages '404 / 405'; **Ll4v** / **Mmm1r**, pages '472 / 473'; **Mmm4v** / **Nnn1r**, pages '480 / 481'; **Zzz2v–Zzz4v**, pages [13]–[17]; con for citat at **Ggg2r** / **v**, pages '435 / 436'; conſtan- for ter at **Ggg3r** / **v**, pages '437 / 438'; barde for bardè at **Qqq4r** / **v**, pages '511 / 512'; *Spiritus* for *Rx Spiritus* at **Rrr1v** / **Rrr2r**, pages '514 / 515'; 3. *Eva-* for 8° *Evacuationes* at **Rrr4r** / **v**, pages '527 / 528'.

Frontispiece: none.

Portrait: none.

Printers' ornament: headpiece (coat of arms) at **A1r**, page [5] {**Fell 1**}.

No decorated initials.

Illustrations: **Pl.19a1**. Plate 19 (images 30–33): [3]68 (headline, left), *Tabula. I.[a]* (headline, right), *Figura. I.[a]*, *Figura. II.[da]*, *Figura. III.[tia]*, *Figura. IIII.[ta]* (headers, above each image); lettering to depict structures (in multiples of ≤ 6) A–D. Folding, 215 × 185 millimetres (sheet); 198 × 154 millimetres (plate marks); 48 × 25 millimetres, 121 × 84 millimetres, 77 × 107 millimetres, 115 × 17 millimetres (figures). Legend: FIGARARUM EXPLICATIO. Tabula prima *continet figuras quaſdam e Malpigio excerptas, quibus Bombicis, aliorumque inſectorum, Organa vitalia repræſentantur. Figura Prima.* Exhibet foramen ovale, cujus bina in lateribus cujuſque ſectionis, ſive annuli (exceptis tribus ſuperioribus) conſita, Trachearum oſtia, ſive aperturæ ſunt. *Figura Secunda.* Trachearum in Bombyce ramificationes quaſdam interiores oſtendit. *Figura Tertia.* Tracheæ ramificationes in Cicada exhibet. *Figura Quarta.* Exprimit Bombycis cor, quod oblongum & inæquale pluribus velut corculis ovalibus conſtare videtur. Inserted after legends for Tabulæ I–IV at **F1r–G2v**, pages '59–68'; see: Figure 123.

Pl.20a1. Plate 20 (images 34–35): *Tabula II.[da]* (headline, centre), *page* [3]68 (headline, right), *Figura. I.[a]*, *Figura. II.[da]* (headers, above each image); lettering to depict structures (in

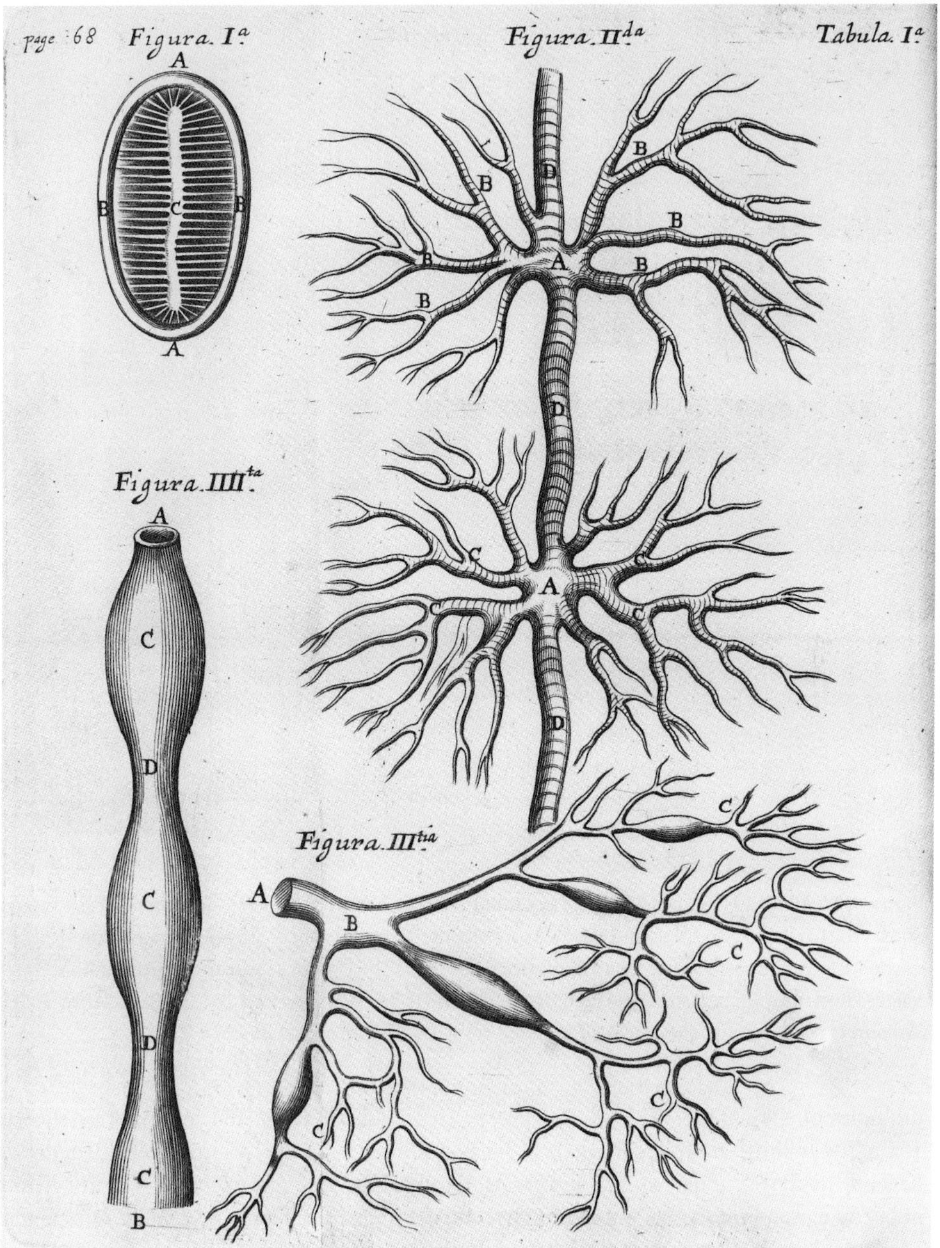

Figure 123 Plate 19 (images 30–33). The Firſt Table, Contains certain Figures taken out of *Malpigius*, in which the Vital Organs of the Silk-Worm and of other Inſects are repreſented. The Firſt Figure Shews the Navil-hole, of which two being planted in the ſides of every Section or little Ring (except in the three uppermoſt) are the Doors or Openings of the Wind-Pipes. The Second Figure Shews ſome interior Branchings in the Silk-Worm. The Third Figure Shews the Ramifications of the *Trachea* or Wind-Pipe in a Graſhopper. The Fourth Figure, Expreſſes the Heart of the Silk-Worm, which ſeems to be made oblong and unequal, as if into too many little oval Hearts. Image from *De anima brutorum* 1672; legend from *Two discourses concerning the soul of brutes* 1683.

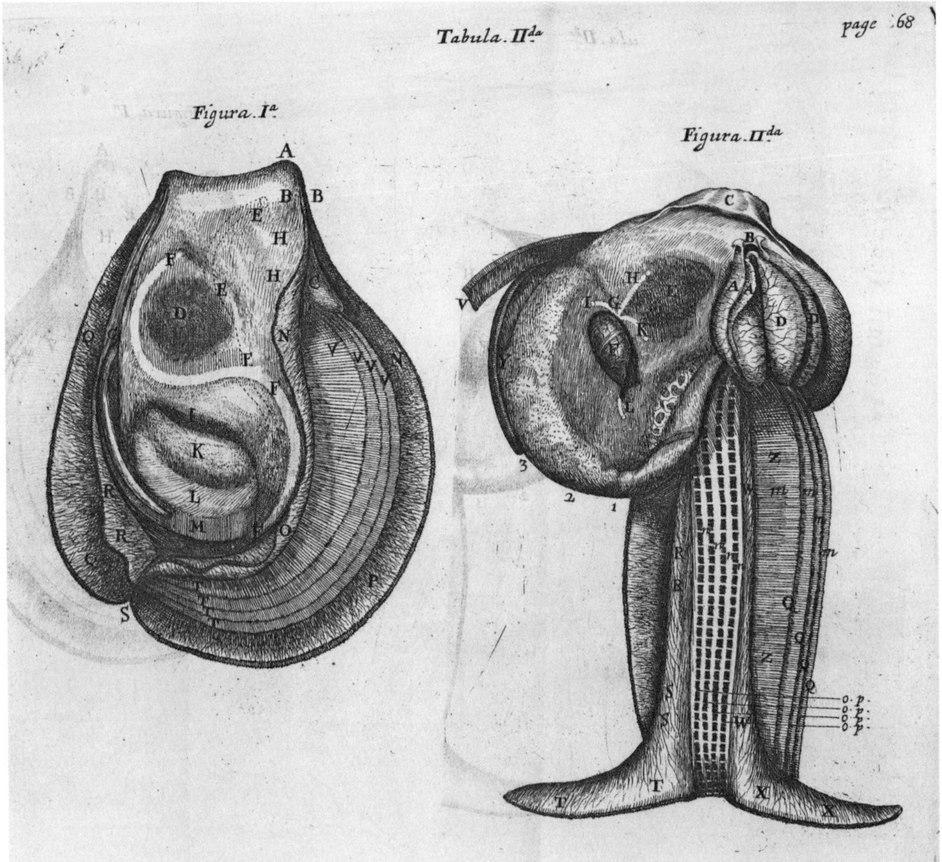

Figure 124 Plate 20 (images 34–35). Legend (1683): The Second Table, of which The Firſt Figure Shews the Oyſter taken forth and whole from the ſhell, that his parts may be ſeen as they are in their natural ſituation. The Second Figure Repreſents the Oyſter open, and unrolled, that its Viſcera and internal parts may be ſeen. Image from *De anima brutorum* 1672; legend from *Two discourses concerning the soul of brutes* 1683.

multiples of ≤ 4) A–I, K–T, V–X, Z, *m*, *o*, *p*, 1–3. Folding, 204 × 254 millimetres (sheet); 184 × 204 millimetres (plate marks); 110 × 86 millimetres, 132 × 95 millimetres (figures). Legend: Tabula Secunda, *cujus Figura prima*. Exhibet Oſtreum teſtâ exemptum, & integrum, ut partes ejus, quomodo habent in ſitu naturali, conſpiciantur. *Figura Secunda*. Repræſentat oſtreum apertum, & evolutum, ut viſcera ejus, & partes internæ conſpiciantur. Inserted after legends for Tabulæ I–IV at **F1r–G2v**, pages '59–68' see: Figure 124.

Pl.21a1. Plate 21 (images 36–38): *Tabula. III.*^{tia} (headline, centre), *page* [*3*]*68* (headline, right), *Figura. 1.*^{ma}, *Figura. II.*^{da}, *Fig. III.*^{tia} (headers, above each image); lettering to depict structures (in multiples of ≤ 4) A–I, K–T, V–X, *d*, *m*, 1–6, *α–γ*, *κ*. Folding, 255 × 187 millimetres (sheet); 249 × 185 millimetres (plate marks); 242 × 103 millimetres, 121 × 92 millimetres, 40 × 18 millimetres (figures). Legend: Tabula Tertia. *Figura Prima* Exhibet Aſtacum in dorſo apertum, ut Cerebrum, viſcera, partes vitales, genitaleſque, aliæque interiores conſpici poſſint. *Figura Secunda.* Exhibet Aſtaci uterum, ejuſque collum & pudendum, ſive aperturam, per foramen pedunculo antepenultimo excuſum, unà cum pedunculo ipſo, & branchiis affixis. *Figura Tertia*. Exprimit Branchiæ portionem abſciſſam, ut illius tres ductus, ſive cavitates appareant. Inserted after legends for Tabulæ I–IV at **F1r–G2v**, pages '59–68'; see: Figure 125.

Pl.22a1. Plate 22 (images 39–41): *Tab. IIII.* (headline, left), *page 68* (headline, right), *Figura. I.^{ma}*, *Figura. II.^{da}*, *Figura. III.^{tia}* (headers, above each image); lettering to depict structures (in multiples of ≤ 5) A–I, K, *a–c*, *e*. Folding, 215 × 186 millimetres (sheet); 197 × 152 millimetres (plate marks); 159 × 68 millimetres, 45 × 17 millimetres, 166 × 16 millimetres (figures). Legend: Tabula Quarta. *Figura prima*. Exhibet Lumbricum terreſtrem ſupinatum, quoad maximum Portionem ejus diſſectum, & apertum, ut Cerebrum, præcordia, viſcera, aliæque partes conſpiciantur. *Figura Secunda*. Exprimit ejuſdem lumbrici portionem cum cauda abſciſſam, ut pedunculorum ſeries, quæ ſunt 4. ſc. a.a.a.a. conſpiciantur. *Figura Tertia*. Exhibet Lumbricum integrum, pronum, ut muſculi annulares, in iiſque tracheæ videantur. Inserted after legends for Tabulæ I–IV at **F1r–G2v**, pages '59–68'; see: Figure 126.

Pl.23a1. Plate 23 (image 42): *page 86* (headline, left), *Tabu. V.* (headline right); lettering to depict structures (in multiples of ≤ 2) A–I, K–T, V, W, *e*. Leaf size, cropped, 204 × 153 millimetres (sheet); 173 × 121 millimetres (plate marks); 160 × 99 millimetres (figure). Legend: FIGARARUM EXPLICATIO. *Tabula Quinta*. Exhibet Figuram cerebri ovine evoluti, & quibuſdam in locis deraſi, & velut excarnati, ut tractus medullares conſpiciantur. Inserted after legends for Tabulæ V–VII at **I2r–I3v**, pages 83–86; see: Figure 127.

Pl.24a1. Plate 24 (image 43): *page 86* (headline, left), *Tabu. VI.* (headline right); lettering to depict structures (in multiples of ≤ 3) A–I, K, L–M, *f*. Leaf size, cropped, 204 × 150 millimetres (sheet); 152 × 109 millimetres (plate marks); 131 × 87 millimetres (figure). Legend: Tabula Sexta. Exhibet ἐγκεφάλου ovini baſin, in cujus partibus quibuſdam deraſis, aliiſque nudè expoſitis, ſtriæ, ſive tractus medullares, quaſi totidem nervi apparent. Inserted after legends for Tabulæ V–VII at **I2r–I3v**, pages 83–6; see: Figure 128.

Pl.25a1. Plate 25 (image 44): *page 86* (headline, left), *Tabu. VII.* (headline right); lettering to depict structures (in multiples of ≤ 2) A–I. Leaf size, cropped, 204 × 153 millimetres (sheet); 152 × 132 millimetres (plate marks); 120 × 106 millimetres (figure). Legend: Tabula Septima. Exhibet prominentias orbicularis, & thalamos opticos eraſos, & velut excarnatos, ut interiores ipſorum compages conſpiciantur. Inserted after legends for Tabulæ V–VII at **I2r–I3v**, pages 83–6; see: Figure 129.

Pl.26a1. Plate 26 (image 45): *page 126* (headline, left), *Tabula. VIII.* (headline right); lettering to depict structures (in multiples of ≤ 2) A–I, K, L–T, V–Z, *s*, *r*, *y*. Folding, 215 × 204 millimetres (sheet); 182 × 185 millimetres (plate marks); 150 × 173 millimetres (figure). Legend: Tabula Octava Continet novam Cerebri Humani Anatomen, ubi ſectione per ſalcem, corpus calloſum, & fornicem factâ, eorumque partibus diductis, & ſepoſitis, corpora ſtriata, nec non prominentiæ opticæ, & orbiculares, unius lateris eraſa, & alterius integra, & plana exhibentur. Plate inserted after legend for Tabula VIII at **O3v**, page 126; see: Figure 130.

Copy: DASC. Recent full calf with blind stamped central panel, floral corners, and alternating ornament (two tools) at the edges, double-lined border, and gilt edges to boards, spine with

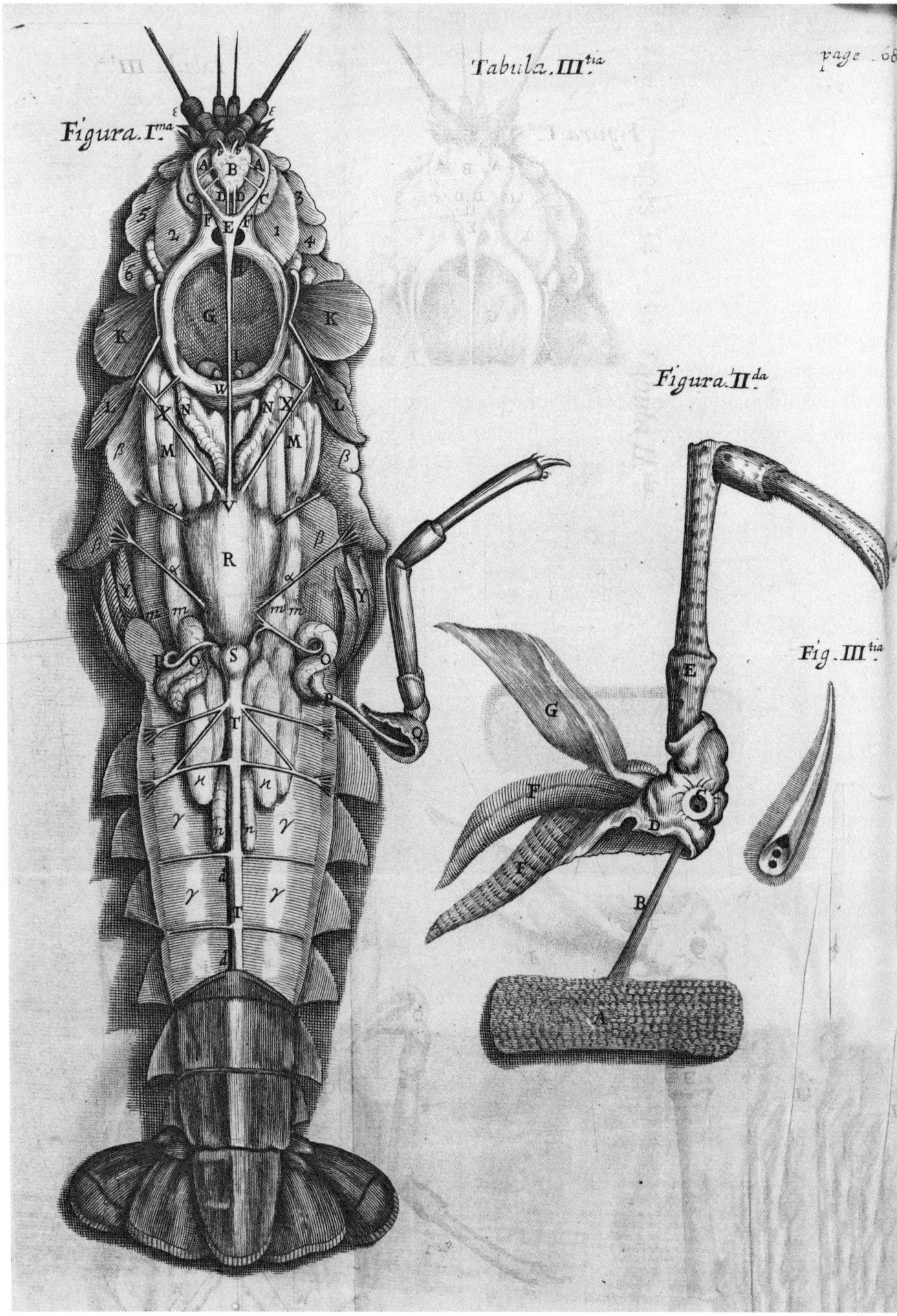

Figure 125 Plate 21 (images 36–38). Legend (1683): The Third Table. The Firſt Figure Shews the Lobſter open in the back, that the Brain, Viſcera, Vital, Genital, and other interior parts may be ſeen. The Second Figure Shews the Womb of the Lobſter, and its neck, and Privy Member, or aperture made thorow the hole in the laſt little Foot but one, together with the little Foot it ſelf, and the affixed Gills. The Third Figure Expreſſes a portion of the Gill cut off, that its three Paſſages or Cavities may appear. Image from *De anima brutorum* 1672; legend from *Two discourses concerning the soul of brutes* 1683.

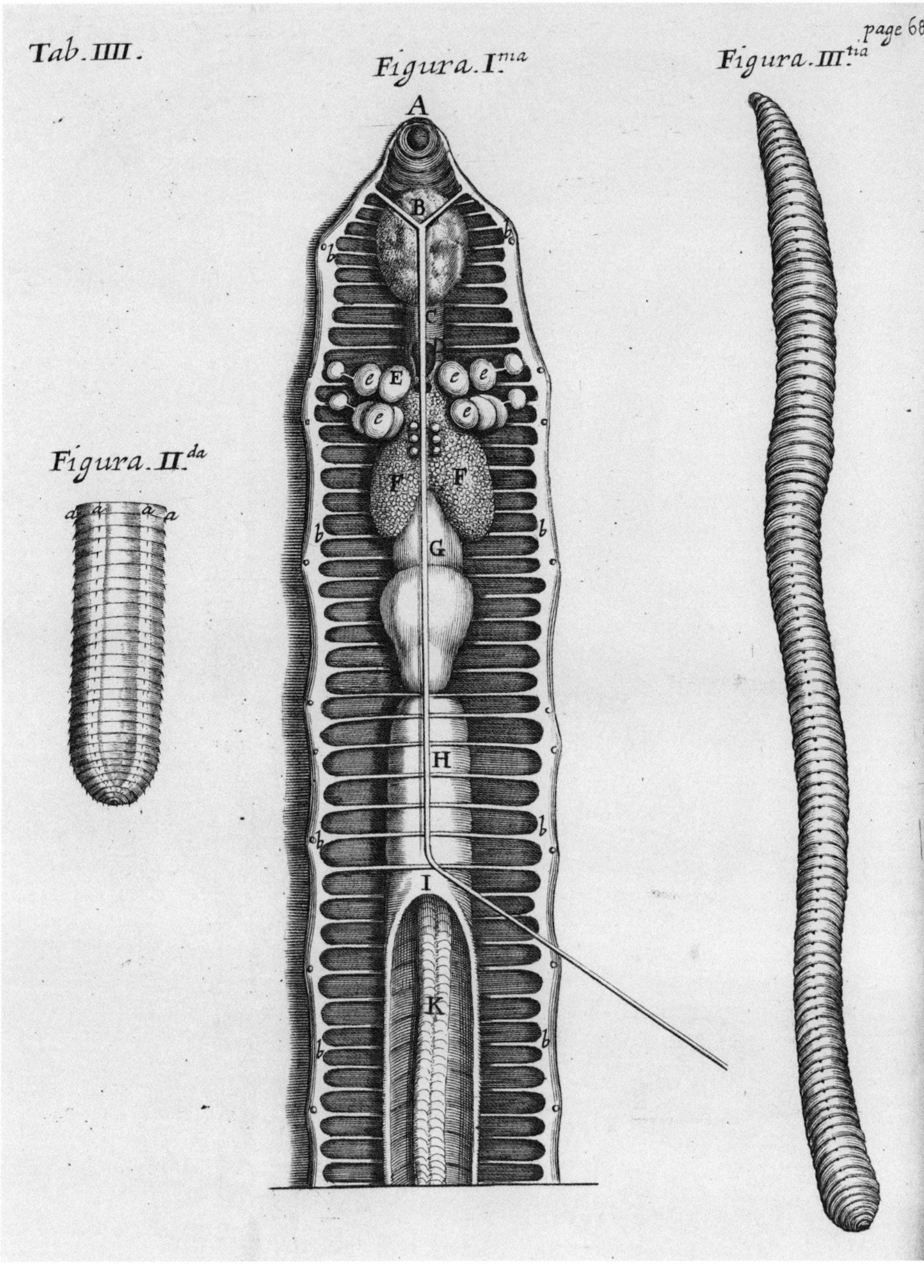

Figure 126 Plate 22 (images 39–41). Legend (1683): The Fourth Table. The Firft Figure Shews an Earth-Worm laid with its belly upwards, the greateft part of it diffected and lay'd open, that the Brain, *Præcordia*, *Vifcera*, and other Parts may be feen. The Second Figure Expreffes a portion of the fame Earth-Worm, with the Tail cut off, that the rowes of the little Feet, which are 4, to wit, *a. a. a. a.* may be feen. Image from *De anima brutorum* 1672; legend from *Two discourses concerning the soul of brutes* 1683.

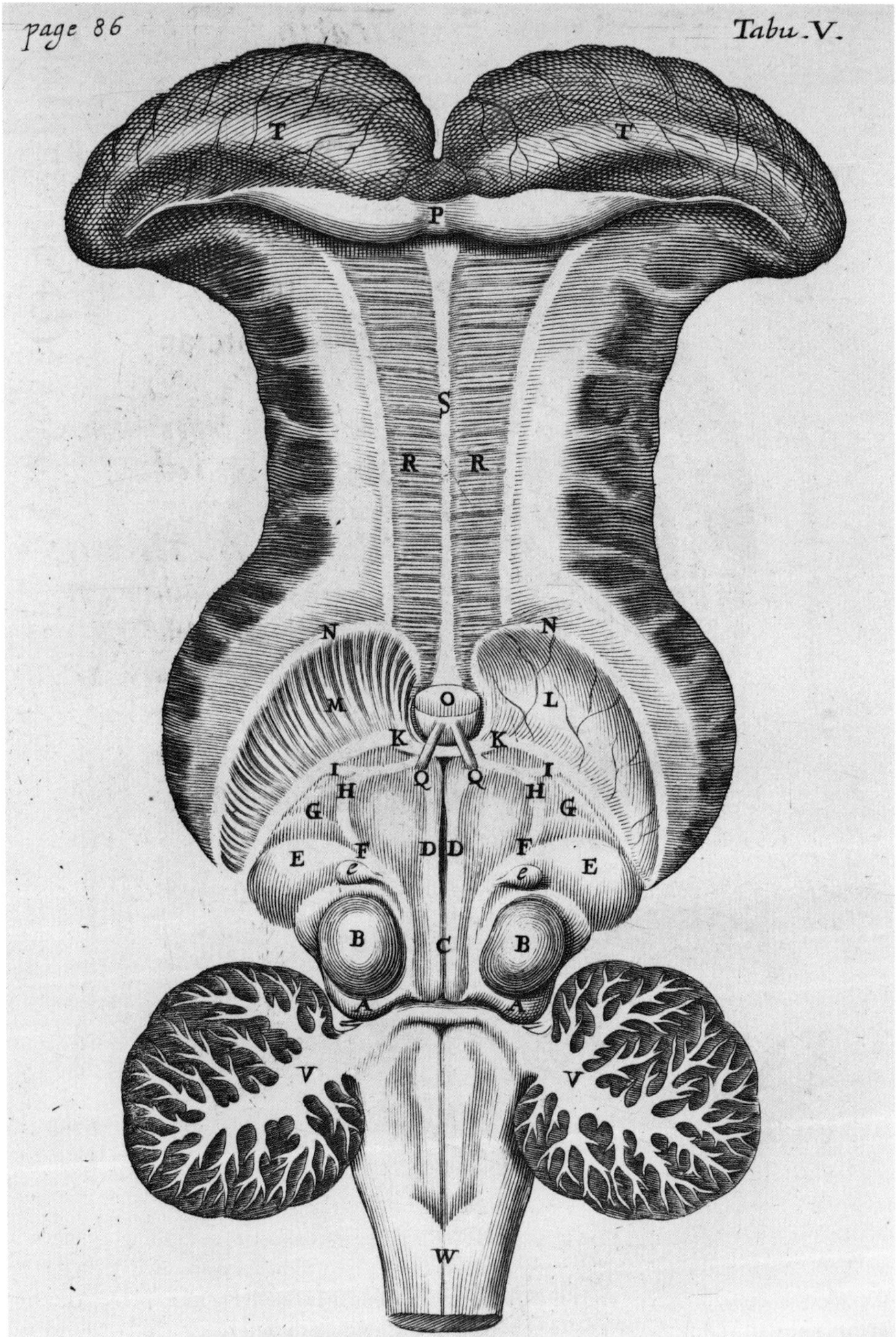

Figure 127 Plate 23 (image 42). Legend (1683): The Fifth Table, Shews the Figure of the Brain of a Sheep roled forth, and derafed, and as it were made bare of the Flefh, in many places, that the Marrowy tracts may be feen. Image from *De anima brutorum* 1672; legend from *Two discourses concerning the soul of brutes* 1683.

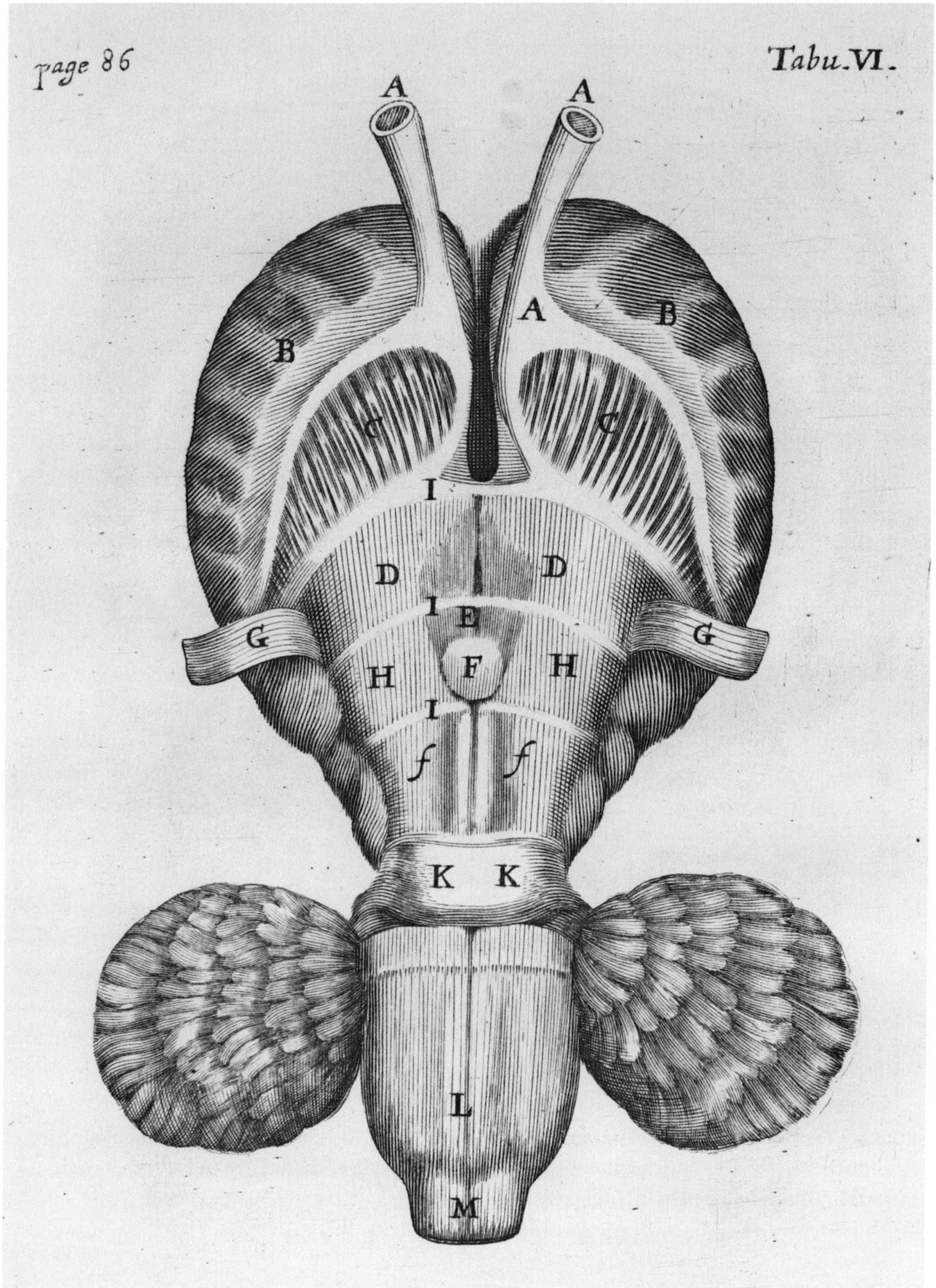

Figure 128 Plate 24 (image 43). Legend (1683): The Sixth Table Shews the Baſis of a Sheeps Head, in certain parts of which Deraſed, and in others Expoſed naked, the Streaks or Medullary Tracts, as ſo many Nerves, appear. Image from *De anima brutorum* 1672; legend from *Two discourses concerning the soul of brutes* 1683.

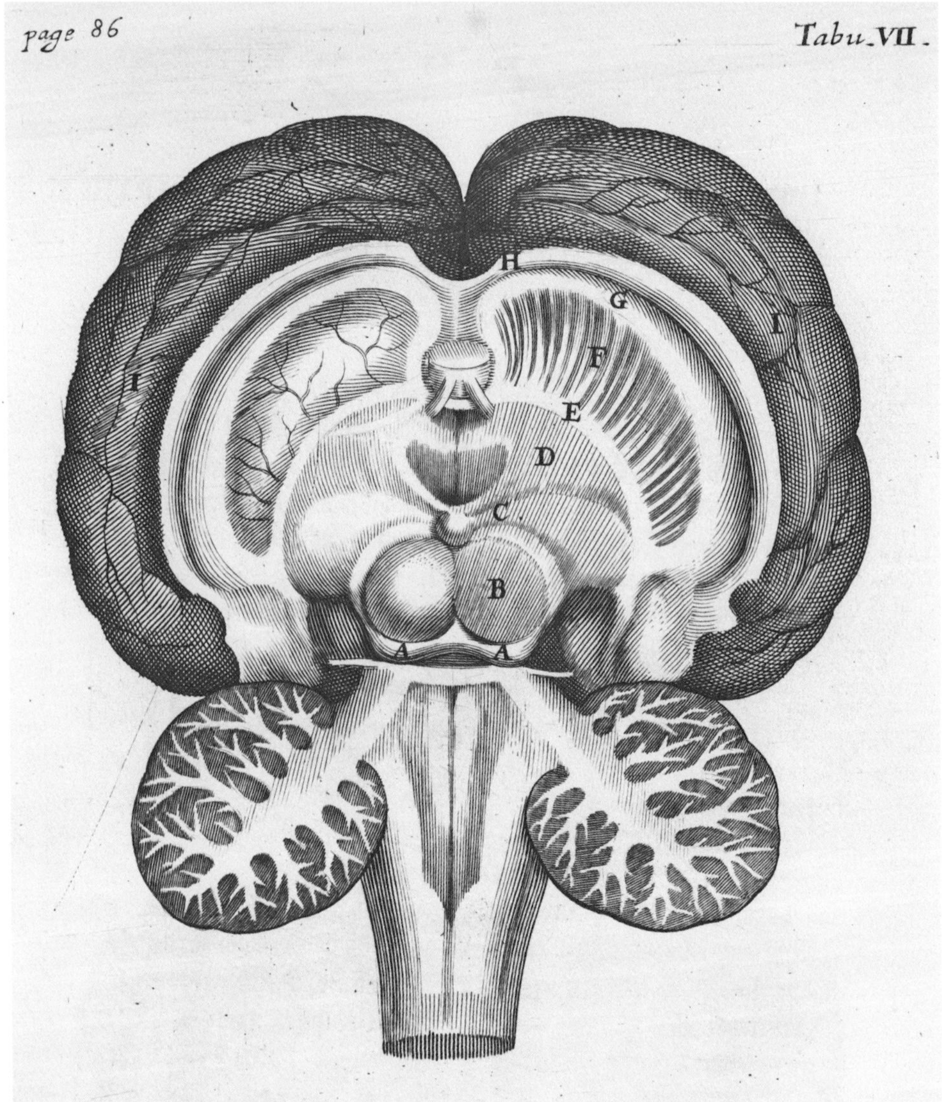

Figure 129 Plate 25 (image 44). Legend (1683): The Seventh Table, Shews the orbicular Prominences, and the Optick Chambers Erafed, and as it were made bare of Flefh that their inward Frames may be beheld. Image from *De anima brutorum* 1672; legend from *Two discourses concerning the soul of brutes* 1683.

five raised bands and gilt decorated panels, labelled WILLIS | DE ANIMA | BRUTORUM, new endpapers. Leaves 214 × 165 millimetres (cropped at upper margin), boards 222 × 168 × 42 millimetres. Inscribed: James Johnstone. Stamped: Birmingham Medical Institute (title page and all plates).[21]

[21] The owner was either James Johnstone (*c.*1730–1802) or, possibly, his son James (1754–1783). The father had studied with Robert Whytt (1714–1766) in Edinburgh and used that experience to write *An essay on the ganglion of the nerves* (1771), which was reprinted with other writings on the nervous system and related topics as *Medical essays and observations* (1795). The son, James, also studied in Edinburgh and was much praised by his teacher

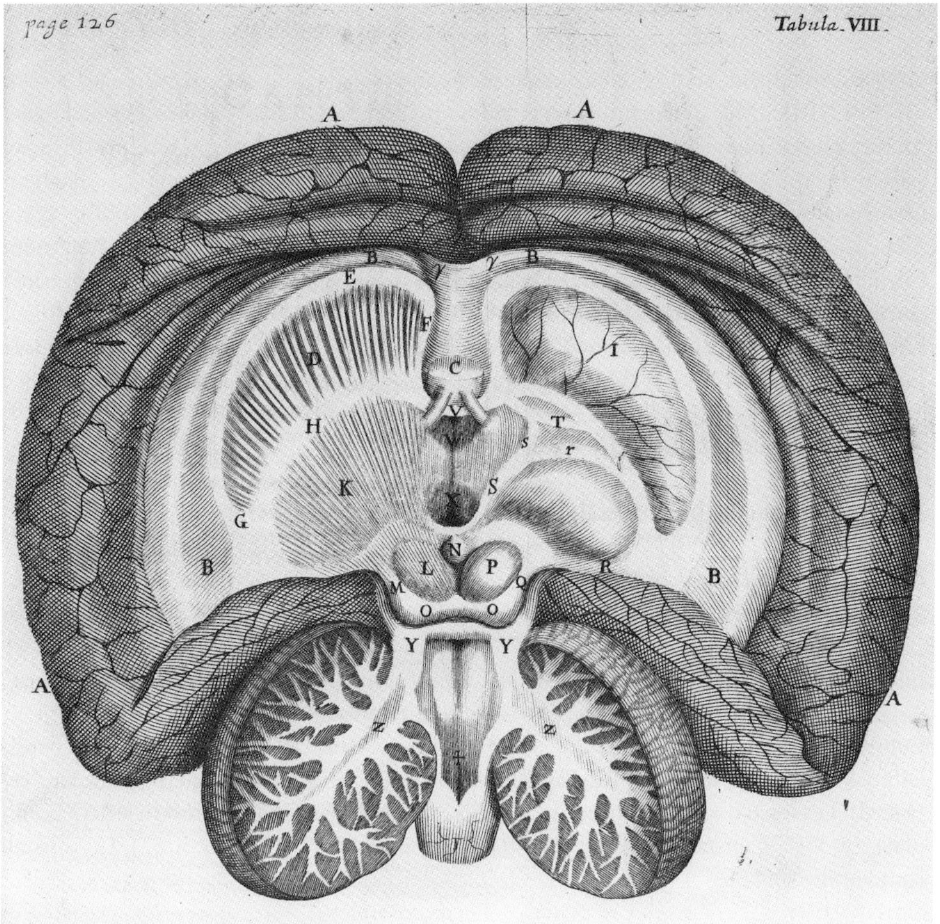

Figure 130 Plate 26 (image 45). Legend (1683): The Eighth Table, Contains a new Anatomy of the Humane Brain, where, by a Diſſection with an Inſtrument made thorow the Bill, the Callous Body, and the Fornix or Arch, and their Parts being taken away and ſeparated; the ſtreaked Bodies, alſo the Optic and Orbicular Prominences, one ſide eraſed, and the other whole and plain, are Exhibited. Inserted after the legend for The Eighth Table at G2v, page 44. Image from *De anima brutorum* 1672; legend from *Two discourses concerning the soul of brutes* 1683.

5A2. DE ANIMA BRUTORUM, Oxford quarto 1672

The ordinary paper issue of the first edition of Willis's fifth book, with the Oxford imprint, imprimatur, second setting of the dedication to Gilbert Sheldon, Oldfield settings BAABAABAB of various headlines, cancellandum after Zzz1, cancellans (signed Zzzz Aaaa), Ric Davis's catalogue and the index but without the errata [not distinguished from HJR Wing 26, Oldfield A1].

William Cullen (1710–1790) for his MD thesis on *De angina maligna* (1773, reprinted 1779). After being appointed physician to the Worcester Infirmary, he agreed to help inmates with gaol fever which he duly contracted, dying aged 27 years. The Birmingham Medical Institute founded in 1875 was initially a library, then a social club and now a conference centre. Many of their books were sold at auction by Dominic Winter in 2012.

As in **5A1** apart from:

Contents: [Oldfield setting B in dedication and epistle] ... **A1r–A2v**, pages [5–8], REVERENDISSIMO In Chriſto Patri & Domino Domino GILBERTO Providentia Divina Archiepiſcopo *Cantuarienſi*, totius *Angliæ* Primati & Metropolitano, & Auguſtiſſimo Principi Carolo II. M. *Britanniæ Franciæ* & *Hiberniæ* Regi, à Secretioribus Conſiliis ... [signed] Clementiæ veſtræ *Cultorem humillimum, ſervum devotiſſimum* THO. WILLIS.; **A3r–A4r**, pages [9–11] ERUDITISSIMIS *ET* VENERABILIBUS VIRIS Mihique æternum colendis D. VICE-CANCELLARIO DOCTORIBUS ET MAGISTRIS Qui in Celeberrimâ Univerſitate Oxonienſi BONAS LITERAS *DILIGENTISSIME EXCOLUNT* Egregie ornant FELICISSIME PROMOVENT. *Salutem*. ... [signed] *Clariſsimi Domini Veſtrum omnium Cultori addictiſſimo* THO. WILLIS.

[*Collation*: Zzz Aaaa1 signed Zzzz Aaaa].

[Cccc1r–v, Errata, 12 lines correcting 21 errors in the text, not present].

Headlines: Oldfield settings: K outer forme, B; K, inner forme, A; Bb signature, A; Cc signature, B; Dd signature, A; Gg signature, A; Ii signature, B; Mm signature, A; Ss signature, B.

Illustrations: as in **5A1** apart from variation in sheet sizes and occasional binding positions.

Copy: DASC. Original calf with double line to borders, spine (relaid) with four raised bands lettered WILLI'S | ANIMA | BRUTOR: (label) | 1672, original endpapers (front free replaced). Leaves 200 × 147 millimetres, boards 208 × 147 × 50 millimetres. Inserted: bookplate of W^{m}. Constable Esqr F.R.S & F.A.S. Inscribed: (1) erased; (2) C Tunstall (unidentified).[22]

5A3. DE ANIMA BRUTORUM, Oxford quarto 1672

The ordinary paper issue of the first edition of Willis's fifth book, with the Oxford imprint, imprimatur, second variant setting of the dedication to Gilbert Sheldon, Oldfield settings ABAAAABAB of various headlines, at least one leaf in a second state, cancellandum after Zzz1, cancellans signed Zzz Aaaa, Ric Davis's catalogue and the index but without the errata [not distinguished from HJR Wing 26, Oldfield A1].

As in **5A2** apart from:

Collation: Zzz Aaaa1 correctly signed.

[Cccc1r–v, Errata, 12 lines correcting 21 errors in the text not present].

[22] William Constable (1721–1791) was a scientist and collector of works of art, numismatics, scientific instruments, and natural history specimens many of which were acquired during a Grand Tour to Italy in 1769. These remain on display in purpose built cabinets of curiosity at Burton Constable Hall. He made attempts at classification of the natural world (pre-Linnaeus) but held that it was possible to cross-breed chickens with rabbits. He was elected FRS on 4 May 1775. Some books with his bookplate were sold at Sotheby's on 14 June 1889.

Headlines: Oldfield settings: K outer forme, A; K inner forme, B; Bb signature, A; Cc signature, A; Dd signature, A; Gg signature, A; Ii signature, B; Mm signature, A; Ss signature, B. Correction of ELENCHUS RRERUM. to ELENCHUS RERUM. at **e2r**, page [39].

Illustrations: as in **5A1** apart from variation in sheet sizes and occasional binding positions.

Copy: DASC. Modern half citron morocco with cloth boards, spine with five raised bands, blind ruling, gilt stamped WILLIS | — | DE | ANIMA BRUTORUM | 1672, new endpapers. Leaves 198 × 157 millimetres, boards 208 × 157 × 52 millimetres. Inscribed: Francis Wrangham 1804. Stamped: Withdrawn from Wellcome Library.[23]

5A4. DE ANIMA BRUTORUM, London quarto 1672

The London issue of the first edition of Willis's fifth book, no imprimatur, second variant setting of the dedication to Gilbert Sheldon, Oldfield settings BAAAAABAA of various headlines, cancellandum after Zzz1, cancellans (signed Zzzz Aaaa), Ric Davis's catalogue, the index, and errata [HJR Wing 27, Oldfield A1a].

Title page: DE | ANIMA BRUTORUM | Quæ Hominis Vitalis ac Senſitiva eſt, | *EXERCITATIONES DUÆ.* | Prior | PHYSIOLOGICA | Ejuſdem Naturam, Partes, Potentias & Affectiones tradit: | Altera | PATHOLOGICA | Morbos qui ipſam, & ſedem ejus Primariam, | NEMPE | Cerebrum & Nervoſum Genus afficiunt, | *explicat, eorúmque Therapeias instituit.* | Studio *THOMÆ WILLIS* M.D. | Philoſophiæ Natural. Profeſſ. Sidleian. *Oxon.* | Nec Non | *Inclyti Med. Coll. Lond. & Societ. Reg. Socii.* | *LONDINI,* | Proſtant apud *Gulielm. Wells* & *Robertum Scott.* | [rule] | Anno Dom. M. DC. LXXII.

Then as in **5A2** apart from:

[*Collation*: Zzz Aaaa1 signed Zzzz Aaaa].

Contents: **π1r**, page [1], ERRATA, eight lines listing 20 errors; **π1v**, page [2], blank (bound after Bbbb2v); **π2r**, page [1], title; **π2v**, page [2], blank.

Headlines: Oldfield settings: K outer forme, B; K inner forme, A; Bb signature, A; Cc signature, A; Dd signature, A; Gg signature, A; Ii signature, B; Mm signature, A; Ss signature, A.

Illustrations: as in **5A1** apart from variation in sheet sizes and occasional binding positions.

Copy: DASC. Original calf boards with gilt coat of arms and crowns at each corner, upper and lower, gilt lines at borders, spine (rebacked) with five raised bands, gilt lines, and label

[23] After studying at Magdalene College and Trinity Hall, Cambridge, Francis Wrangham (1769–1842) was ordained and served as a rector in Yorkshire rising eventually to become archdeacon of the East Riding (1828–1841). As a well-connected cleric who passed most of his ecclesiastical duties to curates, Wrangham was an acknowledged and widely read poet, essayist, and translator of Greek and Latin literature who published scholarly works on biblical themes. His religion was orthodox but he was an advocate for the abolition of slavery, the education of women, free libraries, charity schools, and hospitals and other progressive social reforms. Wrangham was elected FRS on 15 November 1804 and was a member of the Roxburghe Club.

WILLIS | DE ANIMA | BRUTORUM, later endpapers. Leaves 202 × 152 millimetres, boards 213 × 153 × 47 millimetres. Inscribed: (1) ex libris Wm Mussat N° 89; (2) ex libris Wm Mussat 1854 No. (unidentified). Inserted: bookplate of HF NORMAN MD; (2) book label of LIBRARIE JACQUES LECHEVALIER | 23 rue Racine, PARIS VI. Annotated: Lechevalier Cat 47 No 1835. Shelfmarks: (1) 138 (crossed through); (2) 228; (3) *F*.[24]

5A5. DE ANIMA BRUTORUM, London quarto 1672

The London issue of the first edition of Willis's fifth book, no imprimatur, second variant setting of the dedication to Gilbert Sheldon, Oldfield settings BAABAAABB of various headlines, one further leaf in second state, cancellans (signed Zzz Aaaa) after Zzz1, the index and errata but no cancellandum and without Ric Davis's catalogue [not distinguished from HJR Wing 27, Oldfield A1a].[25]

As in **5A4** apart from:

Collation: π^2, A^4, b–f^4, g^2, $2A^4$, B–Z^4, Aa–Zz^4, Aaa^4–Zzz^1, [Zzz2–Zzz4 omitted], Zzz $Aaaa^4$, $Bbbb^2$.

Mispaginated: apart from correction of 358 for 360.

Contents: ... **π1r**, page [1], errata, eight lines listing 20 errors; **π1v**, page [2], blank (bound after A4v) ... **Zzz1r–v**, [text] pages 561–2; **Zzz Aaaa1r**, page '565', cancellans; **Zzz Aaaa1v–Bbbb2v**, pages [1–11], INDEX ALPHABETICUS Rerum & Verborum.

Headlines: Oldfield settings: K outer forme, B; K inner forme, A; Bb signature, A; Cc signature, B; Dd signature, A; Gg signature, A; Ii signature, A; Mm signature, B; Ss signature, B.

Illustrations: as in **5A1** apart from variation in sheet sizes and occasional binding positions.

Copy: DASC, lacking g2, vertical half title. Original calf, spine (relaid) with five raised bands and gilt decorated panels, lettered WILLIS | DE ANIMA | BRVTORUVM, original endpapers. Leaves 202 × 150 millimetres, boards 212 × 155 × 50 millimetres.

[24] This may be Professor Mussat mentioned in the LISTE DES MEMBRES DE LA SOCIÉTÉ BOTANIQUE DE FRANCE for 31 December 1900 as: '1856. MUSSAT, professeur aux Ecoles nationales de Grignon et de Versailles, boulevard Saint-Germain, 11, à Paris, Ve'. Haskell Field Norman (1915–1996) was a psychoanalyst and bibliophile many of whose books were sold at auction in 1384 lots by Christie's, New York, between 18 March and 29 October 1998 (this copy #868). He also founded the Marin County branch of the International Wine and Food Society (1976). Norman wrote *One hundred books famous in medicine*, New York (1995). For a much to be envied account of his collecting, see: 'My Education as a Bibliophile' by Haskell F. Norman, M.D, originally published as an introduction to *The Haskell F. Norman library of science & medicine* (1991). Jacques Lechevalier was a Parisian publisher and bookseller especially of scientific and medical works active in the nineteenth and early twentieth centuries.

[25] Bibliographers may question the inclusion of this copy as a separate issue. The justification is that it suggests that the final signatures of the quarto were eventually simplified with realization that the advertisements for Richard Davis's books were no longer needed and the index was sufficient. Whether the half title g2 was also discarded or missing from this copy is unclear.

5B1. DE ANIMA BRUTORUM, London octavo 1672

The first issue of the second edition of Willis's fifth book, printed in London for sale in Oxford [HJR Wing 28, Oldfield A2].

Title page: De | ANIMA | BRUTORUM | QUÆ | *Hominis* Vitalis ac Senſitiva eſt, | EXERCITATIONES DUÆ. | PRIOR PHYSIOLOGICA | Ejuſdem Naturam, partes, Potentias | & Affectiones tradit; | ALTERA PATHOLOGICA | Morbos qui ipſam, & ſedem ejus Primariam, | NEMPE | CEREBRUM & NERVOSUM | GENUS afficiunt, explicat, eorúmque | THERAPEIAS inſtituit, cum Figuris Æneis. | [rule] | STUDIO | *THOMÆ WILLIS* M.D. Natural. | Philoſophiæ Profeſſ. *OXON.* nec non inclyti | Medic. Colleg. *Londin.* & Societ. Reg. Socii. | [rule] | *LONDINI,* | Typis *E.F.* Impenſis *Ric. Davis, Oxon.* 1672.[26]

Collation: octavo; 23 letter roman alphabet using I and V: A^8, a–b^8, B–Z^8, Aa–Dd^8; $1–4 signed, apart from: -S4.

232 leaves: paginated as [48], 1–176, [177–8], 179–400, [16]. Mispaginated: 283 for 183, 285 for 185, 233 for 221, 240 for 224.

Type: 46 lines; height (20 lines) 53 millimetres, width 65 millimetres (80 millimetres with marginal notes).

Contents: **A1r**, page [1], blank; **A1v**, page [2], Imprimatur, *Sam. Parker Reverend. in Chriſto Patri ac Domino D*[no] Gilberto *Archiep. Cant. à Sac. Dom.*; **A2r**, page [3], title; **A2v**, page [4], blank; **A3r–A4v**, pages [5–8], REVERENDISSIMO in CHRISTO Patri, & Domino, D[no] GILBERTO, PROVIDENTIA DIVINA *Archiepiſcopo Cantuarienſi,* totius ANGLIÆ Primati, & Metropolitano, & Augiſtiſſimo Principi CAROLO II. *M. Britanniæ Franciæ, & Hiberniæ* Regi, à Secretioribus Conſiliis. ... [signed] *Clementiæ Veſtræ Cultorem humillimum, ſervum devotiſſimum* THO. WILLIS.; **A5r–A5v**, pages [9–10], ERUDITISSIMIS, ET VENERABILIBUS VIRIS, Mihíque æternum colendis, D. VICECANCELLARIO, DOCTORIBUS, & MAGISTRIS, Qui in Celeberrimâ Univerſitate *Oxonienſi* BONAS LITERAS Diligentiſſimè excolunt, egregiè ornant, Feliciſſimè promovent, SALUTEM. ... [signed] Clariſſimi Domini Veſtrum omnium Cultori addictiſſimo THO. WILLIS.; **A6r–a1v**, pages [11–18], PRÆFATIO AD LECTOREM.; **a2r–a7v**, pages [19–30], ELENCHUS RERUM, In Tractatu DE ANIMA BRUTORUM, Sive parte primâ.; **a8r–b7r**, pages [31–45], ELENCHUS RERUM. PARS II. PATHOLOGICA.; **b7v**, page [46], blank; **b8r**, page [47] [half title] DE ANIMA BRRUTORUM QUÆ *Hominis* Vitalis ac Senſitiva eſt, Pars Prima PHYSIOLOGICA, Ejuſdem Naturam, partes, Potentias & affectiones tradens.; **b8v**, page [48], blank.

B1r–M8v, pages 1–176, [text] DE ANIMA BRUTORUM; **N1r**, page [177], [half title] PARS SECUNDA *PATHOLOGICA* SIVE De Morbis Quæ ad Animam Corpoream, ejuſque ſubjecta, ſcilicet Cerebrum, & Genus nervoſum ſpectant.; **N1v**, page [178], blank; **N2r–Cc8v**, pages 179–400, [text] PARS SECUNDA.

Dd1r–Dd8v, pages [1–16] INDEX ALPHABETICUS Rerum & Verborum.

[26] EF is Elizabeth Flesher, see chapter 3.

Headlines and *Catchwords*: no CAP at **B1r**, page 1; **D3v**, page 38; **E2v**, page 52; **E5v**, page 58; **N2r**, page 179; **P4r**, page 215; **Q3r**, page 229; **Q7v**, page 238; **R2v**, page 244; **R5r**, page 249; **S4r**, page 263; **T3v**, page 278; **X2v**, page 308; **Z4v**, page 344; **Cc1v**, page 386; no ⁏ after headline at **B7v**, page 14; ⁏ added after headline at **D4v**, page 40; *visu.* for *Visu.* at **K5v**, page 138, **L3r**, page 149; **L6r**, page 155; CAP II for CAP. I. at **O1r**, page 193; no ⁏ after headline at **P4v**, page 216; CAP. VI. for CAP. IV. at **Q6v**, page 236; CAP. IX. for CAP. XI. at **Y5v**, page 330.

No catchword at **A5v** / **A6r**, pages [10] / [11]; **a1v** / **a2r**, pages [18] / [19]; viden- for evidentes at **b1r** / v, pages [33] / [34]; 1 igirur for 1° igitur at **B7r** / v, pages 13 / 14; onibus for tionibus at **N12v** / **O1r**, pages 192 / 193; fecretas for fecretos at **P3r** / **P3v**, pages 213 / 214; cunque for cunq; at **S5v** / **S6r**, pages 266 / 267; cut for ficut at **T12v** / **V1r**, pages 288 / 289; dole for indole at **Y4v** / **Y5r**, pages 328 / 329.

Frontispiece: none.

Portrait: none.

Printers' ornaments: two rows each of 10 fleurons placed horizontally and reversed alternately, separated by ? between ##5 / 6 in each row at **N1r**, page [177]; two rows each of 12 arranged vertically, the lower row inverted, separated by : between ##7 / 8 in each row, at **N2r**, page [179] {**Fell 2**}.

No decorated initials.

Illustrations: as in **5A1** apart from:

Pl.19a2. Plate 19 (images 30–33): *page* [*3*]*68* erased and replaced with *page* 33 (headline, left). Folding, 207 × 155 millimetres (sheet). Inserted within legends for Tabulæ I–IV at **C8v–D3r**, pages 32–7.

Pl.20a2. Plate 20 (images 34–35): *page* [*3*]*68* erased and replaced with *page* 33 (headline, right). Folding, 190 × 216 millimetres (sheet). Inserted within legends for Tabulæ I–IV at **C8v–D3r**, pages 32–7.

Pl.21a2. Plate 21 (images 36–38): *page* [*3*]*68* erased and replaced with *page* 33 (headline, right). Folding, 258 × 195 millimetres (sheet). Inserted within legends for Tabulæ I–IV at **C8v–D3r**, pages 32–7.

Pl.22a2. Plate 22 (images 39–41): *page 68* erased and replaced with *page* 36 (headline, left). Folding, 205 × 166 millimetres (sheet). Inserted within legends for Tabulæ I–IV at **C8v–D3r**, pages 32–7.

Pl.23a2. Plate 23 (image 42): *page 86* erased and replaced with *page 49* (headline, right). 190 × 144 millimetres (sheet). Inserted within legends for Tabulæ V–VII at **E1r–E2r**, pages 49–51.

Pl.24a2. Plate 24 (image 43): *page 86* erased and replaced with *page 50* (headline, left). 161 × 109 millimetres (sheet). Inserted within legends for Tabulæ V–VII at **E1r–E2r**, pages 49–51.

Pl25a2. Plate 25 (image 44): *page 86* erased and replaced with *page 51* (headline, left). 162 × 133 millimetres (sheet). Inserted within legends for Tabulæ V–VII at **E1r–E2r**, pages 49–51.

Pl26a2. Plate 26 (image 45): *page 126* erased and replaced with *page 80* (headline, left). 188 × 188 millimetres (sheet). Inserted within legend for Tabula VIII at **F8v–G1r**, pages 80–1.

Copy: DASC (#1 of 2). Original calf with blind stamped central panel, double-lined borders, and floral ornaments at each corner, double rule to boards, spine (rebacked) with four raised bands, double blind lines to each, labelled in gilt with double-lined birder, DE | ANIMA | BRUTORUM | THO. WILLIS / 1672, original endpapers. Leaves 150 × 95 millimetres, boards 153 × 95 × 37 millimetres. Inscribed: Saul Jarcho, MD College of Physicians and Surgeons Columbia University V–1942 (twice).[27]

5B2.c1. DE ANIMA BRUTORUM, London octavo 1672

The second issue of the second edition of Willis's fifth book, with the title page reset identifying the London imprint in its first state [HJR Wing 29, Oldfield A2a].

Title page: De | ANIMA | BRUTORUM | QUÆ | *Hominis* Vitalis ac Senſitiva eſt, | EXERCITATIONES DUÆ. | PRIOR PHYSIOLOGICA | Ejuſdem Naturam, partes, Potentias | & Affectiones tradit; | ALTERA PATHOLOGICA | Morbos qui ipſam, & ſedem ejus Primariam, | NEMPE | CEREBRUM & NERVOSUM | GENUS afficiunt, explicat, eorúmque | THERAPEIAS inſtituit, cum Figuris Æneis. | [rule] | STUDIO | *THOMÆ WILLIS* M.D. Natural. | Philoſophiæ Profeſſ. *OXON*. nec non inclyti | Medic. Colleg. *Londin*. & Societ. Reg. Socii. | [rule] | *LONDINI*, | Proſtant apud *Gulielm. Wells, & Rob. Scot*, 1672.

Then as in **5B1**.

Copy: DASC. Original calf, spine with five raised bands, gilt decorated panels, labelled DE | ANIMA | BRVTOR, original endpapers. Leaves 157 × 92 millimetres, boards 163 × 98 × 34 millimetres. Stamped: (1) 87 686; (2) INSTITUT CATHOLIQUE DE PARIS.[28]

5B2.c2. DE ANIMA BRUTORUM, London octavo 1672

The second issue of the second edition of Willis's fifth book, with the title page reset identifying the London imprint in its second state [not distinguished from HJR Wing 29, Oldfield A2a].[29]

[27] Saul Wallenstein Jarcho (1906–2000) graduated from Harvard University and took a master's degree in Latin literature at Columbia University. He then trained in medicine at Columbia and studied pathology in Puerto Rica. He taught this subject at Columbia and the Johns Hopkins Hospital. During the Second World War Jarcho was chief medical intelligence officer in the Office of the Surgeon General. In retirement he was fully occupied with research into the history of medicine taking a particular interest in disorders of the heart, serving as president of the American Association for the History of Medicine, and active in the section on historical medicine of the New York Academy of Medicine.

[28] The Catholic University of Paris (founded 1875) has a library with 600 000 volumes that includes 60 000 antiquarian books and 800 manuscripts, many donated by Edmonds de Fel (nd).

[29] As noted by Oldfield (1991): page 20, the differences from **5B2.c1** are on the title page, 'Partes' in place of 'partes' at line 8; and 'affectiones' in place of 'Affectiones' at line 9, each with different spacing.

Title page: De | ANIMA | BRUTORUM | QUÆ | *Hominis* Vitalis ac Senſitiva eſt, | EXERCITATIONES DUÆ. | PRIOR PHYSIOLOGICA | Ejuſdem Naturam, Partes, Potentias | & affectiones tradit; | ALTERA PATHOLOGICA | Morbos qui ipſam, & ſedem ejus Primariam, | NEMPE | CEREBRUM & NERVOSUM | GENUS afficiunt, explicat, eorúmque | THERAPEIAS inſtituit, cum Figuris Æneis. | [rule] | STUDIO | *THOMÆ WILLIS* M.D. Natural. | Philoſophiæ Profeſſ. *OXON*. nec non inclyti | Medic. Colleg. *Londin.* & Societ. Reg. Socii. | [rule] | *LONDINI*, | Proſtant apud *Gulielm. Wells*, & *Rob. Scot*, 1672.

Then as in **5B1**.

Copy: DASC. Original calf, spine with five raised bands, gilt decorated panels, labelled DE ANIMA | BRVTORVM, original endpapers. Leaves 155 × 92 millimetres, boards 163 × 95 × 38 millimetres.

5B3. DE ANIMA BRUTORUM, Amsterdam octavo 1672

The third issue of the second edition of Willis's fifth book, with the title page reset and in the same state as **2B2.c1** apart from indicating the Amsterdam imprint [HJR Wing 30, Oldfield A2b].

Title page: De | ANIMA | BRUTORUM | QUÆ | *Hominis* Vitalis ac Senſitiva eſt, | EXERCITATIONES DUÆ. | PRIOR PHYSIOLOGICA | Ejuſdem Naturam, partes, Potentias | & Affectiones tradit; | ALTERA PATHOLOGICA | Morbos qui ipſam, & ſedem ejus Primariam, | NEMPE | CEREBRUM & NERVOSUM | GENUS afficiunt, explicat, eorúmque | THERAPEIAS inſtituit, cum Figuris Æneis. | [rule] | STUDIO | *THOMÆ WILLIS* M.D. Natural. | Philoſophiæ Profeſſ. *OXON*. nec non inclyti | Medic. Colleg. *Londin.* & Societ. Reg. Socii. | [rule] | *AMSTELODAMI*, | Apud *Joannem Blaeu*, M DC LXXII.

Then as in **5B1**.

Copy: DASC. Original calf, spine (relaid) with four raised bands, four gilt decorated and bordered panels, gilt stamped WILLIS. DE | ANIMA | BRVTORVM, new endpapers. Leaves 154 × 94 millimetres, boards 162 × 98 × 42 millimetres. Inscribed: Naudin.[30]

5C. DE ANIMA BRUTORUM, Amsterdam duodecimo 1674

The third edition of Willis's fifth book, with the type reset and the plates reengraved, published in Amsterdam [HJR Wing 31, Oldfield A3].

[30] Charles Victor Naudin (1815–1899) was a French naturalist and botanist who joined the herbarium of the National Museum of Natural History in 1846 where he studied Brazilian flora, introducing *Jubaea chilensis* into France. He continued private work in horticulture and studying the weather after a neurological disease left him deaf and threatened his eyesight. Naudin was interested in heredity and natural selection, some claiming that his work from 1852 preceded that of Charles Darwin (1809–1882). Naudin explained the process of artificial selection in plants: 'we do not think that Nature has made her species in a different fashion from that in which we proceed ourselves in order to make our variations'. But Darwin held that Naudin did not 'show how selection acts under nature'.

Title page: DE | ANIMA | BRUTORUM | *Quæ* | Hominis Vitalis ac Senſitiva | eſt, Exercitationes Duæ. | PRIOR PHYSIOLOGICA | *Ejuſdem Naturam, partes, Potentias* | *& Affectiones tradit*; | ALTERA PATHOLOGICA | Morbus qui ipſam, & ſedem | ejus Primariam, | NEMPE | *Cerebrum & Nervoſum Genus afficiunt*, | *explicat, eorumque Therapeias inſtituit*, | *cum Figuris Æneis.* | *STUDIO* | THOMÆ WILLIS M.D. Natural. | Philoſophiæ Profeſſ. Oxon. nec non inclyti Medic. | Colleg. Londin. & Societ. Reg. Socii. | [ornaments] | AMSTELODAMI, | Apud JOANNEM à SOMEREN, 1674.

Collation: duodecimo; 23 letter roman alphabet using I and V: $*\text{–}**^{12}$, A–Z^{12}, Aa^{12}; $1–7 signed, apart from: -N3, -P3 [signed in some other copies], -T7.

312 leaves: paginated as [48], 1–240, [241–2], 243–552, [24]. Mispaginated: 224 for 324, 245 for 345.

Type: 41 lines; height (20 lines) 53 millimetres, width 49 millimetres (62 millimetres with marginal notes).

Contents: ***1r**, page [1], title; ***1v**, page [2], blank; ***2r**–***3v**, pages [3–6], *Reverendiſſimo in Chriſto Patri, & Domino*, D[no] GILBERTO, PROVIDENTIA DIVINA Archiepiſcopo Cantuarienſi, totius Angliæ Primati, & Metropolitano, & Augiſtiſſimo Principi CAROLO II. Magnæ Britanniæ, Franciæ, & Hiberniæ Regi, à Secretioribus Conſiliis. ... [signed] *Clementiæ Veſtræ* Cultorem humillimum, *Servum devotiſſimum* THOM. WILLIS; ***4r**–***4v**, pages [7–8], Eruditiſſimis, & venerabilibus VIRIS, *Mihíque æternùm colendis*, D. VICECANCELLARIO, Doctoribus, & Magiſtris, *Qui in* Celeberrimâ Univerſitate Oxonienſi Bonas Literas Diligentiſſimè excolunt, egregiè ornant, Feliciſſimè promovent, SALUTEM. ... [signed] Clariſſimi Domini *Veſtrum omnium Cultori addictiſſimo* THOM. WILLIS.; ***5r**–***9v**, pages [9–18], PRÆFATIO AD LECTOREM.; ***10r**–****3v**, pages [19–30], ELENCHUS RERUM, *In Tractatu* DE ANIMA BRUTORUM, Sive parte primâ.; ****4r**–****11v**, pages [31–46], PARS II. PATHOLOGICA.; ****12r**, page [47], [half title] DE ANIMA BRUTORUM *Quæ* Hominis Vitalis ac Senſitiva eſt, PARS PRIMA PHYSIOLOGICA, *Ejuſdem Naturam, partes, Potentias & affectiones tradens.*; ****12v**, page [48], blank.

A1r–**K12v**, pages 1–240, [text] DE ANIMA BRUTORUM [pars prima]; **L1r**, page [241], [half title] PARS SECUNDA PATHOLOGICA SIVE DE MORBIS Quæ ad Animam Corpoream, ejuſque ſubjecta, ſcilicet Cerebrum, & Genus nervoſum ſpectant.; **L1v**, page [242], blank; **L2r**–**Z12v**, pages 243–552, [text] [De anima brutorum] PARS SECUNDA.

Aa1r–**Aa10v**, pages [1–20], INDEX ALPHABETICUS *Rerum & Verborum.*; **Aa11r**–**Aa12v**, pages [21–4], blank.

Headlines and *Catchwords*: ⁏ for ⁚ after headline at ***10r**, page [19]; *corpoream* for *Corpoream* at **A8r**, page 15; no ⁏ after headline at **C6v**, page 60; **C7v**, page 62; **C8v**, page 64; CAP- for CAP. at **I6r**, page 203; **I9r**, page 209; *De stupiditate* for *sive Marosi* at **X7r**, page 493.

cens for cèns at **H10r** / v, pages 187 / 188; planè for plane at **N2r** / v, pages 291 / 292; mò (letter inverted) for mò at **N8v** / **N9r**, pages 304 / 305; cunque for utcunque at **P6v** / **P7r**, pages 348 / 349.

Frontispiece: none.

Portrait: none.

Printers' ornaments: inverted triangle of 3 fleurons on title page at *__1r__, page [1] {__Someren 1__}; tailpiece at **__12v__, page [46] {__Someren 4__}.

Decorated Q at *__2r__, page [3]; __A1r__, page 1{__Someren 2__}; E at *__5r__, page [9] {__Someren 3__}; A at __Aa1r__, page [1] {__Someren 5__}.

Illustrations: legends as in __5A__.

__Pl.19b1__. Plate 19 (images 30–33): *page. 44* (headline, left), *Tab. I.*^{a} (headline, right), *Fig. I.*^{a}, *Fig. II.*^{da}, *Fig. IIII.*^{ta}, *Fig. III.*^{tia} (headers, above each figure); lettering to depict structures (in multiples of ≤ 6 on any one figure) *a–d*. Folding, 195 × 146 (sheet); printed from a larger plate (plate marks at upper and left borders; no lines); 46 × 25 millimetres, 118 × 88 millimetres, 76 × 104 millimetres, 110 × 17 millimetres (figures). Inserted within legends for Tabulæ I–IV at __B10v–C2v__, pages 44–52.

__Pl.20b1__. Plate 20 (images 34–35): *Tab. II.*^{da} (headline, centre), *page 46* (headline, right), *Fig. I*^{a}, *Fig. II.* ^{da} (headers, above each image), lettering to depict structures (in multiples of ≤ 4) W–Z, *a–h*, *k–r*, *t*, *u*, w, *x*, 1–*3*. Folding, 143 × 190 millimetres (sheet); printed from a larger plate (plate marks at right and lower borders; no lines); 105 × 82 millimetres, 128 × 90 millimetres (figures). Inserted within legends for Tabulæ I–IV at __B10v–C2v__, pages 44–52.

__Pl.21b1__. Plate 21 (images 36–38): *Tab. III.*^{tia} (headline, centre), *pag 50.* (headline, right), *Figura. 1.*^{ma}, *Fig. II.*^{da}., *Fig. III.*^{tia} (headers, above each figure); lettering to depict structures (in multiples of ≤ 4) *a–i*, k, *l–u*, w–*y*, *α–δ*, *κ*, *1–6*. Folding, 243 × 165 millimetres (sheet); printed from a larger plate, >243 × 155 millimetres (plate marks at left border, line at right edge); 241 × 99 millimetres, 120 × 84 millimetres, 46 × 16 millimetres (figures). Inserted within legends for Tabulæ I–IV at __B10v–C2v__, pages 44–52.

__Pl.22b1__. Plate 22 (images 39–41): *Tab. IIII.* (headline, left), *page. 52.* (headline, right), *Fig. I.*^{ma}, *Fig. II.*^{da}, *Fig. III.*^{tia} (headers, above each image), lettering to depict structures (in multiples of ≤ 5) *a–c*, *e–i*, *k*. Folding, 176 × 136 millimetres (sheet); printed from a larger plate 176 × >134 millimetres (plate marks at right and lower borders, line at upper edge); 155 × 65 millimetres, 44 × 17 millimetres, 164 × 15 millimetres (figures). Inserted within legends for Tabulæ I–IV at __B10v–C2v__, pages 44–52.

__Pl.23b1__. Plate 23 (image 42): *page. 69.* (headline, left), *Tab. V.* (headline right); lettering to depict structures (in multiples of ≤ 2) *a–i*, *k*, *l–u*, *w*. Folding, 176 × 115 millimetres (sheet); printed from a larger plate (plate mark at right border, line at upper edge); 155 × 97 millimetres (figure). Inserted within legends for Tabulæ V–VII at __C9v–C11r__, pages 66–9.

__Pl.24b1__. Plate 24 (image 43): *page. 68.* (headline, left), *Tab. VI.* (headline right); lettering to depict structures (in multiples of ≤ 3) *a–i*, *k*, *l–m*. Folding, 135 × 105 millimetres (sheet); printed from a larger plate (no plate marks, line at right edge); 128 × 85 millimetres (figure). Inserted within legends for Tabulæ V–VII at __C9v–C11r__, pages 66–9.

Pl.25b1. Plate 26 (image 44): *page 69.* (headline, left), *Tab. VII.* (headline right); lettering to depict structures (in multiples of ≤ 2) *a–i*. Folding, 135 × 118 millimetres (sheet); printed from a larger plate (no plate marks or lines); 118 × 103 millimetres (figure). Inserted within legends for Tabulæ V–VII at **C9v–C11r**, pages 66–9.

Pl.26b1. Plate 27 (image 45): *page. 209.* (headline, left), *Tab. VIII.* (headline right); lettering to depict structures (in multiples of ≤ 2) *a–i*, *k–u*, *w–z*. Folding, 165 × 192 millimetres (sheet); printed from a larger plate (plate marks at upper and left borders, no lines); 146 × 169 millimetres (figure). Inserted within text of CAP. XV at **I8v**, page 208.

Copy: DASC. Original vellum, spine labelled with double gilt lines WILLIS | DE | ANIMA BRUTOR: | 1674., original endpapers. Leaves 136 × 72 millimetres, boards 147 × 77 × 37 millimetres. Inserted: label B. VII. Inscribed: in Spanish (undeciphered).

10

'The happy curing of cephalick diseases'

Pharmaceutice rationalis (1674–1679)

Willis's twelfth and thirteenth treatises, published as his sixth book in two parts, brought together ideas on how disorders of fermentation might best be treated. The Latin versions were published separately, the second part posthumously. *Pharmaceutice rationalis* part 1 appeared in a quarto edition with issues from Oxford and London (1674). These were followed by duodecimo editions from Oxford, London, and The Hague (1674–1675). Part 2 was published in quarto and duodecimo editions from Oxford (1675), and in duodecimo from The Hague (1677). Dutch translations of each treatise were published in octavo (1677, 1681). As expected, the Oxford quarto editions from 1674 and 1675 are sometimes found together in a contemporary binding. Eventually the two parts were published from Oxford as one book in octavo (1679). No errata sheet was printed but a few corrections to the headlines were made for this final edition.

Pharmaceutice rationalis: part 1

Willis dedicated the first part of *Pharmaceutice rationalis* to the Royal College of Physicians of London and its president, George Ent (1604–1689). This was despite opposition to the doctrine of fermentation and their confidence in remedies based on the principles of Galenic medicine. The treatise was completed well before 1674. In *De anima brutorum* (1672), Willis writes: 'Super his in peculiari tractatu, *de operationibus medicamentorum in corpus humanum* fuse disseruimus.' [We have already discoursed of these things in a particular Tract, *Of the Operations of Medicines on the Humane Body*].[1] Willis presented a copy to the Royal Society, which has the title page inscribed: 'Liber exhibitus Societati Regali ex dono Authoris d. 10. Decemb. 1673'. A few copies of the quarto edition from Oxford were printed on large paper but these are otherwise identical to the ordinary issue (**6A1**). The London issue (**6A2**) retained the setting of the Oxford imprint but added a final line in blank space indicating that this was to be sold (bibliopolam) by Robert Scott (1632–1710), London agent of the Oxford press. In both issues, the imprimatur reads:

> LIBRUM hunc, Authore ſuo, ſagaciſſimo Phyſiologo, Medico peritiſſimo, dignum; olim Symmiſta, ſemper Amicus, libentiſſime Typis mando. Oxon. *Octob.* 31. 1673. *RAD. BATHURST. Vice-Cancel.*

[1] See: Thomas Willis, *De anima brutorum*, Oxford (1672): page 312; *Concerning the soul of brutes* (1683): page 128 referring to *Pharmaceutice rationalis* (1674): part 1, pages 285–303; and chapter 17.

> [This BOOK, worthy of its author, most sagacious physiologist and most able physician; erstwhile a colleague, always a friend, it is with utmost pleasure that I commit it to the printer. Oxford, October 31, 1673. RALPH BATHURST, Vice-Chancellor]

All copies have the 'i' of 'Symmiſta' corrected in pen and ink to 'y'. Some words in the text combine roman and greek type: 'Systolῶν and Diaſtolῶν' at Nn1v, page 282. The occasional English word is interspersed: 'eg vulgo ventris tormina (five noſtro Idiomate) *Griping of the Guts*' at P3v / P4r, pages 118 / 119. Marginal notes are added to the quarto edition (**6A**), and those in duodecimo printed at The Hague (1674 and 1675; **6C** and **6D**). These were omitted from the duodecimo Oxford and London issues (1674; **6B1** and **6B2**) and from the octavo combining both parts of *Pharmaceutice rationalis* (1679; **6I**). The notice in the *Term Catalogue* indicates that the Oxford and London quarto issue sold for 7s and the duodecimo for 2s 6d:

> Easter 1674 May 26th, II Numb 17, I 172, column 2, *Libri Latini.*
>
> *PHARMACEUTICE Rationalis, sive Diatriba de Medicamentorum operationibus in humano corpore.* Authore Tho. Willis, M.D., in Univ. *Oxon.* Prof. *Sedleiano*, nec non Coll. Med. *Lond.* et Societ. Reg. Socio. In Quarto. Price 7s. Printed in a lesser Volume, price 2s 6d. Both sold by R. Scot at the Prince's Arms in *Little Britain.*

Pharmaceutice rationalis: part 2

The second part of *Pharmaceutice rationalis* is dedicated to colleagues in the University of Oxford and to James, 1st Duke of Ormond (1610–1688) who after a turbulent political and military career had been elected chancellor of the University on 4 August 1669:

> This Pharmaceutical Treatise I devote and dedicate to THE ATHENS OF BRITAIN, Most Splendid Light of the Literate World, THE UNIVERSITY OF OXFORD, and there to its MOST ILLUSTRIOUS PRINCIPAL JAMES DUKE OF ORMOND AND MOST HONOURED CHANCELLOR, to RALPH BATHURST, DEAN OF WELLS CATHEDRAL, MOST WORTHY VICE-CHANCELLOR, to the highly respectable and greatly learned DOCTORS, PROCTORS, PROFESSORS of all faculties, prefects of COLLEGES and HALLS, AS WELL AS the venerable Senate of Teachers, with devotion and gratefulness, your alumnus and most indebted beneficiary THOMAS WILLIS.

In his biographical essay from 1741, Browne Willis (1682–1760) made the point that the imprimatur, signed by the vice-chancellor, Ralph Bathurst (1620–1704), is dated 12 November 1675, the day after Willis died:[2]

> AMiciſſimo Authori, poſt tam Immortale opus, nihil mortale facturo, tanquam Lumina morienti claudens, extremum hoc officium præſtat

[2] See: [Browne Willis], 'Willis (Thomas)'. In: [John Bernard, Thomas Birch, John Locke, and other hands] *A general dictionary, historical and critical* etc., volume X, London (1741): pages 171–5.

[This represents the final task for the author, my greatest friend, who was to do nothing more in his mortal existence, after such an immortal work, a work that closed his eyes in death, as it were].

As the postscript by John Fell (1625–1686) indicates: 'While these were printing, the most sad message arrives, that the Author, most worthy of Immortality, oppressed by the irresistible assault of a Pleurisie, is departed from among the Living'. This unexpected event threw the arrangement of preliminary sheets since explanatory text was now needed. Fell was manager of the press in Oxford and in a position to instruct the printer at the Sheldonian Theatre to move quickly and typeset the additional material. This was done before the end of the year (although, until full replacement of the Julian with the Gregorian calendar, the 1675 imprint would have remained valid until Lady Day, 25 March 1676).

Fell's brief biographical notice on his brother-in-law is found in the quarto edition (**6E**) at b2v–c2r, pages [12–19]. Since this begins on the same sheet as Willis's own preface, it follows that the preliminary pages had not been set before he died. Fell's notice was simply printed after b2r, page [11] and its eight pages were followed by William Dawkins's (nd) dedicatory poem. Already written, and extolling the virtues of Willis as physician and friend, this was printed at c3r–c4v, pages [21–4]. The catchword AU at c2r, page [19] links across a blank at c2v, page [20]) to the start of Dawkins's dedicatory verse. This is followed by the Elenchus rerum printed at d1r–g2r, pages [25–51].

But what happened to the remaining half sheet (g3 and g4) is less clear. g2r (unsigned), page [51], has a catchword DE with no obvious link since g2v is blank and the next printed word is PHARMACEUTICE at A1r, page 1.[3] It is possible that text with DE as the first printed word was discarded in rearranging the preliminaries, but nothing obvious is missing. Even less likely is that the first page of the main text, originally starting DE, was reset. The better explanation is that the extravagant dedication by William Dawkins, written when Willis was living, was no longer appropriate and a more sober eulogy in verse was required. Therefore the available half sheet, which might otherwise have been discarded, was used to print 'Querela libri posthumi de obitu autoris'. This was signed (c)1 and [(c)2], possibly because the intention was to replace the existing dedicatory verse printed on c3 and c4 with the hastily written second poem. In the event each is always present, perhaps because Dawkins objected to removal of his original verse, or it seemed sensible to retain both the extravagant and more measured notices of his late friend.

That c^2 is printed on the remaining half of sheet g is consistent with the fact that it is bound after g2v, page [52], in all five copies examined for this bibliography and has watermarks indicating that it is conjugate with the corresponding leaves, g1 and g2. However the more logical place for the obituary in verse by William Dawkins would have been adjacent to Fell's postscriptum after c2v. HJR Wing describes this arrangement and several other variations in the copies he examined. One has much sympathy for any binder trying to organize these leaves and deciding where best to place the half sheet with Dawkins's lament.[4] The *Term Catalogue* indicates that copies of the book sold for 10s:

[3] DE is also without a link in the final page of the preliminaries in the duodecimo edition of *Pharmaceutice rationalis* part 2 (1675: **6F**) at d4v, page [44].

[4] With all these late arrangements, minor changes could be made and some leaves are found in more than one state. For example, the letter used for the 'U' of AULARUM in the dedication at a2r, page [3] varies from swash to non-swash in different copies. Other random uses of type are certain to be present elsewhere in this and other copies, but that level of detail is beyond the scope of this bibliography.

Hilary 1676 February 10th, III Numb 6, I 229, column 1, *Libri Latini.*

Pharmaceutice Rationalis, sive Diatriba de Medicamentorum operationibus in Humano corpore. Pars Secunda. Autore Tho. Willis, M.D., in Univ. *Oxon.* Professore *Sedleiano.* In Quarto. Price, bound, 10s. Printed for R. Davis, G. West, and J. Crosley.

In the event, neither George West (fl.1650-1707) nor John Crosley (fl.1664-1703), booksellers in Oxford, appear on the title page. The quarto edition (1675; 6E), but neither duodecimo (1675, 1677; 6F and 6G) has marginal notes. Generally overlooked are Dutch translations of *Pharmaceutice rationalis* printed in octavo from Middelburg and Amsterdam (1677, part 1: **6H**), and Amsterdam (1681, part 2: **6J**). As with the Dutch versions of *Diatribæ duæ* (**1H, 1J**) and *De scorbuto* (**3C**), the translator [Dr Antonius de Heide (1646–*c.*1702) for both works] added a large number of footnotes as commentary on Willis's works.[5] For the second part of *Pharmaceutice rationalis* (**6J**), but still following the original sequence, he divides Willis's text into three separate 'books': I. Medicines active on the lungs and thorax; II. Medicines active on the organs of the abdomen; and III. External manoeuvres involving surgical procedures.

The *Editio tertia* from Oxford, the only printing of both parts as a single work, has continuous signatures but repeat pagination (**6I**). The title page is dated 1679 on part 1, but 1678 on part 2. It was available from December 1678 for 6s as noted in the *Term Catalogue*:

Michaelmas 1678 December 6th, III Numb 17, I 338, column 2, *Books reprinted.*

Pharmaceutice Rationalis, sive Diatriba de Medicamentorum Operationibus in humano Corpore. Authore Tho. Willis. Editio Tertia. In Octavo. Price, bound, 6s. Printed at the Theatre, and sold by R. Davis, Bookseller in *Oxford.*

The illustrations to *Pharmaceutice rationalis*

The title pages for parts 1 and 2 of the quarto editions of *Pharmaceutice rationalis* went twice through the press in order to combine the text and engraving of Christopher Wren's (1632–1723) Sheldonian theatre. This is shown surrounded by railings with 14 burghers on plinths, as seen from the north aspect looking across from The Broad. It is engraved by David Loggan (1634–1692). The plate used for the Oxford and London issues of part 1 (**6A**) is identical but that for part 2 (**6E**) is different with alterations to the sky, and several aspects of shading and spacing on the building and plinths. The image was redone in a smaller version for the octavo 1679 edition (**6I**) with the engraver showing much less artistry and attention to detail.

The orientation of watermarks indicates that some plates were rotated with respect to arrangement of the images before printing the illustrations, presumably to fit within one forme. Perhaps for the same reason, or possibly because of damage, a few plates used for early copies of *Pharmaceutice rationalis* part 1 were subsequently cut down. The large paper copy in the Royal Society has wider boundaries than the regular issue for Tabula IIII (Pl.30), and possibly also Tabula I (Pl.27), but the engravings are otherwise identical. Page placements are present on the plates in part 1. Those in part 2 are indicated as belonging in *Sect. 1: Cap. I* but with no directions to the binder. As a result, the eight leaves are grouped, not

[5] See chapter 5 for the suggestion that a study is needed of these footnotes by an authority on Dutch medicine in the seventeenth century.

necessarily in sequence, and usually placed away from the legends, which are printed at E1r–E4v, pages 33–40.

Economies were made when the plates were reused for the duodecimo editions from Oxford and London of parts 1 (**6B**) and 2 (**6F**) by printing on the recto and verso of each sheet. This was achieved either by locking single plates together on one forme or, less likely, putting the sheet through the press several times. Since the plate sizes differ, careful arrangement was needed to ensure that those on each side were not cropped when cutting the sheet. It is likely that Tabulæ I, III, and V (Pl.27a2, Pl.29a2, and Pl.31a2) were printed on one side and Tabulæ II, IV, and VI (Pl.28a2, Pl.30a2, and Pl.32a2) on the other for each of the duodecimo 1674 issues of part 1 (**6B1, 6B2**). The original page placements were left untouched at the top right, but blank space used to engrave new details; for example, *12º p. 24* added at the top left corner of Tabula I. For the duodecimo edition of part 2 (**6F**), it is likely that Tabulæ I, III, V, and VII (Pl.33a2, Pl.35a2, Pl.37a2, and Pl.39a2) were printed on one side of the sheet, and Tabulæ II, IV, VI, and VIII (Pl.34a2, Pl.36a2, Pl.38a2, and Pl.40a2) on the other.

The Dutch publishers reengraved the plates for both parts of *Pharmaceutice rationalis*. With the exception of illustrations for the Dutch translation of part 2, these were printed on one side of each sheet from large engraved plates and cut for binding. Several leaves have one deckled edge where the illustration has been torn from the larger sheet, or a jagged cut with the knife. Those engraved for the duodecimo editions of part 1 (1674, **6C**) were reused in an altered state for both the second duodecimo edition (1675, **6D**) and the octavo translation in Dutch (1677, **6H**). The illustrations were also reengraved for part 2 issued from The Hague (1677, **6G**). These are faithful but with slightly different etching and occasional letters omitted (for example, Pl.35b1; Tabula III; Figure 2). In making these changes, the four figures of Tabula VII (Pl.39b1) were engraved as mirror images of those in the Oxford quarto and duodecimo editions (**6E, 6F**). However, the plates were no longer available for the octavo Dutch translation of part 2, for which new engravings were made (1681, **6J**). Unlike the earlier Dutch engravings, the eight leaves were printed from individual plates.

The original engravings were still usable when the Latin edition in one volume was published from Oxford in 1679 (**6I**). The illustrations were bound in groups. Page placements were added but those relevant to part 1 were not distinguished from the plates for part 2. By ill luck, the page numbers were sometimes identical. As a result, it was not clear to the binder which plates belonged in which part and more often than not he got this wrong.[6] This confusion needed to be resolved when the engraved plates were used again for the English translation printed in folio: *Pharmaceutice rationalis* (1679, **9A**). Now, in addition to page placements and the section and chapter indicators for illustrations to part 2, details were added specifying to which part of the complete work each illustration belonged so that, for the first time, these were correctly bound.[7]

[6] HJR Wing suggests that the mistakes mainly relate to Tabs V and VI from each part but this is too simple. Each of the five copies examined for this bibliography has plates belonging to part 2 bound in part 1, and vice versa, or eight in part 1 and six in part 2 rather than six and eight, respectively. Only the copy held by the Royal Society is entirely correct.

[7] As explained in chapter 13, this only became fully apparent after Tabula 1, part 1 (Pl.27a4) had been adjusted to show the new page placement. Confusingly, even though the engraving is therefore in a new state, this might be overlooked since the page number happens to be 16 in both the octavo (**6I**) and folio (**9A**) editions.

6A1. PHARMACEUTIC RATIONALIS (part 1), Oxford quarto 1674

The first issue of the first edition of the first part of Willis's sixth book, published from Oxford [HJR Wing 32].

Title page: PHARMACEUTICE RATIONALIS. | SIVE | DIATRIBA | *DE MEDICAMENTORUM* | Operationibus in humano Corpore. | AUTHORE | *Tho. Willis* M.D. in *Univ. Oxon* Prof. Sedleiano, | Nec non *Coll. Med. Lond.* & Societ. Reg. Socio. | [ornament] | E THEATRO SHELDONIANO. [short rule over date] M. DC. LXXIV.

Collation: quarto; 23 letter roman alphabet using I, V and Uu: a–d^4, A–Z^4, Aa–Tt^4, Uu^2; $1 and 2 signed apart from: -c2, c4 signed c2, V2 signed U2.

186 leaves: paginated as [32], 1–330, [10]. Mispaginated: 216 for 116.

Type: 35 lines; height (20 lines) 94 millimetres, width 99 millimetres (199 millimetres with marginal notes).

Contents: **a1r**, page [1], title; **a1v**, page [2], blank; **a2r**, page [3], CELEBERRIMO *MEDICORUM LONDINENSIUM* COLLEGIO; Et Singulatim VIRO INSIGNISSIMO DOCTISSIMOQUE D^{no} GEORGIO ENT EQUITI AURATO Præſidi Illuſtriſſimo, Nec non CENSORIBUS DIGNISSIMIS, Cæteriſque omnibus, ampliſſimæ hujus Societatis Membris. DIATRIBAM HANC PHARMACEUTICAM Obſervantiæ & Honoris ergo Dicat, Dedicatque, THO. WILLIS.; **a2v**, page [4], [imprimatur] LIBRUM hunc, Authore ſuo, ſagaciſſimo Phyſiologo, Medico peritiſſimo, dignum; olim Symmi[y]ſta, ſemper Amicus, libentiſſime Typis mando. Oxon. *Octob.* 31. 1673. *RAD. BATHURST. Vice-Cancel.*; **a3r–b2v**, page [5–12], *CANDIDO LECTORI* PRÆFATIO.; **b3r–d4r**, page [13–31], ELENCHUS RERUM.; **d4v**, page [32], blank.

A1r–Tt1v, pages 1–330, [text] DE MEDICAMENTORUM OPERATIONIBUS IN Corpore Humano.

Tt2r–Uu2v, page [1–10], INDEX ALPHABETICUS.

Headlines and *Catchwords*: CAP. III for CAP. II., at **K1r**, page 73; **P2r**, page 115; *Formnlæ.* for *Formulæ.* at **P1r**, page 113; *Sudatione* for *Sudore* at **Ff4v**, page 232; *Opiatis.* for *Medicamentis Opiatis.* at **Oo2v**, page 292; and *Nocumentia.* for *nocumentia.* at **Qq3r**, page 309.

debiles for debilis at **Ee4v** / **Ff1r**, pages 224 / 225.

Frontispiece: none.

Portrait: none.

Printers' ornaments: printers' device at **a1r**, page [1] {**Fell 3**}; headpiece at **a3r**, page [5]; **A1r**, page 1 {**Fell 4**}.

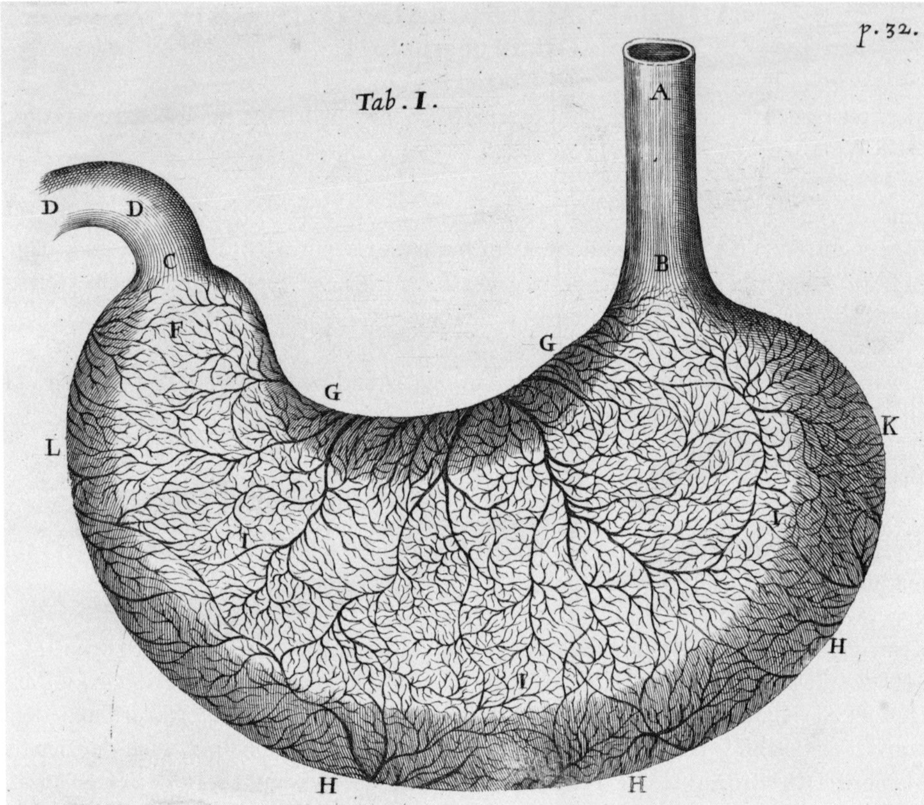

Figure 131 Plate 27 (image 46). The firſt Table repreſents a Mans Stomach taken out and blown up, with the Veſſels full of Bloud; ſo that all the Arteries and Veins, with their branches (which are truly and exactly delineated) may be plainly ſeen. Image from *Pharmaceutice rationalis* part 1 1674; legend from *Dr Willis's practice of physick* 1684.

Decorated Q at **a3r**, page [5] {**Fell 5**}; A at **A1r**, page 1 {**Fell 6**}.

Illustrations: **Pl.27a1**. Plate 27 (image 46): *Tab. I.* (headline, centre), *p. 32.* (headline, right); lettering to depict structures (in multiples of ≤ 3) A–D, F–I, K–L. Folding, 183 × 205 millimetres (sheet); 160 × 202 millimetres (plate marks); 150 × 175 millimetres (figure). Legend: TAbula prima repræſentat Hominis Ventriculum, cum vaſis ſanguine turgidis exemtum, & inflatum, ut Arteriæ & Venæ omnes cum ramificationibus earum, (quæ verè & exactiſſime delineantur) conſpici poſſint. Inserted within legends for Tabula I–VI at **D4v–E2v**, pages 32–6; see: Figure 131.

Pl.28a1. Plate 28 (image 47): *Tab. II.* (headline, centre), *p. 33.* (headline, right); lettering to depict structures (in multiples of ≤ 3) A–G. Folding, 180 × 202 millimetres (sheet); 157 × 198 millimetres (plate marks); 128 × 174 millimetres (figure). Legend: TABULA II. exprimit Ventriculi Humani Tunicam extimam prorſus nerveam, cujus fibræ nervæ per longitudinem ejus ductæ carneas exteriores ſubſtratas ad rectos fere angulos ſecant. Inserted within legends for Tabula I–VI at **D4v–E2v**, pages 32–6; see: Figure 132.

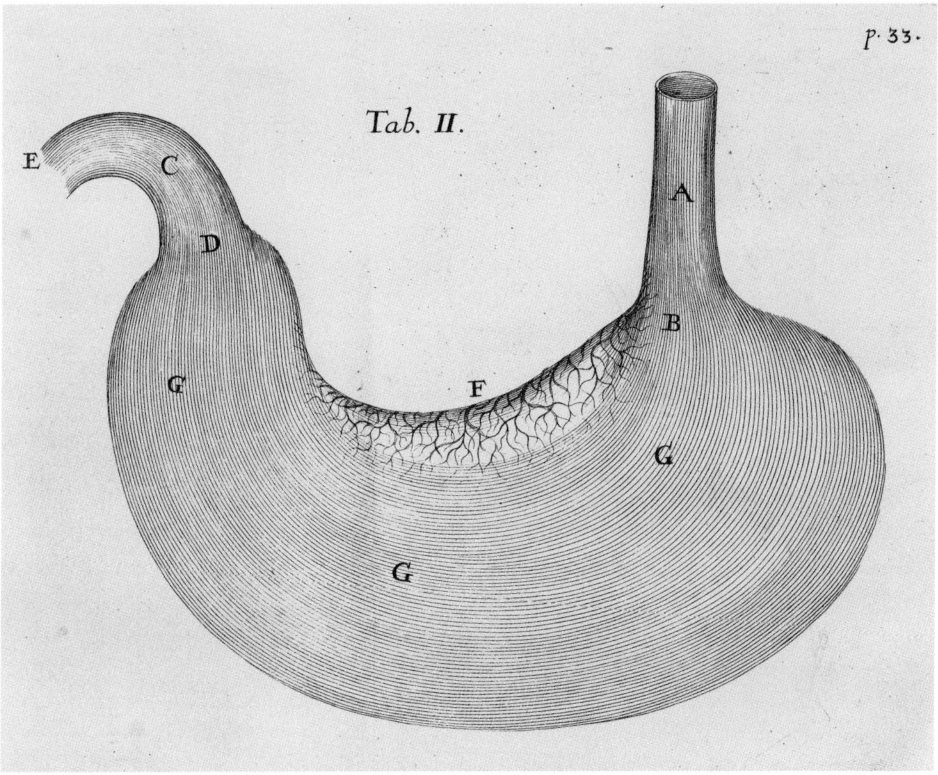

Figure 132 Plate 28 (image 47). The ſecond Table expreſſes the outmoſt coat of a Mans Stomach, which is altogether nervous; whoſe nervous fibres running out the whole length of it, cut the outward fleſhy ones that are under them almoſt at right angles. Image from *Pharmaceutice rationalis* part 1 1674; legend from *Dr Willis's practice of physick* 1684.

Pl.29a1. Plate 29 (image 48): *Tab. III.* (headline, centre), *p. 34.* (headline, right); lettering to depict structures (in multiples of ≤ 3) A–E, a–b. Folding, 182 × 199 millimetres (sheet); 160 × 195 millimetres (plate marks); 143 × 178 millimetres (figure). Legend: TABULA III. exhibit Ventriculú Humanum Turnica extima nervea nudatum, ut Tunicæ mediæ cum fibris ejus carneis ſuperficies exterior ſive convexa appareat. Inserted within legends for Tabula I–VI at **D4v–E2v**, pages 32–6; see: Figure 133.

Pl.30a1. Plate 30 (image 49–51): *Tab. IV.* (headline, left), *p. 34.* (headline, right), *Fig. I.*, *Fig. 2.*, *Fig. 3.* (headers, above each image); lettering to depict structures (in multiples of ≤ 4) A–E. Folding, 190 × 222 millimetres (sheet, cropped); 161 × 232 millimetres (plate marks); 146 × 157 millimetres, 49 × 55 millimetres, 62 × 52 millimetres (figures). Legend: TABULA IV. Cujus figura I. oſtendit Ventriculum inverſum, cum ſuperficie interior & concava in exteriorem & convexam mutata, ut cruſta villoſa cum rugis & plicis ſtomachum obducentibus conſpiciatur. Figura II. repræſentat portionem Tunicæ nervæ, in qua, cruſtâ villoſâ exemptâ, ſuperficies interior ſive concava, cum vaſorum ramificatione denſiſſima apparet. Figura III. exhibet portionem Tunicæ villoſæ, ſive glanduloſæ, in qua ſuperficies ejus exterior, quâ Tunicæ nervæ cohæret, glandulis, & vaſorum oſculis, refertiſſima conſpicitur. Inserted within legends for Tabula I–VI at **D4v–E2v**, pages 32–36; see: Figure 134.

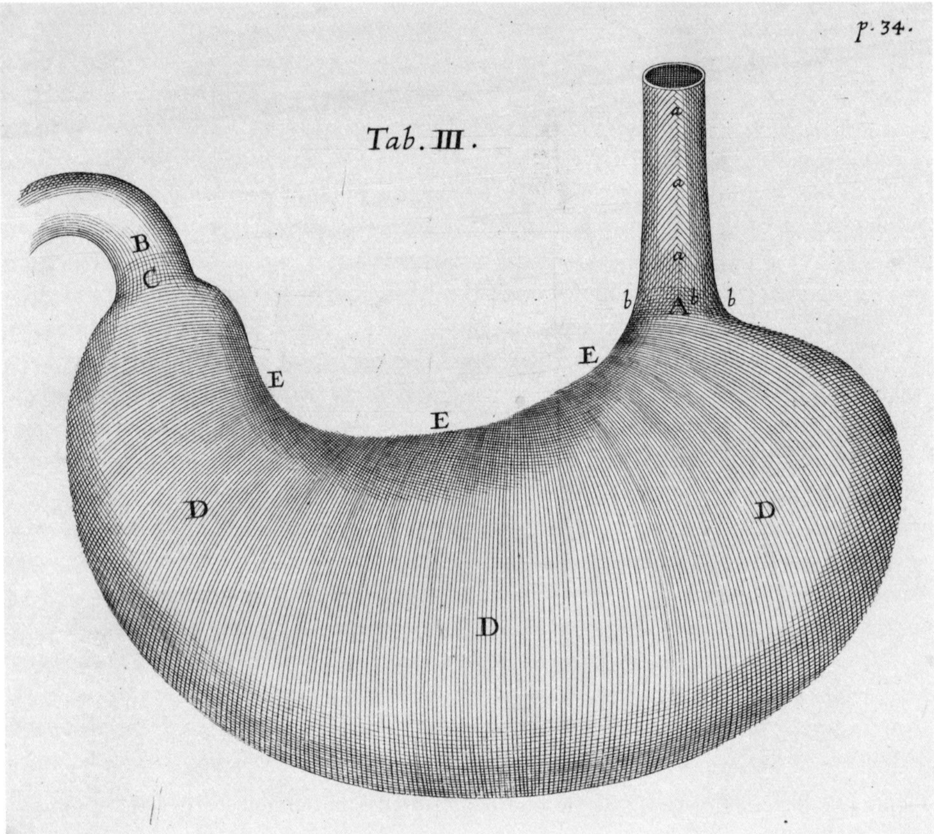

Figure 133 Plate 29 (image 48). The third Table ſhews the Stomach of a Man ſtript of its outmoſt nervous tunick or coat, that the outward or convex ſurface of its middlemoſt coat, together with the fleſhy fibres thereof, may appear. Image from *Pharmaceutice rationalis* part 1 1674; legend from *Dr Willis's practice of physick* 1684.

Pl.31a1. Plate 31 (image 52): *Tab.* V. (headline, centre), *p. 35.* (headline, right); lettering to depict structures (in multiples of ≤ 4) A, B, D–F. Folding, 185 × 195 millimetres (sheet, cropped); 165 × 200 millimetres (plate marks); 150 × 156 millimetres (figure). Legend: TABULA V. exhibet Tunicæ carnæ ſuperficiem interiorem, & concavam exterius inverſam, ut fibrarum motricium ſeries altera conſpiciatur. Inserted within legends for Tabula I–VI at **D4v–E2v**, pages 32–6; see: Figure 135.

Pl.32a1. Plate 32 (images 53–57): *Tab.* VI. (headline, centre), *p. 35.* (headline, right); lettering to depict structures (in multiples of ≤ 4) A–E. Folding, 183 × 216 millimetres (sheet, cropped); 155 × 228 millimetres (plate marks); 115 × 22 millimetres, 114 × 22 millimetres, 114 × 22 millimetres, 115 × 22 millimetres, 113 × 22 millimetres (figures). Legend: TABULA VI. repræſentat inteſtinorum gracilium Tunicas omnes ab invicem ſeparatas, ut fibræ nerveæ cum glandulis & vaſorum ramificationibus, nec non fibrarum motricum ordines, clare & diſtincte obſervari poſſint. Inserted within legends for Tabula I–VI at **D4v–E2v**, pages 32–6; see: Figure 136.

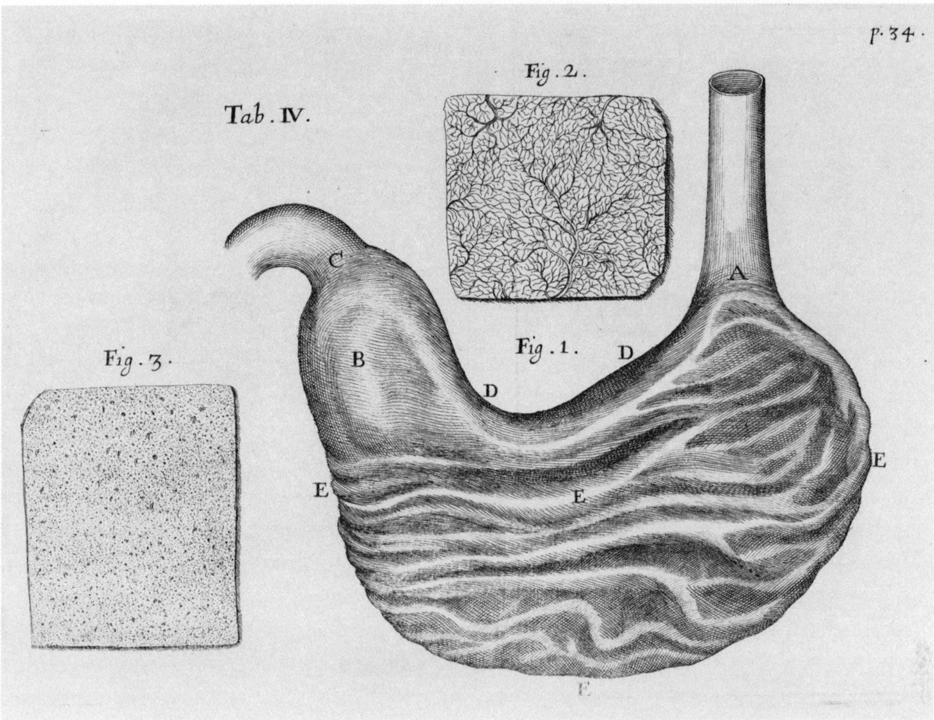

Figure 134 Plate 30 (images 49–51). The fourth Table; whofe firft Figure fhews the whole Stomach, with the inner, concave furface, changed into the outward and convex, that the hairy veil or covering, with thofe wrinkles and folds that go all over the Stomach, may come in view. Figure II. reprefents a part of the Nervous Coat, in which, the hairy covering being taken off, the inner or concave furface, together with a thick and numerous company of branches of Veffels doth appear. Figure III. Shews a part of the hairy or glandulous coat, in which the outward furface, whereby it is connected to the Nervous Coat, is apparently very full of glandules and mouths or orifices of veffels. Image from *Pharmaceutice rationalis* part 1 1674; legend from *Dr Willis's practice of physick* 1684.

Copy: DASC. Original calf with blind stamped central panel, triple-lined borders, and floral corners, edges with triple lines, spine relaid, five raised bands with double-lined borders, original endpapers. Leaves 198 × 142 millimetres, boards 205 × 140 × 52 millimetres. Inscribed: Geo Peyton Col: Balliolem 1693, with occasional annotations in his hand (bound with part 2: **6G**).[8]

[8] George Peyton (c.1676–1742) of Tewkesbury, Gloucestershire was a member of Balliol College, Oxford: he matriculated on 8 April 1693, aged 17, and qualified BA (1696), MA (1699) and Doctor of Medicine (1720). Of his subsequent career, little is known but there is a monument to him in white marble edged with gold on the north side of the chancel of St Mary's Church, Tewkesbury noting 'whose Probity and Piety, will, we hope entitle him to a Joyfull Resurrection': see William Dyde and James Johnstone, *The history and antiquities of Tewkesbury*, London (1790): page 29.

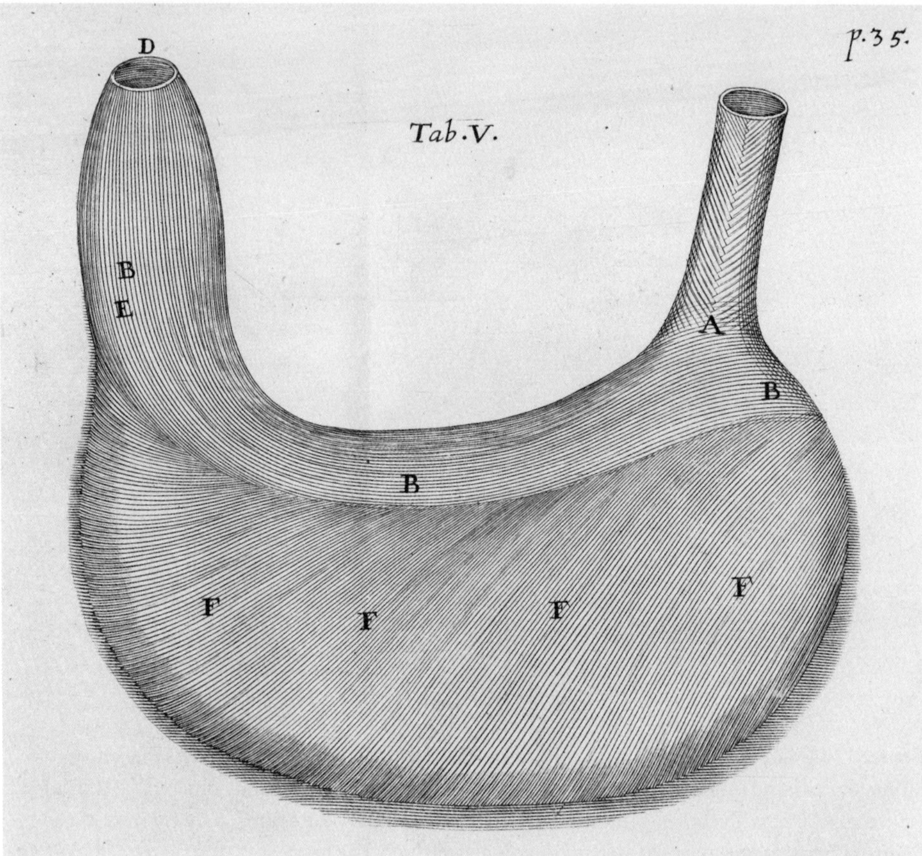

Figure 135 Plate 31 (image 52). The fifth Table ſhews the inner and concave ſurface of the fleſhy coat, turned with the wrong ſide outward, that the other row of moving fibres may come in view. Image from *Pharmaceutice rationalis* part 1 1674; legend from *Dr Willis's practice of physick* 1684.

6A2. PHARMACEUTIC RATIONALIS (part 1), Oxford and London quarto 1674

The second issue of the first edition of the first part of Willis's sixth book, published from Oxford and London [HJR Wing 33].

Title page: PHARMACEUTICE RATIONALIS. | SIVE | DIATRIBA | *DE MEDICAMENTORUM* | Operationibus in humano Corpore, | AUTHORE | *Tho. Willis* M.D. in *Univ. Oxon* Prof. Sedleiano, | Nec non *Coll. Med. Lond.* & Societ. Reg. Socio. | [ornament] | E THEATRO SHELDONIANO. [short rule over date] M. DC. LXXIV. | Proſtant apud *Robertum Scott* Bibliopolam *LONDINENSEM*.

Then as in **6A1** apart from:

Illustrations: variation in sheet sizes and occasional binding positions.

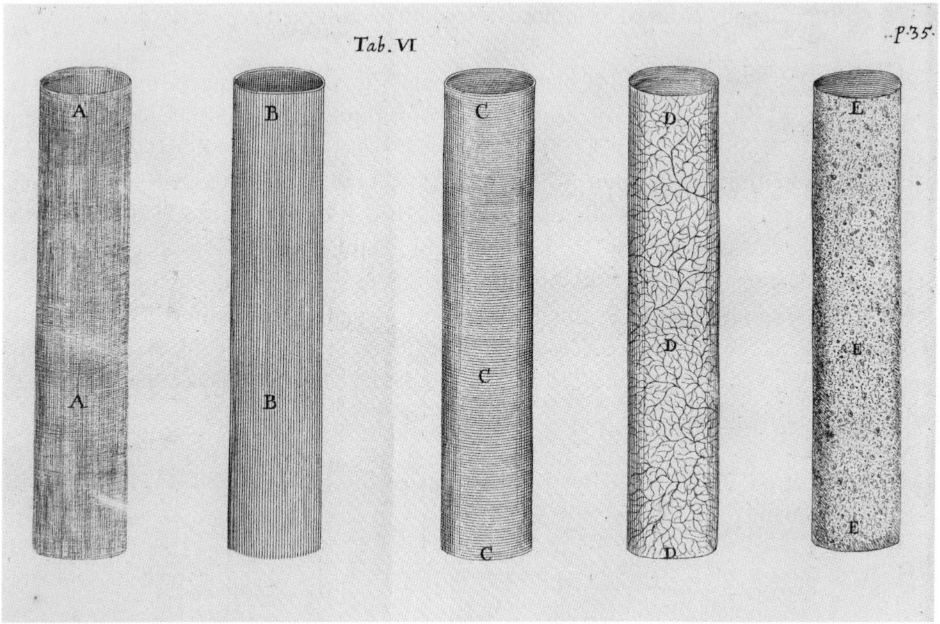

Figure 136 Plate 32 (images 53–57). The fixth Table reprefents all the Coats of the fmall Guts feparated from each other, so that the nervous fibres, with the glandules and branches of Veffels, as alfo the ranks of moving fibres may clearly and diftinctly be obferved. Image from *Pharmaceutice rationalis* part 1 1674; legend from *Dr Willis's practice of physick* 1684.

Copy: DASC (#1 of 2). Original calf, spine with four raised bands, gilt decorated panels, lettered WILL | PHAR, original endpapers. Leaves 210 × 145 millimetres, boards 217 × 145 × 27 millimetres. Inscribed: inked over (unidentified). Stamped: GILLS THOISON (unidentified) throughout.

6B1. PHARMACEUTICE RATIONALIS (part 1), Oxford duodecimo 1674

The first issue of the second edition of the first part of Willis's sixth book, published from Oxford with the illustrations all double-sided [not listed by HJR Wing].

Title page: PHARMACEUTICE RATIONALIS. | SIVE | DIATRIBA | DE | Medicamentorum | OPERATIONIBUS | in | HUMANO CORPORE. | [rule] | AUTHORE | *Tho. Willis* M.D. in *Univ. Oxon* | Prof. Sedleiano, Nec non *Coll.* | *Med. Lond.* & Societ. Reg. | Socio. | [rule] | OXON. | *E. THEATRO SHELDONIANO* | [short rule] | M. DC. LXXIV.

Collation: duodecimo in 6s: 23 letter roman alphabet using I and U: π^4, a–b^6, A–U^6; \$1–4 signed apart from: a2v signed a2; -a4, A4 signed A7, F4 signed E4, -P2, -Q4, U2 signed U3.

136 leaves: paginated as [32], 1–74, 74–80, [8]1, 8[2], 83, 83–94, 93–102, 133, 104–5, [1]06, 170, 108–20, 120–1, 123–44, 1[4]5, 146–64, 159–60, 167–202, 201, 204–6, 203, 208–30, [6]; i.e. [32], 1–234, [6].

Type: 45 lines: height (20 lines) 52 millimetres, width 63 millimetres.

Contents: **π1r–π2v**, pages [1–4] blank; **π3r**, page [5], title; **π3v**, page [6], blank; **π4r**, page [7], CELEBERRIMO *Medicorum Londinenſium* COLLEGIO, Et Singulatim VIRO INSIGNISSIMO DOCTISSIMOQUE D^no^ Georgio Ent EQUITI AURATO Præſidi Illuſtriſſimo, *Nec non CENSORIBUS DIGNISSIMIS*, Ceteriſque omnibus, ampliſſimæ hujus Societatis Membris, DIATRIBAM HANC PHARMACEUTICAM Obſservantiæ & Honoris ergo Dicat, Dedicatque, THO. WILLIS:; **π4v**, page [8], blank; **a1r**, page [9], [imprimatur] LIBRUM hunc, Authore ſuo, ſagaciſſimo Phyſiologo, Medico peritiſſimo, dignum; olim Symmyſta, ſemper Amicus, libentiſſime Typis mando. Oxon *Octob*. 31. 1673. *RAD. BATHURST. Vice-Cancel.*; **a1v**, page [10], blank; **a2r–a6v**, pages [11–20], *CANDIDO LECTORI* PRÆFATIO.; **b1r–b6v**, pages [pages 21–32], *ELENCHUS RERUM*.

A1r–U3v, pages 1–'230' (234) [text] DE MEDICAMENTORUM OPERATIONIBUS IN Corpore Humano.

U3v–U6v, page '230'–[6], *INDEX ALPHABETICUS*.

Headlines and *Catchwords*: *Eletchus.* for *Elenchus.* at **b2r**, page [23]; R*erum* for *Rerum* at **b6v**, page [32]; *Uomitoriorum* for *Vomitoriorum* at **E2r**, page 51; SECT. V. for SECT. IV. at **I4v**, page '100'; CAP. I for CAP. IV. at **L5r**, page '125'; SECT V (left) and 130 (right) for 130 (left) and SECT. V. (right) at **M1v**, page '130'; no SECT. V. at **N4v**, page '148'; SECT. IV. for SECT. V. at **O1v**, page '154'; *medicamentis* for *Medicamentis* at **P3v**, page '170'; SECT. VI. for SECT. VII. at **S1v**, page '202'; **S2v**, page '204', **S3v**, page '206'; no '.' after headline at **U6r**, page [5].

pri- for vatam at **a6r / v**, pages [19] / [20]; appo- for Appo at **O4v / O5r**, pages '160 / 161'.

Frontispiece: none.

Portrait: none.

Printers' ornaments: row of 6 fleurons {**Fell 7**} separated by a single fleuron {**Fell 8**} between ##1–2 and 5–6 at A1r, page 1.

No decorated initials.

Illustrations: as in **6A** apart from:

Pl.27a2. Plate 27 (image 46): *12º p. 24* (added to headline, left); with **Pl.28a2.** Plate 28 (image 47): *12º p. 24* (added to headline, left) on the verso. Folding, 176 × 210 millimetres (sheet). Inserted within legend for Tabula III and IV / V at **B6v–B7r**, pages 24–5.

Pl.29a2. Plate 29 (image 48): *12º p. 24* (added to headline, left); with **Pl.30a2.** Plate 30 (image 49–51): *12º p. 25* (added to headline, left) on the verso. Folding, 172 × 220 millimetres (sheet). Inserted between legend for Tabula III and IV / V at **B6v–B7r**, pages 24–5.

Pl.31a2. Plate 31 (image 52): *12º p. 25* (added to headline, left); with **Pl.32a2**. Plate 32 (images 53–57): *12º p. 26* (added to headline, left) on the verso. Folding, 174 × 212 millimetres. Inserted between legend for Tabula III and IV/V at **B6v–B7r**, pages 24–5.

Copy: Wadham (J 33.2). Original calf, spine with seven panels, lettered WILLIS | MEDICAMEN | OPERATION (faded), lacking free endpapers. Leaves 151 × 75 millimetres, boards 155 × 78 × 20 millimetres. Inscribed: (1) Liber S. Hunt e Coll. Trin. Oxon 1683; (2) Liber Wadham Collegii in Academia Oxoniensi ex Dono Alexandri Thistlethwayte. Inserted: bookplate of Alex Thistlethwayte Esq.[9]

6B2. PHARMACEUTICE RATIONALIS (part 1), Oxford and London duodecimo 1674

The second issue of the second edition of the first part of Willis's sixth book, published from Oxford and London [HJR Wing 35].[10]

Title page: *Pharmaceutice Rationalis*: | SIVE | DIATRIBA | DE | *MEDICAMENTORUM* | OPERATIONIBUS | *IN* | *HUMANO CORPORE.* | [rule] | AUTHORE | *THO. WILLIS* M.D. in *Univ. Oxon* | Prof. Sedleiano, Nec non *Coll.* | *Med. Lond.* & Societ. Reg. | Socio. | [double rule] | *E. THEATRO SHELDONIANO* | *M. DC. LXXIV.* | Proſtant apud *Robertum Scott* Bibliopolam | *LONDINENSEM.*

Then as in **6B1** apart from:

Illustrations: variation in sheet sizes and occasional binding positions.

Copy: DASC. Original calf with blind stamped double-lined border and floral corners, spine (rebacked [Athene Binding 1988]) with four raised bands, gilt lettering WILLIS | PHARMACY | 1674, original endpapers. Leaves 144 × 76 millimetres, boards 146 × 78 × 22 millimetres. Inscribed: (1) Ex Libris Alexandri Arbuthnot; (2) Liber Gulielmi Thompson emptor in Annº Dom 1686/7; (3) Wm Thompson son of G Thompson Esq. of Lytham (×3 in part, also spelled Thomson). Stamped: (1) PRESENTED TO THE LIBRARY BY Dr Harold Bentley 25 June 1947; (2) Withdrawn from [Wellcome] stock. Book label 'HB' pasted in. (all previous owners unidentified).[11]

9 Alexander Thistlethwayte (*c*.1718–1771), MP and owner of a Hampshire estate, was dubbed by Horace Walpole (1717–1797) as that most unpleasant of creatures, 'a country squire'. Thistlewayte amassed a library of over eight thousand books, and made large donations to the libraries of his alma mater Wadham College (prose works), and to Winchester College (mainly poetry). See: Will Poole, *Wadham College books in the age of John Wilkins (1614–1672)* (2014): page 67, footnote 166. For books acquired while Thistlethwayte was studying at Wadham, 1735–1736, see Carly Watson, 'The Legacy of an Eighteenth-Century Gentleman: Alexander Thistlethwayte's Books in Winchester College Fellows' Library', University of Birmingham, PhD. Thesis (2014): appendix 9.

10 HJR Wing appears not to have noticed the Oxford issue (6B1); nor does he mention the missing signature at Q4. Allowing for the erratic pagination, Wing lists 136 leaves (π^4, a–b^6, A–U^6) but his account of the pagination describes 135 leaves and runs across one section as: . . . 83–94, 93–4, 97–105 . . . , etc. This omits pages 96–6 which are printed on I2r–v. This makes his description of item 35 slightly incorrect.

11 Alexander Arbuthnot describes himself as a physician and surgeon from Montrose. He is presumably not Alexander Arbuthnot of Knox MP (1654–1705) who died in Montrose.

6C. PHARMACEUTICE RATIONALIS (part 1), The Hague duodecimo 1674

The third edition of the first part of Willis's sixth book, published at The Hague, with an engraved frontispiece [HJR Wing 37].

Title page: PHARMACEUTICE | RATIONALIS | five | DIATRIBA | de | MEDICAMENTORUM | Operationibus in humano Corpore, | *Authore* | THOMA WILLIS, M.D. | *In Univ. Oxon.* Prof. Sedleiano, Nec non *Coll.* | *Med. Lond.* & *Societ. Reg.* Socio. | [ornament] | *HAGÆ—COMITIS*, | [short rule] | Ex Officinâ ARNOLDI LEERS, Bibliopolæ. | cIↄ Iↄc LXXIV.

Collation: duodecimo; 23 letter roman alphabet using I: $*^{12}$, $**^{8}$, A–0^{12}, P^{2}; $ 1–6 signed apart from: -K3, K4 signed B4.

190 leaves: paginated as [40], 1–330, [10]. Mispaginated: 364 for 264.

Type: 38 lines; height (20 lines) 57 millimetres, width 50 millimetres (59 millimetres with marginal notes).

Contents; ***1r**, page [1], engraved title page; ***1v**, page [2], blank; ***2r**, page [3], title; ***2v**, page [4], blank; ***3r**, page [5], CELEBERRIMO MEDICORUM LONDINENSIUM COLLEGIO; Et Singulatim VIRO INSIGNISSIMO DOCTISIMOQUE D^no. GEORGIO ENT EQUITI AURATO Præſidi Illuſtriſſimo, *Nec non* CENSORIBUS DIGNISSIMIS, Cæteriſſque omnibus, ampliſſimæ hujus Societatis Membris, DIATRIBAM HANC PHARMACEUTICAM *Obſervantiæ & Honoris ergo Dicat, Dedicatque,* THO. WILLIS.; ***3v**, page [6], [imprimatur] *Librum hunc, Authore ſuo, ſagaciſſimo Phyſiologo, Medico peritiſſimo, dignum; olim Symmyſta, ſemper Amicus, libentiſſime Typis mando.* Oxon. Octob. 31. 1673. RAD. BATHURST, *Vice-Cancel.*; ***4r**–***8v**, pages [7–16], CANDIDO LECTORI PRAEFATIO; ***9r**–****8v**, pages [17–40], ELENCHUS RERUM.

A1r–O9v, pages 1–330, [text] DE MEDICAMENTORUM OPERATIONIBUS In CORPORE HUMANO.

O10r–P2r, pages [1–9], INDEX ALPHABETICUS.; **P2v**, page [10], blank.

Headlines and *Catchwords*: *Auglico.* for *Anglico.* at **K8v**, page 232; *Pulſu* for *pulſu* at **M7v**, page 278; *ocumenta* for *nocumenta* at **N11v–N12r**, pages 310–11.

cujuſ- for que at **M12v** / **N1r**, pages 288 / 289; cias for cius at **N12v** / **O1r**, pages 312 / 313.

Frontispiece: **F.3a1**. Engraved title page at *1r, page [1], PHARMACEUTICE RATIONALIS. *Authore.* Thom. Willis. MD. *1674. Romeyn de Hoogh ſecit 1674*; see: Figure 137.

Portrait: none.

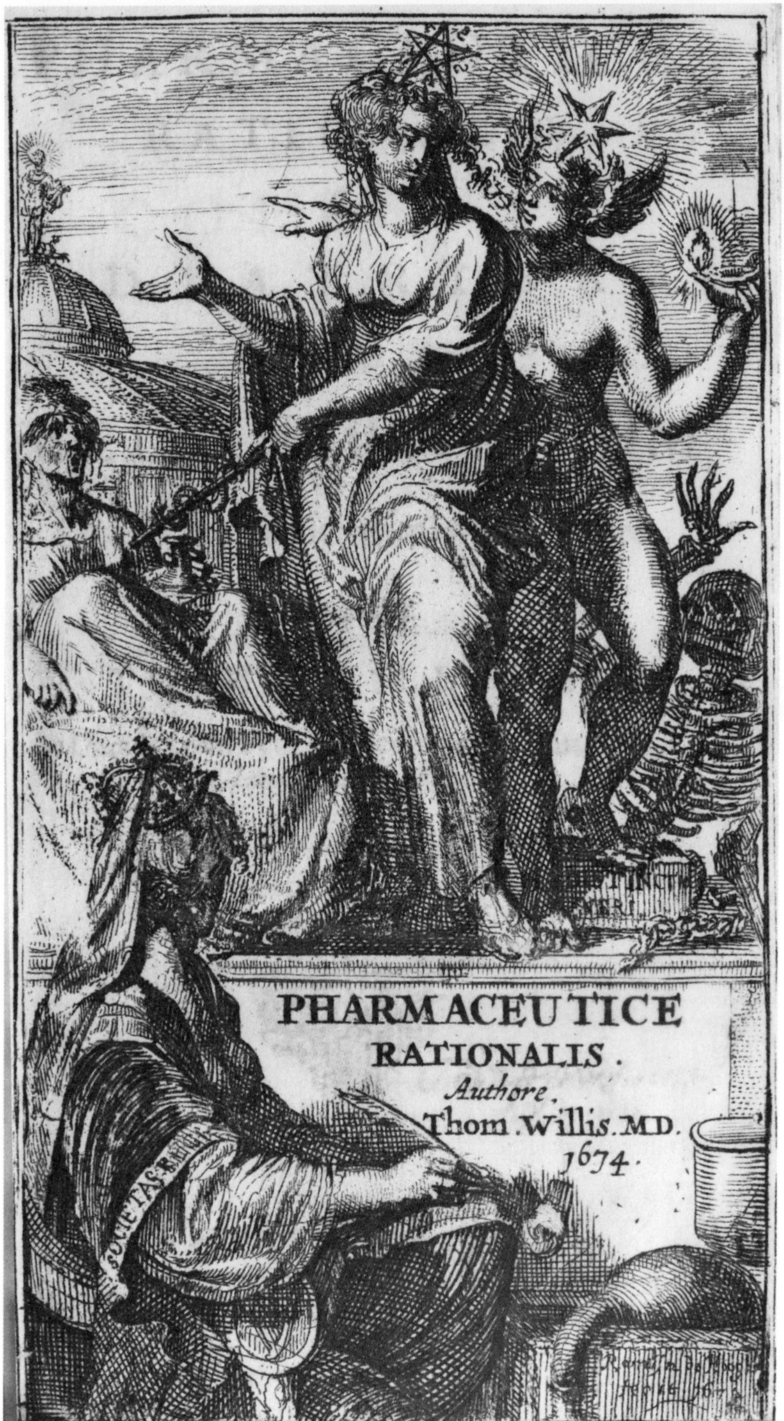

Figure 137 Engraved allegorical frontispiece: *Pharmaceutice rationalis* part 1 1674 (F.3a1).

Printers' ornament: tailpiece on title page at *2r, page [3], *8v, page [16], **8v, page [40] {**Leers 1**}.

Decorated Q at *4r, page [7] {**Leers 2**}; A at A1r, page 1 {**Leers 3**}.

Illustrations: as in **6A** apart from:

Pl.27b1. Plate 27 (image 46): *Tab. I.* (headline, centre), *pag. 33.* (headline, right). Folding, 174 × 206 millimetres (sheet); printed from a larger plate, 163 × >192 millimetres (plate marks at the upper, right, and lower borders, rough edge on the left from tearing); 146 × 170 millimetres (figure). Inserted before legend for Tabula I at **B5r**, page 33.

Pl.28b1. Plate 28 (image 47): *Tab. II.* (headline, centre), *p. 33.* (headline, right). Folding, 146 × 180 millimetres (sheet); printed from a larger plate (jagged cut from a knife at the lower edge, rough edge on the right from tearing), 123 × 161 millimetres (figure). Inserted before legend for Tabula II at **B5r**, page 33.

Pl.29b1. Plate 29 (image 48): *Tab. III.* (headline, centre), *p. 34.* (headline, right). Folding, 158 × 185 millimetres (sheet); printed from a larger plate (rough lower and right edges from tearing); 141 × 170 millimetres (figure). Inserted after legend for Tabula III at **B5v**, page 34.

Pl.30b1. Plate 30 (image 49–51): *Tab.* IV. (headline, left), *Fig. 2.* (headline, centre), *pag. 34.* (headline, right), *Fig. 3* (footer, left), *Fig. I.* (footer, centre). Folding, 162 × 244 millimetres (sheet); printed from a larger plate, >157 × 233 millimetres (plate marks at the upper, left, and right borders); 47 × 53 millimetres, 60 × 52 millimetres, 140 × 153 millimetres (figures). Inserted within legend for Tabula IV at **B5v–B6r**, pages 34–5.

Pl.31b1. Plate 31 (image 52): *Tab.* V. (headline, centre), *p. 35.* (headline, right). Folding, 157 × 184 millimetres (sheet, cropped); printed from a larger plate (rough upper edge from tearing); 146 × 153 millimetres (figure). Inserted before legend for Tabula V at **B6r**, page 35.

Pl.32b1 (images 53–57): *Tab.* VI. (headline, centre), *pag. 35.* (headline, right). Folding, 132 × 186 millimetres (sheet, cropped); printed from a larger plate (rough edge on the right from tearing); 113 × 23 millimetres, 114 × 22 millimetres, 113 × 22 millimetres, 113 × 22 millimetres, 112 × 22 millimetres (figures). Inserted after legend for Tabula VI at **B6v**, page 36.

Copy: DASC. Original vellum, spine lettered in manuscript Willis | pharma | ceutices | pt 1, original endpapers. Leaves 132 × 67 millimetres, boards 137 × 73 × 25 millimetres. Inscribed: ?D'Apples (unidentified).

6D. PHARMACEUTICE RATIONALIS (part 1). Ed. Postrema, The Hague duodecimo 1675

The fourth edition of the first part of Willis's sixth book, published at The Hague, with the engraved frontispiece [HJR Wing 38.].

Title page: PHARMACEUTICE | RATIONALIS | five | DIATRIBA | de | MEDICAMENTORUM | Operationibus in humano Corpore, | *Authore* | THOMA WILLIS, M.D. | *In Univ. Oxon.* Prof. Sedleiano, Nec non *Coll.* | *Med. Lond.* & *Societ. Reg.* Socio. | Editio poſtrema, prioribus emendatior. | [ornament] | *HAGÆ-COMITIS,* | [short rule] | Ex Officinâ ARNOLDI LEERS, Bibliopolæ. | cIↄ Iↄc LXXV.

Collation: duodecimo; 23 letter roman alphabet using I: $*^{12}$, $**^{8}$, A–S^{12}, T^{4}; $1–6 signed apart from: –**6

240 leaves: paginated as [40], 1–426, [14].

Type: 33 lines; height (20 lines) 65 millimetres (9 pts with leading), width 50 millimetres (59 with marginal notes).

Contents; ***1r**, page [1], engraved title page; ***1v**, page [2], blank; ***2r**, page [3], title; ***2v**, page [4], blank; ***3r**, page [5], CELEBERRIMO MEDICORUM LONDINENSIUM COLLEGIO; Et Singulatim VIRO INSIGNISSIMO DOCTISSIMOQUE D^no.^ GEORGIO ENT EQUITI AURATO Præſidi Illuſtriſſimo, *Nec non* CENSORIBUS DIGNISSIMIS, Cæteriſque omnibus, ampliſſimæ hujus Societatis Membris, DIATRIBAM HANC PHARMACEUTICAM *Observantiæ & Honoris ergo Dicat, Dedicatque*, THO. WILLIS.; ***3v**, page [6], [imprimatur] *Librum hunc, Authore ſuo, ſagacisſimo Phyſiologo, Medico peritisſimo, dignum*; *olim Symmyſta, ſemper Amicus, libentisſime Typis mando.* Oxon. Octob. 31. 1673. RAD. BATHURST, *Vice-Cancel.*; ***4r**–***8v**, pages [7–16], CANDIDO LECTORI PRÆFATIO.; ***9r**–****8v**, pages [17–40], ELENCHUS RERUM.

A1r–**S9v**, pages 1–426, [text] De MEDICAMENTORUM OPERATIONIBUS *In* CORPORE HUMANO.

S10r–**T3v**, pages [1–12], INDEX ALPHABETICUS.; **T4r**–**v**, pages [1–2], blank.

Headlines and *Catchwords*: no '.' after headline at **a10r**, page 21; Londinens. for Londinensis. at **G5r**, page 153, **G7r**, page 157; **G8r**, page 159; *pulſu* for *Pulſu* at **P10r**, page 355; **P11v**, page 358.

tæ for ta at **Rr11r** / **v**, pages 405 / 406.

Frontispiece: **F.3a1**. Engraved title page at ***1r**, page [1], PHARMACEUTICE RATIONALIS. *Authore*. Thom. Willis. MD. *1674. Romeyn de Hoogh fecit 1674.*

Portrait: none.

Printers' ornaments: tailpiece on title page ***2r**, page [3] {**Leers 4**}; tailpiece at ***8v**, page [16]; ****8v**, page [40] {**Leers 6**}.

Decorated Q at ***4r**, page [7] {**Leers 5**}; A at **A1r**, page 1 {**Leers 7**}.

Illustrations: as in **6C** apart from:

Pl.27b2. Plate 27 (image 46): *Tab. I.* (headline, centre), *pag. 41.* (headline, right). 165 × 205 millimetres (sheet). Inserted before legends for Tabula I–VI at **B9r–B11r**, pages 41–5.

Pl.28b2. Plate 28 (image 47): *Tab. II.* (headline, centre), *p. 42.* (headline, right). 138 × 190 millimetres (sheet). Inserted before legends for Tabula I–VI at **B9r–B11r**, pages 41–5.

Pl.29b2. Plate 29 (image 48): *Tab. III.* (headline, centre), *p. 42.* (headline, right). 152 × 190 millimetres (sheet). Inserted before legends for Tabula I–VI at **B9r–B11r**, pages 41–5.

Pl.30b2. Plate 30 (image 49–51): *Tab.* IV. (headline, left), *Fig. 2.* (headline, centre), *pag. 44.* (headline, right), *Fig. 3* (footer, left), *Fig. I.* (footer, centre). 162 × 243 millimetres (sheet). Inserted before legends for Tabula I–VI at **B9r–B11r**, pages 41–5.

Pl.31b2. Plate 31 (image 52): *Tab.* V. (headline, centre), *p. 44.* (headline, right). 156 × 185 millimetres (sheet). Inserted before legends for Tabula I–VI at **B9r–B11r**, pages 41–5.

Pl.32b2. Plate 32 (images 53–57): *Tab.* VI. (headline, centre), *pag. 42.* (headline, right). 132 × 185 millimetres (sheet). Inserted before legends for Tabula I–VI at **B9r–B11r**, pages 41–5.

Copy: DASC (#1 of 2). Original vellum, spine WIILIS | PHARM, original endpapers. Leaves 130 × 74 millimetres, boards 137 × 75 × 37 millimetres. Inscribed: (1) Epossess Dav. Grimy. M. Cull. 1687; (2) Consc. I.R. ic 16 Marti: (both unidentified).

6E. PHARMACEUTICE RATIONALIS (part 2), Oxford quarto 1675

The first edition of the second part of Willis's sixth book, published from Oxford [HJR Wing 34].

Title page: PHARMACEUTICE RATIONALIS, | SIVE | DIATRIBA | *DE MEDICAMENTORUM* | Operationibus in humano Corpore | PARS SECUNDA. | *AUTORE* | *Tho. Willis* M.D. in *Univ. Oxon.* Prof. Sedleiano. | [ornament] | E THEATRO SHELDONIANO. [rule over date] M. DC. LXXV.

Collation: quarto; 23 letter roman alphabet using I and V: a–f^4, g^2, (c)^2, A–Z^4, Aa–Zz^4, Aaa–Iii^4, Kkk^2: $1–3 signed apart from:[12] f3 signed f2, -A3, -B3, -C3, -D3, -I3, -K3, -M3, -N3, -Q3, -R3, -S3, -Cc3, Eee3 signed Eee2.

250 leaves: paginated as [56], 1–54, 57–8, 57–176, 185–251 for 177–243, 256–86 for 244–72, 267–308 for 273–312, 306 for 313, 310–64 for 314–66, 367–79, 378 for 380, 381–403, 444–5 for 404–5, 406–25, and 496 for 426; i.e. [56], 1–[426], [12].

Type: 35 lines; height (20 lines) 93 millimetres, width 99 millimetres (119 millimetres with marginal notes).

[12] Designating leaves $3 as 'unsigned' is somewhat arbitrary since most quarto books would be $1–2 signed as are the slight majority here.

Contents: **a1r**, page [1], title; **a1v**, page [2], blank; **a2r**, page [3], ATHENIS BRITANNICIS, Literati Orbis lumini Splendiſſimo, *UNIVERSITATI OXONIENSI*, Et Ibidem ILLUSTRISSIMO PRINCIPI JAC. ORMONDIÆ DUCI CANCEELLARIO HONORATISSIMO, *RAD. BATHURST* DECANO WELLENSI VICECANCELLARIO DIGNISSIMO, Reverendis admodum, & perquam Eruditis DOCTORIBUS, PROCURATORIBUS, Facultatum omnium PROFESSORIBUS, COLLEGIORUM & AULARUM Præſectis, NEC NON Venerabili Magiſtrorum Senatui Diatribam hanc Pharmaceuticam Pietatis & gratitudinis ergo Dicat Dedicatque Alumnus & beneficarius adſtrictiſſimus THO. WILLIS.; **a2v**, page [4], Imprimatur AMiciſſimo Authori, poſt tam Immortale opus, nihil mortale facturo, tanquam Lumina morienti claudens, extremum hoc officium præſtat Oxon. *Novemb.* 12. 1675. *RAD. BATHURST* Vice-Cancel. *Oxonienſis.*; **a3r–b2r**, pages [5–11], *CANDIDO LECTORI* PRÆFATIO.; **b2v–c2r**, pages [12–19], POST SCRIPTUM.; **c2v**, page [20], blank; **c3r–c4v**, pages [21–4], *AUTORI CLARISSIMO, nec non mihi (de quo jure glorior) AMICISSIMO, in illius* Pharmaceutices Rationalis *Partem utramque* ... [signed] *Gul. Dawkins.*; **d1r–g2r**, pages [25–51], ELENCHUS RERUM.; **g2v**, page [52], blank; **(c)1r–(c)2r**, pages [53–5], QUERELA LIBRI POSTHUMI DE OBITU AUTORIS. ... [signed] *Gul. Dawkins.* MED. B.; **(c)2v**, page [56], blank.

A1r–Hhh4v, pages 1–'496' (i.e. 426), [text] Pharmaceuticæ Rationalis, SIVE DE MEDICAMENTORUM OPERATIONIBUS IN Corpore Humano Pars Secunda.

Iii1r–Kkk2v, pages [1–12], INDEX ALPHABETICUS.

Headlines and *Catchwords*: Explicatio. for explicatio. at **E3v**, page 38; *læſæ ſpecies.* for *læſæ variæ ſpecies.* at **F2v**, page 44; *læſa.* for *læſâ.* at **H1r–H2r**, pages '57'–'59'; headline and chapter title *De Exſpiratione læſâ.* for *De Tuſſi.* at **H2v**, page '60'; CAP. III. for CAP. IV. at **H3r**, page '63'; no SECT. I. at **M3v**, page '94'; **M4v**, page '96'; page number in () with no other headline at **Q3r**, page '125'; **X3v**, page '166'; **Z3r**, page '189'; no CAP. VI. at **M4r**, page '95'; *exempla.* for *Exempla.* at **S2v**, page '140'; CAP. VII. for CAP. VIII. at **V4r**, page '159'; *Epyemata.* for *Empyemate.* at **Aa3r**, page '197'; *Empyemate.* for *Pulmonis Vomica.* at **Bb1r–Bb2r**, pages '201–203'; CAP. X. for CAP. XI. at **Bb1r**, page '201'; **Bb2r**, page '203'; additional chapter break headed SECT. 1. CAP. XI. (as at **Aa4r**, page '199') at **Bb2v**, page '204'; CAP. X. for CAP. XI. at **Bb3r**, page '205'; **Bb4r**, page '207'; CAP. II for CAP. I. at **Gg3r**, page '245'; CAP. II. for CAP. III. at **Ii4r**, page '267'; *remediis* for *Remediis* at **Kk2v**, page '272'; *Asciter.* for *Aſcitem.* at **Ll3r**, page '281'; CAP. III. for CAP. IV. at **Aaa3r**, page '367'; **Aaa4r**, page '369'; **Bbb1r**, page '371'; CAP. V. for CAP. IV. at **Ccc1r**, page '379'; '.' after headline at **Ddd4v**, page '394'; CAP.V. for CAP. VI. at **Eee2r**, page '397'; INDEX. for ALPHABETICUS. at **Iii2r**, page [3]; no '.' after headline at **Iii2v**, page [4].

[With one exception, catchwords are present before blanks linking to the next page of print]:[13] nium for tum at **b1r / v**, pages [9] / [10]; DE unlinked at **g2r**, page [51]; no catchword at **(c)1r / A1r**, pages [55] / 1; thema for pathema at **H3v / H4r**, pages '62' / '63'; 2. In- for 2da Ind at **M2r / v**, pages '91' / '92'; Hart- for *Hart* at **Oo2v / Oo3r**, pages '284' / '285'; ſem for menſum at **Zz1r / v**, pages '353' / '354'.

Frontispiece: none.

[13] CAP is used as the catchword linking the end of each chapter to the start of the next irrespective of the first printed word as part of the headline, chapter number, or title: these variations are not listed.

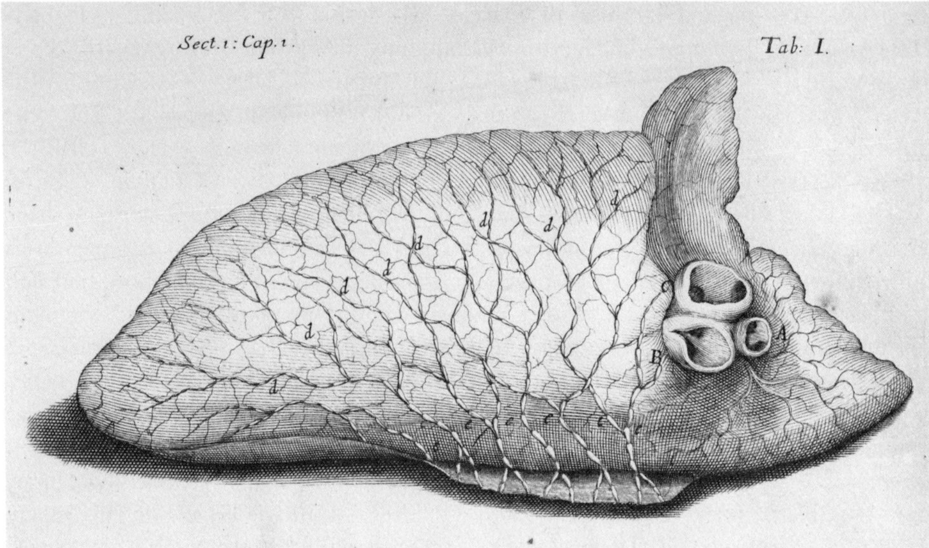

Figure 138 Plate 33 (image 58). The firſt Table ſhews one entire Lobe of the Lungs, upon whoſe ſuperficies the Lymphæducts are ſeen fpread through every where. Image from *Pharmaceutice rationalis* part 2 1675; legend from *Dr Willis's practice of physick* 1684.

Portrait: none.

Printers' ornaments: printers' device at **a1r**, page [1] {**Fell 9**}; headpiece at **a3r**, page [5]; **A1r**, page 1 {**Fell 4**}.

Decorated A at **a3r**, page [5] {**Fell 6**}; I at **A1r**, page 1{**Fell 10**}.

Illustrations:[14] **Pl.33a1**. Plate 33 (image 58): *Sect. i: Cap. i* (headline, left), *Tab: I.* (headline, right); lettering to depict structures (in multiples of ≤ 8) A–C, d, e. Leaf size, 141 × 205 millimetres (sheet); 115 × 192 millimetres (plate marks); 93 × 187 millimetres (figure). Legend: TABULA Prima exhibet pulmonis lobum unum integrum revolutum, in cujus ſuperficie Lymphæductus, huc illuc perreptantes, conſpiciuntur. Inserted before text for Sect. I Cap. I at **A1r**, page 1; see: Figure 138.

Pl.34a1. Plate 34 (image 59): *Tab: II.* (headline, left), *Sect. i: Cap. i.* (headline, right); lettering to depict structures (in multiples of ≤ 5) A–G, f. Folding, 215 × 169 millimetres (sheet); 200 × 141 millimetres (plate marks); 186 × 122 millimetres (figure). Legend: TABULA II exhibet pulmonis Ovini lobum unum in medio ſectum, ut portione ſuperiore (in qua Venæ caudex eſt) amota, & Aſperæ Arteriæ Trunco ſepoſito, Arteriæ Pneumonicæ per totam ejus compagem, ſc. lobulos minores & minimos, ramificatio oſtendatur. Hujus ductus omnes, ſc. propagines & ſurculi, ut minuti, à liquido quodam injecto impleti & colorati, ad vivum delineabantur. Inserted before text for Sect. I Cap. I at **A1r**, page 1; see: Figure 139.

[14] Although all eight figure legends are printed in sequence at E1r–E4v, pages 33–40, the plates lack page placements and are often randomly bound in different copies: apart from that described, in the four other copies examined for this bibliography they are together at A1r, page 1 (2 copies); before the Elenchus rerum at d1r, page 25; or after the final index, at Kkk2v, page [12].

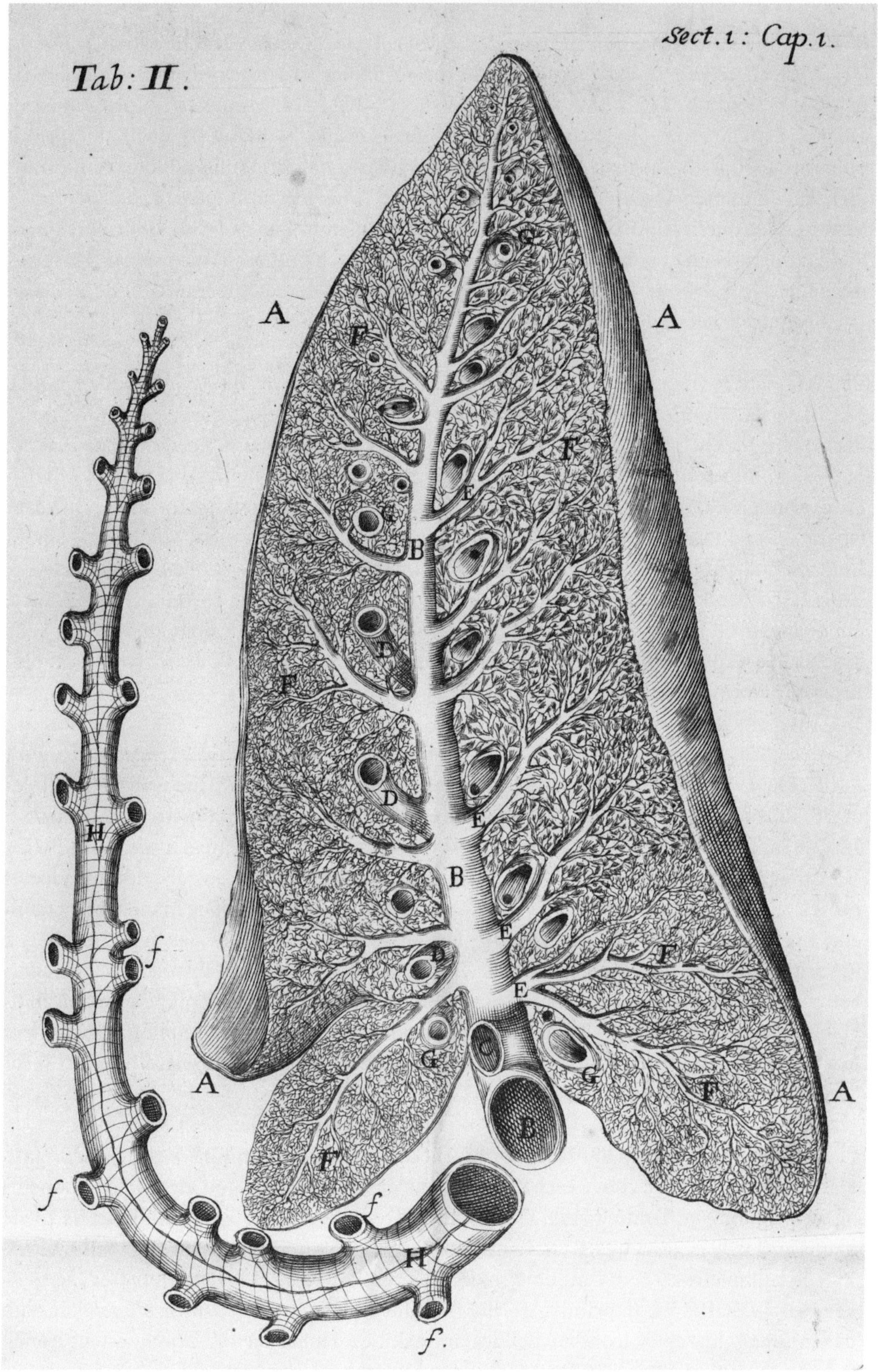

Figure 139 Plate 34 (image 59). The second Table ſhews one Lobe of a Sheeps Lung cut in the midſt, that the upper part (wherein is the trunk of the Vein) being removed, and the trunk of the *Aſpera Arteria* laid by it ſelf, the branching of the Pneumonic Artery is ſhewn throughout its whole frame, *viz*. through the ſmall and leaſt little Lobes. All the paſſages of this, *viz*. the ſlips and twigs how ſmall ſoever, being filled and coloured by any liquid thing caſt into them, are drawn to the life. Image from *Pharmaceutice rationalis* part 2 1675; legend from *Dr Willis's practice of physick* 1684.

Pl.35a1 (images 60–61): *Tab: III.* (headline, left), *Sect. i: Cap. i.* (headline, right), *Fig: 1.*, *Fig: 2.* (headers, left of each image); lettering to depict structures (in multiples of ≤ 5) A–H, a, b. Folding, 215 × 180 millimetres (sheet); 202 × 143 millimetres (plate marks); 183 × 138 millimetres, 44 × 26 millimetres (figures). Legend: TABULA III. Figura I. exprimit pulmonis lobum unum, juxta Aſperæ Arteriæ ramificationes, in lobulos minores & minimos diviſum, cujus vaſis ſurculi & propagines à liquido prius injecto impleti, & deinde quoad lobulos ab invicem ſejuncti, etiam ad vivum delineabantur. Figura II. exprimit portionem lobi pulmonaris, in quo, interſtitiis membranoſis inflatis, lobuli omnes in propria figura apparent, atque Polypodii folium nonnihil repræſentant. Inserted before text for Sect. I Cap. I at **A1r**, page 1; see: Figure 140.

Pl.36a1. Plate 36 (images 62–64): *Tab: IV.* (headline, centre), *Sect. i: Cap. i.* (headline, right), *Fig: 1.*, *Fig: 2.*, *Fig: 3.* (footers, left of each image); lettering to depict structures (in multiples of ≤ 5) A, b–d. Leaf size, 205 × 141 millimetres (sheet); 166 × 116 millimetres (plate marks); 68 × 41 millimetres, 60 × 34 millimetres, 62 × 35 millimetres (figures). Legend: TABULA IV. exprimit vaſa tum Trachealia tum ſanguifera, pro uno lobulo conſtituendo ab invicem ſeparata & diſtincta, nec non cujuſque illorum conformationes peculiares. Figura I repræſentat rami Trachealis intra lobulum unum diſtributi divaricationem, inque Tubos & veſiculas orbiculares ramificationem. Figura II. & III. Arteriæ & Venæ Pneumonicæ intra eundem lobulum pares ramificationes diſtinctim oſtendunt; quæ ambæ cum vaſis Trachealibus complicatæ, compagis pulmonaris texturam maximâ *ex parte* conſtituunt. Inserted before text for Sect. I Cap. I at **A1r**, page 1; see: Figure 141.

Pl.37a1. Plate 37 (images 65–67): *Sect. i: Cap. i:* (headline, left), *Tab: V.* (headline, right), *Fig: 2.*, *Fig: 1.*, *Fig: 3.* (footers, below each image); lettering to depict structures (in multiples of ≤ 8) A, B, a–c. Folding, 232 × 188 millimetres (sheet); 217 × 165 millimetres (plate marks); 78 × 68 millimetres, 76 × 92 millimetres, 141 × 157 millimetres (figures). Legend: TABULA V. exhibet Nervum Pulmonarem ſubſidio microſcopii paulo accuratius deſcriptum: adeo ut plane conſtet truncum ejus fibrillarum innumerabilium unà colligatarum quaſi faſciculum eſſe; quinimo & caudicem ejus, dum in ſerpilli modum pulmones perreptat, ſurculos à ſe varios huc illuc propagare. Figura I. Trunci Nervei portionem abſciſſam refert, cujus extremitas una aperta, & per microſcopium inſpecta, in fibras ferè innumeras explicabilis videtur. Figura II. & III. tum trunci, tum rami cujuſque fibras quaſdam explicatas, ac inſuper ſurculorum è varia ſtirpe propagationes, crebro iteratas oſtendunt. Inserted before text for Sect. I Cap. I at **A1r**, page 1; see: Figure 142.

Pl.38a1. Plate 38 (images 68–75): *Tab: VI.* (headline, left), *Sect. i: Cap. i:* (headline, right), *Fig: 1.*, *Fig: 2.* (headers, above each group of four images); lettering to identify components of each figure 1–4. Folding, 199 × 245 millimetres (sheet); 166 × 216 millimetres (plate marks); 70 × 49 millimetres, 72 × 48 millimetres, 70 × 50 millimetres, 69 × 49 millimetres, 71 × 17 millimetres, 72 × 17 millimetres, 73 × 17 millimetres, 74 × 17 millimetres (figures). Legend: TABULA VI. imprimis Arteriæ ſanguiferæ Anatomen, quam in nupero tractatu deſcripſimus, hic aptis Iconibus delineatam exhibet. Hujus *Figuræ primæ* ac *ſuperiores*, vaſis iſtius quatuor tunicas diſtinctas, ſc. nerveam, muſcularem, glanduloſam & vaſculoſam repræſentant. *Figuræ 2dæ & inferiores*, Venæ Anatomen, ſive quatuor ejus tunicas Iconibus idoneis expreſſas, oſtendunt; quæ tunicæ, ut è vaſis portione quadam (exterius incipiendo) ſucceſſivè eximuntur, integræ apparent. Inserted before text for Sect. I Cap. I at **A1r**, page 1; see: Figure 143.

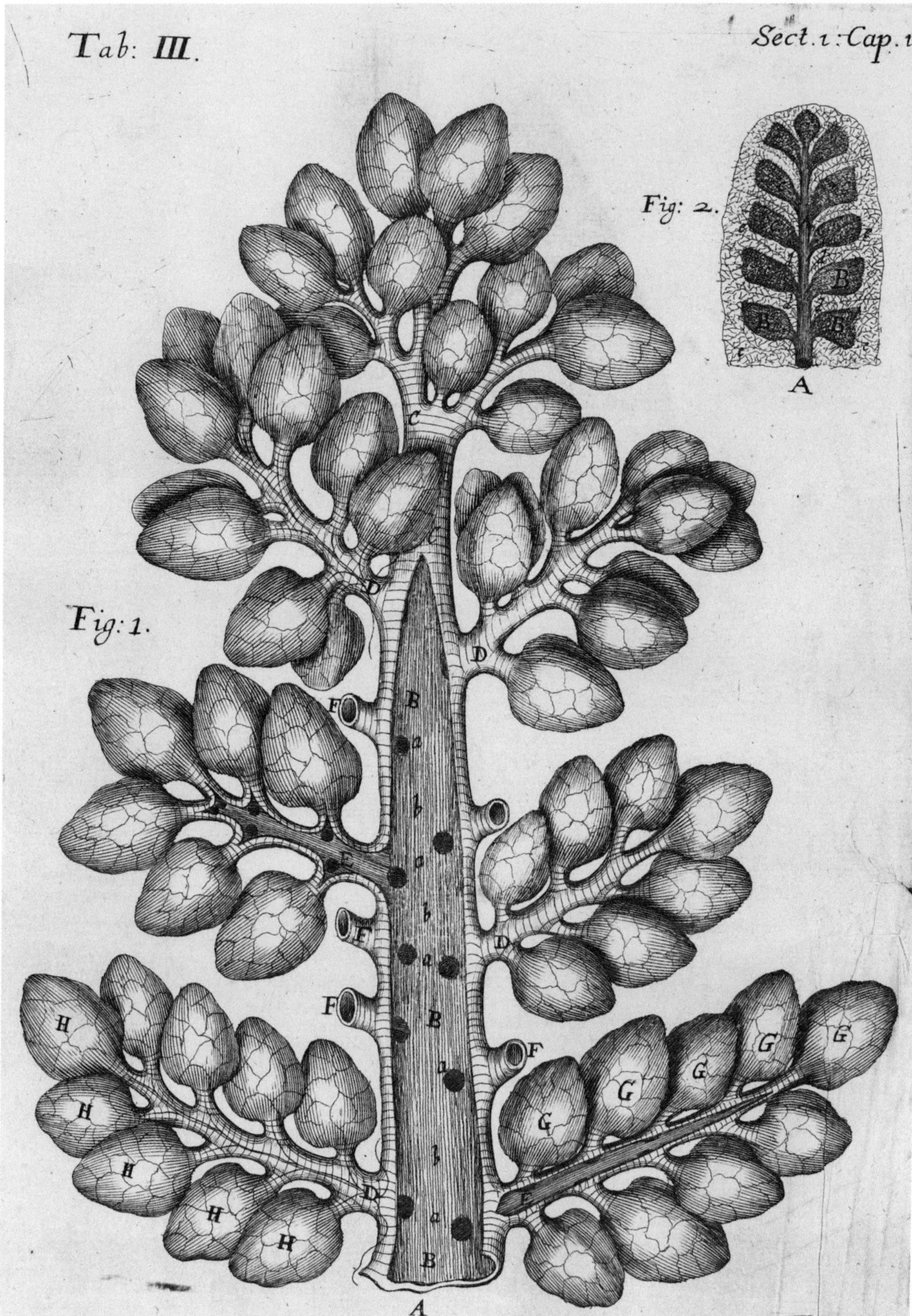

Figure 140 Plate 35 (images 60–61). The firſt Figure of the third Table expreſſes one Lobe of the Lungs, according to the branchings of the *Aspera Arteria* divided into leſſer and leſs Lobes, the twigs and ſlips of which Veſſel being filled by a liquid firſt injected, and afterwards ſeparated from among themſelves towards the little Lobes, are alſo drawn to the life. The ſecond Figure of the third Table expreſſes a part of the pulmonary Lobe, wherein the membranous interſpaces being blown up, all the little Lobes appear in their proper figure, and do ſomewhat repreſent the leaf of Polypody. Image from *Pharmaceutice rationalis* part 2 1675; legend from *Dr Willis's practice of physick* 1684.

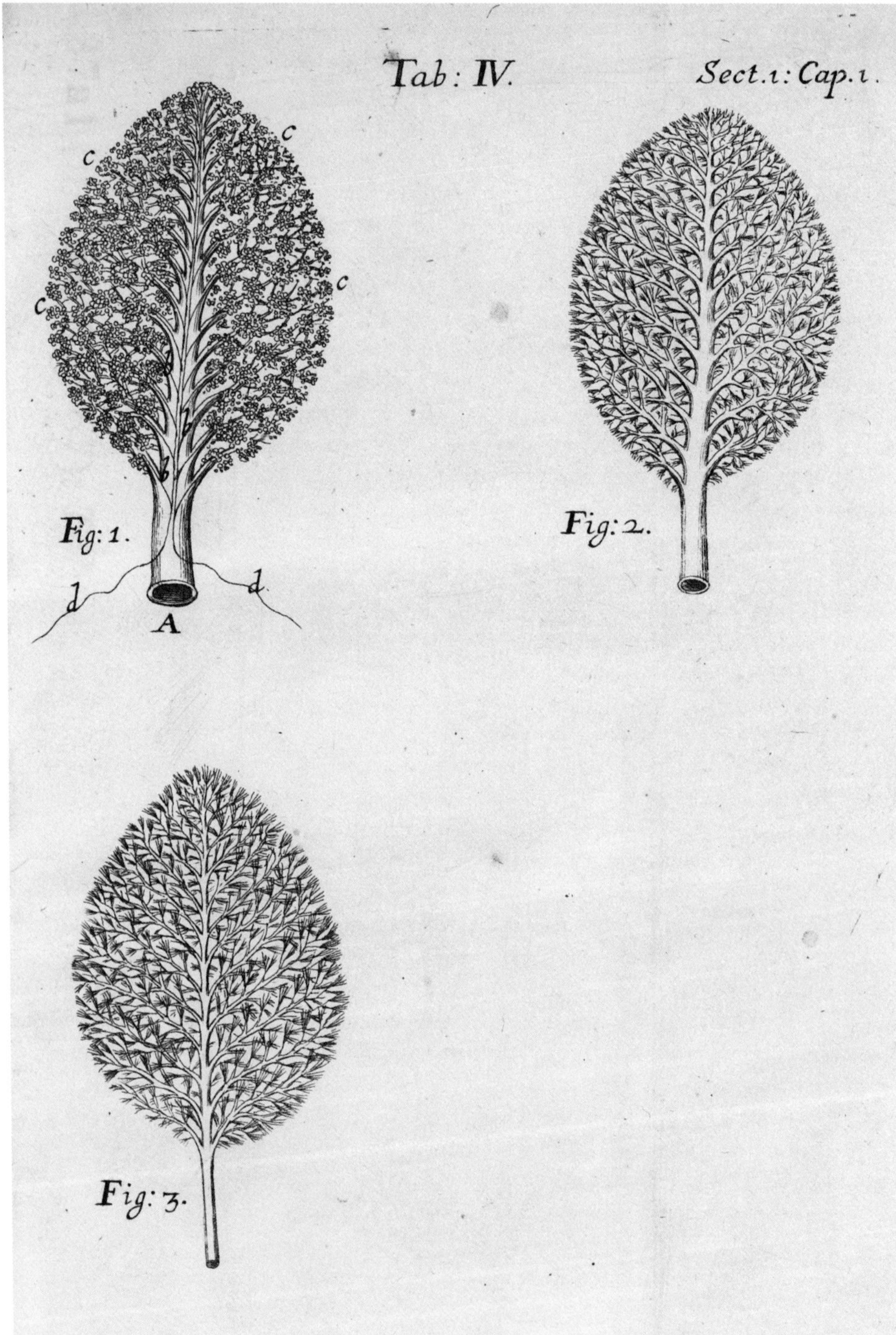

Figure 141 Plate 36 (images 62–64). The fourth Table expreſſes as well the Veſſels belonging to the *Trachea* as thoſe bringing blood, ſeparate and diſtinct one from another, conſtituting one little Lobe, as alſo peculiar framing of every one of them. The firſt Figure repreſents the ſeparating into divers parts the Tracheal branch diſtributed into one little lobe, and the branching into Pipes and orbicular little bladders. The ſecond and third Figure ſhews diſtinctly the equal branchings of the Artery and Pneumonick Veins within the ſame little Lobe; both which being complicated with tracheal Veſſels, do for the moſt part make up the texture of the pulmonary frame. Image from *Pharmaceutice rationalis* part 2 1675; legend from *Dr Willis's practice of physick* 1684.

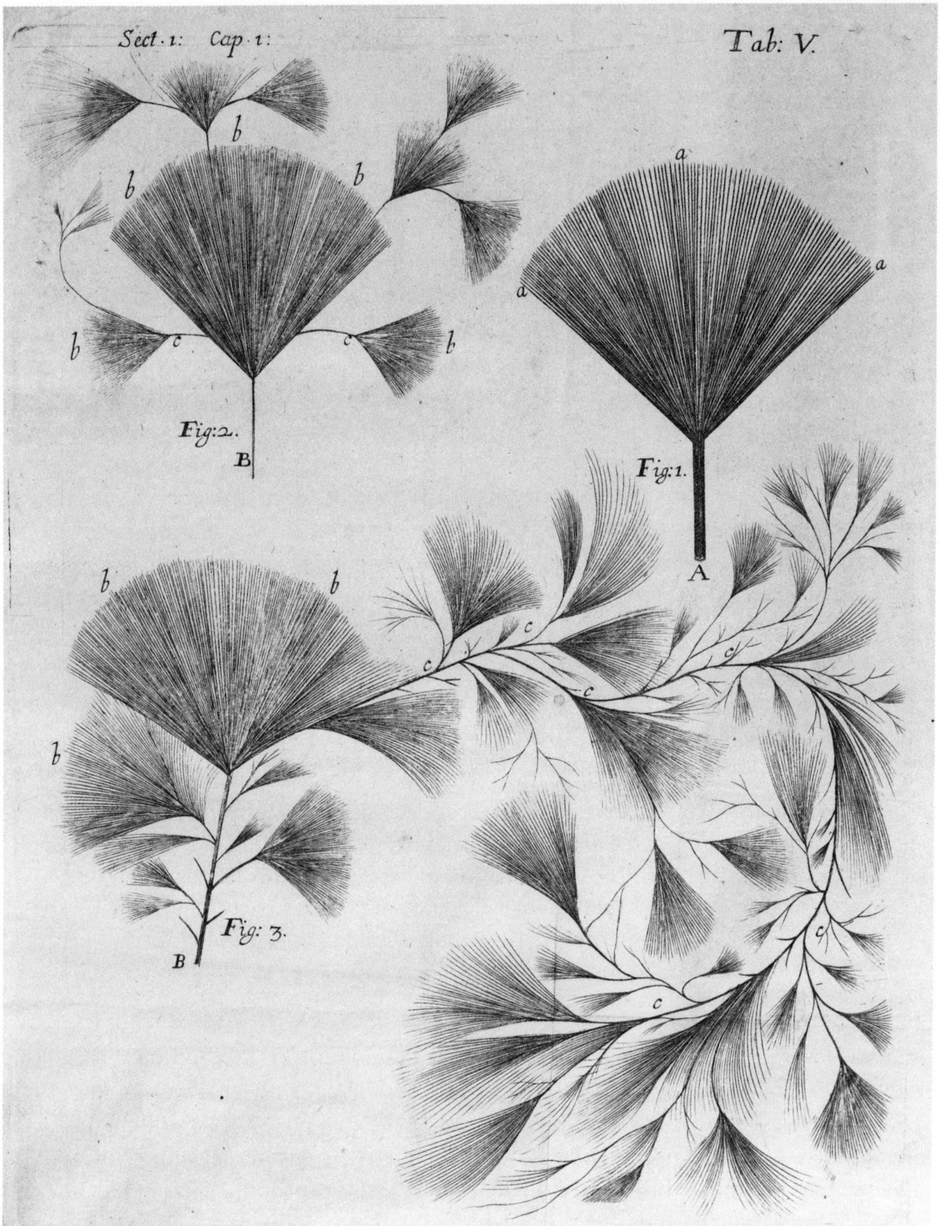

Figure 142 Plate 37 (images 65–67). The fifth Table fets forth the pulmonary Nerve more accurately defcribed by the aid of a Microfcope: fo that it plainly appears that the Trunk is as it were a bundle of innumerable little Fibres bound together; Moreover its Trunk, while it creeps into the Lungs in the likenefs of Mother of Time, doth fpread the various little fprigs every way. Fig. I. refembles a part of the nervous trunk cut away, one end whereof being opened and lookt on by a Microfcope, feems to unfold it felf almoft into innumerable little fibres. The fecond and third figure do fhew fome fibres as well of the trunk as of every branch, and moreover the flips of the little twigs from divers ftemmes often repeated. Image from *Pharmaceutice rationalis* part 2 1675; legend from *Dr Willis's practice of physick* 1684.

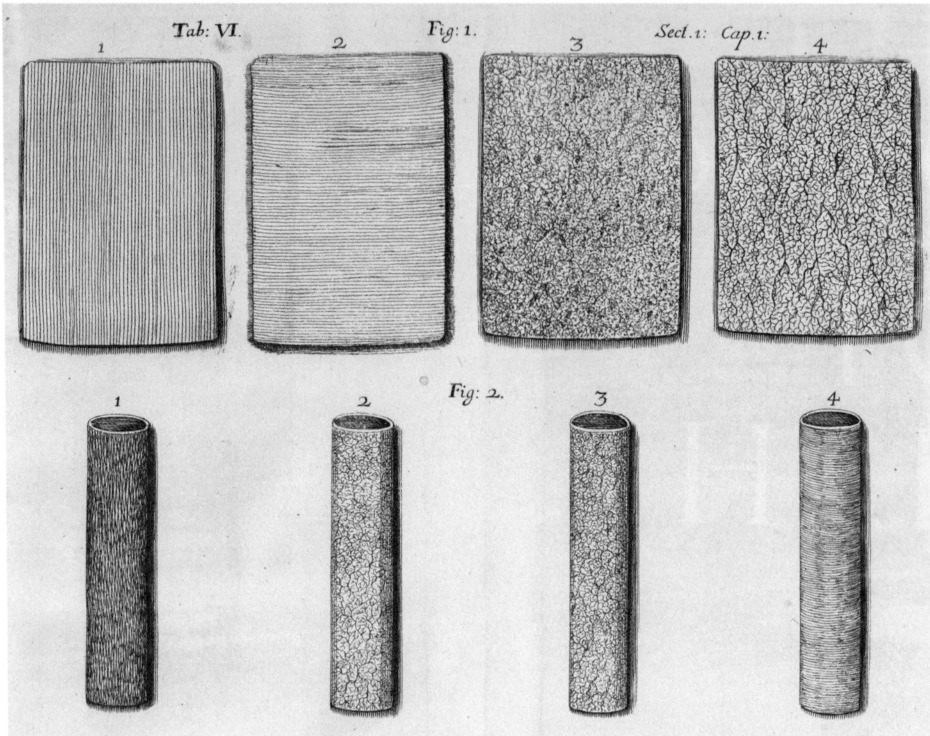

Figure 143 Plate 38 (images 68–75). The ſix Table firſt ſets from the anatomy of the Artery bringing blood drawn in apt figures, which we have deſcribed in a late treatiſe. *The firſt and upper figures hereof*, repreſent the four distinct Coats of that Veſſel, *viz*. the nervous, muſcular, glandulous, and the vaſculous. The *ſecond and lower figures* of the ſixth Table, do ſhew the anatomy of the Vein, or its four coats expreſſed in fit places; which Coats do appear entire as ſucceſſively taken one part from the other (beginning outmoſt.). Image from *Pharmaceutice rationalis* part 2 1675; legend from *Dr Willis's practice of physick* 1684.

Pl.39a1. Plate 39 (images 76–79): *Tab: VII.* (headline, centre), *Sect. i: Cap i*: (headline, right), *Fig 1*, *Fig: 3.*, *Fig: 4.*, *Fig: 2.* (headers, above each image); no lettering. Folding, 192 × 160 millimetres (sheet); 150 × 137 millimetres (plate marks); 57 × 56 millimetres, 58 × 56 millimetres, 56 × 59 millimetres; 57 × 48 millimetres (figures). Legend: TABULA VII. Aſperæ Arteriæ tunicas diſtinctas, & ab invicem ſeparatas exprimit. *Figura prima Tunicam intimam*, fibris muſcularibus rectis, sive longitudinalibus præditam oſtendit. II.III. *Figura* 2da *Tunicam glanduloſam*, & 3^{tia} *vaſculoſam* (quæ pari ſere ritu ac in vaſis ſanguiferis, ac etiam in inteſtinis habent) deſignat. IV. *Figura* 4ta *tunicam exteriorem* (quæ partim cartilagenea, & partim muſcularis eſt) exprimit. Hujus fibræ tranſverſæ, ſive Annulares, cartilaginum interſtitia adimplent & connectunt. Inserted before text for Sect. I Cap. I at **A1r**, page 1; see: Figure 144.

Pl.40a1. Plate 40 (images 80–82): *Sect. i: Cap i.* (headline, left), *Tab: VIII.* (headline, centre), *Fig: 1.*, *Fig: 3.*, *Fig: 2.* (headers, above each image); no lettering. Folding, 158 × 197 millimetres (sheet); 128 × 166 millimetres (plate marks); 50 × 51 millimetres, 24 × 26 millimetres, 52 × 51 millimetres (figures). Legend: TABULA VIII. Tunicæ pulmonaris extimæ, totam ejus

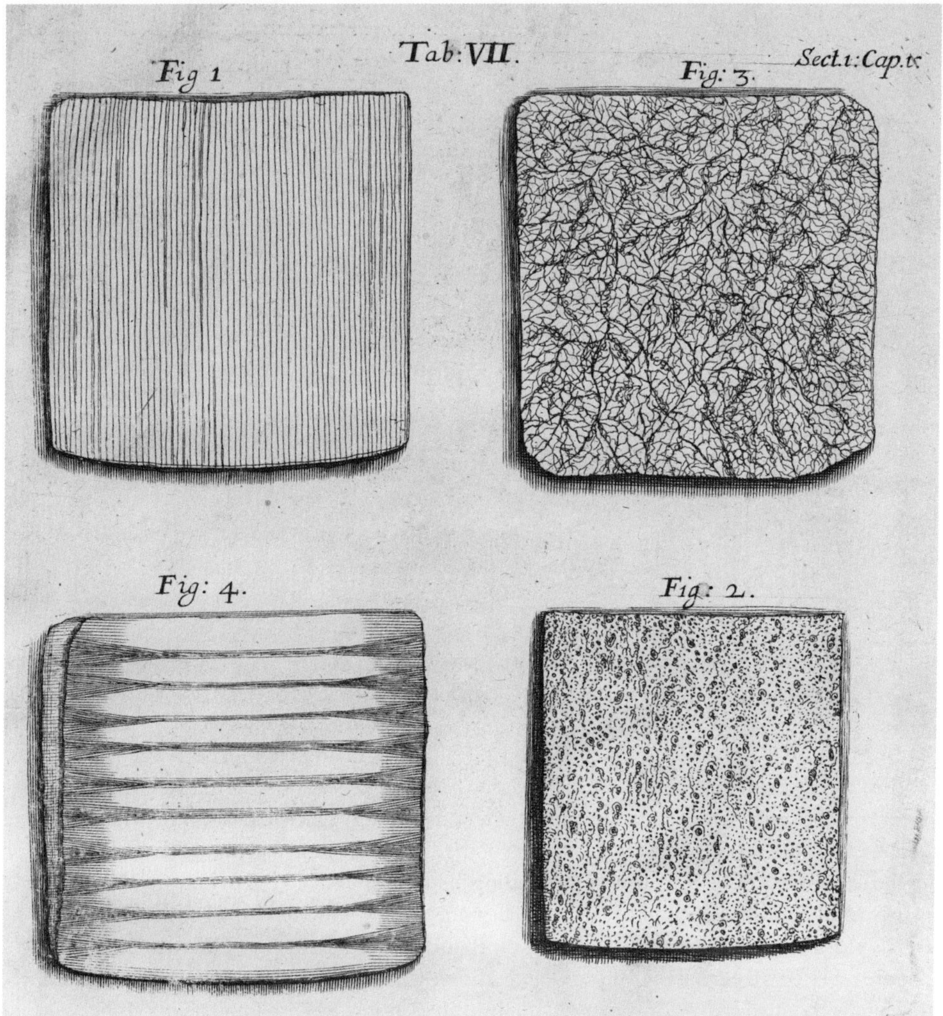

Figure 144 Plate 39 (images 76–79). The ſeventh Table expreſſes the diſtinct Coats of the *aſpera arteria*, and ſeparated one from the other. *The firſt figure ſhews the moſt inward Coat*, endowed with ſtreight or long muſcular fibres. *The ſecond figure deſcribes the glandulous coat*, and the third figure the vaſculous coat (which are almost the ſame as in the veſſels bringing blood, and alſo in the Guts). 4. *The fourth figure expreſſes the outward coat* (which is partly cartilaginous, and partly muſcular.) The tranſverſe or annular fibres hereof do fill up and weave together the interſpaces of the Cartilages. Image from *Pharmaceutice rationalis* part 2 1675; legend from *Pharmaceutice rationalis* 1679.

compagem obducentis, portionem, microscopii ope elegantiſſime ſimulque accuratiſſime deſcriptam exhibet. Figura I. exhibet prædictæ tunicæ portionem, quæ partium ob vaſorum cujuſque generis in ea terminatorum extremitates, foveolis quaſi punctūris denſiſſimis excudi videtur, & partim è vaſorum ſanguiferorum complicationibus, velut corymbeis, veſiculas orbiculares cingentibus, in plures velut areas τραπεζώδεις diſtinguitur. Figura II. repræſentat membranæ extimæ portionem à vaſorum corymbis avulſis ſeparatam, & ſine areis, ſolummodo foveis minutiſſimis quaſi punctūtis inſignitam. Figura III. exprimit Tunicæ

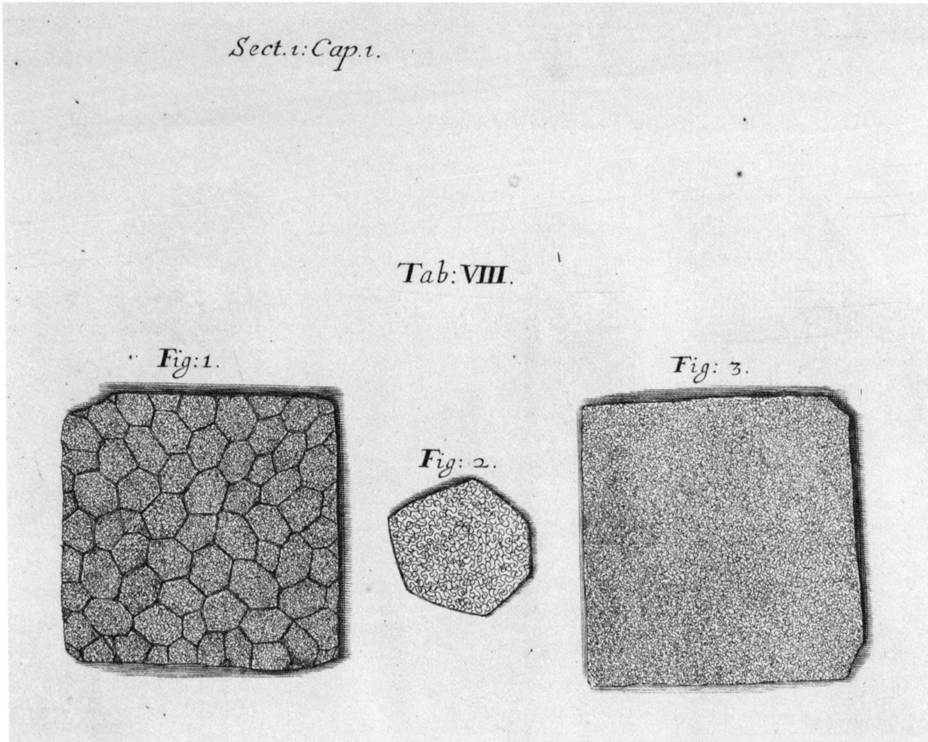

Figure 145 Plate 40 (images 80–82). The eighth Table ſhews a part of the outmoſt pulmonary Coat covering over its whole frame, moſt finely and curiouſly deſcribed by the help of a Microſcope. The firſt Figure ſhews a portion of the above mentioned coat, which partly by reaſon of the extremities of Veſſels of every ſort ending in it, ſeems pricked full of holes as it were, and partly from the complications of the veſſels bringing blood, which like the twining ſprigs of Vines gird about the orbicular bladders, is diſtinguished into many irregular *Area's*. The ſecond Figure repreſents a part of the outermoſt membrane ſeparated from the cluſters of veſſels pull'd off, and without any *Areæ*, only markt with little holes as it were with ſmall pricks. The third Figure expreſſes one ſingular *area* of the Coat above mentioned, augmented in largeneſs by the help of a Microſcope. Image from *Pharmaceutice rationalis* part 2 1675; legend from *Dr Willis's practice of physick* 1684.

prædictæ aream quandam ſingularem, ope microſcopii magnitudine auctam. Inserted before text for Sect. I Cap. I at **A1r**, page 1; see: Figure 145.

Copy: DASC (#1 of 5). Original calf with double-lined borders; spine rebacked, four raised bands with double-lined borders, new endpapers. Leaves 205 × 147 millimetres, boards 213 × 148 × 22 millimetres. Inscribed T Willoughby K2: 9.[15]

[15] Willoughby's signature is present on the copy of Richard Lower's *Diatribæ Thomæ Willisii* (1665) illustrated in John Fulton (1899–1960), *A Bibliography of two Oxford physiologists: Richard Lower 1631–1691, John Mayow 1643–1679*, Oxford (1935): figure 1, after page 13, the implication being that this is Francis Willoughby FRS (1635–1672) ornithologist and ichthyologist. But Francis Willoughby died in 1672. The signature is that of Thomas Willoughby (c1602–1691), 11th Baron Willoughby of Parham (1547) and 1st Baron Willoughby of Parham (1685). As a puritan, Willoughby fought with the parliamentarians during the English Civil War, seeing action at the battles of

6F. PHARMACEUTICE RATIONALIS (part 2), Oxford duodecimo 1675

The second edition of the second part of Willis's sixth book, published from Oxford, with the illustrations all double-sided [HJR Wing 36].

Title page: PHARMACEUTICE RATIONALIS, | SIVE | DIATRIBA | DE | Medicamentorum OPERATIONIBUS | IN | Humano Corpore. | [rule] | PARS SECUNDA. | [rule] | *AUTORE* | *Tho. Willis* M.D. in *Univ. Oxon.* | Prof. Sedleiano. | [rule] | OXONIÆ, | *E THEATRO SHELDONIANO,* | [short rule over date] M. DC. LXXV.

Collation: duodecimo in 6s: 23 letter roman alphabet using I and U; *a*–*b*^{6}, c^6, d^4, A–Z^6, Aa–Ee^6; $1–4 signed apart from: -*b*4, -c4, -A4, -I3, -T2, Bb2 signed Ab2.

190 leaves: paginated as [44], 1–72, 75–161, 138 for 162, 163–70, 173–83, 120 for 184, 185–248, 246 for 249, 250–327; i.e. [44], 1–324, [12].

Type: 45 lines; height (20 lines) 52 millimetres, width 50 millimetres.

Contents: ***a*1a**, page [1], title; ***a*1v**, page [2], blank; ***a*2r**, page [3], ATHENIS BRITANNICIS, Literati Orbis lumini Splendiſſimo, *UNIVERSITATI OXONIENSI*, Et Ibidem ILLUSTRISSIMO PRINCIPI JAC. ORMONDIÆ DUCI CANCELLARIO HONORATISSIMO, *RAD. BATHURST* DECANO WELLENSI VICECANCELLARIO DIGNISSIMO, Reverendis admodum, & perquam Eruditis DOCTORIBUS, PROCURATORIBUS, Facultatum omnium PROFESSORIBUS, Collegiorum & Aularum Profectis, NEC NON Venerabili Magiſtrorum Senatui Diatribam hanc Pharmaceuticam Pietatis & gratitudinis ergo Dicat Dedicatque Alumnus & beneficiarius adſtrictiſſimus THO. WILLIS.; ***a*2v**, page [4], Imprimatur AMiciſſimo Authori, poſt tam Immortale opus, nihil mortale facturo, tanquam Lumina morienti claudens, extremum hoc officium præſtat Oxon. *Novemb.* 12. 1675 *RAD. BATHURST* Vice-Cancellarius. *Oxonienſis.*; ***a*3r–*a*6r**, pages [5–11], *CANDIDO LECTORI* PRÆFATIO.; ***a*6v–*b*4r**, pages [12–19], POSTSCRIPTUM., ***b*4v**, page [20], blank; ***b*5r–v**, pages [21–2], *AUTORI CLARISIMO, nec non mihi (de quo jure glorior) AMICISSIMO, in illius* Pharmaceutices Rationalis *Partem utramque* Carmen Gratulatorium … [signed] *Gul. Dawkins.*; ***b*6r–v**, pages [23–4], QUERELA LIBRI POSTHUMI DE OBITU AUTORIS. … [signed] *GUL. DAWKINS.* Med. Bac.; **c1r–d4v**, pages [25–44], ELENCHUS RERUM.

A1r–Dd6r, pages 1–'327', [text] PHARMACEUTICÆ RATIONALIS, SIVE DE MEDICAMENTORUM OPERATIONIBUS *In Corpore Humano* Pars Secunda.; **Dd6v**, page [324], blank.

Ee1r–Ee5v, pages [1–10], INDEX ALPHABETICUS.; **Ee6r–v**, pages [1–2], blank.

Middlewich (1643) and the Bolton Massacre (1644). His civilian work was in the support of grammar schools. Unable to make contact with the first in line who had migrated to Virginia, in 1679 Thomas succeeded his cousin, Charles Willoughby, 10th Baron Willoughby of Parham. He lived at Old Lord's Farm in Horwich, an area still known as 'Old Lords Estate', and is buried under the chancel by the east window at the old Horwich Parish Church.

Headlines and *Catchwords*: *læſa.* for *læſâ.* at **D3v**, page 42; headline and chapter title *Exſpiratione læſa.* for *Tuſſi.* at **D4r**, page 43; *CAP. V.* for *CAP. VI.* at **E3r**, page '53'; *Tabe* Dorſali. for *Phthyſi Pulmonari.* at **E3r**, page '53'; *CAP. VI.* for *CAP. VII.* at **I2r**, page '101'; *CAP. IX.* for *CAP. XI.* at **M5r**, page '143'; *Asthmate.* for *Aſthmate.* at **N6r**, page '157'; *Aſthmate.* for *pectoris Hydrope.* at **O3v**, page '164'; *CAP. II.* for *CAP. I.* at **P3r**, page '177'; *CAP. III.* for *CAP. IV.* at **T2r**, page '223'; *CAP. IV.* for *CAP. V.* at **U2r**, page '235'; *CAP. V.* for *CAP. I.* at **X3r**, page '246'; *SECT. I* for *SECT. III.* at **X4v**, page '252'; *CAP. III.* for *CAP. IV.* at **Aa3r**, page '285'; *CAP. III.* for *CAP. V.* at **Bb1v**, page '294'; *Eorumque Remediis*, for *De Aſſectibus Cutaneis*, at **Bb2v**, page '296'.

DE unlinked at **d4v**, page [44]; rapeia for peia at **P2r / v**, pages '175 / 176'; *punctum* (letters all inverted) for *punctum* at **S1v / S2r**, pages '210 / 211'; partium for una plurium at **S2r / S2v**, pages '211 / 212'; *ſalvia* for *viæ* at **U2r / v**, pages '235 / 236'; fectum for defectum at **Cc2r / v**, page '307 / 308'; Dimetri- for DIureticorum at **Ee1v / Ee2r**, pages [2] / [3].

Frontispiece: none.

Portrait: none.

Printers' ornaments: none.

No decorated initials.

Illustrations: as in **6E** apart from:

Pl.33a1. Plate 33 (image 58): Folding, 149 × 207 millimetres (sheet); with **Pl.34a1**. Plate 34 (image 59) printed on the verso. Inserted before text for Sect. I Cap. I at **A1r**, page 1.

Pl.35a1. Plate 35 (images 60 and 61): Folding, 212 × 149 millimetres (sheet); with **Pl.36a1**. Plate 36 (images 62–64) printed on the verso. Inserted before text for Sect. I Cap. I at **A1r**, page 1.

Pl.37a1. Plate 37 (images 65–67): Folding, 231 × 193 millimetres (sheet); with **Pl.38a1**. Plate 38 (images 68–75) printed on the verso. Inserted before text for Sect. I Cap. I at **A1r**, page 1.

Pl.39a1. Plate 39 (images 76–79): Folding, 153 × 149 millimetres (sheet); with **Pl.40a1**. Plate 40 (images 80–82) printed on the verso. Inserted before text for Sect. I Cap. I at **A1r**, page 1.

Copy: DASC (#1 of 2). Original calf, spine with five raised bands, gilt decorated panels and edges, lettered WILLIS | OPERA | TO. 2, original endpapers. Leaves 142 × 78 millimetres, boards 155 × 84 × 26 millimetres.

6G. PHARMACEUTICE RATIONALIS (part 2), The Hague duodecimo 1677

The third edition of the second part of Willis's sixth book, published from The Hague [HJR Wing 39].

Title page: PHARMACEUTICE | RATIONALIS | ſive | DIATRIBA | de | MEDICAMENTORUM | Operationibus in humano Corpore. | PARS SECUNDA | *Authore* | THOMA WILLIS, M. D. | *In Univ. Oxon.* Prof, Sedleiano, Nec non *Coll.* | *Med. Lond. &* *Societ. Reg.* Socio | Editio poſtrema emendatior. | [ornament] | *HAGÆ-COMITIS*, | [short rule] | Ex Officinâ ARNOLDI LEERS, Bibliopolæ. | cIↃ IↃc LXXVII.

Collation: duodecimo; 23 letter roman alphabet using I and V; *a*–b[12], A–Y[12]; $1–6 signed apart from: -C6, -F4, +A7, G5 for G4, *I*1 for I1, +M7, +N7, +O7, +P7, +Q7, +R7, +S7, +T7, +V7, +X7.

288 leaves: paginated as [48], 1–518, [10]. Mispaginated: 391 for 291, 490 for 460.

Type: 33 lines: height (20 lines) 63 millimetres, width 55 millimetres.

Contents: ***a*1r**, page [1], title; ***a*1v**, page [2], blank; ***a*2r**, page [3], ATHENIS BRITANNICIS, Literati Orbis lumini Splendiſſimo, *UNIVERSITATI OXONIENSI*, Et Ibidem ILLUSTRISSIMO PRINCIPI JAC. ORMONDIÆ DUCI CANCELLARIO HONORATISSIMO, *RAD. BATHURST* DECANO WELLENSI VICECANCELLARIO DIGNISSIMO, Reverendis admodum, & perquam Eruditis DOCTORIBUS, PROCURATORIBUS, *F*acultatum omnium PROFESSORIBUS, Collegiorum & Aularum Præfectus, NEC NON Venerabili Magiſtrorum Senatui Diatribam hanc Pharmacenticam Pietatis & gratitudinis ergo Dicat Dedicatque Alumnus & beneficarius adſtrictiſſimus THO. WILLIS.; ***a*2v**, page [4], Imprimatur AMiciſſimo Authori, poſt tam Immortale opus, nihil mortale facturo, tanquam Lumina morienti claudens, extremum hoc officium præſtat Oxon. *Novemb.* 12. 1675 *RAD. BATHURST* Vice-Cancellarius *Oxonienſis*.; ***a*3r–*a*6v**, pages [5–12], *CANDIDO LECTORI* PRÆFATIO.; ***a*7r–*a*10v**, pages [13–20], POSTSCRIPTUM., ***a*11r–*a*11v**, pages [21–2], *AUTORI CLARISSIMO, nec non mihi (de quo jure glorior) AMICISSIMO, in illius* Pharmaceutices Rationalis *Partem utramque* Carmen Gratulatorium … [signed] *Gul. Dawkins.*; ***a*12r–*a*12v**, pages [23–4], QUERELA LIBRI POSTHUMI DE OBITU AUTORIS. … [signed] *GUL. DAWKINS*. Med. Bac.; **b1r–b12v**, pages [25–48], ELENCHUS RERUM.

A1r–Y7v, pages 1–518, [Text] PHARMACEUTICÆ RATIONALIS, *Sive* DE MEDICAMENTORUM OPERATIONIBUS *In Corpore Humano* PARS SECUNDA.

Y8r–Y12v, pages [1–10], INDEX. ALPHABETICUS.

Headlines and *Catchwords*: CAP. It. for CAP. I. at **B1r**, page 25; *De respirationis* for Figurarum explicatio at **B9v**, page 42; CAP. I for CAP. III at **C9r**, page 65; CAP. VI. for CAP. IV. at **D2r**, page 75; CAP. I. for CAP. VI. at **D11r**, page 93; CAP. V. for CAP. VI. at **E1r**, page 97; CAP. V. for CAP. VI. at **E7r**, page 109; *Phthiſa in genere* for *Phthiſi Pulmonari* at **E7v**, page 112; CAP. VI. for CAP. VII. at **G7r**, page 157; **G9r**, page 161; **G10r**, page 163; **G12r**, page 167; *Sanguinem* for *Sanguinis* at **G10r**, page 163; *Peripnomonia* for *Peripnemonia* at **H5r**, page 177; *Peripnœmonia* for *Peripnemonia* at **H6v**, page 180; 'e' inverted in *De Peripnemonia* at **H8r**, page 183; *Do* for *De* at **H12v**, page 192; **I2v**, page 196; *Pluritide* for *Pleuritide* at **I7r**, page 207; 213 … SECT. I. for CAP. IX. … 213 at **I11r**, page 213; *Empyemata* for *Empyemete* at **K3v**, page 222; CAA. X for CAP. X. at **K4r**, page 223; CAP. IX. for CAP. XI. at **K7r**, page 229; SECT. I. for CAP. XII. at **K11r**, page 237; CAP. X. for CAP. XII. at **L2r**, page 243; **L7r**, page 253; CAP. XI. for CAP. XII. at **L3r**, page 245; **L4r**, page 247; SECT. I. for CAP. XII. at **L9r**, page 257; *Aſthmate* for *Pectoris Hydrope* at **L10v**, page 260; **L11v**, page 262; CAP. II. for CAP. I. at **M7r**, page 277; **M8r**, page 279; CAP. IV. for CAP. V. at **Q3r**, page 365; CAP. V. for CAP. I. at **R2r**, page 387; ALPHABETICUS. for INDEX. at **Y11v**, page [8]; INDEX. for ALPHABETICUS. at **Y12r**, page [9].

vipe- for rarum at **b12r / v**, pages [47] / [48]; è poris for é poris at **B1r / v**, pages 25 / 26; Pul- for 2. Pul at **E2r / v**, pages 99 / 100; ſtructus- for ctus at **I3r / v**, pages 197 / 198; aut for ant at **I9v / I10r**, pages 210 / 211; dui for du Unc. at **I10r / v**, pages 211 / 212; Vnc for Unc at **L6v / L7r**, pages 252 / 253; copio- for fus in at **L10r / v**, pages 259 / 260; nunquam for nonnunquam at **R9r / v**, pages 401 / 402; and ras for ceteras at **R11r / v**, pages 405 / 406.

Frontispiece: none.

Portrait: none.

Printers' ornaments: tailpiece on title page, ***a*1r**, page [1] {**Leers 1**}; tailpiece at ***a*10v**, page [20] {**Leers 10**}; headpiece (cut down from a larger ornament and inverted) at **b1r**, page [25] {**Leers 11**}; tailpiece at **b12v**, page [48] {**Leers 12**}.

Decorated A at ***a*3r**, page [5] {**Leers 8**}; D at ***a*7r**, page [13] {**Leers 9**}; I at **A1r**, page 1 {**Leers 13**}.

Illustrations: as in **6E** apart from:

Pl.33b1. Plate 33 (image 58): *Sect. i: Cap. i* (headline, left), *Tab: I.* (headline, right); lettering to depict structures (in multiples of ≤ 8) A–C, *d*, *e*. Folding, 128 × 193 millimetres (sheet); 113 × 187 millimetres (plate marks); 93 × 179 millimetres (figure). Inserted after legends for Tabula I–VIII at **B9r–B12v**, pages 41–8.

Pl.34b1. Plate 34 (image 59): *Tab: II.* (headline, left), *Sect. i: Cap. i.* (headline, right); lettering to depict structures (in multiples of ≤ 5) A–G, *f*. Folding, 206 × 132 millimetres (sheet); 195 × 125 millimetres (plate marks); 183 × 115 millimetres (figure). Inserted after legends for Tabula I–VIII at **B9r–B12v**, pages 41–8.

Pl.35b1. Plate 35 (images 60–61): *Tab. III.* (headline, left), *Sect. i: Cap i* (headline, right); lettering to depict structures (in multiples of ≤ 5) A–H, *a*, *b*. Folding, 205 × 148 millimetres (sheet); 202 × 145 millimetres (plate marks, cropped); 177 × 133 millimetres, 43 × 24 millimetres (figures). Inserted after legends for Tabula I–VIII at **B9r–B12v**, pages 41–8.

Pl.36b1. Plate 36 (images 62–64): *Tab: IV.* (headline, centre), *Sect. i: Cap. i.* (headline, right), *Fig: 1.*, *Fig: 2.*, *Fig: 3.* (footers, centre below each image); lettering to depict structures (in multiples of ≤ 5) A, b–d. Folding, 169 × 130 millimetres (sheet); 168 × 126 millimetres (plate marks); 70 × 42 millimetres, 58 × 33 millimetres, 62 × 35 millimetres (figures). Inserted after legends for Tabula I–VIII at **B9r–B12v**, pages 41–8.

Pl.37b1. Plate 37 (images 65–67): *Sect. i: Cap. i*: (headline, left), *Tab: V.* (headline, right), *Fig: 2.*, *Fig: 1.*, *Fig: 3.* (centre, left of each image); lettering to depict structures (in multiples of ≤ 8) A, B, a–c. Folding, 232 × 175 millimetres (sheet); 224 × 172 millimetres (plate marks);

76 × 65 millimetres, 77 × 89 millimetres, 137 × 153 millimetres (figures). Inserted after legends for Tabula I–VIII at **B9r–B12v**, pages 41–8.

Pl.38b1. Plate 38 (images 68–75): *Tab: VI.* (headline, left), *Sect. i: Cap. i*: (headline, right), *Fig: 1.*, *Fig: 2.* (headers, above each group of four images); lettering to identify components of each figure 1–4. Folding, 156 × 225 millimetres (sheet); 144 × 220 millimetres (plate marks); 67 × 49 millimetres, 66 × 47 millimetres, 67 × 47 millimetres, 67 × 48 millimetres, 69 × 18 millimetres, 69 × 17 millimetres, 70 × 16 millimetres, 72 × 17 millimetres (figures). Inserted after legends for Tabula I–VIII at **B9r–B12v**, pages 41–8.

Pl.39b1. Plate 39 (images 76–79): *Sect. i: Cap. i*: (headline, left), *Tab: VII.* (headline, centre), *Fig: 1.*, *Fig: 3.*, *Fig: 4.*, *Fig: 2.* (headers, above each image); no lettering. Folding, 130 × 145 millimetres (sheet); 122 × 138 millimetres (plate marks); 57 × 53 millimetres, 52 × 47 millimetres, 58 × 59 millimetres, 55 × 59 millimetres (figures). Inserted after legends for Tabula I–VIII at **B9r–B12v**, pages 41–8.

Pl.40b1. Plate 40 (images 80–82): *Sect. Cap. i. Fig: 1.* (headline, left), *Tab: VIII.* (headline, centre), *Fig: 1.*, *Fig: 2.*, *Fig: 3.* (headers, above each image); no lettering. Folding, 130 × 155 millimetres (sheet); 62 × 135 millimetres (plate marks); 49 × 49 millimetres, 21 × 26 millimetres, 52 × 50 millimetres (figures). Inserted after legends for Tabula I–VIII at **B9r–B12v**, pages 41–8.

Copy: DASC (bound with #2 of **6D**). Original vellum, spine lettered (in manuscript) THOMÆ WILLIS | PHARMACEUTICE | Rationalis | Pars I & II, original endpapers. Leaves 132 × 74 millimetres, boards 138 × 73 × 60 millimetres. Inserted: bookplate Ex Libris ED. QUANTIN (unidentified). Stamped: Ex Libris J. Derône (unidentified).

6H. [PHARMACEUTICE RATIONALIS (part 1)], Middelburg and Amsterdam octavo 1677

The Dutch translation of the first part of Willis's sixth book, printed in Amsterdam [not listed by HJR Wing].

Title page: d' Algemeene | En byſondere Wercking der | GENEES-MIDDELEN | In s'Menſchen Lichaam, | Door een Wis-konſtige Redeneringh | volgens de Nieuwe gronden der Genees-kunde, nader | als oyt voor deſen verklaart en met PRINT-VER. | BEELDINGEN vertoont, | Door THOMAS WILLIS, | *Hoog-Leeraar in de Genees-oeffening tot Oxfort*: | Uyt het Latijn vertaalt, en met noodighe | aanteyckeningen verrijckt. | *Door A d' HEIDE, M. Doctor.* | [ornament] | Tot MIDDELBURG. | [short rule] | By WILHELMUS GOEREE, Boecke- | verkooper in *Cicero*: en zijn mede te bekomen tot | *Amſterdam*, by *Joh: Janſſonium van* | *Waeſbergen*, 1677.[*16]

[*] Underlined text originally printed in red.

[16] 'The general and specific Action of MEDICAMENTS In the Human Body, Through Rational Reasoning according to the New fundaments of Medicine, closer than ever explained and displayed with PRINTED ILLUSTRATIONS, By THOMAS WILLIS, *Professor of the Practice of Medicine in Oxford*: Translated from Latin, and supplemented with appropriate comments. *By A d' HEIDE, Med. Doctor.* At MIDDELBURG. With

Collation: octavo: 23 letter roman alphabet using I and V: $*^8$, $**^2$ (-**2), A–Z^8, Aa–Ff^8, Gg^8 (-Gg 6, 7, and 8); $1–5 signed.

246 leaves: paginated as [18], 1–454, [20]. Mispaginated: 207 for 107, 109 for 209.

Type: 34 lines; height (20 lines, without footnotes) 69 millimetres, width 62 millimetres (77 with marginal notes).

Contents:[17] ***1r**, page [1], title page; ***1v**, page [2], blank; ***2r–*5v**, pages [3–10], *AAN DEN LESER.*; ***6r–**1v**, pages [11–18], *DEN OVERSETTER TOT DEN LESER.*

A1r–Ff3v, pages 1–454, text [Pharmaceutice rationalis, part 1].

Ff4r–Gg5v, pages [1–20], BLAT–WYSER ... Berigt aen den Boek-binder. Den Binder ſy gewaerſchuwt, dat de Figuren alle agter den anderen volgens Tabula 1. 2. 3. &c. tuſſchen het Regiſter en het eynde van't Boeck moeten ingevoegt worden, en de ſelve ſoo ver voorwaerts uyt laten gaen als mogelijck is.[18]

Headlines and *Catchwords*: *bereidyng.* for *bereiding.* at **E5r**, page 73; *her bereyding.* for *haar bereiding.* at **L1r**, page 161; **L2r**, page 163; *Vande roode en witte Bloed-loop.* for Hoe de Pis afgeſet werd. at **M8r**, page 191; *bereyding.* for *bereiding.* at **O5v**, page 218; **P3v**, page 230; **Z4r**, page 359; **Z5r**, page 361; *De ontleding des Slag-aders.* for *Van de Verdoovende of Slaap-middelen.* at **Bb6r**, page 395.

zcnu- for zenu at **D7v / D8r**, pages 62 / 63; aardge- for aange at **K1r / v** at pages 145 / 146; ge ſtof for ghe ſtof at **K8v / L1r**, pages 160 / 161; 3. Af- for 3de Af- at **L2r / v**, pages 163 / 164; 4. Af- for 4de Af- at **O2r / v**, pages 211 / 212; **P4v / P5r**, pages 232 / 233; 5. Af- for 5de Af- at **V2r / v**, pages 307 / 308; nigende for nighende at **Y5r / v**, pages 345 / 346; 6. Af- for 6de Af- at **Z6v / Z7r**, pages 364 / 365; 7. Af- for 7de Af- at **Dd7v / Dd8r**, pages 430 / 431.

Frontispiece: none.

Portrait: none.

Printers' ornaments: tailpiece at ***1r**, page [1] {**Goeree 9**}; tailpiece at **Gg5v**, page [20] {**Goeree 12**}.

Decorated H at ***2r**, page [3] {**Goeree 10**}; W at ***6r**, page [11] {**Goeree 2**}; D at **A1r**, page 1 {**Goeree 11**}.

WILHELMUS GOEREE, Book-Merchant at *Cicero*: and also available in Amsterdam, at Joh: Janssonius van Waesbergen, 1677'. Jan van Gijn explains that 'Redeneringh' is probably a misprint for 'Redenkundige'; but the translator may have intended the meaning 'mathematical reasoning' rather than the tautology 'rational reasoning' as in the title for *Pharmaceutice rationalis*, part 2 Dutch (**6J**).

[17] As also indicated in the collation pencilled onto the rear pastedown in a copy held in the Amsterdam University Library, the assumption is that (since the catchwords are correct across *8v / **1 and **1v / A1r) **2 was discarded; and the same probably applies to Gg6–Gg8.

[18] 'Message to the book-binder. The binder should take care that all the Figures are inserted in due order as Plate 1. 2. 3. &c. between the Index and the end of the book and to place them as much to the front as possible'.

Illustrations: Legends translated into Dutch, variable use of roman and italic lettering, and as in **6D** apart from:

Pl.27b2. Plate 27 (image 46): Folding, 181 × 205 millimetres (sheet). Inserted within legends for Tabula I–VI at **C5v–C6r**, pages 42–3.

Pl.28b2. Plate 28 (image 47): Folding, 145 × 197 millimetres (sheet). Inserted within legends for Tabula I–VI at **C5v–C6r**, pages 42–3.

Pl.29b2. Plate 29 (image 48): Folding, 152 × 197 millimetres (sheet). Inserted within legends for Tabula I–VI at **C5v–C6r**, pages 42–3.

Pl.30b2. Plate 30 (image 49–51): Folding, 158 × 250 millimetres (sheet). Inserted within legends for Tabula I–VI at **C5v–C6r**, pages 42–3.

Pl.31b2. Plate 31 (image 52): Folding, 152 × 185 millimetres (sheet). Inserted within legends for Tabula I–VI at **C5v–C6r**, pages 42–3.

Pl.32b2. Plate 32 (images 53–57): Folding, 142 × 193 millimetres (sheet). Inserted within legends for Tabula I–VI at **C5v–C6r**, pages 42–3.

Copy: DASC. Original vellum, spine lettered T: willis. | 1 deel, original endpapers. Leaves 153 × 96 millimetres, boards 160 × 100 × 33 millimetres. Inscribed: (1) Dit boek behoort aen N= Heijlma; (2) Dr J. van der Hoeven 1901. Inserted: bookplate of [J] van der Hoeven.[19]

6I. PHARMACEUTICE RATIONALIS (parts 1 and 2), Oxford octavo 1679

The only edition combining both parts of Willis's sixth book as one work, published from Oxford [HJR Wing 40].

Title page: [1]. Pharmaceutice Rationalis. | SIVE | DIATRIBA | *DE MEDICAMENTORUM* | OPERATIONIBUS | IN | Humano Corpore. | [rule] | AUTHORE | *Tho. Willis* M. D. in *Univ. Oxon.* Prof. Sedleiano, nec non | *Coll. Med. Lond.* & Societ. Reg. Socio. | [rule] | *Editio tertia*, | [ornament] | OXONIÆ, | E THEATRO SHELDONIANO, Proftant | apud *Ric. Davis*. 1679.

[19] Nikolaas Arnoldus Heijlma (nd) was a surgeon working in Oud-Beijerland, south of Rotterdam, early in the eighteenth century. Church records indicate that he married Geertruyd, the daughter of Pieter Landmeeter (the surname, land surveyor, presumably reflecting the profession of Pieter or one of his forebears) on 4 February 1731. Jan van der Hoeven (1863–1941) came from a distinguished medical family. After qualifying in 1888, he was appointed to the Sophia Children's Hospital in Rotterdam, founded by his father, Jan van der Hoeven (1834–1900), and then the municipal hospital in Zutphen where he remained until 1934. He wrote extensively on the history of medicine. His grandfather, Jan van der Hoeven (1802–1868), professor of natural history in Rotterdam wrote a Handboek de Dierkunde (zoology) which was translated into English by Reverend William Clark MD FRS (1788–1869) and published by Cambridge University Press (two volumes: 1856–1858).

[2]. PHARMACEUTICE RATIONALIS, | SIVE | DIATRIBA | DE | Medicamentorum | OPERATIONIBUS | IN | Humano Corpore. | [rule] | PARS SECUNDA | [rule] | *AUTORE* | *Tho. Willis* M. D. in *Univ. Oxon.* | Prof. Sedleiano. | [rule] | OXONIÆ, | *E THEATRO SHELDONIANO*, | M. DC. LXXVIII.

Collation: octavo in 4s: 23 letter roman alphabet using I and U: [a]^2, *b*^{4}, c–e^4, A–Z^4, Aa–Zz^4, Aaa–Eee^4; $1–3 signed apart from -b3, -c3, -d3, -e3, -O2, -P3, -S3, -U2, -X3, -Y3, -Z3, -Bb3, -Ff3, -Gg3, -Kk3, -Mm3, -Nn3, -Ss3, Yy2 signed Y2, -Ccc2, -Ddd3.

222 leaves: paginated as [36], 1–164, [20], 1–210, [14].

Type: 55 lines; height (20 lines) 54 millimetres, width 80 millimetres.

Contents: **[a]1r**, page [1], title; **a1v**, page [2], blank; **a2r**, page [3], CELEBERRIMO *MEDICORUM LONDINENSIUM* COLLEGIO, Et Singulatim VIRO INSIGNISSIMO DOCTISSIMOQUE D^{no} Georgio Ent EQUITI AURATO Præſidi Illuſtriſſimo; Nec non CENSORIBUS DIGNISSIMIS, Cæteriſque omnibus, ampliſſimæ hujus Societatis Membris; DIATRIBAM HANC PHARMACEUTICAM Obſervantiæ & Honoris ergo Dicat, Dedicatque, THO. WILLIS.; **a2v**, page [4], [imprimatur] LIBRUM hunc, Authore ſuo, ſagaciſſimo Phyſiologo, Medico peritiſſimo, dignum; olim Symmyſta, ſemper Amicus, libentiſſime Typis mando. Oxon. *Octob*. 31. 1673. *RAD. BATHURST. Vice-Cancel*.; ***b*1r–*b*4r**, pages [5–11], CANDIDO LECTORI PRÆFATIO.; ***b*4v**, page [12], blank; **c1r–d1v**, pages [13–22], ELENCHUS RERUM [part 1]; **d2r–c4v**, pages [23–36], ELENCHUS RERUM [part 2].

A1r–X2v, pages 1–164, [text] DE MEDICAMENTORUM OPERATIONIBUS IN Corpore Humano.

X3r, page [1], title; **X3v**, page [2], Imprimatur. AMiciſſimo Authori, poſt tam Immortale opus, nihil mortale facturo, tanquam Lumina morienti claudens, extremum hoc officium præſtat. Oxon. *Novemb.* 12. 1675, *RAD. BATHURST* Vice-Cancel. *Oxonienſis*.; **X4r**, page [3], ATHENIS BRITANNICIS, Literati Orbis lumini Splendiſſimo, *UNIVERSITATI OXONIENSI*: Et Ibidem ILLUSTRISSIMO PRINCIPI JAC. ORMONDIÆ DUCI, CANCELLARIO HONORATISSIMO, *RAD. BATHURST* DECANO WELLENSI, VICECANCELLARIO DIGNISSIMO; Reverendis admodum, & perquam Eruditis DOCTORIBUS, PROCURATORIBUS, Facultatum omnium PROFESSORIBUS, Collegiorum & Aularum Præfectis, NEC NON Venerabili Magiſtrorum Senatui, Diatribam hanc Pharmaceuticam Pietatis & gratitudinis ergo Dicat Dedicatque Alumnus & Beneficarius adſtrictiſſimus THO. WILLIS.; **X4v**, page [4], blank; **Y1r–Y3r**, pages [5–9], *CANDIDO LECTORI* PRÆFATIO.; **Y3r–Z1v**, pages [9–14], POSTSCRIPTUM.; **Z2r–Z3r**, pages [15–17], *AUTORI CLARISSIMO, nec non mihi (de quo jure glorior) AMICISSIMO, in illius* Pharmaceutices Rationalis *Partem utramque.* Carmen Gratulatorium. ... [signed] *Gul. Dawkins*.; **Z3v–Z4r**, pages [18–19], QUERELA LIBRI POSTHUMI DE OBITU AUTORIS.... [signed] *Gul. Dawkins*. MED. B.; **Z4v**, page [20], blank.

A1r–Ddd1v, pages 1–210, [text] Pharmaceuticæ Rationalis, SIVE DE MEDICAMENTORUM OPERATIONIBUS IN Corpore Humano. PARS SECUNDA.

Ddd2r–Ddd4v, pages [1–6], INDEX PRIMÆ PARTIS.; **Eee1r–Eee3r**, pages [7–13], INDEX PARTIS SECUNDÆ.; **Eee3v**, page [14], blank.

Headlines and *Catchwords*: *Vomitoriorum* for *Vomitorum* at **D2v**, page 28; **D3v**, page 30; **D4v–E2r**, pages 32–5; D*iabete.* for *Diabete.* at **L3v**, page 86; *Species* for *ſpecies* at **N3v**, page 102; *Diaphoresin* for *Diaphoresi* at **O3r**, page 109; *Medicamentiis* for *Medicamentis* at **P4v**, page 120; *ſpecies,.* for *ſpecies* at **Q3v**, page 126; *Pulſu* for *pulſu* at **S1r**, page 137; *Puerorum* for *puerorum* at **Ff4v**, page 48; *Asthmate.* for *Aſthmate.* at **Nn1v**, 98.

PHAR- for DE at **e4v / A1r**, page [36] / 1; XVI. Pri for 1. Pri at **F3v / F4r**, page 46 / 47; XI. Præ for IX. Præ at **K3r / v**, page 77 / 78; pide for trepide at **T4v / U1r**, page 152 / 153; ad præ for prædium at **Y3r / v**, pages [9] / [10]; no catchword at **Z4r / Aa1r**, pages [19] / 1; tur for fatur at **Kk1v / Kk2r**, pages 74 / 75; Secundo for XIV Secundo at **Ll3r / v**, pages 85 / 86; nem for guinem at **Qq4r / v**, pages 127 / 128; hujuf for modi at **Uu1v / Uu2r**, pages 154 / 155.

Frontispiece: none.

Portrait: none.

Printers' ornament: printers' device at **a1r**, page [1] {**Fell 11**}.

Decorated A at **A1r**, page 1{**Fell 12**}.

Illustrations: lettering and legends as in **6A** and **6E** apart from:[20]

Pl.27a3. Plate 27 (image 46): *p. 16.* (added to headline, right). Folding, 177 × 200 millimetres (sheet). Inserted within legends for Tabulæ I–VI at **B4v–C1r**, pages 16–17.

Pl.28a3. Plate 28 (image 47): *p. 16.* (added to headline, right). Folding, 182 × 200 millimetres (sheet). Inserted within legends for Tabulæ I–VI at **B4v–C1r**, pages 16–17.

Pl.29a3. Plate 29 (image 48): *p. 16.* (added to headline, right). Folding, 179 × 194 mm (sheet). Inserted within legends for Tabulæ I–VI at **B4v–C1r**, pages 16–17.

Pl.30a3. Plate 30 (image 49–51): *p. 16.* (added to headline, right). Folding, 180 × 210 millimetres (sheet). Inserted within legends for Tabulæ I–VI at **B4v–C1r**, pages 16–17.

Pl.31a3. Plate 31 (image 52): *p. 17.* (added to headline, right). Folding, 182 × 187 millimetres (sheet). Incorrectly inserted within legends for Tabulæ I–VIII (part 2) at **Bb4v–Cc2r**, pages 16–19.

Pl.32a3. Plate 32 (images 53–57): *p. 17.* (added to headline, right). Folding, 182 × 212 millimetres (sheet, cropped). Incorrectly inserted within legends for Tabulæ I–VIII (part 2) at **Bb4v–Cc2r**, pages 16–19.

[20] The placements given for each plate leaf are as intended by the printer.

Pl.33a2. Plate 33 (image 58): *pag. i6.* (added to headline, left). Folding, 182 × 197 millimetres (sheet). Inserted within legends for Tabulæ I–VIII at **Bb4v–Cc2r**, pages 16–19.

Pl.34a2. Plate 34 (image 59): *pag. i6.* (added to headline, centre). Folding, 195 × 154 millimetres (sheet). Inserted within legends for Tabulæ I–VIII at **Bb4v–Cc2r**, pages 16–19.

Pl.35a2. Plate 35 (images 60 and 61): *ad pag. i7.* (added to headline, left). Folding, 201 × 147 millimetres (sheet). Inserted within legends for Tabulæ I–VIII at **Bb4v–Cc2r**, pages 16–19.

Pl.36a2. Plate 36 (images 62–64): *ad pag. i7* (added to headline, centre). Folding, 177 × 130 millimetres (sheet). Inserted within legends for Tabulæ I–VIII at **Bb4v–Cc2r**, pages 16–19.

Pl.37a2. Plate 37 (images 65–67): *ad pag. i8* (added to headline, centre). Folding, 219 × 169 millimetres (sheet). Incorrectly inserted within legends for Tabulæ I–VI (part 1) at **B4v–C1r**, pages 16–17.

Pl.38a2. Plate 38 (images 68–75): *ad. pag. i8* (added to headline, centre). Folding, 182 × 210 millimetres (sheet, cropped). Incorrectly inserted within legends for Tabulæ I–VI (part 1) at **B4v–C1r**, pages 16–17.

Pl.39a2. Plate 39 (images 76–79): *ad pag. i9* (added to headline, centre). Folding, 182 × 172 millimetres (sheet). Inserted within legends for Tabulæ I–VIII at **Bb4v–Cc2r**, pages 16–19.

Pl.40a2. Plate 40 (images 80–82): *ad pag. i9* (added to centre, right). Folding, 182 × 169 millimetres (sheet). Inserted within legends for Tabulæ I–VIII at **Bb4v–Cc2r**, pages 16–19.

Copy: DASC (#1 of 3). Original calf with blind stamped central panel, triple-lined borders, and floral corners, edges with single line, rebacked, four raised bands with no lettering, original endpapers. Leaves 179 × 107 millimetres, boards 184 × 112 × 34 millimetres. Inscribed: (×2) William Belcher (and annotations probably in a different hand). Shelf mark: (1) i / 134 and i / 136; (2) Gk / 10; (3) 16.549. Bookplate: (rear pastedown; unidentified) 'NIL CONSCIRE SIBI'.[21]

6J. [PHARMACEUTICE RATIONALIS (part 2)], Amsterdam octavo 1681

The Dutch translation of the second part of Willis's sixth book, published from Amsterdam [Not listed by HJR Wing].

Title page: THOMAS WILLIS | Vervolg | OF TWEEDE DEEL, | Der Redenkundige verhandeling van | de kragt en werking | *DER* | GENEES-MIDDELEN, | *ontrent de deelen en ſieketen des menſchen* | *lichaams in 't byſonder*; | VERVAT IN III BOOKEN. | Waar van

[21] The previous owner is unidentified. A possibility is William Belcher (nd) who brushed with the medical profession spending 1778–1795 in a madhouse and making his views known in an *Address to Humanity: containing a letter, to Dr. Thomas Monro; a receipt to make a lunatic and seize his estate; and a sketch of a true smiling hyena*, privately published (1796). Although distinctive, the design elements and motto on the bookplate are used for many coats of arms and are not identified.

het I. ſpreekt van de Genees- | middelen die op de deelen der Borſt werken. Het | II. van de Genees-middelen die op de Buik- | geweijen opſigt hebben. Het III. van het | Bloed-laten, Bloed-ſtempen, de kraght | van Blein-middelen, Fontanellen, | en diergelijke. | *Verligt met verſcheide Kopere Print-verbeeldingen, die | 't maakſel en dienſt der Long met alle haar Buiſen, Aderen, | Zenuwen en Draden naukeurig aanwyſen.* | Uit 't Latijn vertaald, en met noodige aantekeningen verrijkt. | *Door* A. D. H. *Medicinæ Doctor.* | [ornament] | t' AMSTERDAM, | [half-line] | By WILHELMUS GOEREE, Boekverkooper | op't Rokin in Cicero. ANNO 1681.[22]

Collation: octavo; 23 letter roman alphabet using I and V: †^{8}, A–Z^{8}, Aa–Ii^{8}; $1–5 signed.

264 leaves: paginated as [16], 1–500, [12]. Mispaginated: 156 for 157.

Type: 34 lines; height (20 lines, without footnotes) 69 millimetres, width 62 millimetres (75 with marginal notes).

Contents: **†1r**, page [1], title page; **†1v**, page [2], blank; **†2r–†5r**, pages [3–9], THOMAS WILLIS aan den OPMERKENDEN LESER.; **†5v–†6v**, pages [10–12], KORT INHOUD *Van de Hooft-ſtukken* des EERSTEN BOEKS. Handelende van de Borſt-middelen.; **†7r–†7v**, pages [13–14], KORT INHOUD *Van de Hooft-ſtukken* des TWEEDEN BOEKS. Handelende van de Genees-middelen die op de Buik-geweijen opſigt hebben.; **†7v–†8r**, pages [14–15], KORT INHOUD *Van het derde Boek*. Handelende van verſcheidene behandeling en werking der Genees-middelen.; **†8r–†8v**, pages [15–16], BERIGT *aen den* BOEK-BINDER. DEn Binder zy gewaarſchouwd, dat alle de Figuren getekent Tab. 1, II, III, tot VIII incluis ſoondanig volgens d'aanwyſing van de Paginaas, op haar plaats moeten ingevoegt werden, datſe met het aangeſigt tegen derſelver Verklaring konnen opſlaan en nageſien warden[23]

A1r–R8r, pages 1–271, [text] THOMAS WILLIS, Van de kragt ende werking der GENEES-MIDDELEN ontrent de deelen ende ſiecketen des Menſchen Lichaem in 't byſonder: *Het eerſte Boek*. Handelende van de Borſt-middelen.; **R8v–Aa5v**, pages 272–378, II. BOEK, Handelende van de *GENEES-MIDDELEN*, Die op de *Buik-geweijen* opſigt hebben.; **Aa6r–Ii2v**, pages 379–500, III. BOEK, [Handelende van verſcheidene behandeling en werking der Genees-middelen].

Ii3r–Ii8v, pages [1–20], *BLAD-WYSER*.

Headlines and *Catchwords*: *Ademhaling* for *Adem-haling* at **A7r**, page 13; **D5r**, page 57.

22 * Underlined text originally printed in red.
'THOMAS WILLIS Sequel or SECOND VOLUME, of the Rational Treatise of the power and action *OF* MEDICAMENTS, *particularly about the parts and illnesses of the human body;* CONTAINED IN III BOOKS. Of which the Ist speaks about medicines having their action upon the parts of the Chest. The IInd about the medicines related to the entrails of the abdomen. The IIIrd about Blood-letting, Stopping of bleeding, the power of blistering agents, fontanelles, and so on. *Decorated with several Copperplate Illustrations, which illustrate the structure and function of the Lung in great detail, with all her Vessels, Veins, Nerves and Fibres.* Translated from Latin, and supplemented with appropriate comments. *By* A. D. H. *Doctor of Medicine*. At AMSTERDAM, With WILHELMUS GOEREE, Merchant of books, at the Rokin in Cicero. ANNO 1681.'

23 'MESSAGE to the BOOK-BINDER. The Binder should take care that all the Figures marked Plate I. II, III up to and including VIII have to be inserted according to the marking of the pages, in such a way that they are facing the corresponding Explanation and can be found and consulted in this way.'

weinigje for weynigje at **K1r / v**, pages 145 / 146; Des for des at **N7r / v**, pages 205 / 206; ſeer for ſteld at **X7v / X8r**, pages 334 / 335; nen for men at **Aa1r / v**, pages 369 / 370; uitſui for uitzui at **Ee1r / v**, pages 433 / 434; raue for (1) raue at **Hh5r / v**, pages 489 / 490.

Frontispiece: none.

Portrait: none.

Printers' ornaments: tailpiece at †5r, page [9] {**Goeree 14**}; †8v, page [16] {**Leers 4**}.

Decorated N at †2r, page [3] {**Goeree 13**}; S at †5v, page [10] {**Goeree 15**}; I at A1r, page 1 {**Goeree 16**}.

Illustrations: Legends translated into Dutch, variable use of roman and italic lettering, and as in **6E** apart from:

Pl.33c1. Plate 33 (image 58): *TAB. I.* (headline, left), *Sect: 1. Cap: 1.* (headline, centre), *Pag. 45.* (headline, right). Folding, 145 × 195 millimetres (sheet); 100 × 175 millimetres (plate marks); 89 × 173 millimetres (figure). Inserted within legends for Tabulæ I–VIII at **C7r–D2v**, pages 45–52.

Pl.34c1. Plate 34 (image 59): *Sect: 1. Cap: 1.* (headline, left), *TAB. II.* (headline, centre), *Pag. 46.* (headline, right). Folding, 145 × 190 millimetres (sheet); 120 × 190 millimetres (plate marks, cropped); 115 × 176 millimetres (figure). Inserted within legends for Tabulæ I–VIII at **C7r–D2v**, pages 45–52.

Pl.35c1. Plate 35 (images 60 and 61): *Pag. 47.* (headline, left), *TAB. III.* (headline, centre), *Sect: 1 Cap: 1.* (headline, right), *fig. 1.* (header, centre), *fig. 2.* (footer, lower, right). Folding, 145 × 190 millimetres (sheet); 135 × 180 millimetres (plate marks); 132 × 173 millimetres, 24 × 41 millimetres (figures). Inserted within legends for Tabulæ I–VIII at **C7r–D2v**, pages 45–52.

Pl.36c1. Plate 36 (images 62–64): *Sect. 1. Cap. 1.* (headline, left), *TAB. IV.* (headline, centre), *Pag. 48.* (headline, right), *Fig: 1.*, *Fig: 2.*, *Fig: 3.* (headers, left of each image). Folding, 169 × 117 millimetres (sheet); 157 × 104 millimetres (plate marks); 68 × 38 millimetres, 58 × 33 millimetres, 61 × 36 millimetres (figures). Inserted within legends for Tabulæ I–VIII at **C7r–D2v**, pages 45–52.

Pl.37c1. Plate 37 (images 65–67): *Pag. 49.* (headline, left), *TAB. V.* (headline, centre), *Sect 1. Cap: 1.* (headline, right), *fig. 3.*, *fig. 2.*, *fig. 1.* (headers, left of each image). Folding, 166 × 232 millimetres (sheet); 150 × 210 millimetres (plate marks); 149 × 133 millimetres, 85 × 76 millimetres, 66 × 76 millimetres (figures). Inserted within legends for Tabulæ I–VIII at **C7r–D2v**, pages 45–52.

Pl.38c1. Plate 38 (images 68–75): *Pag. 50. Fig: 1.* (headline, centre), *Sect: 1. Cap: 1.*(headline, right), *TAB. VI. Fig: 2.* (header, centre). Folding, 145 × 219 millimetres (sheet); 141 × 202 millimetres (plate marks); 67 × 46 millimetres, 66 × 46 millimetres, 67 × 47 millimetres, 64 ×

47 millimetres, 70 × 17 millimetres, 70 × 16 millimetres, 70 × 16 millimetres, 71 × 17 millimetres (figures). Inserted within legends for Tabulæ I–VIII at **C7r–D2v**, pages 45–52.

Pl.39c1. Plate 39 (images 76–79): *Sect: 1. Cap. 1.* (headline, left), *TAB. VII.* (headline, centre), *Pag. 51.* (headline, right), *Fig: 3.*, *Fig: 1.*, *Fig: 2.*, *Fig: 4.* (headers, above each image). Folding, 145 × 132 millimetres (sheet); 123 × 117 millimetres (plate marks); 60 × 55 millimetres, 58 × 53 millimetres, 52 × 46 millimetres, 56 × 58 millimetres (figures). Inserted within legends for Tabulæ I–VIII at **C7r–D2v**, pages 45–52.

Pl.40c1. Plate 40 (images 80–82): *Pag. 51.* (headline, left), *TAB. VIII.* (headline, centre), *Sect: Cap: 1.* (headline, right), *Fig: 1.*, *Fig: 2.*, *Fig: 3.* (headers, above each image). Folding, 145 × 147 millimetres (sheet); 62 × 127 millimetres (plate marks); 48 × 47 millimetres, 20 × 25 millimetres, 50 × 48 millimetres (figures). Inserted within legends for Tabulæ I–VIII at **C7r–D2v**, pages 45–52.

Copy: DASC. Original vellum, spine lettered 2 deel | Thom. Will:, original endpapers. Leaves 151 × 97 millimetres, boards 160 × 100 × 33 millimetres.

11

'To be avoided as if they were sick'

A plain and easie method for preserving those that are well from the infection of the plague (1691–1721)

For a short work which only went through two editions, the bibliography of *A plain and easie method for preserving those that are well from the infection of the plague*, Willis's fourteenth treatise published as his seventh book, is surprisingly complicated. Written in 1666 but not published until 1691, text sheets of the original edition remained available over the next four years during which several changes were made to the preliminaries and endpages. Thirty years after it first appeared, the second and last edition was published.

Printing of the preliminaries and main text

At first the printer used four whole (B^8–E^8) and three half sheets ([A]^4, a^4, and F^4), providing 44 leaves. The preliminaries are on A^4 which is unsigned. The preface is printed on a^4 and the main text at B^8–F^4. However A4 is folded to the back and used to complete the main text by printing F4 + 1 = A4. This arrangement is maintained in all issues prior to 1721 (**7A1**–**7A4**). Matters then become more complicated.

Although HJR Wing describes the portrait as printed on A2r (or v), this seems unlikely. The plate, engraved by RW (Robert White: 1645–1703) and closely modelled on David Loggan's (1634–1692) version from 1667 (see **3A**), had already been used for *The London practice of physick* (1685: **10A1**). Copies of **7A1** have a stub adjacent to the portrait indicating that a leaf, presumably blank, has been excised. When the need for an errata sheet arose, the blank leaf A2 was retained and used for this purpose. With this change to the preliminaries, the opportunity was also taken of including 'A poem on the virtue of a laurel leaf for the cure of rheumatism'. It is written by W. B. [William Bolton: nd] and, as shown on a footnote at the end of the poem, dated 1690. The poem has no particular bearing on Willis's treatise on the plague, and the best guess is that William Crooke had an unsold stock of the poem available as an independent publication which he wished to sell. It is listed as a separate publication in the *Term Catalogue* for November 1690: '10. A Poem upon a Lawrel leaf. Octavo. Printed for William Crook at the Green dragon, without Temple Bar.'[1]

This added an extra sheet and required setting a new title page for the second issue (**7A2**).[2] However, despite its mention, the poem is lacking from a large number of copies. The

[1] See: Edward Arber, *The term catalogues, 1668–1709 A.D. A Contemporary bibliography of English literature in the reigns of Charles II, William and Mary, and Anne*, London (1903–1906): Michaelmas 1690 November, IV Numb 39, II 336, column 2.

[2] It is confusing that, in describing entry #41 (=**7A1**), HJR Wing collates the first sheet as 'A' but in the second issue, #42 (=**7A2**), rather than describing the additional sheet with the poem as $^2A^4$, switches to π^3 and $F^4 + 1$ for the preliminaries and A^4 for the poem. He retains this collation when describing copies of *A plain and easie method*

probable explanation is that Crooke overestimated his stock and was left with spare sheets of *A plain and easie method*. Rather than resetting the collective title page, he simply sold copies without the final sheet containing the poem. Furthermore, having changed the preliminaries, the decision was also taken no longer to bind in the portrait; or, as with the poem, Crooke may soon have exhausted his supply of the engraving. This all makes for much ambiguity in what constitutes a complete copy of the second issue (**7A2**). HJR Wing makes the point that of the eight examples he examined:[3]

> One at the Bodleian Library has an engraved portrait of Willis facing the title page, on the back of which is pasted on the imprimatur leaf, the errata leaf following the title page. This copy also lacks the poem. One copy at the Wellcome Historical Medical Library has the imprimatur leaf at the end forming leaf F6. This copy also lacks the poem. Another copy has an engraved portrait of Willis facing the title page.

The next change was to issue copies of *A plain and easie method* with *The London practice of physick* (**7A3**). The fact that the portrait had been discarded no longer mattered since that belonging to *The London practice of physick* could be used, bound before the new collective title page. In the copy examined for this bibliography, the subsidiary title page listing both *A plain and easie method* and the poem on a laurel leaf (1691: **7A2**) is retained, with the errata leaf, imprimatur, and final leaf of text (F4 + 1 = A4) but without the (no longer available) poem. The sheets of *The London practice of physick* are those from 1685 (**10A1.c3**).

This was followed by a second collective volume with the title page dated 1695 (**7A4**). This uses sheets of *The London practice of physick* from 1685 in different states (**10A1.c1**). The title of the treatise on the plague is changed to *A treatise of the plague, its nature and cure: Also several receipts to prevent any contagious distemper* but with the same collation as **7A2**.[4] The poem on a laurel leaf is again mentioned and, notwithstanding the suggestion (earlier) that William Crooke's stock of that publication was exhausted, the final sheet with the poem is present in the copy examined for this bibliography. Not for the first time, what binders and booksellers were able to acquire, or held as stock, seems not to have followed an orderly sequence of printing.

A third title was used for the second and final edition printed in 1721: *A preservative from the infection of the plague, or any contagious distemper*. This is entirely reset and published as an independent work. The portrait, imprimatur and errata leaf have gone and there is no mention of the poem on a laurel leaf (**7B**).

A plain and easie method: summary of the four issues of the first edition

The evidence provided by copies of *A plain and easie method* as originally bound, alone or with sheets of *The London practice of physick* in different states, and varying in

which are part of a collective work with *The London practice of physick* (#62, 1692: =**7A3**; and #63, 1695: =**7A4**). See: HJR Wing, *A bibliography of Dr. Thomas Willis (1621–1675)*, privately printed (1962): pages 42–3.

[3] See: HJR Wing (1962): page 43. What HJR Wing does not make explicit is that the item selected for his description of *A plain and easie method* (#42) comes from a collective volume that includes his entry for *The London practice of physick* (#62). This is therefore the same as **7A3** described in the present bibliography.

[4] HJR Wing corrects Donald Wing's description of this book as a folio edition.

inclusion of the portrait, imprimatur, errata leaf, and poem indicates that the various sheets were distributed rather casually for sale during the 1690s. With so many variables, individual copies that lack one or the other leaves, or sheet $^{2}A^{4}$ with the poem on a laurel leaf, should not necessarily be considered imperfect. The situation can best be summarized as:

The distinguishing features of the 1691 edition (**7A1**) are the portrait bound in, the stub of A2, no mention of the poem, and the final leaf of text printed on F4 +1 = A4. The imprimatur dated 5 September 1690, is present, but there is no errata leaf. This issue of *A plain and easie method* may happen to be bound with *The London practice of physick* but they do not belong together as one publication.

The second issue of *A plain and easie method* has the title page reset with 'Colledge' correct to 'College', and space after line 7 used to accommodate extra details indicating the addition of *A poem on the virtue of a laurel leaf for curing of a rheumatism* (**7A2**). The portrait is often lacking. The imprimatur and errata are included and retained in all further issues of the first edition. The poem is printed on the extra sheet, $^{2}A^{4}$. However, when stocks of the poem ran out, copies were released without the final sheet despite this still being mentioned on the collective title page.[5]

A plain and easie method was issued with *The London practice of physick* and a collective title page dated 1692 (**7A3**). Each component work is otherwise independent. The portrait belonging to *The London practice of physick* but may be bound as a preliminary to either of the two works. The subsidiary title page for *A plain and easie method* mentions the poem on a laurel leaf but this is not always present.

Having brought these two works together, *The London practice of physick* was reissued in 1695 with the collective title page reset and now referring to *A Treatise of the plague, its nature and cure: Also several receipts to prevent any contagious distemper* (**7A4**). The collations and text sheets are otherwise unchanged. The subsidiary title page for *A plain and easie method* mentions the poem on a laurel leaf but this is not always present.

The second edition of *A plain and easie method* was again retitled: *A preservative from the infection of the plague or any contagious distemper in city, camp, fleet etc. and for curing such as are infected with it, after the most plain and easy method* (1721: **7B**). The preliminaries and main text are reset in 32 compared to 44 leaves, the imprimatur and errata are now omitted and all mention of the poem has gone.

John Hemming and *A plain and easie method*

Willis had been flattered to believe that he might help in the plague-ridden city. Never intended for publication, his book on the plague is based on compilations for prescriptions prepared and written in about 1666. Amongst his remedies are strong coffee and tobacco—both of which he enjoyed although he seems to have been more abstemious of alcohol. The

[5] A copy in original binding with the poem and separate from *The London practice of physick* has not been identified for the purposes of this bibliography but was present in five of seven examples examined by HJR Wing (1962): page 43.

work was edited by John Hemming (nd) from Willis's manuscripts in response to popular demand. Hemming was Willis's apothecary and amanuensis in London.[6] The book was pronounced worthy of publication on 5 September 1690 by the President and Censors of the Royal College of Physicians of London.

In his preface to the 'good reader', John Hemming explains that, although previously reluctant to publish any of Dr Willis's posthumous works because these lacked his hand in completing them, he had put aside these reservations in presenting *A plain and easie method* after an interval of fifteen years. This was at the request of an old acquaintance on behalf of a friend due to travel to the embassy in Constantinople where the plague 'did frequently rage'. This had reminded Hemming of the short tract that he transcribed from the papers of Dr Willis in 1666 'being then his *Amanuensis*'. He gave his acquaintance a copy on condition that neither he nor the friend did 'make it publick'. Meanwhile a suspicious sickness seized their Majesties armies in Ireland and Hemming's colleague, who had shown the work to several of the most prominent physicians, urged that public good would be served by printing Willis's tract should the Irish condition prove 'pestilential'. This would be a 'charitable instrument in cases of great danger, for such as cannot procure the attendance of Physicians'. No longer able to withstand such persuasive arguments, and still anxious that the regard 'I have always had, and shall still have for the reputation and memory of my dear *Master*, and best *Friend*, will not . . . be thought to lessen, by . . . giving way upon these terms to this Publication; since it is so earnestly desir'd . . .', Hemming proceeded, signing his preface from St Martin's Lane, Sept. 1. 1690.

It seems that doubt arose over the authorship.[7] When the work was last published in 1721 (**7B**) the new preface explained that readers required no stronger a recommendation that Dr Willis was the author than the testimony of the late eminent apothecary, Mr Hemming, which provided sufficient proof. The writer explains that the tract had been printed thirty years ago at Hemming's own expense: '*But upon the present Publication, it has been carefully revis'd with the* Latin *Original. Among* Dr Willis's *Papers; and besides some* Material Additions *throughout the whole, there are Considerable Amendments almost in every* Page'. Perhaps the most tantalizing revelation here is that original manuscripts of Willis's works and his surviving papers were extant and available to publishers in 1721.[8] Their subsequent fate is unknown.

[6] See: Hansruedi Isler, *Thomas Willis. 1621–1675. Doctor and scientist*, New York (1967): pages 24–5 for the suggestion that John Hemming was paid £16, as annual retainer, in 1666 for taking dictation of Willis's treatise on the plague.

[7] See: Lloyd G Stevenson, 'A note on Pordage's translation'. In: Ed. William Feindel, *The anatomy of the brain and nerves*, Montreal (1965): page 64 where, apart from hinting that Willis may not have been the author, Lloyd Stevenson (1918–1988) draws attention to some of the arcane language in the treatise: for example, empty veins 'will readily suck in whatever poisonous Atoms lurk in the outward Pores of the Body, which being admitted, become more prevalent, because Spirits being depauperated are less able to subdue or repel them'. Samuel Pordage (1633–1691) uses 'depauperated' elsewhere: see 'The anatomy of the brain'. In: *The remaining medical works* (1681): page 82, line 30. The term is presumably a faithful translation from Willis's original, qualifying Stevenson's suggestion with respect to the authorship of *A plain and easie method*.

[8] See chapter 18 for discussion of the possibility that other manuscripts, left unpublished at Willis's death in 1675, may have come into the possession of Hemming. If so, these are now lost.

7A1. A PLAIN AND EASIE METHOD FOR PRESERVING THOSE THAT ARE WELL FROM THE INFECTION OF THE PLAGUE, London octavo 1691

The first edition of Willis's seventh book, with the imprimatur but no errata leaf, and without the poem on a laurel leaf [HJR Wing 41].

Title page: [within a double rule] A | Plain and Eaſie Method | FOR | Preſerving [by **God's Bleſſing**] | thoſe that are WELL from the | Infection of the | PLAGUE, | Or any | Contagious Diſtemper, | In | CITY, CAMP, FLEET, &c. | AND | For Curing ſuch as are Infected | with it. | [rule] | Written in the Year 1666. | [rule] | By *Tho. Willis*, M. D. late Sidney Profeſ- | ſor in *Oxford*, and a Member of the | Royal Society and Colledge of Phy- | ſicians in *London*. | [rule] | Never before Printed. | [rule] | *LONDON*, Printed for *W. Crook*, at the *Green-* | *Dragon*, without *Temple-Bar*. 1691.

Collation: octavo; 23 roman letter alphabet: A^4 (-A4), a^4, $B–E^8$, F^4 (F4 +1 = A4); $1–4 signed, apart from: -B4.

44 leaves: paginated as [14], 1–74.

Type: 22 lines; height (20 lines) 115 millimetres, width 73 millimetres.

Contents: **A1r**, page [1], blank; **A1v**, page [2], *Libellum hunc de Peſte, dignum judicamus, qui Imprimatur*. Gault. Charleton, *Præſes Collegii Regalis Medicor. Londinenſ.* Tho. Burwel. J. Gordon. Wil. Dawes. Tho. Gill. [bracketed] *Cenſores*. Dat. *Sepemb.* 5. 1690. *In Comitiis Cenſoriis ex Edibus Collegii noſtri.*; **A2r**, page [3], blank (stub); **A2v**, page [4], blank (stub); **A3r**, page [5], title; **A3v**, page [6], blank; **a1r–a4r**, page [7–13], TO THE READER. ... [signed] *Thy Friend and Servant*, *St.* Martins-Lane, Sept. 1. 1690. *J. Hemming.*; **a4v**, page [14], blank.

B1r–F5v, pages 1–74, [text] A Plain and Eaſie METHOD, &c.

Headlines and *Catchwords*: (14) for [14] at **B7v**, page 14; (30) for [30] at **C7v**, page 30; (46) for [46] at **D7v**, page 46; (60) for [60] at **E6v**, page 60.

of for *of* at **D5r / v**, pages [41] / [42].

Frontispiece: none.

Portrait: **Pt.1f1**: *R. W. ſculp. Thomas Willis M. D.* 173 × 110 millimetres (sheet); 162 × 107 (plate marks); 150 × 95 millimetres (image).

Printers' ornament: none.

No decorated initials.

Illustrations: none.

Copy: DASC (#1 of 2). Original sprinkled calf with blind double-lined border and one double vertical line, spine (relaid) with five double lines in blind tooling, red label with double gilt-lined surround, PLAGUE, original endpapers. Leaves 172 × 109 millimetres, boards 178 × 108 × 17 millimetres.

7A2. A PLAIN AND EASIE METHOD FOR PRESERVING THOSE THAT ARE WELL FROM THE INFECTION OF THE PLAGUE, London octavo 1691

The second issue of Willis's seventh book, with the title page calling for the poem on a laurel leaf, the errata and imprimatur present, often without the portrait, but the poem included together with the advertisement for books sold by William Crook [HJR Wing 42]; see Figure 146.

Title page: [1] [within a double rule] A | Plain and Eaſie Method | FOR | Preserving [by **God's Bleſſing**] | thoſe that are WELL from the | Infection of the | PLAGUE, | OR | Any Contagious Diſtemper in City, | Camp, Fleet, *&c.* | AND | For Curing ſuch as are Infected | with it. | [rule] | Written in the Year 1666. | [rule] | By *Tho. Willis*, M. D. late Sidney Profeſ- | ſor in *Oxford*, and a Member of the | Royal Society and College of Phy- | ſicians in *London.* | [rule] | With a Poem on the virtue of a Laurel | Leaf for curing of a Rheumatiſm. | By *W. B.* | [rule] | Never before Printed. | [rule] | *LONDON*, Printed for *W. Crook*, at the *Green-* | *Dragon*, without *Temple-Bar*. 1691.

[2]. A | POEM | UPON A | Laurel-Leaf. | [rule] | Viris admodum Colendis, | PUBLICÆ SCHOLÆ, | Vulgò dictæ, | *Harrow ſuper Montem*, | GUBERNATORIBUS, | *VIZ.* | Dn° *CAROLO GERARD* Baronetto. | Dn° *EDVARDO WALDO* Militi. | *CHEEK GERARD*, | *DANIELO WALDO*, | *GULIELMO FEN*, | *EDWARDO WALDO*, | [the last four names bracketed] Armigeris. | Hoc qualecunque Poema, *Gulielmus Bolton* M.A. | & ejuſdem Scholæ Archi-didaſcalus, humil- | limè dedicat.

Then as in **7A1** apart from:

Collation: octavo; 23 letter roman alphabet: [1] A^4 (-A4), a^4, B–E^8, F^4, (F4 + 1 = A4). [2] ${}^2A^4$; $1–4 signed, apart from: -B4.

48 leaves; paginated as [14], 1–74, 1–8.

Type: [2]. 38 lines; height (20 lines) 81 millimetres, width 85 millimetres (97 millimetres with marginal notes).

Contents: [1]. **A1r**, page [1], blank; **A1v**, page [2], imprimatur (often lacking); **A2r**, page [3], blank; **A2v**, page [4], ERRATA, 6 lines listing 6 errors; **A3r**, page [5], title; **A3v**, page [6], blank; etc. until:

[2]. **A1r**, page [1], title; **A1v**, **A2v**, and **A3v**, pages (2), (4), and (6), [Text] In LAURUM APPOLLINI dicatam, cujus Foliis (monitu Reverendi Viri Domini *Fiſher*, & juſſu

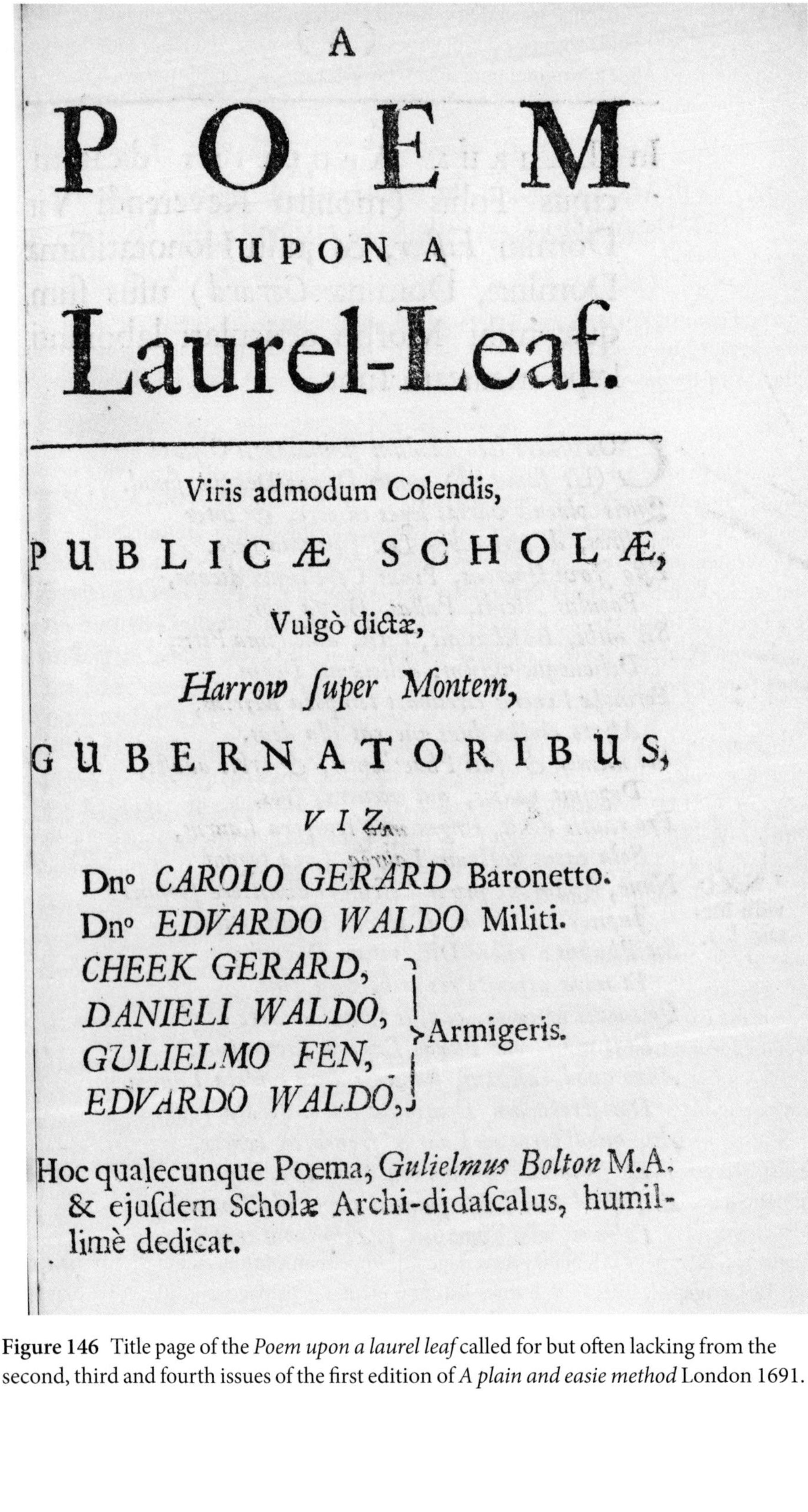

A

POEM

UPON A

Laurel-Leaf.

Viris admodum Colendis,

PUBLICÆ SCHOLÆ,

Vulgò dictæ,

Harrow ſuper Montem,

GUBERNATORIBUS,

VIZ.

Dn° *CAROLO GERARD* Baronetto.
Dn° *EDVARDO WALDO* Militi.
CHEEK GERARD,
DANIELI WALDO,
GULIELMO FEN,
EDVARDO WALDO, } Armigeris.

Hoc qualecunque Poema, *Gulielmus Bolton* M.A. & ejuſdem Scholæ Archi-didaſcalus, humillimè dedicat.

Figure 146 Title page of the *Poem upon a laurel leaf* called for but often lacking from the second, third and fourth issues of the first edition of *A plain and easie method* London 1691.

Honoratiſſimæ Dominæ, Dominæ, *Gerard*) uſus ſum, quæ mihi Morbo articulari laboranti, ſæpe medicate ſunt.; **A2r**, **A3r**, and **A4r**, pages (3), (5), and (7), *Upon the LAUREL, ſacred to* APPOLO, *whoſe Leaves I made uſe of (by the Advice of Mr.* Fiſher, *and the repeated Commands of the Honourable the Lady* Gerard) *which have often cured me of a* Rheumatiſm. Paraphraſtically translated by *T.F.* Gent.; **A4r**, page (7), [footer] *LONDON*, Printed for *W. Crooke* at the *Green Dragon* without *Temple-Bar*. 1690.; **A4v**, page [8], *Books Printed for* W. Crooke.

Printers' ornament: [1]. Single row of 12 fleurons {**Roycroft 11**} separated by : between #6 / 7, with a further identical row (inverted) below text at **A2v**, page [2].

Copy: DASC (#1 of 2). Recent sprinkled calf with double-lined border in blind tooling and one double vertical line, spine with six double lines in blind tooling, red label (horizontal) with double gilt lined surround, PLAGUE. Leaves 178 × 112 millimetres, boards 185 × 115 × 15 millimetres.

7A3. THE LONDON PRACTICE OF PHYSICK, London octavo 1692; with A PLAIN AND EASIE METHOD FOR PRESERVING THOSE THAT ARE WELL FROM THE INFECTION OF THE PLAGUE, London octavo 1691

The third issue of Willis's seventh book, with *The London practice of physick* and a collective title page for the two works, the title page for *A plain and easie method* listing the poem on a laurel leaf, but the poem often lacking [described as part of HJR Wing 62].

Title page: [1]. [within a double rule] The LONDON | **Practiſe of Phyſick**, | BEING THE | PRACTICAL PART | OF | PHYSICK | Contain'd in the | VVORKS | Of the FAMOUS | Dr. WILLIS; | Wherein are | His Definitions, Deſcriptions, and Methods | Of Curing Diſeaſes, with all his RECEIPTS. | To which is now added | His plain and eaſie METHOD for the Preventing | and Curing of the Plague, Publiſhed by Mr. *Flemings*, Amanu- | enſis and Apothecary to the Doctor. | [rule] | *With the allowance of the College of* PHYSICIANS. | [rule] | *LONDON*: | Printed for *T. Baſſett, T. Dring, C. Harper*, and *W. Crook*, and are | to be ſold at the *Flower-de-Luce* in *Fleet-ſtreet*, and at the | *Green Dragon* without *Temple-Bar*. M DC XCII. | Dr. WILLIS's whole Works in *Fol.* With Forty Copper Plates are alſo to | be Sold at the Places above-mentioned.

[2]. [within a double rule] A | Plain and Eaſie Method | FOR | Preserving [by **God's Bleſſing**] | thoſe that are WELL from the | Infection of the | PLAGUE, | OR | Any Contagious Diſtemper in City, | Camp, Fleet, &c. | AND | For Curing ſuch as are Infected | with it. | [rule] | Written in the Year 1666. | [rule] | By *Tho. Willis*, M. D. late Sidney Profeſ- | ſor in *Oxford*, and a Member of the | Royal Society and College of Phy- | ſicians in *London*. | [rule] | With a Poem on the virtue of a Laurel | Leaf for curing of a Rheumatiſm. | By *W. B.* | [rule] | Never before Printed. | [rule] | *LONDON*, Printed for *W. Crook*, at the *Green*- | *Dragon*, without *Temple-Bar*. 1691.

Then as in **7A2** apart from (often) lacking $^{2}A^{4}$.

Copy: DASC, lacking A1 (imprimatur), and $^{2}A^{4}$ (poem on a laurel leaf). Original calf with single lined border, spine (rebacked) with four raised bands and single line at head and foot, original endpapers. Leaves 173 × 107 millimetres, boards 178 × 112 × 48 millimetres. Inserted: bookplate, ALASTAIR ROBB-SMITH'S LIBRARY. Inscribed: (erased and undecipherable). Shelf mark: 5 3 f.[9]

7A4. THE LONDON PRACTICE OF PHYSICK, London octavo 1695; with A PLAIN AND EASIE METHOD FOR PRESERVING THOSE THAT ARE WELL FROM THE INFECTION OF THE PLAGUE, London octavo 1691 [1695]

The fourth issue of Willis's seventh book, with a second collective title page, calling for the poem on a laurel leaf, the errata, and imprimatur both present together with the poem and advertisement for books sold by William Crook [described as part of HJR Wing 63].

Title page: [1] [within a double rule] THE | *LONDON PRACTICE* | OF | PHYSICK: | Or the whole | Practical Part of Phyſick | Contained in the Works of the Learned | Dr. WILLIS, | *Faithfully Engliſhed.* | [rule] | The Second Edition. | [rule] | To which is added a Treatiſe of the Plague, its Na- | ture and Cure: Alſo ſeveral Receipts to prevent | any Contagious Diſtemper in City, Camp, or | Fleet, and for Curing ſuch as are infected with it. | [rule] | *LONDON*, | Printed and are to be Sold by *Richard Wellington,* at | the ſign of the *Lute*, and *Edward Caſtle*, at the *Angel* | and *Crown* in St. *Paul's* Church-Yard. 1695. | *Price Bound Seven Shillings.* | [outside inner lower rule] Where are likewiſe to be had his Works in one Volume in Folio.

[2]. [within a double rule] A | Plain and Eaſie Method | FOR | Preserving [by **God's Bleſſing**] | thoſe that are WELL from the | Infection of the | PLAGUE, | OR | Any Contagious Diſtemper in City, | Camp, Fleet, &c. | AND | For Curing ſuch as are Infected | with it. | [rule] | Written in the Year 1666. | [rule] | By *Tho. Willis*, M. D. late Sidney Profeſ- | ſor in *Oxford*, and a Member of the | Royal Society and College of Phy- | ſicians in *London*. | [rule] | With a Poem on the virtue of a Laurel | Leaf for curing of a Rheumatiſm. | By *W. B.* | [rule] | Never before Printed. | [rule] | *LONDON*, Printed for *W. Crook*, at the *Green-* | *Dragon*, without *Temple-Bar*. 1691.

[3]. A | POEM | UPON A | Laurel-Leaf. | [rule] | Viris admodum Colendis, | PUBLICÆ SCHOLÆ, | Vulgò dictæ, | *Harrow ſuper Montem*, | GUBERNATORIBUS, | *VIZ.* | Dn° *CAROLO GERARD* Baronetto. | Dn° *EDVARDO WALDO* Militi. | *CHEEK GERARD*, | *DANIELO WALDO*, | *GULIELMO FEN*, | *EDWARDO WALDO*, | [the last four names bracketed] Armigeris. | Hoc qualecunque Poema, *Gulielmus Bolton* M.A. | & ejuſdem Scholæ Archi-didaſcalus, humil- | limè dedicat.

Then as in **10A4** and **7A2**.

[9] Alastair Robb-Smith (1908–2000) was a distinguished Oxford pathologist. As a medical student he found the Farringdon Road market with its barrow loads of old books, and thus began his lifelong interest in the history of medicine and bibliography. In 1937 he became Nuffield reader in pathology and head of the University department at the age of 29, where he remained until retirement. See: John Ledingham, *The Times* 15 March 2000 and *Munk's Roll* volume XII (web-based) for further details of this polymath 'remembered for his contributions to medical science, the study of books and his personal qualities of kindness, modesty and consideration for others'.

Copy: Royal Society of Medicine (Marcus Beck Library 32169). Later calf with central blind panels, dotted borders and fleuron corners, upper and lower boards, spine with five raised bands, labelled LONDON | PRACTICE | OF PHYSICK. Leaves 180 × 113 millimetres, boards 190 × 118 × 54 millimetres. Inserted bookplate: (1) Albert J Chalmers (unidentified); (2) Royal Society of Medicine presentation bookplate: THE ROYAL SOCIETY OF MEDICINE, 1870 AJC 1917. 1920 PRESENTED BY M[RS] AJ CHALMERS 1920. Stamped: Royal Society of Medicine 4 SEP 1935. Inscribed: Tho[s] Bennet (unidentified).

7B. A PRESERVATIVE FROM THE INFECTION OF THE PLAGUE, London octavo. 1721

The second edition of Willis's seventh book, retitled, without the imprimatur or errata, and no mention of the poem on a laurel leaf, the contents reset in 32 compared to 44 leaves [HJR Wing 43].

Title page: A | PRESERVATIVE | From the INFECTION of the | PLAGUE, | OR, | Any *Contagious Diſtemper*, in | City, Camp, Fleet, *etc*, | AND | For CURING ſuch as are infected with | it, after the moſt Plain and Eaſy | METHOD. [not centred] | [rule] | *Written in the Year* 1666. | By *THOMAS WILLIS*, M. D. | Late *Sidney-Profeſſor* in *Oxford*, and a | Member of the *Royal Society*, and College | of *Phyſicians* in *London*. | [rule] | *N.B. The* RECEIPTS *in this Book are all Tranſlated* | *into* Engliſh, *for the Uſe of* FAMILIES. | [rule] | *LONDON:* | Printed for A. BETTESWORTH, and J. BATTELY, in *Pater-* | *Noſter-Row*; C. RIVINGTON, in St. *Paul's* Churchyard; | and E. CURLL, in the *Strand*. 1721. *Price* Is.

Collation: octavo in 4s; 23 letter roman alphabet: A^2 (A2 + 1), B–G^4, H^4 (H4 + 1); $1–2 signed.

32 leaves, paginated as [2], iv, 1–58 (all page numbers contained within []).

Type: 24 lines; height (20 lines) 117 millimetres, width 79 millimetres.

Contents: **A1r**, page [1], title; **A1v**, page [2], blank; **A2r**, page [j], PREFACE; **A2v–A3v**, pages [ij]–[iv], Mr. HEMMING's *Advertiſement to the Reader* ... [signed] *Thy Friend and Servant*, St. Martin's-Lane, Sept. 1. 1690. *J. Hemming*.

B1r–H5v, pages 1–58, [text] Dr. *WILLIS*'s PRESERVATIVE AGAINST THE PLAGUE.

Headlines and *Catchwords*: no headlines.

No catchword at **A2+1v / B1r**, pages [iv]–1.

Frontispiece: none.

Portrait: none.

Printers' ornaments: headpiece at **B1r**, page [1] {**Bettesworth 1**}; line of 15 fleurons at **D4v**, page 24, {**Bettesworth 3**}; tailpiece at H5v, page 58 {**Bettesworth 4**}.

Decorated I at **B1r**, page [1] {**Bettesworth 2**}.

Illustrations: none.

Copy: Wellcome (11310666). Original calf with blind stamped central panel, four floral corners, double rule, and central mottling (boards detached), spine with four raised bands, labelled WILLIS | ESSAY | ON | PLAGUE, original endpapers. Leaves 185 × 115 millimetres, boards 193 × 120 × 18 millimetres. Inserted: bookplate of John Phillips F.R.S, St. Mary's Lodge, York. Shelf marks: (1) 54977 | B1, 54978 /B and 54979 / B; (2) 49 / 727; (3) 61. D. 34; (4) 29152 (1). Bound with Richard Mead *A short discourse concerning pestilential contagion*, etc., (1720); and Richard Bradley *The plague at Marseilles consider'd*, etc., (1721).[10]

[10] John Phillips (1800–1874) was a geologist who devised a timescale for fossils based on strata in rock. He also had an interest in lithography. Phillips was keeper of the Yorkshire museum (1826–1840) when this book was acquired. Subsequently he held posts in Oxford and Dublin. Phillips was elected FRS in 1834, president of the Geological Society of London (1859) and of the British Association (1865). He slipped and fell after dining at All Souls College, Oxford, on 23 April 1874 and died the next day. Craters on Mars and the Moon are named after him. His marble bust is in the Oxford University Museum, which he helped to found in 1859.

12

'The whole dowry of all nature'

Opera omnia (1676–1720)

No time was lost in bringing out a collected edition of the printed works in Latin following Willis's death in November 1675. The *Opera medica & physica*, later entitled *Opera omnia*, were published, as Willis's eighth book, in continental Europe between 1676 and 1720. Jean-Antoine Huguetan (1647–*c.*1750)[1] of Lyon, Samuel de Tournes (1628–1695) of Geneva, and Hendrik Wetstein (1649–1726) of Amsterdam produced luxurious quarto editions. From 1694–1720, the *Opera omnia* were printed in folio format from Venice with most illustrations incorporated within the printed page of text. With the exception of Wetstein, each chose to include Croone's essay even though its correct authorship was well known. In his final edition (1695), Tournes added the only Latin translation of *A plain and easie method* (dated 1694). From the bibliographic perspective, these books are relatively uncomplicated. Opinions differ on which is the 'best edition' of Willis's collected works in Latin. HJR Wing suggests Wetstein (1682: **8E**). But few would disagree with his final word: 'a further folio edition from Venice was that of Paulus Monticellus [nd] in 1720 [**8I**]. This is a most beautifully printed edition by Joannes Malachinus' (nd).[2] The text is in two columns each separated by double vertical lines, the printers' ornaments and decorated initials are handsome, and the spacing is generous.

Antonio Huguetan

Huguetan planned his publication as one volume with a collective title page and continuous register. It is in four parts, each of which could probably be purchased separately. Printing of the second part of *Pharmaceutice rationalis*, described as 'Opus posthumum', was completed on 13 June 1676, suggesting that Huguetan was already working on the collected volume when Willis died. Most commentators give him priority although others conclude that the Tournes Geneva imprint (1676), in which both parts of *Pharmaceutice rationalis* were integrated within the second volume, came first.[3] Huguetan forgot initially to set the preface to *De febribus* and so added a bifolium after H3. The first leaf is signed 'H4' with the second unsigned (paginated: 63* and *ibid.* 63 on each recto, respectively). The catchword (CAPVT) on H3v links across the bifolium to the chapter heading for the text of *De febribus* starting at

[1] Although these dates may seem improbable, there is agreement that Huguetan did live to a great age.

[2] HJR Wing (53) describes this as the second Venetian edition with the imprimatur dated 24 August 1719, but in fact it is the third.

[3] See: [Anthony Wood] *Athenæ Oxoniensis. An exact history of all the writers and bishops who have had their education in the most ancient and famous University of Oxford, from the fifteenth year of King Henry the Seventh, Dom. 1500, to the end of the year* 1690, volume 1, London (1690): entries 364–5, column 402; and [Anon] *A new and general biographical dictionary; containing an historical and critical account of the lives and writings of the most eminent persons in every nation; particularly the British and Irish*, volume IV, London (1780): page 133.

H4r, page 63. The bifolium has its own appropriate internal catchwords and DE on the verso of the second leaf, which is correct for the headline of DE FEBRIBUS at H4r, page 63.

Apart from containing all of Willis's treatises published to date, the Latin collected editions are notable for their liberal use of ornaments. Huguetan used red and black to print the collective title page, and also included his printer's device. He added head and tailpieces where space allowed, and incorporated many fleurons. Huguetan's use of decorated initials suggests the involvement of different workshops or craftsmen. Many of the reliefs are small and poorly cut. Others are more elaborate with floral designs, various animals, and scenes involving human and mythical figures.

Huguetan used illustrations that are close in design and engraving to those from earlier Dutch publications of Willis's works. The fifteen plates in *Cerebri anatome* are faithfully copied from those engraved for Caspar Commelin (1636–1693) in 1664, as is the illustration for *De ratione motus musculorum* (**2C2**). Lines used to trace the originals are often visible. Whereas a number of large engravings, each including several illustrations, had been used by Commelin, those copied for Huguetan are all individual with the exception of Tabula IX (Pl.11e1) and Tabula X (Pl.12e1), which may have been engraved together (placed left and right, respectively). Tabula XI (Pl.13e1) and Tabula XIII (Pl.15e1) may also have been on one plate. In some examples, printing of the page placement for Tabula XII (Pl.14e1) has the central '1' of '413' so faint as to be illegible and, with 'I' being a narrow character, not unreasonably the binder placed this plate leaf in the text of *De fermentatione* at page 43. In other copies, the illustration is more clearly imprinted and placed where it belongs at page 413. Huguetan's illustrations for *De anima brutorum* are copied from Joannes Blaeu (1596–1673: 1672, **5B3**), but with some carelessness. The engraver omitted the heading for Tabula II (Pl.20d1); the orientation of the three component figures is reversed on Tabula IIII (Pl.22d1); some of the letters depicting structures in Figura 1 of Tabula V (*b* and *c*) are omitted (Pl.23d1); and Tabula VIII (Pl.26d1) is a mirror image of the original. The illustrations for *De motu musculari* are based on those used by Cornelius Driehuysen (fl.1663–1671) and Felicem Lopez (fl.1664–1693) in 1671 (**4B**). *Pharmaceutice rationalis* parts 1 and 2 use plates from Arnold Leers (1643–1701: 1674, 1677: **6C**; **6G**) as templates for the engravings.

Even though Huguetan's second edition of the *Opera medica & physica* (1681: **8D**) appeared within five years, now entitled *Opera omnia*, everything was reset in two volumes with collective title pages for each. The first volume has a continuous register and pagination, the second contains three treatises each with its own half title, pagination, and separate registers. Huguetan may have underestimated the interest in his 1676 edition and did not have residual sheets for reissue in 1681. The amount of standing type needed for reprinting would have been excessive and breaking up the imposed formes may have been a conscious decision despite the labour involved in resetting the entire book after an interval of only five years. Whatever the reason, it is likely that an existing copy was used and the text reset by slavish transcription without close reading, since many existing errors that would have been easy to correct are carried over to the 1681 edition, and some others introduced.[4]

[4] Neither of the two paper copies examined for this bibliography is complete. HJR Wing correctly points out that in the Wellcome Library, the only example he could find, the text of *Pharmaceutice rationalis* part 2 is lacking from page 97–224 and replaced with sheets of the final sections of *Pharmaceutice rationalis* part I, pages 97–180. Part II therefore runs 1–96. [97–180] [8], and not, as it should, 1–96, 97–224 [4]. This copy also has a letter dropped so that the pagination in part I is 20 for 202; and B3 is signed in part 2. The copy in the Royal Society of Medicine shows further variations in that C3 and D3, part 2, are unsigned. It lacks the conjugate leaf (H4 and H4 + 1) inserted after H3 in part 1. Since, therefore, neither the Wellcome nor Royal Society of Medicine copies are complete, these variations have not been used as the basis for describing a second state of Huguetan's *Opera omnia* (1681: **8D**).

Huguetan incorporated many different printers' ornaments in his 1681 edition. Overall, these are superior to those used in the earlier edition in terms of artistry and complexity of design. The plates had been stored carefully and were reused without alterations of state. The lines are crisp and quality of the printing is maintained. Both in 1676 and 1681, the engraver muddled the page placements for Tabula IX (Pl.11e1) and Tabula X (Pl.12e1) indicating these for pages 410 and 405, respectively. In many copies, the binder followed these instructions so that these two plate leaves are wrongly placed. Old habits die hard and one copy of Huguetan's 1681 edition examined for this bibliography, in which page 413 is clearly printed as the placement for Tabula XII (Pl.14e1), nonetheless still has this leaf bound at page 43.[5]

Samuel de Tournes

Both in 1676 and 1680, Samuel Tournes published the *Opera omnia* from two places: Geneva and Coloniæ Allobrogum, a suburb of that city. HJR Wing, citing JF Fulton (1899–1960), points out that:[6]

> Geneva in the seventeenth century was the centre of protestant propaganda and the Geneva imprint was regarded in Catholic countries as the sign of heretical literature. Various acts of prohibition against the introduction of such books were passed in France which affected the exportation of books. There are on record various official efforts to have these prohibitions removed. Some of them were successful as far as non-theological books were concerned. For the imprint of these, various pseudonymous designations were adopted, such as 'Colonia Allobrogum', 'Colonia Alpina', 'Colonia Alpestra', etc. Cologny is still a suburb of Geneva, as also Saint Gervais. This adoption of the old Roman name led frequently to confusion with Col. Agrippina (Cologne) and Col. Munatiana (Basel). The principal printers of that epoch were the De Tournes who had come from Lyons and Pyramus de Candolle from Provence.

HJR Wing adds that the ordering of leaves varies in the preliminaries of Tournes's 1676 issues (**8B**).[7] This reflects the decision of binders faced with somewhat erratic signing of sheets in which the symbols for each follow neither a numerical nor alphabetical sequence. His point is well taken but could be applied to many of the printings of Thomas Willis's works, individually or in collected editions, through erratic or illogical signatures and text arriving late or forgotten until after some pages had already been typeset. Tournes's pagination is discontinuous across the various treatises, which are grouped into seven parts. Some are found in original paper wrappers indicating that these could be purchased separately. Whereas other printers use different characters for 'ſ' and 's', Tournes has 'ſs' [not available] and 'ſt' ligatures which he uses throughout. As with Huguetan, and presumably working on his book at much the same time, the text for *Pharmaceutice rationalis* part 2 may have arrived late and, dated 1677, this is published only from Geneva in all copies of Tournes's issues of *Opera omnia*. This may indicate that the Coloniæ Allobrogum imprint has priority (**8B2**); however,

[5] As a result, failing to find this at page 43, the Wellcome Library cataloguer has (wrongly) indicated that Tab. XII (Pl.14) is lacking from their copy.

[6] See HJR Wing (1962): page 46, citing EH Gaullieur 'Études sur la typographie genevoise du XVe au XIXe siècles et sur l'introduction de l'imprimerie en Suisse', *Bulletin, Institut National Genevois* (1855) ii: page 211 et seq.; and JF Fulton, *Bibliography of Robert Boyle*, Oxford (1932): page 151.

[7] See HJR Wing (1962): page 55.

plates from that issue are in relatively poor condition, suggesting that the Geneva issue came first (**8B1**).

Tournes reset the text for both his 1680 (**8C**) and 1695 (**8G**) editions, altering details of the preliminaries but retaining the main pagination and most line-by-line arrangements. Some errors from 1676 were corrected, others left unchanged, and a few new mistakes introduced. In general, Tournes's printing is attractive with indulgent use of ornaments and decorated initials. These are more interesting in content than those used by Huguetan. Each component title is listed in the 1676 edition (**8B**). These are separated into those for Tomus priori and Tomus posteriori in 1680 (**8C**). In 1695, the titles are again combined on a single printed leaf, although those in Tomus primus and Tomus secundus are distinguished (**8G**). After 1676, a dedication to Archduke Leopold William of Austria (1614–1662) was added, signed by Christopher Beüer (nd) in 1680 and FEW Bertram (nd) in 1695. With his 1680 edition (**8C**), Tournes adds an explanation for the authorship of William Croone's (1633–1684) treatise. He explains that he had attached the anonymous *De ratione motus musculorum* to Willis's treatises on the brain and nerves partly because it had already been appended to earlier editions, and had been much admired, and on the basis that 'Mr Willis would not object'.[8]

Although the collective title pages for each volume of his final edition are dated 1695, as is the subsidiary title page for *De anima brutorum*, all eight introducing the individual treatises have a 1694 imprint (**8G**). This edition includes the only Latin translation of *A plain and easie method for preserving those that are well from the infection of the plague*, first published in 1691. New ornaments and decorated initials are used. The plates are identical to those used by Tournes in 1676, without changes since 1680 to page placements and other marginal details, but now showing signs of surface wear even if the engraving is intact and the printing still crisp.

By comparison with those published by Huguetan, the illustrations used by Tournes are all relatively crude in their engraving. The plates for *Cerebri anatome* and *De ratione motus musculorum* are closest in design to those used by Commelin (**2C2**). Some are pasted onto the indicated page rather than bound as whole or part leaves (Pl.2f1, Pl.14f1, Pl.15f1 figures 3 and 4). Several are engraved on large individual plates with lines visible indicating where these should be cut. Without direct evidence from single sheets, or fragments of one illustration retained on another, interpretation is speculative. Some images may have been rotated in order to make up a rectangular engraving. It is likely that Figuræ III and the second unnumbered illustration came from the top left of a plate; Figuræ I and VII from the top right; Figuræ II, V, the first unnumbered, and VIII from the lower left; Figuræ IV and VI from the lower right; Tabulæ IX and X from the left and right halves of single sheets; Tabulæ XI and XIII from the upper and lower halves; and Tabula XII from the upper or lower half of another plate. These arrangements on engravings made in Geneva are not the same as those used on large plates made for Dutch publishers.

As with Huguetan, the illustrations for *De motu musculari* are based on the Amsterdam (1671: **4B**) edition. The four figures are engraved on one plate with Figuræ I and II (Pl.17e1) inverted with respect to Figuræ III and IV (Pl.18e1). This arrangement is retained as printed in the copy used for this bibliography (**8B1**), but the two parts are cut and reorientated for binding in the later issues (**8B2**, **8B3**).

The plates for *De anima brutorum* are copied from Johannem à Someren (1632–1678: 1674, **5C**) in terms of engraving, and placement of headings and lettering. The headline is missing

[8] See chapter 6 for more detailed discussion of the print history of *De ratione motus musculorum*.

from Tabula III (Pl.21e1). Again, it seems certain that several images were engraved on one plate although the lack of residual lines makes it difficult to suggest all the configurations. The only certainty is that Tabula IIII (Pl.22e1) was engraved on the same sheet as Tabula VII (Pl.25e1) since these are printed together (although with Tabula IIII, Fig III cut to the left and bound separately). It is likely that Tabula I, III, and VIII came from the top left (or upper part) of a plate; Tabula VI and VII from the lower left; Tabulæ II, IV, and V from the lower right.

The same economies apply, in principle, to the illustrations used for Tournes's printing of *Pharmaceutice rationalis*. It would presumably have been easiest for the engraver to copy existing Dutch editions. Part 1 had been published from The Hague in 1674 and 1675 (**6C**, **6D**), but there was no Dutch edition of part 2 until the year after Tournes published the *Opera omnia*. Whilst in theory he might have had early access to Arnold Leers's (1643–1701) plates for part 2 (**6G**), or passed his own on to Leers, the designs are different. Therefore it seems most likely that Tournes had illustrations copied from the Oxford editions of both parts of *Pharmaceutice rationalis* (**6A**, **6E**). Part 1, Tabula II probably comes from the left or lower half, and Tabula IV from the right or upper half of one plate; Tabula VI is from the lower left, and Tabulæ I, III, and V from the lower right parts of others. For part 2, Tabulæ II, IV, and VIII are from the left or upper halves of separate plates; and Tabulæ 1, III, V, VI, and VII from the right or lower halves of separate plates.

Amongst the collection which forms the basis for this bibliography is a manuscript bound in contemporary calf with an elaborate gilt-decorated spine. Care has been taken to preserve the volume. It is inscribed 'Ex libris J: Primelius Med: Lic: 1756'. Dr Primelius is unidentified. The volume consists of sixty-seven leaves with writing on each side, paginated [2], 1–171, [1], and consists of extracts from Tournes's 1676 edition of *Opera omnia*. The entries are forty-eight pages relating to 'Of fevers of child-bearing women' from *De febribus*; four pages on 'Of an imposthume of the lungs' from *Pharmaceutice rationalis*, part 2; and 119 pages taken from chapters 2, 7, 10, 11, and 12 of *De morbis convulsivis*. The motivation for this exercise in calligraphy is unclear. There is no unifying theme for the extracts, and the printed texts would have been available in 1756 to any serious student of Willis's writings.

Hendrik Wetstein

Wetstein's edition gets off to a spectacular start by adding an elaborate allegorical engraved frontispiece which includes depictions of the practice of medicine, anatomical dissection, and book illustration (F.4a1). The text is edited by Gerard Blasius (1625–1682). HJR Wing points out that, in the many surviving copies, 2π2 is cancelled and often missing. Wetstein omits Croone's treatise, *De ratione motus musculorum*. Unlike Huguetan and Tournes who used reengraved copies of earlier Dutch plates, Wetstein had access to many that had already been used. The engraver made alterations to the original plates, erasing previous indicators for page placements and sections and adding details indicating to which treatise each belongs. Apart from being in second states, the engravings for Wetstein's *Cerebri anatome* are identical to those used by Commelin (1664: **2C2**; Pl.1c2–Pl.15c2).[9] But there is one other difference. Whereas Commelin had large plates engraved with more than one illustration, marks surround each of the fifteen illustrations printed by Wetstein. What seems to have

[9] See chapter 6 for discussion of why Wetstein changed to Schagen's plates for his edition of *Cerebri anatome* (1683: **2F**).

happened is that the original large plates were cut into individual sections, the original lines and page placements erased, and space used outside these old markings to add the new indicators so that the overall boundaries of the metal used to print each illustration are enlarged.[10] Wetstein also had the images for *De motu musculori* engraved on a single plate copied from Driehuysen and Lopez but, unlike Tournes, correctly orientated (1671: **4B**; Pl.17f1 and Pl.18f1). The plates for *De anima brutorum* are borrowed from Someren (1674, **5C**; Pl.19b2–Pl.26b2). The illustrations to *Pharmaceutice rationalis* are new states using the originals from Leers (part 1, 1674: **6C**; Pl.27b3–Pl.32b3; and part 2, 1677: **6G**; Pl.33b2–Pl.40b2).[11]

The Venice folio editions

The text edited by Blasius and issued by Wetstein in quarto (1682: **8E**) was pirated for the first Venice edition in folio published by Gasparis Storti (nd) in 1694 (**8F**). The 'authoris vita' at the beginning of the volume reproduces John Fell's (1625–1686) 'post scriptum' from *Pharmaceutice rationalis* part 2 (1675: **6E**). A second Venice folio edition was published by Storti and Mariae Ruinetti (nd) in 1708 (**8H**).[12] Presumably set from a copy of the 1694 folio, and littered with errors, this takes first place for the sloppiest printing of all Willis's works.

The illustrations for these two editions in folio were newly engraved but most closely modelled on Wetstein; and therefore Commelin, Lopez, Someren, and Leers. They are included on the printed page by passing those sheets twice through the press. For *Cerebri anatome* the second unnumbered figure (Pl.10g1) is reorientated to fit the page, with Figura II on its side but the lettering adjusted. Tabula IX (Pl.11g1) is poorly registered with the text. Tabulæ IX, X, and XI (Pl.11g1, Pl.12g1, and Pl.13g1) have catchwords deftly placed as footers that link to the next page. Tabula XIII (Pl.15g1) is engraved as two plates with Figuræ 1 and 2 on one and Figuræ 3, 4, and 5 on a second page. Unlike Wetstein, *De ratione motus musculorum* is included. The two figures of the plate are engraved in mirror image and reversed in position.

With the illustrations for *De anima brutorum*, the engraver tried a third option, not illogically placing Figura II between Figuræ I and III on Tabula IV (Pl.22f1), whereas the previous Dutch iterations had this ordered as Figuræ II, I, and III (Bleau 1672, **5B3**; Someren 1674, **5C**). The printer added a vertical line separating the two columns of page Cc6r, page 315, and poorly registered the two plates when overprinting the leaf so that the line bisects the left edge of Tabula VII (Pl.25f1) placed to the right.

Unlike earlier sections of the book, the illustrations for *Pharmaceutice rationalis* are not part of the printed page and have no catchwords. These are combined in pairs on single plates for Tabulæ I and II, III and IV, and V and VI (Pl.27g1–Pl.32g1) in part I; and Tabulæ I and II (Pl.33g1, Pl.34g1), III and IV Pl.35g1 and Pl.36g1), V (alone: Pl.37g1), and VI, VIII and VIII (Pl.38g1–Pl.40g1) in part 2. The same plates were reused for the 1708 edition but these had suffered over the fourteen years with the appearance of many cracks and other superficial

[10] See chapter 10 for discussion of reduction in size of printers' plates in contrast to this evidence for cutting up large engravings into individual sections and using marginal space to add new details without altering original details of the image and lettering.

[11] Tabs. VII and VIII (Pl.39b2 and Pl.40b2) are printed on a single sheet but with distinct plate marks for each, although (as with Leers 1677), the images in Pl.39 are reversed from the original arrangement in the Oxford quarto and duodecimo editions.

[12] Having omitted the 1694 folio edition from Venice (**8F**), HJR Wing incorrectly describes the 1708 folio (**8H**) as the first revised version of Wetstein (1682: **8E**).

defects. In placing these on the formes, the registration of plates and text on the printed leaf improved but was still not perfect.

Malachin also printed text and illustrations on the same leaf (1720; **8I**). The plates are as used in 1694 (**8F**) and 1708 (**8H**), some in a further state with revised page placements engraved over the erased earlier markings. Others have deletions of the old page placements and new ones added in pen and ink: Tabulæ I and II (Pl.27g1, Pl.28g1), V and VI (Pl.31g1, Pl.32g1) in *Pharmaceutice rationalis* part 1; and Tabulæ I and II (Pl.33g1, Pl.34g1); V (Pl.37g1); and VI, VII, and VIII (Pl.38g1, Pl.39g1, Pl.40g1) in part 2. The alteration for Tabulæ I and II in part 2 to '240' is incorrect and should be '230'. Those that are in an altered printed state have 'Tomo 2' engraved after the page placements: Tabulæ III and IV in part 1 (Pl.29g2, Pl.30g2); and Tabulæ III and IV in part 2 (Pl.35g2, Pl.36g2). The first plate of two used for Tabula XIII (Pl.15g2) in *Cerebri anatome* is placed on its side to save space. By now many plates are in an even worse state, the impressions pale and poorly imprinted although some, paradoxically, are crisper than in 1708.

Portraits

Without exception, each of the collected editions in Latin has a portrait of Thomas Willis, printed as part of the first sheet (often at *4) or separately bound in.[13] The version used by Wetstein (Pt.1e1) is closest to the original image of David Loggan (1634–1692) included in *Pathologiæ cerebri* (1667: **3A**). The engraving printed by Huguetan in 1676 (**8A**) is reused in 1681 (**8D**). The artist is not identified. Tournes has an image engraved by Fr. Diodati (1647–1690) which appears in two states (1676, **8B**; and 1680, 1695; **8C**, **8G**). The three Venetian editions (**8F**, **8H**, and **8I**) all use a version in the same state, engraved by Isabella Piccini (1644–1734). These various images differ noticeably in the physiognomy. Diodati's is the furthest from Loggan in its likeness. Huguetan's is no more aesthetically appealing.

8A.c1. OPERA MEDICA & PHYSICA, Lyons quarto 1676

The first edition of the collected works of Thomas Willis in Latin, the eighth book, including William Croone's treatise, and with all 40 illustrations [HJR Wing 44, Denham 10, Oldfield B1].

Title page: [1]. CLARISSIMI VIRI THOMÆ | WILLIS, | DOCTORIS MEDICI, | NATURALIS PHILOSOPHIÆ | PROFESSORIS OXON. | Necnon inclyti Medic. Collegij Londin. & Societatis | Regiæ Socij: | Opera Medica & Phyfica, | IN VARIOS TRACTATUS | DISTRIBUTA: | *CUM MULTIS FIGURIS ÆNEIS.* | QUORUM OPERUM SERIEM, PAGINA ELENCHUM | Rerum immediatè præcedens, indicat. | [ornament] | *LUGDUNI,* | Sumptibus JOANNIS ANTONIJ HUGUETAN, & Soc. | [short rule] | *M. D.C. LXXVI.* | CUM SUPERIORUM PERMISSU.*

[2]. CLARISSIMI VIRI THOMÆ | WILLIS, | DOCTORIS MEDICI, | PHOLOSOPHIÆ NATURALIS PROFESSORIS, | Sedleian. Oxon. necnon inclyti Med. Colleg. Londin. | &

[13] See chapter 3 for detailed descriptions.

* Underlined text originally printed in red.

Societatis Regiæ Socij: | DE ANIMA BRUTORUM, | QUÆ HOMINIS VITALIS AC SENSITIVA EST, | EXERCITATIONES DUÆ. | QUARUM PRIOR PHOLOSOPHICA, EJUSDEM | Naturam, Partes, Potentias, & Affectiones tradit: | *ALTERA PATHOLOGICA, MORBOS QUI IPSAM | ſedem ejus primariam, nempe cerebrum & Nervoſum genus afficiunt, explicat, | eorumque Therapeias inſtituit.* | [ornament] | *LUGDUNI,* | Sumptibus JOANNIS ANTONII HUGUETAN, & Soc. | [short rule] | *M. D.C. LXXVI.* | CUM SUPERIORUM PERMISSU.

[3]. CLARISSIMI VIRI THOMÆ | WILLIS, | DOCTORIS MEDICI, | PHILOSOPHIÆ NATURLAIS PROFESSORIS, | Sedleian. Oxon. necnon inclyti Med. Colleg. Londin. | & Societatis Regiæ Socij: | PHARMACEVTICE | RATIONALIS, | SIVE DIATRIBA | DE MEDICAMENTORUM | OPERATIONIBUS IN HUMANO CORPORE. | [ornament] | *LUGDUNI,* | Sumptibus JOANNIS ANTONII HUGUETAN, & Soc. | [short rule] | *M. D.C. LXXVI.* | CUM SUPERIORUM PERMISSU.

[4]. CLARISSIMI VIRI THOMÆ | WILLIS, | DOCTORIS MEDICI, | PHILOSOPHIÆ NATVRALIS | PROFESSORIS OXON. | OPVS POSTHVMVM. | PHARMACEVTICE | RATIONALIS, | *SIVE DIATRIBA* | DE MEDICAMENTORVM | OPERATIONIBVS IN HVMANO CORPORE. | [ornament] | *LVGDVNI,* | Sumptibus JOANNIS ANTONII HVGVETAN, & Soc. | [short rule] | *M. D.C. LXXVI.* | CUM SVPERIORVM PERMISSV.

Collation: quarto, 23 letter roman alphabet using I and V. [1]. $*^4$, $**^2$, $ã^4$, $ẽ^4$, $ĩ^4$, $õ^4$, $ũ^4$, A–G^4, H^4 (H3 + 2; signed H4, -), I–Z^4, Aa–Zz^4, Aaa–Zzz^4, AAaa–$XXxx^4$; $1–3 signed.
388 leaves, paginated as [52], 1–62, [4: paginated as 63*, -, *ibid.* 63, -], 63–694, [26]. Mispaginated: 190 for 160, 156 for 256, 309 for 325, 568 for 580, 226 for 626.

[2]. $ã^4$, $^2ã^4$, $ẽ^4$, A–Z^4, Aa–Qq^4; $1–3 signed apart from: -A3, -B3, -C3, -D3.
168 leaves, paginated as [24], 1–298, [14]. Mispaginated: 227 for 127, 262 for 162.

[3]. $*^4$, $ã^4$, $ẽ^2$, A–Z^4, Aa^2: $1–3 signed apart from: P2 signed O2.
104 leaves, paginated as [20], 1–180, [8].

[4]. $ã^4$, $ẽ^4$, $ĩ^4$, $õ^2$, A–Z^4, Aa–Ee^4, Ff^2; $1–3 signed.
128 leaves, paginated as [28], 1–224, [4]. Mispaginated: 142 for 141.

Type: 46 lines; height (20 lines) 82 millimetres, width ≤ 126 millimetres (≤ 138 millimetres with marginal notes).

Contents: [1]. ***4r**, page [7], blank; ***4v**, page [8], portrait; ***1r**, page [1], title; ***1v**, page [2], blank; ***2r–v**, pages [3–4], REVERENDISSIMO IN CHRISTO PATRI, AC D. DOMINO GILBERTO, EPISCOPO LONDINENSI, & Sacelli Regij Decano.... [signed] *Humillimus, & æternùm addictiſſimus* THOM. WILLIS.; ***3r–v**, pages [5–6], REVERENDISSIMO IN CHRISTO PATRI, ET DOMINO, D. GILBERTO, PROVIDENTIA DIVINA, Archiepiſcopo Cantuarienſi, totius Angliæ Primati, & Metropolitano; & Auguſtiſſimo Principi CAROLO II. M. Britanniæ, Franciæ & Hiberniæ Regi, à ſecretioribus Conſiliis. ... [signed] *Clementiæ veſtræ humillimus cultor, Cliens addictiſſimus* THOM. VUILLIS.; ****1r–**2r**, pages [9–11], AVTHORI, In illius Diatribas Medico-Philoſophicas, CARMEN GRATULATORIUM. ... [signed] PHILIPPVS FELL, *Med. Stud. Oxon.*; ****2v**, page [12],

SERIES OPERVM DOMINI D.THOMÆ VUILLIS, Hac Editione Typis prodeuntium. 1. De Fermentatione. II. De Febribus. III. De Urinis. IV. Cerebri Anatome. V. Nervorum deſcriptio, & uſus. VI. De Morbis Convulſivis. VII. De Scorbuto. VIII. De Affectionibus Hyſtericis, & Hypochondriacis. IX. De Sanguinis incaleſcentia. X. De Motu Muſculari. XI. De Anima Brutorum Exercitationes duæ. XII. Pharmaceutice Rationalis, & de Medicamentorum operationibus in humano corpore, &c.; **ã1r–ã3r**, pages [13–17], ELENCHVS RERVM QUÆ IN TRACTATV DE FERMENTATIONE continentur.; **ã3r–ẽ1v**, pages [17–22]; **ã3r** ELENCHVS RERVM Quæ in Tractatu de FEBRIBVS continentur.; **ẽ1v–ẽ2v**, pages [22–4], ELENCHVS RERVM Quæ in Diſſertatione de VRINIS continentur.; **ẽ2v–ĩ2r**, pages [24–31], ELENCHVS RERVM Quæ in CEREBRI ANATOME continentur.; **ĩ2r–ĩ4r**, pages [31–5], NERVORVM DESCRIPTIO ET VSVS.; **ĩ4r–õ3r**, pages [35–41], ELENCHVS RERVM Quæ in Tractatu de MORBIS CONVVLSIVIS continentur.; **õ3v–ũ1r**, pages [42–5], ELENCHVS RERVM Quæ in Tractatu de SCORBVTO continentur.; **ũ1r–v**, pages [45–6], ELENCHVS MATERIÆ De Affectibus Hyſtericis, & Hypochondriacis.; **ũ1v–ũ2r**, pages [46–7], ELENCHVS MATERIÆ Exercitationis de Accenſione Sanguinis.; **ũ2r–ũ3r**, pages [47–9], ELENCHVS MATERIÆ Exercitationis de Motu Muſculari.; **ũ3v**, page [50], [Imprimatur] *REGII PROCVRATORIS Conſenſus.* PRo Rege aſſentio, ut liceat HVGONI DENOÜALLY, Typographo Lugdunenſi typis mandare Tractatus varios D.D. THOMÆ VVILLIS, ... [with seven further lines listing titles]. ... Datum Lugduni 10. Iulij anni 1675 ... [signed] VAGINAY. [line] *PERMISSIO.* Fiat juxta Concluſiones Procuratoris Regij. Anno & die ſupradictis. [signed] DE SEVE. Prædictus HUGO DENOÜALLY jura ſua pro editione ſupradictorum Operum ceſſit IOANNI-ANTONIO HVGVETAN, Bibliopolæ Lugdunenſi, pacto inter eos inito die 11. Septembris anni 1675. *Regiſtratum in libro Communitatis Bibliopolarum Lugdunenſium, juxta ſententiam in Præſidiali Curia Lugdunenſi latam die* 12. *Ianuarij* 1675. Signatum CELLIER.; **ũ4r–v**, pages [51–2], AMICO LECTORI *PRÆFATIO* [to De Fermentatione].

A1r–H3v, pages 1–62, [text] DE FERMENTATIONE, *SIVE* De MOTV corporum naturalium INORGANICO.

'H4' (= H3 +1) r–'H5' (= H3 + 2) v, pages [1–4], Caput primum de Febribus præ feſtinatione editionis, & incogitanter ante præfationem typis datum, quamvis poſt eam legendum. AMICO LECTORI PRÆFATIO.

H4r–Dd3r, pages 63–213, [text] DE FEBRIBVS.; **Dd3v–Hh2v**, pages 214–44, [text] DE VRINIS Diſſertatio Epiſtolica. *Ad Virum Doctiſsimum mihiquæ amiciſsimum*, D. RADVLPHUM BATHVRST, Med. Doct. & Collegii Sacroſanctæ Trinitatis Oxon. Socium.

Hh3r–Xx3r, pages 245–349, [preface and text] CEREBRI ANATOME, CVI ACCESSIT Nervorum Deſcriptio & Vſus.; **Xx3v–Fff4v**, pages 350–416, [text], NERVORUM Deſcriptio & Vſus.; **Ggg1r–Iii1v**, pages 417–34 [text] DE RATIONE MOTVS MVSCVLORVM; Studio GVLIELMI CROONE, M. D. è Coll. Med. Lond. ac Societatis Regalis Socii. *Ἐν πᾶσι τοῖς φυσικοῖς ἐνεστί τι θαυμαστόν. Ariſt. de Part. Animal.*

Iii2r–BBbb3v, pages 435–566, [preface and text] PATHOLOGIÆ CEREBRI, ET NERVOSI GENERIS SPECIMEN: In quo agitur de MORBIS CONVULSIVIS, & de SCORBUTO.; **BBbb4r–KKkk4v**, pages 567–632, [text] TRACTATVS DE SCORBVTO.

LLlllr–OOoo2r, pages 633–59, [preface and text] AFFECTIONVM HYSTERICARVM, ET HYPOCHONDRIACARVM PATHOLOGIA SPASMODICA VINDICATA; Contra Reſponſionem Epiſtolarem NATHANAELIS HIGMORI M. D. *Cui acceſſerunt Exercitationes duæ Medico-Phyſicæ.* I. *De Sanguinis Accenſione.* II. *De Motu Muſculari.*; **OOoo2v–PPpp4v**, pages 660–72, EXERCITATIO. I. MEDICO-PHYSICA. *De Sanguinis Incaleſcentia, ſive Accenſione.*; **QQqq1r–SSss3v**, pages 673–94, [text] EXERCITATIO II. MEDICO-PHYSICA. *De Motu Muſculari.*

SSss4r–Xxx3v, pages [1–12], INDEX ALPHABETICVS Rerum Notabilium.; **XXxx4r–v**, pages [13–14], blank.

[2]. **1ã1r**, page [1], title; **ã1v**, page [2], blank; **ã2r–v**, pages [3–4], REVERENDISSIMO IN CHRISTO PATRI ET DOMINO GILBERTO PROVIDENTIA DIVINA ARCHIEPISCOPO CANTVARIENSI, totius *Angliæ* Primati & Metropolitano, & Auguſtiſſimo Principi Carolo II. M. *Britanniæ, Franciæ* & *Hiberniæ* Regi, à Secretioribus Conſiliis. ... [signed] *CLEMENTIÆ VESTRÆ,* Cultorem humillimum, ſervum devotiſſimum THO. VVILLIS.; **ã3r**, page [5], ERUDITISSIMIS ET VENERABILIBUS VIRIS, MIHIQUE ÆTERNUM COLENDIS D. VICE-CANCELLARIO, DOCTORIBUS ET MAGISTRIS QUI IN CELEBERRIMA UNIVERSITATE Oxonienſi bonas literas diligentiſſimè excolunt, egregiè ornant, feliciſſimè promovent ... [signed] *CLARISSIMI DOMINI,* Veſtrum omnium Cultori addictiſſimo THO. WILLIS.; **ã3v–ã4v**, pages [6–8], PRÆFATIO AD LECTOREM.; **2ã1r–ã4r**, pages [9–15], ELENCHVS RERVM Quæ in Tractatu. DE ANIMA BRVTORUM. Sive in Parte prima continentur.; **ã4v–ẽ4r**, pages [16–23], ELENCHVS RERVM QUÆ IN PARTE II. PATHOLOGICA Continentur.; **ẽ4v**, page [24], [Imprimatur] *Regij Procuatoris conſenſus.* ... then as in part I.

A1r–R1v, pages 1–130, [text] DE ANIMA BRVTORVM [part 1]; **R2r**, page [131] [half title] PARS SECVNDA PATHOLOGICA *SIVE* DE MORBIS QVI AD ANIMAM CORPOREAM, euiſque ſubjecta, ſcilicet Cerebrum, & Genus Nervoſum ſpectant.; **R2v**, page [132], blank; **R3r–Pp1v**, pages 133–298, [text] PARS SECVNDA.

Pp2r–Qq3v, pages [1–12], INDEX ALPHABETICVS Rerum & Verborum.; **Qq4r–v**, pages [13–14], blank.

[3]. ***1r**, page [1], title [Pharmaceutice rationalis]; ***1v**, page [2], blank; ***2r**, page [3], CELEBERRIMO MEDICORUM LONDINENSIUM COLLEGIO; ET SINGULATIM VIRO INSIGNISSIMO DOCTISSIMOQUE DOMINO GEORGIO ENT EQUITI AURATO PRÆSIDI ILLUSTRISSIMO, *NEC NON* CENSORIBUS DIGNISSIMIS, CÆTERISQUE OMNIBUS, ampliſſimæ hujus Societatis Membris. *DIATRIBAM HANC Pharmaceuticam Obſervantiæ & Honoris ergo Dicat, Dedicatque,* THO. WILLIS.; ***2v**, page [4], blank; ***3r–*4v**, pages [5–8]; CANDIDO LECTORI PRÆFATIO.; **ã1r–ẽ2r**, pages [9–19], ELENCHVS RERVM QVÆ IN PHARMACEVTICE RATIONALI CONTINENTVR.; **ẽ2v**, page [20], [Imprimatur] *REGII PROCVRATORIS CONSENSVS.* ... then as in Part I.

A1r–Z2v, pages 1–180, [text] DE MEDICAMENTORVM OPERATIONIBVS IN COPRORE HVMANO.

Z3r–Aa1v, page [1–6], INDEX ALPHABETICVS Rerum Notabilium.; **Aa2r–v**, pages [7–8], blank.

[4]. **ã1r**, page [1], title; **ã1v**, page [2], blank; **ã2r**, page [3], ATHENIS BRITANNICIS, Literati Orbis lumini Splendidiſſimo, *VNIVERSITATI OXONIENSI*, Et Ibidem ILLVSTRISSIMO PRINCIPI IAC. ORMONDIÆ DVCI CANCELLARIO HONORATISSIMO, RAD. BATHVRST *DECANO WELLENSI* VICECANCELLARIO DIGNISSIMO, Reuerendis admodum, & perquam Eruditis DOCTORIBVS, PROCVRATORIBVS, Facultatum omnium PROFESSORIBVS, COLLEGIORVM & AVLARVM Præfectis, *NECNON* Venerabili Magiſtrorum Senatui, Diatribam hanc Pharmaceuticam Pietatis & gratitudinis ergo Dicat Dedicatque Alumnus & beneficarius adſtrictiſſimus THO. WILLIS.; **ã2v**, page [4], *IMPRIMATVR* AMiciſſimo Authori, poſt tam Immortale opus, nihil mortale facturo, tanquam Lumina morienti claudens, extremum hoc officium præſtat. Oxon. *Novemb.* 12. 1675. *RAD. BATHVRST Vice-Cancel. Oxonienſis.* [rule] *Achevé d'imprimatur à Lyon ce* 13. *Iuin* 1676.; **ã3r–ã4v**, pages [5–8], CANDIDO LECTORI PRÆFATIO; **ã4v–ẽ2v**, pages [8–12], *POST SCRIPTVM.*; **ẽ3r–v**, pages [13–14], *AVTORI CLARISSIMO, necnon mihi (de quo jure glorior) AMICISSIMO*, IN ILLIVS PHARMACEVTICES RATIONALIS Partem vtramque, *Carmen Gratulatorium.* ... [signed] *GVL. DAVVKINS.*; **ẽ4r–v**, pages [15–16], QVERALA LIBRI POSTHVMI *DE OBITV* AVTORIS ... [signed] *GVL. DAWKINS* MED. B.; **ĩ1r–õ2v**, pages [17–28], ELENCHVS RERVM.

A1r–Ee4v, page 1–224, [text] DE MEDIMENTORVM OPERATIONIBVS IN CORPORE HVMANO.

Ff1r–Ff2v, pages [1–4], INDEX ALPHABETICVS.

Headlines and *Catchwords*: [1]. materiæ. for Materiæ. at **ũ1v**, page [46]; *Caput XVI.* for *Caput XVII.* at **Bb3r**, page 199; *Caput IV.* for *Caput VI.* at **Mm4r**, page 279; *uſus.* for *Uſus.* at **Yy3v**, page 358; **Aaa3v**, page 374; **Ccc1v**, page 386, **Ccc3v**, page 390; **Ddd2v**, page 398; **Eee2v**, page 404; **Eee3v**, page 406; **Fff1v**, page 410; **Fff2v**, page 412; **Fff4v**, page 416; *Motus* for *motus* at **Ggg2**, page 419; **Hhh1r**, page 425; ⁏ for ⁚ after headline at **Iii3v**, page 438; **Iii4v**, page 440; **Kkk2v**, page 442; **Kkk3v**, page 446; **Kkk4v**, page 448; *Motu* for *motu* at **QQqq1v–4r**, pages 674–9; **SSss1v–SSss2r**, pages 690–1.

vtraque for utraque at **H2v** / **H3r**, page 60 / 61; cum for cùm at **N4r** / **v**, page 79 / 80; **Z4r** / **v**, page 183 / 184; ſimoda for diverſimoda at **Ff2v** / **Ff3r**, page 228 / 229; cia for mercia at **Tt1v** / **Tt2r**, page 330 / 331; unde for niſi at **Hhh3v** / **Hhh4r**, page 430 / 431; corde for de at **HHhh2r** / **v**, page 611 / 612.

[2]. No CAP. II. at **A3v**, page 6; **A4v**, page 8; no CAP. IV. at **D2v**, page 28; *corpoream &* for *Corpoream* at **A4r**, page 7; no ⁏ after headline at **D3v**, page 30; *Rationali* for *Brutali* at **H1r**, page 57; **H2r**, page 59; *Genere.* for *genere.* at **K2r**, page 75; **K3v**, page 78; CRP. V II. for CAP. VII. at **Aa3v**, page 190; CAP. VII. for CAP. VIII. at **Bb4r**, page 199; no ⁚ after headline at **Ee2r**, page 219; **Ee3v**, page 222; CAP. XI. for CAP. X. at **Gg1r**, page 233; INDEX ALPHABETICUS for RERVM ET VERBORVM. at **Qq2r**, page [9].

No catchword at **ã2v** / **ã3r**, pages [4] / [5]; **ã3r** / **v**, pages [5] / [6]; byce for Bombyce at **B1v** / **B2r**, page 10 / 11; Tabula for TABVLA at **D1v** / **D2r**, pages 26 / 27; FIGVAA for FIGVRA at **E2v** / **E3r**, page 36 / 37; impreſſio for impleſſio at **K2r** / **v**, page 75 / 76; facile for facilè at **M4r** / **v**, page 95 / 96; ad for ſpiritus at **P3v** / **P4r**, page 118 / 119; vòrum for vorum at **S2r** / **v**, page 139 / 140; *mores* for *tremores* at **Y1v** / **Y2r**, page 170 / 171; CAP. VII for CAPVT at **Z4r** / **v**, page 183 / 184; *culas* for *ticulas* at **Ee4v** / **Dd1r**, page 208 / 209; 1° Quoad for Quoad at **Ll1r** / **v**, page 265 / 266; que for *lem* at **Mm2r** / **v**, page 275 / 276; 2da for *Secunda* at **Nn1r** / **v**, page 283 / 284.

[3]. CAP. IV. for CAP. II. at '**O**'[**P**]**2**, page 115; CAP. II. for CAP. III. at **Q2r**, page 123; SECT. III. For SECT. VII. at **Y2v**, page 172.

Apart from SECT. for SECTIO at each section break, no catchword at ***3r** / **v**, pages [5] / [6]; nibus for uibus at **Q2v** / **Q3r**, page 124 / 125; tuo for tus at **V4r** / **v**, page 159 / 160.

[4]. CAP. III. for CAP. IV. at **E1r**, page 33; Medicamentorum ad Phthiſin, for *Species & Formulæ*. at **G1v**, page 50; CAP. X. for CAP. XI. at **N4r**, page 103; CAP. II. for CAP. I. at **Q3r**, page 125; SECT. III. for SECT. II. at S3v, page 142; CAP. III. for CAP. IV. at **Bb2r**, page 195; *De Pſora, ſive Scabie* for *cum Pruritu*. at **Dd3r**, page 213.

No catchword at **A1v** / **A2r**, pages 2 / 3; CAP for SECT at **X3v** / **X4r**, page 166 / 167; **Aa1v** / **Aa2r**, page 186 / 187; **Bb1r** / **v**, page 193 / 194; perfluum for perfidum at **Y1r** / **v**, page 169 / 170; nantru for minantur at **Aa3v** / **Aa4r**, page 190 / 191.

Frontispiece: none.

Portrait: **Pt.1c1**: THOMAS WILLIS MEDIC · PROFESSOR · COLLEGII MED · LONDON · ET SOCIET · REG · SOCIVS, [with] ÆTATIS SVÆ, 45·. 228 × 172 millimetres (sheet); 172 × 130 millimetres (plate marks); 168 × 127 millimetres (image); see: Figure 147.

Printers' ornaments: [1]. Printers' device at ***1r**, page [1] {**Huguetan 1**}; headpiece at ***2r**, page [3]; **A1r**, page 1 {**Huguetan 2**}; headpiece at ***3r**, page [5] {**Huguetan 4**}; row of 23 fleurons at ****1r**, page [9]; 22 fleurons separated by : between ##2 / 3, 5 / 6, 7 / 8 at ****2v**, page [12] {**Huguetan 6**}; tailpiece at ****2r**, page [11] {**Huguetan 8**}; extensive use of {**Huguetan 9**} alone or in combination with other ornaments: row of 23 fleurons with : between ##11 / 12 at **ẽ2v**, page [24]; **ũ1r**, page [45]; 23 separated by : between ##17 / 18, 21 / 22 at **ĩ2r**, page [31]; two rows each of 23, lower inverted, separated by :) between ##12 / 13, 13 / 14 (upper) and ##14 / 15 (lower) at **ũ3v**, page [50]; two rows of 23 (each separated by : between ##11 / 12, 12 / 13), lower inverted with row between of 23 fleurons (printed fragment between ##7 / 8) {**Huguetan 10**} at **ã1r**, page [13]; **ũ4r**, page [51]; row of 20 with : between ##9 / 10, and 4 fleurons {**Huguetan 12**} between ##7 / 8, 11 / 12, 14 / 15, 16 / 17 at **ã3r**, page [17]; **ẽ1v**, page [22]; **ĩ4r**, page [35], **õ3v**, page [42]; row of 23 with single fleuron {**Huguetan 12**} between ##11 / 12, above identical (inverted) row at **H4r**, page 63; **Dd3v**, page 214; **Hh3r**, page 245; **Xx3v**, page 350; **Ggg1r**, page 417; **Iii2r**, page 435; **BBbb4r**, page 567; **LLll1r**, page 633; row of 22 with one fleuron {**Huguetan 10**} placed vertically between ##11 / 12, : between ##16 / 17, and a further space between ##19 / 20 at **LLll2r**, page 635; single row with the same fleuron at **OOoo2v**, page 660; **QQqq1r**, page 673; **SSss4r**, page [1]; row of 22 flanked at each end by 2 fleurons {**Huguetan 12**} above a similar row (inverted), separated by a row of 22 fleurons {**Huguetan 10**} at **ũ4r**, page [51]; tailpiece at **ũ3r**, page [49], **Hh2v**, page 244; **Fff4v**,

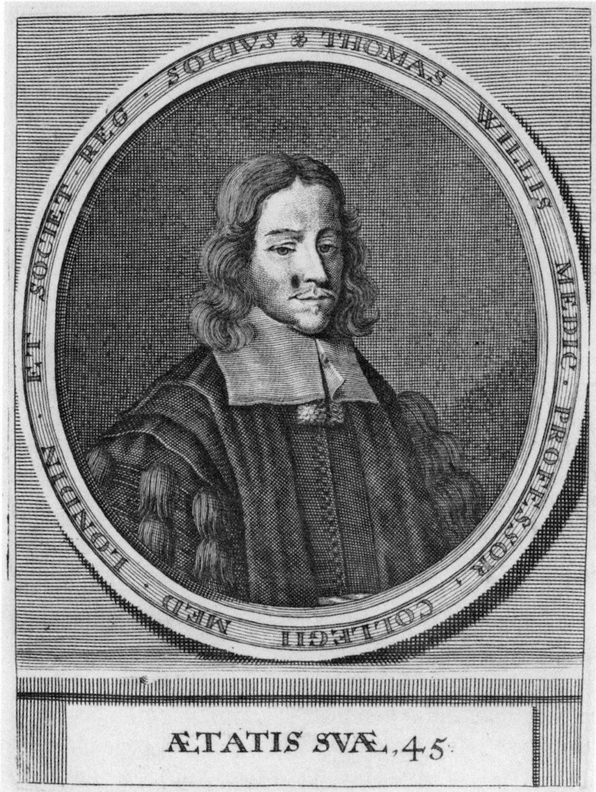

Figure 147 Portrait of Thomas Willis engraved: *Opera Omnia*, Lyon 1676 (Pt.1.c1).

page 416 {**Huguetan 22**}; tailpiece at **ũ4v**, page [52] {**Huguetan 25**}; row of 12 fleurons separated by : between ##4 / 5, 6 / 7, 7 / 8, 8 / 9 over similar row (inverted) at 'H4' (= H3 + 1) r, page 63*{**Huguetan 27**}; tailpiece at 'H5' (= H3 + 2) v, page [4 = *ibid.* 63v] {**Huguetan 29**}.

Decorated S at ***2r**, page [3] {**Huguetan 3**}; I at ***3r**, page [5] {**Huguetan 5**}; A at ****1r**, page [9] {**Huguetan 7**}; F at **ã1r**, page [13] {**Huguetan 11**}; F at **ã3r**, page [17] {**Huguetan 13**}; V at **ẽ1v**, page [22] {**Huguetan 14**}; C at **ẽ2v**, page [24] {**Huguetan 15**}; V at **ĩ2r**, page [31] {**Huguetan 16**}; Q at **ĩ4r**, page [35] {**Huguetan 17**}; I at **õ3v**, page [42]; **OOoo2v**, page 660 {**Huguetan 18**}; O at **ũ1r**, page [45]; **Dd3v**, page 214 {**Huguetan 19**}; I at **ũ1v**, page [46] {**Huguetan 20**}; A at **ũ2r**, page [47] {**Huguetan 21**}; P at **ũ3v**, page [50] {**Huguetan 23**}; D at **ũ4r**, page [51]; **Ggg1r**, page 417 {**Huguetan 24**}; I at **A1r**, page 1; **BBbb4r**, page 567 (inverted) {**Huguetan 26**}; D at 'H4' (= H3 + 1) r, page 63* {**Huguetan 28**}; E at **H4r**, page 63 {**Huguetan 30**}; A at **Hh3r**, page 245 {**Huguetan 31**}; N at **Xx3v**, page 350 {**Huguetan 32**}; Q at **Iii2r**, page 435; **LLll1r**, page 633 {**Huguetan 33**}; R at **LLll2r**, page 635 {**Huguetan 34**}; A at **SSss4r**, page [1] {**Huguetan 35**}.

[2]. Printers' device on title page at **ã1r**, page [1] {**Huguetan 1**}; headpiece at **ã2r**, page [3] {**Huguetan 2**}; row of 22 fleurons separated by : between ##2 / 3, 4 / 5, 7 / 8 at **ã3r**, page [5]; two rows, each of 22, upper with : between ##5 / 6, 6 / 7, 17 / 18, lower inverted

with : between ##7 / 8, 15 / 16, 18 / 19 at **ã3v**, page [6]; two rows each of 23 fleurons, lower inverted at **Pp2r**, page [1] {**Huguetan 6**}; two rows, upper of 23 and lower (inverted) {**Huguetan 6**} with middle row of 22 fleurons {**Huguetan 10**} at **2ã4v**, page [16]; row of 12 symmetrical designs each made up of 4 fleurons arranged in rotation at **2ã1r**, page [9] {**Huguetan 38**}; row of 22 fleurons at **e4v**, page [24] {**Huguetan 10**}; headpiece at **A1r**, page 1 {**Huguetan 41**}; row of 32 fleurons separated by : at ##15 / 16, 16 / 17 at **C4v**, page 24; **3r**, page 37 {**Huguetan 12**}; headpiece at **R3r**, page 133 {**Huguetan 43**}; tailpiece at **Pp1v**, page 298 {**Huguetan 45**}.

Decorated Q at **ã2r**, page [3] {**Huguetan 36**}; I at **ã3r**, page [5] {**Huguetan 5**}; E at **ã3v**, page [6] {**Huguetan 37**}; A at **2ã1r**, page [9]; **Pp2r**, page [1] {**Huguetan 39**}; C at **2ã4v**, page [16] {**Huguetan 40**}; Q at **A1r**, page 1 {**Huguetan 42**}; I at **R3r**, page 133 {**Huguetan 44**}.

[3]. Printers' device on title page at ***1r**, page [1] {**Huguetan 1**}; headpiece at ***3r**, page [5] {**Huguetan 2**}; tailpiece at *4v, page [8] {**Huguetan 46**}; headpiece at **ã1r**, page [9]; **A1r**, page 1 {**Huguetan 41**}; row of 22 fleurons above similar row (inverted) at **Z3r**, page [1] {**Huguetan 6**}.

Decorated Q at ***3r**, page [5] {**Huguetan 36**}; M at **ã1r**, page [9] {**Huguetan 47**}; A at **A1r**, page 1 {**Huguetan 48**}.

[4]. Printers' device on title page at **ã1r**, page [1] {**Huguetan 1**}; headpiece at **ã3r**, page [5]; í1r, page [17]; **A1r**, page 1 {**Huguetan 41**}; tailpiece at ẽ4v, page [16] {**Huguetan 49**}; õ2v, page [28] {**Huguetan 51**}; row of 24 fleurons at **P4v**, page 120; row of 27 at **Ff1r**, page [1] {**Huguetan 9**}.

Decorated A at **ã3r**, page [5] {**Huguetan 48**}; A at **ĩ1r**, page [17] {**Huguetan 50**}; I at **A1r**, page 1 {**Huguetan 52**}; H at **P4v**, page 120 {**Huguetan 53**}; A at **Ff1r**, page [1] {**Huguetan 54**}.

Illustrations: lettering and legends as **2A**, **2C**, **4A**, **5A**, **6A**, and **6E**.

[1]. **Pl.14e1**. Plate 14 (image 18): *Tab.* XII (headline, left), *Pag. 4*[1]3. (headline, right). Folding, 252 × 80 millimetres (sheet); 230 × 55 millimetres (plate marks); 215 × 37 millimetres (figure). Inserted at [1] **F2r**, page 43.

Pl.1e1. Plate 1 (image 1): *Fig. I.* (headline, centre), *Pag. 256* (headline, right), *de medio T vid pag. 401 402* (footer, right). Folding, 228 × 194 (sheet); 210 × 170 millimetres (plate marks); 186 × 166 millimetres (figure). Inserted within legends for Figuræ I and II at **Ii4v–Kk2v**, pages 256–8.

Pl.2e1. Plate 2 (image 2): *Fig. II.*[da.] (headline, centre), *Pag. 257* (headline, right), *de medio S vid pag. 401. 402.* (footer, right). Leaf size, 228 × 172 millimetres (sheet); 142 × 117 millimetres (plate marks); 132 × 102 millimetres (figure). Inserted within legends for Figuræ I and II at **Ii4v–Kk2v**, pages 256–8.

Pl.3e1. Plate 3 (image 3): *Fig. III* (headline, centre), *Pag. 265* (headline, right). Folding, 228 × 205 millimetres (sheet); 220 × 183 millimetres (plate marks); 193 × 172 millimetres (figure). Inserted before legends for Figuræ III and IIII at **Ll1r–Ll2r**, pages 265–7.

Pl.4e1. Plate 4 (image 4): *Fig. IIII.* (headline, centre), *Pag. 266.* (headline, right). Leaf size, 228 × 172 millimetres (sheet); 132 × 98 millimetres (plate marks); 112 × 92 millimetres (figure). Inserted within legends for Figuræ III and IIII at **Ll1r–Ll2r**, pages 265–7.

Pl.6e1. Plate 6 (image 6): *Fig. VI* (headline, centre), *Pag 271* (headline, right). Leaf size, 228 × 172 millimetres (sheet); 174 × 140 millimetres (plate marks); 172 × 126 millimetres (figure). Inserted before legends for Figuræ V and VI at **Ll4r–v**, pages 271–2.

Pl.5e1. Plate 5 (image 5): *Fig. V.* (headline, left), *Pag. 271.* (headline, right). Leaf size, 228 × 172 millimetres (sheet); 184 × 132 millimetres (plate marks); 177 × 130 millimetres (figure). Inserted before legends for Figuræ V and VI at **Ll4r**, page 271.

Pl.7e1. Plate 7 (images 7–10): [unnumbered 1] *Pag. 287* (headline, right), *Fig. 1, Fig. 11.*; *Fig. 111.*, (headers, above each image), *Fig. 1111.* (header, right of image). Leaf size, 228 × 172 millimetres (sheet); 145 × 112 millimetres (plate marks); 25 × 93 millimetres, 73 × 93 millimetres, 34 × 28 millimetres, 72 × 30 millimetres (figures). Inserted before legend at **Nn4r–v**, pages 287–8.

Pl.8e1. Plate 8 (image 11): *Fig.* VII (headline, centre), *Pag. 297* (headline, right). Leaf size, 228 × 172 millimetres (sheet); 197 × 117 millimetres (plate marks, cropped); 190 × 103 millimetres (figure). Inserted before legend at **Pp1r**, page 297.

Pl.9e1. Plate 9 (image 12): *Fig.* VIII (headline, centre), *Pag. 310* (headline, right). Leaf size, 228 × 172 millimetres (sheet); 134 × 105 millimetres (plate marks); 109 × 95 millimetres (figure). Inserted within legend at **Qq3v–Qq4r**, pages 310–11.

Pl.10e1. Plate 10 (images 13–14): [unnumbered 2] *Fig. I.* (headline, centre), *Pag. 359* (headline, right), *Fig. II.* (header, centre above image). Leaf size, 228 × 172 millimetres (sheet); 185 × 113 millimetres (plate marks); 122 × 114, 50 × 109 millimetres (figures). Inserted before legend at **Yy4r–v**, pages 359–60.

Pl.12e1. Plate 12 (image 16): *Tab. X.* (headline, centre), *Pag. 405* (headline, right). Folding, 312 × 210 millimetres (sheet); printed from a larger sheet, 287 × >185 millimetres (plate marks at upper, right, and lower borders); 272 × 180 millimetres (figure). Inserted before legends for Tabulæ IX–XIII at **Eee3r–Fff4r**, pages 405–15.

Pl.11e1. Plate 11 (image 15): *Pag. 409* (headline, left), *Tab. IX.* (headline, right). Folding, 315 × 170 millimetres (sheet); printed from a larger sheet, lines 285 × 165 millimetres (plate marks upper, left, and lower borders, line at the right edge); 272 × 149 millimetres (figure). Inserted within legends for Tabulæ IX–XIII at **Eee3r–Fff4r**, pages 405–15.

Pl.13e1. Plate 13 (image 17): *Pag. 410* (headline, left), *Tab. X1.^{ma}* (headline, right). Folding, 314 × 158 millimetres (sheet); printed from a larger sheet, lines 293 × 135 millimetres (plate marks at upper, left, and lower borders, line at the right edge); 275 × 125 millimetres (figure). Inserted within legends for Tabulæ IX–XIII at **Eee3r–Fff4r**, pages 405–15.

Pl.15e1. Plate 15 (images 19–23): *Pag. 414* (headline, centre), *Tab.* XIII (headline, right), *Fig. I ^{ma}, Fig. 2 $^{da.}$, Fig. 3 ^{tia}, Fig. 4 $^{ta.}$, Fig. 5 $^{ta.}$* (centre above each image, figures 3 and 4 placed horizontally). Folding, 260 × 327 millimetres (sheet); printed from a larger sheet, lines 240 × 293 millimetres (plate marks at left, right and lower borders, line at the upper edge); 163 × 77 millimetres, 169 × 68 millimetres, 283 × 31 millimetres, 268 × 35 millimetres, 73 × 24 millimetres (Figures). Inserted within legends for Tabulæ IX–XIII at **Eee3r–Fff4r**, pages 405–15.

Pl.16b1. Plate 16 (images 24–25) *Pag. 434.* (headline, left), *Fig. 2* (header, above image), *Fig. 1.* (header, left of image). Leaf size, 228 × 172 millimetres (sheet); 140 × 132 millimetres (plate marks); 112 × 66 millimetres, 127 × 56 millimetres (figures). Inserted at **Iii4v**, page 434.

Pl.17d1. Plate 17 (images 26–27): *Pag. 693.* (headline, right), *Fig. I.*, *Fig. II.* (headers, above each image). Leaf size, 172 × 228 millimetres (bound horizontally), 110 × 165 millimetres (plate marks); 28 × 139 millimetres, 48 × 158 millimetres (figures). Inserted before legends for Figuræ I–IV at **SSss3r–v**, pages 693–4.

Pl.18d1. Plate 18 (images 28–29): *Pag. 694.* (headline, right), *Fig. III.*, *Fig. IV.* (headers, above each image). Leaf size, 172 × 228 millimetres (sheet); 100 × 170 millimetres (plate marks); 30 × 151 millimetres, 42 × 159 millimetres (figures). Inserted after legends for Figuræ I–IV at **SSss3r–v**, pages 693–4.

[2]. **Pl.19d1**. Plate 19 (images 30–33): *Pag. 24.* (headline, left), *Tab. I$^{a.}$* (headline, right), *Fig. I.^{a}*, *Fig. II.$^{da.}$*, *Fig. IIII.$^{ta.}$*, *Fig. III.$^{tia.}$* (headers, above each image). Leaf size, 228 × 172 millimetres (sheet); 193 × 135 millimetres (plate marks); 47 × 25 millimetres, 120 × 86 millimetres, 113 × 16 millimetres, 76 × 106 millimetres (Figures). Inserted within legends for Tabulæ I–IIII at **C4v–D3r**, pages 24–9.

Pl.20d1. Plate 20 (images 34–35): *Pag. 24.* (headline, right), *Fig. I.^{a}*, *Fig. II.^{da}* (headers, above each image). Leaf size, 172 × 228 millimetres (sheet); 155 × 185 millimetres (plate marks); 109 × 84 millimetres, 132 × 96 millimetres (figures). Inserted within legends for Tabulæ I–IIII at **C4v–D3r**, pages 24–9.

Pl.21d1. Plate 21 (images 36–38): *Tab. III.$^{tia.}$* (headline, centre), *Pag. 26.* (headline, right), *Fig. 1ma.* (header, left of the image), *Fig. II^{da}*, *Fig. III.^{tia}.* (headers, above each image). Folding, 267 × 190 millimetres (sheet); 245 × 163 millimetres (plate marks) 239 × 97, 120 × 90 and 40 × 17 millimetres (figures). Inserted within legends for Tabulæ I–IIII at **C4v–D3r**, pages 24–9.

Pl.22d1. Plate 22 (images 39–41): *Pag. 26* (headline, left), *Tab. IIII.* (headline, right), *Fig. III ^{tia}*, *Fig. I.^{ma}*, *Fig II. ^{da}.* (headers, above each image). Leaf size, 228 × 172 millimetres (sheet); 175 × 126 millimetres (plate marks); 164 × 20 millimetres, 157 × 68 millimetres, 44 × 16 millimetres (figures). Inserted within legends for Tabulæ I–IIII at **C4v–D3r**, pages 24–9.

Pl.23d1. Plate 23 (image 42): *Pag. 36.* (headline, left), *Tab.V.* (headline right), [letters *b* and *c* not reengraved]. Leaf size, 228 × 172 millimetres (sheet); 167 × 112 millimetres (plate marks); 158 × 96 millimetres (figure). Inserted within legends for Tabulæ V–VII at **E3r–E4r**, pages 37–9.

Pl.24d1. Plate 24 (image 43): *Tab. VI.* (headline, left), *Pag. 38* (headline, right). Leaf size, 228 × 172 millimetres (sheet); 136 × 98 millimetres (plate marks); 130 × 88 millimetres (figure). Inserted within legends for Tabulæ V–VII at **E3r–E4r**, pages 37–9.

Pl.25d1. Plate 25 (image 44): *Pag. 38.* (headline, left), *Tab. VII.* (headline right). Leaf size, 228 × 172 millimetres (sheet); 128 × 119 millimetres (plate marks); 119 × 106 (figure). Inserted within legends for Tabulæ V–VII at **E3r–E4r**, pages 37–9.

Pl.26d1. Plate 26 (image 45): *Tab. VIII.* (headline, left), *Pag. 59.* (headline, right). Leaf size, 172 × 228 millimetres (sheet); 152 × 175 millimetres (plate marks); 146 × 170 millimetres (figure). Inserted before legend at **H2r–v**, pages 59–60.

[3]. **Pl.27e1**. Plate 27 (image 46): *Tab. I.* (headline, centre), *Pag. 18* (headline, right). Folding, 228 × 205 millimetres (sheet); 160 × 180 millimetres (plate marks); 147 × 174 millimetres (figure). Inserted within legends for Tabulæ I–VI at **C1v–C2v**, pages 18–20.

Pl.28e1. Plate 28 (image 47): *Tab. II* (headline, centre), *Pag. 19.* (headline, right). Folding, 228 × 205 millimetres (sheet); 142 × 178 millimetres (plate marks); 130 × 175 millimetres (figure). Inserted within legends for Tabulæ I–VI at **C1v–C2v**, pages 18–20.

Pl.29e1. Plate 29 (image 48): *Tab III* (headline, centre), *Pag. 19.* (headline, right). Folding, 228 × 205 millimetres (sheet); 153 × 185 millimetres (plate marks); 143 × 175 millimetres (figure). Inserted within legends for Tabulæ I–VI at **C1v–C2v**, pages 18–20.

Pl.30e1. Plate 30 (image 49–51): *Tab. IV* (headline, left), *Pag. 19* (headline, right), *Fig. 3.*, *Fig. 2.*, *Fig. I.* (headers, above each image). Folding, 228 × 205 millimetres (sheet); 152 × 205 millimetres (plate marks); 48 × 54 millimetres, 65 × 55 millimetres, 140 × 157 millimetres (figures). Inserted within legends for Tabulæ I–VI at **C1v–C2v**, pages 18–20.

Pl.31e1. Plate 31 (image 52): *Tab. V.* (headline, centre), *Pag. 19.* (headline, right). Folding, 228 × 205 millimetres (sheet); 157 × 163 millimetres (plate marks); 148 × 153 millimetres (figure). Inserted within legends for Tabulæ I–VI at **C1v–C2v**, pages 18–20.

Pl.32e1. Plate 32 (images 53–57): *Tab. VI.* (headline, centre), *Pag. 20.* (headline, right). Folding, 228 × 225 millimetres (sheet); 125 × 206 millimetres (plate marks); 113 × 23 millimetres, 115 × 22 millimetres, 115 × 22 millimetres, 113 × 22 millimetres, 113 × 23 millimetres (figures). Inserted within legends for Tabulæ I–VI at **C1v–C2v**, pages 18–20.

[4]. **Pl.33e1**. Plate 33 (image 58): *Sect. i: Cap. i. pag: 18.* (headline, left), *Tab: I.* (headline, right). Leaf size, 176 × 220 millimetres (sheet); 99 × 189 millimetres (plate marks); 94 × 178 millimetres (figure). Inserted within legends for Tabulæ I–VIII at **C1v–C3r**, pages 18–21.

Pl.35e1. Plate 35 (images 60–61): *Tab: III.* (headline, left), *Sect. i: Cap. i. pag. 19.* (headline, right), *Fig: 1.*, *Fig: 2.* (headers, left of each image). Leaf size, 228 × 172 millimetres (sheet); 190 × 135 millimetres (plate marks); 181 × 132 millimetres, 43 × 25 millimetres (figures). Inserted within legends for Tabulæ I–VIII at **C1v–C3r**, pages 18–21.

Pl.34e1. Plate 34 (image 59): *Tab: II.* (headline, left), *Sect. i: Cap. i. pag: 18 &c 19.* (headline, right). Leaf size, 228 × 172 millimetres (sheet); 190 × 120 millimetres (plate marks); 184 × 116 millimetres (figure). Inserted within legends for Tabulæ I–VIII at **C1v–C3r**, pages 18–21.

Pl.36e1. Plate 36 (images 62–64): *Tab: IV.* (headline, centre), *Sect. i Cap: i. p: 19 &c 20* (headline, right), *Fig: i.*, *Fig: 2.*, *Fig: 3* (headers, left of each image). Leaf size, 222 × 172 millimetres (sheet); 152 × 103 millimetres (plate marks); 68 × 40 millimetres, 58 × 33 millimetres, 61 × 34 millimetres (figures). Inserted within legends for Tabulæ I–VIII at **C1v–C3r**, pages 18–21.

Pl.37e1. Plate 37 (images 65–67): *Sect. i Cap. i.* (headline, left), *Tab. V–pag: 20.* (headline, right), *Fig 2*, *Fig. 1.*, *Fig. 3.* (footers, below each image). Folding, 228 × 192 millimetres (sheet); 212 × 158 millimetres (plate marks); 76 × 87 millimetres, 78 × 67 millimetres, 138 × 155 millimetres (figures). Inserted within legends for Tabulæ I–VIII at **C1v–C3r**, pages 18–21.

Pl.38e1. Plate 38 (images 68–75): *Tab: VI* (headline, left), *Sect: i: Cap. i: pag. 20 &c. 21.* (headline, right), *Fig: 1.*, *Fig. 2* (headers, above each group of four images). Folding, 228 × 235 millimetres (sheet); 156 × 218 millimetres (plate marks); 69 × 47 millimetres, 69 × 48 millimetres, 67 × 49 millimetres, 65 × 48 millimetres, 72 × 17 millimetres, 73 × 18 millimetres, 74 × 17 millimetres, 74 × 17 millimetres (figures). Inserted within legends for Tabulæ I–VIII at **C1v–C3r**, pages 18–21.

Pl.39e1. Plate 39 (images 76–79): *Tab: VII.* (headline, centre), *Sect i. Cap: i. pag: 21.* (headline, right), *Fig: 1.*, *Fig: 3.*, *Fig: 4.*, *Fig: 2.* (headers, above each image). Leaf size, 200 × 142 millimetres (sheet); 150 × 140 millimetres (plate marks); 56 × 56 millimetres, 58 × 56 millimetres, 56 × 59 millimetres, 57 × 48 millimetres (figures). Inserted within legends for Tabulæ I–VIII at **C1v–C3r**, pages 18–21.

Pl.40e1. Plate 40 (images 80–82): *Sect I: Cap. I. pag. 21.* (headline, left), *Tab: VIII.* (headline, centre), *Fig: 1.*, *Fig: 2.*, *Fig: 3.* (headers, above each image). Leaf size, 228 × 172 millimetres (sheet); 143 × 95 millimetres (plate marks); 50 × 50 millimetres, 23 × 26 millimetres, 51 × 50 millimetres (figures). Inserted within legends for Tabulæ I–VIII at **C1v–C3r**, pages 18–21.

Copy: DASC, lacking XXxx4, blank. Early vellum, spine lettered WILLIS | OPERA MEDIC: | 100, original endpapers. Leaves 228 × 172 millimetres, boards 239 × 180 × 105 millimetres. Inscribed Jo. Ger. Wagneri M.D.[14]

8A.c2. OPERA MEDICA & PHYSICA, Lyons quarto 1676

The first edition of the collected works of Thomas Willis in Latin, the eighth book, with one leaf in a second state [not distinguished from HJR Wing 44, Denham 10, Oldfield B1].

As in **8A.c1** parts [1]–[3].

[4]. *Collation*: pagination corrected at 141.

Copy: DASC (#1 of 3). Parts 1–3: original calf, spine with five raised bands, gilt tooled panels, lettered WILLIS | OPERA, original endpapers. Leaves 222 × 175 millimetres, boards

[14] This may be Johannes Wagner listed in the catalogue of alumni as having matriculated at Yale College in 1812 and subsequently associate professor in the Medical Collge of Charleston, South Carolina. See: *Catalogue of the officers and students of Yale College 1842–1843*, New Haven (1842): page 53.

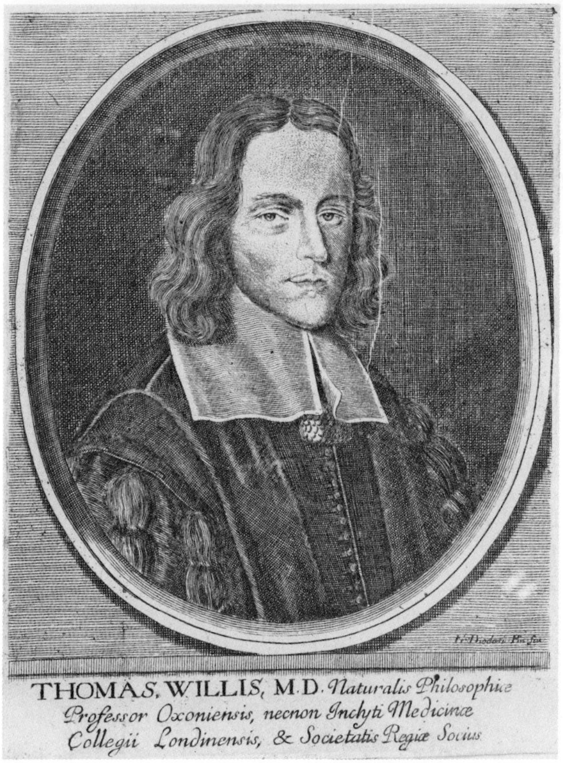
THOMAS WILLIS, M.D. Naturalis Philosophiæ
Professor Oxoniensis, necnon Inclyti Medicinæ
Collegii Londinensis, & Societatis Regiæ Socius

Figure 148 Portrait of Thomas Willis engraved by François Diodati: *Opera Omnia*, Geneva 1676 (Pt.1.d1).

233 × 173 × 83 millimetres. Inscribed: ×3 (each scored through; unidentified). Part 4: original calf, gilt edges, spine with five raised bands, gilt tooled panels, lettered WILLI | OPUS, original endpapers. Leaves 232 × 173 millimetres, boards 242 × 175 × 25 millimetres. Stamped: DOMUS LUGDIENSIS SOC. JESU.

8B1. OPERA OMNIA, Geneva quarto 1676

The first issue of the second edition of the collected works of Thomas Willis in Latin, the eighth book, with William Croone's treatise, and all 40 illustrations [HJR Wing 46, Denham 11, Oldfield B3].

Title page: [1a]. THOMÆ | WILLIS | MEDICINÆ DOCTORIS, | NATVRALIS PHILOSOPHIÆ | PROFESSORIS OXONIENSIS, | *Nec non* | INCLYTI MEDICORVM COLLEGII | Londinenſis, & SOCIETATIS REGIÆ Socii, | OPERA OMNIA, | *Quorum poſthac exſtat Catalogus*. | Cum ELENCHIS RERVM & INDICIBVS neceſſariis, ut & multis FIGVRIS æneis. | [printers' device: lettered, QVOD TIBI | FIERI NON | VIS, ALTERI | NEFECERIS] | *GENEVÆ*, | Apud SAMVELEM DE TOVRNES. | [short rule] | *M. DC. LXXVI*. | Cum SVPERIORVM Permiſſu.*

* Underlined text originally printed in red.

[1b]. DIATRIBÆ DVÆ | MEDICO-PHILOSOPHICÆ | *Quarum* PRIOR *agit* | DE FERMENTATIONE | *Sive de* MOTV *Inteſtino Particularum in quovis Corpore* | ALTERA | DE FEBRIBVS, | *Sive* de MOTV earundem in ſanguine Animalium | *His acceſſit* | DISSERTATIO Epiſtolica de VRINIS. | *Studio* | THOMÆ WILLIS, M.D. | Natural. Philoſoph. *Profeſſ.* Oxon. nec non Inclyti Medic. | Colleg. Londin. & Societatis Regiæ *Socii.* | [ornament: lettered, QUOD TIBI | FIERI NON | VIS, ALTERI | NEFECERIS] | *GENEVÆ,* | Apud SAMVELEM DE TOVRNES. | [short rule] | *M. DC. LXXVI.*

[2]. CEREBRI | ANATOME | NERVORVMQUE | DESCRIPTIO ET VSVS. | *Studio* | THOMÆ WILLIS, M. D. | Natural. Philoſoph. *Profeſſ.* Oxon. nec non Inclyti Medic. | Colleg. Londin. & Societ. Reg. *Socii.* | *Accesſit* VIRI *cujuſdam Clariſsimi* | *De* | RATIONE MOTVS MVSCVLORUM | *Tractatus Singularis.* | [ornament: lettered, QUOD TIBI | FIERI NON | VIS, ALTERI | NEFECERIS] | *GENEVÆ,* | Apud SAMVELEM DE TOVRNES. | [short rule] | *M. DC. LXXVI.*

[3]. PATHOLOGIÆ | CEREBRI | *ET* | NERVOSI GENERIS | SPECIMEN. | *In quo agitur* | De Morbis Convulſivis & de Scorbuto. | *Studio* | THOMÆ WILLIS, M.D. | Natural. Philoſoph. *Profeſſ.* Oxon. nec non Inclyti Medic. | Colleg. Londin. & Societ. Reg. *Socii.* | [printers' device: lettered, QUOD TIBI | FIERI NON | VIS, ALTERI | NEFECERIS] | *GENEVÆ,* | Apud SAMVELEM DE TOVRNES. | [short rule] | *M. DC. LXXVI.*

[4]. AFFECTIONVM | *Quæ dicuntur* | HYSTERICÆ | ET HYPOCHONDRIACÆ | PATHOLOGIA SPASMOCIA VINDICATA, | *Contra Reſponſionem Epiſtolarem* NATH. HIGHMORI *M. D.* | Cui acceſſerunt Exercitationes Medico-Phyſicæ Duæ. | I. *De* SANGVINIS ACCENSIONE. | II *De* MOTV MVSCVLARI. | *Studio* | THOMÆ WILLIS, M. D. | Natur. Philoſoph. *Profeſſ.* Oxon. nec non Inclyti Medic. | Colleg. Londin. *&* Societatis Regiæ *Socii.* | [printers' device: lettered, QUOD TIBI | FIERI NON | VIS, ALTERI | NEFECERIS] | *GENEVÆ,* | Apud SAMVELEM DE TOVRNES. | [short rule] | *M. DC. LXXVI.*

[5]. DE ANIMA | BRVTORVM | *Quæ* HOMINIS *Uitalis ac Senſitava eſt,* | EXERCITATIONES DVÆ. | PRIOR PHYSIOLOGICA | *Ejuſdem* Naturam, Partes, Potentias *&* Affectiones *tradit;* | ALTERA PATHOLOGICA | Morbos qui ipſam & Sedem ejus Primariam, | *Nempe* CEREBRVM *&* NERVOSVM GENVS *afficiunt, explicitat; eorúmque* | *Therapeias inſtituit, cum Figuris æneis.* | STVDIO | THOMÆ WILLIS, M. D. | Natural. Philoſoph. *Profeſſ.* Oxon. nec non Inclyti Medic. | Colleg. Londin. & Societatis Regiæ *Socii.* | [printers' devicet: lettered, QUOD TIBI | FIERI NON | VIS, ALTERI | NEFECERIS] | *GENEVÆ,* | Apud SAMVELEM DE TOVRNES. | [short rule] | *M. DC. LXXVI.*

[6]. PHARMACEVTICE | RATIONALIS | *Sive* | DIATRIBA | *De* | MEDICAMENTORVM | OPERATIONIBVS | In Humano CORPORE, | *Studio* | THOMÆ WILLIS, M. D. | Natural. Philoſoph. *Profeſſ.* Oxon. nec non Inclyti Medic. | Colleg. Londin. & Societatis Regiæ *Socii.* | [printers' device: lettered, QUOD TIBI | FIERI NON | VIS, ALTERI | NEFECERIS] | *GENEVÆ,* | Apud SAMVELEM DE TOVRNES. | [short rule] | *M. DC. LXXVI.*

[7]. PHARMACEVTICES | RATIONALIS | *Sive* | DIATRIBÆ, | *De* | MEDICAMENTORVM | OPERATIONIBVS | In Humano CORPORE, | PARS SECVNDA. | *Opus Poſthumum* | THOMÆ WILLIS, M. D. | Natural. Philoſoph. *Profeſſ.* Oxon. nec non Inclytic Medic. | Colleg. Londin. & Societatis Regiæ *Socii.* | [printers' device: lettered, QUOD TIBI | FIERI NON |

VIS, ALTERI | NEFECERIS] | *GENEVÆ,* | Apud SAMVELEM DE TOVRNES. | [short rule over date] | *M. DC. LXXVII.*

Collation: quarto, 23 letter alphabet using i and u, and *v* and V. [1]. ¶^{4}, §–§§§^{4}, a–z^{4}, aa–ii^{4}; $1–3 signed.
144 leaves, paginated as [32], 1–254, [2].

[2]. ¶^{4}, ¶¶^{4}, A–Z^{4}, Aa–Bb^{4}; $1–3 signed.
108 leaves, paginated as [16], 1–176, [2] 3–21 [22], [2].

[3]. *–**^{4}; *A–*Z^{4}, *Aa–*Dd^{4}; $1–3 signed apart from: *I3 signed I3.
116 leaves, paginated as [16], 1–214, [2].

[4]. *^{2}, a–h^{4}, i^{2}; $1–3 signed.
36 leaves, paginated as [4], 1–63, [5].

[5]. †–††††^{4}, *a–z*^{4}, *aa–uu*^{4}; $1–3 signed apart from: +*d*4.
188 leaves, paginated as [32], 1–333, [11].

[6]. (*)–(**)^{4}, *A–Z*^{4}, *Aa–Cc*^{4}; $1–3 signed apart from: -*I*3.
112 leaves, paginated as [16], 1–204, [4].

[7]. ¶–¶¶¶¶^{4}, A–Z^{4}, Aa–Ll^{4}; $1–3 signed apart from: -¶2, +G4.
152 leaves, paginated as [32], 1–266, [6]. Mispaginated: 35 for 53, 203 for 103, 279 for 179, 218 for 217.

Type: 43 lines; height (20 lines) 81 millimetres, width 119 millimetres (126 millimetres with marginal notes).

Contents: [1]. **¶4r**, page [1], blank; **¶4v**, page [2], [portrait]; **¶1r**, page [3], title; **¶1v**, page [4], blank; **¶2r–v**, pages [5–6], BENEVOLO LECTORI TYPOGRAPHVS *SALVTEM*.; **¶3r–v**, pages [7–8], OPERVM THOMÆ WILLIS CATALOGVS.; **§1r**, page [9], title; **§1v**, page [10], blank; **§2r–v**, page [11–12], *Reverendiſſimo in* CHRISTO PATRI, ET DOMINO, D. GILBERTO, *Epiſcopo* Londinensi, & *Sacelli Regii Decano...* [signed] *Humillimus & æternum Addictiſsimus,* THOM. WILLIS.; **§3r–§3v**, pages [13–14], AMICO LECTORI PRÆFATIO. [De Fermentatione]; **§4r–§§1v**, pages [15–18], AMICO LECTORI PRÆFATIO. [De Febribus]; **§§2r–v**, pages [19–20], AVTHORI *In illius Diatribas Medico-Philoſophicas*, Carmen gratulatorium ... [signed] PHILIPPVS FELL, Med. Stud. Oxon.; **§§3r–§§4v**, pages [21–4], ELENCHVS RERVM IN TRACTATV *DE* FERMENTATIONE.; **§§§1r–§§§3r**, pages [25–9], ELENCHVS RERVM IN TRACTATV *DE* FEBRIBVS.; **§§§3v–§§§4r**, pages [30–1], ELENCHVS RERVM IN DISSERTATIONE *DE* VRINIS.; **§§§4v**, pages [32], blank.

a1r–h4v, pages 1–64, [text] *DE* FERMENTATIONE, *Sive* DE MOTV CORPORVM NATVRALIVM INORGANICO.; **i1r–ee3v**, pages 65–222, [text] DE FEBRIBVS.; **ee4r–v**, pages 223–4, DE VRINIS DISSERTATIO EPISTOLICA, *Ad Virum Doctiſsimum, mihiq; Amiciſsimum* D. RVDOLPHVM BATHVRST, Med. Doct. & Collegii S. Sanctæ Trinitatis Oxon. Socium.; **ff1r–ii3v**, pages 225–54, [text] DE URINIS.; **ii4r–v**, pages [1–2], blank.

[2]. **¶1r**, page [1], title; **¶1v**, page [2], blank; **¶2r–¶3v**, pages [3–6], AMICO LECTORI PRÆFATIO.; **¶4r–¶¶3r**, pages [7–13], ELENCHVS RERVM IN ANATOME CEREBRI.; **¶¶3r–¶¶4v**, pages [13–16], ELENCHVS RERVM IN NERVORVM DESCRIPTIONE ET VSV.

A1r–O2r, pages 1–107, [text] CEREBRI ANATOME.; **O2v–Y4v**, page 108–76, [text] NERVORVM DESCRIPTIO ET VSVS.; **Z1r**, page [1], [half title] DE RATIONE MOTVS MVSCVLORVM. *Ἐν πᾶσι τοῖς φυσικοῖς ἔνεστί τι θαυμαστόν.* Arift. de Part. Animal.; **Z1v**, page 2, BENEVOLIS LECTORIBVS TYPOGRAPHVS S. TRACTATVM De Ratione Motus Mufculorum (*etfi Authoris Anonymi*) Anatomiæ Cerebri, Nervorumque Defcriptioni *ab* Excellentifs. Viro D. THOMA WILLIS M.D. Celeberrimo *inftitutæ, fubnectere non incongruum duxi; vel eâ potiffimum ratione* (*ut alias, tum à Materiæ affinitate, tum ab Operis præfentiâ petitas, miffas faciam,*) *quòd in prioribus Editionibus magno cum Doctorum applaufu, & fine ullâ, quod fciam*, Clariffimi D. WILLIS *querelâ, appofitus reperiatur.* Valete.

Z2r–Bb4r, pages 3–21, [text] *DE* RATIONE MOTVS MVSCVLORVM.; **Bb4v**, page [22], blank.

[3]. ***1r**, page [1], title; ***2r–v**, pages [3–4], *Reverendiffimo in* CHRISTO PATRI, ET DOMINO, D. GILBERTO, PROVIDENTIA DIVINA, *Archiepifcopo Cantuarienfi, totius Angliæ Primati, & Metropolitano; & Auguftiffimo Principi* CAROLO II. M. *Britanniæ, Franciæ* & *Hiberniæ Regi, à Secretioribus Confiliis....* [signed] CLEMENTIÆ VESTRÆ, *Humillimus Cultor, Cliens addictiffimus* THOM. WILLIS.; ***3r–v**, pages [5–6], AMICO LECTORI PRÆFATIO.; ***4r–**2v**, pages [7–12], ELENCHVS RERVM IN TRACTATV *De* MORBIS CONVVLSIVIS.; ****3r–**4v**, pages [13–16], ELENCHVS RERVM IN TRACTATV *DE* SCORBVTO.

***A1r–*S3v**, pages 1–142, [text] TRACTATVS PRIMVS *DE* MORBIS CONVVLSIVIS.; ***S4r–*Dd3v**, pages 143–214, [text] TRACTATVS SECVNDUS *DE* SCORBUTO.; ***Dd4r–v**, pages [1–2], blank.

[4]. ***1r**, page [1], title; ***2r–v**, pages [3–4], AMICO LECTORI PRÆFATIO.

a1r–d2r, pages 1–27, [text] AFFECTIONVM *Quæ dicuntur* HYSTERICÆ ET HYPOCHONDRICÆ PATHOLOGIA SPASMODICA VINDICATA.; **d2v–f1r**, pages 28–41, [text] DE SANGVINIS INCALESCENTIA SIVE ACCENSIONE EXERCITATIO MEDICO-PHYSICA.; **f1v–h4r**, pages 42–[63], [text] DE MOTV MVSCVLARI EXERCITATIO MEDICO-PHYSICA.; **h4v–i1r**, pages [1–2], ELENCHVS MATERIÆ *DE* AFFECTIBVS HISTERICIS *ET* HYPOCHONDRIACIS.; **i1r–v**, pages [2–3], ELENCHVS MATERIÆ EXERCITATIONIS *De* ACCENSIONE SANGVINIS.; **i1v–i2r**, pages [3–4], ELENCHVS MATERIÆ EXERCITATIONIS *De* MOTV MVSCVLARI; **i2v**, page [5], blank.

[5]. **†1r**, page [1], title; **†1v**, page [2], blank; **†2r–v**, pages [3–4], *Reverendiffimo in* CHRISTO PATRI, ET DOMINO, D. GILBERTO, PROVIDENTIA DIVINA, *Archiepifcopo Cantuarienfi, totius Angliæ Primati & Metropolitano, & Auguftiffimo Principi* CAROLO II. *Magnæ Britanniæ, Franciæ* & *Hiberniæ Regi, à Secretioribus Confiliis.* ... [signed] CLEMENTIÆ VESTRÆ, *Cultorem humillimum, Servum devotiffimum* THOM. WILLIS.;

†3r–v, pages [5–6], *Eruditiſsimis, & Venerabilibus* VIRIS, *Mihique æternùm colendis,* D. VICECANCELLARIO, DOCTORIBVS, ET MAGISTRIS, *Qui in Celeberrima* VNIVERSITATE OXONIENSI *Bonas Literas Diligentiſsimè excolunt, Egregiè ornant, Feliciſsimè promovent,* SALVTEM. ... [signed] CLARISSIMI DOMINI *Veſtrum omnium Cultori additiſſimo,* THOM. WILLIS.; **†4r–††2v**, pages [7–12], PRÆFATIO *AD* LECTOREM.; **††3r–†††2v**, pages [13–20], ELENCHVS RERVM IN TRACTATV *DE* ANIMA BRVTORVM. Sive Parte Phyſiologica.; **†††3r–††††4r**, pages [21–31], ELENCHVS RERVM IN TRACTATV *DE* ANIMA BRVTORVM, Sive Parte Pathologica.; **††††4v**, page [32], blank.

***a*1r–*ſ*4r**, pages 1–143, [text] *DE* ANIMA BRVTORVM *Quæ* Hominis Vitalis ac Senſitiva eſt, PARS PRIMA PHYSIOLOGICA, *Ejuſdem* Naturam, Partes, Potentias & Affectiones *tradens.*; ***ſ*4v**, page [144], blank; ***t*1r–*tt*3r**, pages 145–333, [text] PARS SECVNDA PATHOLOGICA *SIVE* DE MORBIS Quæ Ad Animam Corpoream, eiuſq; ſubjecta, ſcilicet Cerebrum, & Genus nervoſum ſpectant.; ***tt*3v–*uu*4v**, pages [1–11], INDEX ALPHABETICVS Rerum & Verborum.

[6]. **(*)1r**, page [1], title; **(*)1v**, page [2], *CELEBERRIMO* MEDICORVM LONDINENSIVM COLLEGIO; *Et singulatim* VIRO INSIGNISSIMO DOCTISSIMOQVE DOMINO GEORGIO ENT EQVITI Aurato PRÆSIDI Illuſtriſſimo, *Nec non* CENSORIBVS DIGNISSIMIS, *Cæteriſq; omnibus,* Ampliſſimæ *hujus* Societatis *Membris.* DIATRIBAM HANC PHARMACEVTICAM *Obſervantiæ & Honoris ergo Dicat, Dedicatq;* THO. WILLIS.; **(*)2r–(*)3r**, pages [3–5], CANDIDO LECTORI PRÆFATIO.; **(*)3v–(**)4v**, pages [6–16], ELENCHVS RERVM IN PHARMACEVTICA RATIONALI.

***A*1r–*Cc*2v**, pages 1–204, [text] *DE* MEDICAMENTORVM OPERATIONIBVS *IN* CORPORE HVMANO SECTIO PRIMA.; ***Cc*2v–*Cc*4v**, pages 204–[4], INDEX ALPHABETICVS.

[7]. **¶1r**, page [1], title; **¶1v**, page [2], blank; **¶2r**, page [3], ATHENIS BRITANNICIS, *Literati Orbis Lumini Splendidiſſimo,* VNIVERSITATI OXONIENSI. *Et Ibidem* ILLVSTRISSIMO PRINCIPI IAC. ORMONDIÆ DVCI CANCELLARIO HONORATISSIMO, RAD. BATHVRST *DECANO WELLENSI* VICECANCELLARIO DIGNISSIMO, *Reverendis admodum, & perquam Eruditis* DOCTORIBVS, PROCVRATORIBVS, FACVLTATVM *omnium* PROFESSORIBVS, COLLEGIORVM & AVLARVM PRÆFECTIS. *NEC NON* VENERABILI MAGISTRORVM SENATVI, Diatribam hanc Pharmaceuticam Pietatis & gratitudinis ergo *Dicat Dedicatque* Alumnus & Beneficarius adſtrictiſſimus THO. WILLIS.; **¶2v**, page [4], *Imprimatur* AMiciſſimo Authori, poſt tam Immortale Opus, nihil mortale facturo, tanquam Lumina morienti claudens, extremum hoc officium præſtat. *Oxon. Novemb.* 12. 1675. *RAD. BATHVRST Vice-Cancel. Oxonienſis.*; **¶3r–4v**, pages [5–8], CANDIDO LECTORI PRÆFATIO.; **¶¶1r–¶¶2v**, pages [9–12], POST-SCRIPTVM.; **¶¶3r–¶¶4r**, pages [13–15], AVTORI CLARISSIMO *Nec non mihi* (*de quo jure glorior*) AMICISSIMO, *in illius* PHARMACEVTICES RATIONALIS PARTEM VTRAMQVE *Carmen Gratulatorium.* ...[signed] *Gul. Dauukins.*; **¶¶4r–v**, pages [15–16], QVERELA LIBRI POSTHVMI DE OBITV AVTORIS. ... [signed] *Gul. Dauukins. Med. B.*; **¶¶¶1r–¶¶¶¶4v**, pages [17–32], ELENCHVS RERVM SECVNDÆ PARTIS, PHARMACEVTICES RATIONALIS.

A1r–Ll1v, pages 1–266, [text] *DE* MEDICAMENTORVM OPERATIONIBVS *IN* CORPORE HVMANO, PARS SECVNDA.; **Ll2r–Ll4v**, pages [1–8], INDEX ALPHABETICVS SECVNDÆ PARTIS PHARMACEVTICES RATIONALIS.

Headlines and *Catchwords*: [1]. FFEBRIBVS. for FEBRIBVS. at **l3r**, page 85; **o2r**, page 107; **t1r**, page 145.

No catchword at **f3r / v**, page 45 / 46; **g3r / v**, page 53 / 54; buſdam for quſdam at **ii1v / ii2r**, page 250 / 251.

[2]. Headlines correct.

interea for tali at **A1r / v**, page 1 / 2; no catchword at **B2r / v**, page 11 / 12; APUT for CAPUT at **V1r / v**, page 153 / 154.

[3]. *Caput* VII. for *Caput* VIII. at [*]**I3r**, page 69; *Caput* XI. for *Caput* IX. at ***N3r**, page 101; SCOBVTO. for SCORBVTO. at ***X1v**, page 162; *Caput* III. for *Caput* IV. at ***X3r**–***X4v**, pages 165–168, reflecting CAPVT III. for CAPVT IV. in chapter heading at ***X3r**, page 165; *Caput* IX. for *Caput* X. at ***Cc3r**, page 205.

No catchword at ***2v / *3r**, page [4] / [5]; æquabile for ęquabile at ***E1v / *E2r**, page 36 / 37; affectum for affectũ at ***H1v / *H2r**, page 58 / 59; fęce for fæce at ***Q3r / v**, page 125 / 126.

[4]. Headlines correct.

No catchword at *2v / a1r, pages [4] / 1.

[5]. Cap. III. for Cap. VIII. at ***aa*1v**, page 218; *Phenetide.* for *& Phenetide.* at ***kk*4r**, page 263; Cap. XI. for Cap. XII. at ***nn*3r**, page 285; *De Stupidate.* for *De Stupidate sive Moroſi.* at ***pp*1r**, page 297.

No catchword at **†2v / †3r**, pages [4] / [5]; tum for cum at ***nn*2r / v**, page 283 / 284.

[6]. *explicationes.* for *Explicationes* at **C3r**, page 21; *De Vomitoriorum* for *Vomitoriorum* at ***E*2v**, page 36; *Vomitiorium.* for *Vomitoriorum.* at **F2r**, page 43; *Vomitorium.* for *Vomitoriorum.* at ***F*2v**, page 44; *Hyperchartharſeos* for *Hypercatharſeos* at ***I*4v**, page 72; *Hypercartharſeos* for *Hypercatharſeos* at ***K*1v**, page 74; *medicamentis* for *Medicamentis* at **P4r**, page 119; *de* for *De* at ***T*4r**, page 151; *Opiatis.* for *Medicamentis Opiatis.* at ***Z*3r**, page 181; *nocumentia.* for *Nocumentia.* at ***Aa*2v–Aa3r**, pages 188–9.

No catchword at (*) **1v** / (*) **2r**, pages [2] / [3]; Dragm for Drag. J at ***V*4r / v**, page 159 / 160; tum for Verum at **X1r / v**, page 161 / 162.

[7]. PRÆFATIO. for POST-SCRIPTVM at **¶¶1v–¶¶2v**, pages [10–12]; *De Reſpirationis organis & uſu.* for *Reſpirationis læsæ variæ species.* at **D1v**, page 26; CAP. I. for CAP. II. at **E1r**, page 33; SECTIO. I. for SECT I. at **F4v**, page 52; **K3v**, page 78; *ſputo.* for *Sputo.* at **K4r**, page 79; no SECT. I. at **P4v**, page 120; *De Ictero.* for *De Ictero eiuſque remediis.* at **T3v**, page 150; *remediis ad Aſciten.* for *Remediis ad Aſciten.* at **V4v**, page 160; *de* for *De* at **X1v**, page 162; CAPVT. V. for

CAP. V. at **Z4r**, page 183; **Aa2r**, page 187; **Cc4r**, page 207; **Dd3r**, page 213; De *Hæmorrhagia, eiuſque de Remedio.* for *Hæmorrhagia, eiuſque Remedio.* at **Dd4v**, page 216; CAP. III. for CAP. IV. at **Ff4r**, page 231; **Gg1r**, page 233; *Fonticulis ſive Pontanellis.* for *Fonticulis, ſive Fontanellis.* at **Gg3r**, page 237; *Pſora ſive* for *Pſora, ſive* at **Hh3v**, page 246; '*u*' of *siue* inverted at **Kk2v**, page 260.

No catchword at **¶2r / ¶2v**, pages [3] / [4]; **¶2v / ¶3r**, pages [4] / [5]; **T4r / T4v**, page 151 / 152; Medendi for 3^{tia} Medendi at **M4v / N1r**, page 96 / 97; *Radic* for Rx *Radic* at **N2r / v**, page 99 / 100; CAP. XII for SECTIO at **Q1v / Q2r**, page 122 / 123; Rx Urinæ for Rx Vrinæ at **X3r / v**, page 165 / 166.

Frontispiece: none.

Portrait: **Pt.1d1**: THOMAS WILLIS, M. D. *Naturalis Philosophiæ Professor Oxoniensis, necnon Inclyti Medicinæ Collegii Londinensis, & Societatis Regiæ Socius*, [signed] *Fr: Diodoti Pin. ſcu.* 208 × 163 millimetres (sheet); 205 × 153 millimetres (plate marks); 202 × 150 millimetres (image); see: Figure 148.

Printers' ornaments: [1]. Printers' device at title page **¶1r**, page [3]; **§1r**, page [9] {**Tournes 1**}; headpiece at **¶2r**, page [5]; **§1r**, page [11]; **a1r**, page 1, {**Tournes 2**}; headpiece at **¶3r**, page [7]; **§3r**, page [13]; **i1r**, page 65 {**Tournes 4**}; two rows each of 29 fleurons, the lower inverted {**Tournes 7**} with middle row of 16 fleurons {**Tournes 8**} at **§4r**, page [15]; two rows each of 29 fleurons, the lower inverted {**Tournes 7**} at **§§§1r**, page [25]; single row of 16 fleurons {**Tournes 8**} at **§§2r**, page [19]; tailpiece at **§§1v**, page [18] {**Tournes 10**}; row of 13 fleurons {**Tournes 11**} flanked at left end by two fleurons horizontally at **§§3r**, page [21]; **§§§3v**, page [30] {**Tournes 12**}; tailpiece at **ee3v**, page 222 {**Tournes 17**}; double row of 25 fleurons {**Tournes 18**} each flanked at both ends by one fleuron {**Tournes 19**} at **ee4r**, page 223; row of 27 fleurons {**Tournes 7**} over row of 25 fleurons {**Tournes 18**} each flanked at both ends by another fleuron {**Tournes 19**}, over row of 27 fleurons (inverted) {**Tournes 7**}, the upper and lower rows each flanked by (, or), at **ff1r**, page 225; tail piece at **ii3v**, page 254 {**Tournes 22**}.

Decorated E at **¶2r**, page [5] {**Tournes 3**}; S at **§2r**, page [11] {**Tournes 5**}; D at **§3r**, page [13] {**Tournes 6**}; D at **§4r**, page [15] {**Tournes 9**}; F at **§§3r**, page [21]; **§§§1r**, page [25] {**Tournes 13**}; V at **§§§3v**, page [30] {**Tournes 14**}; I at **a1r**, page 1. {**Tournes 15**}; E at **i1r**, page 65{**Tournes 16**}; V at **ee4r**, page 223 {**Tournes 20**}; C at **ff1r**, page 225 {**Tournes 21**}.

[2]. Printers' device at **¶1r**, page [1] {**Tournes 1**}; two rows each of 29 fleurons, lower inverted, at **¶2r**, page [3]; **¶4r**, page [7] {**Tournes 7**}; tailpiece at **¶3v**, page [6] {**Tournes 17**}; row of 16 fleurons at **¶¶3r**, page [13] {**Tournes 8**}; headpiece at **A1r**, page 1 {**Tournes 2**}; headpiece at **O2v**, page 108 {**Tournes 26**}; two rows each of 25 fleurons {**Tournes 18**} flanked at both ends by a fleuron {**Tournes 19**} at **Z1v**, page 2; headpiece at **Z2r**, page 3 {**Tournes 4**}.

Decorated A at **¶2r**, page [3] {**Tournes 23**}; C at **¶4r**, page [7] {**Tournes 24**}; V at **¶¶3r**, page [13] {**Tournes 14**}; I at **A1r**, page 1 {**Tournes 25**}; N at **O2v**, page 108 {**Tournes 27**}; T at **Z1v**, page 2 {**Tournes 28**}; D at **Z2r**, page 3 {**Tournes 29**}.

[3]. Printers' device at ***1r**, page [1] {**Tournes 1**}; headpiece at ***2r**, page [3] {**Tournes 2**}; single row of 5 fleurons, ##1, 2, 4, 34, 35 {**Tournes 12**} with 30, odd ##3–33 correctly

orientated and even ##6–32 reversed, fleurons {**Tournes 31**} interspersed at ***3r**, page [5]; row of 16 fleurons at ***4r**, page [7] {**Tournes 8**}; two rows each of 29 fleurons, lower inverted, at ****3r**, page [13] {**Tournes 7**}; headpiece at ***A1r**, page 1; ***S4r**, page 143 {**Tournes 35**}.

Decorated I at ***2r**, page [3] {**Tournes 30**}; Q at ***3r**, page [5] {**Tournes 32**}; Q at ***4r**, page [7] {**Tournes 33**}; I at ****3r**, page [13] {**Tournes 34**}; I at ***A1r**, page 1 {**Tournes 36**}; I at ***S4r**, page 143 {**Tournes 37**}.

[4]. Printers' device at ***1r**, page [1] {**Tournes 1**}; headpiece at ***2r**, page [3] {**Tournes 2**}; **a1r**, page 1 {**Tournes 39**}; two rows each of 27 fleurons at **d2v**, page 28 {**Tournes 18**}; two rows each of 27 fleurons {**Tournes 18**} with two central rows each of 42 fleurons, alternate numbers reversed {**Tournes 42**} at **f1v**, page 42; **h4v**, page [1].

Decorated Q at ***2r**, page [3] {**Tournes 38**}; R at **a1r**, page 1 {**Tournes 40**}; I at **d2v**, page 28 {**Tournes 41**}; C at **f1v**, page 42 {**Tournes 43**}.

[5]. Printers' device at **†1r**, page [1] {**Tournes 1**}; headpiece at **†2r**, page [3]; **†3r**, page [5] {**Tournes 2**}; **†4r**, page [7]; ***a*1r**, page 1 {**Tournes 4**}; row of 13 fleurons {**Tournes 11**} flanked at the left by 2 fleurons {**Tournes 12**} at **††3r**, page [13]; two rows each of 29 fleurons, lower inverted, at **†††3r**, page [21]; ***tt*3v**, page [1] {**Tournes 7**}; tailpiece at **††††4r**, page [31] {**Tournes 17**}; headpiece at ***t*1r**, page 145 {**Tournes 35**}.

Decorated A at **†2r**, page [3] {**Tournes 44**}; I at **†3r**, page [5] {**Tournes 30**}; E at **†4r**, page [7] {**Tournes 16**}; A at **††3r**, page [13]; ***tt*3v**, page [1] {**Tournes 45**}; C at **†††3r**, page [21] {**Tournes 24**}; Q at ***a*1r**, page 1 {**Tournes 38**}; I at ***t*1r**, page 145 {**Tournes 15**}.

[6]. Printers' device at **(*)1r**, page [1] {**Tournes 1**}; row of 16 fleurons at **(*)2r**, page [3] {**Tournes 8**}; two rows each of 29 fleurons, lower inverted, at **(*)3v**, page [6] {**Tournes 7**}; headpiece at ***A*1r**, page 1 {**Tournes 39**}; row of 27 fleurons {**Tournes 18**} separated by 2 fleurons {**Tournes 42**} placed at right angles between ##2 / 3, 15 / 16 at ***Cc*2v**, page 204.

Decorated Q at **(*)2r**, page [3] {**Tournes 32**}; M at **(*)3v**, page [6] {**Tournes 46**}; A at ***A*1r**, page 1 {**Tournes 47**}.

[7]. Printers' device at **¶1r**, page [1] {**Tournes 1**}; headpiece at **¶3r**, page [5] {**Tournes 2**}; tailpiece at **¶4v**, page [8] {**Tournes 10**}; headpiece at **¶¶1r**, page [9] {**Tournes 4**}; two rows each of 28 fleurons, lower inverted, flanked by: at each end at **¶¶3r**, page [13]; row of 28 with : between ##9 / 10, 14 / 15, 15 / 16 at **¶¶4r**, page [15] {**Tournes 7**}; two rows each of 29, lower inverted, {**Tournes 7**} with row between of 28 fleurons {**Tournes 18**} at **¶¶¶1r**, page [17]; similar arrangement but with : between ##9 / 10, 14 / 15, 15 / 16, lower row, at **Ll2r**, page [1]; headpiece at **A1r**, page 1 {**Tournes 39**}.

Decorated A at **¶3r**, page [5] {**Tournes 48**}; D at **¶¶1r**, page [9] {**Tournes 9**}; O at **¶¶¶1r**, page [17] {**Tournes 49**}; I at **A1r**, page 1 (inverted) {**Tournes 41**}; A at **Ll2r**, page [1] {**Tournes 50**}.

Illustrations: lettering and legends as **2A**, **2C**, **4A**, **5A**, **6A**, and **6E**.

[2]. **Pl.1f1**. Plate 1 (image 1): *Figura. 1ª·* (headline, centre), *pag 10* (headline, right), *de medio T. vid pag 162* (footer, right). Leaf size, 214 × 168 millimetres (sheet, cropped); printed from a larger plate (plate marks, upper and right borders); 187 × 165 millimetres (figure). Inserted between legends for Figuræ I–II at **B1v–B2r**, pages 10–11.

Pl.2f1. Plate 2 (image 2): *pag 11* (headline, left), *Fig II da·* (headline, centre), *de medio S: vid. pag. 162* (footer, right). Leaf size cropped, 183 × 147 millimetres (sheet); printed from a larger plate, lines 132 × 103 millimetres (plate marks, lower and right borders, lines at upper and left edges); 130 × 100 millimetres (figure). Pasted onto legend for Figura II at **B2r**, page 11.

Pl.3f1. Plate 3 (image 3): *pag 20.* (headline, left), *Fig III* (headline, centre). Folding, 222 × 190 (sheet); printed from a larger plate, lines 207 × >173 millimetres (plate marks, upper and left borders, line at lower edge); 192 × 170 millimetres (figure). Inserted within legends for Figuræ III–IV at **C2r–C3r**, pages 19–21.

Pl.4f1. Plate 4 (image 4): *Fig IIII.* (headline, centre), *pag 20* (headline, right). Cropped Leaf size, 208 × 163 millimetres (sheet); printed from a larger plate, lines 132 × 103 millimetres (plate marks, lower and right borders, lines at upper and left edges); 113 × 92 millimetres (figure). Inserted within legends for Figuræ III–IV at **C2r–C3r**, pages 19–21.

Pl.5f1. Plate 5 (image 5): *Fig V.* (headline, left), *pag 25* (headline, right). Leaf size, 208 × 163 millimetres (sheet); printed from a larger plate, lines 182 × 138 millimetres (plate marks, lower and left borders, lines at upper and right edges); 178 × 132 millimetres (figure). Inserted before legends for Figuræ V–VI at **D1r–v**, pages 25–6.

Pl.6f1. Plate 6 (image 6): *Fig VI.* (headline, left), *pag 26* (headline, right). Leaf size, 208 × 163 millimetres (sheet); printed from a larger plate, lines 178 × 133 millimetres (plate marks, lower and right borders, lines at upper and left edges); 171 × 126 millimetres (figure). Inserted before legends for Figuræ V–VI at **D1r–v**, pages 25–2.

Pl.7f1. Plate 7 (images 7–10): [Unnumbered 1] *pag 42* (headline, right), *Fig 1, Fig 11, Fig 111,* (centre above each image), *Fig 1111* (right of image). Cropped Leaf size, 165 × 130 millimetres (sheet); printed from a larger plate, lines 132 × 103 millimetres (plate marks, lower and left borders, lines at upper and right edges); 21 × 93 millimetres, 76 × 93 millimetres, 34 × 28 millimetres, 71 × 25 millimetres (figures). Inserted within legend at **F1v–F2r**, pages 42–3.

Pl.8f1. Plate 8 (image 11): *Fig VII.ª* (headline, centre), *pag 52* (headline, right). Leaf size, 203 × 163 millimetres (sheet); printed from a larger plate, lines 192 × 132 millimetres (plate marks, upper and right borders, lines at left and lower edges); 190 × 104 millimetres (figure). Inserted within legend at **G2v–G3r**, pages 52–3.

Pl.9f1. Plate 9 (image 12): *Fig VIII* (headline, centre), *pag 66* (headline, right). Cropped Leaf size, 185 × 148 millimetres (sheet); printed from a larger plate, lines 132 × 102 millimetres (plate marks, lower and left borders, lines at upper and right edges); 109 × 95 millimetres (figure). Inserted within legend at **I1v–I2r**, pages 66–7.

Pl.10f1. Plate 10 (images 13–14): [Unnumbered 2] *Fig I* (headline, centre), *pag 118* (headline, right), *Fig II* (header, centre above image). Cropped Leaf size, 196 × 153 millimetres (sheet); printed from a larger plate, lines 183 × 139 millimetres (plate marks, upper and left borders, lines at right and lower edges); 125 × 111 millimetres, 47 × 112 millimetres (figures). Inserted within legend at **P3r–P4r**, pages 117–19.

Pl.11f1. Plate 11 (image 15): *Tabula. IX. / p. 166.* (headline, right). Folding, 293 × 172 millimetres (sheet); printed from a larger plate, lines 273 × 155 millimetres (plate marks, upper, lower, and left borders, line at right edge); 272 × 148 millimetres (figure). Inserted within legends for Tabulæ IX–XIII at **X3v–Y4v**, pages 166–76.

Pl.12f1. Plate 12 (image 16): *Tabula. X* ^{ma} */ p. 170* (headline, right). Folding, 298 × 200 millimetres (sheet); printed from a larger plate, 277 × >185 millimetres (plate marks, upper, right, and lower borders, no line); 270 × 178 millimetres (figure). Inserted within legends for Tabulæ IX–XIII at **X3v–Y4v**, pages 166–76.

Pl.13f1. Plate 13 (image 17): *Tabula. X1.* ^{ma} */ pag 170.* (footer, right). Folding, 303 × 143 millimetres (sheet); printed from a larger plate, lines 284 × 132 millimetres (plate marks, upper, left, and lower borders, line at right edge); 275 × 123 millimetres (figure). Inserted within legends for Tabulæ IX–XIII at **X3v–Y4v**, pages 166–76.

Pl.14f1. Plate 14 (image 18): *Tabula XII / pag 174* (headline, right). Folding, 265 × 58 millimetres (sheet); printed from a larger sheet >240 × 49 millimetres (plate mark, right, line at left edge); 212 × 38 millimetres (figure). Pasted onto **Y4r**, page 175.

Pl.15f1. Plate 15 (images 19–23): bound as two sheets: [1] *Tabula XIII / pag 174* (headline, left), *Fig. I* ^{ma}, *Fig 5.* ^{ta} *pag 176.* (headline, centre), *pag 175 Fig 2* $^{da.}$ (headline, right). Folding, 175 × 293 millimetres (sheet); printed from a larger plate (plate mark, left border, lines at upper and lower edges and separating each figure); 163 × 78 millimetres, 73 × 28 millimetres, 165 × 68 millimetres (figures). Inserted within legends for Tabulæ IX–XIII at **X3v–Y4v**, pages 166–76. [2] *page 176.* (headline, centre), *Fig 3.* $^{tia..}$, *Fig 4.* $^{ta.}$ (header, above each figure). Folding, 295 × 80 millimetres (sheet); printed from a larger plate (plate marks, upper, right, and lower borders); 283 × 30 millimetres, 269 × 34 millimetres (figures). Pasted onto **Y4v**, page 176.

Pl.16c1. Plate 16 (images 24–25) *Fig 1.*, *Fig 2.* (header, above each image). Folding, 213 × 170 millimetres (sheet); 140 × 130 millimetres (plate marks); 122 × 54 millimetres, 113 × 66 millimetres (figures). Printed on **Bb4r**, page [1].

[4]. **Pl.17e1**. Plate 17 (images 26–27): *p. 62* (headline, left), *Fig I*, *Fig II* (header, above each image). Folding, 200 × 270 millimetres (sheet); 165 × 110 millimetres (plate marks); 26 × 143 millimetres, 50 × 158 millimetres (figures); with **Pl.18e1**. Plate 18 (images 28–29): *p. 62* (headline, left), *Fig III*, *Fig IV* (headline, centre); 117 × 163 millimetres (plate marks); 30 × 152 millimetres, 42 × 160 millimetres (figures, rotated). Inserted after legend at **h3v**, page 62.

[5]. **Pl.19e1**. Plate 19 (images 30–33): *page 27.* (headline, left), *Tab. I.* ^{a} (headline, right), *Fig. 1* ^{a}, *Fig. II.* ^{da}, *Fig IIII.* ^{ta}, *Fig III.* ^{tia} (headers, above each image). Cropped Leaf size, 195 × 132 millimetres (sheet); printed from a larger plate, >191 × 128 millimetres (plate marks,

upper, left, and right borders); 44 × 26 millimetres, 114 × 86 millimetres, 106 × 16 millimetres, 75 × 103 millimetres (figures). Inserted within legends for Tabulæ I–IV at ***d*2r–*d*4v**, pages 27–32.

Pl.20e1. Plate 20 (images 34–35): *Tab. II.^{da}* (headline, centre), *pag 28* (headline, right), *Fig I^{a}*, *Fig. II.^{da}* (header, above each image). Folding, 152 × 193 millimetres (sheet); printed from a larger plate (plate marks, lower and right borders); 104 × 80 millimetres, 129 × 82 millimetres (figures). Inserted within legends for Tabulæ I–IV at ***d*2r–*d*4v**, pages 27–32.

Pl.21e1. Plate 21 (images 36–38): *pag 30* (headline, right), *Figura. 1.ma* (header, left of image), *Fig II^{da}*, *Fig. III ^{tia}*. (headers, above images). Folding, 260 × 185 millimetres (sheet); printed from a larger plate, >247 × 148 millimetres (plate marks, upper and left borders, line at the right edge); 240 × 97 millimetres, 122 × 81 millimetres, 39 × 15 millimetres (figures). Inserted within legends for Tabulæ I–IV at ***d*2r–*d*4v**, pages 27–32.

Pl.22e1. Plate 22 (images 39–41): *Tab IIII* (headline, left), *pag 31* (headline, right), *Fig II^{da}*, *Fig I ^{ma}*, *Fig III^{tia}* (headers, above each image). Cropped Leaf size, 190 × 140 millimetres (sheet); printed from a larger plate (plate marks, lower and right); 154 × 38 millimetres, 153 × 20 millimetres, 43 × 17 millimetres (figures). Inserted within legends for Tabulæ I–IV at ***d*2r–*d*4v**, pages 27–32.

Pl.23e1. Plate 23 (image 42): *pag 40* (headline, left), *Tab.V* (headline right). Cropped Leaf size, 180 × 155 millimetres (sheet); printed from a larger plate (plate marks, lower and right); 153 × 96 millimetres (figure). Inserted within legends for Tabulæ V–VII at ***e*4v–*f*1v**, pages 40–2.

Pl.24e1. Plate 24 (image 43): *pag 41* (headline, left), *Tab. VI.* (headline, right). Cropped Leaf size, 145 × 120 millimetres (sheet); printed from a larger plate, lines 132 × 115 millimetres (plate marks, left and lower borders, lines at upper and right edges); 127 × 85 millimetres (figure). Inserted within legends for Tabulæ V–VII at ***e*4v–*f*1v**, pages 40–2.

Pl.25e1. Plate 25 (image 44): *pag 42* (headline, left), *Tab. VII.* (headline, right). Cropped Leaf size, 160 × 129 millimetres (sheet); printed from a larger plate, lines 134 × 128 millimetres (plate marks, lower and left borders, lines at upper and right edges); 118 × 100 millimetres (figure). Inserted within legends for Tabulæ V–VII at ***e*4v–*f*1v**, pages 40–2.

Pl.26e1. Plate 26 (image 45): *pag 65.* (headline, left), *Tab VIII.* (headline, right). Folding, 165 × 185 millimetres (sheet); printed from a larger plate (plate marks, upper and left); 145 × 166 millimetres (figure). Inserted before legend at ***i*1r–v**, page 65–6.

[6]. **Pl.27f1**. Plate 27 (image 46): *Tab. I.* (headline, centre), *pag 20* (headline, right). Folding, 175 × 215 millimetres (sheet); printed from a larger plate, lines 157 × >189 millimetres (plate marks, lower and right borders, line at upper edge); 145 × 170 millimetres (figure). Inserted between legends at **C2v–C3v**, pages 20–2.

Pl.28f1. Plate 28 (image 47): T*ab. II.* (headline, centre), *p. 21 (*headline, right). Folding, 162 × 190 millimetres (sheet); printed from a larger plate, >146 × 157 millimetres (plate marks, left, right, and lower borders), 128 × 147 millimetres (figure). Inserted between legends at **C2v–C3v**, pages 20–2.

Pl.29f1. Plate 29 (image 48): *Tab. III.* (headline, centre), *p. 21.* (headline, right). Folding, 160 × 188 millimetres (sheet); printed from a larger plate (plate marks, lower and right); 138 × 163 millimetres (figure). Inserted between legends at **C2v–C3v**, pages 20–2.

Pl.30f1. Plate 30 (image 49–51): *Tab IV* (headline, left), *pag 21* (headline, right), *Fig* 2, *Fig 3*, *Fig* I. (headers, above each image). Folding, 168 × 225 millimetres (sheet); printed from a larger plate, 144 × >205 millimetres (plate marks, upper, right, and lower borders); 47 × 53 millimetres, 60 × 52 millimetres, 137 × 153 millimetres (figures). Inserted between legends at **C2v–C3v**, pages 20–2.

Pl.31f1. Plate 31 (image 52): *Tab. V.* (headline, centre), *p. 22* (headline, right). Folding, 161 × 170 millimetres (sheet); printed from a larger plate, lines 140 × >153 millimetres (plate marks, lower and right, lines upper, incorrectly straddling the image, and left); 140 × 150 millimetres (figure). Inserted after legends at **C3v**, page 22.

Pl.32f1. Plate 32 (images 53–57): *Tab*: *VI.* (headline, centre), *p: 22* (headline, right). Folding, 153 × 190 millimetres (sheet); printed from a larger plate, lines 142 × >170 millimetres (plate marks, lower and left, line at upper edge); 112 × 21 millimetres, 112 × 21 millimetres, 112 × 21 millimetres, 114 × 21 millimetres, 112 × 21 millimetres (figures). Inserted after legends at **C3v**, page 22.

[7]. **Pl.33f1**. Plate 33 (image 58): *pag. 20. Sect. i: Cap: i.* (headline, left), *Tab: I.* (headline, right). Cropped Leaf size, 140 × 205 millimetres (sheet); printed from a larger plate, lines 107 × >193 millimetres (plate marks, lower and left borders, line at upper edge); 93 × 182 millimetres (figure), rotated. Inserted before legends at **C3r–D1r**, pages 21–5.

Pl.34f1. Plate 34 (image 59): *Tab: II. pag. 22:* (headline, left), *Sect. i: Cap. i.* (headline, right). Cropped Leaf size, 203 × 155 millimetres (sheet); 182 × >136 millimetres (plate marks, left, right and upper borders); 180 × 122 millimetres (figure). Inserted before legends for Tabulæ I–VIII at **C3r–D1r**, pages 21–5.

Pl.35f1. Plate 35 (images 60–61): *pag 22 Tab: III.* (headline, left), *Sect. i: Cap. i* (headline, right), *Fig: 1.*, *Fig: 2.* (headers, left of each image). 203 × 155 millimetres (sheet); printed from a larger plate, 186 × >153 millimetres (plate marks, upper, right, and lower, with corner detached); 179 × 136 millimetres, 43 × 25 millimetres (figures). Inserted within legends for Tabulæ I–VIII at **C3r–D1r**, pages 21–5.

Pl.36f1. Plate 36 (images 62–64): *pag 22* (headline, left), *Tab. IV.* (headline, centre), *Sect. i: Cap. i.* (headline, right), *Fig: 1.*, *Fig: 2.*, *Fig: 3.* (headers, left of each image). Cropped Leaf size, 203 × 146 millimetres (sheet); printed from a larger plate, lines 188 × 114 millimetres (plate marks, upper, left and lower borders, line at the right edge); 67 × 40 millimetres, 58 × 34 millimetres, 61 × 36 millimetres (figures). Inserted within legends for Tabulæ I–VIII at **C3r–D1r**, pages 21–5.

Pl.37f1. Plate 37 (images 65–67): *Sect. i: Cap. i.* (headline, left), *pag 24. Tab: V.* (headline, right), (centre, left), *Fig 1.*, *Fig: 2* (headers, left of each image), *Fig 3* (footer, below image). Folding, 233 × 181 millimetres (sheet); printed from a larger image, lines 213 × 175 millimetres (plate marks, upper, lower, and left borders, line at right edge); 74 × 86 millimetres,

75 × 67 millimetres, 138 × 155 millimetres (figures). Inserted within legends for Tabulæ I–VIII at **C3r–D1r**, pages 21–5.

Pl.38f1. Plate 38 (images 68–75): *pag 24. Tab VI* (headline, left), *Sect. i. Cap. i:* (headline, right), *Fig. 1:*, *Fig 2* (headers above each group of four images). Folding, 183 × 242 millimetres (sheet); printed from a larger plate, lines 175 × 213 millimetres (plate marks, left, right and lower borders, line at upper edge); 70 × 49 millimetres, 72 × 48 millimetres, 70 × 49 millimetres, 70 × 48 millimetres, 72 × 18 millimetres, 72 × 18 millimetres, 72 × 17 millimetres, 74 × 19 millimetres (figures). Inserted within legends for Tabulæ I–VIII at **C3r–D1r**, pages 21–5.

Pl.39f1. Plate 39 (images 76–79): *pag. 24.* (headline, left), *Tab. VII.* (headline, centre), *Sect. i. Cap. i.* (headline, right), *Fig. 1.*, *Fig* 3, *Fig.* 4., *Fig:* 2. (headers, above each image). Folding, 170 × 179 millimetres (sheet); printed from a larger plate, lines 155 × >140 millimetres (plate marks, upper, lower, and right, line at left edge); 56 × 56 millimetres, 58 × 56 millimetres, 56 × 59 millimetres, 57 × 49 millimetres (figures). Inserted within legends for Tabulæ I–VIII at **C3r–D1r**, pages 21–5.

Pl.40f1. Plate 40 (images 80–82): *pag 24. Sect i: Cap. i.* (headline, left), *Tab. VIII.* (headline, centre), *Fig: 1.*, *Fig. 2.*, *Fig: 3.* (headers, above each image. Cropped Leaf size, 170 × 162 millimetres (sheet); 140 × >147 millimetres (plate marks, upper, left, and lower borders); 50 × 52 millimetres, 25 × 26 millimetres, 52 × 51 millimetres (figures). Inserted within legends for Tabulæ I–VIII at **C3r–D1r**, pages 21–5.

Copy: DASC, section 4 misbound, lacking [2] Pl.5, Pl.6, Pl.7 and Pl.10. Original vellum with illegible faded script above, original endpapers. Leaves 215 × 172 millimetres, boards 224 × 170 × 115 millimetres. Inscribed: ex libris Fr. Angelici Breng[?]. Stamped: (1) CAPUCIN COLMAR; (2) Bibliotheca P. P. CAPUCHINUM??LSHEIM. Shelf marks: (1) Varia a6 (corrected in manuscript to a4) x2; (2) N.12.[15]

8B2. OPERA OMNIA, Coloniæ Allobrogum quarto 1676

The second issue of the second edition of the collected works of Thomas Willis in Latin, the eighth book, identical to 8B1 apart from title pages showing COLONIÆ ALLOBROGVM as the place of publication [HJR Wing 47, Denham 12, Oldfield B3a].

Title page: [1a]. THOMÆ | WILLIS | MEDICINÆ DOCTORIS, | NATVRALIS PHILOSOPHIÆ | PROFESSORIS OXONIENSIS, | *Nec non* | INCLYTI MEDICORVM COLLEGII | Londinenſis, & SOCIETATIS REGIÆ Socii, | OPERA OMNIA, | *Quorum poſthac exſtat Catalogus.* | Cum ELENCHIS RERVM & INDICIBVS neceſſariis, ut & multis FIGVRIS æneis. | [printers' device: lettered, QVOD TIBI | FIERI NON | VIS, ALTERI |

[15] The Convent of Colmar in the French department of Haut-Rhin was built in 1700 by the Capuchins. They were previously installed in Vieux-Brisach but left in 1697 following attachment of this region to the Holy Empire. The community of *c.*30 members was dissolved during the revolution of 1789, and the property sold in 1796 with the church transformed into a shed which contained a press in the choir. It became the property of the bishop of Strasbourg in 1857 who installed an episcopal institute which lapsed in 1871. The building now accommodates the College and Lycée Épiscopal Saint-André.

NEFECERIS] | *COLONIÆ ALLOBROGVM*, | Apud SAMVELEM DE TOVRNES. | [short rule] | *M. DC. LXXVI.* | Cum SVPERIORVM Permiſſu.*

[1b] [2] [3] [4] [5] [6]. As in **8B1** apart from:

... | *COLONIÆ ALLOBROGVM,* | Apud SAMVELEM DE TOVRNES. | [short rule] | *M. DC. LXXVI.*

[7]. As in **8B1**.

Then as in **8B1** apart from:

Headlines: [7]. *Aſcen.* for *Aſciten.* at **X4r**, page 167.

Illustrations: variation in sheet sizes and occasional binding positions.

Copy: DASC. Original vellum, spine lettered (on red background) Tho Willis | Opera Medici, and E 37, original endpapers. Leaves 208 × 163 millimetres, boards 218 × 164 × 98 millimetres. Inserted: bookplate of Ignatius Dominicias SR (unidentified). Shelf mark: *y y y 1*.

8B3. OPERA OMNIA, Coloniæ Allobrogum quarto 1676

The third issue of the second edition of the collected works of Thomas Willis in Latin, the eighth book, identical to 8B2 apart from resetting of the collective title page [Oldfield B3b, not distingushed from HJR Wing 47, Denham 12].

Title page: [1a]. THOMÆ | WILLIS | MEDICINÆ DOCTORIS, | Natvralis philoſophiæ Profeſſoris Oxonienſis | *Nec non* | INCLYTI MEDICORVM COLLEGII | Londinenſis, & SOCIETATIS REGIÆ Socii, | OPERA OMNIA, | *Quorum poſthac exſtat Catalogus.* | Cum ELENCHIS RERVM & INDICIBVS neceſſariis, ut & multis FIGVRIS æneis. | [ornament: lettered, QVOD TIBI | FIERI NON | VIS, ALTERI | NEFECERIS] | *COLONIÆ ALLOBROGVM,* | Apud SAMVELEM DE TOVRNES. | [short rule] | *M. DC. LXXVI.* | Cum SVPERIORVM Permiſſu.

Then as in **8B2** apart from:

Illustrations: variation in sheet sizes and occasional binding positions.

Copy: Wellcome (27687775). Later sprinkled calf and new endpapers. Leaves 208 × 165 millimetres (volume 1) and 212 × 155 millimetres (volume 2), boards 223 × 162 × 70 millimetres and 222 × 159 × 75 millimetres. Inserted bookplate: The library of the Wellcome Institute for the History of Medicine MEDICAL SOCIETY OF LONDON DEPOSIT. Stamped: Medical

* Underlined text originally printed in red.

Society Of London. Accession number 63467/B Vol 1 and Vol 2. Inscribed: David Clipham (unidentified) with seven lines of Latin script.

8C1. OPERA OMNIA, Geneva quarto 1680

First issue of the third edition of the collected works of Thomas Willis in Latin, the eighth book, with William Croone's treatise and all the illustrations, planned as two volumes with an extra bifolium, the type reset but retaining the same format as the second edition and with the use of some different ornaments and decorated initials [HJR Wing 48, Denham 13, Oldfield B4].

Title page: [1a]. THOMÆ | WILLIS | MEDICINÆ DOCTORIS, | NATVRALIS PHILOSOPHIÆ | PROFESSORIS OXONIENSIS, | *Nec non* | INCLYTI MEDICORVM COLLEGII | Londinenſis, & SOCIETATIS REGIÆ Socii, | OPERA OMNIA. | TOMVS PRIOR. | Cum ELENCHIS RERVM & INDICIBVS Neceſſariis, ut & multis FIGVRIS Æneis. | [printers' device: lettered, QVOD TIBI | FIERI NON | VIS, ALTERI | NEFECERIS] | *GENEVÆ,* | Apud SAMVELEM DE TOVRNES. | [short rule] | *M. DC. LXXX.* | Cum Privilegio S. CÆSAREÆ MAIESTATIS.[*]

[1b]. DIATRIBÆ DVÆ | MEDICO-PHILOSOPHICÆ | *Quarum* PRIOR *agit* | DE FERMENTATIONE, | *Sive de* MOTV *Inteſtino Particularum in quovis Corpore*; | ALTERA | DE FEBRIBVS, | *Sive* de MOTV earundem in ſanguine Animalium: | *His acceſſit* | DISSERTATIO Epiſtolica de VRINIS. | *Studio* | THOMÆ WILLIS, M.D. | Natural. Philoſoph. *Profeſſ.* Oxon. nec non Inclyti Medic. | Colleg. Londin. & Societatis Regiæ *Socii.* | [printers' device: lettered, QUOD TIBI | FIERI NON | VIS, ALTERI | NEFECERIS] | *GENEVÆ,* | Apud SAMVELEM DE TOVRNES. | [short rule] | *M. DC. LXXX.*

[2]. CEREBRI | ANATOME | NERVORVMQVE | DESCRIPTIO ET VSVS. | *Studio* | THOMÆ WILLIS, M. D. | Natural. Philoſoph. *Profeſſ.* Oxon. nec non Inclyti Medic. | Colleg. Londin. & Societ. Reg. *Socii.* | *Acceſsit* VIRI *cujuſdam Clariſsimi* | *De* | RATIONE MOTVS MVSCVLORVM | *Tractatus Singularis.* | [printers' device: lettered, QUOD TIBI | FIERI NON | VIS, ALTERI | NEFECERIS] | *GENEVÆ,* | Apud SAMVELEM DE TOVRNES. | [short rule] | *M. DC. LXXX.*

[3]. PATHOLOGIÆ | CEREBRI | *ET* | NERVOSI GENERIS | SPECIMEN. | *In quo agitur* | De Morbis Convulſivis & de Scorbuto. | *Studio* | THOMÆ WILLIS, M.D. | Natural. Philoſoph. *Profeſſ.* Oxon. nec non Inclyti Medic. | Colleg. Londin. & Societatis Regiæ *Socii.* | [printers' device: lettered, QUOD TIBI | FIERI NON | VIS, ALTERI | NEFECERIS] | *GENEVÆ,* | Apud SAMVELEM DE TOVRNES. | [short rule] | *M. DC. LXXX.*

[4]. AFFECTIONVM | *Quæ dicuntur* | HYSTERICÆ | ET HYPOCHONDRIACÆ | PATHOLOGIA SPASMOCIA VINDICATA, | *Contra Reſponſionem Epiſtolarem* NATH. HIGHMRORI *M. D.* | Cui acceſſerunt Exercitationes Medico-Phyſicæ Duæ. | I. *De* SANGVINIS ACCENSIONE. | II *De* MOTV MVSCVLARI. | *Studio* | THOMÆ WILLIS,

[*] Underlined text originally printed in red.

M. D. | Natural. Philoſoph. *Profeſſ.* Oxon. nec non Inclyti Medic. | Colleg. Londin. & Societatis Regiæ *Socii.* | [printers' device: lettered, QUOD TIBI | FIERI NON | VIS, ALTERI | NEFECERIS] | *GENEVÆ,* | Apud SAMVELEM DE TOVRNES. | [short rule] | *M. DC. LXXX.*

[5a]. THOMÆ | WILLIS | MEDICINÆ DOCTORIS, | NATVRALIS PHILOSOPHIÆ | PROFESSORIS OXONIENSIS, | *Nec non* | INCLYTI MEDICORVM COLLEGII | Londinenſis, & SOCIETATIS REGIÆ Socii, | OPERA OMNIA. | TOMVS POSTERIOR. | Cum ELENCHIS RERVM & INDICIBVS Neceſſariis, ut & multis FIGVRIS Æneis. | [printers' device: lettered, QUOD TIBI | FIERI NON | VIS, ALTERI | NEFECERIS] | *GENEVÆ,* | Apud SAMVELEM DE TOVRNES, | [short rule] | *M. DC. LXXX.* | Cum Privilegio S. CÆSAREÆ MAIESTATIS.

[5b]. DE ANIMA | BRVTORVM | *Quæ* HOMINIS *Vitalis ac Senſitava eſt,* | EXERCITATIONES DVÆ. | PRIOR PHYSIOLOGICA | *Ejuſdem* Naturam, Partes, Potentias & Affectiones *tradit;* | ALTERA PATHOLOGICA | Morbos qui ipſam & Sedem ejus Primariam, | *Nempe* CEREBRVM *&* NERVOSVM GENVS *afficiunt, explicitat; eorúmque* | *Therapeias inſtituit, cum Figuris æneis.* | STVDIO | THOMÆ WILLIS, M. D. | Natural. Philoſoph. *Profeſſ.* Oxon. nec non Inclyti Medic. | Colleg. Londin. & Societatis Regiæ *Socii.* | [printers' device: lettered, QUOD TIBI | FIERI NON | VIS, ALTERI | NEFECERIS | *GENEVÆ,* | Apud SAMVELEM DE TOVRNES. | [short rule] | *M. DC. LXXX.*

[6]. PHARMACEVTICE | RATIONALIS | *Sive* | DIATRIBA | *De* | MEDICAMENTORVM | OPERATIONIBVS | In Humano CORPORE, | *Studio* | THOMÆ WILLIS, M. D. | Natural. Philoſoph. *Profeſſ.* Oxon. nec non Inclyti Medic. | Colleg. Londin. & Societatis Regiæ *Socii.* | [printers' device: lettered, QUOD TIBI | FIERI NON | VIS, ALTERI | NEFECERIS] | *GENEVÆ,* | Apud SAMVELEM DE TOVRNES. | [short rule] | *M. DC. LXXX.*

[7]. PHARMACEVTICES | RATIONALIS | *Sive* | DIATRIBÆ, | *De* | MEDICAMENTORVM | OPERATIONIBVS | In Humano CORPORE, | PARS SECVNDA. | *Opus Poſthumum* | THOMÆ WILLIS, M. D. | Natural. Philoſoph. *Profeſſ.* Oxon. nec non Inclyti Medic. | Colleg. Londin. & Societatis Regiæ *Socii.* | [printers' device: lettered, QUOD TIBI | FIERI NON | VIS, ALTERI | NEFECERIS] | *GENEVÆ,* | Apud SAMVELEM DE TOVRNES. | [short rule] | *M. DC. LXXX.*

Collation: quarto, 23 letter alphabet using i and u, and *v* and V. [1]. ¶^{4}, §–§§§^{4}, a–z^4, aa–ii^4; $1–3 signed.
144 leaves, paginated as [32], 1–254, [2].

[2]. ¶^{4}, ¶¶^{4}, A–Z^4, Aa–Bb^4; $1–3 signed.
108 leaves, paginated as [16], 1–176, [2] 3–21 [22], [2].

[3]. *–**^{4}; *A–*Z^4, *Aa–*Dd^4; $1–3 signed apart from: *I3 signed I3.
116 leaves, paginated as [16], 1–214, [2]. Mispaginated: 186 for 168.

[4]. *^{2}, a–h^4, i^2; $1–3 signed.
36 leaves, paginated as [4], 1–63, [5].

[5]. †^{2}, ^{2}†^{4}, †††–††††^{4}, *a*–*z*^{4}, *aa*–*uu*^{4}; $1–3 signed.

190 leaves, paginated as [36], 1–333, [11].

[6]. (*)–(**)^4, *A–Z*^{4}, *Aa–Cc*^{4}; $1–3 signed.
112 leaves, paginated as [16], 1–204, [4].

[7]. ¶–¶¶¶¶^{4}, A–Z^4, Aa–Ll^4; $1–3 signed apart from: -¶2.
152 leaves, paginated as [32], 1–266, [6].

Type: 43 lines; height (20 lines) 82 millimetres, width 117 millimetres (128 with marginal notes).

Contents: [1]. **¶4r**, page [1], blank; **¶4v**, page [2], [portrait]; **¶1r**, page [3], title; **¶1v**, page [4], blank; **¶2r**, page [5], TYPOGRAPHVS LECTORI *SALVTEM.*; **¶2v**, page [6], CONTENTA *IN* PRIORI TOMO. I. Diatribæ duæ Medico-Philoſophicæ, *quarum* Prior *agit de* FERMENTATIONE, Altera de FEBRIBVS; *quibus acceſſit* Diſſertatio *de* VRINIS. II. CEREBRI ANATOME, NERVORVMQUE DESCRIPTIO & VSVS; *quibus acceſſit VIRI cujuſdam Clariſſimi* De RATIONE MOTVS MVSCVLORVM *Tractatus Singularis.* III. PATHOLOGIÆ CEREBRI & NERVOSI GENERIS SPECIMEN, *in quo agitur de* MORBIS CONVULSIVIS *& de* SCORBUTO. IV. AFFECTIONUM *quæ dicuntur* HYSTERICÆ *&* HYPOCHONDRIACÆ PATHOLOGIA SPASMODICA VINDICATA, *contra* Reſponſionem Epiſtolarem NATHAN. HIGHMORI M.D. *cui acceſſerunt* Exercitationes Medico-Phyſicæ Duæ. I. *De* SANGUINIS ACCENSIONE. II. *De* MOTU MUSCULARI.; **¶3r–v**, pages [7–8], PRIVILEGIVM SACRÆ CÆSAREÆ MAIESTATIS. … [signed] LEOPOLDUS, M. D. (L.S.) Vidit LEOPOLDVS GVILIELMVS Comes in Kinigſeggs, m.p. *Ad Mandatum Sac. Cæſ. Maieſtatis proprium.* Chriſtoph. Beüer. m. p.; **§1r**, page [9], title; **§1v**, page [10], blank; **§2r–v**, pages [11–12], *Reverendiſſimo in* CHRISTO PATRI, ET DOMINO, D. GILBERTO, *Epiſcopo* Londinensi, & *Sacelli Regii Decano* … [signed] *Humillimus & æternum addictiſsimus,* THOM. WILLIS.; **§3r–§3v**, pages [13–14], AMICO LECTORI PRÆFATIO. [De Fermentatione]; **§4r–§§1v**, pages [15–18], AMICO LECTORI PRÆFATIO. [De Febribus]; **§§2r–v**, pages [19–20], AVTHORI *In illius Diatribas Medico-Philoſophicas,* Carmen Gratulatorium... [signed] PHILIPPVS FELL, Med. Stud. Oxon.; **§§3r–§§4v**, pages [21–4], ELENCHVS RERVM IN TRACTATV *DE* FERMENTATIONE.; **§§§1r–§§§3r**, pages [25–9], ELENCHVS RERVM IN TRACTATV *DE* FEBRIBVS.; **§§§3v–§§§4r**, pages [30–1], ELENCHVS RERVM IN DISSERTATIONE *DE* VRINIS.; **§§§4v**, pages [32], blank.

a1r–h4v, pages 1–64, [text] *DE* FERMENTATIONE, *Sive* DE MOTV CORPORVM NATVRALIVM INORGANICO.; **i1r–ee3v**, pages 65–222, [text] DE FEBRIBVS.; **ee4r–v**, pages 223–4, DE VRINIS DISSERTATIO EPISTOLICA, *Ad Virum Doctiſsimum, mihiq́ Amiciſsimum* D. RVDOLPHVM BATHVRST, Med. Doct. & Collegii S. Sanctæ Trinitatis Oxon. Socium.; **ff1r–ii3v**, pages 225–54, [text] DE URINIS.; **ii4r–v**, pages [1–2], blank.

[2]. **¶1r**, page [1], title; **¶1v**, page [2], blank; **¶2r–¶3v**, pages [3–6], AMICO LECTORI PRÆFATIO.; **¶4r–¶¶3r**, pages [7–13], ELENCHVS RERVM IN ANATOME CEREBRI.; **¶¶3r–¶¶4v**, pages [13–16], ELENCHVS RERVM IN NERVORUM DESCRIPTIONE ET VSV.

A1r–O2r, pages 1–107, [text] CEREBRI ANATOME.; **O2v–Y4v**, page 108–76, [text] NERVORVM DESCRIPTIO ET VSVS.; **Z1r**, page [1], [half title] DE RATIONE MOTUS

MUSCULORUM. *Ἐν πᾶσι τοῖς φυσικοῖς ἔνεστί τι θαυμαστόν.* Arift. de Part. Animal.; **Z1v**, page 2, BENEVOLIS LECTORIBUS TYPOGRAPHVS, S. TRACTATVM De Ratione Motus Mufculorum (*etfi Authoris Anonymi*) Anatomiæ Cerebri, Nervorumque Defcriptioni *ab* Excellentifs. Viro D. THOMA WILLIS M.D. Celeberrimo *inftitutæ, fubnectere non incongruum duxi; vel eâ potiffimum ratione (ut alias, tum à Materiæ affinitate, tum ab Operis præfentiâ petitas, miffas faciam,) quòd in prioribus Editionibus magno cum Doctorum applaufu, & fine ullâ, quod fciam*, Clariffimi D. WILLIS *querelâ, appofitus reperiatur.* Valete.

Z2r–Bb4r, pages 3–21, [text] *DE* RATIONE MOTUS MUSCULORUM.; **Bb4v**, page [22], blank.

[3]. ***1r**, page [1], title; ***2r–v**, pages [3–4], *Reverendiffimo in* CHRISTO PATRI, ET DOMINO, D. GILBERTO, PROVIDENTIA DIVINA, *Archiepifcopo Cantuarienfi, totius Angliæ Primati, & Metropolitano; & Auguftiffimo Principi* CAROLO II. M. *Britanniæ, Franciæ & Hiberniæ Regi, à Secretioribus Confiliis....* [signed] CLEMENTIÆ VESTRÆ, *Humillimus Cultor, Cliens addictiffimus* THOM. WILLIS.; ***3r–v**, pages [5–6], AMICO LECTORI PRÆFATIO.; ***4r–**2v**, pages [7–12], ELENCHVS RERVM IN TRACTATV *De* MORBIS CONVVLSIVIS.; ****3r–**4v**, pages [13–16], ELENCHVS RERVM IN TRACTATV *DE* SCORBVTO.

***A1r–*S3v**, pages 1–142, [text] TRACTATVS PRIMVS *DE* MORBIS CONVVLSIVIS.; ***S4r–*Dd3v**, pages 143–214, [text] TRACTATVS SECVNDUS *DE* SCORBUTO.; ***Dd4r–v**, pages [1–2], blank.

[4]. ***1r**, page [1], title; ***2r–v**, pages [3–4], AMICO LECTORI PRÆFATIO.

a1r–d2r, pages 1–27, [text] AFFECTIONVM *Quæ dicuntur* HYSTERICÆ ET HYPOCHONDRICÆ PATHOLOGIA SPASMODICA VINDICATA.; **d2v–f1r**, pages 28–41, [text] DE SANGVINIS INCALESCENTIA SIVE ACCENSIONE EXERCITATIO MEDICO-PHYSICA.; **f1v–h4r**, pages 42–63, [text] DE MOTV MVSCVLARI EXERCITATIO MEDICO-PHYSICA.; **h4v–i1r**, pages [1–2], ELENCHVS MATERIÆ *DE* AFFECTIBVS HYSTERICIS *ET* HYPOCHONDRIACIS.; **i1r–v**, pages [2–3], ELENCHVS MATERIÆ EXERCITATIONIS *De* ACCENSIONE SANGVINIS.; **i1v–i2r**, pages [3–4], ELENCHVS MATERIÆ EXERCITATIONIS *De* MOTV MVSCVLARI; **i2v**, page [5], blank.

[5]. **†1r**, page [1], title; **†1v**, page [2], blank; **†2r**, page [3], CONTENTA *IN* POSTERIORI TOMO. I. *De* ANIMA BRVTORUM; *quæ* HOMINIS *Vitalis ac Senfitiva est*, Exercitationes Duæ, *quarum* Prior PHYSIOLOGICA *eft*, Altera PATHOLOGICA *Morbos qui Ipfam*, Cerebrum, & Nervofum Genus *afficiunt, explicans.* II. PHARMACEVTICE RATIONALIS, *five* Diatriba *de* MEDICAMENTORVM OPERATIONIBVS *in* Humano Corpore. III. PHARMACEVTICES RATIONALIS, *five* Diatribæ *de* MEDICAMENTORVM OPERATIONIBVS *in* Humano Corpore, *Pars Secunda.*; **†2v**, page [4], blank; **2†1r**, page [5], title; **2†1v**, page [6], blank; **2†2r–v**, pages [7–8], *Reverendiffimo in* CHRISTO PATRI, ET DOMINO, D. GILBERTO, PROVIDENTIA DIVINA, *Archiepifcopo Cantuarienfi, totius Angliæ Primati & Metropolitano, & Auguftifsimo Principi* CAROLO II. *Magnæ Britanniæ, Franciæ & Hiberniæ Regi, à Secretioribus Confiliis. ...* [signed] CLEMENTIÆ VESTRÆ, *Cultorem humillimum, Servum devotiffimum* THOM. WILLIS.; **2†3r–v**, pages [9–10], *Eruditifsimis*, & *Venerabilibus* VIRIS, *Mihíque æternùm colendis*, D. VICECANCELLARIO, DOCTORIBVS, ET MAGISTRIS, *Qui in Celeberrima* VNIVERSITATE OXONIENSI *Bonas*

Literas Diligentiſsimè excolunt, Egregiè ornant, Feliciſsimè promovent, SALVTEM.... [signed] CLARISSIMI DOMINI *Veſtrûm omnium Cultori addictiſſimo,* THOM. WILLIS.; **2†4r–v–††2v**, pages [11–16], PRÆFATIO *AD* LECTOREM.; **††3r–†††2v**, pages [17–24], ELENCHVS RERVM IN TRACTATV *DE* ANIMA BRVTORVM. Sive Parte Phyſiologica.; **†††3r–††††4r**, pages [25–35], ELENCHVS RERVM IN TRACTATV *DE* ANIMA BRVTORVM, Sive Parte Pathologica.; **††††4v**, page [36], blank

***a*1r–*ſ*4r**, pages 1–143, [text] *DE* ANIMA BRVTORVM *Quæ* Hominis Vitalis ac Senſitiva eſt, PARS PRIMA PHYSIOLOGICA, *Ejuſdem* Naturam, Partes, Potentias & Affectiones *tradens.*; ***ſ*4v**, page [144], blank; ***t*1r–*tt*3r**, pages 145–333, [text] PARS SECVNDA PATHOLOGICA *SIVE* DE MORBIS Quæ Ad Animam Corpoream, eiuſq; ſubjecta, ſcilicet Cerebrum, & Genus nervoſum ſpectant.; ***tt*3v–*uu*4v**, pages [1–11], INDEX ALPHABETICVS Rerum & Verborum.

[6]. **(*)1r**, page [1], title; **(*)1v**, page [2], *CELEBERRIMO* MEDICORVM LONDINENSIVM COLLEGIO; *Et singulatim* VIRO INSIGNISSIMO DOCTISSIMOQVE DOMINO GEORGIO ENT EQVITI Aurato PRÆSIDI Illuſtriſſimo, *Nec non* CENSORIBVS DIGNISSIMIS, *Cæteriſq; omnibus*, Ampliſſimæ *hujus* Societatis *Membris*. DIATRIBAM HANC PHARMACEVTICAM *Obſervantiæ & Honoris ergo Dicat, Dedicatq;* THO. WILLIS.; **(*)2r–(*)3r**, pages [3–5], CANDIDO LECTORI PRÆFATIO.; **(*)3v–(**)4v**, pages [6–16], ELENCHVS RERVM IN PHARMACEVTICA RATIONALI.

***A*1r–*Cc*2v**, pages 1–204, [text] *DE* MEDICAMENTORVM OPERATIONIBVS *IN* CORPORE HVMANO SECTIO PRIMA.; ***Cc*2v–*Cc*4v**, pages 204–[4], INDEX ALPHABETICVS.

[7]. **¶1r**, page [1], title; **¶1v**, page [2], blank; **¶2r**, page [3], ATHENIS BRITANNICIS, *Literati Orbis Lumini Splendidiſſimo*, VNIVERSITATI OXONIENSI. *Et Ibidem* ILLVSTRISSIMO PRINCIPI IAC. ORMONDIÆ DVCI CANCELLARIO HONORATISSIMO, RAD. BATHVRST *DECANO WELLENSI* VICECANCELLARIO DIGNISSIMO, *Reverendis admodum, & perquam Eruditis* DOCTORIBVS, PROCVRATORIBVS, FACVLTATVM *omnium* PROFESSORIBVS, COLLEGIORVM & AVLARVM PRÆFECTIS. *NEC NON* VENERABILI MAGISTRORVM SENATVI, Diatribam hanc Pharmaceuticam Pietatis & Gratitudinis ergo *Dicat Dedicatque* Alumnus & Beneficarius adſtrictiſſimus THO. WILLIS.; **¶2v**, page [4], *Imprimatur* AMiciſſimo Authori, poſt tam Immortale Opus, nihil mortale facturo, tanquam Lumina morienti claudens, extremum hoc officium præſtat. *Oxon. Novemb.* 12. 1675. *RAD. BATHVRST Vice-Cancel. Oxonienſis.*; **¶3r–4v**, pages [5–8], CANDIDO LECTORI PRÆFATIO.; **¶¶1r–¶¶2v**, pages [9–12], POST-SCRIPTVM.; **¶¶3r–¶¶4r**, pages [13–15], AVTORI CLARISSIMO *Nec non mihi* (*de quo jure glorior*) AMICISSIMO, *in illius* PHARMACEVTICES RATIONALIS PARTEM VTRAMQVE *Carmen Gratulatorium*.... [signed] *Gul. Davvkins.*; **¶¶4r–v**, pages [15–16], QVERELA LIBRI POSTHVMI DE OBITV AVTORIS.... [signed] *Gul. Davvkins. Med. B.*; **¶¶¶1r–¶¶¶¶4v**, pages [17–32], ELENCHVS RERVM SECVNDÆ PARTIS, PHARMACEVTICES RATIONALIS.

A1r–Ll1v, pages 1–266, [text] *DE* MEDICAMENTORVM OPERATIONIBVS *IN* CORPORE HVMANO, PARS SECVNDA.; **Ll2r–Ll4v**, pages [1–8], INDEX ALPHABETICVS SECVNDÆ PARTIS PHARMACEVTICES RATIONALIS.

Headlines and *Catchwords*: [1]. Headlines correct.

cipiunt for excipiunt at **e4v** / **f1r**, pages 40 / 41; CAPUT for CAPVT at **m4v** / **n1r**, pages 96 / 97; no catchword at **x4v** / **y1r**, pages 168 / 169; bus for ribus at **y4r** / **v**, pages 175 / 176; Variolarum for Uariolarum at **bb1v** / **bb2r**, pages 194 / 195; busdam for quibusdam at **ii1v** / **ii2r**, pages 250 / 251.

[2]. *Cap.* for *Caput.* at **A3r**, page 5; **E3r**, page 37; **K1r**, page 73.

CAP. for CAPVT at **E3v** / **Er4r**, pages 38 / 39; Itaque for Jtaque at **M4v** / **N1r**, pages 96 / 97; ragitur for agitur at **O3v** / **O4r**, pages 110 / 111.

[3]. *Caput* VII. for *Caput* VIII. at [*]**I3r**, page 69; *Caput* XI. for *Caput* IX. at ***N3r**, page 101; *Caput II.* for *Caput III.* at ***X1r**–***X2v**, pages 161–4; *Caput* III. for *Caput* IV. at ***X3r**–***X4v**, pages 165–'186' [168], reflecting CAPVT III. for CAPVT IV. in chapter heading at ***X3r**, page 165.

No catchword at ***2v** / ***3r**, page [4] / [5]; velut for velnt at ***D1r** / **v**, page 25 / 26; CAP. for CAPVT at ***Y3r** / **v**, pages 173 / 174.

[4]. Headlines correct.

No catchword at ***2v** / **a1r**, pages [4] / 1; fæpius for Sæpius at **c1v** / **c2r**, pages 18 / 19.

[5]. Cap. II. for Cap. XII. at ***m*4r**, page 95; Cap. III. for Cap. VIII. at ***aa*1v**, page 218; *De Stupidate.* for *De Stupidate sive Morofi.* at ***pp*1r**, page 297.

No catchword at **†2v** / **†3r**, pages [8] / [9]; B. *Pars* for A. *Pars* at **d2r** / **v**, pages 27 / 28.

[6]. *explicationes.* for *Explicationes.* at **C3r**, page 21; *Hyperchatharfeos* for *Hypercatharfeos* at ***I*4v**, page 72; *de* for *De* at ***T*4r**, page 151; *Cardiacis.* for *Opiatis.* at **Z1v**, page 178; *Nocumentia.* for *nocumentia.* at ***Aa*3v**–***Aa*4v**, 190–2.

No catchword at **(*) 1v** / **(*) 2r**, pages [2] / [3]; tum for Verum at **X1r** / **v**, pages 161 / 162.

[7]. PRÆFATIO. for POST-SCRIPTUM at **¶¶1v**–**¶¶2v**, pages [10–12]; *læfæ fpecies.* for *læfæ variæ fpecies* at **D2v**, page 28; *fputo.* for *Sputo.* at **K3v**–**K4r**, pages 78–79; *Vomicâ.* for *Vomica.* at **P4r**–**v**, pages 119–20; *Ictero.* for *Ictero euifque remediis.* at **T3v**, page 150; *remediis* for *Remediis* at **V4v**, page 160; CAPUT. V. for CAP. V. at **Aa2r**, page 187; **Cc4r**, page 207; CAP. III. for CAP. IV. at **Ff4r**, page 231; **Gg1r**, page 233; *Fonticulis five* for *Fonticulis, five* at **Gg3r**, page 237; *Pfora five* for *Pfora, five* at **Hh3v**, page 246.

No catchword at **¶2r** / **¶2v**, pages [3] / [4]; and **¶2v** / **¶3r**, pages [4] / [5]; CAP. XII for SECTIO at **Q1v** / **Q2r**, pages 122 / 123; no catchword at **S4r** / **v**, pages 143 / 144; uent for vent at **V3r** / **v**, pages 157 / 158.

Frontispiece: none.

Portrait: **Pt.1d2**: THOMAS WILLIS, M. D. *Naturalis Philosophiæ Professor Oxoniensis, necnon Inclyti Medicinæ Collegii Londinensis, & Societatis Regiæ Socius,* [signed] *Fr: Diodoti Pin. fcu.* 208 × 163 millimetres (sheet); 202 × 153 millimetres (plate marks); 202 × 150 millimetres (image).

Printers' ornaments: [1]. Printers' device at **¶1r**, page [3]; **§1r**, page [9] {**Tournes 51**}; headpiece at **¶2r**, page [5]; **§2r**, page [11]; **a1r**, page 1{**Tournes 2**}; headpiece at **¶2v**, page [6]; **§3r**, page [13]; **i1r**, page 65 {**Tournes 4**}; two rows each of 27 fleurons {**Tournes 18**} flanked at each end by a single fleuron {**Tournes 19**} with a row between of 16 fleurons (inverted) {**Tournes 8**} flanked at each end by a single fleuron {**Tournes 53**} at **¶3r**, page [7]; two rows of 29 fleurons {**Tournes 7**} with a single row between of 16 fleurons (#15 inverted) {**Tournes 8**} flanked at the right hand end by a single fleuron {**Tournes 53**} at **§4r**, page [15]; tailpiece at **§§1v**, page [18] {**Tournes 10**}; single row of 16 fleurons {**Tournes 8**} at **§§2r**, page [19]; row of 13 fleurons {**Tournes 11**}, flanked by a single fleuron at the left {**Tournes 7**} and another, rotated, at the right hand end {**Tournes 18**} at **§§3r**, page [21]; **§§§1r**, page [25]; **§§§3v**, page [30]; tailpiece at **ee3v**, page 222 {**Tournes 17**}; two rows each of 25 fleurons {**Tournes 18**} flanked at both ends by another {**Tournes 19**} at **ee4r**, page 223; two rows of 27 fleurons separated by: between ##12 / 13, 17 / 18, lower inverted separated by : between ##9 / 10, 19 / 20, {**Tournes 7**}, with row between of 25 fleurons {**Tournes 18**} flanked at both ends by another fleuron {**Tournes 19**}, at **ff1r**, page 225; tailpiece at **ii3v**, page 254 {**Tournes 22**}.

Decorated E at **¶2r**, page [5] {**Tournes 3**}; L at **¶3r**, page [7] {**Tournes 52**}; S at **§2r**, page [11] {**Tournes 5**}; D at **§3r**, page [13] {**Tournes 6**}; D at **§4r**, page [15] {**Tournes 9**}; F at **§§3r**, page [21]; **§§§1r**, page [25] {**Tournes 13**}; V at **§§§3v**, page [30] {**Tournes 54**}; I at **a1r**, page 1 {**Tournes 36**}; E at **i1r**, page 65{**Tournes 55**}; V at **ee4r**, page 223 {**Tournes 20**}; C at **ff1r**, page 225 {**Tournes 56**}.

[2]. Printers' device at **¶1r**, page [1] {**Tournes 51**}; two rows each of 29 fleurons, lower inverted, at **¶2r**, page [3]; **¶4r**, page [7] {**Tournes 7**}; tailpiece at **¶3v**, page [6] {**Tournes 17**}; row of 16 fleurons at **¶¶3r**, page [13] {**Tournes 8**}; headpiece at **A1r**, page 1 {**Tournes 2**}; **O2v**, page 108 {**Tournes 26**}; two rows each of 25 fleurons {**Tournes 18**} each flanked at both ends by another fleuron {**Tournes 19**} at **Z1v**, page 2; headpiece at **Z2r**, page 3 {**Tournes 4**}.

Decorated A at **¶2r**, page [3] {**Tournes 23**}; C at **¶4r**, page [7] {**Tournes 24**}; V at **¶¶3r**, page [13] {**Tournes 54**}; I at **A1r**, page 1 {**Tournes 25**}; N at **O2v**, page 108 {**Tournes 27**}; T at **Z1v**, page 2 {**Tournes 57**}; D at **Z2r**, page 3 {**Tournes 9**}.

[3]. Printers' device at ***1r**, page [1] {**Tournes 51**}; head piece at ***2r**, page [3] {**Tournes 2**}; row of 26 fleurons {**Tournes 18**} flanked at each end by a single fleuron {**Tournes 19**} at ***3r**, page [5]; row of 16 fleurons at ***4r**, page [7] {**Tournes 8**}; two rows each of 29 fleurons, lower inverted, at ****3r**, page [13] {**Tournes 7**}; headpiece at **A1r**, page 1; **S4r**, page 143 {**Tournes 35**}.

Decorated I at ***2r**, page [3] {**Tournes 30**}; Q at ***3r**, page [5] {**Tournes 32**}; Q at ***4r**, page [7] {**Tournes 33**}; I at ****3r**, page [13] {**Tournes 34**}; I at **A1r**, page 1; **S4r**, page 143 {**Tournes 15**}.

[4]. Printers' device at ***1r**, page [1] {**Tournes 51**}; headpiece at ***2r**, page [3]; **a1r**, page 1 {**Tournes 2**}; two rows each of 25 fleurons {**Tournes 18**} flanked at each end by a single fleuron {**Tournes 19**} at **d2v**, page 28; two rows each of 26 fleurons separated by : between ##13 / 14, upper; ##12 / 13, 19 / 20, lower {**Tournes 18**} with a row between of 27 fleurons {**Tournes 7**} at **f1v**, page 42; two rows each of 27 fleurons, lower inverted, {**Tournes 7**} at **h4v**, page [1].

Decorated Q at ***2r**, page [3] {**Tournes 38**}; R at **a1r**, page 1 {**Tournes 58**}; I at **d2v**, page 28 {**Tournes 41**}; C at **f1v**, page 42 {**Tournes 21**}.

[5]. Printers' device at **†1r**, page [1]; **2†1r**, page [5] {**Tournes 51**}; headpiece at **†2r**, page [3]; **†4r**, page [11]; ***a*1r**, page 1 {**Tournes 4**}; **2†2r**, page [7]; **†3r**, page [9] {**Tournes 2**}; row of 13 fleurons {**Tournes 11**} with flanked at each end by a single fleuron {**Tournes 12**} at **††3r**, page [17]; two rows each of 29 fleurons, lower inverted, at **†††3r**, page [25]; ***tt*3v**, page [1] {**Tournes 7**}; tailpiece at **††††4r**, page [35] {**Tournes 17**}; headpiece at ***t*1r**, page 145 {**Tournes 35**}.

Decorated A at **2†2r**, page [7] {**Tournes 44**}; I at **†3r**, page [9] {**Tournes 30**}; E at **†4r**, page [11] {**Tournes 16**}; A at **††3r**, page [17] {**Tournes 50**}; C at **†††3r**, page [25] {**Tournes 24**}; Q at ***a*1r**, page 1 {**Tournes 32**}; I at ***t*1r**, page 145 {**Tournes 15**}; A at ***tt*3v**, page [1] {**Tournes 45**}.

[6]. Printers' device at **(*)1r**, page [1] {**Tournes 51**}; row of 16 fleurons at **(*)2r**, page [3] {**Tournes 8**}; two rows each of 29 fleurons, lower inverted at **(*)3v**, page [6] {**Tournes 7**}; headpiece at ***A*1r**, page 1 {**Tournes 4**}; row of 27 fleurons {**Tournes 18**} flanked at each end by a single fleuron {**Tournes 19**} at ***Cc*2v**, page 204.

Decorated Q at **(*)2r**, page [3] {**Tournes 38**}; M at **(*)3v**, page [6] {**Tournes 46**}; A at ***A*1r**, page 1 {**Tournes 23**}.

[7]. Printers' device at **¶1r**, page [1] {**Tournes 51**}; headpiece at **¶3r**, page [5]; **A1r**, page 1 {**Tournes 2**}; tailpiece at **¶4v**, page [8] {**Tournes 10**}; headpiece at **¶¶1r**, page [9] {**Tournes 4**}; two rows each of 29 fleurons, lower inverted, flanked by] at right hand end at **¶¶3r**, page [13]; single row of 29 fleurons with: at the right hand end at **¶¶4r**, page [15] {**Tournes 7**}; two rows each of 29 fleurons, lower inverted, {**Tournes 7**}, each flanked by] at right hand end, with row between of 28 fleurons {**Tournes 18**} at **¶¶¶1r**, page [17]; **Ll2r**, page [1] with: at right hand end {**Tournes 7**}; headpiece at **A1r**, page 1 **Tournes 2**}.

Decorated A at **¶3r**, page [5] {**Tournes 48**}; D at **¶¶1r**, page [9] {**Tournes 6**}; O at **¶¶¶1r**, page [17] {**Tournes 49**}; I at **A1r**, page 1{**Tournes 37**}; A at **Ll2r**, page [1] {**Tournes 50**}.

Illustrations: as in **8B** apart from variation in sheet sizes and occasional binding positions.

Copy: DASC, lacking [1] ii4 and [3] *Dd4 (both blanks): with another copy of part 2 only in original printers' marbled paper covers. Original vellum, spine lettered *Thoma Willis MD | Opera omnia* | 1680, floral decoration to foreedges, original endpapers. Leaves 214 × 170 millimetres, boards 223 × 170 × 110 millimetres. Inscribed: (1) Ludwig Edinger Frankfurt Main; (2) Ex libris Ludwig Edinger Frankfurt / M; (3) Wm Feindel Montréal. Shelf marks: W735 1680 C662. Bookseller's label: Heinrich Lesser Antiquariat & Bookhandlung Breslau Elizabethstrasse 1.[16]

[16] Ludwig Edinger (1855–1918) was a German anatomist who cofounded the University of Frankfurt. His interest in the nervous system developed whilst working as a physician in Giessen (1877–1882). He lived in Frankfurt am Main from 1883 and was appointed the first German professor of neurology (1914). A victim of anti-semitism, Edinger financed the Institute where he worked through the large inheritance, in 1906, to his wife Anna Goldschmidt, the daughter of a family of traditional Jewish bankers in Frankfurt. Edinger described tracts and nuclei in the hindbrain and introduced Greek terms into neurology: for example, agnosia and apraxia. Edinger died suddenly of coronary thrombosis having left instructions that his brain was to be examined in his own Institute. Edinger bought this copy (subsequently a gift to the present owner from William Feindel) from the shop of Heinrich Lesser (nd). Sigismund Schletter (d.1876) had founded a publishing house and antiquarian bookstore in Breslau (1833), which was acquired in 1855 and expanded by Hugo Skutsch (d.1873). His widow sold the business to Eugen Franck, whose partner Heinrich Lesser continued to run the antiquarian bookshop under his own name from 1889. After further changes in ownership, the bookstore and publishing house became the property of Alfred Kurtze (d.1932), whose predecessor Ruth Kurtze had focused the firm almost exclusively on Jewish literature written in German and Polish.

8C2. OPERA OMNIA, Coloniæ Allobrogum quarto 1680

Second issue of the third edition of the collected works of Thomas Willis in Latin, the eighth book, identical to 8C1 apart from variant title pages showing COLONIÆ ALLOBROGVM as the place of publication [HJR Wing 49, Denham 14, Oldfield B4a].

Title page: [1a]. THOMÆ | WILLIS | MEDICINÆ DOCTORIS, | NATVRALIS PHILOSOPHIÆ | PROFESSORIS OXONIENSIS, | *Nec non* | INCLYTI MEDICORVM COLLEGII | Londinenſis, & SOCIETATIS REGIÆ Socii, | OPERA OMNIA, | TOMVS PRIOR | Cum ELENCHIS RERVM & INDICIBVS Neceſſariis, ut & multis FIGVRIS Æneis. | [ornament: lettered, QVOD TIBI | FIERI NON | VIS, ALTERI | NEFECERIS] | *COLONIÆ ALLOBROGVM,* | Apud SAMVELEM DE TOVRNES. | [short rule] | *M. DC. LXXX.* | Cum Privilegio S.CAESAREÆ MAIESTATIS.*

[1b] [2] [3] [4] [5a] [5b] [6] [7]. As in **8C1** apart from:
... | *COLONIÆ ALLOBROGVM,* | Apud SAMVELEM DE TOVRNES. | [short rule] | *M. DC. LXXX.*

Then as in **8C1**:

Illustrations: as in **8B** apart from variation in sheet sizes and occasional binding positions.

Copy: DASC. Two volumes, original full calf, spines (rebacked) lettered WILLIS'S | OPERA OMNIA | TOM I [&] TOM II | 1680, original endpapers. Leaves 220 × 165 millimetres, boards 230 × 175 × 55 millimetres. Inscribed: (1) Wm Mcleod (unidentified); (2) (undeciphered).

8D. OPERA OMNIA, Lyons quarto 1681

Fourth edition of the collected works of Thomas Willis in Latin, the eighth book, with William Croone's treatise, and all the illustrations, and retaining the same format as the first edition but with the type reset, and the use of some different ornaments and decorated initials [HJR Wing 45, Denham 15, Oldfield B2].[17]

Title page: [1]. CLARISSIMI VIRI THOMÆ | WILLIS, | MEDICINÆ DOCTORIS, | Naturalis Philoſophiæ Profeſſoris Oxonienſis, | *NECNON* | INCLYTI MEDICORUM COLLEGIJ | Londinenſis & Societatis Regiæ Socij; | OPERA OMNIA: | TOMUS PRIOR. | CUM ELENCHIS RERUM ET INDICIBUS | neceſſariis, ut & multis Figuris æneis. | [printers' device: lettered UNIVERSITAS RERVM VT PVLSIS IN MANVIE HOVÆ] | *LUGDUNI.* | Sumptibus JOANNIS ANTONIJ HUGUETAN, & Soc. | [short rule] | *M. DC. LXXXI.* | CUM SUPERIORUM PERMISSU.

* Underlined text originally printed in red.

[17] See footnote 2 for discussion of other copies that may constitute a further state of this edition.

[2]. CLARISSIMI VIRI THOMÆ | WILLIS, | MEDICINÆ DOCTORIS, | Naturalis Philoſophiæ Profeſſoris Oxonienſis, | *NECNON* | INCLYTI MEDICORUM COLLEGIJ | Londinenſis & Societatis Regiæ Socij; | OPERA OMNIA: | TOMUS POSTERIOR. | *CUM ELENCHIS RERUM ET INDICIBUS* | *neceſſariis, ut & multis Figuris æneis.* | [printers' device: lettered UNIVERSITAS RERVM VT PVLSIS IN MANVIE HOVÆ] | *LVGDVNI,* | Sumptibus JOANNIS ANTONII HUGUETAN, & Soc. | [short rule] | *M. DC. LXXXI.* | CUM SUPERIORUM PERMISSU.

Collation: quarto, 23 letter roman alphabet using I and V. [1]. ❡^{4}, **^{2}, ã^4, ẽ^4, ĩ^4, õ^4, ũ^4, A–G^4, H^4 (H3 + 2, signed H4, –), I–Z^4, Aa–Zz^4, Aaa–Zzz^4, Aaaa–Xxxx^4; $1–3 signed apart from: -ũ3, +'H4' (= H3 + 1).
388 leaves, paginated as [52], 1–62, [4: paginated 63*, -, *ibid.* 63, -], 63–694, [26]. Mispaginated: 151 for 551.

[2]. ã^4, 2ã^4, ẽ ^{4}, A–Z^4, Aa–Qq^4; $1–3 signed apart from: -A3, -B3.
168 leaves, paginated as [24], 1–298, [14].

[3]. ❡^{4}, ã^4, ẽ ^{2}, A–Z^4, Aa^2: $1–3 signed.
104 leaves, paginated as [20], 1–180, [8].

[4]. ã^4, ẽ^4, ĩ^4, õ^2, A–Z^4, Aa–Ee^4, Ff^2; $1–3 signed.
128 leaves, paginated as [28], 1–224, [4].

Type: 46 lines; height (20 lines) 84 millimetres, width ≤ 118 millimetres (≤ 129 millimetres with marginal notes).

Contents: [1]. **❡1r**, page [1], title; **❡1v**, page [2], blank; **❡2r–v**, pages [3–4], REVERENDISSIMO IN CHRISTO PATRI, AC D. DOMINO GILBERTO, EPISCOPO LONDINENSI, & Sacelli Regij Decano. … [signed] *Humillimus, & æternùm addictiſsimus* THOMAS VVILLIS.; **❡3r–v**, pages [5–6], REVERENDISSIMO IN CHRISTO PATRI, ET DOMINO, D. GILBERTO, PROVIDENTIA DIVINA, Archiepiſcopo Cantuarienſi, totius Angliæ Primati, & Metropolitano; & Auguſtiſſimo Principi CAROLO II. M. Britanniæ, Franciæ & Hiberniæ Regi, à ſecretioribus Conſiliis. … [signed] *Clementiæ veſtræ humillimus cultor, Cliens addictiſſimus* THOMAS VVILLIS.; **❡4r**, page [7], blank; **❡4v**, [page 8], portrait; ****1r–**2r**, pages [9–11], AUTHORI, In illius Diatribas Medico-Philoſophicas, CARMEN GRATULATORIUM. … [signed] PHILIPPUS FELL; *Med. Stud. Oxon.*; ****2v**, page [12], SERIES OPERUM DOMINI D.THOMÆ VVILLIS, Hac Editione Typis prodeuntium. *TOMI PRIORIS.* 1. De Fermentatione. II. De Febribus. III. De Urinis. IV. Cerebri Anatome. V. Nervorum deſcriptio, & uſus. VI. De Morbis Convulſivis. VII. De Scorbuto. VIII. De Affectionibus Hyſtericis, & Hypochondriacis. IX. De Sanguinis incaleſcentia. X. De Motu Muſculari. *TOMI POSTERIORIS.* I. De Anima Brutorum Exercitationes duæ. II. Pharmaceutice Rationalis, & de Medicamentorum operationibus in humano corpore, &c.; **ã1r–ã3r**, pages [13–17], ELENCHUS RERUM QUÆ IN TRACTATU DE FERMENTATIONE CONTINENTUR.; **ã3r–ẽ1v**, pages [17–22], ELENCHUS RERUM Quæ in Tractatu de FEBRIBUS continentur.; **ẽ1v–ẽ2v**, pages [22–4], ELENCHUS RERUM Quæ in Diſſertatione de URINIS continentur.; **ẽ2v–ĩ2r**, pages [24–31], ELENCHUS RERUM Quæ in CEREBRI ANATOME continentur.; **ĩ2r–ĩ4r**, pages [31–5], NERVORUM

DESCRIPTIO ET USUS.; ĩ4r–õ3r, pages [35–41], ELENCHUS RERUM Quæ in Tractatu de MORBIS CONVULSIVIS continentur.; õ3v–ũ1r, pages [42–5], ELENCHUS RERUM Quæ in Tractatu de SCORBUTO continentur.; ũ1r–v, pages [45–6], ELENCHUS MATERIÆ De Affectibus Hyſtericis, & Hypochondriacis.; ũ1v–ũ2r, pages [46–7], ELENCHUS MATERIÆ Exercitationis de Accenſione Sanguinis.; ũ2r–ũ3r, pages [47–9], ELENCHUS MATERIÆ Exercitationis de Motu Muſculari.; ũ3v, page [50], [Imprimatur] *Regii Procuratoris Conſensus.* PRO Rege aſſentio, ut liceat HUGONI DENOÜALLY Typographo Lugdunenſi typis mandare Tractatus varios D.D. *Thomae Vuillis*, ... [and 7 further lines listing titles]. ... Conceſſis imperanti inhibitionibus conſuetis per triennium duraturis. Datum Lugduni 10. Julii anni 1675 ... [signed] VAGINAY. [line] *Permiſſio*. FIat juxta Concluſiones Procuratoris Regii. Anno & die ſupradictis. [signed] DESEVE. Prædictus HUGO DENOÜALLY jura ſua pro editione ſupradictorum Operum ceſſit JOANNI-ANTONIO HUGUETAN, Bibliopolæ Lugdunenſi, pacto inter eos inito die ll. Septembr. anni 1675. *Regiſtratum in libro Communitatis Bibliopolarum Lugdunenſium, juxta ſententiam in Præſidiali Curia Lugdunenſi latam die* 12. *Ianuarii* 1675. *Signatum* CELLIER.; **ũ4r–v**, pages [51–2], AMICO LECTORI *PRÆFATIO* [to De Fermentatione].

A1r–H3v, pages 1–62, [text] DE FERMENTATIONE, SIVE De MOTU corporum naturalium INRGANICO.

'H4' (= H3 + 1)r–'H5' (= H3 + 2)v, pages [*63r–*ibid.* 63v: = 1–4], Caput primum de Febribus præ feſtinatione editionis, & incogitanter ante præfationem typis datum, quamvis poſt eam legendum. AMICO LECTORI PRÆFATIO.

H4r–Dd3r, pages 63–213, [text] DE FEBRIBUS; **Dd3v–Hh2v**, pages 214–44, [text] DE URINIS Diſſertatio Epiſtolica. *Ad Virum Doctiſsimum mihíquæ amiciſsimum*, D. RADULPHUM BATHURST, Med. Doct. & Collegii Sacroſanctæ Trinitatis Oxon. Socium.

Hh3r–Xx3r, pages 245–349, [preface and text] CEREBRI ANATOME, CUI ACCESSIT Nervorum Deſcriptio & Uſus. PRÆFATIO.; **Xx3v–Fff4v**, pages 350–416, [text], NERVORUM Deſcriptio & Uſus.; **Ggg1r**–Iii1v, pages 417–34, [text] DE RATIONE MOTUS MUSCULORUM; Studio GULIELMI CROONE, M. D. è Coll. Med. Lond. ac Sociatatis Regalis Socii. *Ἐν πᾶσι τοῖς φυσικοῖς ἐνεστί τι θαυμαστόν. Ariſt. de Part. Animal.*

Iii2r–Bbbb3v, pages 435–566, [preface and text] PATHOLOGIÆ CEREBRI, ET NERVOSI GENERIS SPECIMEN: In quo agitur de MORBIS CONVULSIVIS, & de SCORBUTO. *PRÆFATIO.*; **Bbbb4r–Kkkk4v**, pages 567–632, [text] TRACTATUS DE SCORBUTO.

Llll1r–v, pages 633–34; AFFECTIONUM HYSTERICARUM, ET HYPOCHONDRIACARUM PATHOLOGIA SPASMODICA VINDICATA; Contra Reſponſionem Epiſtolarem NATHANAELIS HIGMORI M.D. *Cui acceſſerunt Exercitationes duæ Medico-Phyſicæ*. I. *De Sanguinis Accenſione*. II. *De motu Muſculari. PRÆFATIO.*; **Llll2r–Oooo2r**, page 635–59, [text] AD VIRUM NATHANAEL. HIGHMORI, M. D.; **Oooo2v–Pppp4v**, pages 660–72, EXERCITATIO. I. MEDICO-PHYSICA. *De Sanguinis Incaleſcentia, ſive Accenſione.*; **Qqqq1r–Sſſſ3v**, pages 673–94, [text] EXERCITATIO II. MEDICO-PHYSICA. *De Motu Muſculari.*; **Sſſſ4r–Xxxx3v**, pages [1–24], INDEX ALPHABETICUS Rerum Notabilium.; **Xxxx4r–v**, pages [25–6], blank.

[2]. **1ã1r**, page [1], title; **ã1v**, page [2], blank; **ã2r–v**, page [3–4], REVERENDISSIMO IN CHRISTO PATRI, ET DOMINO, D. GILBERTO, PROVIDENTIA DIVINA, Archiepiſcopo Cantuarienſi, totius Angliæ Primati, & Metropolitano; & Auguſtiſſimo Principi CAROLI II. M. Britanniæ, Franciæ & Hiberniæ Regi, à Secretioribus Conſiliis.... [signed] *CLEMENTIÆ VESTRÆ,* Cultorem humillimum, ſervum devotiſſimum THOMAM VVILLIS.; **ã3r**, page [5], ERUDITISSIMIS ET VENERABILIBUS VIRIS, MIHIQUE ÆTERNUM COLENDIS D. VICE-CANCELLARIO, DOCTORIBUS ET MAGISTRIS QUI IN CELEBERRIMA UNIVERSITATE Oxonienſi bonas literas diligentiſſimè excolunt, egregiè ornant, feliciſſimè promovent; *SALUTEM.* ... [signed] *CLARISSIMI DOMINI,* Veſtrum omnium Cultori addictiſſimo THOMÆ VVILLIS.; **ã3v–ã4v**, page [6–8], PRÆFATIO AD LECTOREM.; **2ã1r–ã4r**, pages [9–15], ELENCHUS RERUM, Quæ in Tractatu DE ANIMA BRUTORUM. Sive in Parte prima continentur.; **ã4v–ẽ4r**, pages [16–23], ELENCHUS RERUM, QUÆ IN PARTE II. PATHOLOGICA Continentur.; **ẽ4v**, page [24], [Imprimatur: as in part 1]

A1r–R1v, pages 1–130, [text] DE ANIMA BRUTORUM [Part I]; **R2r**, page [131] [half title] PARS SECUNDA PATHOLOGICA *SIVE* DE MORBIS QUI AD ANIMAM CORPOREAM, ejuſque ſubjecta, ſcilicet Cerebrum, & Genus Nervoſum ſpectant.; **R2v**, page [132], blank; **R3r–Pp1v**, pages 133–298, [text] PARS SECUNDA.; **Pp2r–Qq3v**, pages [1–12], INDEX ALPHABETICUS Rerum & Verborum.; **Qq4r–v**, pages [13–14], blank.

[3]. ***¶1r**, page [1], [half title] THOMÆ WILLIS PHARMACEUTICES RATIONALIS, Sivè Diatribæ de Medicamentorum operationibus in Corpore Humano; PARS PRIMA.; **¶1v**, page [2], blank; **¶2r**, page [3], CELEBERRIMO MEDICORUM LONDINENSIUM COLLEGIO, ET SINGULATIM VIRO INSIGNISSIMO DOCTISSIMOQUE DOMINO GEORGIO ENT EQUITI AURATO PRÆSIDI ILLUSTRISSIMO, *NEC NON* CENSORIBUS DIGNISSIMIS, CÆTERISQUE OMNIBUS, ampliſſimæ hujus Societatis Membris, *DIATRIBAM HANC Pharmaceuticam Obſervantiæ & Honoris ergo Dicat, Dedicatque,* THO. VVILLIS.; **¶2v**, page [4], blank; **¶3r–¶4v**, pages [5–8]; CANDIDO LECTORI PRÆFATIO.; **ã1r–ê2r**, pages [9–19], ELENCHUS RERUM QUÆ IN PHARMACEUTICE RATIONALI CONTINENTUR.; **ê2v**, page [20], [Imprimatur as in part 1].

A1r–Z2v, pages 1–180, [text] DE MEDICAMENTORUM OPERATIONIBVS IN CORPORE HVMANO.; **Z3r–Aa1v**, page [1–6], INDEX ALPHABETICUS Rerum Notabilium.; **Aa2r–v**, pages [7–8], blank.

[4]. **ã1r**, page [1], [half title] THOMÆ WILLIS PHARMACEUTICES RATIONALIS, Sivè Diatribæ de Medicamentorum operationibus in Corpore Humano; PARS SECUNDA, OPUS POSTHUMUM.; **ã1v**, page [2], blank; **ã2r**, page [3], ATHENIS BRITANNICIS, Literati Orbis lumini Splendidiſſimo, *UNIVERSITATI OXONIENSI,* Et Ibidem ILLUSTRISSIMO PRINCIPI JAC. ORMONDIÆ DUCI CANCELLARIO HONORATISSIMO, RAD. BATHURST *DECANO VVELLENSI* VICECANCELLARIO DIGNISSIMO, Reverendis admodum, & perquam Eruditis DOCTORIBUS, PROCURATORIBUS, Facultatum omnium PROFESSORIBUS, COLLEGIORUM & AULARUM Præfectis, *NECNON* Venerabili Magiſtrorum Senatui, Diatribam hanc Pharmaceuticam Pietatis & gratitudinis ergo Dicat Dedicatque Alumnus & beneficarius adſtrictiſſimus THO. VVILLIS.; **ã2v**, page [4], blank; **ã3r–ã4v**, pages [5–8], CANDIDO LECTORI PRÆFATIO; **ã4v–ẽ2v**, pages [8–12], *POST SCRIPTUM.*; **ẽ3r–v**, pages [13–14], *AVTORI CLARISSIMO, necnon mihi* (*de quo jure glorior*)

AMICISSIMO, IN ILLIUS PHARMACEUTICES RATIONALIS Partem utramque, *Carmen Gratulatorium.* .... [signed] *GVL. DAVVKINS.*; **ẽ4r–v**, pages [15–16], QUERALA LIBRI POSTHUMI *DE OBITV* AUTORIS ... [signed] *GVL. DAVVKINS.* MED. B.; **ĩ1r–õ2v**, pages [17–28], ELENCHUS RERUM.

A1r–Ee4v, pages 1–224, [text] DE MEDICAMENTORUM OPERATIONIBVS IN CORPORE HVMANO.; **Ff1r–Ff2v**, pages [1–4], INDEX ALPHABETICUS.

Headlines and *Catchwords*: [1]. (where chapters change on a given page, this is indicated as *Caput. I & II*): *Caput VII.* for *Caput VI.* at **N1r**, page 97; **N3r**, page 101; *Caput IV.* for *Caput III & IV.* at **Ll2r**, page 267; *Caput IX.* for *Caput X.* at **Oo4r**, page 295; *Caput XXIX.* for *Caput XXVIII.* at **Ddd3r**, page 397; *Caput X.* for *Caput X & XI.* at **Zzz1r**, page 545; *Caput VI.* for *Caput VII.* at **Ffff4r**, page 599; *Caput VIII.* for *Caput VII & VIII.* at **Gggg4r**, page 607.

cum for cùm at **Krr / v**, pages 79 / 80; **Z4e / v**, pages 183 / 184; subitâ for subita at **Cc4r / v**, pages 207 / 208; ſimoda for diverſimoda at **Ff2v / Ff3r**, pages 228 / 229; ritus for spiritus at **Rr4v / Ss1r**, pages 320 / 321; minime for minimè at **Xxx1v / Xxxx2r**, pages 530 / 531; cum for vertigo at **Xxx2r / v**, pages 531 / 532; &c for & at **Eeee2v / Eeee3r**, pages 588 / 589; no catchword at **Iiii4r / v**, pages 623 / 624; pabulo for pabulò at **Pppp1r / v**, pages 665 / 666.

[2]. (where chapters change on a given page, this is indicated by the next CAP.); variable use of ';' in place of ':' between **B1v–C4v**, pages 10–24: no CAP. III. at **D2v**, page 28; *ſive Membra.* for *Animæ partes,* at **E1v**, page 34; *diſpoſitiones,* for *Diſpoſitiones,* at **F1v**, page 42; *Rationali* for *Brutali* at **H1r**, page 57; **H2r**, page 59; CAP. XI. for CAP. X. at **K2r**, page 75; *Viſu.* CAP. XV. for *Somno & Vigilia.* CAP. XVI. at **P3r**, page 117; *De Cephalgia.* for *Cephalgiæ Curatio.* at **S4v**, page 144; *Caro.* CAP. IV. for *Pervigilio.* CAP. V. at **Y4r**, page 175; *Vertigine.* CAP. VII. for *Apoplexia.* CAP. VIII. at **Bb1v**, page 194; *Paralyſi.* CAP. IX. for *Delirio & Phrenitide.* CAP. X. at **Ff2r**, page 227; CAP. XI. for CAP. X. at **Gg1r**, page 233; *Mania.* for *Stupidate.* at **Ll1r**, page 265; *De Stupidate.* for *ſive Moroſi.* at **Ll2r**, page 267; *Stupidate.* CAP. XIII for *Arthritide.* CAP. XIV. at **Ll4v**, page 272; *Arthritide.* CAP. XIV. for *Colica.* CAP. XV. at **Nn3v**, page 286.

ERVDI for ERUDI at **ã2v / ã3r**, page [4] / [5]; no catchword at **ã3r / v**, page [5] / [6]; TABVLA for TABULA at **E3r / v**, page 37 / 38; adeo for facilè at **M4r / v**, page 95 / 96; Qnam for Quam at **Z3r / v**, page 181 / 182; 1. Quoad for Quoad at **Ll1r / v**, page 265 / 266; que for *lem* at **Mm2r / v**, page 275 / 276; *In* for *Secunda* at **Nn2r / v**, page 283 / 284; *Diſpo* for 2. *Diſpoſitio* at **Oo2r / v**, page 291 / 292.

[3]. *& Formulae.* for *ac Formulæ.* at **O3v**, page 110; CAP. IV. for CAP. II. at **P2r**, page 115; CAP. II. for CAP. III. at **Q2r**, page 123; **Y2r**, page 171; SECT. III. for SECT. VII. at **Y2v**, page 172.

No catchword at **¶3r / v**, page [5] / [6]; **M2v / M3r**, page 92 / 93; tuo for tus at **V4r / v**, page 159 / 160; imo for mo at **X4v / Y1r**, page 168 / 169; matum for mentum at **X3r / v**, page 173 / 174; Helmontus for Helmontius at **Y4r / v**, page 175 / 176.

[4]. CAP. III. for CAP. IV. at **E1r**, page 33; *Medicamentorum ad Phthiſin,* for *Species & Formulæe.* at **G1v**, page 50; CAP. X. for CAP. XI. at **N4r**, page 103; CAP. II. for CAP. I. at **Q3r**,

page 125; SECT. II. for SECT. III. at **X4v**, page 168; *Remediis.* for *Remedio.* at **Aa1v**, page 186; CAP. III. for CAP. IV. at **Bb2r**, page 195; *Fontanellis* for *Fonticulis*, at **Bb4v**, page 200; *cum* for *Cum.* at **Cc4r**, page 207; CAP. IV. for CAP. VI, at **Dd3r**, page 213; *De Pſora, ſive Scabie* for *Cum Pruritu.* at **Dd3r**, page 213.

Cafuæ for Cauſæ at **D4v / E1r**, page 32 / 33; Cap. for SECT. at **S3v / S4r**, page 142 / 143; flatus for atus at **T2v / T3r**, page 148 / 149; perfluum for perfidium at **Y1r / v**, page 169 / 170.

Frontispiece: none.

Portrait: **Pt.1c1**: THOMAS WILLIS MEDIC· PROFESSOR · COLLEGII MED· LONDON · ET SOCIET· REG · SOCIVS [with] ÆTATIS SVAE, 45. 228 × 172 millimetres (sheet); 171 × 130 millimetres (plate marks); 168 × 127 millimetres (image).

Printers' ornaments: [1]. Printers' device on title page at **¶1r**, page [1] {**Huguetan 1**}; headpiece at **¶2r**, page [3] {**Huguetan 55**}; headpiece at **¶3r**, page [5] {**Huguetan 4**}; extensive use of one fleuron: row of 22 at ****1r**, page [9]; row of 22 separated by *t* between ##4 / 5, *o* between ##7 / 8, and *l* between ##9 / 10 at ****2v**, page [12]; 24 separated by : between ##4 / 5 at **ĩ2r**, page [31]; 24 separated by O between ##12 / 13 at **ĩ4r**, page [29]; 24 separated by *r* between ##7 / 8, 12 / 13 at **õ3v**, page [42]; double row each of 24 separated by *t* between ##7 / 8, 13 / 14, the lower row inverted at **ũ4r**, page [51]; 24 separated by O between ##10 / 11 and t between 19 / 20 at **ẽ1v**, page [22]; **ẽ2v**, page [24]; **ũ1r**, page [45]; row of 19 arranged horizontally with base alternating to the right at ##1, 3, 5, 7, 9, 11, 13, 15, and 17, others to the left, at **ũ3v**, page [50]; double row each of 22 separated by c between ##7 / 8, and O between ##12 / 13 (upper), and by r between ##7 / 8, and O between ##12 / 13 (lower, unverted) at **'H4' (= H3 + 1)r**, page 63*; double row each of 22 separated by & between ##11 / 12, lower row inverted, at **H4r**, page 63; **Dd3v**, page 214; **Hh3r**, page 245; **Xx3v**, page 350; **Ggg1r**, page 417; double row each of 23 separated by : between ##7 / 8, 16 / 17, the lower row inverted at **Iii2r**, page 435; double row each of 21, the lower row inverted at **Bbbb4r**, page 567; **Llll1r**, page 633; single row of 21 separated by · between ##10 / 11 at **Llll2r**, page 635 {all **Huguetan 9**}; single row of 21 at **Qqqq1r**, page 673; double row each of 22 {**Huguetan 9**}, the lower inverted, each separated by another fleuron {**Huguetan 59**} between ##11 / 12 at **Sfff4r**, page [1]; tailpiece at ****2r**, page [11]; **ũ3r**, page [49]; **Hh2v**, page 244; **Fff4v**, page 416 {**Huguetan 57**}; complex design made up of 40 random fleuron arrangements in squares of 4 each {**Huguetan 58**} surrounded by 5 vertical at each end and 33 horizontal ornaments {**Huguetan 59**} #14 inverted in the upper row at **ã1r**, page [13]; tailpiece at **ũ4v**, page [52] {**Huguetan 49**}; headpiece at **A1r**, page 1{**Huguetan 2**}; tailpiece at **'H5' (= H3 +2)v**, page [*ibid.* 63v] {**Huguetan 29**}.

Decorated S at **¶2r**, page [3] {**Huguetan 3**}; I at **¶3r**, page [5] {**Huguetan 26**}; A at ****1r**, page [9] {**Huguetan 56**}; F at **ã1r**, page [13] {**Huguetan 60**}; F at **ã3r**, page [17] {**Huguetan 61**}; V at **ẽ1v**, page [22]; **ĩ2r**, page [31]{**Huguetan 62**}; Q at **ĩ4r**, page [35] {**Huguetan 63**}; I at **õ3v**, page [42] {**Huguetan 64**}; O at **ũ1r**, page [45] {**Huguetan 65**}; I at **ũ1v**, page [46] {**Huguetan 66**}; A at **ũ2r**, page [47] {**Huguetan 67**}; D at **ũ4r**, page [51]; **'H4' (= H3 + 1)r**, page 63*{**Huguetan 68**}; I at **A1r**, page 1 {**Huguetan 69**}; E at **H4r**, page 63 {**Huguetan 70**}; O at **Dd3v**, page 214; {**Huguetan 65**: inverted}; A at **Hh3r**, page 245 {**Huguetan 56**}; N at **Xx3v**, page 350 {**Huguetan 71**}; D at **Ggg1r**, page 417 {**Huguetan 72**}; Q at **Iii2r**, page 435;

Lllll**r**, page 633 {**Huguetan 36**}; I at **Bbbb4r**, page 567 **Huguetan** 73}; R at **Llll2r**, page 635 {**Huguetan 74**}; C at **Qqqq1r**, page 673 {**Huguetan 75**}; A at **Sfff4r**, page [1] {**Huguetan 76**}.

[2]. Printers' device on title page at **ã1r**, page [1] {**Huguetan 1**}; headpiece at **ã2r**, page [3] {**Huguetan 55**}; extensive use of one fleuron: row of 23 separated by : between ##13 / 14, 18 / 19 at **ã3r**, page [5]; double row of 23, the lower inverted, separated by : between ##1 / 2, 22 / 23 at **ã3v**, page [6]; row of 19 arranged horizontally facing alternately right and left apart from ##18 / 19 (both left) at **ẽ4v**, page [24]; row of 21 at **E3r**, page 37; double row of 23, the lower inverted at **Pp2r**, page [1] {all **Huguetan 9**}; complex ornament made up of 40 fleurons randomly arranged in squares of 4 each {**Huguetan 58**} at **2ã1r**, page [9]; design made up of 40 fleurons symmetrically arranged in squares of 4 each {**Huguetan 80**} at **2ã4v**, page [16]; headpiece at **A1r**, page 1; **R3r**, page 133 {**Huguetan 2**}; tailpiece at **Pp1v**, page 298 {**Huguetan 57**}.

Decorated Q at **ã2r**, page [3] {**Huguetan 77**}; I at **ã3r**, page [5] {**Huguetan 78**}; E at **ã3v**, page [6] {**Huguetan 79**}; A at **2ã1r**, page [9]; **Pp2r**, page [1] {**Huguetan 67**}; Q at **A1r**, page 1 {**Huguetan 36**}; and I at **R3r**, page 133 {**Huguetan 73**}.

[3]. Headpiece at **¶3r**, page [5]; **A1r**, page 1 {**Huguetan 2**}; tailpiece at ***4v**, page [8] {**Huguetan 81**}; headpiece at **ã1r**, page [9] {**Huguetan 82**} with one other headpiece at each end {**Huguetan 83**}; row of 19 fleurons arranged horizontally facing alternately left and right apart from #19 (right) at **ẽ2v**, page [24]; double row of 23 fleurons, the lower inverted at **Z3r**, page [1] {**Huguetan 9**}.

Decorated Q at **¶3r**, page [5] {**Huguetan 77**}; M at **ã1r**, page [9] {**Huguetan 84**}; A at **A1r**, page 1 {**Huguetan 56**}; A at **Z3r**, page [1] {**Huguetan 67**}.

[4]. Headpiece at **ã3r**, page [5] {**Huguetan 4**}; extensive use of one fleuron {**Huguetan 9**}; row of 19 arranged horizontally facing alternately left and right apart from #9 (right), separated by [] between ##4 / 5 and O between ##17 / 18 at **ẽ3r**, page [13]; row of 19 arranged horizontally facing alternately left and right apart from #19 (right), separated by O between ##8 / 9 and 12 / 13 at **ẽ4r**, page [15]; row of 22 separated between ##11 / 12 by ⅃ at **P4v**, page 120; row of 26 at **Ff1r**, page [1]; tailpiece at **ẽ4v**, page [16]; **õ2v**, page [28] {**Huguetan 49**}; headpiece at **ĩ1r**, page [17]; **A1r**, page 1{**Huguetan 2**}.

Decorated A at **ã3r**, page [5] {**Huguetan 85**}; A at **ĩ1r**, page [17] {**Huguetan 86**}; I at **A1r**, page 1 {**Huguetan 69**}; H at **P4v**, page 120 {**Huguetan 87**}; A at **Ff1r**, page [1] {**Huguetan 76**}.

Illustrations: as in **8A** apart from variation in sheet sizes and occasional binding positions.

Copy: Royal Society of Medicine. Original calf (badly worn), spine with five raised bands, gilt decorated panels, labeled OPERA | OMNIA | WILLIS, original endpapers. Leaves 229 × 170 millimetres, boards 242 × 185 × 82 millimetres. Inserted bookplate: (1) Albert J Chalmers (unidentified); (2) Royal Society of Medicine presentation bookplate: THE ROYAL SOCIETY OF MEDICINE, 1870 AJC 1917. 1920, PRESENTED BY M^RS^ AJ CHALMERS 1920]; stamped Royal Society of Medicine 4 SEP 1935. Shelf mark 32167.

8E. OPERA OMNIA, Amsterdam quarto 1682

Fifth edition of the collected works of Thomas Willis in Latin, the eighth book, the only one not to include William Croone's treatise, and with an engraved title page [HJR Wing 51, Denham 16, Oldfield B6].

Title page: THOMÆ | WILLIS | MED. DOCT. | OPERA OMNIA, | Nitidius quàm unquam hactenus edita, plurimum emendata, | Indicibus rerum copiofiffimis, ac diftinctione characterum | exornata. | *Studio & Opera* | GERARDI BLASII, M D. | *Et in Ill. Amftelæd. Gymnafio Prof. Publ. Bibliothecarii, etc.* | [printers' device: lettered CONSULTORIBUS ISTIS] | *AMSTELÆDAMI,* | Apud HENRICUM WETSTENIUM. | [short rule] | CIↃ IↃC LXXXII.

Collation: quarto, 23 letter alphabet using I and V. [1]. π^2; $^2\pi^4$, $*^4$, A–Y^4, Z^2: $1–3 signed.
100 leaves, paginated as [20], 1–176, 179–182 [ie 1–180]; misnumbered 236 for 136.

[2]. $*^2$, *A–P*^{4}, *Q*^{2}: $1–3 signed apart from: L2 for *L*2, O1–P4 for *O*1–*P*4.
64 leaves, paginated as [4], 1–124.

[3]. †^{2}, (*A*)–(*T*)^4; $1–3 signed as (*A*)1–(*E*)2 and then (*E*3)–(*T*3).
78 leaves, paginated as [4], 1–146, [6]. Mispaginated: 238 for 138.

[4]. $*^2$, A–E^4, F^2.
24 leaves, paginated as [4], 1–41, [3].

[5]. $*^4$, A^4, *b*–*z*^{4}, *aa*–*dd*^{4}, *ee*1: $1–3 signed apart from –A3, *e*2 signed e2, *f*2 signed *s*2, -*bb*3.
113 leaves, paginated as [8], 1–210, [8]: page 209 not paginated.

[6]. $*^4$, *A*–*Z*^{4}, *Aa*–*Pp*^{4}: $1–3 signed apart from -*Mm*3.
156 leaves paginated as [8], 1–264, 263–295, 295 [ie 1–298], [6].

Type: ≤ 55 lines; height (20 lines) 69 millimetres, width 129 millimetres (two columns, each 63 millimetres, apart from preliminaries: 141 millimetres with marginal notes).

Contents: [1]. **π1r**, page [1], blank; **π1v**, page [2], portrait; **π2r**, page [3], [engraved title page] TH WILLIS OPERA OMNIA *AMSTELÆDAMI*. Apud HENRICUM WETSTENIUM CIↃ IↃ CLXXXII.; **π2v**, page [4], blank; **2π1r**, page [5], title; **2π1v**, page [6], blank; **2π2r**, page [7], VIRIS NATALIUM SPLENDORE, ERUDITIONIS FAMA, HUMANITATIS LAUDE EXCELLENTISSIMIS D^{n}. JOH. JACABO HARDERO, PHIL. ET MED. DOCTORI, RHETORICES PROFESSORI, IN ACADEMIA BASILIENSI FACULTATIS PHILOSOPHICÆ DECANO SPECTABILI, SER. PRINCIPIS BADENSIS MEDICO, ET S. R. I. NATURÆ CURIOSORUM SOCIO PÆONI DICTO, ET D$^{N.}$. JOH. CONRADO PEYERO, APUD SCAFUSIENSES MEDICO CELEBERRIMO, S. R. I. NATURÆ CURIOSORUM SOCIO DICTO PYTHAGORÆ; **2π2v**, page [8], AMICIS CONJUNCTISSIMIS; DEVOTI ANIMI TESTANDI CAUSA OPERA MEDICORUM HOC SECULO FACILE PRINCIPIS A SE NITIDIORE CULTU ORBI LITERARIO EXHIBITA CUM VOTO OMNIGENÆ PROSPERITATIS D. D. C. HENRICUS

WETSTENIUS BIBLIOPOLA AMSTELÆDAMENSIS KAL. VIIBRIS [short rule above] AN. SAL. PARTÆ CIↃ IↃC LXXXII.; **2π3r**, page [9], GERARDUS BLASIUS LECTORI BENEVOLO *Salutem & Officia*.; **2π3v–2π4r**, pages [10–11], AUCTORIS VITA.; **2π4v**, page [12], CONTENTA HUJUS OPERIS. I. Diatribæ duæ *de* FERMENTATIONE, & FEBRIBUS; *quibus acceſſit* Diſſertatio *de* URINIS. II. CEREBRI ANATOME, NERVORUMQUE DESCRIPTIO *&* USUS; III. PATHOLOGIÆ CEREBRI & NERVOSI GENERIS SPECIMEN, *in quo agitur de* MORBIS CONVULSIVIS *&* SCORBUTO. IV. AFFECTIONUM *quæ dicuntur* HYSTERICÆ *&* HYPOCHONDRIACÆ PATHOLOGIA SPASMODICA VINDICATA, *contra* Reſponſionem Epiſtolarem NATHAN. HIGHMORI M.D. *cui acceſſerunt* Exercitationes Medico-Phyſicæ Duæ. I. *De* SANGUINIS ACCENSIONE. II. *De* MOTU MUSCULARI. V. *De* ANIMA BRUTORUM; *quæ* HOMINIS *Vitalis ac Senſitiva eſt*, Exercitationes Duæ, *quarum* Prior PHYSIOLOGICA *eſt*, Altera PATHOLOGICA, *Morbos, qui* Ipſam, Cerebrum, & Nervoſum Genus *afficiunt, explicans* VI. PHARMACEUTICE RATIONALIS, *ſive* Diatriba *de* MEDICAMENTORUM OPERATIONIBUS *in* Humano Corpore.; ***1r**, page [13] [half title] THOMÆ WILLIS DIATRIBÆ DUÆ *Prior agit* DE FERMENTATIONE, Sive de MOTU Inteſtino Particularum in quovis Corpore; *Altera* DE FEBRIBUS, Sive de MOTU earundem in ſanguine Animalium: *His accesſit* DISSERTATIO Epiſtolica DE URINIS.; ***1v**, page [14], blank; ***2r**, page [15], AD TRACTATUM DE FERMENTATIONE PRÆFATIO.; ***2v–*3r**, pages [16–17], AD TRACTATUM DE FEBRIBUS PRÆFATIO.; ***3v–*4a**, pages [18–19] AD TRACTATUM DE URINIS PRÆFATIO EPISTOLICA, *Ad Virum Doctisſimum, Amicisſimum* D. RUDOLPHUM BATHURST, Med. Doct. & Collegii S. Sanctæ Trinitatis Oxon. Socium.; ***4v**, page [20], INDEX CAPITUM TRACTATUS DE FERMENTATIONE.... DE FEBRIBUS.... DE URINIS.

A1r–F3r, pages 1–45 [text], *DE* FERMENTATIONE, *Sive* DE MOTU CORPORUM NATURALIUM INORGANICO.; **F3r–T4v**, pages 45–152, [text] DE FEBRIBUS.; **T4v–Y2v**, pages 152–72, [text] DE URINIS.; **Y3r–Z1r**, pages 173–'179', INDEX Rerum & verborum TRACTATUS DE FERMENTATIONE.; **Z1r–Z2v**, pages '179'–'182', *Index Rerum & Verbotum Tractatus de* FEBRIBUS.; **Z2v**, page 182, *Index Rerum & Verbotum Tractatus de* URINIS.

[2]. ***1r**, page [1], [half title] THOMÆ WILLIS CEREBRI ANATOME, NERVORUMQUE DESCRIPTIO & USUS.; ***1v–*2r**, pages [2–3], AD CEREBRI & NERVORUM ANATOMEN PRÆFATIO.; ***2v**, page [4], INDEX CAPITUM ANATOMES CEREBRI. ... INDEX CAPITUM TRACTATUS DE NERVIS.

***A*1r–*K*1r**, pages 1–73, [text] CEREBRI ANATOME.; ***K*1r–*P*4r**, pages 73–119, [text] NERVORUM DESCRIPTIO ET USUS; ***P*4v–*Q*2r**, pages 120–3, INDEX *Rerum & Verborum* Tractatu DE CEREBRI ANATOME *Contentorum*.; **Q2v**, page [124], blank.

[3]. **†1r**, page [1] [half title] THOMÆ WILLIS PATHOLOGIÆ CEREBRI *ET* NERVOSI GENERIS SPECIMEN *In quo agitur*. De Morbis Convulſivis, & Scorbuto.; **†1v–†2r**, pages [2–3] AD CEREBRI & NERVOSI GENERIS PATHOLOGIAM PRÆFATIO.; **†2v**, page [4], INDEX CAPITUM TRACTATUS De Morbis convulſivis. ... INDEX CAPITUM TRACTATUS *De ſcorbuto*.

(*A*)**1r**–(*M*)**4v**, pages 1–96, [text] TRACTATUS PRIMUS DE MORBIS CONVULSIVIS.; (*N*)**1r**–(*T*)**1v**, pages 97–146, [text] TRACTATUS SECUNDUS DE SCORBUTO.; (*T*)**2r**–(*T*)**3v**, pages [1–4], INDEX RERUM & VERBORUM TRACTATU DE MORBIS CONVULSIVIS, ET SCORBUTO CONTENTORUM.; (*T*)**4r–v**, pages [5–6], blank.

[4]. ***1r**, page [1], [half title] THOMÆ WILLIS AFFECTIONUM *Quæ dicuntur* HYSTERICÆ ET HYPOCHONDRIACÆ PATHOLOGIA SPASMODICA VINDICATA *Contra Reſponſionem Epiſtolarem* NATHANAELIS HIGHMORI, *M. D.* Cui acceſſerunt Exercitationes Medico-Phyſicæ *De* SANGUINIS ACCENSIONE, ET MOTU MUSCULARI.; ***1v**, page [2], blank; ***2r–v**, pages [3–4], AD TRACTATUM DE AFFECTIONIBUS HYSTERICIS, &c. PRÆFATIO.

A1r–C1r, pages 1–17, [text] AFFECTIONUM *Quæ dicuntur* HYSTERICÆ ET HYPOCHONDRIACÆ PATHOLOGIA SPASMODICA VINDICATA.; **C1v–D1v**, pages 18–26, [text: double columns], DE SANGUINIS INCALESCENTIA SIVE ACCENSIONE, EXERCITATIO MEDICO-PHYSICA.; **D2r–F1r**, pages 27–41, [text], DE MOTU MUSCULARI EXERCITATIO MEDICO-PHYSICA.; **F1v**, page [1], ELENCHUS MATERIÆ DE AFFECTIBUS HYSTERICIS ET HYPOCHONDRIACIS.; **F1v**, page [1], ELENCHUS MATERIÆ EXERCITATIONIS DE ACCENSIONE SANGUINIS.; **F2r–v**, pages [2–3], ELENCHUS MATERIÆ EXERCITATIONIS DE MOTU MUSCULARI.

[5]. ***1r**, page [1], [half title] THOMÆ WILLIS DE ANIMA BRUTORUM *Quæ Hominis Vitalis ac Senſitiva eſt*, EXERCITATIONES DUÆ, QUARUM PRIOR PHYSIOLOGICA *Ejus* Naturam, Partes, Potentias, & Affectiones *tradit*; ALTERA PATHOLOGICA, *Morbos, qui ipſam & Sedem ejus primarium, Cerebrum nempe* & *Nervoſum Genus afficiunt, explicat*; *eorumque Therapeias inſtituit.*; ***1v**, page [2], blank; ***2r–*4r**, pages [3–7], PRÆFATIO IN EXCITATIONES De Anima Brutorum.; ***4v**, page [8], INDEX CAPITUM Tractatus de Anima Brutorum. PHYSIOLOGICI. … INDEX CAPITUM Tractatus de Anima Brutorum PATHOLOGICI.

A1r–*m*2r, pages 1–91, [text] DE ANIMA BRUTORUM *Quæ* Hominis Vitalis ac Senſitiva eſt, PARS PRIMA PHYSIOLOGICA, *Ejuſdem* Naturam, Partes, Potentias, & Affectiones *tradens*.; ***m*2v–*dd*1v**, pages 92–210, [text: double columns] PARS SECUNDA PATHOLOGICA *SIVE* DE MORBIS Quæ ad Animam Corpoream, ejuſque ſubjecta, ſcilicet Cerebrum, & Genus nervoſum ſpectant.; ***dd*2r–*ee*1v**, pages [1–8], INDEX RERUM & VERBORUM TRACTATU DE ANIMA BRUTORUM CONTENTORUM.

[6]. ***1r**, page [1], THOMÆ WILLIS PHARMACEUTICE RATIONALIS, SIVE DIATRIBA DE MEDICAMENTORUM OPERATIONIBUS IN HUMANO CORPORE. [half title]; ***1v**, page [2], blank; ***2r–*3r**, pages [3–5], IN PHARMACEUTICES RATIONALIS PARTEM PRIMAM PRÆFATIO.; ***3v–*4r**, pages [6–7], IN PHARMACEUTICES RATIONALIS PARTEM SECUNDEM PRÆFATIO.; ***4v**, page [8], INDEX CAPITUM Partis primæ Pharmaceutices Rationalis. … INDEX CAPITUM Secundæ Partis Pharmaceutices Rationalis.

***A*1r–*R*1v**, pages 1–130, [text] DE MEDICAMENTORUM OPERATIONIBUS IN CORPORE HUMANO SECTIO PRIMA.; ***R*2r–*Pp*1v**, pages 131–'295', [text] DE MEDICAMENTORUM OPERATIONIBUS IN CORPORE HUMANO PARS SECUNDA.; **Pp2r–Pp4v**, pages

[1–6], INDEX RERUM & VERBORUM TRACTATU DE MEDICAMENTORUM OPERATIONIBUS IN CORPORE HUMANO CONTENTORUM.

Headlines and *Catchwords*: [1]. CAP. I. missing at **A1v**, page 2; CAP. II. missing at **A2r**, page 3; **A3v**, page 6, **A4r**, page 7; CAP. IV. for CAP. V. at **B3v**, page 14; CAP. IV. for CAP. VI. **B4v**, page 16; FREMENTATIONE for FERMENTATIONE at **C3v**, page 22; CAP. IX. for CAP. VIII. at **D1r**, page 25; CAP. XI. for CAP. X. at **E3r**, page 37; CAP. XI. for CAP. XII. at **F2v**, page 44; CAP. IV. for CAP. III. at **H1r**, page 57; **H2v**, page 60; CAP. III. for CAP. IV. at **H3v**, page 62; CAP. V. for CAP. VI. at **I2v**, page 68; CAP. IV. for CAP. VI. at **I3v**, page 70; CAP. VII. for CAP. VIII. at **K1v**, page 74; CAP. XI. for CAP. X. at **L3v**, page 86; CAP. X. for CAP. XI. at **L4v**, page 88; CAP. XI. for CAP. XII. at **N2r**, page 99; CAP. XIII. for CAP. XIV. at **O3v**, page 110; no CAP. IV. at **V4v**, page 160; CAP. VI. for CAP. IV. at **X1r**, page 161; CAP. V. for CAP. IV. at **X1v**, page 162; CAP. IV. for CAP. V. at **X2r**, page 163; **X2v**, page 164; **X3r**, page 165; DE UIRNIS. for. DE URINIS. at **Y1r**, page 169.

solent for solet at **A4v** / **B1r**, pages 8 / 9; *Erit* for Erit at **D4r** / **v**, pages 31 / 32; Hu- for *Hu-* at **F1r** / **v**, pages 41 / 42; indu;it for inducit at **H4r** / **v**, pages 63 / 64; te for poterit at **P4v** / **Q1r**, pages 120 / 121; CAP. XVII for CAPUT at **S1r** / **v**, pages 137 / 138; hijus fe for febris at **S3r** / **v**, pages 141 / 142; accef for ceſſione **T3r** / **v**, pages 149 / 150.

[2]. GEREBRI for CEREBRI at ***B*1v**, page 10; NERVORUM DESCRIPTIO for ET USUS. at ***N*3r**, page 101; DESCRIPTIO NERVORUM for NERVORUM DESCRIPTIO. at **P1v**, page 114.

No catchword at ***2v** / ***A*1r**, pages [4] / 1; **O4v** / **P1r**, pages 112 / 113; qui- for - dam at ***A*4v** / ***B*1r**, pages 8 / 9.

[3]. Cap. II. for Cap. I. at **(*A*)2r**, page 3; D for DE at **(*A*)3v**, page 6; MORBUS for MORBIS at **(*B*)3v**, page 14; **(*B*)4v**, page 16; Cap. VI. for Cap. IV. at **(*D*)1r**, page 25; **(*D*)2r**, page 27; Cap. X. for Cap. XI. at **(*M*)1r**, page 89; Cap. II. for Cap. III. at **(*O*)1r**, page 105; Cap. III. for Cap. IV. at **(*O*)4r–(*P*)1r**, pages 111–113; Cap. VIII. for Cap. IX. at **(*S*)1v**, page '238'.

No catchword at **†2v** / **(*A*1)r**, pages [4] / 1; ferui for ruimus at **(*B*1)r** / **v**, pages 9 / 10; incli- for clinato at **(*D*3)r** / **v**, pages 29 / 30; Quoad for Quod at **(*S*2)r** / **v**, pages 139 / 140.

[4]. MOYU for MOTU at **D4v**, page 32.

No catchword at ***2v** / **A1r**, pages [4] / 1; **D1v** / **D2r**, pages 26 / 27.

[5]. CAP. I. for CAP. II. at **A2v**, page 4; BRU*T*{inverted}ORUM for BRUTORUM at ***b*2v**, page 12; CAP. III. for CAP. IV. at ***c*2v**, page 20; CAP. IV. for CAP. V. at ***d*2r**, page 27; SCIENTIA for ANIMA at ***e*1v**, page 34; ***e*2r**, page 35; ***e*3v**, page 38, ***e*4r**, page 39; CAP. VI. for CAP. VII. at ***e*3v**, page 38; CAP. VII. for CAP. VIII. at ***f*1v**, page 42; CAP. VIII. for CAP. IX. at ***f*3v**, page 46; '.' after headline at ***g*4v**, page 56; ***m*3v**, page 94; ***n*3v**, page 102; ***r*1v**, page 130; ***t*3v**, page 150; CAP. III. for CAP. XII. at ***b*4r**, page 63; CAP. IX. for CAP. XV. at ***i*4r**, page 71; ';' after headline at ***l*2v**, page 84; ***p*3v**, page 118; CAP. VXI. for CAP. XVI. at ***m*2r**, page 91; CAP. XV. for CAP. III. at ***p*1r**, page 113; CAP. XVI. for CAP. III. at ***p*2v**, page 116; CAP. IV. for CAP. V. at ***q*2r**, page 123; VII. for CAP. IX. at ***t*1r**, page 145; CAP. IX. for CAP. XI. at ***x*4v**, page 168; ***y*2v**,

page 170; ***y*2r**, page 171; CAP. VII. for CAP. XI. at ***y*4r**, page 175; CAP. VII. for CAP. XIV. at ***bb*2r**, page 195; CAP. XIN. for CAP. XIV. at ***bb*2v**, page 196; CAP. XV. for CAP. XIV. at ***cc*1r**, page 201; CAP. XV. (right not left) at ***dd*1r**, page [209]; ***dd*1v**, page 210; DE COLICA. for PARS PATHOLOGICA. at ***dd*1r**, page [209]; DE COLICA. for DE ANIMA BRUTORUM at ***dd*1v**, page 210.

No catchword at ***4v / A1r**, pages [8] / 1; eaſ- for conſcii at ***f*2r / v**, pages 43 / 44; & in- for adeo at ***i*4v / *k*1r**, pages 72 / 73; 2. Se for 2. *Serum* at ***m*3v / *m*4r**, page 94 / 95; avo- for *avocant* at ***n*4v / *o*1r**, pages 104 / 105.

[6]. Sect. II. for Sect. I. at ***B*2v**, page 12; Cap. II. for Cap. I. at ***B*4r**, page 15; ***C*3r**, page 21; CAP. III. for Cap. II and numbering of chapter CAPUT III. for CAPUT II. at ***C*4r**, page 23; Cap. I. for Cap. II. at ***D*1r**, page 25; CAP. I. for Cap. III. at ***G*2r**, page 51; Cap. II. for Cap. I. at ***G*3r**, page 53; Cap. IV. for Cap. II. at ***H*2r**, page 59 (reflecting numbering of chapter CAPUT IV. for CAPUT II. at ***H*1v**, page 58); Sect. III. for Sect. IV. at ***H*3v**, page 62; ***H*4v**, page 64; ***I*1v**, page 66; Cap. IV. for Cap. II. at ***H*4r**, page 63; Sect. III. for Sect. V. at ***K*3v**, page 78; Cap. II. for Cap. III. at ***O*4r**, page 111; no Sect. VII. at ***R*1v**, page 130; Sect. VII. for Sect. I. at ***R*3v**, page 134; Cap. VIII. for Cap.VII. at ***Aa*1r**, page 185; OPERATIONIBU for OPERATIONIBUS at ***Bb*1r**, page 193; Cap. VIII. for Cap. IX. at ***Bb*3r**, page 197; Cap. VI. for Cap. XI. at ***Cc*2r**, page 203; Sect. III. for Sect. II. at ***Gg*2v**, page 236; ***Gg*3v**, page 240; ***Hh*1v**, page 242 (reflecting misnumbering of chapter heading SECTIO III. for SECTIO II. at ***Gg*2v**, page 236); Cap. VI. for Cap. IV. at ***Hh*1r**, page 241; ***Hh*2r**, page 243; Cap. I. for Cap. II at ***Kk*4r**, page 263; Cap. III. for Cap. IV. at ***Mm*3r**, page '275'; Cap. VI. for Cap. VII. at ***Oo*2r**, page '289'.

3. Quoud for 3. *Quoad* at **Bb3v / Bb4r**, pages 198 / 199; *Iala* for *Jalapium* at ***Ff*4v / *Gg*1r**, pages 232 / 233.

Frontispiece: **F.4a1**: Engraved allegorical title page within a double ruled border, lettered TH WILLIS OPERA OMNIA *AMSTELÆDAMI* Apud HENRICUM WETSTEINIUM CIↃ IↃ CLXXXII. 235 × 194 millimetres (sheet); 223 × 176 millimetres (plate marks); 220 × 168 millimetres (image); see: Figure 149.

Portrait: **Pt.1e1**: [*Thomas Willis, M.D* added in pen and ink]. 235 × 194 millimetres (sheet); 213 × 158 millimetres (plate marks); 204 × 154 millimetres (image); see: Figure 150.

Printers' ornaments: [1]. Printers' device at **2π1r**, page [5] {**Wetstein 1**}; headpiece at **2π3v**, page [10] {**Wetstein 3**}; tailpiece at **2π4v**, page [12] {**Wetstein 5**}; **Y2v**, page 172 {**Wetstein 10**}.

Decorated S at **2π3r**, page [9] {**Wetstein 2**}; T at **2π3v**, page [10] {**Wetstein 4**}; D at ***2r–v**, pages 15–16 {**Wetstein 6**}; I at **A1r**, page 1 {**Wetstein 7**}; E at **F3r**, page 45 {**Wetstein 8**}; C at **T4v**, page 152 {**Wetstein 9**}.

[2]. No ornaments.

Decorated A at ***1v**, page [2] {**Wetstein 11**}; I at ***A*1r**, page 1 {**Wetstein 7**}.

[3]. Tailpiece at **†2r**, page [3] {**Schagen 17**}; **(*M*)4v**, page 96 {**Wetstein 13**}; **(*T*1)v**, page 146 {**Wetstein 5**}.

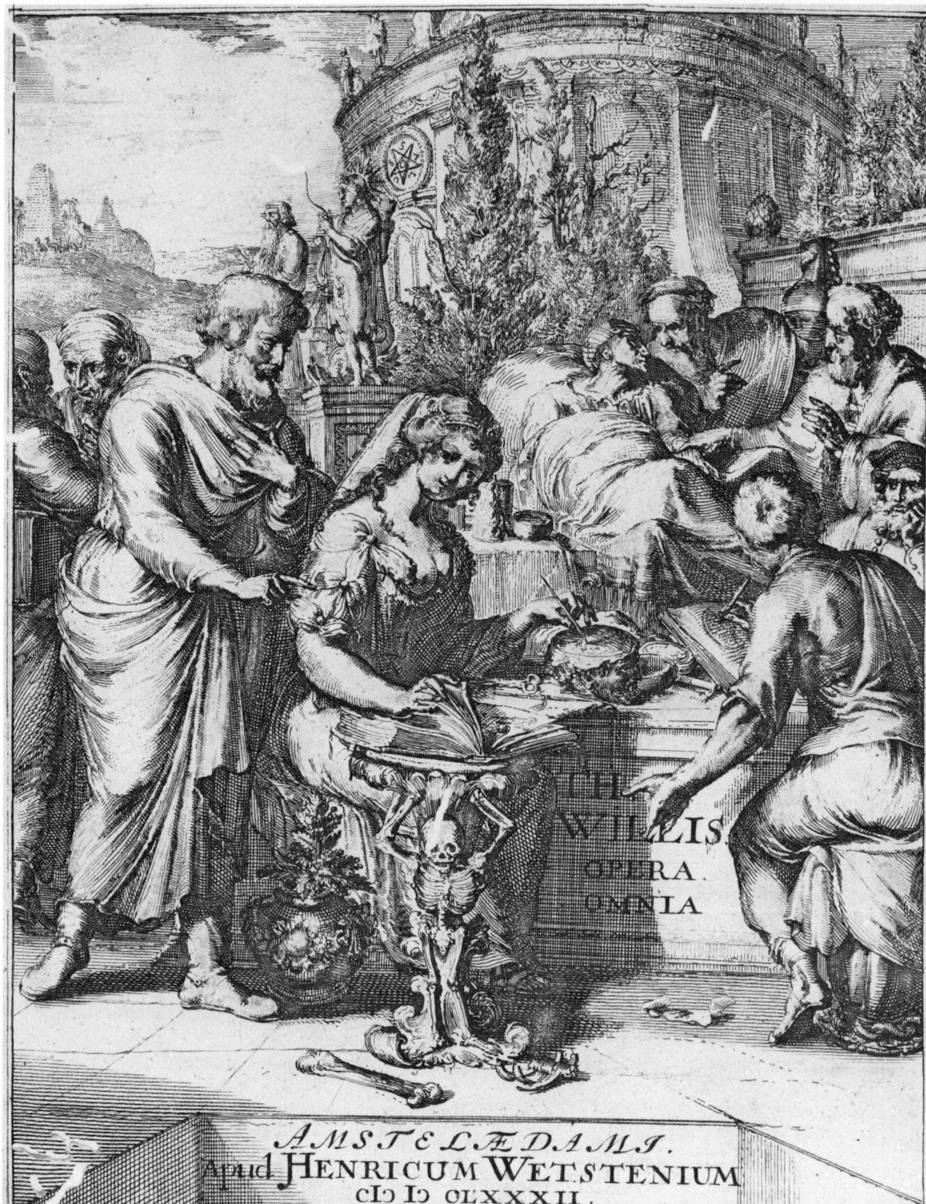

Figure 149 Engraved allegorical frontispiece: *Opera Omnia*, Amsterdam, 1682 (F.3a1).

Decorated Q at †**1v**, page [2] {**Wetstein 12**}; I at (*A*)**1r**, page 1; (*N)***1r**, page 97 {**Wetstein 7**}; A at (*T*2)**r**, page [1] {**Wetstein 14**}.

[4]. Tailpiece at **F1r**, page 41 {**Wetstein 16**}; F2v, page [3] {**Wetstein 10**}.

Decorated Q at *2**r**, page [3] {**Wetstein 12**}; R at **A1r**, page 1 {**Wetstein 15**}; I at **C1v**, page 18 {**Wetstein 7**}; C at **D2r**, page 27 {**Wetstein 9**}.

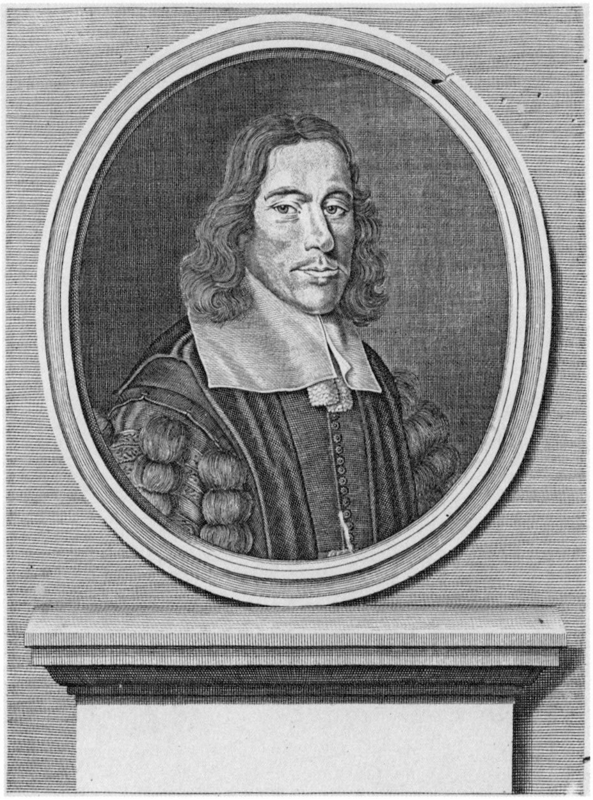

Figure 150 Portrait of Thomas Willis: *Opera Omnia*, Amsterdam, 1682 (Pt.1e1).

[5]. Tailpiece at *4**r**, page [7] {**Wetstein 5**}; ***dd*1v**, page 210 {**Schagen 17**}.

Decorated E at ***2r**, page [3] {**Wetstein 8**}; Q at **A1r**, page 1 {**Wetstein 17**}; I at ***m*2v**, page 92 {**Wetstein 7**}.

[6]. Headpiece at ***2r**, page [3] {**Wetstein 18**}; tailpiece at ***3r**, page [5]; ***R*1v**, page 130; ***Pp*1v**, page '295' {**Wetstein 13**}; headpiece at ***3v**, page [6] {**Wetstein 3**}; tailpiece at ***4r**, page [7] {**Wetstein 19**}; ***Ee*1v**, page 218 {**Wetstein 5**}.

Decorated Q at ***2r**, page [3] {**Wetstein 12**}; A at ***3v**, page [6] {**Wetstein 11**}; A at ***A*1r**, page 1{**Wetstein 20**}; I at ***R*2r**, page 131 {**Wetstein 7**}; A at ***Pp*2r**, page [1] {**Wetstein 14**}.

Illustrations: lettering and legends as in **2A**, **4A**, **5A**, **6A**, and **6E**: figure sizes as in **2C2**, **5C**, **6C**, and **6G**.[18]

[18] With the exception of plates 17 and 18, which are newly engraved, each of the illustrations is an altered state of those used in earlier Dutch editions of Willis's works: Caspar Commelin (**2C2**; *Cerebri anatome* 1664: plates 1–15), Someren (**5C**; *De anima brutorum* 1674: plates 19–26), Arnold Leers (**6C**; *Pharmaceutice rationalis* part I,

[2]. **Pl.1c2**. Plate 1 (image 1): Figura 1.[a] (headline, centre), *Cerebri anat. Pag. 7.* (headline, right). Leaf size, 235 × 194 millimetres (sheet); 220 × 184 millimetres (plate marks). Inserted before legends for Figuræ I–II at ***A*4r–v**, pages 7–8.

Pl.2c2. Plate 2 (image 2): Fig. II.[da.] (headline, centre), *Cerebri anat. Pag. 8.* (headline, right). Leaf size, 235 × 194 millimetres (sheet); 165 × 135 millimetres (plate marks). Inserted after legends for Figuræ I and II at ***A*4r–v**, pages 7–8.

Pl.3c2. Plate 3 (image 3): Fig. III. (headline, centre), *Cerebri anat. Pag. 13.* (headline, right). Leaf size, 235 × 184 millimetres (sheet); 225 × 188 millimetres (plate marks). Inserted before legends for Figuræ III–IV at ***B*3r**–v, pages 13–14.

Pl.4c2. Plate 4 (image 4): Fig. IIII. (headline, centre), *Cerebri anat. Pag. 14.* (headline, right). Cropped Leaf size, 215 × 163 millimetres (sheet); 165 × 135 millimetres (plate marks). Inserted after legends for Figuræ III–IV at ***B*3r**–v, pages 13–14.

Pl.5c2. Plate 5 (image 5): Fig. V. (headline, left), *Cerebri anat. Pag. 17.* (headline, right). Leaf size, 235 × 178 millimetres (sheet); 185 × 157 millimetres (plate marks). Inserted before legends for Figuræ V–VI at **C1r–v**, pages 17–18.

Pl.6c2. Plate 6 (image 6): Fig. VI. (headline, centre), *Cerebri anat. Pag. 17.* (headline, right). Leaf size, 235 × 194 millimetres (sheet); 180 × 145 millimetres (plate marks). Inserted before legends for Figuræ V–VI at **C1r–v**, pages 17–18.

Pl.7c2. Plate 7 (images 7–10): [Unnumbered 1] *Cerebri anat. Pag. 29.* (headline, right), Fig. 1, Fig. 11.; Fig. 111., (headers, centre above each image), *Fig. 1111.* (header, right of image). Leaf size, 235 × 194 millimetres (sheet); 164 × 135 millimetres (plate marks). Inserted before legend at **D3r–v**, pages 29–30.

Pl.8c2. Plate 8 (image 11): *Fig* VII[a] (headline, centre), *Cerebri anat. Pag. 36.* (headline, right). Leaf size, 235 × 194 millimetres (sheet); 198 × 143 millimetres (plate marks). Inserted after legend at ***E*2v**, page 36.

Pl.9c2. Plate 9 (image 12): Fig. VIII (headline, centre), *Cerebri anat. Pag. 45.* (headline, right). Leaf size, 235 × 194 millimetres (sheet); 165 × 135 millimetres (plate marks). Inserted before legend at ***F*3r–v**, pages 45–6.

Pl.10c2. Plate 10 (images 13–14): [Unnumbered 2] *Cerebri anat. Pag. 80.* (headline, right), Fig. I., Fig. II. (headers, above each image): 235 × 194 millimetres (sheet); 192 × 150 millimetres (plate marks). Inserted after legend at ***K*4r–v**, pages 79–80.

Pl.11c2. Plate 11 (image 15): *Cerebri anat. Pag. 115.* (headline, centre), *Tabula IX[a]*. (headline, right). Folding, 318 × 229 millimetres (sheet); 296 × 173 millimetres (plate marks). Inserted within legends for Tabulæ IX–XIII at ***O*4v–*P*4r**, pages 112–19.

1674: plates 27–32) and Arnold Leers (**6G**; *Pharmaceutice rationalis*, part 2, 1677: plates 33–40). Plate and figure sizes are given with the original descriptions in chapters 6, 9, and 10.

Pl.12c2. Plate 12 (image 16): *Cerebri anat. Pag. 115* (headline, centre), *Tabula X^{ma}*. (headline, right). Folding, 316 × 227 millimetres (sheet); 298 × 200 millimetres (plate marks). Inserted within legends for Tabulæ IX–XIII at **O4v–P4r**, pages 112–19.

Pl.13c2. Plate 13 (image 17): *Cerebri anat. Pag. 116* (headline, left), *Tabula X1.^{ma}* (footer, right). Folding, 344 × 203 millimetres (sheet); 298 × 140 millimetres (plate marks). Inserted within legends for Tabulæ IX–XIII at **O4v–P4r**, pages 112–19.

Pl.14c2. Plate 14 (image 18): *Cerebri anat. Pag. 117* (headline, centre right), *Tabula* XII. (headline, right). Folding, 270 × 139 millimetres (sheet); 260 × 72 millimetres (plate marks). Inserted within legends for Tabulæ IX–XIII at **O4v–P4r**, pages 112–19.

Pl.15c2. Plate 15 (images 19–23): *Cerebri anat. Pag. 118* (headline, centre), Tab. XIII. (headline, right), *Fig: I.^{ma}.*, *Fig. 2.da*, *Fig. 3.$^{tia.}$*, *Fig. 4.$^{ta.}$*, *Fig. 5ta*. (centre above each image). Folding, 270 × 343 millimetres (sheet); 240 × 295 millimetres (plate marks). Inserted within legends for Tabulæ IX–XIII at **O4v–P4r**, pages 112–19.

[4]. **Pl.17f1** (images 26–27) with **Pl.18f1** (images 28–29): *De affect hyster.* (headline, left), *Fig.* I., *Fig.* II., *Fig.* III., *Fig.* IV. (header, above each image). Leaf size, 235 × 194 millimetres (sheet); 190 × 170 millimetres (plate marks). Inserted within legend at **E4v–F1r**, pages 40–1.

[5]. **Pl.19b2**. Plate 19 (images 30–33): *de anima brut. Pag. 18* (headline, left), *Tab. I.^{a}* (headline, right), *Fig. I.^{a}*, *Fig. II.^{da}*, *Fig. IIII.^{ta}*, *Fig. III.^{tia}* (header, above each image). Leaf size 235 × 194 millimetres (sheet); 200 × 160 millimetres (plate marks). Inserted within legends for Tabulæ I–IV at **c1v–c2v**, pages 18–20.

Pl.20b2. Plate 20 (images 34–35): *Tab. II.^{da}* (headline, centre), *de anima brut. Pag. 18.* (headline, right), *Fig. I^{a}* and *Fig. II.^{da}* (header, above each image). Folding, 235 × 194 millimetres (sheet); 145 × 200 millimetres (plate marks). Inserted within legends for Tabulæ I–IV at **c1v–c2v**, pages 18–20.

Pl.21b2. Plate 22 (images 36–38): *Tab. III.^{tia}* (headline, centre), *de anim brut. Pag. 20.* (headline, right), *Figura. 1.ma*, *Fig. II.^{da}*, *Fig. III.^{tia}*. (header, above each image). Folding, 290 × 194 millimetres (sheet); 280 × 157 millimetres (plate marks). Inserted after legends for Tabulæ I–IV at **c1v–c2v**, pages 18–20.

Pl.22b2. Plate 22 (images 39–41): *Tab. IIII.*, *de anima brut. Pag. 20.* (headline, left), *Fig II.^{da}*, *Fig. I.^{ma}*, *Fig. III.^{tia}* (header, above each image). Leaf size, 235 × 194 millimetres (sheet); 176 × 142 millimetres (plate marks). Inserted after legends for Tabulæ I–IV at **c1v–c2v**, pages 18–20.

Pl.23b2. Plate 23 (image 42): *de anima brut. Page 26.* (headline, left), *Tab.V.* (headline right). Leaf size, 235 × 194 millimetres (sheet); 190 × 122 millimetres (plate marks). Inserted within legends for Tabulæ V–VII at **d1v–d2r**, pages 26–7.

Pl.24b2. Plate 24 (image 43): *de anima brut. Pag. 26* (headline, left), *Tab. VI.* (headline, right). Cropped Leaf size, 190 × 184 millimetres (sheet); 138 × 118 millimetres (plate marks). Inserted within legends for Tabulæ V–VII at **d1v–d2r**, pages 26–7.

Pl.25b2. Plate 25 (image 44): *de anima brut. Pag. 27.* (headline, left), *Tab. VII.* (headline right). Cropped leaf size, 228 × 172 millimetres (sheet); 140 × 133 millimetres (plate marks). Inserted within legends for Tabulæ V–VII at ***d*1v–*d*2r**, pages 26–7.

Pl.26b2. Plate 26 (image 45): *de anima brut. Pag. 42.* (headline, left), *Tab. VIII.* (headline, right). Folding, 200 × 225 millimetres (sheet); 159 × 204 millimetres (plate marks). Inserted after legend at ***f*1v**, page 42.

[6]. **Pl.27b3**. Plate 27 (image 46): *Tab. I.* (headline, centre), *Pharmac. Pag. 13* (headline, right). Folding, 212 × 229 millimetres (sheet); 165 × 193 millimetres (plate marks). Inserted before legends for Tabulæ I–VI at ***B*3r–v**, pages 13–14.

Pl.28b3. Plate 28 (image 47): *Pharmac. Pag. 13* (headline, left), *Tab. II.* (headline, centre). Folding, 198 × 229 millimetres (sheet); 140 × 192 millimetres (plate marks). Inserted before legends for Tabulæ I–VI at ***B*3r–v**, pages 13–14.

Pl.29b3. Plate 29 (image 48): *Pharmac. Pag. 13.* (headline, left), *Tab. III.* (headline, centre). Folding, 203 × 229 millimetres (sheet); 155 × 188 millimetres (plate marks). Inserted before legends for Tabulæ I–VI at ***B*3r–v**, pages 13–14.

Pl.30b3. Plate 30 (image 49–51): *Pharmac. Pag. 13., Tab.* IV. (headline, left), *Fig.* 2., *Fig. 3., Fig.* I. (headers, above each image. Folding, 235 × 263 millimetres (sheet); 158 × 234 millimetres (plate marks). Inserted before legends for Tabulæ I–VI at ***B*3r–v**, pages 13–14.

Pl.31b3. Plate 31 (image 52): *Tab. V.* (headline, centre), *Pharmac. Pag. 14.* (headline, right). Leaf size, 232 × 194 millimetres (sheet); 157 × 184 millimetres (plate marks). Inserted after legends for Tabulæ I–VI at ***B*3r–v**, pages 13–14.

Pl.32b3. Plate 32 (images 53–57): *Tab.* VI. (headline, centre), *Pharmac. Pag. 14.* (headline, right). Folding, 235 × 209 millimetres (sheet) 140 × 204 millimetres (plate marks). Inserted after legends for Tabulæ I–VI at ***B*3r–v**, pages 13–14.

Pl.33b2. Plate 33 (image 58): *Pharmaceutic. Pag. 144.* (headline, left), *Tab: I.* (headline, right). Folding, 235 × 219 millimetres (sheet); 124 × 195 millimetres (plate marks). Inserted within legends for Tabulæ I–VIII at **S4v–*T*1r**, pages 144–5.

Pl.34b2. Plate 34 (image 59): *Tab: II.* (headline, left), *Pharmac. Pag. 144.* (headline, right). Leaf size, 235 × 167 millimetres (sheet); 197 × 123 millimetres (plate marks). Inserted within legends for Tabulæ I–VIII at **S4v–*T*1r**, pages 144–5.

Pl.35b2. Plate 35 (images 60–61): *Tab: III.* (headline, left), *Pharmac. Pag. 144.* (headline, right), *Fig: 1., Fig: 2.* (headers, left of each image). Leaf size, 235 × 179 millimetres (sheet); 205 × 148 millimetres (plate marks). Inserted within legends for Tabulæ I–VIII at **S4v–*T*1r**, pages 144–5.

Pl.36b2. Plate 36 (images 62–64): *Tab: IV.* (headline, centre), *Pharmac. Pag. 144.* (headline, right), *Fig: 1., Fig: 2., Fig: 3.* (headers, left of each image). Leaf size, 235 × 179 millimetres (sheet); 173 × 135 millimetres (plate marks). Inserted within legends for Tabulæ I–VIII at **S4v–*T*1r**, pages 144–5.

Pl.37b2. Plate 37 (images 65–67): *Pharmac. Pag. 144.* (headline, centre), *Tab: V.* (headline, right), *Fig: 2., Fig: 1., Fig: 3.* (heads, below each image). Leaf size, 225 × 194 millimetres (sheet); 224 × 177 millimetres (plate marks). Inserted within legends for Tabulæ I–VIII at **S4v–*T*1r**, pages 144–5.

Pl.38b2. Plate 38 (images 68–75): *Pharmac. Pag. 146. Tab. VI.* (headline, left), *Tab. VI. Fig: 1., Fig: 2.* (headers, above each group of four images [printed vertically]). Leaf size, 235 × 179 millimetres (sheet); 225 × 145 millimetres (plate marks). Inserted after legends for Tabulæ I–VIII at **S4v–*T*1r**, pages 144–5.

Pl.39b2. Plate 39 (images 76–79): *Pharmac. Pag. 146.* (headline, left), *Tab: VII.* (headline, centre), *Fig: 3., Fig: 1., Fig: 2., Fig: 4.* (headers, above each image). Leaf size 126 × 140 millimetres (plate marks); 235 × 194 millimetres (sheet); printed above **Pl.40b2.** Plate 40 (images 80–82): *Pharmac. Pag. 146.* (headline, centre), *Tab: VIII.* (headline, centre), *Fig: 1., Fig: 2., Fig: 3.* (headers, above each image). Leaf size, 235 × 187 millimetres (sheet); 62 × 140 millimetres (plate marks). Inserted within legends for Tabulæ I–VIII at **S4v–*T*1r**, pages 144–5.

Copy: DASC (#1 of 2). Later half calf with buckram boards, spine with five raised bands, labelled WILLIS | OPERA OMNIA | and lettered 1682, new endpapers. Leaves 235 × 194 millimetres, boards 245 × 195 × 60 millimetres. Inscribed: (1) Wm Feindel MONTREAL; (2) M Emmett Coll. Mer Oxon 1693; (3) Ex Libris Societatis Medica Ediniensis.[19]

8F. OPERA OMNIA, Coloniæ folio 1694

Sixth edition of the collected works of Thomas Willis in Latin, the eighth book, the first in folio format, with William Croone's treatise, and all the illustrations [not listed by HJR Wing, Denham 17, Oldfield B7].

Title page: THOMÆ | WILLIS | MED. DOCT. | OPERA OMNIA, | Nitidius quàm vnquam hactenus edita, plurimùm emendata, Indice | rerum copiofifsimo, ac diftinctione characterum exornata. | *Studio & Opera* | GERARDI BLASII, M. D. | Et in Illuft. Amftelæd. Gymnafio Prof. Publ. Bibliothecarij, &c. | *Hac tandem nouiffima Editione accuratiffimè recognita, ac exploita.* | EXCELLENTISSIMO DOMINO | ANTONIO MASTINI | MEDICORVM CORYPHÆO PRÆSTANTISSIMO | *DICATA.* | [printers' device: lettered FORTITVDO OMNIA VINCIT] | COLONIÆ, M. DC. XCIV. | [rule] | Sumptibus Gafparis Storti. | *CVM SVPERIORVM FACVLTATE.**

[19] Maurice Emott (Emmett) was born in London and matriculated at Merton College on 15 May 1691, aged 15. He was a student of the Inner Temple in the same year. Nothing is known of his subsequent career. He was the second son of Maurice Emmett, gentleman of St Margaret's parish, Westminster. *British History Online* suggests a connection with Maurice Emmett (d.1692) and his son Maurice (1646–1694), master brick builder mentioned in the Annals as having provided carving and brickwork for the Inner Temple, and Master Bricklayer to the Office of Works whose projects included building for Sir Christopher Wren at Hampton Court. These Emmetts are commemorated in a memorial on the north wall of St Margaret's church, Westminster, by William Emmett (nd), another brother who was a sculptor and woodcarver who had worked with Grinling Gibbons (1648–1721).

* Underlined text originally printed in red.

Collation: folio in 6s, 23 letter roman alphabet using I and V. †^{8}, A–Z^6, Aa^8, Bb–Zz^6, Aaa–Ddd^6. $1–3 signed apart from: Mm2 signed Nm2, Yy2 signed Vy2, Ccc3 signed Cc3. Also with *VVillis Tom. I.* or *VVillis Tom. II.* (footer, left) on all signed text sheets.

310 leaves, paginated as [16], 1–586, [18]. Mispaginated: 102 for 101. Illustrations all within the printed page apart from 3 additional leaves, unsigned, between Nn3 / Nn4, pages 430 / 431, and 4 additional leaves between Tt3 / Tt4, pages 502 / 503.

Type: ≤ 80 lines; height (20 lines) 70 millimetres, width 80 millimetres (each of two columns, together 165 millimetres, apart from preliminaries: 93 millimetres in each column with marginal notes, present to the left or right of the text).

Contents: **†1r**, page [1] [half title] THOMÆ WILLIS OPERA OMNIA.; **†1v**, page [2], blank; **†2r**, page [3] title; **†2v**, page [4], blank; **†3r–v**, page [5–6] EXCELLENTISSIME ET PRÆSTANTISSIME UIR, . . . [signed] *Excellentiſs.^{me} Dominat.^{nis} Tuæ* Venetijs die 15. Augusti 1694 *Deuinctiſs.^{mus} & Obſequentiſs.^{mus} Seruus* Gaſpar Storti.; **†4r**, page [7] GERARDUS BLASIUS LECTORI BENEUOLO *Salutem & Officia*,; **†4v**, page [8], portrait; **†5r–v**, pages [9–10] AVTHORIS VITA.

†6r, page [11] CONTENTA HVIVS OPERIS. I. Diatribæ duæ *de* FERMENTATIONE, *et* FEBRIBVS; *quibus acceſſit* Diſsertatio *de* VRINIS.; II. CEREBRI ANATOME, NERVORVMQUE DESCRIPTIO et VSVS.; III. *De* RATIONE MOTVS MVSCVLORVM ſtudio GVIELMI CROONE M.D. Londin. ac. Soc. Reg. Socij.; IV. PATHOLOGIÆ CEREBRI *et* NERVOSI GENERIS SPECIMEN, *in quo agitur de* MORBIS CONVVLSIVIS *et* SCORBVTO.; V. AFFECTIONVM *quæ dicuntur* HYSTERICAE *et* HYPOCHONDRIACAE PATHOLOGIA SPASMODICA VINDICATA, *contra* Reſponſionem Epiſtolarem NATHAN. HIGMORI M.D. *cui acceſserunt* Exercitationes Medico-Phyſicæ duæ. I. *De* SANGVINIS ACCENSIONE. II. *De* MOTV MVSCVLARI.; VI. *De* ANIMA BRVTORVM, *quæ* HOMINIS *Vitalis ac Senſitiva eſt*, Exercitationes duæ, *quarum* Prior PHYSIOLOGICA *eſt*, Altera PATHOLOGICA, *Morbos, qui* Ipſam, Cerebrum, *et* Neruoſum Genus *afficiunt, explicans*; VII. PHARMACEVTICE RATIONALIS, *ſiue* Diatriba *de* MEDICAMENTORVM OPERATIONIBVS *in* Humano Corpore.; VIII. PHARMACEVTICES RATIONALIS, *ſiue* Diatribæ *de* MEDICAMENTORVM OPERATIONIBVS *in* Humano Corpore Pars altera: *opus poſthumum*.; **†6v–†8r**, pages [12–15] ELENCHVS TOTIVS OPERIS.; **†8v**, page [16], AD TRACTATUM DE FERMENTATIONE PRÆFATIO.

A1r–C1v, pages 1–26, [text] DE FERMENTATIONE, SIUE DE MOTU CORPORUM NATURALIUM INORGANICO.

C2r–v, pages 27–28, DE FEBRIBUS PRÆFATIO.

C2v–H3v, pages 28–90, [text] [De Febribus].

H4r–v, pages 91–2, DE URINIS, DISSERTATIO EPISTOLICA. *Ad Virum Doctiſsimum mihique amiciſsimum*, D. RODULPHUM BATHURST, Med. Doct. & Colleg. Sacroſanctæ Trinitatis Oxon. Socium.; **H4v–I3v**, pages 92–102, [text] [De urinis]

I4r–I4v, page 103–4, CEREBRI ANATOME, CVI ACCESSIT NERUORVM DESCRIPTIO ET USVS. PRÆFATIO.; **I3v–N3r**, pages 104–49, [text] [Cerebri Anatome].

N3r–P6v, pages 149–180, [text] NERUORVM DESCRIPTIO ET USVS.

Q1r–Q4v, pages 181–8, DE RATIONE MOTVS MUSCULORUM; Studio GVLIELMI CROONE, M. D. è Coll. Med. Lond. ac Societatis Regalis Socii. *Ἐν πᾶσι τοῖς φυσικοῖς ἐνεστί τι θαυμαστόν. Ariſt. de Part. Animal.*

Q5r–v, pages 189–90, PATHOLOGIÆ CEREBRI, ET NERVOSI GENERIS SPECIMEN: In quo agitur de MORBIS CONVULSIVIS, & de SCORBUTO. PRÆFATIO.; **Q5v–V6v**, pages 190–240, [text] [De morbis convulsivis]; **X1r–Z1v**, pages 241–66, [text] TRACTATVS DE SCORBUTO.

Z2r, page 267, AFFECTIONUM HYSTERICARUM ET HYPOCHONDRIACARUM PATHOLOGIA SPASMODICA VINDICATA; Contra Reſponſionem Epiſtolarem NATHANAELIS HIGHMORI M.D. *Cui acceſſerunt Exercitationes duæ Medico-Phyſicæ. I. De Sanguinis Accenſione. II. De Motu Muſculari.* PRÆFATIO.; **Z2v–Aa1r**, page 268–77, AD VIRVM DOCTISSIMVM NATHANAEL HIGHMORUM M.D., [text] [Affectionum hystericarum etc.]; **Aa1r–Aa3v**, pages 277–82, EXERCITATIO PRIMA MEDICO-PHYSICA. *De Sanguinis Incaleſcentia, ſive Accenſione.*; **Aa4r–Aa8v**, pages 283–92, EXERCITATIO SECVNDA MEDICO-PHYSICA. *De Motu Muſculari.*

Bb1r, page 293, [half title] THOMÆ WILLIS OPERUM MEDICO-PHYSICORUM TOMVS SECVNDVS: *CONTINENS* De Anima Brutorum Exercitationes duas, Pharmaceuticæ Rationalis Partes duas.; **Bb1v**, page 294, blank; **Bb2r–v**, pages 295–6, PRÆFATIO AD LECTOREM.

Bb3r–Ff6v, pages 297–352, [text] DE ANIMA BRUTORUM.; **Gg1r–Mm4v**, pages 353–420, DE ANIMA BRVTORVM PARS SECVNDA, PATHOLOGICA, *SIVE* DE MORBIS Qui ad Animam Corpoream, euiſque ſubjecta, ſcilicet Cerebrum & Genus Neruoſum, ſpectant.

Mm5r–v, pages 421–2, PHARMACEUTICE RATIONALIS, Siue Diatriba de Medicamentorum operationibus in Corpore Humano. PARS PRIMA. PRÆFATIO.; **Mm5v–Ss5v**, pages 422–94, [text] [Pharmaceutice Rationalis, part 1]; **Ss6r–v**, pages 495–6, PHARMACEUTICES RATIONALIS, Siue Diatriba de Medicamentorum operationibus in Corpore Humano, PARS SECVNDA. OPVS POSTHVMVM. PRÆFATIO.; **Ss6v–'Cc'3v**, pages 496–586, [text] [Pharmaceutice Rationalis, part 2].

Ccc4r–Ddd6r, pages [1–17], INDEX ALPHABETICVS RERVM ET UERBORVM, quæ in toto hoc Opere occurrunt, notabilium.; **Ddd6v**, blank.

Headlines and *Catchwords*: (these normally identify the next section or chapter when the number changes on a given page): Caput II. for Caput III. at **A3r**, page 5; Caput IV. for Caput V. at **A4r**, page 7; Caput V. for Caput VI. at **A5r**, page 9; Caput VII. for Caput VIII. at **B1r**, page 13; Caput I. for Caput II. at **C4r**, page 31; Caput II. for Caput III. at **C5r**, page 33; Caput V. for Caput VI. at **D3r**, page 41; Caput XI. for Caput XII. at **E6r**, page 59; Caput II. for Caput III. at **H5r**, page 93; CAPUT IV. for CAPUT VI. in chapter title at **I2v**, page 100; Caput V. for Caput VI. at **K6r**, page 119; Caput IX. for Caput XI. at **L5r**, page 129; Caput III. for Caput IV. at **X5r**, page 249; Caput VIII. for Caput IX. at **Dd6r**, page 327; Caput II. for Caput III. at **Ff6r**, page 363; Caput III. for Caput IV. at **Hh2r**, page 367; Caput X. for Caput XI. at **Kk4r**, page 395;

De Arthritide for De Passione Colica at **Mm4v**, page 420; Cap. I for Cap. II. at **Mm6r**, page 423; Cap. I. for Cap. II. at **Nn6r**, page 435; Cap. I. for Cap. II. at **Oo5r**, page 445; Cap. II. for Cap. II at **Qq5r**, page 469; Cap. VI. for Cap. VII. at **Xx1r**, page 521; Cap. IX. for Cap. X. at **Yy1r**, page 533; Cap. X. for Cap. XI. at **Yy2r**, page 535; Cap. XI. for Cap. XII. at **Yy3r**, page 537; Cap. XII. for Cap. XIII. at **Yy5r**, page 541; Sectio I. Cap. XIII. for Sectio II. Cap. I. at **Yy6r**, page 543; Cap. VI. for Cap. IV. at **Aaa1r**, page 557; Cap. I. for Cap. II. at **Aaa6r**, page 567.

No catchword at **†3v** / **†4r**, page [6] / [7]; pedi- for Peditant at **E1v** / **E2r**, pages 50 / 51; quę for quæ at **Bb4v** / **Cc1r**, pages 304 / 305; caufæ for caufę at **ee3v** / **Ee4r**, pages 338 / 339; sit for fit at **Ee4r** / **v**, pages 339 / 340; ricæ for ricę at **Ff1r** / **v**, pages 341 / 342; IN for PHARMACEUTICE at **Mm4v** / **Mm5r**, pages 420 / 421; cęteras for cæteras at **Mm4v** / **Nnr1**, pages 426 / 427; hęc for hæc at **Qq2v** / **Qq3r**, pages 464 / 465; **Xx4r** / **v**, pages 527 / 528; gręnæ for gręnę at **Aaa3r** / **v**, pages 561 / 562.

Frontispiece: none.

Portrait: **Pt.1g1**: THOMAS WILLIS MEDIC. PROFESSOR. COLLEGII MED. LONDIN. ET SOCIET. REG. SOCI.VS, *suor Isabella Piccini Scolpì*, ÆTATIS SVÆ. 45. 327 × 212 millimetres (sheet); 262 × 171 millimetres (plate marks); 258 × 167 millimetres (image); see: Figure 151.

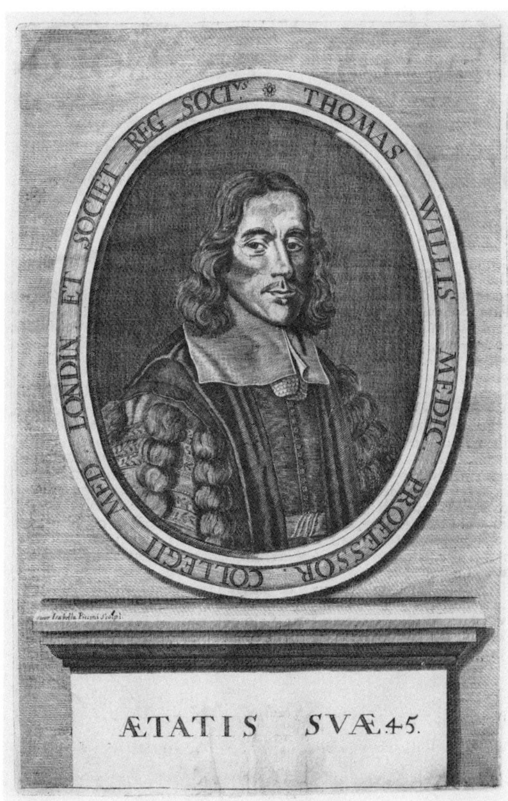

Figure 151 Portrait of Thomas Willis engraved by Isabella Piccini: *Opera Omnia*, Coloniæ, 1694 (Pt.1g1).

Printers' ornaments: printers' device at **†2r**, page [3] {**Storti 1**}; tailpiece at **†4r**, page [7]; **C1v**, page 26 {**Storti 4**}; **†5v**, page [10], **I3v**, page 102; **P2r**, page 171; **Ss5v**, page 494 {**Storti 6**}; **†6r**, page [11]; **Nn3r**, page 429 {**Storti 7**}; **†8r**, page [15] {**Storti 9**}; **†8v**, page [16] {**Storti 11**}; headpiece at **A1r**, page 1 {**Storti 12**}; tailpiece at **H3v**, page 90; **Mm4v**, page 420 {**Storti 14**}; **P4r**, page 175; **Ddd6r**, page [17] {**Storti 17**}; 16 fleurons arranged in squares to make 4 repeating blocks at **V6v**, page 240; **Z1v**, page 266; **Aa3v**, page 282; **Aa7v**, page 290; **Bb2v**, page 296 {**Storti 20**}; tailpiece at **Aa8v**, page 292; **Cc[c]3v**, page 586 {**Storti 24**}; headpiece at **Bb2r**, page 295; **Bb3r**, page 297 {**Storti 25**}.

Decorated C at **†3r**, page [5] {**Storti 2**}; S at **†4r**, page [7] {**Storti 3**}; T at **†5r**, page [9] {**Storti 5**}; C at **†6v**, page [12] {**Storti 8**}; D at **1π2v**, page [16]; **C2r**, page 27 {**Storti 10**}; I at **A1r**, page 1 {**Storti 13**}; O at **H4r**, page 91 {**Storti 15**}; A at **I4r**, page 103; **Ss6r**, page 495 {**Storti 16**}; D at **Q1r**, page 181 {**Storti 18**}; Q at **Q5r**, page 189; **Z2r**, page 267; **Mm5r**, page 421 {**Storti 19**}; I at **X1r**, page 241; **Aa1r**, page 277; **Ss6v**, page 496 {**Storti 21**}; R at **Z2v**, page 268 {**Storti 22**}; C at **Aa4r**, page 283 {**Storti 23**}; E at **Bb2r**, page 295 {**Storti 26**}; Q at **Bb3r**, page 297 {**Storti 27**}; A at **Mm5v**, page 422; **Ccc4r**, page [1] {**Storti 28**}.

Illustrations: lettering and legends as in **2A**, **2C**, **4A**, **5A**, **6A**, and **6E**. All illustrations apart from the seven added sheets (leaf size) in *Pharmaceutice rationalis* parts 1 and 2 are on the printed page which measures 327 × 212 millimetres; registration is not perfect with illustrations occasionally overlapping the text.

Pl.1g1. Plate 1 (image 1): *Fig: I* (headline, centre), *Pag: 108* (headline, right). 195 × 165 millimetres (plate marks); 183 × 160 millimetres (figure). Printed on **I6v**, page 108.

Pl.2g1. Plate 2 (image 2): Fig. II.$^{da.}$ (headline, centre), *Cerebri anat. Pag. 109.* (headline, right). 143 × 100 millimetres (plate marks); 132 × 98 millimetres (figure). Printed on **K1r**, page 109.

Pl.3g1. Plate 3 (image 3): *Fig. III* (headline, centre), *Pag. 113.* (headline, right).[20] 196 × 177 millimetres (plate marks); 190 × 168 millimetres (figure). Printed on **K3r**, page 113.

Pl.4g1. Plate 4 (image 4): *Fig. IV.* (headline, centre), *Pag. 114.* (headline, right). 120 × 95 millimetres (plate marks); 115 × 92 millimetres (figure). Printed on **K3v**, page 114.

Pl.5g1. Plate 5 (image 5): *Fig. V.* (headline, left), *Cerebri anat. Pag. 116.* (headline, right). 182 × 134 millimetres (plate marks); 179 × 129 millimetres (figure). Printed on **K4v**, page 116.

Pl.6g1. Plate 6 (image 6): *Fig. VI.* (headline, centre), *Cerebri anat. Pag. 117.* (headline, right). 175 × 135 millimetres (plate marks); 170 × 125 millimetres (figure). Printed on **K5r**, page 117.

Pl.7g1. Plate 7 (images 7–10): [Unnumbered 1] *Cerebri anat.* (headline, left), *Pag. 124.* (headline, right), *Fig. 1*, *Fig. 11*, *Fig. 111.* (header, above each image), *Fig. 1111* (header, right of the image). 142 × 102 millimetres (plate marks); 24 × 93 millimetres, 75 × 92 millimetres, 36 × 22 millimetres, 72 × 25 millimetres (figures). Printed on **L2v**, page 124.

[20] The registration of Figura III in the three copies examined for this bibliography differs. It is shifted upwards in the copy used for the description, leaving 'Pag. 113' buried in the last line of the legend.

Pl.8g1. Plate 8 (image 11): *Fig* VII^{a} (headline, left), *Cerebri anat. Pag. 128.* (headline, right). 195 × 98 millimetres (plate marks); 190 × 95 millimetres (figure). Printed on **L4v**, page 128.

Pl.9g1. Plate 9 (image 12): *Cerebri anat.* (headline, left), *Fig.* VIII (headline, centre), *Pag. 133.* (headline, right). 119 × 92 millimetres (plate marks); 110 × 91 millimetres (figure). Printed on **M1r**, page 133.

Pl.10g1. Plate 10 (images 13–14): [Unnumbered 2] Fig. I. (headline, left), *Cerebri anat. Pag. 153.* (headline, centre), Fig. II. (headline, right). 130 × 175 millimetres (plate marks); 122 × 108 millimetres, 110 × 48 millimetres (orientated horizontally with lettering adjusted) (figures). Printed on **N5r**, page 153.

Pl.11g1. Plate 11 (image 15): *Cerebri anat. Pag. 172* (headline, centre), *Tabula IX*^{a} (headline, right). 268 × 173 millimetres (plate marks); 270 × 150 millimetres (figure). Printed on **P2v**, page 172.

Pl.12g1. Plate 12 (image 16): *Cerebri anat. Pag. 174* (headline, centre), *Tabula X.*^{ma} (headline, right). 280 × 190 millimetres (plate marks); 270 × 180 millimetres (figure). Printed on **P3v**, page 174.

Pl.13g1. Plate 13 (image 17): *Cerebri anat. Pag. 176* (headline, right), *Tabula X1.*^{ma} (footer, right). 280 × 140 millimetres (plate marks); 273 × 125 millimetres (figure). Printed on **P4v**, page 176.

Pl.14g1. Plate 14 (image 18): *Cerebri anat. Pag. 178* (headline, centre), *Tabula XII.* (headline, right). 221 × 72 millimetres (plate marks); 216 × 36 millimetres (figure). Printed on **P5v**, page 178.

Pl.15g1. Plate 15 (images 19–23): (1) *Pag. 179* (headline, centre), Tab. XIII. (headline, right), *Fig. I.*^{ma} (header, above the image), *Fig. 2.*^{da} (header, within the image). 166 × 170 millimetres (plate marks); 161 × 76 and 165 × 62 millimetres (figures). Printed on **P6r**, page 179. (2) *Pag. 180* (headline, right), *Fig 3.*$^{tia.}$, *Fig. 5.*^{ta}, *Fig. 4.*^{ta} (headers, above each image). 287 × 96 millimetres (plate marks); 280 × 29 millimetres, 74 × 23, 267 × 33 millimetres (Figures). Printed on **P6v**, page 180.

Pl.16d1. Plate 16 (images 24–25) *Pag. 188* (headline, left), *Fig 2, Fig 1* (header, above each image). 141 × 150 millimetres (plate marks); 109 × 64 millimetres, 122 × 46 millimetres (figures). Printed on **Q4v**, page 188.

Pl.17g1. Plate 17 (images 26–27) with **Pl.18g1**. Plate 18 (images 28–29): *De affect hyster.* (headline, left), *Pag.* [291] (headline right), *Fig. I.*, *Fig. II.*, *Fig. III.*, *Fig. IV.* (headers, above each image). 188 × 168 millimetres (plate marks); 27 × 135 millimetres, 45 × 148 millimetres, 30 × 148 millimetres, 41 × 158 millimetres (figures). Printed on **Aa8r**, page 291.

Pl.19f1. Plate 19 (images 30–33): *de anima brut. Pag. 307* (headline, centre), *Tab. I.*^{a} (headline, right), *Fig. I.*^{a}, *Fig. II.*^{da}, *Fig. IIII.*^{ta}, *Fig. III.*^{tia} (headers, above each image). 194 × 148 millimetres (plate marks); 47 × 25 millimetres, 118 × 84 millimetres, 111 × 15 millimetres, 75 × 103 millimetres (figures). Printed on **Cc2r**, page 307.

Pl.20f1. Plate 20 (images 34–35): *Tab. II.^{da}* (headline, centre), *de anima brut. Pag. 308* (headline, right), *Fig. I^{a}*, *Fig. II^{da}* (header, above each image). 143 × 185 millimetres (plate marks); 104 × 82 millimetres and 129 × 83 millimetres (figures). Printed on **Cc2v**, page 308.

Pl.21f1. Plate 21 (images 36–38): *Tab. III.^{tia}* (headline, centre), *de anim brut. pag. 309* (headline, right), *Figura. 1ma*, *Fig. II.^{da}*, *Fig. III.^{tia}* (header, above each image): 239 × 153 millimetres (plate marks) 238 × 100 millimetres, 119 × 85 millimetres, 38 × 16 millimetres (figures). Printed on **Cc3r**, page 309.

Pl.22f1. Plate 22 (images 39–41): *de anima bru. Page 310.* (headline, centre), *Tab. IV.* (headline, right), *Fig. I.^{ma}*, *Fig II.^{da}*, *Fig. III.^{tia}* (headers, above each image). 170 × 92 millimetres (plate marks); 156 × 42 millimetres, 44 × 16 millimetres, 162 × 18 millimetres (figures). Printed on **Cc3v**, page 310.

Pl.23f1. Plate 23 (image 42): *de anima brut. Pag 314.* (headline, left and centre), *Tab.V.* (headline right). 156 × 96 millimetres (plate marks); 154 × 94 millimetres (figure). Printed on **Cc5v**, page 314.

Pl.24f1. Plate 24 (image 43): *de Anima Brut. Pag. 315* (headline, left), *Tab. VI.* (headline, right). 129 × 86 millimetres (plate marks); 126 × 85 millimetres (figure). Printed on **Cc4r**, page 315.

Pl.25f1. Plate 25 (image 44): *de anima brut. Pag. 315* (headline, left), *Tab. VII.* (headline right). 124 × 112 millimetres (plate marks); 116 × 101 millimetres (figure). Printed on **Cc4r**, page 315.

Pl.26f1. Plate 26 (image 45): *de anima brut. Pag. 324.* (headline, left), *Tab. VIII.* (headline, right). 147 × 180 millimetres (plate marks); 143 × 167 millimetres (figure). Printed on **Dd4v**, page 324.

Pl.27g1. Plate 27 (image 46): *Pharmac. Pag. 430* (headline, right), *Tab.* I. (headline, centre). 286 × 184 millimetres (plate marks); 148 × 168 millimetres (figure); with **Pl.28g1**. Plate 28 (image 47): *Tab.* II. (headline, centre). 125 × 159 millimetres (figure). Inserted after legends for Tabulæ I–VI at **Nn3v**, page 430.

Pl.29g1. Plate 29 (image 48): *Pharmac. Pag. 430.* (headline, left), *Tab.* III. (headline, centre). 294 × 200 millimetres (plate marks); 141 × 171 millimetres (figure); with **Pl.30g1**. Plate 30 (image 49–51): *Tab.* IV. (headline, left), *Fig. 2.*, *Fig. 3.*, *Fig. I.* (headers, above each image). 47 × 52 millimetres, 60 × 50 millimetres, 138 × 152 millimetres (figures). Inserted after legends for Tabulæ I–VI at **Nn3v**, page 430.

Pl.31g1. Plate 31 (image 52): *Pharmac. Pag. 430* (headline, right), *Tab. V.* (headline, centre). 272 × 174 millimetres (plate marks); 142 × 152 millimetres (figure); with **Pl.32g1**. Plate 32 (images 53–57): *Tab.* VI. (headline, centre). 112 × 23 millimetres, 112 × 22 millimetres, 112 × 22 millimetres, 113 × 22 millimetres, 110 × 21 millimetres (figures). Inserted after legends for Tabulæ I–VI at **Nn3v**, page 430.

Pl.33g1. Plate 33 (image 58): *Pharmaceutic. Pag. 503.* (headline, left), *Tab: I.* (headline, right). 285 × 190 millimetres (plate marks); 92 × 176 millimetres (figure); with **Pl.34g1**. Plate 34 (image 59): *Tab: II.* (headline, left). 184 × 120 millimetres (figure). Inserted before legend at **Tt4r–v**, pages 503–4.

Pl.35g1. Plate 35 (images 60–61): *Tab: III.* (headline, left), *Pharmac. Pag.ª 503.* (headline, right), *Fig: 2*, *Fig: 1* (headers, left of each image). 280 × 165 millimetres (plate marks); 177 × 130 millimetres, 44 × 25 millimetres (figures); with **Pl.36g1**. Plate 36 (images 62–64): *Tab. IV.* (headline, centre), *Fig: 1.*, *Fig: 2.*, *Fig: 3* (headers, left of each image). 67 × 40 millimetres, 57 × 33 millimetres, 61 × 34 millimetres (figures). Inserted before legend at **Tt4r–v**, pages 503–4.

Pl.37g1. Plate 37 (images 65–67): *Pharmac. Pag.ª 503.* (headline, centre), *Tab: V.* (headline, right), *Fig: 2.*, *Fig: 1.*, *Fig: 3.* (headers, left of each image). 240 × 180 millimetres (plate marks); 75 × 88 millimetres, 75 × 66 millimetres, 135 × 153 millimetres (figures). Inserted before legend at **Tt4r–v**, pages 503–4.

Pl.38g1. Plate 38 (images 68–75): *Pharmac.* (headline, left), *Tab: VI.* (headline, centre), *Pag. 503.* (headline, right), *Fig: 1.* (header, right above the top group of four inages), *Fig: 2.* (header, centre above the second group of four images). 288 × 200 millimetres (plate marks); 68 × 47 millimetres, 67 × 46 millimetres, 68 × 48 millimetres, 65 × 48 millimetres, 70 × 17 millimetres, 70 × 17 millimetres, 72 × 17 millimetres, 72 × 17 millimetres (figures); with **Pl.39g1**. Plate 39 (images 76–79): *Tab: VII.* (headline, centre), *Fig: 3.*, *Fig: 1.*, *Fig: 2.*, *Fig: 4.* (headers, above each image). 57 × 55 millimetres, 56 × 54 millimetres, 55 × 47 millimetres, 60 × 59 millimetres; with **Pl.40g1**. Plate 40 (images 80–82): *Tab: VIII.* (headline, centre), *Fig: 1.*, *Fig: 2.*, *Fig: 3.* (headers, above each image). 53 × 50 millimetres, 29 × 27 millimetres, 53 × 49 millimetres (figures). Inserted before legend at **Tt4r–v**, pages 503–4.

Copy: DASC (#1 of 3). Original vellum, spine lettered Willis Opera Medica, original endpapers. Leaves 322 × 222 millimetres, boards 326 × 220 × 53 millimetres. Book label: Prof. Dr. Vincenzo Gallucci (1935–1991), with presentation letter from Professor Giancarlo Leoncilli Massi, Spoleto, February 1985.[21]

8G. OPERA OMNIA, Coloniæ Allobrogum quarto 1695

Seventh edition of the collected works of Thomas Willis in Latin, the eighth book, with William Croone's treatise, the only Latin translation of *A plain and easie method* (see: Figure 152), the type reset and using different printers' ornaments but retaining the same format as the third and fourth editions [HJR Wing 50, Denham 18, Oldfield B5].

[21] This edition is omitted by HJR Wing (1962). Denham (1965): page 98, #17, concludes that 'The rarity of the 1694 edition today suggests that it met with an indifferent reception from the contemporary medical public'. Of the three copies considered for this bibliography, one was bought from Japan and two from Italian collections. Vincenzo Maria Gallucci (1935–1991) was an Italian cardiac surgeon based in Padua who, in 1978, carried out the first heart transplant in Italy declaring his frustration at the bureaucratic delays in gaining permission for the procedure: 'heart transplantation is not a difficult operation, it requires a commitment of two, three hours at most . . . Despite the apparent calm, the whole hospital knows that something fantastic is about to happen. . . . an inevitable, though exhausting, passage towards history. God wants it. He masterfully embedded the building blocks of life'. Professor Gallucci died in a road traffic accident returning from operating in Milan. Giancarlo Leoncilli Massi (1938–2007) was professor of architecture at the University of Florence.

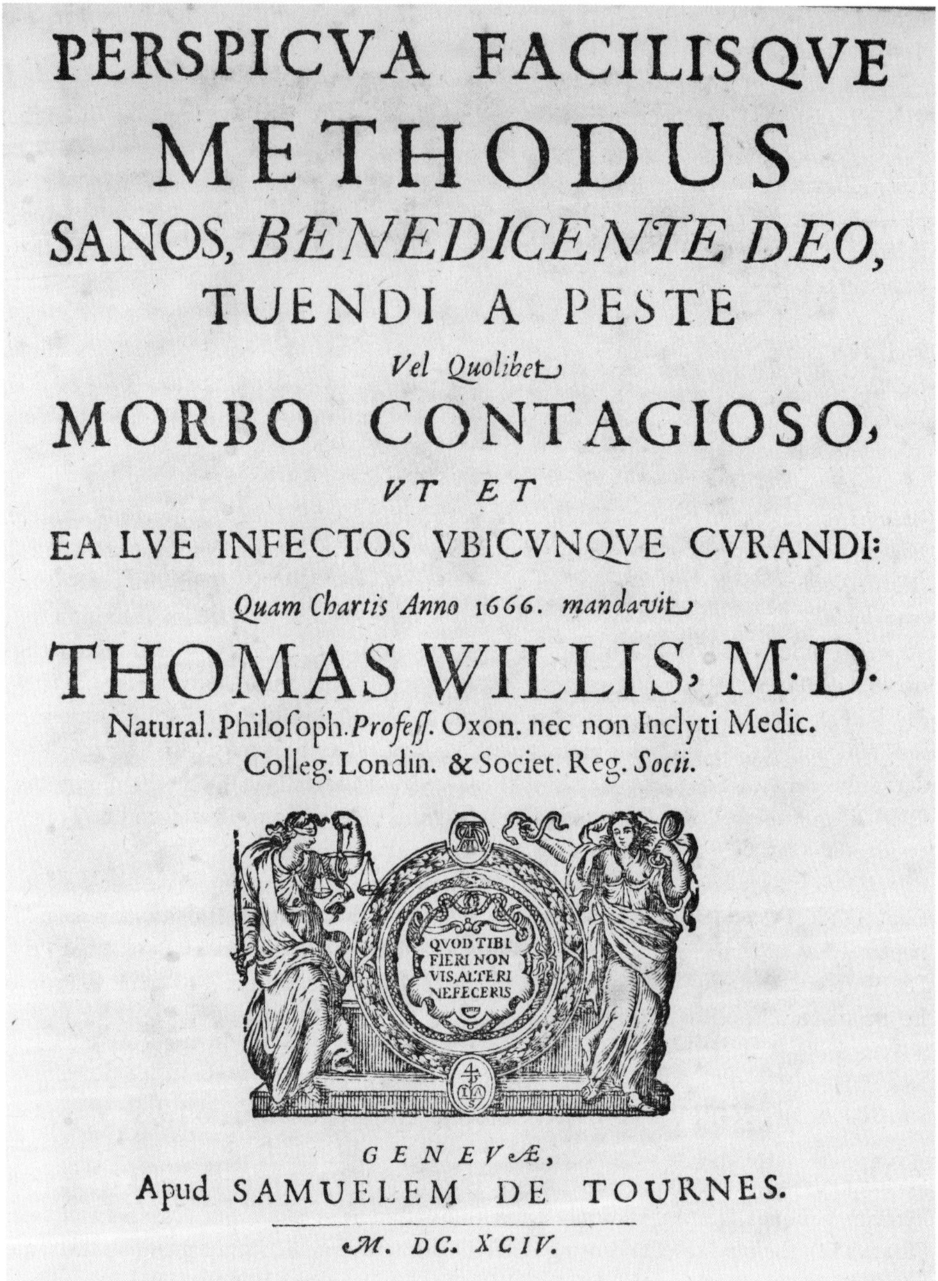

PERSPICVA FACILISQVE
METHODUS
SANOS, *BENEDICENTE DEO,*
TUENDI A PESTE
Vel Quolibet
MORBO CONTAGIOSO,
VT ET
EA LVE INFECTOS VBICVNQVE CVRANDI:
Quam Chartis Anno 1666. mandavit
THOMAS WILLIS, M.D.
Natural. Philosoph. *Profess.* Oxon. nec non Inclyti Medic.
Colleg. Londin. & Societ. Reg. *Socii.*

GENEVÆ,
Apud SAMUELEM DE TOURNES.

M. DC. XCIV.

Figure 152 Title page of the only translation into Latin of 'A plain and easie method' in *Opera Omnia*: Geneva, 1694.

Title page: Volume I: [1a]. THOMÆ | WILLIS | MEDICINÆ DOCTORIS, | NATURALIS PHILOSOPHIÆ | PROFESSORIS OXONIENSIS, | *Nec non* | INCLYTI MEDICORVM COLLEGII | Londinensis, & SOCIETATIS REGIÆ Socii, | OPERA OMNIA. | EDITIO NOVA Emendatior & TRACTATU DE PESTE Auctior. | TOMVS PRIMVS. | *Cum*

ELENCHIS RERUM & INDICIBUS *Neceſſariis, ut & multis* FIGURIS *Æneis.* | [printers' device: lettered, QUOD TIBI | FIERI NON | VIS, ALTERI | NEFECERIS] | *COLONIÆ ALLOBROGVM,* | Apud SAMUELEM DE TOURNES. | [short rule] | *M. DC. XCV.* | Cum Privilegio S.CÆSAREÆ MAIESTATIS.*

[1b]. DIATRIBÆ DUÆ | MEDICO-PHILOSOPHICÆ | *Quarum PRIOR agit* | DE FERMENTATIONE, | Sive de MOTU Inteſtino Particularum in quovis Corpore; | *POSTERIOR* | DE FEBRIBUS, | Sive de MOTU earundem in Sanguine Animalium | *His acceſſit* | DISSERTATIO EPISTOLICA *De* VRINIS. | *Studio* | THOMÆ WILLIS, M.D. | Natural. Philoſoph. *Profeſſ.* Oxon. nec non Inclyti Medic. | Colleg. Londin. & Societ Reg. *Socii.* | [printers' device: lettered, QUOD TIBI | FIERI NON | VIS, ALTERI | NEFECERIS] | *GENEVÆ,* | Apud SAMUELEM DE TOURNES. | [short rule] | *M. DC. XCIV.*

[2]. CEREBRI | ANATOME | NERVORVMQUE | DESCRIPTIO ET VSVS. | *Studio* | THOMÆ WILLIS, M. D. | Natural. Philoſoph. *Profeſſ.* Oxon. nec non Inclyti Medic. | Colleg. Londin. & Societ Reg. *Socii.* | *Acceſsit* VIRI *cujuſdam Clariſsimi* | *De* | RATIONE MOTVS MVSCVLORUM | *Tractatus Singularis.* | [printers' device: lettered, QUOD TIBI | FIERI NON | VIS, ALTERI | NEFECERIS] | *GENEVÆ,* | Apud SAMUELEM DE TOURNES. | [short rule] | *M. DC. XCIV.*

[3]. PATHOLOGIÆ | CEREBRI | *ET* | NERVOSI GENERIS | SPECIMEN. | *In quo agitur* | De Morbis Convulſivis, & de Scorbuto. | *Studio* | THOMÆ WILLIS, M.D. | Natural. Philoſoph. *Profeſſ.* Oxon. nec non Inclyti Medic. | Colleg. Londin. & Societatis. Regiæ *Socii.* | [printers' device: lettered, QUOD TIBI | FIERI NON | VIS, ALTERI | NEFECERIS] | *GENEVÆ,* | Apud SAMUELEM DE TOURNES. | [short rule] | *M. DC. XCIV.*

[4]. AFFECTIONUM | *Quæ dicuntur* | HYSTERICÆ | ET HYPOCHONDRIACÆ | PATHOLOGIA SPASMOCIA VINDICATA, | *Contra Reſponſionem Epiſtolarem* NATH. HIGHMORI *M. D.* | Cui acceſſerunt Exercitationes Medico-Phyſicæ Duæ. | I. *De* SANGUINIS ACCENSIONE. | II *De* MOTU MUSCULARI. | *Studio* | THOMÆ WILLIS, M. D. | Natural. Philoſoph. *Profeſſ.* Oxon. nec non Inclyti Medic. | Colleg. Londin. & Societatis Regiæ *Socii.* | [printers' device: lettered, QUOD TIBI | FIERI NON | VIS, ALTERI | NEFECERIS] | *GENEVÆ,* | Apud SAMUELEM DE TOURNES. | [short rule] | *M. DC. XCIV.*

[Volume 2] [1a]. THOMÆ | WILLIS | MEDICINÆ DOCTORIS, | NATURALIS PHILOSOPHIÆ | PROFESSORIS OXONIENSIS, | *Nec non* | INCLYTI MEDICORVM COLLEGII | Londinenſis, & SOCIETATIS REGIÆ Socii, | OPERA OMNIA. | EDITIO NOVA Emendatior & TRACTATU DE PESTE Auctior | TOMVS SECUNDVS. | Cum ELENCHIS RERUM & INDICIBUS *Neceſſariis, ut & multis* FIGURIS *Æneis.* | [printers' device: lettered, QUOD TIBI | FIERI NON | VIS, ALTERI | NEFECERIS] | *GENEVÆ,* | Apud SAMUELEM DE TOURNES. | [short rule] | *M. DC. XCV.* | Cum Privilegio S.CÆSAREÆ MAIESTATIS.

* Underlined text originally printed in red.

[1b]. DE ANIMA | BRUTORUM | *Quæ* HOMINIS *Uitalis ac Senſitava eſt,* | EXERCITATIONES DVÆ, | PRIOR PHYSIOLOGICA | *Ejuſdem* Naturam, Partes, Potentias & Affectiones *tradit*; | ALTERA PATHOLOGICA | Morbos qui ipſam & Sedem ejus Primariam, | *Nempe* CEREBRUM *&* NERVOSUM GENUS *afficiunt, explicitat; eorumque* | *Therapeias inſtituit. Cum Figuris æneis.* | STUDIO | THOMÆ WILLIS, M. D. | Natural. Philoſoph. *Profeſſ.* Oxon. nec non Inclyti Medic. | Colleg. Londin. & Societatis Regiæ *Socii.* | [printers' device: lettered, QUOD TIBI | FIERI NON | VIS, ALTERI | NEFECERIS] | *GENEVÆ,* | Apud SAMUELEM DE TOURNES. | [short rule] | *M. DC. XCV.*

[2]. PHARMACEUTICE | RATIONALIS: | *Sive* | DIATRIBA | *De* | MEDICAMENTORUM | OPERATIONIBUS | In Humano CORPORE: | *Studio* | THOMÆ WILLIS, M. D. | Natural. Philoſoph. *Profeſſ.* Oxon. nec non Inclyti Medic. | Colleg. Londin. & Societatis Regiæ *Socii.* | [printers' device: lettered, QUOD TIBI | FIERI NON | VIS, ALTERI | NEFECERIS] | *GENEVÆ,* | Apud SAMUELEM DE TOURNES. | [short rule] | *M. DC. XCIV.*

[3]. PHARMACEUTICES | RATIONALIS | *Sive* | DIATRIBÆ, | *De* | MEDICAMENTORUM | OPERATIONIBUS | In Humano CORPORE, | PARS SECUNDA. | *Opus Poſthumum* | THOMÆ WILLIS, M. D. | Natural. Philoſoph. *Profeſſ.* Oxon. nec non Inclyti Medic. | Colleg. Londin. & Societatis Regiæ *Socii.* | [printers' device: lettered, QUOD TIBI | FIERI NON | VIS, ALTERI | NEFECERIS] | *GENEVÆ,* | Apud SAMUELEM DE TOURNES. | [short rule] | *M. DC. XCIV.*

[4]. PERSPICVA FACILISQVE | METHODUS | SANOS, *BENEDICENTE DEO,* | TUENDI A PESTE | *Vel Quolibet* | MORBO CONTAGIOSO, | *VT ET* | EA LVE INFECTOS VBICVNQVE CVRANDI: | *Quam Chartis Anno* 1666. *mandavit* | THOMAS WILLIS, M.D. | Natural. Phil*oſoph. Profeſſ.* Oxon. nec non Inclyti Medic. | Colleg. Londin. & Societ. Reg. *Socii.* | [printers' device: lettered, QUOD TIBI | FIERI NON | VIS, ALTERI | NEFECERIS] | *GENEVÆ,* | Apud SAMUELEM DE TOURNES. | [short rule] | *M. DC. XCIV.*

Collation: quarto, 23 letter roman alphabet using i and u, ſ, and *V* and V. Volume 1: [1]. $+^4$, $++^2$, §–$§§^4$, $§§§^2$, a–z^4, aa–ii^4; \$1–3 signed apart from: cc2 signed Cc2.
144 leaves, paginated as [32], 1–254, [2]. Mispaginated: 132 for 130, 166 for 196.

[2]. ¶^{4}, ¶¶^{4}, A–Z^4, Aa–Bb^4; \$1–3 signed.
108 leaves, paginated as [16], 1–176, [1]–22, [2]. Mispaginated: 10 for 101, 107^s for 107.

[3]. *–$**^4$; *A–*Z^4, *Aa–*Dd^4; \$1–3 signed apart from: *I3 signed I3.
116 leaves, paginated as [16], 1–214, [2]. Mispaginated: 19 for 9, 31 for 11.

[4]. $§^2$, a–h^4, i^2; \$1–3 signed.
36 leaves, paginated as [4], 1–63, [5].

Volume 2: [5]. †–††††^{4}, *a*–*z*^{4}, *aa*–*uu*^{4}; \$1–3 signed apart from *Z*1 for *z*1, and *Z*3 for *z*3.
188 leaves, paginated as [32] 1–333 [1–11]. Mispaginated: 239 for 329.

[6]. (*)–(**)^4, *A*–*Z*^{4}, *Aa*–*Cc*^{4}; \$1–3 signed.
112 leaves, paginated as [16], 1–204, [4]: page 83 not paginated.

[7]. ¶–¶¶¶^{4}, A–Z^4, Aa–Ll^4; $1–3 signed apart from: PARS II added to numerical signing at G1r, M1r, N1r, O1r, P1r, Q1r, S1r, X1r, Z1r, Ee1r, Gg1r, Hh1r and Kk1r.
148 leaves, paginated as [24], 1–266, [6]. Mispaginated: 17 for 14, 179 for 197.

[8]. A–B^4, C^2; $1–3 signed.
10 leaves, paginated as 1–19, [1].

Type: 43 lines; height (20 lines) 82 millimetres, width 119 millimetres (126 millimetres with marginal notes).

Contents: Volume 1. [1]: +**1r**, page [1], title; +**1v**, page [2], blank; +**2r–v**, pages [3–4], TYPOGRAPHVS LECTORI *SALUTEM*.; +**3r**, page [5], CONTENTA TOTIUS OPERIS. TOM. PRIM. I. Diatribæ duæ Medico Philoſophicæ, *quarum* Prior *agit de* FERMENTATIONE, Altera *de* FEBRIBUS; *quibus acceſſit* Diſſertatio *de* URINIS. II. CEREBRI ANATOME, NERVORUMQUE DESCRIPTIO *&* USUS; *quibus acceſſit* VIRI *cujuſdam Clariſſimi* De RATIONE MOTUS MUSCULORUM Tractatus Singularis. III. PATHOLOGIÆ CEREBRI & NERVOSI GENERIS SPECIMEN, *in quo agitur de* MORBIS CONVULSIVIS *& de* SCORBUTO.; IV. AFFECTIONUM *quæ dicuntur* HYSTERICÆ *&* HYPOCHONDRIACÆ PATHOLOGIA SPASMODICA VINDICATA, *contra* Reſponſionem Epiſtolarem NATHAN. HIGHMORI M.D. *cui acceſſerunt* Exercitationes Medico—Phyſicæ Duæ. I. *De* SANGUINIS ACCENSIONE. II. *De* MOTU MUSCULARI.; +**3v**, page [6], TOM. SECVND. I. *De* ANIMA BRUTORUM; *quæ* HOMINIS *Vitalis ac Senſitiva eſt*, Exercitationes Duæ, *quarum* Prior PHYSIOLOGICA *eſt*, Altera PATHOLOGICA, *Morbos, qui* Ipſam, Cerebrum, & Nervoſum Genus *afficiunt, explicans*; II. PHARMACEUTICE RATIONALIS, *ſive* Diatriba *de* MEDICAMENTORUM OPERATIONIBUS *in* Humano Corpore, *Pars Prima*.; III. PHARMACEUTICES RATIONALIS, *ſive* Diatribæ *de* MEDICAMENTORUM OPERATIONIBUS *in* Humano Corpore, *Pars Secunda*.; IV. PERSPICUA FACILISQUE METHODUS Sanos à PESTE vel quolibet MORBO CONTAGIOSO tuendi, ut & ea LUE Infectos ubicunque currandi.; +**4r**, page [7], blank; +**4v**, page [8], [portrait]; ++**1r–v**, pages [9–10], AUTORIS VITA.; ++**2r–v**, pages [11–12], PRIVILEGIUM SACRÆ CÆSARÆ MAIESTATIS.... [signed] LEOPOLDUS, (L.S.) Vidit LEOPOLDVS GVILLIELMVS Comes in Königſeggs, m.p. *Ad Mandatum Sac. Cæſ. Maieſtatis proprium* F.W.E Bertram, m.p.; §**1r**, page [13], title; §**1v**, page [14], blank; §**2r–v**, pages [15–16], *Reverendiſſimo in* CHRISTO PATRI, ET DOMINO, D. GILBERTO, *Epiſcopo* LONDINENSI, & *Sacelli Regii Decano*. ... [signed] *Humillimus & æternùm addictiſſimus,* THOMAS WILLIS.; §**3r**, page [17], AMICO LECTORI PRÆFATIO. [De Fermentatione]; §**3v**–§**4v**, pages [18–20], AMICO LECTORI PRÆFATIO. [De Febribus]; §§**1r–v**, pages [21–2], AVTHORI *In illius Diatribas Medico-Philoſophicas*, Carmen Gratulatorium. ... [signed] PHILIPPUS FELL, Med. Stud. Oxon.; §§**2r**–§§**3v**, pages [23–6], ELENCHUS RERUM IN TRACTATU DE FERMENTATIONE.; §§**4r**–§§§**2r**, pages [27–31], ELENCHUS RERUM IN TRACTATU DE FEBRIBUS.; §§§**2r**–§§§**2v**, pages [31–32], ELENCHUS RERUM IN DISSERTATIONE DE URINIS.

[2–6]. As in **8B**.

[7]. ¶**1r**, page [1], title; ¶**1v**, page [2], ATHENIS BRITANNICIS, *Literati Orbis Lumini Splendidiſſimo*, UNIVERSITATI OXONIENSI, *Et Ibidem* ILLUSTRISSIMO PRINCIPI JAC. ORMONDIÆ DUCI CANCELLARIO HONORATISSIMO, RAD. BATHVRST *DECANO WELLENSI* VICECANCELLARIO DIGNISSIMO, *Reverendis admodum, &*

perquam Eruditis DOCTORIBVS, PROCVRATORIBVS, FACULTATUM *omnium* PROFESSORIBUS, COLLEGIORUM & AULARUM PRÆFECTIS. *NEC NON* VENERABILI MAGISTRORUM SENATUI, Diatribam Hanc Pharmaceuticam Pietatis & Gratitudinis ergo *Dicat, Dedicatque* Alumnus & Beneficiarius Adſtrictiſſimus THO. WILLIS.; **¶2r–v**, pages [3–4], CANDIDO LECTORI PRÆFATIO.; **¶3r–¶4r**, pages [5–7], AUTORI CLARISSIMO *Nec non mihi (de quo jure glorior)* AMICISSIMO, *in Illius* PHARMACEVTICES RATIONALIS PARTEM UTRAMQUE *Carmen Gratulatorium*. ... [signed] *Gul. Dauukins.*; **¶4r–¶4v**, pages [7–8], QUERELA LIBRI POSTHUMI DE OBITV AVTORIS. ... [signed] *Gul. Dauukins Med. B.*; **¶4v**, page [8], *Imprimatur* AMiciſſimo Authori, poſt tam Immortale Opus, nihil mortale facturo, tanquam Lumina morienti claudens, extremum hoc officium præſtat. *Oxon. Novemb.* 12. 1675. RAD. BATHURST Vice-Cancel. Oxonienſis; **¶¶1r–¶¶¶4v**, pages [9–24]. ELENCHVS RERVM SECVNDÆ PARTIS, PHARMACEVTICES RATIONALIS.

A1r–Ll1v, pages 1–266, [text] *DE* MEDICAMENTORVM OPERATIONIBVS *IN* CORPORE HVMANO, PARS SECVNDA.; **Ll2r–Ll4v**, pages [1–8], INDEX ALPHABETICUS SECUNDÆ PARTIS PHARMACEVTICES RATIONALIS.

[8]. **A1r**, page 1, title; **A1v**, page 2, blank; **A2r–v**, pages 3–4, PRÆFATIO. AMICE LECTOR. ... [signed] Studioſiſſimo & obſequentiſſimo famulo tuo J. HEMMING. In via S. Martini Kal. Sept. 1690.

A3r–C2r, pages 5–19, [text] PERSPICUA FACILISQUE METHODUS SANOS, *BENEDICENTE DEO*, TUENDI A PESTE, *vel Quolibet* MORBO CONTAGIOSO. *VT ET* EA LVE INFECTOS VBICVNQVE CURANDI.; **C2v**, page 20, blank.

Headlines and *Catchwords*: [Volume 1] [1]. Variable use of DE FEBRIBVS. and DE FEBRIBUS. from **i1r–ee3v**, pages 65–222; and DE URINIS. for DE VRINIS from **ee4r–ii3v**, pages 223–54.

No catchword at **§§§2v / a1r**, pages [32] /1; cipiunt for excipient at **e4v / f1r**, pages 40 / 41; ut for at at **g4v / h1r**, pages 56 / 57; DE for *DE* at **h4v / i1r**, pages 64 / 65; CAPVT for CAPUT at **k3v / k4r**, pages 78 / 79; CAPUT for CAPVT at **m4v / n1r**, pages 96 / 97; **o2r / v**, pages 107 / 108; **t4v / u1r**, pages 152 / 153; nitudinem for nituiddem at **n4v / o1r**, pages 104 / 105; DE VRI for DE URINIS at **ee3v / ee4r**, pages 222 / 223; tur, ut for tur: ut at **ff3r / v**, pages 229 / 230.

[2]. *Caput* II. for *Caput* III. at **B4v**, page 16; *Caput* XVIII. for *Caput* XIX. at **M2v**, page 92; *Caput* XXIX. for *Caput* XXII. at **P1r**, page 113.

Catchwords correct.

[3]. Variable use of CONVVLSIVIS. and CONVULSIVIS., throughout; CONWLSIVIS. for CONVVLSIVIS. at ***D1r**, page 25; ***D3r**, page 29; *Caput* VII. for *Caput* VIII. at [*]**I3r**, page 69; *Chap.* XI for *Caput* XI. at ***Q3r**, page 125; *Caput* IX. for *Caput* XI. at ***R2r**, page 131; ***R3r**, page 133; SCORBUTO. for DE SCORBUTO. at ***V1r**, page 153; ***V3r**, page 157; ***Z1r**, page 177; *Caput* II. for *Caput* III. at ***X1r–*X2v**, pages 161–4; *Caput* III. for *Caput* IV. at ***X3r–*X4v**, pages 165–8, reflecting misnumbering of chapter heading as CAPUT III. for CAPUT

IV. at ***X3r**, page 165; *Caput* II. for *Caput* VII. at ***Z1r**, page 177; DF SCORCVTO. for DE SCORBVTO. at ***Aa1v**, page 186; *Caput* VII. for *Caput* VIII. at ***Aa3v**, page 190.

No catchword at ***2v** / ***3r**, page [4] / [5]; ***P1v** / ***P2r**, pages 114 / 115; Cap. for CAP. at ***4v** / ****1r**, page [8] / [9]; *usti* for *uſti* at ***Z4r** / **v**, pages 183 / 184.

[4]. SEU for SIVE at **c1r**, page 33.

No catchword at §**2v** / **a1r**, pages [4] / 1.

[Volume 2] [5]. Variable use of ELENCHVS and ELENCHUS, throughout; EENCHVS for ELENCHVS at ††**3v**, page [14]; ††††**3v**, page [30]; *diſpoſitiones &* for *Diſpoſitiones, &* at ***f*2v**–***f*3r**, pages 44–5; CAP. XIV. for CAP.XV. at ***p*3r**, page 113; CAP. XV. for CAP. XVI. at ***r*2r**, page 131; Caput I. for Cap. I. at ***t*4r**–**v**, pages 151–2; *Cephalgiæ* for *De Cephalgiæ* at ***u*3r**–***x*4v**, pages 159–68; ***y*1v**–***y*3v**, pages 170–4; *Lethargo.* for *De Lethargo.* at ***z*1v**, page 178; Cap. III. for Cap. VIII. at ***cc*1v**, page 218; Cap. VII. for Cap. VIII. at ***cc*4r**, page 223; *Melancholia.* for *De Melancholia.* at ***ll*3r**, page 269; Cap. XI. for Cap. XII. at ***oo*1v**, page 290; *Stupiditate.* for *Stupiditate sive Moroſi.* at ***pp*1r**, page 297; *Paralyſi.* for *Arthritide.* at ***qq*3r**, page 309; Cap. IX. for Cap. XIV. at ***rr*3r**, page 317.

No catchword at †**3v** / †**4r**, pages [6] / [7]; FIGURARUM for FIGURARVM at ***d*1v** / ***d*2r**, pages 26 / 27; PARS SECUNDA for PARS SECVNDA at ***ſ*4r** / ***t*1r**, pages 143 / 145; *Uir illuſtris* for *Vir illuſtris* at ***aa*4v** / ***bb*1r**, pages 192 / 193; Cree for Cerebri at ***tt*4v** / ***uu*1r**, pages [3] / [4].

[6]. Variable use of ELENCHVS and ELENCHUS, throughout; *hyperchatharſeos* for *Hypercatharſeos* at ***I*4v**, page 72; *Londinen ſis* for *Londinenſis* at ***L*2r**, page '83'; *de* for *De* at ***T*4r**, page 151; *Cardiacis.* for *Opiatis.* at **Z1v**, page 178; *effectus* for *Effectus* at ***Aa*2r**, page 187; *nocumentia.* for *Nocumentia.* at ***Aa*2v**–***Aa*3r**, pages 188–9; *Formula.* for *formula.* at **Cc1r**, page 201.

No catchword at (*)**1v** / (*)**2r**, pages [2] / [3]; *DE* MEDICA for DE MEDICA at (**)**2v** / **A1r**, page [16] / 1; tum for Verum at **X1r** / **v**, pages 161 / 162.

[7]. *Respirationis læſæ* for *Reſpirationis læſæ varia* at **D2v**, page 28; *Ob Sanguinem in pulmone impeditum.* for *Sanguinis in pulmone impedimenta.* at **D3r**, page 29; CAP. V. for CAP. VI. at **G4r**, page 55; *ſputo.* for *Sputo.* at **K3v**–**K4r**, pages 78–9; **L3r**, page 85; CAP. X. for CAP. XI. at **P3r**, page 117; [additional chapter break SECTI I. CAPUT XII. in text at **P4v**, page 120]; *Aſtmate.* for *Aſthmate.* at **R1v**, page 130; *ictero, ejuſque Remedis.* for *ictero ejusque remedis.* at **T1v**, page 146; CAP. II. for CAP. I. at **T2r**, page 147; *De Ictero.* for *De Ictero euiſque remediis.* at **T3v**, page 150; CAP. II. for CAP. III. at **V3r**, page 157; *remediis* for *Remediis* at **V4v**, page 160; CAP. III. for CAP. IV. at **X4r**, page 167; CAP. IV. for CAP. V. at **Z3r**, page 181; CAP. III. for CAP. IV. at **Ff4r**, page 231; **Gg1r**, page 233; *ſeu* for *ſive* at **Ff3v**, page 232; **Gg2v**, page 236; *ſive Scabie.* for *ſive.* at **Ii4v**, page 256; *Impetigine.* for *Impetigine, ſive.* at **Ll1v**, page 266.

No catchword at ¶**1v** / ¶**2r**, pages [2] / [3]; ¶**4v** / ¶¶**1r**, pages [8] / [9]; **S4r** / **v**, pages 143 / 144; Poteſt for poteſt at **O1v** / **O2r**, page 106 / 107; erecto ffor recto at **S4r** / **v**, pages 127 / 128;

tantum for tantùm at **V4v / X1r**, pages 160 / 161; ſterilitta for ſterilitatem at **Gg3r / v**, pages 237 / 238.

[8]. *Pestis.* for *Peſtis.* at **B4v**, page 16; **C2r**, page 19.

Catchwords correct.

Frontispiece: none.

Portrait: **Pt.1d2**: THOMAS WILLIS, M. D. *Naturalis Philosophiæ Professor Oxoniensis, necnon Inclyti Medicinæ Collegii Londinensis, & Societatis Regiæ Socius,* [signed] *Fr: Diodoti Pin. ſcu.* 208 × 163 millimetres (sheet); 202 × 153 millimetres (plate marks); 202 × 150 millimetres (image).

Printers' ornaments: Volume 1: [1]. Printers' device at **+1r**, page [1]; **++3r**, page [13] {**Tournes 51**}; headpiece at **+2r**, page [3] {**Tournes 39**}; headpiece at **+3r**, page [5]; **§2r**, page [15]; **a1r**, page 1{**Tournes 2**}; two rows each of 34 fleurons, the lower inverted at **++1r**, page [9]; **ee4r**, page 223 {**Tournes 59**}; two rows each of 33 rosettes with single rosette {**Tournes 61**} at right end of central row of 44 fleurons placed horizontally and alternating left and right {**Tournes 62**} at **++2r**, page [11]; two rows each of 30 fleurons, the lower inverted, at **§3r**, page [17]; two rows each of 44 fleurons placed horizontally and alternating left and right at **§§2r**, page [23] {**Tournes 62**}; row of 22 interlocking fleurons (##1, 7 / 8, 11 / 14, 16 / 19 rotated) at **§3v**, page [18]; row of 22 (with #7 rotated) at **§§1r**, page [21] {**Tournes 64**}; row of 21 fleurons at **§§4r**, page [27] {**Tournes 18**}; row of 33 fleurons at **§§§2r**, page [31] {**Tournes 61**}; headpiece at **i1r**, page 65 {**Tournes 4**}; tailpiece at **ee3v**, page 222 {**Tournes 10**}; two rows each of 34 fleurons {**Tournes 59**} with row of 47 fleurons {**Tournes 69**} at **ff1r**, page 225; tailpiece at **ii3v**, page 254 {**Tournes 71**}.

Decorated E at **+2r**, page [3] {**Tournes 3**}; T at **++1r**, page [9] {**Tournes 60**}; L at **++2r**, page [11] {**Tournes 52**}; S at **§2r**, page [15] {**Tournes 5**}; D at **§3r**, page [17] {**Tournes 63**}; **§3v**, page [18] {**Tournes 65**}; F at **§§2r**, page [23] {**Tournes 13**}; F at **§§4r**, page [27] {**Tournes 66**}; V at **§§§2r**, page [31] {**Tournes 14**}; I at **a1r**, page 1 {**Tournes 15**}; E at **i1r**, page 65{**Tournes 67**}; V at **ee4r**, page 223 {**Tournes 68**}; C at **ff1r**, page 225 {**Tournes 70**}.

[2]. Printers' device at **¶1r**, page [1] {**Tournes 51**}; headpiece at **¶2r**, page [3]; **Z2r**, page 3 {**Tournes 4**}; tailpiece at **¶3v**, page [6] {**Tournes 17**}; two rows each of 44 fleurons placed horizontally and alternating left and right at **¶4r**, page [7] {**Tournes 62**}; row of one fleuron {**Tournes 61**} and 42 fleurons {**Tournes 62**} at **¶¶3r**, page [13]; headpiece at **A1r**, page 1 {**Tournes 2**}; **O2v**, page 108 {**Tournes 26**}; two rows each of 34 fleurons, the lower inverted at **Z1v**, page 2 {**Tournes 59**}.

Decorated A at **¶2r**, page [3] {**Tournes 23**}; C at **¶4r**, page [7] {**Tournes 24**}; V at **¶¶3r**, page [13] {**Tournes 14**}; I at **A1r**, page 1 {**Tournes 37**}; N at **O2v**, page 108 {**Tournes 27**}; T at **Z1v**, page 2 {**Tournes 57**}; D at **Z2r**, page 3 {**Tournes 6**}.

[3]. Printers' device at ***1r**, page [1] {**Tournes 51**}; headpiece at ***2r**, page [3] {**Tournes 2**}; row of 20 fleurons {**Tournes 18**} flanked at right hand end by one fleuron (rotated) {**Tournes 59**} at ***3r**, page [5]; row of 44 fleurons placed vertically and alternating left and right at ***4r**, page

[7] {**Tournes 62**}; two rows each of 16 fleurons at ****3r**, page [13] {**Tournes 72**}; headpiece at **A1r**, page 1; **S4r**, page 143 {**Tournes 35**}.

Decorated I at ***2r**, page [3] (inverted) {**Tournes 30**}; Q at ***3r**, page [5] {**Tournes 32**}; Q at ***4r**, page [7] {**Tournes 33**}; I at ****3r**, page [13] {**Tournes 34**}; I at **A1r**, page 1 {**Tournes 15**}; I at **S4r**, page 143 {**Tournes 37**}.

[4]. Printers' device at **§1r**, page [1] {**Tournes 51**}; headpiece at **§2r**, page [3]; **a1r**, page 1 {**Tournes 2**}; tailpiece at **d2r**, page 27; **f1r**, page 41 {**Tournes 10**}; two rows each of 36 fleurons, lower inverted, at **d2v**, page 28, {**Tournes 59**}; two rows of 36 rosettes fleurons, lower inverted, {**Tournes 59**} with row of 47 fleurons {**Tournes 69**} at **f1v**, page 42; two rows each of 10 fleurons (##2 and 10 reversed) {**Tournes 73**}, each row flanked at each end by one fleuron {**Tournes 59**} at **h4v**, page [1].

Decorated Q at **§2r**, page [3] {**Tournes 38**}; R at **a1r**, page 1 {**Tournes 58**}; I at **d2v**, page 28 {**Tournes 37**}; C at **f1v**, page 42 {**Tournes 70**}.

Volume 2 [5]. Printers' device at **†1r**, page [1]; **†2r**, page [3] {**Tournes 51**}; headpiece at **†3r**, page [5]{**Tournes 39**}; **†4r**, page [7] {**Tournes 2**}; **††1r**, page [9]; ***a*1r**, page 1{**Tournes 4**}; two rows each of 44 fleurons placed vertically, rotated alternately right and left at **††3r**, page [13]; **†††3r**, page [21] {**Tournes 62**}; tailpiece at **††††4r**, page [31] {**Tournes 17**}; headpiece at ***t*1r**, page 145 {**Tournes 35**}; two rows each of 16 fleurons at ***tt*3v**, page [1] {**Tournes 72**}.

Decorated A at **†3r**, page [5] {**Tournes 23**}; I at **†4r**, page [7] {**Tournes 30**}; E at **††1r**, page [9] {**Tournes 67**}; A at **††3r**, page [13]; ***tt*3v**, page [1] {**Tournes 45**}; C at **†††3r**, page [21] {**Tournes 24**}; Q at ***a*1r**, page 1 {**Tournes 38**}; I at ***t*1r**, page 145 {**Tournes 37**}.

[6]. Printers' device at **(*)1r**, page [1] {**Tournes 51**}; row of 42 fleurons, reversed alternately, {**Tournes 62**} flanked by one fleuron {**Tournes 61**} and : at the left and right, at **(*)2r**, page [3]; two rows each of 36 fleurons, lower inverted, at **(*)3v**, page [6] {**Tournes 59**}; headpiece at ***A*1r**, page 1 {**Tournes 4**}; row of 27 fleurons {**Tournes 18**} with (between ##19 / 20, flanked at each end by one fleuron {**Tournes 19**} at ***Cc*2v**, page 204.

Decorated Q at **(*)2r**, page [3] {**Tournes 32**}; M at **(*)3v**, page [6] {**Tournes 46**}; A at ***A*1r**, page 1 {**Tournes 44**}.

[7]. Printers' device at **¶1r**, page [1] {**Tournes 51**}; two rows each of 32 fleurons {**Tournes 61**} separated by two each of 29 fleurons, placed horizontally {**Tournes 62**} at **¶2r**, page [3]; double row each of 20 fleurons {**Tournes 18**} flanked at the right-hand end by one fleuron {**Tournes 19**} at **¶3r**, page [5]; single row of 35 fleurons at **¶4r**, page [7] {**Tournes 59**}; single row of 15 fleurons {**Tournes 72**} with one other fleuron between ##1 / 2 {**Tournes 74**} at **¶4v**, page [8]; double row each of 36 fleurons, lower inverted, {**Tournes 59**} separated by single row of 28 fleurons {**Tournes 18**} at **¶¶1r**, page [9]; headpiece at A1r, page 1 {**Tournes 2**}; two rows each of 44 fleurons, reversed alternately, {**Tournes 62**}, separated by single row of 33 fleurons {**Tournes 61**}, at **Ll2r**, page [1].

Decorated A at **¶2r**, page [3] {**Tournes 23**}; O (inverted) at **¶¶1r**, page [9] {**Tournes 49**}; I at **A1r**, page 1{**Tournes 15**}; A at **Ll2r**, page [1] {**Tournes 50**}.

[8]. Printers' device at **A1r**, page 1 {**Tournes 1**}; headpiece at **A2r**, page 3 {**Tournes 2**}; **A3r**, page 5 {**Tournes 4**}.

Decorated Q at **A2r**, page 3 {**Tournes 32**}; Q at **A3r**, page 5 {**Tournes 38**}.

Illustrations: As in **8B** apart from variation in sheet sizes and occasional binding positions.

Copy: DASC. Original calf, spine relaid (and partly defective), with five raised bands, panels and bands gilt decorated, lettered WILLIS | OPERA | TOM I / II, later endpapers. Leaves 222 × 163 × 52 millimetres, 233 × 173 × 65 millimetres. Inserted: bookplate of M. GONZALEZ-ULLOA MEXICO. Stamped: BIBLIOTHECA GONZALEANA LES MARIÓDES, vertical lettering alongside profile GONZALEZ-ULLOA, 1968. Inscribed: Ex Libris ?AM Grasan D. csse (unidentified).[22]

8H.c1. OPERA OMNIA, Venice folio 1708

Eighth edition of the collected works of Thomas Willis in Latin, the eighth book, the second in folio, reset with new printers' ornaments but following the format of 8F and using illustrations in the same states [HJR Wing 52, Denham 19, Oldfield B8].

Title page: THOMÆ | WILLIS | MED. DOCT. | OPERA OMNIA, | Nitidiùs quàm unquam hactenus edita, plurimùm emendata, Indice | rerum copiofiffimo, ac diftinctione characterum exornata. | *Studio, & Opera* | GERARDI BLASII, M. D. | Et in Illuft. Amftelod. Gymnafio Prof. Publ. Bibliothecarii, &c. | *Hac noviffima Editione accuratiffimè recognita, exploita, ac Dicata* | ILLUSTRISSIMO DOMINO | LAURENTIO ROSMARINO | VERONENSI, M. D. PRÆSTANTISSIMO | Veronenfium Practico feliciffimo. | [printers' device: lettered FORTITVDO OMNIA VINCIT] | VENETIIS; M.DCCVIII. | [rule] | Sumptibus Ruinetti, & Storti. | *CUM SUPERIORUM FACULTATE.*[*]

Collation: folio in 6s, 23 letter roman alphabet using I and V. $†^8$, A–Z^6, Aa^8, Bb–Zz^6, Aaa–Ddd^6. \$1–3 signed apart from: L1 signed D1, -Z2, Z5 signed Z2, Kk3 signed Kk2, Yy2 signed Vv2, Ccc3 signed Cc3. Also with *VVillis Tom. I.* or *VVillis Tom. II.* (footer, left) on all signed text sheets apart from: -A2, -A3, -H3, -P3, -Oo2, -Qq2; *VVillis I. Tom.* for *VVillis Tom. I.* at G1, O1, O2; *VVilis* for *VVillis* at P1, Q3, R1, V1, Cc2; *VVillie* for *VVillis* at **Aa4**; *Tom II.* for *Tom I.* at T2, T3, Z3; *Tom I.* for *Tom II.* at **Mm2, Zz1**.

310 leaves, paginated as [16], 1–586, [18]. Mispaginated: 59 for 65, 296 for 196, 107 for 207, 526 for 226, 168 for 268, 91 for 291, 195 for 295, 360 for 306, 434 for 334, 438 for 338, 585 for 583. Illustrations all on the printed page apart from 3 additional leaves, unsigned, between Nn3 / Nn4, pages 430 / 431, and 4 additional leaves between Tt3 / Tt4, pages 502 / 503.

[22] Mario Gonzalez-Ulloa (1913–1995) was a Mexican doctor who developed services in plastic surgery. His experience included work in British military hospitals during the Second World War. Working at the Dalinde Hosiital in Mexico City, he established the Dalinde Seminars on Aesthetic Surgery which took as their principle the concept that, with hands trained to operate in general surgery, the aesthetic sense of plastic surgery is a craft based on maturity, wisdom, and personal fulfilment.

[*] Underlined text originally printed in red.

Type: ≤ 80 lines; height (20 lines) 70 millimetres, width 77 millimetres (each of two columns, together 160 millimetres, apart from preliminaries: ≤ 90 millimetres in each column with marginal notes, present to the left or right of the text).

Contents: (although with one register and continuous pagination, the book is structured in two parts separated by a half title) [1]. **†1r**, page [1] [half title] THOMÆ WILLIS OPERA OMNIA:; **†1v**, page [2], blank; **†2r**, page [3] title; **†2v**, page [4], blank; **†3r–v**, page [5–6] ILLVSTRISSIME VIR... [signed] Venetiis VIII. Kalend. Mart. M.DCCVIII. *In ſignum Obſequii* N.N. M.D.; **†4r**, page [7] GERARDUS BLASIUS LECTORI BENEVOLO Salutem & Officia,; **†4v**, page [8] [portrait]; **†5r–v**, pages [9–10] AUTHORIS VITA.; **†6r**, page [11] CONTENTA HUJUS OPERIS. I. Diatribæ duæ *de* FERMENTATIONE, *&* FEBRIBUS; *quibus acceſsit* Diſſertatio *de* VRINIS.; II. CEREBRI ANATOME, NERVORVMQUE DESCRIPTIO *&* VSVS.; III. De RATIONE MOTVS MVSCVLORVM ſtudio GVLIELMI CROONE M.D. Londin. ac. Soc. Reg. Socii.; IV. PATHOLOGIÆ CEREBRI *&* NERVOSI GENERIS SPECIMEN, *in quo agitur de* MORBIS CONVVLSIVIS *&* SCORBVTO.; V. AFFECTIONVM *quæ dicuntur* HYSTERICÆ *et* HYPOCHONDRIACÆ PATHOLOGIA SPASMODICA VINDICATA, *contra* Reſponſionem Epiſtolarem NATHAN. HIGMORI M.D. *cui acceſſerunt* Exercitationes Medico-Phyſicæ duæ. I. *De* SANGVINIS ACCENSIONE. II. *De* MOTV MUSCVLARI.; VI. *De* ANIMA BRVTORVM, *quæ* HOMINIS *Vitalis ac Senſitiva eſt*, Exercitationes duæ, *quarum* Prior PHYSIOLOGICA *eſt*, Altera PATHOLOGICA, *Morbos, qui* Ipſam, Cerebrum, *&* Neruoſum Genus *afficiunt, explicans*; VII. PHARMACEVTICE RATIONALIS, *ſive* Diatriba *de* MEDICAMENTORVM OPERATIONIBVS *in* Humano Corpore.; VIII. PHARMACEVTICES RATIONALIS, *ſiue* Diatribæ *de* MEDICAMENTORVM OPERATIONIBVS *in* Humano Corpore Pars altera: *opus poſthumus*.; **†6v–†8r**, pages [12–15] ELENCHVS TOTIVS OPERIS.; **†8v**, page [16] AD TRACTATUM DE FERMENTATIONE PRÆFATIO.

A1r–C1v, pages 1–26, [text] DE FERMENTATIONE, SIUE *DE MOTV CORPORVM* NATURALIUM INORGANICO.

C2r–v, pages 27–8, DE FEBRIBVS PRÆFATIO.

C2v–H3v, pages 28–90, [text] [De Febribus].

H4r–v, pages 91–2, DE VRINIS, DISSERTATIO EPISTOLICA. *Ad Virum Doctiſsimum mihique amiciſsimum*, D. RODULPHUM BATHURST, Med. Doct. & Colleg. Sacroſanctæ Trinitatis Oxon. Socium.; **H4v–I3v**, pages 92–102, [text] [De urinis]

I4r–I4v, pages 103–4, CEREBRI ANATOME, CUI ACCESSIT NERVORUM DESCRIPTIO ET USUS. *PRÆFATIO*.; **I3v–N3r**, pages 104–49, [text] [Cerebri Anatome].

N3r–P6v, pages 149–80, [text] NERVORVM DESCRIPTIO ET USUS.

Q1r–Q4v, pages 181–8, DE RATIONE MOTVS MUSCULORUM; Studio GULIELMI CROONE, M. D. è Coll. Med. Lond. ac Societatis Regalis Socii. *Ἐν πᾶσι τοῖς φυσικοῖς ἐνεστί τι θαυμαστόν. Ariſt. de Part. Animal.*

Q5r–v, pages 189–90, PATHOLOGIÆ CEREBRI, ET NERUOSI GENERIS SPECIMEN: *In quo agitur de MORBIS CONVULSIVIS, & de SCORBUTO*. PRÆFATIO; **Q5v–V6v**, pages

190–240, [text] [De morbis convulsivis]; **X1r–Z1v**, pages 241–66, [text] TRACTATUS DE SCORBUTO.

Z2r, page 267, AFFECTIONVM HYSTERICARVM ET HYPOCHONDRIACARUM PATHOLOGIA SPASMODICA VINDICATA; Contra Reſponſionem Epiſtolarem Nathanaelis Highmori M.D. *Cui acceſſerunt Exercitationes duæ Medico-Phycæ. I. De Sanguinis Accenſione. II. De Motu Muſculari.* PRÆFATIO.; **Z2v–Aa1r**, page 268–77, AD VIRVM DOCTISSIMVM NATHANAEL HIGHMORVM M.D., [text] [Affectionum hystericarum etc.]; **Aa1r–Aa3v**, pages 277–82, EXERCITATIO PRIMA MEDICO-PHYSICA. *De Sanguinis Incaleſcentia, ſive Accenſione.*; **Aa4r–Aa8v**, pages 283–92, EXERCITATIO II. MEDICO-PHYSICA. *De Motu Muſculari.*

[2.] **Bb1r**, page 293, [half title] THOMÆ WILLIS OPERUM MEDICO-PHYSICORUM TOMVS SECVNDVS: *CONTINENS* De Anima Brutorum Exercitationes duas, Pharmaceuticæ Rationalis Partes duas.; **Bb1v**, page 294, blank; **Bb2r–v**, page '195'–296, PRÆFATIO AD LECTOREM.

Bb3r–Ff6v, pages 297–352, [text] DE ANIMA BRUTORUM.; **Gg1r–Mm4v**, pages 353–420, DE ANIMA BRUTORUM PARS SECUNDA, PATHOLOGICA, *SIVE* DE MORBIS Qui ad Animam Corpoream, euiſque ſubjecta, ſcilicet Cerebrum & Genus Nervoſum, ſpectant.

Mm5r–v, pages 421–2, PHARMACEUTICE RATIONALIS, Sive Diatriba de Medicamentorum operationibus in Corpore Humano. PARS PRIMA PRÆFATIO.; **Mm5v–Ss5v**, pages 422–94, [text] [Pharmaceutice Rationalis, part 1]; **Ss6r–v**, pages 495–6, PHARMACEUTICES RATIONALIS, Sive Diatriba de Medicamentorum operationibus in Corpore Humano, PARS SECUNDA. OPUS POSTHUMUM. PRÆFATIO.; **Ss6v–'Cc'3v**, pages 496–586, [text] [Pharmaceutice Rationalis, part 2].

Ccc4r–Ddd6r, pages [1–17], INDEX ALPHABETICUS RERUM ET VERBORUM, quæ in toto hoc Opere occurrunt, notabilium.; **Ddd6v**, page [18], blank.

Headlines and *Catchwords*: [1]. (Headings in *Diatribæ duæ* identify the current section or chapter when the number changes on a given page; in *Cerebri anatome* and thereafter headings identify the next section or chapter when the number changes on a given page); Caput XI. for Caput VII. at **B1r**, page 13; Caput XI. for Caput X. at **B6r**, page 23; Caput XII. for Caput XI. at **C1r**, page 25; Caput VIII. for Caput VII. at **D5r**, page 45; Caput X. for Caput IX. at **E1r**, page 49; Caput XI. for Caput X. at **E3r**, page 53; Caput XIII. for Caput XII. at **F2r**, page 63; De Urinis, for De Vrinis. at **H4v**, page 92; Caput VII. for Caput VI. at **I3r**, page 101 [CAPUT VI. misnumbered CAPUT IV. at **I2v**, page 100]; Caut I. for Caput I. at **I6r**, page 107; Caput V. for Caput VI. at **E6r**, page 119; Caput XVII. for Caput XIII. at **L6r**, page 131; Caput VIII. for Caput XIII. at **M1r**, page 133; [chapter title CAPUT VX for CAPUT XV at **M2v**, page 136]; Caput XXII. for Caput XXI. at **N3r**, page 149; Vuſus. for Vſus. at **N4v**, page 152; [chapter title CAPUT XXVI. for CAPUT XXIV at **N6r**, page 155]; [chapter title CAPUV XXVIII. for CAPUT XVIII at **O6r**, page 167]; Caput XIII. for Caput VIII. at **S6r**, page 215; Caput VIII. for Caput IV. at **X5r**, page 249; Hyſter: & Hypoch: for Hyſtericis & Hypocond. at **Z3r**, page 269; Hiſter. & Hypoch: for Hyſtericis & Hypocond. at **Z3v**, page 270; Affectionibns for Affectionibus at **Z4r**, page 271; no '.' after headline at **Z4v**, page 272; Affection. for

Affectionibus at **Z5r**, page 273; Affectibus for Affectionibus at **Z5v**, page 274; &c. for & Hypocond. at **Z6r–v**, page 275–6; Motus for Motu at **Aa6r–2π1v**, pages 287–90.

No catchword at **†3v** / **†4r**, pages [6] / [7]; Ui- for Vitrificationis at **C1r** / **v**, pages 25 / 26; iccpa- for occupatus at **C2r** / **v**, pages 27 / 28; GA for CAPUT at **D5r** / **v**, pages 45 / 46; pedi for Pedicant at **E1v** / **E2r**, pages 50 / 51; vit- for uit; at **L6v** / **M1r**, pages 132 / 133; TACU for TABU at **P2r** / **v**, pages 171 / 172; *Nervi* for A. *Nervi* at **P3v** / **P4r**, pages 174 / 175; cos for tos at **X5r** / **v**, pages 249 / 250; CA for *CATHARSIS* at **X4v** / **Y1r**, pages 252 / 253; no catchword at **Z2r** / **v**, pages 267 / '168'.

[2]. Caput IV. for Caput III. at **Cc3r**, page 309; Captu IV. for Caput IV. at **Cc4r**, page 311; Caput VIII. for Caput IX. at **Dd6r**, page 327; Caput XVI. for Caput XV. at **Ff3r**, page 345; Caput II. at Caput III. at **Gg6r**, page 363; Caput III. for Caput IV. at **Hh2r**, page 367; Caput X. for Caput XI. at **Kk3r**, page 395; Capnt XV. for Caput XV. at **Mm2r**, page 415; Arthridite. for Passione Colica. at **Mm4v**, page 420; Cap. I. for Cap. II. at **Mm6r**, page 423; Cap. I. for Cap. II at **Oo5r**, page 445; Sect. IV. for Sect. VI. at **Rr6r**, page 483; Cap. I. for Cap. III. at **Tt6r**, page 507; Cap. VI. for Cap. VII. at **Xx1r**, page 521; Cap. IX. for Cap. X. at **Yy1r**, page 533; Cap. X. for Cap. XI. at **'Vv2'r**, page 535; Cap. XI. for Cap. XII. at **Yy3r**, page 537; Cap. XII. for Cap. XIII. at **Yy5r**, page 541; Sect. I. Cap. XIII. for Sect. II. Cap. I. at **Yy6r**, page 543; Cap. IV. for Cap. II. at **Zz2r**, page 547; Cap. VI. for Cap. IV. at **Aaa1r**, page 557; Hæmorrhagia, & for Hæmorrhagia & at **Aaa4v**, page 564; Cap. I. for Cap. II. at **Aaa4r**, page 567; Cap. VI. for Cap. VII. at **Ccc2r**, page 585.

fiue for five at **Bb3v** / **Bb4r**, pages 298 / 299; ptatis for aptatis at **Dd4r** / **v**, pages 327 / 328; pru for profint at **Gg4r** / **v**, pages 359 / 360; nificem for nifices at **Mm5r** / **v**, pages 421 / 422; mufcu- for mafculam at **Mm6r** / **v**, pages 423 / 424; Quòd for Quod at **Nn6r** / **v**, pages 435 / 436; rate for arteriosum at **Rr6r** / **v**, pages 483 / 484; quam for quàm at **Tt6v** / **Vu1r**, pages 508 / 509; gærnæ for grænæ at **Aaa3r** / **v**, pages 561 / 562.

Frontispiece: none.

Portrait: as in **8F**.

Printers' ornaments: [1]. Printers' device at **†2r**, page [3] {**Storti 1**}; tailpiece at **†4r**, page [7] {**Ruinetti 3**}; headpiece at **†5r**, page [9] {**Ruinetti 4**}; tailpiece at **†5v**, page [10]{**Ruinetti 6**}; **†6r**, page [11]{**Ruinetti 7**}; **†8r**, page [15] {**Ruinetti 8**}; **†8v**, page [16] {**Ruinetti 10**}; headpiece at **A1r**, page 1 {**Ruinetti 11**}; tailpiece at **H3v**, page 90; **Aa8v**, page 292 {**Ruinetti 14**}; **P2r**, page 171; **Aa7v**, page 290 {**Ruinetti 17**}; **P4r**, page 175 {**Ruinetti 18**}; **V6v**, page 240; **Ddd6r**, page [17] {**Storti 24**}; **Aa3v**, page 282 {**Ruinetti 24**}.

Decorated C at **†3r**, page [5] {**Ruinetti 1**}; S at **†4r**, page [7] {**Ruinetti 2**}; T at **†5r**, page [9] {**Ruinetti 5**}; D at **†8v**, page [16]{**Ruinetti 9**}; I at **A1r**, page 1 {**Ruinetti 12**}; D at **C2r**, page 27 {**Ruinetti 13**}; O at **H4r**, page 91 {**Ruinetti 15**}; A at **I4r**, page 103 {**Ruinetti 16**}; D at **Q1r**, page 181 {**Ruinetti 19**}; Q at **Q5r**, page 189 {**Ruinetti 20**}; Q at **Z2r**, page 267 {**Ruinetti 21**}; R at **Z2v**, page '168' {**Ruinetti 22**}; I at **Aa1r**, page 277 {**Ruinetti 23**}; C at **Aa4r**, page 283 {**Ruinetti 25**}.

[2] Headpiece at **Bb3r**, page 297 {**Storti 25**}; tailpiece at **Mm4v**, page 420 **Ruinetti 28**}; **Ss5v**, page 494 {**Ruinetti 31**}; **Cc[c]3v**, page 586 {**Ruinetti 34**}.

Decorated E at **Bb2r**, page '195' {**Ruinetti 26**}; Q at **Bb3r**, page 297 {**Ruinetti 27**}; Q at **Mm5r**, page 421{**Ruinetti 29**}; A at **Mm5v**, page 422{**Ruinetti 30**}; A at **Ss6r**, page 495 {**Ruinetti 32**}; I at **Ss6v**, page 496 {**Ruinetti 33**}.

Illustrations: as in **8F**.

Copy: DASC. Original quarter calf with paper covered boards, spine lettered Willif | Opera | Omnia, original endpapers. Leaves 323 × 226 millimetres, boards 329 × 222 × 42 millimetres. Inscribed: C.A.M.P. 1709 on title page (unidentified). From the library of Warren G. Smirl.[23]

8H.c2. OPERA OMNIA, Venice folio 1708

Eighth edition of the collected works of Thomas Willis in Latin, the eighth book, with one leaf in a second state [not distinguished by HJR Wing, Denham, or Oldfield].

As in **8H.c1** apart from:

Collation: Mispaginated (296 for 196, 107 for 207, 526 for 226, 168 for 268, 91 for 291, 195 for 295, 360 for 306, 434 for 334, 585 for 583), 438 for 338 corrected.

Copy: DASC, Ddd1, and Ddd6 reprinted on contemporary paper, lacking †8. Recent full vellum (by Bernard Middleton) with gold tooled border to upper and lower boards, spine with six compartments labelled WILLIS | OPERA | OMNIA, recent endpapers. Leaves 312 × 222 millimetres, boards 320 × 218 × 52 millimetres.

8H.c3. OPERA OMNIA, Venice folio 1708

Eighth edition of the collected works of Thomas Willis in Latin, the eighth book, with one sheet cancelled [not distinguished by HJR Wing, Denham, or Oldfield].[24]

As in **8H.c1** apart from:

Collation: †1 and †8 (conjugate), cancelled.

[23] After training at Columbia University Medical School, Warren G. Smirl (1921–2000) underwent post-graduate study at the University of Vienna and, after serving in the US Air Force following the Second World War, was for many years a general surgeon in Waukesha. He started collecting books as a medical student and his library—strong in anatomy, surgery, and obstetrics—was sold at auction by Sotheby's, London, on 11 November 1994. This copy was item 379 of 384 lots.

[24] It is not clear why and when †1 and its conjugate leaf †8 were reset. The earlier version of †8r lacks the 'D' of 'DE' in line 1, for which the catchword on †7v is correct, and the 'P' of 'PATHOLOGICI' in line 2 of column 1. But correcting these printing errors would not seem a sufficient reason for resetting the entire sheet. The cancellans is itself imperfect in that it lacks the catchword 'DE' at †8v. Whereas, being the exposed outer leaf, the half-title (†1r) and its conjugate leaf might have been damaged during storage or discarded, it is unlikely that the sheet would have been reset in order to make up one or more copies for sale. It would be instructive if other copies with this cancelled sheet are known. Whatever the reason for cancellation, it is most likely that this occurred some years after 1708 since the decorated initial 'D' at †8v is that used by Malachin in the *Opera omnia* 1720 (**8I**: see [2] T6r, page 227) for which the designation Malachin 10 has been adopted rather than attributing this ornament to Ruinetti.

Type: †1r, reset with larger type; †8, reset in 56 lines; height (20 lines) 97 millimetres, width 80 millimetres (each of two columns, together 165 millimetres); †8v, height (20 lines) 97 millimetres, width 168 millimetres.

Contents: †1r; †8r–v, as in **8H.c1**.

Printers' ornaments: [I]. No tailpiece at **†8r**, page [15].

Decorated D at **†8v**, page [16] {**Malachin 10**}.

Copy: DASC. Original full vellum, spine lettered Willis | Opera | Medica, original endpapers (defective). Leaves 322 × 225 millimetres, boards 328 × 228 × 50 millimetres. Inscribed (title-page and portrait) Doct. Sr. Physic. Aloysius Labini 1763 (unidentified).

8I. OPERA OMNIA, Venice folio 1720

Ninth edition of the collected works of Thomas Willis in Latin, the eighth book, the third in folio, with William Croone's treatise, several of the illustrations engraved in combination, and most printed with the text but imperfectly registered [HJR Wing 53, Denham 20, Oldfield B9].

Title page: THOMÆ | WILLIS | MEDICINÆ DOCTORIS, | NATURALIS PHILOSOPH. PROFES. OXONIENSIS, | *NEC NON* | INCLYTI MEDICORUM COLLEGII | Londinenſis, & Societatis Regiæ Socii; | OPERA OMNIA, | Ex nupera editione graviſſimis undequaque, atque ad publicam perniciem | erroribus ſcatente tamquam ab excidio ſummo labore, eximioque ſtu- | dio vindicata, atque ad priſtinam puritatem, integritatemque reſtituta. | *EXCELLENTISSIMO DOMINO* | PAULO MONTICELLO | VENETO MEDIC. DOCT. PRÆSTANTISSIMO, | Celebratiſſimo, Feliciſſimo Dicata. | TOMUS PRIOR. | [ornament] | VENETIIS, | [short rule] | Apud Joannem Malachinum, ſub ſigno D. Ignatii. | Impenſis Julii de Maphæis. M. DCC. XX | *CUM SUPERIORUM LICENTIA, AC PRIVILEGIO.*[*]

Collation: folio in 6s, 23 letter roman alphabet using I and V. [1]. $+^{10}$, A–Z^{6}, Aa–Cc^{6}, Dd^{4}, Ee^{6}. $1–3 signed apart from: B3 signed A3, Ee2 signed E2.

[2]. A–S^{6}, T^{8}, V–Z^{6}, Aa–Dd^{6}, Ee^{8}. $1–3 signed apart from: A3 signed A2, X3 signed 3X.

Leaves 1 and 2 of each sheet with *Vuillis Tom. I.* and *Vuillis Tom. II.* (footer, left) apart from: [1]. -A3; *Uuillis* for *Vuillis* at F1, H1, L1, M1, N1, O1, Q1, R3, S3, T2, V1, V3, X2, Y1, Y3, Z2, Aa1–Aa3, Cc3; *Vuilis* for *Vuillis* at N3, O2, P2, Q2, R1, S2, T3, V2, X3; [2]. Correct.

348 leaves, double columns separated by two vertical lines, paginated as: [1]. [20], 1–320, [12]. [2]. [1]–334, [10]. Mispaginated: 82 for 28, 230 for 240.

Type: ≤ 79 lines; height (20 lines) 69 millimetres, width 76 millimetres (each of two columns, together 159 millimetres, apart from preliminaries: 90 millimetres in each column with marginal notes, present to the left or right of the text).

[*] Underlined text originally printed in red.

Contents: [1]. **+1r**, page [1], [half title] THOMÆ WILLIS OPERA OMNIA.; **+1v**, page [2], blank; **+2r**, page [3], title; **+2v**, page [4], blank; **+3r–+4v**, pages [5–8] EXCELLENTISSIME DOMINE. ... [signed] Dominat. Tuæ Excellentiſs. *Addictiſſimus, Obſequentiſſimus Servus* Joannes Malachinus Bibliopola.; **+5r**, page [9] AUTORI, In illius Diatribas Medico-Philoſophicas, CARMEN GRATULATORIUM. ... [signed] PHILIPUS FELL, *Med. Stud. Oxon.*; **+5v**, page [10] SERIES OPERUM *DOMINI D.* THOMÆ VVILLIS, Hac Editione Typi prodeuntium, *TOMI PRIORIS*. 1. De Fermentatione. II. De Febribus. III. De Urinis. IV. Cerebri Anatome. V. Nervorum deſcriptio, & uſus. VI. De Morbis Convulſivis. VIII. De Scorbuto. VIII. De Affectionibus Hyſtericis, & Hypochondriacis. IX. De Sanguinis incaleſcentia. X. De Motu Muſculari. *TOMI POSTERIORIS*. I. De Anima Brutorum Exercitationes duæ. II. Pharmaceutice Rationalis, & de Medicamentorum operationibus in humano corpore, &c.; **+6r**, page [11] AD LECTOREM; **+6v**, page [12], portrait; **+7r–+8r**, pages [13–15], ELENCHUS PRIMI TOMI.; **+8v–+9r**, pages [16–17] ELENCHUS SECUNDI TOMI.; **+9v**, page [18] AD TRACTATUM DE FERMENTATIONE PRÆFATIO.; **+10r**, page [19] NOI REFORMATORI Dello Studio di Padoa. COncediamo licenza à Gioanni Malachini Stampatore, che poſſi riſtampare il Libro intitolato *Thomæ Villis Med. Doct. Opera Omnia*, ſecondo l'eſſemplare ſtampato in Venetia nell' Anno 1708. *Dat, li* 24. *Agoſto* 1719. [Alviſe Piſani K. P. Ref. [Gio: Pietro Paſqualigo Ref. [Michele Moroſini Ref. Agoſtino Galdaldini Segretario.;[25] **+10v**, page [20] blank.

A1r–C2r, pages 1–27, [text] DE FERMENTATIONE, SIVE DE MOTU CORPORUM NATURALIUM INORGANICO.

C2v–C3r, pages 28–9, DE FEBRIBUS PRÆFATIO.; **C3r–H5v**, pages 29–94, [text] [De Febribus].

H6r–H6v, pages 95–108, DE URINIS DISSERTATIO EPISTOLICA. *Ad Virum Doctiſſimum, mihique amiciſſimum* D. RODULPHUM BATHURST, Med. Doct. & Colleg. Sacroſanctæ Trinit. Oxon. Socium.

K1r–K1v, pages 109–10, CEREBRI ANATOME CUI ACCESSIT NERVORUM DESCRIPTIO, ET USUS *PRÆFATIO.*; **Kiv–O3r**, pages 110–61, [text] [Cerebri anatome].; **O3r–R3r**, pages 161–97, [text] NERVORUM DESCRIPTIO, ET USUS.; **R3r–S1r**, pages 197–205, DE RATIONE MOTUS MUSCULORUM; Studio GULIELMI CROONE M. D. è Coll. Med. Lond,. ac Societatis Regalis Socii. *Ἐν πᾶσι τοῖς φυσικοῖς ἐνεστί τι θαυμαστόν. Ariſtoteles de Partibus Animalium.*

S1v–S2r, pages 206–7, PATHOLOGIÆ CEREBRI, ET NERVOSI GENERIS SPECIMEN, *In quo agitur de MORBIS CONVULSIVIS, & de SCOBURTO*. PRÆFATIO.; **S2r–Y5v**, pages 207–62, [text] [Pathologiæ cerebri]; **Y6r–Bb2v**, pages 263–92, [text] TRACTATUS DE SCORBUTO.; **Bb3r**, page 293, AFFECTIONUM HYSTERICARUM, ET HYPOCHONDRIACARUM PATOLOGIA SPASMODICA VINDICATA Contra Reſponſionem Epiſtolarem Nathanaelis Highmori Medicinæ Doctoris. *Cui acceſſerunt Exercitationes duæ Medico-Phyſicæ*. I. De Sanguinis Accenſione. II. De Motu Muſculari. PRÆFATIO.; **Bb3v–Cc2v**, pages 294–304, *AD VIRUM DOCTISS.*^{M} NATHANAEL HIGHMORUM M. D.; **Cc2v–Cc5v**, pages 304–10, EXERCITATIO I. MEDICO-PHYSICA. *De Sanguinis Incaleſcentia, ſive Accenſione.*;

[25] BOARD MEMBERS of the University of Padua. We grant permission to Gianni Malachini, printer, to reprint the book entitled *Dr. Thomas Villis, Collected Works*, according to the edition printed in Venice in the year 1708. Dated 24 August 1719. Members: Alvise Pisani, K.P, Gio: Pietro Pasqualigo, Michele Morosini; and Agostino Galdaldini, secretary.

Cc5v–Dd4v, pages 310–20, EXERCITATIO II. MEDICO-PHYSICA. *De Motu Muſculari.*; **Ee1r–Ee6r**, pages [1–11], INDEX ALPHABETICUS RERUM ET VERBORUM, quæ in Tomo I. occurrunt, notabilium.; **Ee6v**, page [12], blank.

[2]. **A1r**, page 1, [half title] THOMÆ WILLIS OPERUM MEDICO-PHYSICORUM Tomus Secundus *CONTINENS* I. De Anima Brutorum Exercitationes duas, II. Pharmaceuticæ Rationalis Partes duas.; **A1v**, page 2, blank; **A2r–v**, pages 3–4, PRÆFATIO AD LECTOREM.

A[3]r–F3v, pages 5–66, [text] De ANIMA BRUTORUM.; **F4r–M5r**, pages 67–141, DE ANIMA BRUTORUM *PARS SECUNDA* PATHOLOGICA SIVE DE MORBIS *Qui ad Animam Corpoream, ejuſque ſubjecta, ſcilicet, Cerebrum, & Genus Nervoſum ſpectant.*

M5v–M6r, pages 142–3, PHARMACEUTICES RATIONALIS, Sive Diatribæ de Medicamentorum operationibus in Corpore Humano. PARS PRIMA *PRÆFATIO.*
M6r–T4v, pages 143–224, SECTIO PRIMA CAPUT PRIMUM. *DESIGNATIO TOTIUS OPERIS.*

T5r–T8v, pages 225–32, PHARMACEUTICES RATIONALIS, Sive Diatribæ de Medicamentorum operationibus in Corpore Humano. PARS SECUNDA. OPUS POSTHUMUM. *PRÆFATIO.*; **T6r–T7r**, pages 227–9, POST SCRIPTUM; **T7v–T8r**, pages 230–1, *AUTORI CLARISSIMO, necnon mihi (de quo jure glorior) Amiciſſimo,* IN ILLIUS PHARMACEUTICES RATIONALIS PARTEM UTRAMQUE *Carmen Gratulatorium.* … [signed] *GUL. DAVVKINS.*; **T8v**, page 232, QUERALLA LIBRI POSTUMI *DE OBITU* AUTORIS... [signed] *GUL. DAVVKINS* MED. B.

V1r–Ee3v, pages 233–4, [text] [Pharmaceutices Rationalis Part II].

Ee4r–Ee8v, pages [1–10], INDEX ALPHABETICUS RERUM ET VERBORUM, quæ in Tomo II. occurrunt, notabilium.

Headlines and *Catchwords*: [1]. (These normally identify the next section or chapter when the number changes on a given page): Febribus. for Fermentatione. at **C1v**, pages 26; Caput X. for Caput XI. at **E4r**, page 55; Caput XII. for Caput XIII. at **F3r**, page 65; Caput IX. for Caput X. at **M2r**, page 135; Caput XII. for Caput XIII. at **M5r**, page 141; Caput XXII. for Caput XXI. at **O3r**, page 161; Caput XXI. for Caput XXII. at **O4r**, page 163; Caput XXIX. for De Ratione motus Muſculorum. at **R3r**, page 197.

(No catchwords at pages with illustrations reaching the foot of the leaf): no catchword at **+4v / +5r**, pages [8] / [9]; lefa for calefactis at **G6v / H1r**, pages 84 / 85; sola for & *Autumno* at **S6v / T1r**, page 216 / 217; Suman- for *Sumantur* at **Z6v / Aa1r**, pages 276 / 277.

[2]. Caput III. for Caput IV. at **G6r**, page 83; Cap. I. for Cap. II. at **N4r**, page 151; Sect. III. Cap. I for Sect. II. Cap. I. at **O1r**, page 157; Sect. II. Cap. III. for Sect. III. Cap, I. at **O4r**, page 163; Formulæ. for formulæ. at **T2v**, page 220; Cap. II for Cap. III. at **X1r**, page 245; Cap. VII. for Cap. VIII. at **Y6r**, page 267; Cap. III. for Cap. IV. at **Bb3r**, page 297; Cap. I. for Cap. II. at **Cc5r**, page 313; Cap. IV. for Cap. V. at **Dd4r**, page 323; Cap. VII. for Cap. VI. at **Ee1r**, page 329.

Catchwords correct.

Frontispiece: none.

Portrait: **Pt.1g1**: as in **8H** apart from: 337 × 224 millimetres (sheet).

Printers' ornaments: [1]. Printers' device on title page at **+2r**, page [3] {**Malachin 1**}; tailpiece at **+9r**, page [17]; **Ee6r**, page [11] {**Malachin 3**}; headpiece at **A1r**, page 1 {**Malachin 4**}; tailpiece at D at **C2r**, page 27; **K6v**, page 120; **Bb2v**, page 292 {**Storti 24**}; **I6v**, page 108 {**Malachin 6**}; K3v, page 114 {**Storti 6**}; L2v, page 124 {**Ruinetti 18**}.

Decorated N at **+3r**, page [5] {**Malachin 2**}; I at **A1r**, page 1 {**Malachin 5**}; D at **C2v**, page 28 {**Ruinetti 13**}; O at **H5r**, page 95 {**Ruinetti 15**}; A at **K1r**, page 109 {**Malachin 7**}; Q at **S1v**, page 206 {**Ruinetti 20**}; Q at **Bb3r**, page 293 {**Malachin 8**}.

[2]. Headpiece at **A2r**, page 5 {**Malachin 4**}; tailpiece at **N4r**, page 151; **T4v**, page 224; **Ee3v**, page 334 {**Malachin 3**}; **T7r**, page 229 {**Storti 6**}.

Decorated E at **A2r**, page 3 {**Malachin 9**}; Q at **A[3]r**, page 5 {**Ruinetti 21**}; Q at **M5v**, page 142 {**Ruinetti 20**}; A at **T5r**, page 225 {**Ruinetti 16**}; D at **T6r**, page 227 {**Malachin 10**}.

Illustrations: as in **8H** apart from:

[1]. **Pl.1g2**. Plate 1 (image 1): *Fig I* (headline, centre), *Pag: ii5* (headline, right). Printed on **K4r**, page 115.

Pl.2g2. Plate 2 (image 2): *Fig. II.^da.^* (headline, centre), *Cerebri anat. Pag. ii6* (headline, right). Printed on **K4v**, page 116.

Pl.3g2. Plate 3 (image 3): *Fig. III* (headline, centre), *Pag. i2i* (headline, right). Printed on **L1r**, page 121.

Pl.4g2. Plate 4 (image 4): *Fig. IV.* (headline, centre), *Pag. i22* (headline, right). Printed on **L1v**, page 122.

Pl.5g2. Plate 5 (image 5): *Fig. V.* (headline, left), *Cerebri anat. Pag. i25* (headline, right). Printed on **L3r**, page 125.

Pl.6g2. Plate 6 (image 6): *Fig: VI.* (headline, centre), *Cerebri anat. Pag. i26* (headline, right). Printed on **L3v**, page 126.

Pll.7g2. Plate 7 (images 7–10): [Unnumbered 1] *Cerebri anat.* (headline, left), *Pag. 133* (headline, right), *Fig. 1*, *Fig. 11*, *Fig. 111*, (header, above each image), *Fig. 1111* (header, right of the image). Printed on **M1r**, page 133.

Pl.8g2. Plate 8 (image 11): *Fig VII^a^* (headline, centre), *Cerebri anat. Pag. 138.* (headline, right). Printed on **M3v**, page 138.

Pl.9g2. Plate 9 (image 12): *Cerebri anat.* (headline, left), *Fig. VIII.* (headline, centre), *Pag 144* (headline, right). Printed on **M4v**, page 144.

Pl.10g2. Plate 10 (images 13–14): [Unnumbered 2] *Cerebri anat. Pag 166* (headline, centre), *Fig. I.*, *Fig. II.* (header, above each image). Printed on **O5v**, page 166.

Pl.11g2. Plate 11 (image 15): *Cerebri anat. Pag. 187.* (headline, centre), *Tabula IX.*^{a} (headline, right). Printed on **Q4r**, page 187.

Pl.12g2. Plate 12 (image 16): *Cerebri anat. Pag. 190* (headline, centre), *Tabula X.*^{ma} (headline, right). Printed on **Q5v**, page 190.

Pl.13g2. Plate 13 (image 17): *Cerebri anat. Pag. 192* (headline, right), *Tabula X1.*^{ma} (footer, right). Printed on **Q6v**, page 192.

Pl.14g2. Plate 14 (image 18): *Cerebri anat. Pag. 194* (headline, centre), *Tabula XII* (headline, right). Printed on **R1v**, page 194.

Pl.15g2. Plate 15 (images 19–23): *Pag. 195* (headline, centre), *Tab: XIII* (headline, right), *Fig. I.*^{ma} (header, above the image), *Fig. 2.*$^{da..}$(header, within the image). Printed horizontally on **R2r**, page 195; and *Pag 196* (headline, right), *Fig. 3.*$^{tia.}$, *Fig. 5.*^{ta}, *Fig. 4.*$^{ta.}$ (header, above each image). Printed on **R2v**, page 196.

Pl.16d2. Plate 16 (images 24–25) *Pag: 205* (headline, left), *Fig 2*, *Fig 1.* (header, above each image). Printed on **S1r**, page 205.

Pl.17g2. Plate 17 (images 26–27) and **Pl.18g2**. Plate 18 (images 28–29): *De affect hyster.* (headline, left), *Pag. 319* (headline right), *Fig. I.*, *Fig. II.*, *Fig. III.*, *Fig. IV.* (header, above each image). Printed on **Dd4r**, page 319.

[2]. **Pl.19.f2**. Plate 19 (images 30–33): *de anima brut. Pag: i6 T*^{o} *2* (headline, centre), *Tab. I.*^{a} (headline, right), *Fig. I.*^{a}, *Fig. II.*^{da}, *Fig. IIII.*^{ta}, *Fig. III.*^{tia} (headers, above each image). Printed on **B2v**, page 16.

Pl.20f2. Plate 20 (images 34–35): *Tab. II.*^{da} (headline, centre), *de animâ brut. Pag: 17 T:*^{o} *2* (headline, right), *Fig. I.*^{a}, *Fig. II.*^{da} (header, above each image). Printed on **B3r**, page 17.

Pl.21f2. Plate 21 (images 36–38): *Tab. III.*^{tia} (headline, centre), *de anim. brut. pag. i8 T*^{o} *2* (headline, right), *Figura. 1.*^{ma}, *Fig. II.*^{da}, *Fig. III.*^{tia} (headers, above each image). Printed on **B3v**, page 18.

Pl.22f2. Plate 22 (images 39–41): *de anima bru. Pag i9 T*^{o} *2* (headline, centre), *Tab. IV.* (headline, right), *Fig. I*^{ma}, *Fig II.*^{da}, *Fig. III.*^{tia} (header, above each image). Printed on **B4r**, page 19.

Pl.23f2. Plate 23 (image 42): *de Anim. brut.* (headline, left), *Pag. 24 T:*^{o} *2* (headline, centre), *Tab.V.* (headline right). Printed on **B6v**, page 24.

Pl.24f2. Plate 24 (image 43): *de Anima Brut. Pag. 25* (headline, left), *Tomo. 2* (headline, right) [Tabula VI omitted]. Printed on **C1r**, page 25.

Pl.25f2. Plate 25 (image 44): *de Anima Brut. Pag. 25* (headline, left), *Tomo. 2* (headline, right) [Tabula VII omitted]. Printed on **C1r**, page 25.

Pl.26f2. Plate 26 (image 45): *de anima brut. Pag. 35* (headline, left), *Tomo. 2* (headline, right) [Tabula VIII omitted]. Printed on **C6r**, page 35.

Pl.27g1. Plate 27 (image 46): *Tab. I.* (headline, centre). *Pharmac. Pag. 430* [altered in pen and ink to 152] (headline, right); with **Pl.28g1**. Plate 28 (image 47): *Tab. II.* (headline, centre). Inserted after legends for Tabulæ I–VI at **N4v**, page 152.

Pl.29g2. Plate 29 (image 48): *Pharmac. Pag. 152: Tomo: 2.* (headline, left), *Tab. III.* (headline, centre); with **Pl.30g2**. Plate 30 (image 49–51): *Tab.* IV. (headline, left), *Fig.* 2., *Fig. 3.*, *Fig.* I. (headers, above each image). Inserted after legends for Tabulæ I–VI at **N4v**, page 152.

Pl.31g1. Plate 31 (image 52): *Tab. V.* (headline, centre), *Pharmac. Pag. 430.* [altered in pen and ink to 152] (headline, right); with **Pl.32g1**. Plate 32 (images 53–57): *Tab.* VI. (headline, centre). Inserted after legends for Tabulæ I–VI at **N4v**, page 152.

Pl.33g1. Plate 33 (image 58): *Pharmaceutic. Pag. 503.* [altered in pen and ink to 240] (headline, left), *Tab. I.* (headline, right); with **Pl.34g1**. Plate 34 (image 59): *Tab: II.* (headline, centre). Inserted before legends for Tabulæ I–VIII at **V5r–v**, pages 241–2.

Pl.35g2. Plate 35 (images 60–61): *Tab: III.* (headline, left), *Pharmac. Pag.*[a] *240: Tomo. 2* (headline, right), Fig: *1*, *Fig: 2* (headers, left off each image); with **Pl.36g2**. Plate 36 (images 62–64): *Tab: IV.* (headline, centre), *Fig: 1.*, *Fig: 2.*, *Fig: 3* (headers, left of each image). Inserted before legends for Tabulæ I–VIII at **V5r–v**, pages 241–2.

Pl.37g1. Plate 37 (images 65–67): *Pharmac. Pag.*[a] *503.* [altered in pen and ink to 240] (headline, centre), *Tab: V.* (headline, right), *Fig: 2.*, *Fig: 1.*, *Fig: 3.* (lheaders, below each image). Inserted before legends for Tabulæ I–VIII at **V5r–v**, pages 241–2.

Pl.38g1. Plate 38 (images 68–75): *Pharmac Tab: VI.* (headline, left), *Pag. 503.* [altered in pen and ink to 240] (headline, right), *Fig: 1.*, *Fig: 2.* (headers, above each group of four images); with **Pl.39g1**. Plate 39 (images 76–79): with *Tab: VII.* (headline, centre), *Fig: 3*, *Fig: i.*, *Fig: 2.*, *Fig: 4.* (headers, below each image); with **Pl.40g1**. Plate 40 (images 80–82): *Tab. VIII.* (headline, centre), *Fig: i.*, *Fig: 2.*, *Fig: 3.* (headers, above each image). Inserted before legends for Tabulæ I–VIII at **V5r–v**, pages 241–2.

Copy: DASC. Original vellum, spine with five raised bands, labelled THOMAE WILL | IS | OPERA. OMNI, original endpapers. Leaves 337 × 224 millimetres, boards 352 × 228 × 75 millimetres. Shelf mark ??6-3 cofɔæŭh BS. Inscribed: Franc:[s] Monticelli Medicina Professor 1729.[26]

[26] The Archive of the State of Venice and that of the Venice Health Magistracy indicate that one or more physicians named Monticelli were working in Venice between March 1696 and December 1746 but their forenames are not documented. Presumably Franciscus Monticelli who owned the book from 1729, nine years after publication, was a close relative of Paolo Monticelli (nd). Paolo was working in Venice in August 1724 and selected as one of a group of physicians entitled to conduct post-mortems in May 1732. See: MG Levi, *Ricordi intorno agli medici chirurghi e farmacisti che praticarono loro arte in Venezia dopo il 1740*, Venice (1835): pages 20B and 74A.

13

'Satisfying a mind desirous of truth'

Dr Willis's practice of physick (1679–1684)

Four years after his death in November 1675, the decision was taken by printers and booksellers not previously involved with the editions written in Latin to publish Thomas Willis's works in English. From the outset, the intention was a single folio edition containing all of the treatises and their illustrations. The error of adding William Croone's *De ratione motus musculorum* was avoided. *Affectionum quæ dicuntur hystericæ et hypochondriacæ* addressed to Nathanael Highmore (1613–1685) was not to be included. The manuscript of *A plain and easy method* was as yet unknown. The plan was therefore to gather in the vernacular twelve treatises: *Of fermentation*, *Of feavers*, *Of urines*, *Of the accension of the blood*, *Of musculary motion*, *Of the anatomy of the brain*, *Of the description and use of the nerves*, *Of convulsive diseases*, *Of the scurvy*, *Two discourses concerning the soul of brutes*, and the two parts of *Pharmaceutice rationalis*, The project evolved slowly. The two parts of *Pharmaceutice rationalis* with separate title pages and discontinuous signatures and pagination appeared first, together with *A tract of the scurvy* individually signed and paginated but without a separate title page (1679: **9A**). Aptly named, *The remaining medical works* containing eight treatises was next published (1681: **9B**). These two publications were then combined as the first edition of *Dr Willis's practice of physick* (1681: **9C**). Once *Two discourses concerning the soul of brutes* had appeared (1683: **9D**), this was incorporated with existing and some newly set sheets to make up the second edition of *Dr Willis's practice of physick* (1684: **9E**). The original plan concluded with publication of the third and final edition in which treatises making up *The remaining medical works* were also revised and reset (1684: **9F**).[1]

Samuel Pordage

Pharmaceutice rationalis (1679) was licensed to R. L'Estrange (1616–1704) on 31 October 1678. Some commentators have therefore assumed that he was the translator.[2] From what is known of L'Estrange this seems unlikely. But that he captured the rights and perhaps commissioned putting the work into English is not surprising. *The remaining medical works* was 'Englished' by S.P. The dedication to Sir Theophilus Biddulph at A2r–v, pages [7–8], laying out in the usual oleaginous terms the many achievements and virtues of his patron, is signed *S. Pordage*. A note added to the sale by Sotheran's of *Dr Willis's practice of physick* (1681: **9C**; see next) states that 'the translator was the dramatist S[amuel] P[ordage] and the verses "On

[1] Carrying over sheets from an earlier printing to a new edition is reflected in the bibliographic descriptions that follow. The reader is asked to refer back to identical accounts of individual sections of the collective works. Apart from avoiding much repetition, this serves to show how the various editions were put together from existing material.

[2] See: Robert Watt, *Bibliotheca Britannica; or a general index to British and foreign literature*. Volume II. Edinburgh and London (1824): page 971.

the Author's Medical-Philosophical Discourses" preceding the text are also supposed to be by him'. Samuel Pordage (1633–1691) is named as the translator of the only English edition of *Two discourses concerning the soul of brutes* (1683).[3]

William Feindel (1918–2014) considers Pordage 'an obscure choice as translator from the Latin of Willis's publications'.[4] Described on the title page of *Two discourses concerning the soul of brutes* as 'Student in PHYSICK', the details of his medical education (if any) are unknown. Pordage wrote a volume of poems and several Restoration plays but his literary successes were few. He was critical of John Dryden (1631–1700), who responded by dubbing Pordage a 'lame Mephibosheth, the wizard's son'. It seems that Willis thought out his text in English and put this into unpretentious Latin, making Pordage's task of making the writings accessible to 'my Countrymen' easier than it might otherwise have been. Lloyd Stevenson (1918–1988) quotes Professor JF Leddy (1911–1998) who had himself started a translation of *Cerebri anatome*:[5]

> Willis's Latin prose is direct and unpretentious, conforming to the basic rules of composition and word order, but in no degree attempting a high style or exhibiting even a markedly personal manner ... Pordage usually had a straightforward course to pursue. However, Willis's vocabulary does often pose a problem. His exposition is often ... surprisingly vague, as if he himself despaired of finding an altogether satisfactory Latin word for the detailed description of his dissections and experiments. When this happens, the English of Pordage is of little assistance.

Pordage's efforts at moving Willis's technical phrases from Latin to English were often uninformed. Where Willis found difficulty in coining a Latin word, Pordage was no more successful in English and often retained the Latin versions. He uses English words that were well understood in his day but have now altered or lost their meaning. In other contexts, Pordage forced translation on terms that have since reverted to the Latin: for example, 'the oblong marrow' for the medulla oblongata. But, for Stevenson, Pordage on Willis is 'with rare exceptions ... an accurate, vigorous translation, forthright and full of life. Thomas Willis is well served by his translator'.

Publication of the individual treatises in English

There are two issues of the English edition of *Pharmaceutice rationalis* (1679). Both identify the involvement of Thomas Dring (*c*.1644–1695), Charles Harper (*c*.1643–1714) and John Leigh (d.1685); one also lists Robert Clavell (*c*.1633–1711) on the title page of part 1 but not part 2. Notices appearing in the *Term Catalogue* indicate that there were delays in publication:

> Hilary 1679 February 18th, III Numb 18, I 341, column 2, *Physick*.
>
> *PHARMACEUTICE Rationalis*, or An Exercitation of the Operations of Medicines in humane Bodies. Shewing the Signs, Causes, and Cures, of most distempers incident thereunto.

[3] See: Philip M Oldfield, *A bibliography of Thomas Willis's De anima brutorum*, unpublished manuscript (1991): page 24 for reference to papers in Sloane MS 630, ff 121 at the British Library containing extracts in English translation of *De anima brutorum* by Dr Samuel Bellingham (nk) in the seventeenth century, including text 'on lethargy' and 'on gout' not intended for publication.

[4] See: *Thomas Willis. The anatomy of the brain and nerves*, volume 1. Ed. William Feindel, Montreal (1965): pages 45–7.

[5] See: Lloyd G Stevenson, 'A note on Pordage's translation'. In: Feindel (1965), volume I: pages 61–5.

In Two Parts. As also a Treatise of the Scurvy, and the several sorts thereof; with their Symptomes, Causes, and Cure. By Thos. Willis, M.D., and Sedley Professour in the University of *Oxford*, also one of the Colledge of Physitians in *London*, and Fellow of the Royal Society. In Folio. Printed for T. Dring at the Harrow, C. Harper at the Flower de Luce, and J. Leigh at the Bell, in *Fleet street*.

Easter 1679 May, III Numb 19, I 355, column 2, *Advertisements*.

Dr Willis' *Pharmaceutice Rationalis*, or An Exercitation of the Operations of Medicines in humane Bodies; shewing the Signs, Causes, and Cures, of most diseases incident thereunto. Also A Treatise of the Scurvy. In Folio. / This Book was in the last Catalogue; but not being finished, is now sold by R. Clavell at the Peacock in St. Paul's Churchyard.

In the copies examined for this bibliography, the pagination errors at R4v, page 124 for 128 (part 1), and S1v, 132 for 130 (part 2) are always present; but those at O2v–O3r, pages 100–1 (101 for 100, and 102 for 101: part 2), are correct in some copies of the issue published without Robert Clavell. It follows that leaves in different states were randomly distributed and therefore copies bound with both variant title pages may have either the correct or incorrect paginations at O2v and O3r.

The remaining medical works (1681: **9B**) is also found in two issues distinguished by the title page adding the bookseller Robert Clavell to the list of the four others for whom the book was printed: Thomas Dring, Charles Harper, John Leigh, and S Martyn (nd). The setting without Robert Clavell has different spacing in order to accommodate one extra line, 'The firſt part, though laſt published', with a rule above and below but without adding to the overall height of the text and surrounding double rule (263 millimetres). This does not of itself establish priority, although a case can be made for the reference to the first part but last published being added as an after-thought. More compelling, as discussed next, is evidence from two states of the first unnumbered illustration in the treatise 'Of the anatomy of the brain' (Pl.7). The second state with the page placement at the top left corner is seen only in the issue without Robert Clavell, suggesting that the issues listing him as bookseller are the earlier.

The English edition of *Two discourses concerning the soul of brutes* (1683) has no sheet O between the two parts, and the pagination moves from 96 to 105 even though the text is continuous across this interval. The printer either miscalculated the number of sheets and pages in assigning 'pars secunda' to a different typesetter from the compositor for the first part; or preliminaries such as a table were originally intended for part 1 but amended during preparation of the text and moved to the table for 'pars secunda' at the end of the book. If so, the four text leaves of the table for which sheet O might have been used eventually were printed at Hh2, Ii1 and Ii2, and Kk1. The Latin version of *De anima brutorum* (1672) has no text between the two parts identifying what might have been intended for signature O, pages 97–104, in the English translation.

Dr Willis's practice of physick

A note printed at the end of the table listing contents of *Two discourses concerning the soul of brutes*, draws attention to the collected works.[6] This was not the first such advertisement.

6 See description of **9E.c1** (next) for full text.

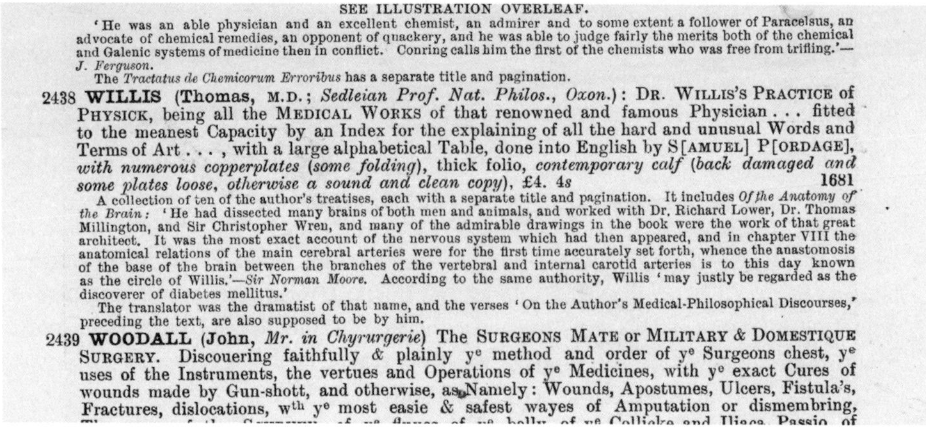

SEE ILLUSTRATION OVERLEAF.

'He was an able physician and an excellent chemist, an admirer and to some extent a follower of Paracelsus, an advocate of chemical remedies, an opponent of quackery, and he was able to judge fairly the merits both of the chemical and Galenic systems of medicine then in conflict. Conring calls him the first of the chemists who was free from trifling.'—*J. Ferguson.*

The *Tractatus de Chemicorum Erroribus* has a separate title and pagination.

2438 **WILLIS** (Thomas, M.D.; *Sedleian Prof. Nat. Philos., Oxon.*): DR. WILLIS'S PRACTICE of PHYSICK, being all the MEDICAL WORKS of that renowned and famous Physician . . . fitted to the meanest Capacity by an Index for the explaining of all the hard and unusual Words and Terms of Art . . . , with a large alphabetical Table, done into English by S[AMUEL] P[ORDAGE], *with numerous copperplates (some folding)*, thick folio, *contemporary calf (back damaged and some plates loose, otherwise a sound and clean copy)*, £4. 4s 1681

A collection of ten of the author's treatises, each with a separate title and pagination. It includes *Of the Anatomy of the Brain*: 'He had dissected many brains of both men and animals, and worked with Dr. Richard Lower, Dr. Thomas Millington, and Sir Christopher Wren, and many of the admirable drawings in the book were the work of that great architect. It was the most exact account of the nervous system which had then appeared, and in chapter VIII the anatomical relations of the main cerebral arteries were for the first time accurately set forth, whence the anastomosis of the base of the brain between the branches of the vertebral and internal carotid arteries is to this day known as the circle of Willis.'—*Sir Norman Moore.* According to the same authority, Willis 'may justly be regarded as the discoverer of diabetes mellitus.'

The translator was the dramatist of that name, and the verses 'On the Author's Medical-Philosophical Discourses,' preceding the text, are also supposed to be by him.

2439 **WOODALL** (John, *Mr. in Chyrurgerie*) The SURGEONS MATE or MILITARY & DOMESTIQUE SURGERY. Discouering faithfully & plainly ye method and order of ye Surgeons chest, ye uses of the Instruments, the vertues and Operations of ye Medicines, with ye exact Cures of wounds made by Gun-shott, and otherwise, as Namely: Wounds, Apostumes, Ulcers, Fistula's, Fractures, dislocations, wth ye most easie & safest wayes of Amputation or dismembring,

Figure 153 Entry from catalogue of Henry Sotheran, Ltd., 43, Piccadilly, London, W.1, *c.*1935, offering *Dr Willis's practice of physick* 1681 at £4. 4s.

An entry in the Term Catalogue during 1681 had already made clear that the various English translations had always been planned as one publication:

> Hilary 1681 February, IV Numb 2, I 431, column 1/2, *Physick.*
>
> DR· Willis's practice of Physick: being all the medical Works of that renowned and famous Physician; containing these ten several Treatises, viz. I. of Fermentation. 2. of Fevers. 3. of Urines. 4. of the Ascension of the Blood. 5. of Musculary Motion. 6. of the Anatomy of the Brain. 7. of the description and use of the Nerves. 8. of Convulsive Diseases. [9. *Pharmaceutice Rationalis*, First and Second Part. 10. of the Scurvey]. Wherein most of the Diseases belonging to the Body of Man are treated of, with excellent Methods and Receipts for the cure of the same; fitted to the meanest Capacity by an Index for explaining of all the hard and unusual words and terms of Art derived from the Greek, Latin, or other Languages, for the Benefit of the English Reader With a large alphabetical Table to the whole. With thirty-two Copper plates. Done into English by S. P., Esquire. Folio.

What happened in 1681 is that sheets of *Pharmaceutice rationalis* unsold from 1679 and those of the recently printed *The remaining medical works* were bound as one volume with a collective title page and sold as *Dr Willis's practice of physick* (1681: **9C**). Whilst the two component works are sometimes bound together, copies that also have the 1681 collective title page are very rare. Possibly only a single example survives.[7] Henry Sotheran Ltd. (founded in York, 1761, and based in London from 1815) sold a copy from their premises at 43 Piccadilly, London, before the Second World War for £4. 4s (see: Figure 153). The example now in the Huntington Library, San Marino, was handled by Raphael King (fl 1924–1954; d.1955) at his shop in Museum Street, London, in May 1942 (Catalogue 38: #410); and bought from the San Francisco bookseller,

[7] At the time of writing, the English Short Title Catalogue lists copies in seven United Kingdom libraries and eight in the United States but, of these, all except one are 'virtual' and relate to online e-book access to the Huntington Library copy. This appears to lack two leaves (A1 and A3). It is incorrectly collated in the catalogue as: [12], 178, [4], 191, [5], 106, [42], 155, [9], 179, [1], 56, [16], i.e. 477 leaves and 952 pages despite having only 5 preliminary leaves [10] in the first section.

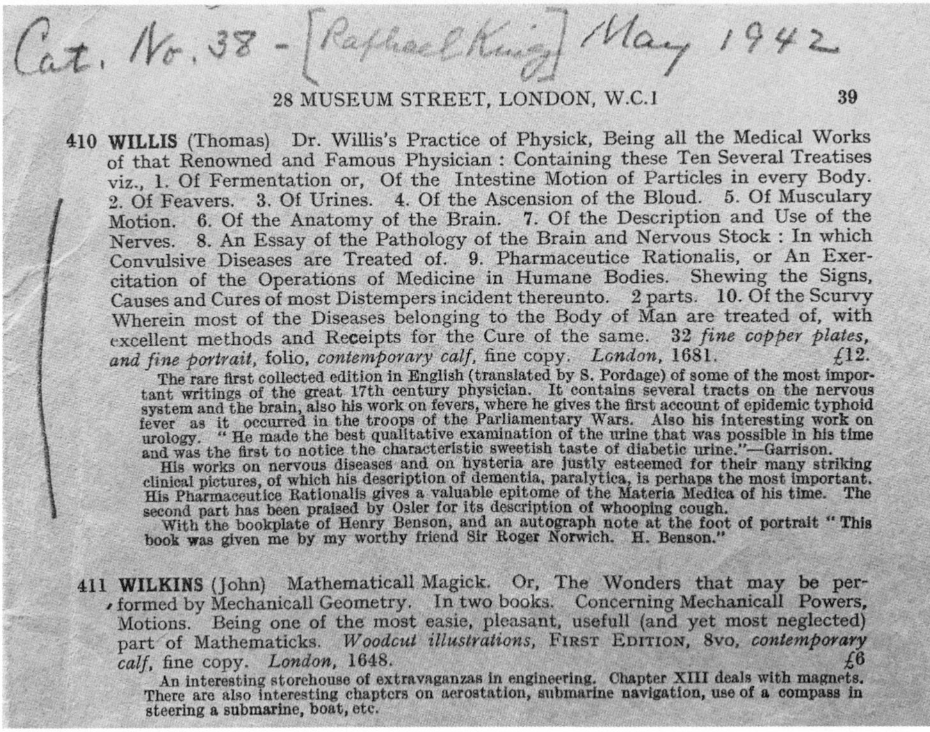

Cat. No. 38 - [Raphael King] May 1942

28 MUSEUM STREET, LONDON, W.C.1 39

410 **WILLIS** (Thomas) Dr. Willis's Practice of Physick, Being all the Medical Works of that Renowned and Famous Physician : Containing these Ten Several Treatises viz., 1. Of Fermentation or, Of the Intestine Motion of Particles in every Body. 2. Of Feavers. 3. Of Urines. 4. Of the Ascension of the Bloud. 5. Of Musculary Motion. 6. Of the Anatomy of the Brain. 7. Of the Description and Use of the Nerves. 8. An Essay of the Pathology of the Brain and Nervous Stock : In which Convulsive Diseases are Treated of. 9. Pharmaceutice Rationalis, or An Exercitation of the Operations of Medicine in Humane Bodies. Shewing the Signs, Causes and Cures of most Distempers incident thereunto. 2 parts. 10. Of the Scurvy Wherein most of the Diseases belonging to the Body of Man are treated of, with excellent methods and Receipts for the Cure of the same. 32 *fine copper plates, and fine portrait,* folio, *contemporary calf,* fine copy. *London,* 1681. £12.

The rare first collected edition in English (translated by S. Pordage) of some of the most important writings of the great 17th century physician. It contains several tracts on the nervous system and the brain, also his work on fevers, where he gives the first account of epidemic typhoid fever as it occurred in the troops of the Parliamentary Wars. Also his interesting work on urology. " He made the best qualitative examination of the urine that was possible in his time and was the first to notice the characteristic sweetish taste of diabetic urine."—Garrison.

His works on nervous diseases and on hysteria are justly esteemed for their many striking clinical pictures, of which his description of dementia, paralytica, is perhaps the most important. His Pharmaceutice Rationalis gives a valuable epitome of the Materia Medica of his time. The second part has been praised by Osler for its description of whooping cough.

With the bookplate of Henry Benson, and an autograph note at the foot of portrait " This book was given me by my worthy friend Sir Roger Norwich. H. Benson."

411 **WILKINS** (John) Mathematicall Magick. Or, The Wonders that may be performed by Mechanicall Geometry. In two books. Concerning Mechanicall Powers, Motions. Being one of the most easie, pleasant, usefull (and yet most neglected) part of Mathematicks. *Woodcut illustrations,* FIRST EDITION, 8vo, *contemporary calf,* fine copy. *London,* 1648. £6

An interesting storehouse of extravaganzas in engineering. Chapter XIII deals with magnets. There are also interesting chapters on aerostation, submarine navigation, use of a compass in steering a submarine, boat, etc.

Figure 154 Entry from catalogue of Raphael King, 28 Museum St., London, WC1, May 1942, offering *Dr Willis's practice of physick* 1681 at £12.

Glen Dawson (1912–2016), on 24 April 1961 for $200 (see: Figure 154). The booksellers' descriptions do not suggest that this is the copy handled by Henry Sotheran Ltd. The Huntington Library copy has title pages for each component work in the states that do not list Clavell as one of the booksellers. Why there are so few surviving copies remains unclear. Although sheets of *The remaining medical works* were still available, those for *Pharmaceutice rationalis* (1679) may have run out, preventing further sales of the collective volume. Whatever happened in 1681, within two years *Two discourses concerning the soul of brutes* (1683) was available, making the earlier collection incomplete and no longer of commercial interest. Although it made sense to use existing sheets of *The remaining medical works* for the next edition of *Dr Willis's practice of physick* (1684: **9E**), the view was taken that the translation of *Pharmaceutice rationalis* from 1679, licensed to Roger L'Estrange, the supply of which may in any case have been exhausted, could be improved upon. This was now redone by Pordage. Anthony Wood (1632–1695) wrote: 'This *Pharmaceutice* was translated into *English* by *Anon*. Lond. 1679. Fol. But being not well done it was corrected by *S. P.* Esq.; before mention'd and involved in the former Translation of 1681'.[8]

[8] See: [Anthony Wood] *Athenæ Oxoniensis. An exact history of all the writers and bishops who have had their education in the most ancient and famous University of Oxford, from the fifteenth year of King Henry the Seventh, Dom. 1500, to the end of the year 1690. Representing the birth, fortune, preferment, and death of all those authors and prelates, the great accidents of their lives, and the fate and character of their writings. To which are added, the Fasti or Annals, of the said University, for the same time,* volume 1, London (1690): page 403.

The second edition of *Dr Willis's practice of physick* (1684: **9E**) is made up of unsold sheets of *The remaining medical works* (1681), the newly translated *Pharmaceutice rationalis* (redated 1684), and copies of *Two discourses concerning the soul of brutes* (1693). Whereas the 1681 edition retained the title page for *The remaining medical works* on π1r, printing the new collective title page on *1r, the former was omitted when the second edition was published in 1684. Therefore this edition has fewer preliminary leaves.

Later that year, the decision was taken also to correct and amend the eight treatises of *The remaining medical works*. The third edition of Willis's collected works in English, published in 1684 (**9F**), therefore contains texts of *The remaining medical works* corrected and reset in 1684; the second translation of *Pharmaceutice rationalis*; and the sheets of *Two discourses concerning the soul of brutes*. This final 1684 edition has subsidiary title pages for *A medical-philosophical discourse* (Of fermentation and Of fevers), *An essay of the pathology of the brain and nervous stock in which convulsive diseases are treated of* (both with 1681 redated 1684), *each part of Pharmaceutice rationalis* (1684) and *Two discourses concerning the soul of brutes* (1683). The title page for the Five treatises is omitted. The third edition is the book usually referred to as Dr Willis's practice of physick (1684). Although never reissued, a large number of copies survive indicating that the print run was considerable, and the book valued by contemporary readers, libraries, and collectors and therefore preserved.

The table of hard words

Pordage had a popular readership in mind and understood that his text might prove difficult for the general reader. His problem was that English words did not exist for many of the Latin terms to which physicians and medical scientists were accustomed. Therefore he included an explanatory table of hard words:[9]

> Since nothing could so well express the meaning and intention of the Author, as the very *Latin* and *Greek* words used in these tracts, we have continued them expressly, and though in many places I have given their meanings by *Synonymas*, yet for the benefit of the meer *English* Readers, we have here composed a Table Alphabetically of all the hard *Greek* and *Latin* words, used in the whole Volume; as also of all Terms of Art, and many other words derived from the *Latin* and *Greek*, though usual among Scholars, yet not frequently known to the vulgar, and therefore we have fully explained them and rendred them intelligible to the meanest Capacity in the following Table.

[9] The earliest example of an explanatory table for the general reader is in the cleric Robert Cawdrey's (*c.*1538–*c.*1604) *A table alphabeticall conteyning and teaching the true writing, and vnderstanding of hard usuall English words, borrowed from the Hebrew, Greeke, Latine, or French, &c. With the interpretation thereof by plaine English words, gathered for the benefit & helpe of ladies, gentlewomen, or any other vnskilfull persons. Whereby they may the more easilie and better vnderstand many hard English wordes, vvhich they shall heare or read in scriptures, sermons, or elswhere, and also be made able to vse the same aptly themselues*, London (1604). This has 2500 entries 'for the benefit and help of Ladies, gentlewomen or any other unskilful persons. Whereby they may more easily and better understand many hard English words, which they shall heare or read in the Scriptures, Sermons or elsewhere, and also be made able to vse the same aptly themselves'. After working as a teacher in Oakham, Rutland, Cawdrey was ordained and, on 22 October 1571, made rector of South Luffenham. His sympathy for Puritan teachings created difficulties with his bishop, Richard Howland (1540–1600), and, in 1588, Cawdrey was deprived of his living and returned to teaching.

Separately signed and unpaginated, the binder struggled to know where this table was best placed. Most copies of *The remaining medical works* (1681) have the table of hard words and that for the contents as a final section at (a)1r–(d)1r, pages [3–15], preceded by a blank (3P2, pages [1–2], often lacking), which separates these tables from the last leaf of *An essay of the pathology of the brain*. But it was less clear where best to place the tables when the last two editions of *Dr Willis's practice of physick* were assembled in 1684. Harold Denham (1917–1999) sought to explain the matter:[10]

> They occur in one place, e.g. preceding all the texts or split into sections, e.g. Table of Hard Words preceding and the rest following the texts of Fermentation and Feavers. The way in which they have been printed with continuous signatures and with some of the individual indexes combined suggests to me that they were intended to be bound together and the most logical place would be before the texts (as in my description). As far as I know they are not found at the end of the section to which they belong, i.e. after Convulsive Diseases nor at the end of the volume. The former would be confusing as Convulsive Diseases is treated as a separate part and there is no indication that the section ends here and the latter would involve a complete separation from the works to which they apply. Evidently the lines On the Authors Medical-Philosophical Discourses were printed on the blank leaf at the end of the Table of Hard Words to save using another sheet. I have left it in this position in my description but presumably it was intended that this leaf should be cut off and bound in after the preface as the catchword indicates and in some copies it does occur in this position.

This analysis needs qualification. When everything was finally reset for *Dr Willis's practice of physick* (1684, **9F**), the preliminaries contained material relevant to the whole volume and text that related specifically to the first three treatises, originally published as *Diatribæ duæ*. The table of hard words applied throughout the book. However, the tables of contents for the two parts of *Pharmaceutice rationalis* and for *Two discourses concerning the soul of brutes* were printed and bound separately from contents for the treatises that had previously made up *The remaining medical works*.

As a result the ordering of general and specific preliminary material is erratic, and no arrangement fully reconciles the signatures, catchwords, and flow of text. The main problem relates to the sheets, (a)–(g), containing the table of hard words and the list of contents for the first eight treatises. The verse 'On the Authors Medical-Philosophical Discourses' had been printed at A4r–v, pages [11–12] in *The remaining medical works*. Now it was printed on (d)2r–v, between the end of 'A TABLE of all the hard words' at (d)1r, page [23]—with (d)1v, page [24], blank—and 'The TABLE To the Treatises of FERMENTATION and FEAVERS' at (e)1r, page[25], as indicated by Denham. This is clearly inappropriate. The catchword on B2v, and the headline ('PREFACE') on the second page of the verse indicate that it was intended to follow the preface printed on B2r–v. The catchword at (d)2v ('OF') links this to the first page of text at 2B1r. The catchword on B1 is consistent with this preceding B2.

There are no catchwords linking to the start of the table of hard words at (a)1r. The catchword at end of the table of hard words, (d)1r 'THE', links to the start of the table of contents which ends at (g2)v with 'FINIS'. This therefore has no catchword. Stripped of (d)2, the two tables remain orphan and can be placed wherever seems most appropriate. Taken together,

[10] In an undated letter to a former owner of *Dr Willis's Practice of Physick* (1684, now **9F**) subsequently identified by Mr Denham as Mrs Strachan of New Zealand and dating the correspondence as 5 November [1984].

the best arrangement for the preliminaries is: π1, A1, A2, (a)1–(d)1, (e)1–(g)2, B1, B2, (d)2, 2B1, etc.

Illustrations to the English editions

If the evolution and organization of the texts was erratic, the story of the illustrations is no less complicated, both in terms of which plates were used in their various states and how many were included in each publication. One has only to read the different title pages to sense the confusion:[11]

Pharmaceutice rationalis (1679) part I, makes no mention of plates although there are twelve images engraved on six plates printed on six sheets.

Pharmaceutice rationalis part II (1679) has 'Copper Plates' and contains twenty five images, eight plates and eight sheets.

The remaining medical works (1681) mentions 'Eighteen copper plates' but has twenty seven images, seventeen plates and sixteen sheets.

Dr Willis's practice of physick (1681) describes 'Thirty two Copper Plates' and contains sixty-four figures, thirty-one plates and thirty sheets.

The advertisement for *Dr Willis's practice of physick* (1683) promises 'With Thirty Copper Plates'.

Two discourses concerning the soul of brutes (1683) is 'With Copper Cuts' and has sixteen figures, eight plates and seven sheets.

Dr Willis's practice of physick (1684, second edition) claims 'With Forty Copper Plates' but contains eighty images, thirty-eight plates and thirty-five sheets.

Dr Willis's practice of physick (1684, third edition) is also published 'With Forty Copper Plates' and has eighty images, thirty-seven plates and thirty-four sheets.

The title page of *The London practice of physick* (1692) advertises Dr WILLIS'S whole works in *Fol.* 'with Forty Copper Plates'.

Although the same plates are used for *Pharmaceutice rationalis* in Latin (1674, 1675) and the folio edition in English (1679: **9A**), these are in different states in order to amend the page placements. When insufficient blank space was available, the new indicators were engraved over the old page numbers, traces of which remain visible. But it was clear that the confusion of correctly binding the illustrations in parts 1 and 2 also needed to be resolved. This only became apparent after Tabula 1, part 1 (Pl.27a4) had been amended to show the new placement, by chance at page 16 for both the 1674 and 1679 editions. It seemed sensible thereafter to engrave 'part 1' or 'part 2' on each plate so that this was bound into the correct section of the 1679 English edition. The Latin editio tertia (1679) appeared before the English translation and retained the original ambiguities. Storage of the original plates was evidently careless with damage occurring in the intervals from 1674 / 1675 to 1679. Although identical in terms of the engraving and figure sizes, the plate margins for Tabula I, part I (Pl.27a4) and Tabula VIII part II (Pl.40a3) are reduced in the English folio 1679 (**9A**); and Tabula VI, part I (Pl.32a4) has lost its top left corner. In some copies a minor alteration to the page placement

[11] See also chapter 3 for other details relating to these plates.

is made in the top right corner of Tabula I, part 1, from '*p.i6.*' to '*p. i6* .', creating two states of this plate leaf.

The remaining medical works (1681) contains the illustrations for *Cerebri anatome* (1664) and *De motu musculari* (1670). HJR Wing writes that: 'most of the illustrations to the Anatomy of the brain and Description and use of the nerves are printed from the same plates that were used in the original quarto edition of *Cerebri anatome* in 1664. Some of the original numbers of the facing pages engraved on the plates are still visible'. This is a slight simplification. Since the cost of engraving was considerable, many of the original plates were retained but extensively reworked after 1664. Several suffered in the process. Eventually Tabula XI and Tabula XII (Pl.13 and Pl.14) had to be replaced. An additional problem arose with the first unnumbered illustration (Pl.7). The indication (*pag. 56*) had been added for the London octavo in space that was previously blank at the top right corner. The first issue of *The remaining medical works* (**9B1**) has the new number '*pag. 86*' engraved over this old placement (Pl.7a3). The plate is already showing various cracks and stains and after some sheets had been printed, but before the second issue was published without Robert Clavell as bookseller, the top right corner fell off. The engraver therefore put '*pag. 86*' in blank space at the top left corner (Pl.7a4).

Engravings from 1670 for the four figures on two plates in *De motu musculari* (1670) containing Figures I and II (Pl.17) and Figures III and IV (Pl.18) were still available and printed on one leaf but at some point the margins of these plates were reduced from 127 × 171 millimetres and 129 × 172 millimetres to 113 × 160 millimetres and 114 × 165 millimetres, respectively.[12] Each was altered to show the new page placements (Pl.17a2, Pl.18a2). However, the plate leaf is found in two states: one has Figures III and IV printed above Figures I and II, and the other (less common) with Figures I and II above Figures III and IV. Judging by their frequency, both were readily available and each is found in copies of *The remaining medical works* as issued in 1681 or as part of *Dr Willis's practice of physick* (1684: **9E**).

With one exception, the plates bound in *Dr Willis's practice of physick* (1681: **9C**) are identical to those in copies of *Pharmaceutice rationalis* (1679) and *The remaining medical works* (1681) in the issues published without Robert Clavell (**9A2** and **9B2**). Tabula I from part 1 of *Phamaceutice rationalis* has, as expected for the second issue, the altered lettering, '*p. 16* .' in the top right corner (Pl.27a5). But the first unnumbered plate of 'The anatomy of the brain' in *The remaining medical works* is the first state with '*pag. 86*' in the top right corner (Pl.7a3). It differs from other copies of that plate leaf in that 'VII' has been added in manuscript at the top left. In the only available copy, the plate leaf for Pl.17 and Pl.18 has Figures III and IV above Figures I and II.

The eight illustrations for *Two discourses concerning the soul of brutes* (1683) were newly engraved. In general, whilst retaining the same arabic or roman type, different characters were used and occasional changes made or letters omitted: for example, the corpora quadrigemina in Tabu. V in *Two discourses concerning the soul of brutes* (1683) are labelled '*a B b*' (Pl.23c1) whereas the same illustration in *De anima brutorum* (1672: **5A**) has only '*B*' (Pl.23a1); and the 'A' at the top of the heart of the silkworm in *De anima brutorum* (1672: Pl.19a1) is omitted in *Two discourses concerning the soul of brutes* (1683: Pl.19c1).

[12] The probability that the corner fell away during printing of illustrations for later issues of *The remaining medical works*, not naming Robert Clavell, is suggested by copies in the Dorchester Library of the Royal College of Physicians: one without Robert Clavell has the first unnumbered illustration with 'p. 86' in the intact top right corner; another (bound with *Pharmaceutice rationalis*) has *The remaining medical works* without Clavell but the first unnumbered illustration in its second state, with 'p. 86' top left and the corner lost at top right.

Tabu VI (Pl.24) and Tabu VII (Pl.25) are on a single sheet in *Two discourses concerning the soul of brutes* (1683) but still printed from two plates.

Matters changed again in 1684. The second edition of *Dr Willis's practice of physick* (1684: **9E**) used illustrations for *Pharmaceutice rationalis* that were newly engraved. Those for *The remaining medical works* remained as in the original issues with the first unnumbered illustration in its second state (Pl.7a4). For the third edition of *Dr Willis's practice of physick* (1684: **9F**), just as the text of the treatises forming *The remaining medical works* was entirely reset, with two exceptions the plates also were reengraved. Tabula XI and Tabula XII had already been redone in 1681 and were still serviceable. Their old page placements were left untouched but details added to indicate the new pagination (Pl.13d2 and Pl.14d2). The unhappy first unnumbered illustration (Pl.7), which had experienced such an awkward history since its first appearance in the 1664 quarto edition, eventually reached its final state, printed in pristine condition and with all the information made clear (Pl.7d1). But despite all this new work, the opportunity to update the numbering and identify all fifteen illustrations in sequence was never taken and, twenty years on, the two late arrivals from 1664 remained unnumbered. All four figures for the illustrations to 'Of musculary motion' (Pl.17c1 and Pl.18c1) were now engraved on a single plate. The engraver also combined Figures I (Pl.1) and Figure II (Pl.2) from 'Of the anatomy of the brain' with a line indicating where the images were to be cut, even though the binder retained these on the same single folio sheet. As a result, the number of illustrations in the third edition of *Dr Willis's practice of physick* (1684) is reduced to eighty images, engraved on thirty-seven plates bound as thirty-four sheets.[13]

9A1. PHARMACEUTICE RATIONALIS, London folio 1679

The first issue of the first edition of both parts of Willis's sixth book in English, the ninth publication, using the first of four titles, with pagination errors [HJR Wing 54].

Title page: [1]. [within a double rule] PHARMACEUTICE RATIONALIS: | OR, AN | EXERCITATION | OF THE | OPERATIONS | OF | MEDICINES | IN | Humane Bodies. | SHEWING | The Signs, Caufes, and Cures of moft Diftempers inci- | dent thereunto. | [rule] | In Two PARTS. | [rule] | AS ALSO | A Treatife of the SCURVY, and the feveral forts | thereof, with their Symptoms, Caufes, and Cure. | [rule] | By *Tho. Willis* M.D. and *Sidley* Profeffor in the Univerfity of *Oxford*: Alfo | one of the College of Phyficians in *London*, and Fellow of the Royal Society. | [rule] | *Licenfed, October* 31. 1678. R. L' Eftrange. | [rule] | *LONDON,* | Printed for *T. Dring, C. Harper,* and *J. Leigh* in | *Fleetftreet*: And are to be fold by *R. Clavell* at the | Peacock, at the Weft End of St. *Paul's*: 1679.

[2]. [within a double rule] *PHARMACEUTICE RATIONALIS*: | OR, THE | OPERATIONS | OF | MEDICINES | IN | Humane Bodies. | [rule] | The Second Part. | With Copper Plates defcribing the feveral Parts treated of in this Volume. | [rule] | By *THO. WILLIS*, M. D. and *Sedley* Profeffor | in the Univerfity of *OXFORD*. | [rule] | [printers' ornament] | [double

[13] See chapter 3 for further details.

rule] | *LONDON*, | Printed for *Thomas Dring*, *Charles Harper*, and | *John Leigh*, Bookſellers in *Fleet-ſtreet*, 1679.

[3]. [No title page].

Collation: folio in 4s; 23 letter roman alphabet using I and U: [1]. A^4, a–b^4, B–U^4, X^2; \$1–2 signed.
90 leaves, paginated as [24], 1–155 [156]. Mispaginated: 101 for 100, 102 for 101, 124 for 128.

[2]. A–Z^4, Aa^2; \$1–2 signed.
94 leaves, paginated as [8], 1–179 [180]. Mispaginated: 132 for 130.

[3]. A–G^4, H1; \$1–2 signed.
29 leaves, paginated as 1–56, [2].

Type: 61 lines; height (20 lines) 81 millimetres, width 125 millimetres (146 millimetres with marginal notes).

Contents: [1]. **A1r**, page [1], title; **A1v**, page [2], blank; **A2r–A4v**, pages [3–8], THE PREFACE TO THE READER.; **a1r–b1r**, pages [9–17], THE TABLE TO THE Firſt Part.; **b1v–b4v**, pages [18–24], The TABLE to the Second PART.

B1r–X2r, pages 1–155, [text] THE FIRST PART OF Pharmaceutice Rationalis, OR OF THE OPERATIONS OF MEDICINES IN Humane Bodies.; **X2v**, page [156], blank.

[2]. **A1r**, page [1], title; **A1v**, page [2], blank; **A2r–A3r**, pages [3–5], THE PREFACE TO THE READER.; **A3v–A4v**, pages [6–8], POSTSCRIPT.

B1r–Aa2r, pages 1–179, [text] THE SECOND PART OF *PHARMACEUTICE RATIONALIS*, OR OF THE OPERATIONS OF MEDICINES IN HUMANE BODIES.; **Aa2v**, page [180], blank.

[3]. **A1r–G4v**, pages 1–56, [text] A TRACT OF THE SCURVY.; **H1r–v**, pages [1–2], THE TABLE to the Tract of the SCURVY.

Headlines and *Catchwords*: [1]. No '.' after headline at **b4v**, page [24]; **exceſſive** for **Exceſſive** at **I1r**, page 57; **Flux.** for **Dyſentery.** at **I4r**, page 63; **K1r**, page 65; Chap. I. for Chap. II. at **O3r**, page '102'.

Bottom for bottom at **B4v / C1r**, page 8 / 9; nough for enough at **D4v / E1r**, page 24 / 25; cinnamon for Cinamon at **I4r / v**, page 63 / 64; other for another at **S1r / v**, page 129 / 130.

[2]. **Impediments** for **The Impediments** at **D2r**, page 19; **the Phthiſis** for **a Conſumption** at **E3r**, page 29; **thoſe that ſpit blood.** for **perſons Spitting Blood.** at **I1v**, page 58; Chap. IX. for Chap. VIII. at **K1r**, page 65; Chap. XI. for Chap. XII. at **M2r**, page 83; Chap. XIII. for Chap. XII. at **N1r**, page 89.

(whhic for (which at **C4v** / **D1r**, pages 16 / 17; There for 3. There at **D3r** / **v**, pages 21 / 22; quently for frequently at **F2r** / **v**, pages 35 / 36; CHAP for SECT at **I2r** / **v**, pages 59 / 60; 3. Against for 3$^{\text{ly,}}$ Against at **K1r** / **v**, pages 65 / 66; alone: for alone at **K3v** / **K4r**, pages 70 / 71; 1. *Sul* for *Sul* at **Aa1r** / **v**, pages 177 / 178.

[3]. No “. after headline at **A1v**, page 2; **A2v**, page 4; no CHAP. II. at **A3v**, page 6; **A4v**, page 8; CHAP. I for CHAP. II at **A4r**, page 7.

CHAP. I for CHAP. II at **A3r** / **v**, pages 5 / 6; ved for depraved at **A3v** / **A4r**, pages 6 / 7; Melancholy for melancholy at **B4v** / **C1r**, pages 16 / 17.

Frontispiece: none.

Portrait: none.

Printers’ ornaments: [1]. Composite of four fleurons at **A2r**, page [3] {**Dring 1**}.

Decorated W at **A2r**, page [3] {**Dring 2**}.

[2]. Printers’ device at **A1r**, page [1] {**Dring 3**}.

Illustrations: as in **6A** and **6E** apart from:

[1]. **Pl.27a4**. Plate 27 (image 46): *Tab.I.* (headline, centre), *p.16.* (headline, right). Leaf size, 318 × 188 millimetres (sheet). Legend: The firſt Table repreſents the Ventricle of a Man with its Veſſels ſtrutting with Blood, enptied, and blown up that all the Arteries and Veins with their Ramifications (which are truly and moſt exactly delineated) may be ſeen. Inserted within THE EXPLICATION OF THE FIGURES at **C4v–D1v**, pages 16–18.

Pl.28a4. Plate 28 (image 47): *Tab. II. part i.st* (headline, centre). Leaf size, 318 × 198 millimetres (sheet) Legend: The ſecond table expreſſes altogether the outmoſt nervous Coat of the humane Ventricle, whoſe nervous Fibres being carried the length of it, do cut the underlying exterior fleſhy Fibres almoſt in right Angles. Inserted within THE EXPLICATION OF THE FIGURES at **C4v–D1v**, pages 16–18.

Pl.29a4. Plate 29 (image 48): *Tab. III. part i.st* (headline, centre). Leaf size, 318 × 198 millimetres (sheet). Legend: The third Table exhibits the humane Ventricle naked without its outward nervous Coat, that the exterior or Convex ſuperficies of the middle Coat with its fleſhy Fibres may appear. Inserted within THE EXPLICATION OF THE FIGURES at **C4v–D1v**, pages 16–18.

Pl.30a4. Plate 30 (images 49–51): *Tab.* IV. *part i.st* (headline, left), *Fig. 2.*, *Fig. 3*, *Fig. I.* (headers, above each image). Leaf size, 318 × 198 millimetres (sheet). Legend: The Fourth Table whoſe firſt Figure ſhews the Ventricle turned inſide out, with the interior and concave Superficies changed into the exterior and convex, that the hairy Cruſt, with its Wrinkles and Folds covering the Stomach, may be ſeen. The Second Figure repreſents a Portion of the nervous Coat in which the hairy Cruſt being taken away, the interior or concave ſuperficies, with the moſt thick Ramification of the Veſſels appears. The Third Figure ſhews a Portion of the hairy Coat, or glandulous, in which its exterior ſuperficies whereby it ſticks to the nervous Coat repleniſhed with glandulas and little Mouths of the Veſſels, is beheld. Inserted within THE EXPLICATION OF THE FIGURES at **C4v–D1v**, pages 16–18.

Pl.31a4. Plate 31 (image 52): *Tab.* V. *part. i.st* (headline, centre). Leaf size, 318 × 198 millimetres (sheet). Legend: The Fifth Table ſhews the interior ſuperficies of the fleſhy Coat, and the concave inverted or turned outwards that one of the Series of the moving Fibres may be ſeen. Inserted within THE EXPLICATION OF THE FIGURES at **C4v–D1v**, pages 16–18.

Pl.32a4. Plate 32 (images 53–57): *Tab.* VI. *part. i.ts* (headline, centre). Leaf size, 318 × 198 millimetres (sheet). Legend: The Sixth Table repreſents all the Coats of the ſmall Guts ſeparated one from another, that the nervous Fibres with the Glandulas and Ramifications of the Veſſels, alſo the orders of the moving Fibres may be clearly and diſtinctly obſerved. Inserted within THE EXPLICATION OF THE FIGURES at **C4v–D1v**, pages 16–18.

[2]. **Pl.33a3**. Plate 32 (image 58): *Sect. i: Cap. i. part.2.ist* (headline, left), *Tab: I.* (headline, right). Leaf size, 318 × 198 millimetres (sheet). Legend: THe firſt Table ſhews one entire lobe of the Lungs, upon whoſe ſuperficies the Lymphæducts are ſeen ſpread through every where. Inserted within *The Explication of the Figures* at **C3v–D1r**, pages 14–17.

Pl.34a3. Plate 34 (image 59): *Tab: II.* (headline, left), *part.2.ist* (headline, centre), *Sect. i: Cap. i.* (headline, right). Leaf size, 318 × 198 millimetres (sheet). Legend: The ſecond Table ſhews one lobe of a Sheeps Lung cut in the midſt, that the upper part (wherein is the trunk of the Vein) being removed, and the trunk of the *Aſpera Arteria* laid by it ſelf, the branching of the Pneumonic Artery is ſhewn throughout its whole frame, *viz.* through the ſmall and leaſt little Lobes. All the paſſages of this, *viz.* the ſlips and twigs how ſmall ſoever, being filled and coloured by any liquid thing caſt into them, are drawn to the life. Inserted within *The Explication of the Figures* at **C3v–D1r**, pages 14–17.

Pl.35a3. Plate 35 (images 60–61): *Tab. III.* (headline, left), *part 2.ist Sect. i: Cap i* (headline, right). Leaf size, 318 × 198 millimetres (sheet). Legend: The firſt Figure of the third Table expreſſes one lobe of the Lungs, according to the branchings of the *Aſpera Arteria* divided into leſſer and leſs lobes, the twigs and ſlips of which Veſſel being filled by a liquid firſt injected, and afterwards ſeparated from among themſelves towards the little lobes, are alſo drawn to the life. The ſecond Figure of the third Table expreſſes a part of the pulmonary lobe, wherein the membraneous interſpaces being blown up, all the little lobes appear in their proper figure, and do ſomewhat repreſent the leaf of Polypody. Inserted within *The Explication of the Figures* at **C3v–D1r**, pages 14–17.

Pl.36a3. Plate 36 (images 62–64): *Tab: IV.* (headline, centre), *Sect. i: Cap. i.* (headline, right), *Fig: 1.*, *Fig: 2.*, *Fig: 3.* (headers, left of each image). Leaf size, 318 × 198 millimetres (sheet). Legend: The fourth Table expreſſes as well the Veſſels belonging to the *Trachea* as thoſe bringing blood, ſeparate and diſtinct one from another, conſtituting one little Lobe, as alſo peculiar framing of every one of them. The firſt Figure repreſents the ſeparating into divers parts the Tracheal branch diſtributed into one little lobe, and the branching into Pipes and orbicular little bladders. The ſecond and third Figure ſhews diſtinctly the equal branchings of the Artery and Pneumonic Veins within the ſame little Lobe; both which being complicated with Tracheal Veſſels, do for the moſt part make up the texture of the pulmonary frame. Inserted within *The Explication of the Figures* at **C3v–D1r**, pages 14–17.

Pl.37a3. Plate 37 (images 65–67): *Sect. i: Cap. i*: (headline, left), *part 2.ist* (headline, centre), *Tab: V.* (headline, right), *Fig: 2.*, *Fig: 1.*, *Fig: 3.* (headers, below each image). Leaf size, 318 × 198 millimetres (sheet). Legend: The fifth Table ſets forth the pulmonary Nerve more accurately deſcribed by the aid of a Microſcope: ſo that it plainly appears that the Trunk is as it were a bundle of innumerable little Fibres bound together; moreover its Trunk, while it creeps into the lungs in the likeneſs of Mother of Time, doth ſpread the various little ſprigs every way. Fig. I. reſembles a part of the nervous trunk cut away, one end whereof being opened and lookt on by a Microſcope, ſeems to unfold it ſelf almoſt into innumerable little fibres. The ſecond and third figure do ſhew ſome fibres as well of the trunk as of every branch, and moreover the ſlips of the little twigs from divers ſtemmes often repeated. Inserted within *The Explication of the Figures* at **C3v–D1r**, pages 14–17.

Pl.38a3. Plate 38 (images 68–75): *Tab: VI. part 2.ist* (headline, left), *Sect. i: Cap. i*: (headline, right), *Fig: 1.*, *Fig: 2.* (header, above each set of four images). Leaf size, 318 × 198 millimetres (sheet). Legend: The ſixth Table firſt ſets forth the anatomy of the Artery bringing blood drawn in apt figures, which we have deſcribed in a late treatiſe. *The firſt and upper figures hereof*, repreſent the four diſtinct Coats of that Veſſel, *viz.* the nervous, muſcular, glandulous, and the vaſculous. The *ſecond and lower figures* of the ſixth Table, do ſhew the anatomy of the Vein, or its four coats expreſſed in fit places; which Coats do appear entire as ſucceſſively taken one part from the other (beginning outmoſt). Inserted within *The Explication of the Figures* at **C3v–D1r**, pages 14–17.

Pl.39a3. Plate 39 (images 76–79): *Tab: VII. part. 2.ist* (headline, centre), *Sect. i: Cap i*: (headline, right), *Fig: 1.*, *Fig: 3.*, *Fig: 4.*, *Fig: 2.* (headers, above each image). Leaf size, 318 × 198 millimetres (sheet). Legend: The ſeventh Table expreſſes the diſtinct Coats of the *aſpera arteria*, and ſeparated one from the other. *The firſt figure ſhews the moſt inward Coat*, endowed with ſtreight or long muſcular fibres. *The ſecond figure deſcribes the glandulous coat*, and the third figure the vaſculous coat (which are almost the ſame as in the veſſels bringing blood, and alſo in the Guts). 4. *The fourth figure expreſſes the outward coat* (which is partly cartilaginous, and partly muſcular.) The tranſverſe or annular fibres hereof do fill up and weave together the interſpaces of the Cartilages. Inserted within *The Explication of the Figures* at **C3v–D1r**, pages 14–17.

Pl.40a3. Plate 40 (images 80–82): *Sect. i: Cap i.* (headline, left), *Tab: VIII part 2.ist* (headline, centre), *Fig: 1.*, *Fig: 2.*, *Fig: 3.* (headers, above each image). Leaf size, 318 × 198 millimetres (sheet). Legend: The eighth Table ſhews a part of the outmoſt pulmonary Coat covering over its whole frame, moſt finely and curiouſly deſcribed by the help of a Microſcope. The first Figure ſhews a portion of the above mentioned coat, which partly by reaſon of the extremities of Veſſels of every ſort ending in it, ſeems pricked full of holes as it were, and partly from the complications of the veſſels bringing blood, which like the twining sprigs of Vines gird about the orbicular bladders, is diſtinguished into many irregular *Area's*. The ſecond Figure repreſents a part of the outermoſt membrane ſeparated from the cluſters of veſſels pull'd off, and without any *Areæ*, onely markt with little holes as it were with ſmall pricks. The third Figure expreſſes one ſingular *area* of the Coat above mentioned, augmented in largeneſs by the help of a Microſcope. Inserted at **C3v–D1r**, pages 14–17 within *The Explication of the Figures*.

Copy: DASC (#1 of 2). Original calf, spine (rebacked) with five raised bands, each with double gilt rules at top and bottom, gilt panels, red label WILLIS | PHARMACEUTICE | RATIONALIS / 1679. Leaves 318 × 198 millimetres, boards 330 × 200 × 46 millimetres. Inscribed: THO: GREGORY. MDCC ƆCƆCIII [1723] (unidentified).

9A2.c1. PHARMACEUTICE RATIONALIS, London folio 1679

The second issue of the first edition of both parts of Willis's sixth book in English, the ninth publication, using the first of four titles, with variant title page and all pagination errors retained [HJR Wing 55].

Title page: [1]. [within a double rule] PHARMACEUTICE RATIONALIS: | OR, AN | EXERCITATION | OF THE | OPERATIONS | OF | MEDICINES | IN | Humane Bodies. | SHEWING | The Signs, Cauſes, and Cures of moſt Diſtempers inci- | dent thereunto. | [rule] | In Two PARTS. | [rule] | AS ALSO | A Treatiſe of the SCURVY, and the ſeveral ſorts | thereof, with their Symptoms, Cauſes, and Cure. | [rule] | By *Tho. Willis* M.D. and *Sidley* Profeſſor in the Univerſity of *Oxford*: Alſo | one of the College of Phyſicians in *London*, and Fellow of the Royal Society. | [rule] | *Licenſed, October* 31. 1678. R. L'Eſtrange. | [rule] | *LONDON*, | Printed for *Thomas Dring* at the Harrow, *Charles Harper* | at the Flower *de Luce*, and *John Leigh* at the Bell | in *Fleetſtreet*. 1679.

[2]. [within a double rule] *PHARMACEUTICE RATIONALIS:* | OR, THE | OPERATIONS | OF | MEDICINES | IN | Humane Bodies. | [rule] | The Second Part. | With Copper Plates deſcribing the ſeveral Parts treated of in this Volume. | [rule] | By *THO. WILLIS*, M. D. and *Sedley* Profeſſor | in the Univerſity of *OXFORD*. | [rule] | [printers' ornament] | [double rule] | *LONDON*, | Printed for *Thomas Dring*, *Charles Harper*, and | *John Leigh*, Bookſellers in *Fleet-ſtreet*, 1679.

Then as in **9A1** apart from:

Illustrations: [1]. **Pl.27a5**. Plate 27 (image 46): *Tab. I.* (headline, centre), *p. 16* . (headline, right: page placement reengraved). Leaf size, 300 × 191 millimetres (sheet).

Copy: DASC, Tabulæ I and II for part 1 in facsimile on contemporary paper. Original boards with blind tooling, spine relaid with five raised bands and gilt decorated panels (by Bernard Middleton),[14] label WILLIS ON | MEDICINES IN | HUMANE BODIES, new endpapers.

[14] This is one of several volumes described in this bibliography, restored or rebound by Bernard Middleton (1924–2019). After training at the Central School of Arts and Crafts and the British Museum and teaching at the Royal College of Art and London School of Printing, Middleton worked at Zaehnsdorf's before establishing his own bindery in Soho and then Clapham. Bernard Middleton was active as a bookbinder for 78 years. He wrote *A history of English craft bookbinding technique*, New Castle (1963) and *The restoration of leather bindings*, Chicago (1972). At an early stage in his career, Middleton had acquired a large amount of blank paper from the early centuries of printing on which he reproduced missing leaves often by having made a lithographic plate of the original from which the facsimile was printed, as in this example. On the occasion that this restored copy of Willis's book

Leaves 307 × 185 millimetres, boards 317 × 190 × [68] millimetres. Bound with *The remaining medical works* (1681; **9B2**).

9A2.c2. PHARMACEUTICE RATIONALIS, London folio 1679

The second issue of the first edition of both parts of Willis's sixth book in English, the ninth publication, using the first of four titles, with variant title page and some pagination errors corrected [not distinguished from HJR Wing 55.].

As in **9A2.c1** apart from:

Collation: [1]. 90 leaves, paginated as [24], 1–[156]. Mispaginated: [1]. 124 for 128; [2]. 132 for 130 only (101 for 100, 102 for 101 corrected).

Copy: DASC (#1 of 2). Nineteenth-century half calf with marbled paper boards, new spine with five raised bands, three gilt lines above and below each, with additional gilt at head and tail, gilt decorated panels, red label PRACTICE | OF | PHYSIC. Leaves 300 × 190 millimetres, boards 313 × 197 × 38 millimetres. Shelf mark: (1) H 2 6; (2) B 6. Stamped: Manchester Infirmary (x2) on title page.

9B1.c1 THE REMAINING MEDICAL WORKS, London folio 1681

The first issue of the first edition of Willis's first, second, third (one treatise), and fourth (two treatises) books in English, the ninth publication, using the second of its four titles [HJR Wing 56, Denham 21].

Title page: [1a]. [within a double rule] THE | REMAINING | MEDICAL WORKS | OF THAT | FAMOUS AND RENOWNED | PHYSICIAN | Dr Thomas Willis | OF | *Chriſt-Church* in OXFORD, and *Sidley* Profeſſor of | Natural Philosophy in that famous UNIVERSITY. | *VIZ.* | I. Of Fermentation. | II. Of Feavours. | III. Of Urines. | IV. Of the Accenſion of the Bloud. | V. Of Muſculary Motion. | VI. Of the Anatomy of the Brain. | VII. Of the Deſcription and Uſe of the Nerves. | VIII. Of Convulſive Diſeaſes. | With large Alphabetical Tables for the whole, and an Index for the Ex- | plaining all the hard and unuſual Words and Terms of Art, derived from the | Latine, Greek, or other Languages, for the benefit of the meer Engliſh Reader, | and meaneſt capacity. | [rule] | *With Eighteen Copper Plates.* | [rule] | Engliſhed by *S.P.* Eſq; | [double rule] | *LONDON,* | Printed for *T. Dring*, *C. Harper*, *J. Leigh*, and *S. Martyn*, and | are to be ſold by *Robert Clavell*, at the *Peacock* in St *Paul's* | *Church=Yard*, MDCLXXXI.

[1b]. A | Medical-Philoſophical Diſcourſe | OF | FERMENTATION | OR, | Of the Inteſtine Motion of | PARTICLES | IN EVERY | BODY. | [rule] | BY | Dr. *THOMAS WILLIS* of Chriſt-Church in | *Oxford*, and *Sidley* Profeſſor of Natural Philosophy | in that Famous

was collected from his home in Clapham, Middleton's cat 'Caxton' was sitting astride a copy of the Shakespeare first folio that had been sent for restoration.

Univerſity. | [rule] | Translated into Engliſh by *S. P.* | [rule] | *LONDON*: | Printed for *T. Dring, C. Harper, J. Leigh*, and *S. Martin*. | MDCLXXXI.

[2]. FIVE | TREATISES, | VIZ. | 1. *Of Urines.* | 2. *Of the Accenſion of the Blood.* | 3. *Of Muſculary Motion.* | 4. *The Anatomy of the Brain.* | 5. *The Deſcription and uſe of the Nerves.* (contained by single {) | [rule] | BY | *THOMAS WILLIS*, M. D. | [double rule] | [printers' device: NOSCE TE IPSUM / LOVE AND LIVE / NE QVID NEMIS / D] | [double rule] | *LONDON*: | Printed for *T. Dring, C. Harper, J. Leigh*, and *S. Martin*. | MDCLXXXI.

[3]. AN | ESSAY | OF THE | PATHOLOGY | OF THE | BRAIN | AND | Nervous Stock: | In Which | Convulſive Diſeaſes | Are Treated of: | [rule] | Being the Work of *THOMAS WILLIS* | of *Chriſt-Church* in *Oxford*, Doctor in Phyſick, and | *Sidly*-Profeſſor of Natural Philoſophy in that | Famous Academy. | [rule] | Translated out of *Latine* into *Engliſh*, By *S. P.* | [rule] | *LONDON*, | Printed by *J. B.* for *T. Dring*, at the Signe of the *Harrow* | at *Chancery-Lane-End* in *Fleet-ſtreet*. 1681.[15]

Collation: [1]. Folio in 4s, 23 letter alphabet using I and V. [1]: π^2, A–Z^4, Aa1; \$1–2 signed apart from: A1 signed A2.
95 leaves, paginated as [12], 1–178.

[2]. [A]1, B–Z^4, Aa–Bb^4, Cc1: \$1–2 signed.
98 leaves, paginated as [4], 1–49 [50], [4], 55–192.

[3]. $[A]^2$, B–O^4, P^2, (a)–$(g)^2$, (h)1: \$1–2 signed apart from: +B3, +C3, -(d)2.
71 leaves, paginated as [4], 1–106, [32].

Type: 61 lines; height (20 lines) 81 millimetres, width 125 millimetres.

Contents: [1]. **π1r**, page [1] collective title; **π1v**, page [2] blank; **π2r**, page [3], title; **π2v**, page [4], blank; **A[1]r–v**, pages [5–6], TO THE Moſt Reverend Father in Chriſt And the Right Honorable HIS GRACE, GILBERT: By Divine Providence Arch-Biſhop of *Canterbury*, Primate and Metropolitan of all *England*, and one of His Majeſties moſt Honorable Privy-Councellors. … [signed] Your Graces moſt Humble And for ever obliged Servant, *T. W.*; **A2r–v**, pages [7–8], TO THE RIGHT WORSHIPFUL Sr Theophilus Biddulph KNIGHT and BARONET. … [signed] Honoured Sir, Your moſt humble and faithful Servant, *S. PORDAGE.*; **A3r–v**, pages [9–10], THE PREFACE. [Of Fermentation]; **A4r–v**, pages [11–12], ON THE AUTHORS Medical-Philoſophical Diſcourſes.

B1r–H2v, pages 1–52, [text] OF FERMENTATION, OR THE Inorganical Motion OF *NATURAL BODIES.*

H3r–H4r, pages 53–5, THE PREFACE [Of Feavers]; **H4v**, page [56], blank.

[15] Henry Plomer, *A dictionary of the booksellers and printers who were at work in England, Scotland and Ireland from 1668 to 1725*, Oxford (1922) lists three individuals with the initials J.B who were active in 1681: John Bagford (1650–1716), Joseph Bennett (fl 1675–1691), and John Bringhurst (fl 1680–1684), none of whom is known to have worked with Thomas Dring.

I1r–Aa1v, pages 57–178, [text] OF FEAVERS.

[2]. **Aa2r**, page [1], title; **Aa2v**, page [2], blank; **B1r–v**, pages [3–4], THE AUTHORS EPISTLE TO D[r] BATHURST. [Of Urines].

B2r–E1r, pages 1–23, [text] OF URINES.

E1v–F2r, pages 24–33, [text] Two Phyſical and Medical EXERCITATIONS, *VIZ.* 1. Of the Accenſion of the Blood. II. Of Muſculary Motion. The firſt Medical and Phyſical DISCOURSE. *Of the growing hot or inkindling of the Blood.*; **F2v–H2r**, pages 34–49, [text] The ſecond medical and Phyſical DISCOURSE. *Of Muſculary Motion.*; **H2v**, page [50], blank.

H3r–v, page [51–2], THE ANATOMY OF THE BRAIN. *The Authors Epiſtle Dedicatory to his Grace* Gilbert *Archbiſhop of* Canterbury, *&c.* ... [signed] YOUR GRACES *Moſt humble and obliged Servant*, THO. WILLIS.; **H4r–v**, pages [53–4], The Preface to the Reader.

I1r–T1v, pages 55–136, [text] THE ANATOMY OF THE BRAIN.; **T2r–Cc1v**, pages 137–92, [text] The Deſcription and Uſe OF THE NERVES.

[3]. **A1r**, page [1], title; **A1v**, page [2], blank; **A2r–v**, pages [3–4], The Authours Epiſtle Dedicatory. *To the Moſt Reverend Father in Chriſt, His Grace*, Gilbert, *by Divine Providence, Archbiſhop of* Canterbury, *Primate and Metropolitan of all* England, *and one of His Sacred Majeſties moſt Honourable Privy Council.* ... [signed] Your Graces moſt humble and Devoted Servant, *T. W.*

B1r–P1v, pages 1–106, [text] *Of Convulſve Diſeaſes.*; **P2r–v**, pages [1–2], blank.

(a)1r–(d)1r, pages [3–15], A TABLE of all the hard words derived from the *Greek* and *Latin*, of all Terms of Art and other words not vulgarly received, with the explanation of them.;[16] **(d)1v**, page [16], blank; **(d)2r–(e)1v**, page [17–20], THE FIRST INDEX or TABLE, WHEREIN IS Alphabetically digeſted the principal matters contained in the Treatiſes of Fermentation and Feavers. (in two columns); **(e)1v–(g)1r**, pages [20–7], THE SECOND INDEX or TABLE, WHEREIN IS Alphabetically digeſted the principal matters contained in the Treatiſes 1. *Of Urines*, 2. *Of the Accenſion of the Blood.* 3. *Of muſculary motion.* 4. *Of the Anatomy of the Brain*: *and* 5. *Of the deſcription and uſe of the Nerves.*; **(g)1v–(h)1v**, pages [28–32], THE THIRD INDEX or TABLE, WHEREIN IS Alphabetically digested all the principal matters contained in the Treatiſe of Convulſive Diſeaſes.

Headlines and *Catchwords*: [1]. Chap. VIII. for Chap. IX. at **E4r**, page 31; **Intermitting** for **Of Intermitting** at **L1r**, page 73; **M2r**, page 83; Chap. IX. for Chap. VII. at **N1r**, page 89; Chap. VIII. for Chap. IX. at **N4v**, page 96; Chap. XI. for Chap. X. at **P1r**, page 105; **peſtilential** for **putrid** at **Q1r**, page 113; Chap. X. for Chap. XI. at **Q3v**, page 118; Chap. XIV. for Chap. XIII. at **S1r**, page 129; **a peſtilential feaver.** for **the Meaſles and Small=pox.** at **T2r**, page 141; **Small=pox and Meaſles.** for **Meaſles and Small=pox.** at **T4r**, page 143; **Small pox and the**

16 See introductory notes for more detailed discussion and transcription of text.

Meafils. for **Meafles and Small=pox**. at **V1r**, page 145; **Lying in**. for **in Child=bed**. at **V4r**, page 151.

No catchword at **A2v**, page 6; **H2v / H3r**, pages 52 / 53; **N2v / N3r**, pages 92 / 93; the for proper at **B2v / B3r**, page 4 / 5; night for and at **P4v / Q1r**, page 112 / 113; The for the at **Z1v / Z2r**, pages 170 / 171.

[2]. **Urine**. for **Urines**. at **B3v**, page 4; **B4v**, page 6; **The Actions** for **Of the Actions** at **O4r**, page 101.

Catchwords correct.

[3]. Chap. II. for Chap. I. at **C1r**, page 9; **C1v**, page 10; **the Epilepfie**, for **Convulfive Difeafes**. at **C1v**, page 10; **Falling Sickneffe**. for **the Epilepfie**, at **C3r**, page 13; **Convulsive Diseases**. for **the Epilepsie**. at **C4r**, page 15; Chap IX for Chap. IX. at **I4r**, page 63; **K2r**, page 67; **L1r**, page 73; or, **Fits** for **Fits** at **N1r**, page 89; **O1r**, page 97; **O2r**, page 99; Chap. X for Chap. XI. at **N2r**, page 91; **N3v**, page 94.

by for dy at **E1v / E2r**, pages 26 / 27; *Chervil*, for *chervill* at **F4r / v**, pages 39 / 40; *nutts* for *nuts* at **F4v / G1r**, page 40 / 41; found for people at **I4v / K1r**, pages 64 / 65; convulsions for it at **L2r / v**, page 75 / 76; nores for notes at **L3r / v**, pages 77 / 78; Parotide for Parotida at **(b2)v / (c1)**, pages [10] / [11].

Frontispiece: none.

Portrait: **Pt.1a1**: *D: Loggan: delin: et fculpt*: *ÆTATIS SUÆ, 45.* 195 × 150 millimetres (sheet); 187 × 139 millimetres (plate marks); 184 × 135 millimetres (image).

Printers' ornament: printers' device at **2[A]1r**, page [1] {**Dring 8**}.

Decorated T at **A2r**, page [5], **B1r**, page 1 {**Dring 4**}; T at **A3r**, page [9] {**Dring 5**}; T at **H3r**, page 53 {**Dring 6**}; T at **I1r**, page 57 {**Dring 7**}.

Illustrations: as in **4A** and **2A** apart from:

Pl.18a2. Plate 18 (images 28 and 29): *P. 49.* (headline, left), *Fig. III.*, *Fig. IV.*, (headers, above each image). Leaf size, 313 × 192 millimetres (sheet). Legend: The Third Figure *Exhibits a certain Mufcle lefs compounded, to whofe two flefhy* Bellies *two compounded Tendons alfo (equal to four fimple ones) are deftinated.* The Fourth Figure *Shews a regular compounded Mufcle, divided and opened in the middle, fo that the interiour face of either Belly may appear.*; printed above **Pl.17a2** (images 26 and 27): *P. 49.* (headline, left), *Fig. I.*, *Fig. II.* (headers, above each image). Legend: The Firft Figure *SHews a fimple regular mufcle, defcribed according to its natural appearance, in the Belly of which the Flefhy fibres being opened, are diduced one from another, that the membranaceous Fibrils may be the better beheld.* The Second Figure *Shews a fimple Mufcle cleft in the middle, after the Tendon being cut off, and portions of it pulled away, that the interiour feries of the fleffhy Fibres, or their commixtures or mingling with the Tendons, may appear.* Inserted before The Explication of the Figures at [2] **H2r**, page 49.

Pl.2a3. Plate 2 (image 2): *p. 63.* (headline, left), *Figura II.*[da.] (headline, centre), [*pag: 27* (headline, right, erased)], *de medio S vid pag; 414* (footer, right). Leaf size, 314 × 192 millimetres (sheet). Legend: The Second Figure *Shews the Bafis of a Sheeps Brain taken out of the Skull, and the Roots of the Veſſels cut off, where all the Arteries, by Ink being injected into one of the Carotides, are made black and more conspicuous.* Inserted within legends Figuræ I–II at **I4v–K1r**, pages 62–3.

Pl.1a3. Plate 1 (image 1): *Figura 1*[a]. (headline, centre), *p. 63.* (headline, left), [*pag: 25* (headline, right: partly erased)], *de medio T vid pag: 414* (footer, right). Leaf size, 314 × 192 millimetres (sheet). Legend: The Firſt Figure *SHews the Baſis of an humane Brain taken out of the Skull, with the Roots of the Veſſels cut off.* Inserted within legends Figuræ I–II at **I4v–K1r**, pages 62–3.

Pl.3a3. Plate 3 (image 3): *p. 69* (headline, left), *Fig: III.* (headline, centre), [*pag: 49.* (headline, right, partly erased)]. Leaf size, 314 × 192 millimetres (sheet). Legend: The Third Figure *SHews the outmoſt or ſuperior Superficies of the humane Brain taken out of the Skull; where the border of the Brain being looſned from the knitting of the other Parts, made by the Membranes, is elevated and turned outward, that the ſhanks of the oblong Marrow, the* Fornix *or arched Vault, the* Nates *and* Teſtes, *with the pineal Kernel, and other Proceſſes, may be clearly and diſtinctly beheld.* Inserted before legends for Figuræ III–IV at **K4r–v**, page 69–70.

Pl.4a3. Plate 4 (image 4): *p. 70.* (headline, left), *Fig: IIII.* (headline, centre), [*pag: 51* (headline, right, partly erased)]. Leaf size, 314 × 192 millimetres × (sheet). Legend: The Fourth Figure. *The Effigies of an humane Brain of a certain Youth that was fooliſh from his birth, and of that ſort which are commonly termed Changelings; the bulk of whoſe brain, as it was thinner and leſſer than is uſual, its border could be farther lifted up and turned back, that all the more interior parts might be more deeply beheld together.* Inserted after legends for Figuræ III–IV at **K4r–v**, page 69–70.

Pl.5a3. Plate 5 (image 5): *p: 73* (headline, left), *Figura V.* (headline, centre), [*pag: 63* (headline, right, partly erased)]. Leaf size, 314 × 192 millimetres (sheet). Legend: *The Fifth Figure* SHews the interior Baſis of an humane Skull; where is ſhewn after what manner the Veſſels of every kind cut off from the Brain, and about to go out of the Skull, are hid or laid up under the *dura Mater*. Inserted before legends for Figuræ V–VI at **L2r–v**, pages 73–4.

Pl.6a3. Plate 6 (image 6): *p. 74.* (headline, left), *Fig: VI*[a] (headline, centre), [*pag: 64* (headline, right) erased]. Leaf size, 314 × 192 millimetres (sheet). Legend: The Sixth Figure Shews the Baſis of a Calfs Skull; where is ſhewn after what manner the Veſſels cut off from the Brain, and about to go out from the Skull, are drowned under the *dura Mater*. Inserted after legends for Figuræ V–VI at **L2r–v**, pages 73–4.

Pl.7a3. Plate 7 (images 7–10): [Unnumbered 1] *pag: 86.* (headline, right), *Fig: 1*, *Fig: 11*; *Fig: 111* (header, above each image), *Fig: 1111* (header, left of the image). Leaf size, 314 × 192 millimetres (sheet). Legend: *The Firſt Figure* Shews the aſcent of the Carotidick Artery, and its ſituation within an humane Skull, before it is carried toward the Brain. The Second Figure Shews the aſcent of the Carotidick Arteries, and their ſituation in a Horſes Skull.; The Third Figure Shews the wonderful Net with the pituitary Kernel in a Calfs Skull. The Fourth Figure

Shews after what manner the lateral Boſom goes into the Jugular Vein with a diverting place hanging to it. Inserted within legend at **M4v–N1r**, pages 86–7.

Pl.8a3. Plate 8 (image 11): *p: 94.* (headline, left), *Fig: VII^a.* (headline, centre), [*pag: 131* (headline, right, erased; right upper corner missing)]. Leaf size, 314 × 192 millimetres (sheet). Legend: *The Seventh Figure* SHews the Brain of a Sheep bent back and cut a little open in the places where they ſtick together near the ſtreaked bodies, that its interior ſubſtance may be turned the inſide out, and unfolded on a plain. Inserted after legend at **N4v**, page 94.

Pl.9a3. Plate 9 (image 12): *Fig: VIII^a.* (headline, centre), [*pag: 167* (headline, right erased)], *pag: 105.* (headline, right). Leaf size, 314 × 192 millimetres (sheet). Legend: *The Eighth Figure* REpresents the oblong Marrow taken out of the Head of a Sheep with the Brain cut off and removed, and with the Cerebel and one ſtreaked Body cut in two in the middle, and the other things chiefly belonging to the medullar Trunk. Inserted before legend at **P2r**, page 105.

Pl.10a3. Plate 10 (images 13 and 14): [Unnumbered 2] *p. 144.* (headline, left), [*pag: 302* headline, right: corner detached], *Fig: I.*, *Fig: II* (headers, above each image). Leaf size, 314 × 192 millimetres. Legend: This figure ſhews the Branchings of the fifth and ſixth pair of Nerves. The Second Figure ſhews all the Nerves, which being carried from the Nerves of the third, fourth, fifth and ſixth Pair, are beſtowed upon the Muſcles and other parts of the Eye. Inserted within legend for second unnumbered figure at **V1v–V2r**, pages 144–5.

Pl.11a3. Plate 11 (image 15): *p: 183:* (headline, left), *Tabula IX^a.* (headline, right). Folding, 406 × 228 millimetres (sheet). Legend: *The Ninth Table* Shews the beginnings of the fifth and ſixth pair of Nerves, and the Roots of the Intercoſtal Nerve proceeding from them; moreover, the Origines and Branchings out of the ſame Intercoſtal nerve and the wandring Pair, and of the accessory Nerve produced out of the Spine to the wandering Pair carried to the Region of the Ventricle. Beſides, here are repreſented the beginnings and diſtributions of the ſeventh, ninth, tenth Pair of Nerves, and of the Nerve of the Diaphragma; alſo the beginnings of the Vertebral Nerves in their whole Tract from the Region of the Nerves inſerted in the *Præcordia* and *Viſcera* are deſcribed, and their Communications with the former. All this whole following Table ſhews how it is found in Man different from other living Creatures. Inserted before legends for Tabulæ IX–XIII at **Bb1r–Cc1r**, pages 183–91.

Pl.12a3. Plate 12 (image 16): *P: 186:* (headline, left), *Tabula X^ma.* (headline, right). Folding, 405 × 282 millimetres (sheet). Legend: *The Tenth Table* Shews the beginnings and Branchings out of the ſame Nerves which were deſcribed in the former Table, as ſome of them are found in brute Beaſts otherwiſe than in Man / The other Nerves and their Branchings out are as in the other Figure, which ſhews the pattern of them in Man. Inserted within legends for Tabulæ IX–XIII at **Bb1r–Cc1r**, pages 183–91.

Pl.13d1. Plate 13 (image 17): *p. 187.* (headline, left). Folding, 389 × 192 millimetres (sheet). Legend: *The Eleventh Table* Shews the lower Branchings out of the wandring and the Intercoſtal Pair diſtributed to the Ventricle and the *Viſcera* of the Abdomen; alſo the beginnings of the Vertebral Nerves, which are placed over againſt the former, and are ingraffed into ſome of them. The figure of theſe in Man and in the four-footed Beaſts is almoſt alike, ſo that this Table may be common for both. Inserted within legends for Tabulæ IX–XIII at **Bb1r–Cc1r**, pages 183–91.

Pl.14d1. Plate 14 (image 18): *P. 189.* (headline, left). Leaf size, 314 × 192 millimetres (sheet). Legend: *The Twelfth Table* Shews the Spinal Marrow whole taken out of its bony Den, and half taken from the Membrane cloathing it, being diſſected, that the beginnings and productions of all the Vertebral Nerves might be ſeen together. Inserted within legends for Tabulæ IX–XIII at **Bb1r–Cc1r**, pages 183–91.

Pl.15a3. Plate 15 (images 19–23): *P. 191.* (headline, left), *TABVL. XIII* (headline, right), *fig. 3*$^{tia..}$, *fig: I,*^{ma}, *fig 4*$^{ta.}$, *fig. 2*$^{da..}$, *fig 5*$^{ta.}$ (headers, above each image). Folding, 378 × 225 millimetres (sheet). Legend: *The Thirteenth Table*. FIGURE I. Shews the branchings forth of the Vertebral Artery reaching out, on both ſides into the ſuperiour part of the Spinal Marrow, and into the hinder Region of the oblong Marrow. FIGURE II. Shews the Vertebral Veins which are Companions to the aboveſaid Arteries; alſo the upper portion of the Vertebral Boſom and the communications of either among themſelves and lateral Boſoms of the Head, and between the Jugular Veins. FIGURE III. Shews the Spinal Artery which is produced within the bony Den nigh the more inward Superficies of the Marrow, from the hinder part of the Head to the *Os Sacrum*, in the ſhape of a Net-work purl. FIGURE IV. Shews the Branchings out of the Spinal Boſom in its whole paſſage. FIGURE V. Shews the Image of the Spinal Boſom in a Dog, which hath not joynings together in its whole paſſage, as it is in a Calf, Sheep, Hog, and many others, but only in the loweſt and uppermoſt part, where it communicates with it ſelf by three or four croſs Proceſſes. Inserted within legends for Tabulæ IX–XIII at **Bb1r–Cc1r**, pages 183–91.

Copy: DASC (#1 of 2). Original calf with two blind stamped central panels each with double lines and additional tooling, lined borders, spine (restored) with five raised bands, red label DR WILLIS'S | MEDICAL | WORKS, original endpapers. Leaves 313 × 192 millimetres; boards 323 × 195 × 50 millimetres. Inscribed: (1) Matthias Blackwall (unidentified); (2) Ant. Johnson (unidentified); (3) Arthur F Hurst, 1926.[17]

9B1.c2 THE REMAINING MEDICAL WORKS, London folio 1681

The first issue of the first edition of Willis's first, second, third (one treatise), and fourth (two treatises) books in English, the ninth publication, using the second of four titles, with one plate and one plate leaf in second states [not distinguished from HJR Wing 56, Denham 21].

As in **9B1.c1** apart from:

Illustrations: **Pl.7a4**. Plate 7 (images 7–10): [Unnumbered 1] *pag 86.* (headline, left), [*pag: 86.* headline, right, partly erased and corner missing]. Leaf size, 300 × 188 millimetres (sheet).

Pl.17a2. (images 26 and 27) printed on plate leaf above **Pl.18a2**. Plate 18 (images 28 and 29).

[17] Sir Arthur Frederick Hurst (1879–1944: born Hertz) was appointed assistant physician to Guy's Hospital with responsibility for the neurological department in 1907. He used his military experience in Salonika to treat shell shock and civilian neuroses after the First World War. His wide range of physiological and medical interests led Hurst to found, with others, the British Society of Gastroenterology. He was considered a fine judge of pictures, furniture, and books, and was an artist and a skilful modeller in clay. Hurst was knighted in 1937 as was his brother Sir Gerald Berkeley Hurst QC (1877–1957) in 1929.

Copy: DASC. Original calf, spine (relaid) with five raised bands, each with double gilt rules at top and bottom, gilt panels, red label WILLIS | OF. | HUM: BODIE. Leaves 300 × 185 millimetres, boards 313 × 195 × [78] millimetres. Bound with *Pharmaceutice rationalis* (1679: **9A1**, copy #2). Inscribed: (1) Ferrers Chartley 1843; (2) Wm Ffranceys (unidentified). Inserted bookplate: (1) The Right Honorable Washington Sewallis Earl Ferrers; (2) Ex libris B.E.J. Pagel. Stamped: with a crown and F underneath.[18]

9B2. THE REMAINING MEDICAL WORKS, London folio 1681

The second issue of the first edition of Willis's first, second, third (one treatise), and fourth (two treatises) books in English, the ninth publication, using the second of four titles, with the title page reset [HJR Wing 57, not distinguished from Denham 21].

Title page: [1]. [within a double rule] THE | REMAINING | MEDICAL WORKS | OF THAT | FAMOUS AND RENOWNED | PHYSICIAN | Dr Thomas Willis | OF | *Chriſt-Church* in OXFORD, and *Sidley* Profeſſor of | Natural Philoſophy in that famous UNIVERSITY. | *VIZ.* | I. Of Fermentation. | II. Of Feavours. | III. Of Urines. | IV. Of the Accenſion of the Bloud. | V. Of Muſculary Motion. | VI. Of the Anatomy of the Brain. | VII. Of the Deſcription and Uſe of the Nerves. | VIII. Of Convulſive Diſeaſes. | [rule] | **The firſt part, though laſt publiſhed.** | [rule] | With large Alphabetical Tables for the whole, and an Index for the Explain- | ing all the hard and unuſual Words and terms of Art, derived from the Latine, | Greek, or other Languages, for the benefit of the meer Engliſh Reader, and | meaneſt capacity. | [rule] | *With Eighteen Copper Plates.* | [rule] | Engliſhed by *S.P.* Esq; | [double rule] | *LONDON*, | Printed for *T. Dring, C. Harper, J. Leigh*, and *S. Martyn*, and are to be | ſold at the corner of *Chancery-lane*, and the *Flower-de-Luce* over | againſt St *Dunſtans* Church in *Fleet-ſtreet*, MDCLXXXI.

Then as in **9B1.c1** apart from:

Illustrations: **Pl.7a4.** Plate 7 (images 7–10): [Unnumbered 1] *pag 86.* (headline, left), [*pag: 86.* headline, right, partly erased and corner missing]. Leaf size, 306 × 186 millimetres (sheet).

Copy: DASC, Tabulæ IX, X, and XI in facsimile on contemporary paper. Original calf with blind stamped central panels, floral tooling at corners, double-lined edges, spine (rebacked) with five raised bands and five elaborate gilt panels, label WILLIS ON | MEDICINES IN | HUMANE BODIES, new endpapers (restored by Bernard Middleton). Leaves 306 × 185

[18] Washington Sewallis Shirley (1822–1859), styled Hon. Washington Shirley from 1827 to 1830 and Viscount Tamworth from 1830 to 1842, became ninth Earl Ferrers in 1842. He was appointed deputy lieutenant of Leicestershire (1852) and Staffordshire (1857). His bookplate, measuring 167 × 123 millimetres and on a leaf 215 × 180 millimetres, has as its crest a Saracen's head in profile wreathed about the temples above a coronet and helmet with elaborate scroll work supported by a talbot and reindeer, both with coronets, the central arms in six parts, and the motto **honor virtutis præmium** (honour is rewarded). It is signed 'B. Warwick Sculp^t 124 Regent S^t.' printed above '**The Right Honorable Washington Sewallis Earl Ferrers**'. Acquired when he was aged 21, Ferrers annotated the age of his copy as: 1843–1679 = 164 (years). Bernard Ephraim Julius Pagel FRS (1930–2007) was a British astrophysicist who worked on the measurement and interpretation of elemental abundances in stars and galaxies. This book came from his father Walter Pagel (1898–1983), professor of medicine in Heidelberg (1931–1933) who became pathologist to the Central Middlesex Hospital (1939–1956) and Clare Hall Hospital (1956–1967). A notable historian of medicine, Walter Pagel wrote on Theophrastus von Hohenheim (Paracelsus: *c.*1493–1541) and Jan Baptist van Helmont (1580–1644), both of whose works were especially relevant to Thomas Willis.

millimetres, boards 316 × 190 × 73 millimetres. Bound with *Pharmaceutice rationalis* (1679; **9A2.c1**).

9C. DR WILLIS'S PRACTICE OF PHYSICK, London folio 1681

The first edition with the collective title *Dr Willis's practice of physick*, containing Willis's first, second, third, fourth, and sixth books in English, the ninth publication, using the third of four titles, made up from the sheets and illustrations of *Pharmaceutice rationalis* (1679: **9A2.c1**) and *The remaining medical works* (1681: **9B2**), but without *Two discourses concerning the soul of brutes* [not listed by HJR Wing or Denham]; see Figure 155.

Title page: [1a]. [within a double rule] DR WILLIS'S | Practice of Phyfick, | Being all the | MEDICAL WORKS | OF THAT | RENOWNED and FAMOUS | PHYSICIAN: | CONTAINING | Thefe Ten feveral Treatifes, *viz.* | I. Of Fermentation. | II. Of Feavours. | III. Of Urines. | IV. Of the Accenfion of the Bloud. | V. Of Mufculary Motion. | VI. Of the Anatomy of the Brain. | VII. Of the Defcription and Ufe of the Nerves. | VIII. Of Convulfive Difeafes. | IX. Pharmaceutice Rationalis, the 1st and 2^{d} Part. | X. Of the Scurvy. | Wherein moft of the Difeafes belonging to the Body of Man are Treated of, | with excellent methods and Receipts for the Cure | of the fame. | Fitted to the meaneft Capacity by an Index for the Explaining of all the | hard and unufual Words and Terms of Art derived from the Greek, Latine, or | other Languages, for the benefit of the Englifh Reader, with a large Alpha- | betical Table to the whole. | [rule] | *With Thirty two Copper Plates.* | [rule] | Done into Englifh by *S.P* Esq; | [double rule] | *LONDON,* | Printed for *T. Dring, C. Harper,* and *J. Leigh,* and are to be fold at the | Corner of *Chancery-lane*, and the *Flower-de-Luce* over againft | St. *Dunftans* Church in *Fleet-ftreet*, MDCLXXXI.

Then as for **9B2** followed by **9A2.c1** apart from:

Collation: [1]. *1, π^2, A–Z^4 etc.; and (a)1r–(d)1v bound after **H1v** in part [3].

Contents: [1]. ***1r**, page [1], collective title page; ***1v**, page [2], blank then preliminaries for **9B2** (without **A1**, **A3**) etc.

Copy: Huntington Library (347768). Original calf with blind double fillets at the edges, rebacked, original endpapers. Leaves, 315 × 197 millimetres, boards 325 × 215 × 73 millimetres. Inscribed: Henry Benson, Dodford, Northants., with (in pen and ink): 'This book was given me by my worthy ffrend Sr Roger Norwich'. Bookplates: (1) Benson; (2) Fawsley (unidentified).[19]

[19] This copy appears to be unique and has not been directly examined. Details were resolved through correspondence between 8 February 2018 and 16 March 2019 with Stephen Tabor, curator of rare books at the Huntington Library. He confirmed the collation and provenance of this copy bought from Dawson's bookshop in Los Angeles on 24 April 1961 for $200. An earlier inscription reads: 'Cat. 38: 410 (May 1942); pencil inscription: JHZ from CSZ Christmas 1942'. It is unclear whether A1 and A3 are lacking or were never bound into this assembly of 9B2 and 9A2.c1 with its additional collective title page. Henry Benson (1653–1725) of Dodford, Northamptonshire, was Gentleman of the Privy Chamber to King Charles II, and sheriff of Northamptonshire (1685). A monument to him is in the church of St Mary the Virgin in Dodford. The activities of Sir Roger Norwich (1636–1691), of Brampton Ash, Northamptonshire, resonate closely with those of his contemporary Thomas

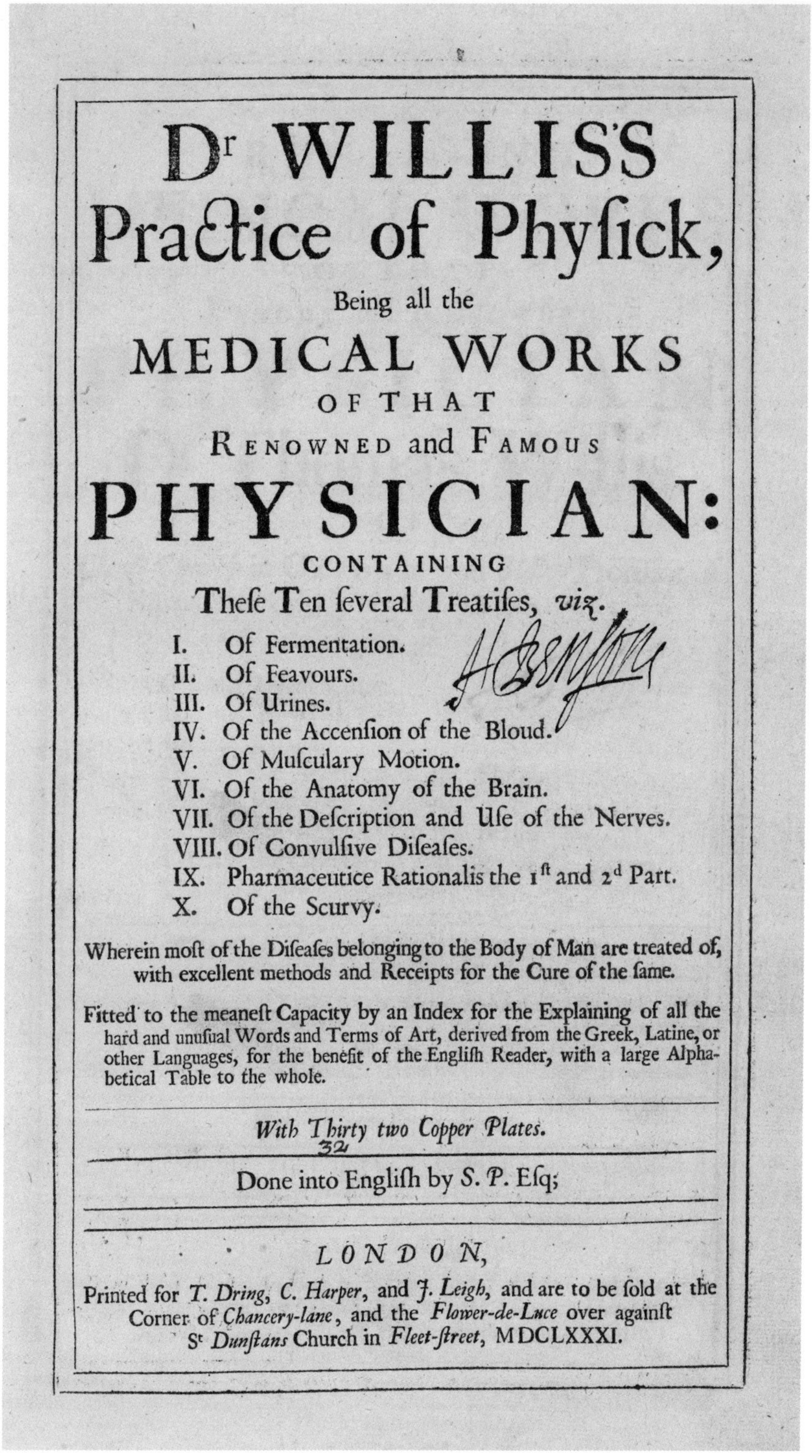

Dr WILLIS'S
Practice of Phyſick,
Being all the
MEDICAL WORKS
OF THAT
RENOWNED and FAMOUS
PHYSICIAN:
CONTAINING
Theſe Ten ſeveral Treatiſes, *viz.*

I. Of Fermentation.
II. Of Feavours.
III. Of Urines.
IV. Of the Accenſion of the Bloud.
V. Of Muſculary Motion.
VI. Of the Anatomy of the Brain.
VII. Of the Deſcription and Uſe of the Nerves.
VIII. Of Convulſive Diſeaſes.
IX. Pharmaceutice Rationalis the 1ſt and 2d Part.
X. Of the Scurvy.

Wherein moſt of the Diſeaſes belonging to the Body of Man are treated of, with excellent methods and Receipts for the Cure of the ſame.

Fitted to the meaneſt Capacity by an Index for the Explaining of all the hard and unuſual Words and Terms of Art, derived from the Greek, Latine, or other Languages, for the benefit of the Engliſh Reader, with a large Alphabetical Table to the whole.

With Thirty two Copper Plates.

Done into Engliſh by *S. P.* Eſq;

LONDON,

Printed for *T. Dring*, *C. Harper*, and *J. Leigh*, and are to be ſold at the Corner of *Chancery-lane*, and the *Flower-de-Luce* over againſt St *Dunſtans* Church in *Fleet-ſtreet*, MDCLXXXI.

Figure 155 Title page of the first edition of *Dr Willis's practice of physick* 1681.
Reproduced courtesy of the Huntington Library, San Marino, California.

9D. TWO DISCOURSES CONCERNING THE SOUL OF BRUTES, London folio 1683

The only issue in English of Willis's fifth book, the ninth publication, using the fourth of four titles [HJR Wing 58, Oldfield A4].

Title page: [within a double rule] TWO | DISCOURSES | CONCERNING | The Soul of Brutes, | Which is that of the | Vital and Senſitive of Man. | The Firſt is PHYSIOLOGICAL, ſhewing the NATURE, | PARTS, POWERS, and AFFECTIONS of the ſame. | The Other is PATHOLOGICAL, which unfolds the | DISEASES which Affect it and its Primary Seat; to wit, The | *BRAIN* and *NERVOUS STOCK*, And Treats of their CURES: | With Copper Cuts. | [rule] | By *THOMAS WILLIS* Doctor in PHYSICK, Profeſſor | of Natural Philoſophy in *OXFORD*, and alſo one of the Royal So- | ciety, and of the renowned College of Phyſicians in *LONDON*. | [rule] | Engliſhed | By *S. PORDAGE*, Student in PHYSICK. | [rule] | *LONDON*, | Printed for *Thomas Dring* at the *Harrow* near *Chancery-Lane End* in *Fleet-* | *ſtreet*, *Ch. Harper* at the *Flower=de-Luce* againſt St. *Dunſtan*'s Church | in *Fleet-ſtreet*, and *John Leigh* at *Stationers=Hall*. 1683.

Collation: folio in 4s: 23 letter roman alphabet using I and V; A–N^4, P–Z^4, Aa–Gg^4, Hh–Ii^2, Kk1; $1–2 signed apart from: [lacking O^4], P2 signed B2, V2 signed U2.

121 leaves, paginated as [8], 1–96, 105–234, [8]. Mispaginated: 88 for 68, 89 for 69.

Type: 64 lines; height (20 lines) 80 millimetres, width 139 millimetres (158 millimetres with marginal notes).

Contents: **A1r**, page [1], title; **A1v**, page [2], blank; **A2r–A2v**, pages [3–4], To the moſt Reverend Father in God GILBERT (By Divine Providence) **Arch=Biſhop of Canterbury**, Primate and Metropolitan of all *ENGLAND*, and one of the Privy Council to His Sacred Majeſty *CHARLES* the Second, King of *Great Britain*, *France*, and *Ireland*, &c. … [signed] Your Graces Moſt humble and devoted Servant *Tho. Willis*.; **A3r**, page [5], To the Moſt LEARNED and WORSHIPFUL By me ever Reſpected *The* Vice-Chancellor, Doctors, *and* Maſters, *who diligently Profeſs, greatly Adorn, and happily Promote good Letters in the moſt Famous Univerſity of* Oxford, *Health*. … [signed] *Honored Sirs, the Admirer of you all*, THO. WILLIS.; **A3v–A4v**, pages [6–8], THE PREFACE TO THE READER.

B1r–N4v, pages 1–96, [text] OF **The Soul of the Brutes**, the Firſt Part PHYSIOLOGICAL, SHEWING, Its NATURE, PARTS, POWERS, AND AFFECTIONS.; **P1r–Hh1v**, pages '105–234', THE SECOND PART PATHOLOGICAL: OR Of the DISEASES which belong to the Corporeal Soul and its Subjects, *viz*. The Brain and the Nervous Stock.

Willis. An Anglican and Royalist, Norwich was involved in demolishing the defences of Northampton during the Civil War. Not without controversy, in 1666 Norwich's estate had become liable to forfeiture for murder, but presumably he was pardoned. Norwich disliked sending young women to prison for interrupting Anglican services, but the violence of his methods provoked resentment and threats against his life. He stood for parliament and was involved in reestablishing government control after the dissolution of the Oxford Parliament (1681: the year in which his surviving copy of *Dr Willis's practice of physick* was published). In 1683 he was responsible for demanding the suppression of coffee houses and the tendering of the oaths to Roman Catholic and Protestant nonconformists. Norwich's political career ended in 1685. He died of the palsy.

Hh2r–Kk1v, pages [1–8], A TABLE.; **Kk1v**, page [8], *Advertiſement.* DOctor *Willis's* Practice of Phyſick, being all the Medical Works of that Renowned and Famous Phyſician, Containing theſe Ten Treatiſes following, *viz.* I. Of Fermentation. II. Of Feavers. III. Of Urines. IV. Of the Accenſion of the Blood. V. Of Muſculary Motion. VI. Of the Anatomy of the Brain. VII. Of the Deſcription and Uſe of the Nerves. VIII. Of Convulſive Diſeaſes. IX. Pharmaceutice Rationalis, the first and ſecond Part. X. Of the Scurvey. Wherein moſt of the Diſeaſes belonging to the Body of Man are Treated of, with excellent methods and Receipts for the Cure of the ſame. Fitted to the meaneſt Capacity by an Index for the Explaining of all the hard and unuſual Words and Terms of Art, derived from the Greek, Latin, or other Languages, for the benefit of the Engliſh Reader. With a large Alphabetical Table to the Whole. With Thirty Copper Plates. Done into Engliſh by *S. Pordage* Student in Phyſick. Printed for *T. Dring,* and *C. Harper* in *Fleetſtreet,* and *J. Leigh* at Stationers Hall. Price Thirty Shillings.

Headlines and *Catchwords*: *That the Soul of the Brute is Corporeal and Fiery.* for *The Species and differences of Brutes.* at **B4v**, page 8; *The Explanation of the Figures.* for *According to their Vital Parts.* at **D1r**, page 17; *An Explanation* for *The Explanation* at **D1v**, page 18; **D2v**, page 20; **D3r**, page 21; *Parts and Members* for *Parts or Members* at **E1r–E2r**, pages 25–27; *Of the Science of Brutes.* for *A Comparing the Soul of the Brutes with the Rational.* at **F4v**, page 40; *of the Rational Soul with the Brutal.* for *the Soul of the Brutes with the Rational.* at **G1v**, page 42; *Affections in General.* for *Affections of the Corporeal Soul in General.* at **G3r**, page 45; *Affections* for *Paſſions* at **H2v**, page 52; *Senſe* for *the Senſe* at **I2r**, page 59; *Caros.* for *Carus.* at **S4v**, page 136.

(excepting for excepting at **F4r / v**, pages 39 / 40; no catchword at **N4v / P1r**, pages 96 / 105; narily for ordinarily at **R4r / v**, pages 127 / 128; fulneſs for fullneſs at **Gg2r / v**, pages 227 / 228.

Frontispiece: none.

Portrait: none.

Printers' ornaments: none.

Decorated I at **A2r**, page [3] {**Dring 9**}.

Illustrations: As in **5A** apart from:

Pl.19c1. Plate 19 (images 30–33): *page. 18.*, *Tabula I^{a}* (headline, right), *Figura. I^{a}*, *Figura. II^{da}*, *Figura. IIII.^{ta}*, *Figura III.^{tia}* (headers, above each image). Leaf size, 312 × 194 millimetres (sheet). Legend: The Firſt Table, Contains certain Figures taken out of *Malpigius*, in which the Vital Organs of the Silk-Worm and of other Inſects are repreſented. The Firſt Figure Shews the Navil-hole, of which two being planted in the ſides of every Section or little Ring (except in the three uppermoſt) are the Doors or Openings of the Wind-Pipes. The Second Figure Shews ſome interior Branchings in the Silk-Worm. The Third Figure Shews the Ramifications of the *Trachea* or Wind-Pipe in a Graſhopper. The Fourth Figure, Expreſſes the Heart of the Silk-Worm, which ſeems to be made oblong and unequal, as if into many little oval Hearts. Inserted within legends for Tabulæ I–IV at **D1v–D3r**, pages 18–21.

Pl.20c1. Plate 20 (images 34–35): *Tabula II.*^{da} (headline, centre), *page. 19.* (headline, right), *Figura. I.*^{a}, *Figura. II.*^{da} (header, above each image). Leaf size, 312 × 194 millimetres (sheet). Legend: The Second Table, of which The Firſt Figure Shews the Oyſter taken forth and whole from the ſhell, that his parts may be ſeen as they are in their natural ſituation. The Second Figure Repreſents the Oyſter open, and unrolled, that its Viſcera and internal parts may be ſeen. Inserted within legends for Tabulæ I–IV at **D1v–D3r**, pages 18–21.

Pl.21c1. Plate 21 (images 36–38): *Tabula III* ^{tia} (headline, centre), *page. 20.* (headline, right), *Figura 1*^{ma}, *Figura II*^{da}., *Fig III*^{tia} (headers, above each image). Leaf size, 312 × 194 millimetres (sheet). Legend: The Third Table. The Firſt Figure Shews the Lobſter open in the back, that the Brain, Viſcera, Vital, Genital, and other interior parts may be ſeen. The Second Figure Shews the Womb of the Lobſter, and its neck, and Privy Member, or aperture made thorow the hole in the laſt little Foot but one, together with the little Foot it ſelf, and the affixed Gills. The Third Figure Expreſſes a portion of the Gill cut off, that its three Paſſages or Cavities may appear. Inserted within legends for Tabulæ I–IV at **D1v–D3r**, pages 18–21.

Pl.22c1. Plate 22 (images 39–41): *Tab IIII* (headline, left), *page*^{21} (headline, right), *Figura II*^{da}, *Figura. I*^{ma}, *Figura III*^{tia} (header, above each image). Leaf size, 312 × 194 millimetres (sheet). Legend: The Fourth Table. The Firſt Figure Shews an Earth-Worm laid with its belly upwards, the greateſt part of it diſſected and lay'd open, that the Brain, *Præcordia*, *Viſcera*, and other Parts may be ſeen. The Second Figure Expreſſes a portion of the ſame Earth-Worm, with the Tail cut off, that the rowes of the little Feet, which are 4, to wit, *a. a. a. a.* may be ſeen. The Third Figure Shews the whole Earth-Worm prone, or with its back uppermoſt, that the ringie Muſcles, and the Wind-Pipes in them, may be ſeen. Inserted within legends for Tabulæ I–IV at **D1v–D3r**, pages 18–21.

Pl.23c1. Plate 23 (image 42): *page. 27.* (headline, left), *Tabu V.* (headline right). Leaf size, 312 × 194 millimetres (sheet). Legend: The Fifth Table, Shews the Figure of the Brain of a Sheep roled forth, and deraſed, and as it were made bare of the Fleſh, in many places, that the Marrowy Tracts may be ſeen. Inserted before the legends for Tabulæ V–VII at **E2r–E3r**, pages 27–9.

Pl.24c1. Plate 24 (image 43): *page 28* (headline, left), *Tabu.* VI. (headline right). Leaf size, 312 × 194 millimetres (sheet). Legend: The Sixth Table Shews the Baſis of a Sheeps Head, in certain parts of which Deraſed, and in others Expoſed naked, the Streaks or Medullary Tracts, as ſo many Nerves, appear.; printed above **Pl25c1** (image 44): *page 28* (headline, left), *Tabu. VII.* (headline right). Legend: The Seventh Table, Shews the orbicular Prominences, and the Optick Chambers Eraſed, and as it were made bare of Fleſh that their inward Frames may be beheld. Inserted before the legends for Tabulæ V–VII at **E2r–E3r**, pages 27–9.

Pl.26c1. Plate 26 (image 45): *page 44* (headline, left), *Tabula VIII* (headline right). Leaf size, 312 × 194 millimetres (sheet). Legend: The Eighth Table, Contains a new Anatomy of the Humane Brain, where, by a Diſſection with an Inſtrument made thorow the Bill, the Callous Body, and the Fornix or Arch, and their Parts being taken away and ſeparated; the ſtreaked Bodies, alſo the Optic and Orbicular Prominences, one ſide eraſed, and the other whole and plain, are Exhibited. Inserted after the legend for Tabula VIII at **G2v**, page 44.

Copy: DASC (#1 of 3). Original calf with two central panels, double-lined borders and edges, spine (rebacked) with six raised bands and six panels with gilt floral tooling, lettered

WILLIS | ON | BRUTES, later endpapers. Leaves 313 × 195 millimetres, boards 318 × 196 × 26 millimetres. Inscribed: (1) H.D... (unidentified); (2) R. Bradley Saturday Feby 26th 1780 Cost 8 / 11d (unidentified). From the library of Robert Lenkiewicz.[20]

9E.c1 DR WILLIS'S PRACTICE OF PHYSICK, London folio 1684

The second edition with the collective title *Dr Willis's practice of physick*, containing Willis's first, second, third, fourth, fifth, and sixth books in English, the ninth publication, using the third of four titles, made up from the sheets *The remaining medical works* (1681: **9B2**) and *Two discourses concerning the soul of brutes* (1683: **9D**), *Pharmaceutice rationalis* parts 1 and 2 newly translated and the plates to that treatise reengraved [not distinguished from HJR Wing 59, Denham 22].

Title page: [1a]. [within a double rule] DR WILLIS'^S | Practice of Phyſick, | Being the Whole | WORKS | OF THAT | RENOWNED and FAMOUS | PHYSICIAN: | CONTAINING | Theſe Eleven Several Treatiſes, *viz.* | I. Of Fermentation. | II. Of Feavers. | III. Of Urines. | IV. Of the Accenſion of the Blood. | V. Of Muſculary Motion. | VI. Of the Anatomy of the Brain. | VII. Of the Deſcription and Uſe of the Nerves. | VIII. Of Convulſive Diſeaſes. | IX. Pharmaceutice Rationalis, the Firſt and Second Part. | X. Of the Scurvy. | XI. Two Diſcourſes concerning the Soul of Brutes. | Wherein moſt of the Diſeaſes belonging to the Body of | Man are Treated of, with excellent Methods and Receipts for the Cure | of the ſame. | Fitted for the meaneſt Capacity by an Index for the Explaining of all the | hard and unuſual Words and Terms of Art derived from the Greek, Latine, | or other Languages, for the benefit of the Engliſh Reader. | [rule] | *With Forty Copper Plates.* | [rule] | The Pharmaceutice new Tranſlated, and the Whole | carefully Corrected and Amended. | [rule] | *LONDON,* | Printed for *T. Dring, C. Harper,* and *J. Leigh*, and are to be Sold at the | Corner of *Chancery-Lane*, and the *Flower-de-Luce* over againſt St. *Dunſtan*'s | Church in *Fleetſtreet*, MDCLXXXIV.

[1b] and [2]. As in **9B**.[21]

[4]. [within a double rule] Pharmaceutice Rationalis: | OR, AN | EXERCITATION | OF THE | OPERATIONS | OF | MEDICINES | IN | Humane Bodies: | SHEWING | The Signs, Cauſes, and Cures of moſt | Diſtempers incident thereunto. | [rule] | In Two PARTS. | [rule] | AS ALSO | A Treatiſe of the SCURVY, and the ſeveral ſorts | thereof, with their Symptoms, Cauſes, and Cure. | [rule] | By *Tho. Willis*, M.D. and *Sidley* Profeſſor in the Univerſity of

[20] Robert Oscar Lenkiewicz (1941–2002) was a prolific artist, popular with his public but only recognized by the art establishment posthumously. His topics were macabre as was his lifestyle. After moving from London, where he trained at Saint Martin's School of Art and the Royal Academy, his home and studios in Devon became a refuge for vagrants, criminals, alcoholics, and the mentally ill. At his death, the embalmed corpse of a tramp was found hidden behind panelling at the bottom of a bookcase. Many of his paintings portray states of human physiology that drew upon the books in in his library: 25 000 items on art, the occult, demonology, magic, and witchcraft. He died impoverished and in debt but left a valuable estate now managed by the Lenkiewicz Foundation. This copy of *Two discourses concerning the soul of brutes* was item 757 in the Lyon and Turnbull sale, 10 May 2007.

[21] In both copies of **9E** examined for this bibliography, the title page and author's dedicatory epistle for *An essay of the pathology of the brain* ($^{3}A^{2}$) are not present. The decision has been taken that these are not called for and therefore excluded from the description that follows. However, they may be lacking by chance from each, and it would be instructive if a copy is identified that otherwise matches the collation of **9E** and does contain these leaves.

Oxford; Alſo | one of the College of Phyſicians in *London*, and Fellow of the *Royal Society*. | [rule] | *LONDON*: | Printed for *T. Dring*, *C. Harper*, and *J. Leigh* and are to be Sold at | the Corner of *Chancery-Lane*, and the *Flower-de-Luce* over againſt | St *Dunſtan*'s-Church in *Fleet-ſtreet*, M DC LXXX IV.

[5]. [within a double rule] *PHARMACEUTICE RATIONALIS*: | OR, THE | OPERATIONS | OF | MEDICINES | IN | Humane Bodies. | [rule] | [The Second Part. | With Copper Plates deſcribing the ſeveral Parts treated of in this Volume. | [rule] | By *THO. WILLIS*, M.D. and *Sedley* Profeſſor | in the Univerſity of *OXFORD*. | [rule] | [ornaments in two rows] | [double rule] | *LONDON*, | Printed for *Thomas Dring*, *Charles Harper*, Bookſel- | lers in *Fleet=ſtreet*, and *John Leigh* at *Stationers*-Hall, 1684.

[6]. As in **9D**.

Then as in **9B** apart from:

Collation: [1]. π^2 (-π1 = *1); [3] A^2 (-A1, -A2) etc., to:

[4]. A–T^4, U–Z^2.
84 leaves, paginated as [8], 1–160. Mispaginated (part 1): 83 for 93.

[5]. A–Ee^4, Ff1.
113 leaves, paginated as [8], 1–218.

[6]. As in **9D**.

Contents: [1]. ***1r**, page [1], title page; ***1v**, page [2], blank; etc., then as in **9B** to:

[4]. **A1r**, page [1], title page; **A1v**, page [2], blank; **A2r–A4v**, pages [3–8], THE PREFACE TO THE READER.

B1r–T4r, pages 1–143, [text] SECT. I. Of the Operations of Medicins in Mans Body.; **T4v**, page [144], blank.

U1r–X1v, pages 145–50, THE TABLE To the Firſt Part of *PHARMACEUTICE RATIONALIS*.; **X2r–Z1v**, pages 151–8, THE TABLE To the Second Part of *PHARMACEUTICE RATIONALIS*.; **Z1v–Z2v**, pages 158–60, THE TABLE To the TRACT of The *SCURVEY*.

[5]. **A1r**, page [1], title page; **A1v**, page [2], blank; **A2r–A3r**, pages [3–5], THE PREFACE TO THE READER.; **A3v–A4v**, pages [6–8], POSTSCRIPT.

B1r–Ff1v, pages 1–218, [text] THE SECOND PART OF *PHARMACEUTICE RATIONALIS*, OR OF THE OPERATIONS OF MEDICINES IN HUMANE BODIES.

[6]. As in **9D**.

Headlines and *Catchwords*: as in **9B** to: [4]. No CHAP. I. at **B1r**, page 1; *Operation* for *Operations* at **B1v**, page 2; **B4r**, page 7; **C1v**, page 10; **C2v–C3r**, pages 12–13; **C4r**, page 15;

D1r, page 17; **D2v–D3r**, pages 20–1; **D4v**, page 24; **E1v**, page 26; **E2r**, page 27; **E3v–E4r**, pages 30–1; **F1r–F1v**, pages 33–34; **F2v–F3r**, pages 36–7; **F4r–G1r**, pages 39–41; **G2r**, page 43; **G3v**, page 46; **G4v**, page 48; **H1v–H2r**, pages 50–1; **H3v–H4r**, pages 54–5; **I1r**, page 57; **I2r**, page 59; **I3v**, page 62; **I4v–K1r**, pages 64–5; **K2r**, page 67; **K3v**, page 70; **K4v–L1r**, pages 72–3; **L2r**, page 75; **L3r–L3v**, pages 77–8; **L4v–M1r**, pages 80–1; **M2r–M3v**, pages 83–6; **M4v–N1r**, pages 88–9; **N2r**, page 91; **N3v**, page 94; **N4v**, page 96; **O1v**, page 98; **O2v–O3r**, pages 100–1; **O4r**, page 103; **P1r**, page 105; **P2r**, page 107; **P3v**, page 110; **P4v–Q1r**, pages 112–13; **Q2r**, page 115; **Q3v**, page 118; **Q4v**, page 120; **R1v**, page 122; **R2v–R3r**, pages 124–5; **R4r**, page 127; **S1v**, page 130; **S2v–S3r**, pages 132–3; **S4r**, page 135; **T1r**, page 137; **T2v–T3r**, pages 140–1.

ration for teration at **P4v / Q1r**, pages 112 / 113.

[5]. Chap. III. for Chap. II. at **D1r**, page 17; Chap. V. for Chap. VI. at **E4r**, page 31; **F2r**, page 35; *confirmed* for *beginning* at **G2v**, page 44; Chap. VII. for Chap. VI. at **G4r**, page 47; Chap. VI. for Chap. VII. at **H2r**, page 51; *Examples* for *Of Examples* at **H4r**, page 55; *Examples of thoſe that ſpit Blood.* for *Of Examples of Perſons Spitting Blood.* at **H4v**, page 56; Chap. X. for Chap. IX. at **K2r**, page 67; Chap. XI. for Chap. XII. at **M2r**, page 83; Sect. I. for Sect. II. at **N2v**, page 92; **N3v**, page 94; Chap. IV. for Chap. III. at **P1r**, page 105; *Phlebotomy.* for *Phlebotomie.* at **R3r**, page 125; *Hæmorrhagie.* for *Hæmorrhage.* at **S3v**, page 134; *Veſicatores.* for *Veſicatories.* at **U1r**, page 145; Chap. IV. for Chap. VI. at **X3r**, page 157; Chap. I. for Chap. II. at **Z4r–v**, pages 175–176; Chap. VII. for Chap. VIII. at **Cc4v**, page 200; Chap. XI. for Chap. IX. at **Dd2v**, page 204.

the for 1. The at **D3r / v**, pages 21 / 22; 3. Against for 3ly, Against at **I3v / I4r**, pages 62 / 63; it for the at **N3v / N4r**, pages 94 / 95; And for An at **Q4r / v**, pages 119 / 120; tion for is at **Aa2r / v**, pages 179 / 180; or for of at **Dd3r / v**, pages 205 / 206.

Frontispiece: none.

Portrait: **Pt.1a1**: *D: Loggan: delin: et ſculpt*: ÆTATIS SUÆ, 45. 195 × 150 millimetres (sheet); 187 × 139 millimetres (plate marks); 184 × 135 millimetres (image).

Printers' ornaments: [4]. No ornaments or decorated initials

[5]. Two rows of five (upper) and four (lower) fleurons at **A1r**, page [1] {**Dring 10**}.

No decorated initials.

Illustrations: [2]. As in **9B2** [ie **Pl.7a4**; and **Pl.18a2** printed above **Pl.17a2**] until, lettering as in **6A** and **6E**:

[4]. **Pl.27c1**. Plate 27 (image 46): *Tab. I. part 1.st* (headline, centre), *Oq: P. 14.* (headline, right). Leaf size, 314 × 190 millimetres (sheet); 159 × 198 millimetres (plate marks); 145 × 178 millimetres (figure). Legend: The firſt Table repreſents a Mans Stomach taken out and blown up, with the Veſſels full of Bloud; ſo that all the Arteries and Veins, with their branches (which are truly and exactly delineated) may be plainly ſeen. Inserted within *The Explications of the Figures* at **C3r–C4r**, pages 13–15.

Pl.28c1. Plate 28 (image 47): *Tab. II part I.st* (headline, centre), *RR. P. 14.* (headline, right). Leaf size, 314 × 190 millimetres (sheet); 158 × 206 millimetres (plate marks); 125

× 174 millimetres (figure). Legend: The ſecond Table expreſſes the outmoſt coat of a Mans Stomach, which is altogether nervous; whoſe nervous fibres running out the whole length of it, cut the outward fleſhy ones that are under them almoſt at right angles. Inserted within *The Explications of the Figures* at **C3r–C4r**, pages 13–15.

Pl.29c1. Plate 29 (image 48): *Tab. III. part I.*st (headline, centre), *Ss. P. 14.* (headline, right). Leaf size, 314 × 190 millimetres (sheet); 159 × 195 millimetres (plate marks); 140 × 176 millimetres (figure). Legend: The third Table ſhews the Stomach of a Man ſtript of its outmoſt nervous tunick or coat, that the outward or convex ſurface of its middlemoſt coat, together with the fleſhy fibres thereof, may appear. Inserted within *The Explications of the Figures* at **C3r–C4r**, pages 13–15.

Pl.30c1. Plate 30 (images 49–51): *Tab.* IV. *part I.*st (headline, left), *T.t. P. 14.* (headline, right), *Fig. 2.*, *Fig. 3.*, *Fig. I.* (header, above each image). Leaf size, 314 × 190 millimetres (sheet); 157 × 198 millimetres (plate marks); 142 × 157 millimetres, 49 × 55 millimetres, 61 × 52 millimetres (figures). Legend: The fourth Table; whoſe firſt Figure ſhews the whole Stomach, with the inner, concave ſurface, changed into the outward and convex, that the hairy veil or covering, with thoſe wrinkles and folds that go all over the Stomach, may come in view. Figure II. repreſents a part of the Nervous Coat, in which, the hairy covering being taken off, the inner or concave ſurface, together with a thick and numerous company of branches of Veſſels doth appear. Figure III. Shews a part of the hairy or glandulous coat, in which the outward ſurface, whereby it is connected to the Nervous Coat, is apparently very full of glandules and mouths or orifices of veſſels. Inserted within *The Explications of the Figures* at **C3r–C4r**, pages 13–15.

Pl.31c1. Plate 31 (image 52): *Tab.* V. *part. I.*st (headline, centre), *V.u. P. 14.* (headline, right). Leaf size, 314 × 190 millimetres (sheet); 157 × 198 millimetres (plate marks); 146 × 150 millimetres (figure). Legend: The fifth Table ſhews the inner and concave ſurface of the fleſhy coat, turned with the wrong ſide outward, that the other row of moving fibres may come in view. Inserted within *The Explications of the Figures* at **C3r–C4r**, pages 13–15.

Pl.32c1. Plate 32 (images 53–57): *Tab.* VI. *part I.*st (headline, centre), *X.x. P. 15.* (headline, right). Leaf size, 314 × 190 millimetres (sheet); 152 × 231 millimetres (plate marks); 113 × 22 millimetres, 112 × 22 millimetres, 112 × 21 millimetres, 113 × 21 millimetres, 111 × 22 millimetres (figures). Legend: The ſixth Table repreſents all the Coats of the ſmall Guts ſeparated from each other, so that the nervous fibres, with the glandules and branches of Veſſels, as alſo the ranks of moving fibres may clearly and diſtinctly be obſerved. Inserted within *The Explications of the Figures* at **C3r–C4r**, pages 13–15.

[5]. **Pl.33d1**. Plate 33 (image 58): *Sect. I. Cap. I. part. 2.* (headline, left), *Tab: I. Y.y P. 14* (headline, right). Leaf size, 314 × 190 millimetres (sheet); 116 × 183 millimetres (plate marks); 90 × 184 millimetres (figure). Legend: THe first Table ſhews one entire Lobe of the Lungs, upon whoſe ſuperficies the Lymphæducts are ſeen ſpread through every where. Inserted within *The Explication of the Figures* at **C3v–C4v**, pages 14–16.

Pl.34d1. Plate 34 (image 59): *Tab: II.* (headline, left), *part. 2*^{d}. (headline, centre), *Zz. P. 14. / Sect. 1. Cap. 1.* (headline, right). Leaf size, 314 × 190 millimetres (sheet); 200 × 140 millimetres (plate marks); 191 × 118 millimetres (figure). Legend: The second Table ſhews one Lobe of a Sheeps Lung cut in the midſt, that the upper part (wherein is the trunk of the

Vein) being removed, and the trunk of the *Afpera Arteria* laid by it felf, the branching of the Pneumonic Artery is fhewn throughout its whole frame, *viz.* through the fmall and leaft little Lobes. All the paffages of this, *viz.* the flips and twigs how fmall foever, being filled and coloured by any liquid thing caft into them, are drawn to the life. Inserted within *The Explication of the Figures* at **C3v–C4v**, pages 14–16.

Pl.35d1. Plate 35 (images 60–61): *Tab. III.* (headline, left), *Aaa. P. 14.* (headline, right), *Fig. j.*, *Fig. 2.* (headers, left of each image). Leaf size, 314 × 190 millimetres (sheet); 197 × 134 millimetres (plate marks); 181 × 131 millimetres, 43 × 25 millimetres (figures). Legend: The firft Figure of the third Table expreffes one Lobe of the Lungs, according to the branchings of the *Afpera Arteria* divided into leffer and leff Lobes, the twigs and flips of which Veffel being filled by a liquid firft injected, and afterwards feparated from among themfelves towards the little Lobes, are alfo drawn to the life. The fecond Figure of the third Table expreffes a part of the pulmonary Lobe, wherein the membranous interfpaces being blown up, all the little Lobes appear in their proper figure, and do fomewhat reprefent the leaf of Polypody. Inserted within *The Explication of the Figures* at **C3v–C4v**, pages 14–16.

Pl.36d1. Plate 36 (images 62–64): *Tab. IV.* (headline, centre), *B.bb. P. 15. Sect. 1. Cap. 1.* (headline, right), *Fig: 1.*, *Fig: 2.*, *Fig: 3.* (headers, left of each image). Leaf size, 314 × 190 millimetres (sheet); 163 × 118 millimetres (plate marks); 69 × 40 millimetres, 60 × 34 millimetres, 63 × 35 millimetres (figures). Legend: The fourth Table expreffs as well the Veffels belonging to the *Trachea* as thofe bringing blood, feparate and diftinct one from another, conftituting one little Lobe, as alfo the peculiar framing of every one of them. The firft Figure reprefents the feparating into divers parts the Tracheal branch diftributed into one little Lobe, and the branching into Pipes and orbicular little bladders. The fecond and third Figure fhews distinctly the equal branchings of the Artery and Pneumonick Veins within the fame little Lobe; both which being complicated with Tracheal Veffels, do for the moft part make up the texture of the pulmonary frame. Inserted within *The Explication of the Figures* at **C3v–C4v**, pages 14–16.

Pl.37d1. Plate 37 (images 65–67): *Sect. 1. Cap. 1*: (headline, left), *part 2.*[d] (headline, centre), *Tab: V. C.cc P. 15.* (headline, right), *Fig. 2.*, *Fig. 1.*, *Fig. 3.* (headers, left of each image). Leaf size, 314 × 190 millimetres (sheet); 213 × 164 millimetres (plate marks); 75 × 66 millimetres, 73 × 90 millimetres, 137 × 155 millimetres (figures). Legend: The fifth Table fets forth the pulmonary Nerve more accurately defcribed by the aid of a Microfcope: fo that it plainly appears that the Trunk is as it were a bundle of innumerable little Fibres bound together; Moreover its Trunk, while it creeps into the Lungs in the likenefs of Mother of Time, doth fpread the various little fprigs every way. Fig. I. refembles a part of the nervous trunk cut away, one end whereof being opened and lookt on by a Microfcope, feems to unfold it felf almoft into innumerable little fibres. The fecond and third figure do fhew fome fibres as well of the trunk as of every branch, and moreover the flips of the little twigs from divers ftemmes often repeated. Inserted within *The Explication of the Figures* at **C3v–C4v**, pages 14–16.

Pl.38d1. Plate 38 (images 68–75): *Tab. VI part 2.*[d] (headline, left), *Sect. 1. Cap. 1. Ddd. P. 15.* (headline, right), *Fig. 1.*, *Fig. 2.* (headers, above each group of four images). Leaf size, 314 × 190 millimetres (sheet); 163 × 215 millimetres (plate marks); 69 × 49 millimetres,

73 × 47 millimetres, 70 × 49 millimetres, 71 × 49 millimetres, 72 × 16 millimetres, 72 × 16 millimetres, 74 × 16 millimetres, 75 × 16 millimetres (figures). Legend: The ſix Table firſt ſets from the anatomy of the Artery bringing blood drawn in apt figures, which we have deſcribed in a late treatiſe. *The firſt and upper figures hereof*, repreſent the four diſtinct Coats of that Veſſel, *viz.* the nervous, muſcular, glandulous, and the vaſculous. 1. *The firſt inward nervous coat*, which perhaps is ſomewhat muſculous, conſiſting of ſtreight or long fibres, which being contracted ſhorten the Pipe of the Artery. 2. *The coat properly muſcular*, conſiſting of a heap of ſmall circular fibres, which when they are contracted ſucceſſively under the ſtream of blood, do make its circuit to be ſhortened. It is from the motion of theſe that the arteries beat. 3. *The glandulous coat*, which (like that in the guts) being placed over the muſculous coat, is weaved together of very ſmall and moſt numerous glandules. 4. *The outward vaſculous coat*, which variously folded together and wreathed, of Veſſels bringing blood, and with ſlips and nervous fibres, ſeems like a certain little net. The *ſecond and lower figures* of the ſixth Table, do ſhew the anatomy of the Vein, or its four coats expreſſed in fit places; which Coats do appear entire as ſucceſſively taken one part from the other (beginning outmoſt). I. *The outward coat* conſiſting of nervous fibres (which perhaps are ſomewhat muſcular) and as it were ſtreight or ſtretch'd out in length, although not orderly. II. & III. *The vaſculous and glandulous coat*, which are the ſame as in an Artery. IV. *The moſt inward muſcular coat*, conſiſting alſo of circular fibres as in an Artery, which being contracted behind the ſtream of blood, haſtens its returning courſe. Inserted within *The Explication of the Figures* at **C3v–C4v**, pages 14–16.

Pl.39d1. Plate 39 (images 76–79): *Sect. 1. Cap 1*: (headline, left), *Tab. VII part 2^{d}.* (headline, centre), *E.ee. P. 15.* (headline, right), *Fig: 1.*, *Fig: 2.*, *Fig: 3.*, *Fig: 4.* (headers, above each image). Leaf size, 314 × 190 millimetres (sheet); 207 × 145 millimetres (plate marks); 56 × 54 millimetres, 50 × 45 millimetres, 56 × 55 millimetres, 55 × 58 millimetres (figures). Legend: The ſeventh Table expreſſes the diſtinct Coats of the *aſpera arteria*, and ſeparated one from the other. *The firſt figure ſhews the moſt inward Coat*, endowed with ſtreight or long muſcular fibres. *The ſecond figure deſcribes the glandulous coat*, and the third figure the vaſculous coat (which are almoſt the ſame as in the veſſels bringing blood, and alſo in the Guts). 4. *The fourth figure expreſſes the outward* coat (which is partly cartilaginous, and partly muſcular). The tranſverſe or annular fibres hereof do fill up and weave together the interſpaces of the Cartilages.; printed above **Pl.40d1**. Plate 40 (images 80–82): *Sect.1. Cap. 1.* (headline, left), *Tab: VIII. part 2.^{d}* (headline, centre), *Fig. 1.* (centre, left), *Fig: 3.* (centre, right), *Fig: 2.* (lower, centre), no lettering. 48 × 49 millimetres, 23 × 24 millimetres and 50 × 48 millimetres (figures). Legend: The eighth Table ſhews a part of the utmoſt pulmonary Coat covering over its whole frame, moſt finely and curiouſly deſcribed by the help of a Microſcope. The firſt figure ſhews a portion of the above mentioned coat, which partly by reaſon of the extremities of Veſſels of every ſort ending in it, ſeems pricked full of holes as it were, and partly from the complications of the veſſels bringing blood, which like the twining ſprigs of Vines gird about the orbicular bladders, is diſtinguished into many irregular *Area*'s. The ſecond Figure repreſents a part of the outermoſt membrane ſeparated from the cluſters of veſſels pull'd off and without any *Areæ*, only markt with little holes as it were with ſmall pricks. The third Figure expreſſes one ſingular *area* of the Coat above mentioned, augmented in largeneſs by the help of a Microſcope. Inserted within *The Explication of the Figures* at **C3v–C4v**, pages 14–16.

[6]. As in **9D**.

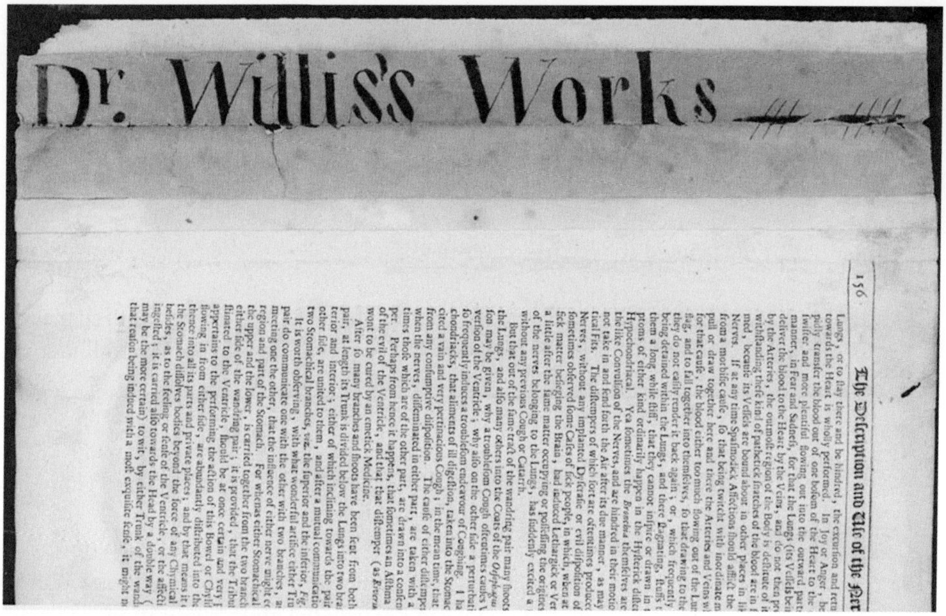

Figure 156 Previous owner's vertical half title in pen and ink pasted onto a central section of *Dr Willis's practice of physick* 1684. This copy previously owned by HJR Wing.

Copy: DASC, may lack [3] A². Later full calf, spine with six raised bands, labelled DR. WILLIS'S | PRACTICE OF | PHYSICK, with gilt borders and tooling, new endpapers. Leaves 316 × 194 millimetres, boards 323 × 195 × 87 millimetres. Inscribed: (1) Robert Smith Bunney; (2) John Smith Bunney Notts (×4) with annotations in his hand. John Smith has pasted a vertical half title in pen and ink, DR WILLIS'S WORKS, folded into the book at [4] X3v, page 156 (see: Figure 156).[22]

9E.c2. DR WILLIS'S PRACTICE OF PHYSICK, London folio 1684

The second edition with the collective title *Dr Willis's practice of physick*, containing Willis's first, second, third, fourth, fifth, and sixth books in English, the ninth publication, using the

[22] This copy was previously owned by HJR Wing. He wrote in correspondence dated 27 October 2003: 'Soon after completing my bibliography I acquired what is probably the earliest state of the *Practice of physick*. It was unbound as issued with contemporary endpapers before the frontispiece and at the end. Similarly between the end of *An essay of the pathology of the brain* and *Pharmaceutice rationalis* there is another contemporary blank leaf. All the blank leaves have inscriptions by members of the Smith Bunney family of Nottinghamshire. I had it bound in full leather in the late 1960s. Unfortunately it lacks the title page to *An essay of the pathology of the brain* and its epistle dedicatory to Gilbert Sheldon ... In the eighteenth century a former owner pasted a strip of paper on the edge of pages 155–6 ... and wrote on it *Dr Willis's Works* so that when the volume was shelved with the foreedge to the front the strip of paper was visible. It was probably used as a working copy as it contains a couple of remedies written in manuscript. It has the full complement of 39 plates but the folding ones are torn.' See above for whether John Wing's comment on the missing subsidiary title page and dedicatory epistle is correct. The annotations include advice in a footnote at [3: *Of urines*] D1v, page 16, 'For the stone take 1. Ounce of Elicant sage every Day and drink plenty of Lime water made of Oyster or cockle shells. For the gravell only Drink Lime water made of Oyster or Cockell shells.' The rear free endpaper (recto) is inscribed: 'Penny Worth. A Gumborge to cure the Bad Disorder. Boiled in 2 or 3 neat spoonful of Spring Water and mixed with neat Clover. Make it in Pils take 5 or 6 night and morning.'

third of four titles, made up from the sheets *The remaining medical works* (1681: **9B2**) and *Two discourses concerning the soul of brutes* (1683: **9D**), *Pharmaceutice rationalis* parts 1 and 2 newly translated and the plates to that treatise reengraved, and one plate leaf in a second state [not distinguished from HJR Wing 59, Denham 22].

As in **9E.c1** apart from:

Illustrations: **Pl.17a2** printed above **Pl.18a2** (as in **9B1.c2**).

Copy: DASC. Later quarter calf with buckram boards, spine with six raised bands, labelled DR. WILLIS'S | PRACTICE OF | PHYSICK, new endpapers. Leaves 314 × 195 millimetres, boards 325 × 200 × 90 millimetres. From the library of Edwin Clarke.[23]

9F. DR WILLIS'S PRACTICE OF PHYSICK, London folio 1684

The third edition with the collective title *Dr Willis's practice of physick*, containing Willis's first, second, third, fourth, fifth, and sixth books in English, the ninth publication, using the third of four titles, made up from the sheets and illustrations of *Pharmaceutice rationalis* parts 1 and 2 (**9E**) and *Two discourses concerning the soul of brutes* (**9D**), the treatises originally published in *The remaining medical works* corrected and reset, with their plates newly engraved [HJR Wing 59, Denham 22].

Title page: [1a]. [within a double rule] DR WILLIS'S | Practice of Phyſick, | Being the whole | WORKS | OF THAT | RENOWNED and FAMOUS | PHYSICIAN: | CONTAINING | Theſe Eleven Several Treatiſes, *viz.* | I. Of Fermentation. | II. Of Feavers. | III. Of Urines. | IV. Of the Accenſion of the Blood. | V. Of Muſculary Motion. | VI. Of the Anatomy of the Brain. | VII. Of the Deſcription and Uſe of the Nerves. | VIII. Of Convulſive Diſeaſes. | IX. Pharmaceutice Rationalis, the Firſt and Second Part. | X. Of the Scurvy. | XI. Two Diſcourſes concerning the Soul of Brutes. | Wherein moſt of the Diſeaſes belonging to the Body of | Man are Treated of, with excellent Methods and Receipts for the Cure | of the ſame. | Fitted to the meaneſt Capacity by an Index for the Explaining of all the | hard and unuſual Words and Terms of Art derived from the Greek, Latine, | or other Languages, for the Benefit of the Engliſh Reader. | [rule] | *With Forty Copper Plates.* | [rule] | The Pharmaceutice new Tranſlated, and the Whole | carefully Corrected and Amended. | [double rule] | *LONDON*, | Printed for *T. Dring*, *C. Harper*, and *J. Leigh*, and are to be Sold at | the Corner of *Chancery-Lane*, and the *Flower-de-Luce* over againſt | St *Dunſtans* Church in *Fleet-ſtreet*, M DC LXXXIV.

[23] Edwin Clarke (1919–1996) trained in neurology in Oxford and worked as a consultant at the Hammersmith Hospital but switched to a career in medical history, becoming director of the Wellcome Institute for the History of Medicine and editor of *Medical History* (1973–1979). This copy of *Dr Willis's practice of physick* is one that seems to have escaped the Sherrington Room, University of Oxford, where the core collection is based on Clarke's library. Reference is made in other chapters to *The human brain and spinal cord. A historical study illustrated by writings from antiquity to the twentieth century* (1968) written with CD O'Malley, and the *Illustrated history of brain function* (1972) with Kenneth Dewhurst, who used this copy when writing *Willis's Oxford Casebook*, Oxford (1981). William Bynum comments that: 'Although [Clarke] played a seminal role in the evolution of academic medical history in Britain, he was never entirely comfortable with the social-historical emphasis which characterizes the modern discipline. Any diffidence was entirely inappropriate, for his scholarship possessed the timeless qualities of accuracy and care'.

[1b]. A | Medical=Philofophical Difcourfe | OF | FERMENTATION. | OR, OF THE | Inteftine Motion | OF | PARTICLES | IN EVERY | BODY. | [rule] | BY | Dr. *THOMAS WILLIS* of Chrift-Church in | *Oxford*, and *Sidley* Profeffor of Natural Philofophy in that | Famous Univerfity. | [rule] | Translated into *Englifh*, by *S.P.* | [rule] | *LONDON:* | Printed by *H. Clark*, for *T. Dring*, *C. Harper*, and *J. Leigh*. | M DC LXXXIV.

[2]. [within a double rule] AN | ESSAY | OF THE | PATHOLOGY | OF THE | BRAIN | AND | Nervous Stock: | In Which | Convulfive Difeafes | Are Treated of. | [rule] | Being the Work of *THOMAS WILLIS* of *Chrift-Church* | in *Oxford*, Doctor in Phyfick, and *Sidly*-Profeffor of | Natural Philofophy in that Famous Academy. | [rule] | Tranflated out of *Latine* into *Englifh*, By *S.P.* | [rule] | *LONDON:* | Printed by *A. M.* and *R. R.* for *T. Dring*, *J. Leigh*, and *C. Harper*; | 1684.

[3]. Pharmaceutice rationalis part 1, as in **9E.c1** [4].

[4]. Pharmaceutice rationalis part 2, as in **9E.c1** [5].

[5]. Two discourses concerning the soul of Brutes; as in **9D**.

Collation: folio in 4s; 23 letter roman alphabet using I and V: [1]. π1; A–B^2; (a)–(g)^2, ^{2}B^4–V^4, ^{3}B^4–X^4; $1–2 signed apart from: -B2, -d2, -e2, -f2, -g2, 3X3 signed X2
175 leaves, paginated as: [38], 1–152, [2], 1–40, [41–4], 45–158. Mispaginated: (section 1) 137 for 139, 138 for 140, 139 for 141, 140 for 142.

[2]. [A]^2, B–N^4; $1–2 signed.
50 leaves, paginated as [4] 1–96.

[3] and [4]. As in **9E.c1** (parts [4] and [5]).

[5]. As in **9D**.

Contents: [1]. **π1r**, page [1], title; **π1v**, page [2], blank; **A1r–v**, pages [3–4], TO THE Moft Reverend Father in Chrift, And the Right Honorable HIS GRACE, GILBERT, **By Divine Providence**, Arch-Bifhop of CANTERBURY, Primate and Metropolitan of all *England*, and one of His Majefties moft Honourable Privy-Councellors. … [signed] *Your Graces moft Humble And for ever Obliged Servant*, T. W.; **A2r**, page [5], sub-title; **A2v**, page [6], blank; **B1r–v**, pages [7–8], TO THE RIGHT WORSHIPFUL S[r] Theophilus Biddulph, KNIGHT and BARONET. … [signed] Honoured Sir, Your moft humble and faithful Servant, *S. PORDAGE.*; **B2r–v**, pages [9–10], THE PREFACE.; **(a)1r–(d)1r**, pages [11–23], A TABLE of all the hard words derived from the *Greek* and *Latin*, of all Terms of Art and other words not vulgarly received, with the Explanation of them.; **(d)1v**, page [24], blank; **(d)2r–v**, pages [25–6], ON THE AUTHORS Medical-Philofophical Difcourfes.; **(e)1r–(e)2r**, pages [27–9], THE TABLE To the Treatifes of FERMENTATION and FEAVERS.; **(e)2r–(g)1r**, pages [29–35], THE TABLE To the Treatifes of 1. *Of Urins*. 2. *Of the Accenfion of the Blood*. 3. *Of Mufculary Motion*. 4. *Of the Anatomy of the Brain:* &. 5. *Of the Defcription and Ufe of the Nerves*. (in two columns); **(g)1r–(g)2v**, pages [35–8], THE TABLE To the Treatife of CONVULSIVE DISEASES.

2B1r–G2v, pages 1–44, [text] OF FERMENTATION, OR THE Inorganical Motion OF NATURAL BODIES.

G3r–v, pages 45–6, THE PREFACE TO THE Treatiſe of Feavers.

G4r–V4v, pages 47–152, [text] OF FEAVERS.

3B1r–v, pages [1–2], THE AUTHORS EPISTLE (To the *Treatiſe of Urines*) TO Dr. Bathurſt.

B2r–D3r, pages 1–19, [text] OF URINES.; **D3v–E3r**, pages 20–7, [text] TWO Phyſical and Medical EXERCITATIONS, *VIZ.* 1. Of the Accenſion of the Blood. II. Of Muſculary Motion. THE FIRST Medical and Phyſical DISCOURSE. *Of the growing hot or inkindling of the Blood.*; **E3v–G1v**, pages 28–40, [text] THE SECOND Phyſical & Medical DISCOURSE. *Of Muſculary Motion.*

G2r–v, pages [41–2], THE ANATOMY OF THE BRAIN. *The Authors Epiſtle Dedicatory to his Grace* Gilbert *Arch-biſhop of* Canterbury, *&*. … [signed] YOUR GRACES *moſt humble and obliged Servant*, THO. WILLIS.; **G3r–v**, pages [43–4], THE PREFACE TO THE READER.

G4r–Q1r, pages 45–111, [text] THE ANATOMY OF THE BRAIN.; **Q1v–X4v**, pages 112–58, [text] THE Deſcription and uſe OF THE NERVES.

[2]. **[A]1r**, page [1], sub-title; **[A]1v**, page [2], blank; **[A]2r–[A]2b**, pages [3–4],], The Authors Epiſtle Dedicatory, *To the Moſt Reverend Father in Chriſt, His Grace*, Gilbert, *By Divine Providence Archbiſhop of* Canterbury, *Primate and Metropolitan of all* England, *and one of His Sacred Majeſties moſt Honourable Privy Council.* … [signed] Your Graces moſt humble and Devoted Servant, *T. W.*

B1r–N4v, pages 1–96, [text] *Of Convulſive Diſeaſes.*

[3] and [4]. As in **9E.c1** (parts [4] and [5]).

[5]. As in **9D**.

Headlines and *Catchwords*: [1]. ⁚ for ; after headline at **B1v**, page 2; **B2v**, page 4; **B3v**, page 6; **B4v**, page 8; **C3v**, page 14; Chap. IX. for Chap. VIII. at **E1r**, page 25; *a Intermitting* for *Of Intermitting* at **K1r**, page 65; *Quartan Feavers or Agues.* for *a Quartan Feaver or Ague.* at **K3r**, page 69; *Feaver* for *Quartan Feaver* at **L1r**, page 73; Chap. VIII. for Chap. IX. at **L4v**, page 80; Chap. XI. for Chap. X. at **M4v**, page 88; *a Putrid Feaver.* for FEAVERS. at **O1v**, page 98; FEAVERS. for *a Putrid Feaver.* at **O4r**, page 103; Chap. XIII. for Chap. XII. at **P1r**, page 105; FEAVERS. for *the Small Pox and Meaſles* at **R1r**, page 121; **R2r**, page 123; *the Small Pox and Meaſles.* for FEAVERS. at **R1v**, page 122; *the Feavers in Women Lying in.* for FEAVERS. at **R3v**, page 126; **R4v**, page 128; FEAVERS. for *the Feavers in Women Lying in.* at **R4r**, page 127; Chap. XVII. for Chap. XVI. at **T1v**, page 138; Chap. XVI. for Chap. XVII. at **T4r**, page 143; *the Quantity and Colour in Urines of ſick People.* for *Urines.* at **2B4v**, page 6; *The Quantity and Colour of ſick peoples Urines.* for *Of the Contents in the Urines of ſick People.* at **C4r**, page 13; *the accenſion of the Blood.* for *Judgments by Urines.* at **D1r**, page 15; *Judgments by Urines.* for *Urines.* at **D1v**, page 16; *the Examination of Urines.* for *Urines.* at **D2v**, page 18; *Urines.* for *the Accenſion of the Blood.* at **D4v**, page 22.

No catchword at **A1v / A2r**, pages [4] / [5];[24] Cribrous for Cribrious at **(a2)r / v**, pages [13] / [14]; Paenchima for Parotida at **(b2)v / (c1)r**, pages [18] / [19]; **2C3v / D1r**, pages 12 / 13, which, for which; THE for The at **G1r / v**, pages 39 / 40; CHAP. for The at **I1v / I2r**, pages 56 / 57.

[2]. *Of the wonderful Net.* for *The Anatomy of the Brain.* at **L1v**, page 72; *Anatomy of the Brain.* for *ufes of the Brain properly so called.* at **L4r**, page 77; *The Anatomy of the Brain.* for *Of the Nervous Juyce.* at **Q1r**, page 111; *Of the Eighth or wandering Pair.* for *The Defcription and Ufe of the Nerves.* at **R1v**, page 120; *The Defcription and Ufe of the Nerves.* for *Of the Intercoftal Nerve.* at **S2r**, page 129; *Of the Intercoftal Nerve.* for *The Defcription and Ufe of the Nerves.* at **S2v**, page 130.

ions for tions at **K1v / K2r**, pages 66 / 67; Tumour for Tumor at **L1r / v**, pages 73 / 74; mefentery for Mefentery at **L2r / v**, pages 75 / 76.

[3] and [4]. As in **9E.c1** (parts [4] and [5]).

[5]. As in **9D**.

Frontispiece: none.

Portrait: none.

Printers' ornaments: none.

Decorated T at **A1r**, page [3]; **B1r**, page 1 {**Dring 11**}; T at **G4r**, page 47 {**Dring 12**}; then [3] and [4] as in **9E**; [5] as in **9D**.

Illustrations: lettering as in **2A** and **4A**:

[1]. **Pl.17c1** (images 26 and 27) engraved with **Pl.18c1**. Plates 17 and 18 (images 28 and 29): *A A. p. 40.* (headline, right), *Fig. I.*, *Fig. II.*, *Fig. III.*, *Fig. IV* (headers, above each image). Leaf size, 312 × 193 millimetres (sheet); 244 × 164 millimetres (plate marks); 28 × 140 millimetres, 44 × 157 millimetres, 30 × 152 millimetres, 42 × 160 millimetres (figures). Legend: The Firft Figure *SHews a fimple regular Mufcle, defcribed according to its natural appearance, in the Belly of which the flefhy Fibres being opened, are diduced one from another, that the membranaceous Fibrils may be the better beheld.* The Secod Figure *Shews a simple Mufcle cleft in the middle, after the Tendon being cut off, and portions of it pulled away, that the interiour feries of the flefhy Fibres, or their commixtures or mingling with the Tendons may appear.* The Third Figure. *Exhibits a certain Mufcle lefs compounded, to whofe two flefhy Bellies two compounded Tendons alfo (equal to four fimple ones) are deftinated.* The Fourth Figure. *Shews a regular compounded Mufcle, divided and opened in the middle, fo that the interiour face of either Belly may appear.* Inserted after The Explication of the Figures at **G1v**, page 40.

[24] See introductory notes for resolution of apparent discontinuities resulting from erratic organization of the preliminaries. By any analysis, A1v has no catchword.

Pl.1d1. Plate 1 (image 1) engraved with **Pl.2d1**. Plate 2 (image 2): *Fig. 1.*[a] (headline, left), *Fig. II*[d]. (headline, centre), *B B. p. 51.* (headline, right), *de medio S vid pag* (number erased) (footer, right). Leaf size, 312 × 193 millimetres (sheet); 160 × 279 millimetres (plate marks); 151 × 136 millimetres, 135 × 102 millimetres (figure, bound horizontally). Legend: The Firſt Figure. *SHews the Baſis of an humane Brain taken out of the Skull, with the Roots of the Veſſels cut off.* The Second Figure. *Shews the Baſis of a Sheeps Brain taken out of the Skull, and the Roots of the Veſſels cut off, where all the Arteries, by Ink being injected into one of the Carotides, are made black and more conſpicuous.* Inserted before legends for Figuræ I–II at **H3r**, page 51.

Pl.3d1. Plate 3 (image 3): *Fig. III* (headline, centre), *C C. p. 57.* (headline, right). Leaf size, 312 × 193 millimetres (sheet); 220 × 164 millimetres (plate marks); 183 × 160 millimetres (figure). Legend: The Third Figure. *SHews the outmoſt or ſuperiour Superficies of the humane Brain taken out of the skull; where the border of the Brain being looſned from the knitting of the other Parts, made by the Membranes, is elevated and turned outward, that the ſhanks of the oblong Marrow, the* Fornix *or arched Vault, the* Nates *and* Teſtes, *with the pineal Kernel, and other Proceſſes, may be clearly and diſtinctly beheld.* Inserted before legends for the Third and Fourth Figures at **I2r**, page 57.

Pl.4d1. Plate 4 (image 4): *Fig. IIII.* (headline, centre), *D D. p. 57.* (headline, right). Leaf size, 312 × 193 millimetres (sheet); 150 × 116 millimetres (plate marks); 118 × 92 millimetres (figure). Legend: The Fourth Figure. *The Effigies of an humane Brain of a certain Youth that was fooliſh from his birth, and of that ſort which are commonly termed Changelings; the bulk of whoſe brain, as it was thinner and leſſer than is uſual, its border could be farther lifted up and turned back, that all the more interior parts might be more deeply held together.* Inserted before legends for the Third and Fourth Figures at **I2r**, page 57.

Pl.5d1. Plate 5 (image 5): *Fig. V.* (headline, centre), *E E p. 60* (headline, right). Leaf size, 312 × 193 millimetres (sheet); 214 × 135 millimetres (plate marks); 182 × 131 millimetres (figure). Legend: The Fifth Figure. *SHews the interior Baſis of an humane Skull; where is ſhewn after what manner the Veſſels of every kind cut off from the Brain, and about to go out of the Skull, are hid or laid up under the* dura Mater. Inserted within legends for Figuræ V–VI at **I3v–I4r**, pages 60–1.

Pl.6d1. Plate 6 (image 6): *Fig. VI.* (headline, centre), *F F. p. 61.* (headline, right). Leaf size, 312 × 193 millimetres (sheet); 214 × 138 millimetres (plate marks); 196 × 129 millimetres (figure). Legend: The Sixth Figure. *SHews the Baſis of a Calfs Skull; where is ſhewn after what manner the Veſſels cut off from the Brain, and about to go out from the Skull, are drowned under the* dura Mater. Inserted within legends for Figuræ V–VI at **I3v–I4r**, pages 60–1.

Pl.7d1. Plate 7 (images 7–10): [Unnumbered 1] *G G. p. 71.* (headline, right), *Fig. 1.*, *Fig. 11.*, *Fig. 111.*, (header, above each image), *Fig. 1111.* (header, left of the image). Leaf size, 312 × 190 millimetres (sheet); 203 × 140 millimetres (plate marks); 29 × 97 millimetres, 83 × 93 millimetres, 36 × 28 millimetres, 74 × 26 millimetres (figures). Legend: The Firſt Figure *Shews the aſcent of the Carotidick Artery, and its ſituation within an humane Skull, before it is carried towards the Brain.* The Second Figure *Shews the aſcent of the Carotidick Arteries, and their ſituation in a Horſes Skull.* The Third Figure *Shews the wonderful Net with the pituitary Kernel in a Calfs Skull.* The Fourth Figure *Shews after what manner the lateral Boſom goes into* *the Jugular Vein with a diverting place hanging to it.* Inserted before legend for the first unnumbered figure at **L1r**, page 71.

Pl.8d1. Plate 8 (image 11): *Fig. VII.* (headline, centre), *H H. p. 77.* (headline, right). Leaf size, 312 × 193 millimetres (sheet); 232 × 130 millimetres (plate marks); 198 × 105 millimetres (figure). Legend: *The Seventh Figure* SHews the Brain of a Sheep bent back and cut a little open in the places where they ſtick together near the ſtreaked bodies, that its interior ſubstance may be turned the inſide out, and unfolded on a plain. Inserted before legend at **L4r**, page 77.

Pl.9d1. Plate 9 (image 12): *Fig. VIII.* (headline, centre), *II. p. 86* (headline, right). Leaf size, 312 × 193 millimetres (sheet); 137 × 97 millimetres (plate marks); 111 × 92 millimetres (figure). Legend: The Eighth Figure. REpreſents the oblong Marrow taken out of the Head of a Sheep with the Brain cut off and removed, and with the Cerebel and one ſtreaked Body cut in two in the middle, and the other things chiefly belonging to the medullar Trunk. Inserted after legend at **M4v**, page 86.

Pl.10d1. Plate 10 (images 13 and 14): [Unnumbered 2] *KK. p. 118* (headline, right), *Fig. I.*, *Fig. II.* (header, above each image). Leaf size, 312 × 193 millimetres (sheet); 200 × 138 millimetres (plate marks); 126 × 113 millimetres, 49 × 111 millimetres (figures). Legend: This figure ſhews the Branchings of the fifth and ſixth pair of Nerves. The Second Figure ſhews all the Nerves, which being carried from the Nerves of the third, fourth, fifth and ſixth Pair, are beſtowed upon the Muſcles and other parts of the Eye. Inserted within legend at **Q4v–R1r**, pages 118–19.

Pl.11d1. Plate 11 (image 15): *Tab. IX.* (headline, centre), *LL p 149* (headline, right). Leaf size, 312 × 193 millimetres (sheet); 280 × 164 millimetres (plate marks); 268 × 155 millimetres (figure). Legend: *The Ninth Table.* Shews the beginnings of the fifth and ſixth pair of Nerves, and the Roots of the Intercoſtal Nerve proceeding from them; moreover, the Origines and Branchings out of the ſame Intercoſtal Nerve and the wandring Pair, and of the acceſſory Nerve produced out of the Spine to the wandring Pair carried to the Region of the Ventricle. Beſides, here are repreſented the beginnings and diſtributions of the ſeventh, ninth, tenth Pair of Nerves, and of the Nerve of the Diaphragma; alſo the beginnings of the Vertebral Nerves in their whole Tract from the Region of the Nerves inſerted in the *Præcordia* and *Viſcera* are deſcribed, and their Communications with the former. All this whole following Table ſhews how it is found in Man different from other living Creatures. Inserted before legends at **V4r–X1r**, pages 149–51.

Pl.12d1. Plate 12 (image 16): *Tab. X.* (headline, centre), *MM. p.152* (headline, right). Leaf size, 312 × 193 millimetres (sheet); 280 × 164 millimetres (plate marks); 266 × 156 millimetres (figure). Legend: *The Tenth Table.* Shews the beginnings and Branchings out of the ſame Nerves which were deſcribed in the former Table, as ſome of them are found in brute Beaſts otherwiſe than in Man. / The other Nerves and their Branchings out are as in the other Figure, which ſhews the pattern of them in Man. Inserted after legend at **X1v**, page 152.

Pl.13d2. Plate 13 (image 17): *p. 187.* (headline, left), *NN p 153* (headline, right). Folding, 407 × 190 millimetres (sheet); 368 × 169 millimetres (plate marks); 356 × 162 millimetres (figure). Legend: *The Eleventh Table.* Shews the lower Branchings out of the wandring and the Intercoſtal Pair, diſtributed to the Ventricle and the *Viſcera* of the Abdomen; alſo the beginning of the Vertebral Nerves, which are placed over againſt the former, and are ingraffed into ſome of them. The Figure of theſe in Man and in four-footed Beaſts is almoſt alike, ſo that this Table may be common for both. Inserted before legend for *The Eleventh Table* at **X2r–v**, page 153–54.

Pl.14d2. Plate 14 (image 18): *P. 189.* (headline, left), *OO. p. 155* (headline, right). Leaf size, 312 × 193 millimetres (sheet); 232 × 80 millimetres (plate marks); 221 × 36 millimetres (figure). Legend: *The Twelfth Table*. Shews the Spinal Marrow whole taken out of its bony Den, and half taken from the Membrane cloathing it, being diſſected, that the beginnings and productions of all the Vertebral Nerves might be ſeen together. Inserted before legends for Tabulæ XII–XIII at **X[2]r–X4r**, pages 155–7.

Pl.15d1. Plate 15 (images 19–23): *Tab. XIII.* (headline, left), *PP. p. 156* (headline, right), *Fig. III.*, Fig. *I.*, *Fig. II.*, *Fig.* IV., Fig. *V* (headers, above each image). Leaf size, 312 × 193 millimetres (sheet); 280 × 163 millimetres (plate marks); 118 × 53 millimetres, 122 × 52 millimetres, 232 × 28 millimetres, 222 × 32 millimetres, 59 × 21 millimetres (figures). Legend: *The Thirteenth Table*. FIGURE I. Shews the branchings forth of the Vertebral Artery reaching out on both ſides into the ſuperiour part of the Spinal Marrow, and into the hinder Region of the oblong Marrow. FIGURE II. Shews the Vertebral Veins which are Companions to the abovesaid Arteries; alſo the upper portion of the Vertebral Boſom and the communications of either among themſelves and lateral Boſoms of the Head, and between the Jugular Veins. FIGURE III. Shews the Spinal Artery which is produced within the bony Den nigh the more inward Superficies of the Marrow, from the hinder part of the Head to the *Os Sacrum*, in the ſhape of a Net-work purl. FIGURE IV. Shews the Branchings out of the Spinal Boſom in its whole paſſage. FIGURE V. Shews the Image of the Spinal Boſom in a Dog, which hath not joynings together in its whole paſſage, as it is in a Calf, Sheep, Hog, and many others, but only in the loweſt and uppermoſt part, where it communicates with it ſelf by three or four croſs Proceſſes. Inserted before legends for Tabulæ XII–XIII at **X[2]r–X4r**, pages 155–7.

[3] and [4]. **Pl.27c1–Pl.32.c1**; **Pl.33d1–Pl.40d1** (images 46–82) as in **9E.c1**.

[5]. **Pl.19c1–Pl.26c1**. Plates 19–26 (images 30–45) as in **9D**.

Copy: DASC (#1 of 3). Original calf, spine (rebacked) with five raised bands, lettered WILLIS's | PRACTICE | OF | PHYSICK | 1684, original endpapers. Leaves 312 × 190 millimetres, boards 320 × 195 × 83 millimetres.

14

'Of drudgery in pursuit of lucre'

The London practice of physick (1685–1695)

The London practice of physick was published between 1685 and 1695. It was intended to provide extracts in English from the published treatises that informed the practice of medicine. The text was newly translated from the Latin by 'Eugenius Φιλιατρος'.[1] There seems no reason to doubt HJR Wing's statement: 'This is most likely J. Hemming, Willis's apothecary and amanuensis, who had Willis's *A plain and easie method for preserving those that are well from the plague* published in 1691'.[2] Eugenius advises those who read Latin to study Dr Willis's works in the original rather than suffer the existing English translations. Nor does he spare himself in criticising his predecessor, Samuel Pordage (1633–1691):

> *As for the way of Translation us'd in this Work, any Man who pleases to compare a Leaf of what is here done with a Leaf of the former Translation, will easily find that this is no Transcript; the way of expression being very differing; and we often disagreeing as to the sense of Dr* Willis; *in which others will judge who has done him most right: and as I do not doubt but now and then there may be found a more apt expression than what I have us'd, so I conceive there is no very material errour in what I have written; and without Animadversion, or Insisting on particulars, I shall take freedom to say that I believe what I have here Translated will be judg'd by all Men to be more easy, correct and clear, than what has been done before.*

The contents of *The London practice of physick*

Quoting from the preface to *The London practice of physick*, in a summary copied but rephrased by Browne Willis (1682–1760), Anthony Wood (1632–1695) explains:[3]

> What are therein made *English* of his Works are (1) His first and second Parts of the *Pharmaceutice rationalis.* (2) His Tract of *Convulsive Diseases.* (3) His Tract of the *Scurvey.* (4) His Tr. of the *Diseases of the Brain*, and *Genus nervosum.* (5) His Tr. of *Fevers*: The other Parts of his Works being Theoretical are therein omitted. This Translation is said to be

[1] Stephen Anderson advises that the correct form is Φιλίατρος, i.e. doctor-lover' or 'friend of medicine'. The Latin form of the Greek name Εὐγένιος meaning 'well born', a name formed from the word εὐγενής, was not much used in the seventeenth century but became popular through Prince Eugene of Savoy (1663–1736), a French-born general who served the Austrian Empire.

[2] See: HJR Wing, *A bibliography of Dr. Thomas Willis (1621–1675)*, unpublished manuscript (1962): page 86.

[3] See: [Anthony Wood] *Athenæ Oxoniensis. An exact history of all the writers and bishops who have had their education in the University of Oxford. To which are added, the Fasti or Annals, of the said University*, volume 3, London (1817) [1813–1820]: entry 550, pages 1052; and [Browne Willis], 'Willis (Thomas)'. In: [John Bernard, Thomas Birch, John Locke, and other hands] *A general dictionary, historical and critical*, volume X, London (1741): pages 171–5.

different from that containing the same Pieces, contained in his former translations of all his Works in fol.

Eugenius describes his purpose as providing a 'Portative Manual to direct [physicians] in Practice on all occasions'. Eugenius's defence against 'all Cavillations, which any Man shall pretend to make against [the] Work, as imperfect' is that he has limited himself to setting out the definitions and descriptions of diseases and symptoms, methods of curing, and every 'Recipe'. He promotes the 'cheapness and portableness' of the volume and avoidance of the Latin tongue with which some readers will be unfamiliar. He has 'omitted what [he] considered too Prolix' and sections that deal at excessive length with 'the Pathology of Diseases, and in the Ætiology of Symptoms'. And he has assisted readers by avoiding 'a deal of Theory, consisting of large Anatomical and Physiological Discourses, and the like, which though never so clearly delivered in England, cannot be comprehended under some years study'.

He does not deal with the five tracts in the order as originally published and doubts that Dr Willis would have written in this sequence, had he in mind a comprehensive and logical account of his work. Specifically, Eugenius argues that *Pharmaceutice rationalis* is a general work that introduces Willis's ideas on particular diseases. The tracts on convulsive diseases and scurvy serve as 'prævious and introductory' to his work on 'Diseases of the Brain and Genus Nervosum' and everything ends with his work on fevers. 'As for the Head Title prefix to [the] volume where it is call'd the London Practice of Physick', no one acquainted with Willis's work would disagree that most of the medicines were described in 'Consultations, practice and most rationally prescribed … here', even though some parts of the relevant works were written in Oxford.

The errors of pagination

The title pages show four different dates: 1685, 1689, 1692, and 1695 during which the typesetting of most sheets did not change. However, some leaves are found in one of two states that differ in their pagination. Because there is no perfect copy, nor a move towards systematic correction of errors, it follows that these are stop press alterations. It seems that the entire stock of printed material, in all states, was available across the 10 year period of publication and gathered erratically for binding. Apart from the change of date, setting of the title page was unaltered from 1685 to 1689 (**10A1–10A2**) but this changed in 1692 when *The London practice of physick* was issued with *A plain easie method for cure of the plague* (**10A3**). But still, an erratic mixture of the original printed sheets continued to be bound as individual copies. For example, the last issue (dated 1695: **10A4**) uses sheets from the first (1685: **10A1.c1**), retaining errors that were partly corrected in sheets used subsequently. With the proviso that these should be regarded as merely a sample of the likely permutations in circulation at one time, the items in this bibliography indicate that:

Copies with the title page dated 1685 (**10A1.c1–10A1.c3**) appear with some leaves in two different states. Each is paginated: 1–376, 367–486, 489–672 (ie 680 pages). Page 239 is always unnumbered and there are mispaginations of 347 for 257, and 263 for 363. Two have mispaginations at 420 for 520, 422 for 522, 423 for 523, 426 for 526, and 427 for 527 (**10A1.c1** and **10A1.c2**), of which one also has no page number at 224 (**10A1.c2**). In a third copy (**10A1.c3**), the errors up to page '520' (ie 420) are retained and page 224 is numbered. Thereafter the mispaginations are corrected but with new errors introduced: 421 for 521, 424 for 524, 425 for 525, and 428 for 528.

The sheets of **10A1.c3** are retained in some copies of the second issue with the title page dated 1689 (**10A2.c1**). In two others the pagination is corrected to 1–680 (**10A2.c2–10A2.c3**). In one, page 239 remains unnumbered as does 347 for 257, and 374 for 474. The individual errors between pages 520–528 are all corrected but the new page 677 is numbered 675 (**10A2.c2**). Another copy from 1689 has all these imperfections but also uses the unnumbered page 224 (**10A2.c3**).

When a new issue was published in 1692, bound with the 1691 edition of *A plain and easie method* (**10A3.c1**), the mispaginations in sheets for *The London practice of physick* reflect those found in **10A1.c3** and **10A2.c1**. Another copy (**10A3.c2**) has the sheets from 1689 (**10A2.c2**) with pages in sequence as 1–680 and retaining the individual mispaginations.

The 1695 issue (**10A4**) uses sheets from 1685 (**10A1.c1**) with all its many errors of pagination.

It follows that no copy of *The London practice of physick* has correct pagination. This bibliography therefore lists four separate issues: 1685 (three copies), 1689 (three copies), 1692 (two copies), and 1695 (one copy). Other combinations are certain to be found.

The advance notice for *The London practice of physick* (**10A1**) in the *Term Catalogue* listed the two booksellers who intended to issue this newly translated work:

Michaelmus 1684 November, IV numb 17, II 97, column 1/2, *Physick*. 2.

The *London* Practise of Physick, or The whole Practical part of Physick contained in the Works of Dr. Willis. Faithfully made English, and printed together for public good. Octavo. Printed for T. Basset at the George in *Fleet street*; and Will. Crook at the Green Dragon, without Temple Bar.

Consistent with the analysis that sheets with leaves in different states were distributed and randomly gathered over time, is a notice in the 1685 *Term Catalogue* for the issue, listing four London booksellers, which was not published until 1689 (**10A2**):

Easter 1685 May, IV numb 19, II 125, column 2, *Physick*. 2.

The *London* Practise of Physick or The whole Practical part of Physick contained in the Works of Dr. Willis. Faithfully made English; and printed together for public good. In Octavo. Printed for T. Basset, W. Crook, T. Dring, and C. Harper, in *Fleet street*.

A notice for the third issue (**10A3**) with the collective title page also listing *A plain and easie method* appeared in the *Term Catalogue* in the year before this was first published in 1692:

Michaelmas 1691 November, IV Numb 43, II 386, column 1, *Reprinted*. 6.

The *London* Practice of Physick; being the practical part of Physick, contained in the works of the famous Dr. Willis: wherein are his definitions, descriptions, and methods of curing diseases: with all his Receipts. To which is now added, his plain and easie method for the preventing and curing of the Plague. Published by Mr. J. Hemming, Amanuensis and Apothecary to the Doctor. Octavo. Sold by C. Harper at the Flower de luce in *Fleet street*; and W. Crook at the Green Dragon, without Temple Bar.

Only with the notice in the *Term Catalogue* for the final issue of *The London practice of physick* published with *A treatise on the plague* (**10A4**), designated a reprint of the 'second edition', and with the poem on a laurel leaf, do we learn that bound copies were priced at 7s:

> Easter 1695 May, IV Numb 57, II 552, column 2, *Reprinted*. 13.
>
> The *London* Practice of Physick, or The whole Practical part of Physick; Contained in the Works of the Learned Dr. Willis: faithfully Englished. The Second Edition. To which is added, A Treatise of the Plague, its nature and cure: also several receipts to prevent any contagious Distemper in City, Camp, or Fleet; and for curing such as are infected. Sold by R. Wellington at the Lute, and E. Castle at the Angel and Crown, in St. *Paul's* Churchyard. Price, bound, 7s. Where are likewise to be had his Works in one Volume. Folio.

Extracts on practical medicine and therapeutics

The other extract from the works of Thomas Willis, *Dr. Willis's receipts for the cure of all distempers* (1701: **10B**) was published in a single edition with no further issues (see: Figure 157). HJR Wing assumes the translator to be John Hemming. He had already drawn attention to

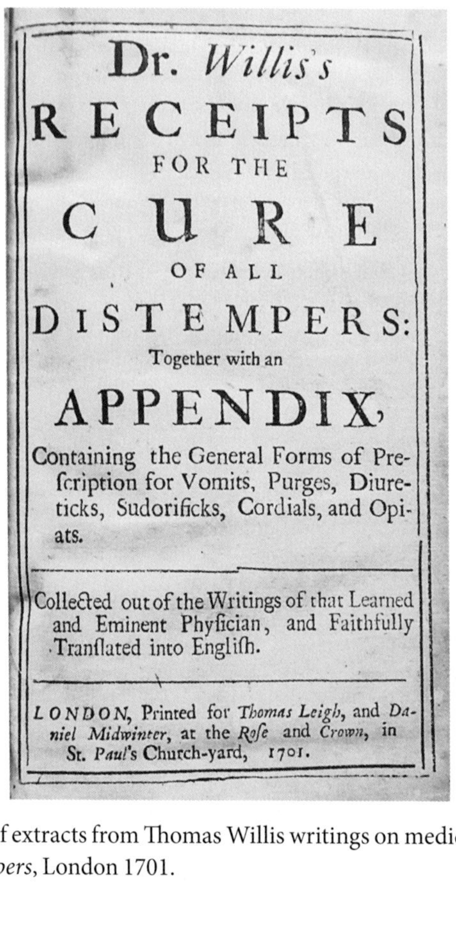

Dr. *Willis's*
RECEIPTS
FOR THE
CURE
OF ALL
DISTEMPERS:
Together with an
APPENDIX,
Containing the General Forms of Prefcription for Vomits, Purges, Diureticks, Sudorificks, Cordials, and Opiats.

Collected out of the Writings of that Learned and Eminent Phyfician, and Faithfully Tranflated into Englifh.

LONDON, Printed for *Thomas Leigh*, and *Daniel Midwinter*, at the *Rofe* and *Crown*, in St. *Paul's* Church-yard, 1701.

Figure 157 Title page of extracts from Thomas Willis writings on medicines, *Dr Willis's receipts for the cure of all distempers*, London 1701.

Willis's 'recipes' in the preface to *The London practice of physick*. The bibliography is straightforward. The book was noted in the *Term Catalogue*:

3. 16971709: Michaelmas 1701 November, V Numb 24, III 273, column 2, *Physick*. 5.

Dr. Willis's Receipts for the Cure of all Distempers; together with an Appendix containing the general Forms of Prescription for Vomits, Purges, Diureticks, Sudorificks, Cordials, and Opiats. Collected out of the Writings of that Learned and Eminent Physician; and faithfully translated into English. Twelves. Both [ie, with 4. A new and Rational Anatomy... By Daniel Tauny, a Member of the College of Physicians in Paris...] printed for D. Midwinter and T. Leigh at the Rose and Crown in St. Paul's Churchyard.

10A1.c1. THE LONDON PRACTICE OF PHYSICK, London octavo 1685

The first issue of the single edition, dated 1685, containing extracts from Willis's first, third, fifth, and sixth books, the tenth publication, using the first of two titles, with extensive pagination errors [HJR Wing 60].

Title page: [within a double rule] THE | *LONDON PRACTICE* | OF | PHYSICK: | Or the whole | Practical part of Phyfick | Contained in the Works of | D$^{r.}$ WILLIS. | [rule] | Faithfully made Englifh, and Printed | together for the Publick Good. | [rule] | *LONDON*, | Printed for *Thomas Baffet at* the *George* in *Fleet-* | *ftreet*, and *William Crooke*, at the *Green-Dragon* | without *Temple-Bar*. 1685.

Collation: octavo in 4s; 23 letter roman alphabet using I and V, Ii and Uu, Iii and Uuu, Iiii: π1; A–Z^4, Aa–Zz^4, Aaa–Zzz^4, Aaaa–Tttt^4; \$1–2 signed apart from: +B3, +B4.

353 leaves: paginated as [10], 1–376, 367–486, 489–672 (= 1–680), [16]. Mispagination: in addition to errors after 376; 239 unnumbered, 347 for 257, 263 for 363, '420' for '520', '422' for '522', '423' for '523', '426' for '526', '427' for '527'.

Type: 45 lines; height (20 lines) 67 millimetres, width 88 millimetres.

Contents: **π1r**, page [1], title; **π1v**, page [2], blank; **A1r–A4v**, pages [3–10], THE PREFACE.... [signed] Eugenius Φιλιατρος.

B1r–K3r, pages 1–69, [text] THE *LONDON PRACTICE* OF PHYSICK, Contained in the *Firft Part* of the Pharmaceutice Rationalis of Dr. *WILLIS*.; **K3v–Hh3r**, pages 70–237, [text] THE *LONDON PRACTICE* OF PHYSICK, Contained in the *Second Part* of the Pharmaceutice Rationalis of Dr. *WILLIS*.; **Hh3v–Tt3r**, pages 238–325, [text] THE *LONDON PRACTICE* OF PHYSICK, Contained in Dr. *WILLIS'S* Tract OF CONVULSIVE DISEASES.; **Tt3v–Ccc2r**, pages 326–'369', [text] The Practice of PHYSICK, Contained in Dr. *WILLIS's* TRACT OF THE SCURVY.; **Ccc2v–Xxx3v**, pages '370'–'518', [text], The *London* Practice OF PHYSICK, CONTAINED in *Dr.* Willis's *Tract of the Difeases that regard the Corporeal Soul, and its fubjects, viz. the Brain and* Genus nervofum.;

Xxx4r–Rrrr4v, pages '519'–'672', [text] THE PRACTISE OF PHYSICK, CONTAINED *In Dr.* Willis's *Tract* of Fevers.

Ssss1r–Tttt3v, pages [1–14] THE TABLE.; **Tttt4r–v**, pages [15–16], ERRATA, in 55 lines listing 139 errors; **Tttt4v**, page [16], *Books Printed for* T. Baſſet, *at the* George *in* Fleet-ſtreet, *and* W. Crook, *at the* Green Dragon *without* Temple-Bar.

Headlines and *Catchwords*: ⁏ for ⁚ after header at **F2r**, page 35; *Phthiſiek.* for *Phthiſick.* at **NN2v**, page 92; *Of the Dropſie of the Breſt.* for *On the Dropſie of the Breaſt.* at **T1r**, page 137; no ⁚ after header at **z1r**, page 169; **Dd1v**, page 202; **Ee2r**, page 211; **Ff3r**, page 221; *Perſous.* for *Perſons.* at **Ll3v**, page 262; *Frenſy.* for *Phrenſy.* at **Ooo1r–v**, pages '455'–'456'; *Melancholy.* for *Madneſs.* at **Rrr3v**, page '484'; *Intermittng* for *Intermitting* at **Yyy3v**, page '426'; *tertian* for *Tertian* at **Zzz4r**, page '535'; *Qartan* for *Quartan* at **Aaaa3r**, page '541'; *Putrid* for *putrid* at **Bbbb4v**, page '552'; *Meaſles.* for *Small Pox.* at **Llll3v**, page '622'.

Take for *The* at **I2r / v**, pages 59 / 60; ſick for Phyſick at **Z3r / v**, pages 173 / 174; mical for Cacochymical at **Bb2r / v**, pages 187 / 188; ous for dangerous at **Bb2v / Bb3r**, pages 188 / 189; celebrate for accelerate at **Bb3v / Bb4r**, pages 190 / 191; *A* for *An* at **Mm4v / Bn1r**, pages 272 / 273; the for Breaſt at **Oo4v / Pp1r**, pages 288 / 289; *off* for *of* at **Uu4v / Xx1r**, pages 336 / 337; These for Of at **Ttt3v / Ttt4r**, pages 502 / 503; cian for ſician at **Xxx2r / v**, pages 515 / 516.

Frontispiece: none.

Portrait: **Pt.1f1**: *R. W. ſculp. Thomas Willis M. D.* 173 × 110 millimetres (sheet); 162 × 107 (plate marks); 150 × 95 millimetres (image): see Figure 158.

Printers' ornaments: none.

No decorated initials.

Illustrations: none.

Copy: DASC (#1 of 2). Original full calf with lined border, spine (rebacked) with four raised bands, label WILLIS | PRACTICE | OF | PHYSICK, original endpapers. Leaves 183 × 115 millimetres, boards 189 × 119 × 50 millimetres.

10A1.c2. THE LONDON PRACTICE OF PHYSICK, London octavo 1685

The first issue of the single edition, dated 1685, containing extracts from Willis's first, third, fifth, and sixth books, the tenth publication, using the first of two titles, retaining all the original pagination errors and with one newly introduced [not distinguished from HJR Wing 60].

As in **10A1.c1** apart from:

Collation: Mispagination: 224 unnumbered, in addition to all errors in 10A1.c1.

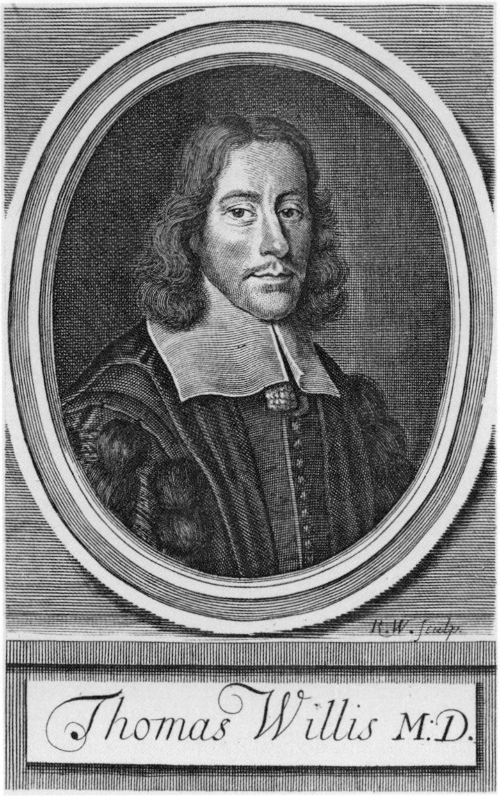

Figure 158 Portrait of Thomas Willis engraved by Robert White: *The London practice of physick*, London, 1685 (Pt.1f1).

Copy: DASC. Original full calf with lined and blind tooled border, spine (rebacked) with four raised bands, no lettering, original endpapers. Leaves 183 × 112 millimetres, boards 188 × 116 × 47 millimetres.

10A1.c3. THE LONDON PRACTICE OF PHYSICK, London octavo 1685

The first issue of the single edition, dated 1685, containing extracts from Willis's first, third, fifth, and sixth books, the tenth publication, using the first of two titles, with some pagination errors corrected and others newly introduced [not distinguished from HJR Wing 60].

As in **10A1.c1** apart from:

Collation: Mispagination: retaining all errors up to page '519'; then '421' for '521', '424' for '524', '425' for '525', '428' for '528' but correcting '422' for '522', '523' for '423', '526' for '426', '527' for '427'.

Copy: DASC. Original full calf with double-lined spine (rebacked) with four raised bands, labelled WILLIS | [short rule] | PHYSICK | 1685, original endpapers. Leaves 178 × 112 millimetres, boards 186 × 116 × 49 millimetres. Inserted bookplate: [1] Henry Hooper.; [2]

Gordon M. Jones M.D. Falmouth Virginia (unidentified). Inscribed: Henry Hooper (crossed out). Stamped: Amory Gale M.D.[4]

10A2.c1. THE LONDON PRACTICE OF PHYSICK, London octavo 1689

The second issue of the single edition, dated 1689, containing extracts from Willis's first, third, fifth, and sixth books, the tenth publication, using the first of two titles, retaining one combination of earlier pagination errors [not distinguished from HJR Wing 61].

Title page: [within a double rule] THE | *LONDON PRACTICE* | OF | PHYSICK: | Or the whole | Practical part of Phyfick | Contained in the Works of | D^r. WILLIS. | [rule] | Faithfully made Englifh, and Printed | together for the Publick Good. | [rule] | *LONDON*, | Printed for *T. Baffet*, *T. Dring*, *C. Harper*, | *W. Crooke*, and *S. Leigh*, at their Shops in | *Fleet-ftreet*, and without *Temple-Bar*. 1689.

Then as in **10A1.c3**.

Copy: DASC. Twentieth century full calf, spine with four raised bands and single line at head and foot, labelled LONDON | PRACTICE | OF PHYSICK / THOMAS WILLIS | 1689, original front free endpaper bound in. Leaves, 177 × 112 millimetres, boards 192 × 118 × 48 millimetres. Bookplate: Birmingham Medical Institute, presented by Dr C Hackall (?).[5]

10A2.c2. THE LONDON PRACTICE OF PHYSICK, London octavo 1689

The second issue of the single edition, dated 1689, containing extracts from Willis's first, third, fifth, and sixth books, the tenth publication, using the first of two titles, with extensive revision of the pagination errors, some errors retained and one newly introduced [HJR Wing 61].

As in **10A1** apart from:

Collation: 353 leaves: paginated as [10], 1–680, [16]. Mispagination: page 239 unnumbered, 347 for 257, 263 for 363, 374 for 474, 677 for 675.

Copy: Wellcome (20189869). Original calf, rebacked in morocco, four raised bands, lettered LONDON | PRACTICE | OF PHYSICK | WILLIS | 1689, new endpapers. Leaves 185 × 113 millimetres, boards 190 × 112 × 42 millimetres.

[4] This volume seems to have been in the USA from early in the eighteenth century. Of the three previous owners, one may be Dr Henry Hooper (1685–1757) mentioned as a witness for the Arnold family in Elaine Forman Crane, *The Poison Plot: A Tale of Adultery and Murder in Colonial Newport*, Ithaca and London (2018); and an Amory Gale (1800–1872) who practised medicine in Massachusetts but was ordained for the Unitarian Ministry in 1844, preaching for several years before resuming the practice of medicine.

[5] See chapter 9, footnote to **5A1** for details of the Birmingham Medical Institute. Dr C Hackall (?) is unidentified.

10A2.c3. THE LONDON PRACTICE OF PHYSICK, London octavo 1689

The second issue of the single edition, dated 1689, containing extracts from Willis's first, third, fifth, and sixth books, the tenth publication, using the first of two titles, with extensive revision of the pagination errors, some errors retained and one other newly introduced [HJR Wing 61].

As in **10A2.c2** apart from:

Collation: Mispagination: 224 unnumbered, in addition to errors at page 239 unnumbered, 347 for 257, 263 for 363, 374 for 474, 677 for 675.

Copy: Wellcome (20189869), lacking portrait, π1 and A1. Later half vellum with crude cloth repair to spine, lettered WILLIS | 1666 {erased} 1689, new endpapers. Leaves 174 × 107 millimetres, boards 181 × 108 × 45 millimetres. Inscribed: Wm Williams (unidentified).

10A3.c1. THE LONDON PRACTICE OF PHYSICK *with* A PLAIN AND EASIE METHOD FOR PRESERVING THOSE THAT ARE WELL FROM THE PLAGUE, London octavo 1692 [1691]

The third issue of the single edition, dated 1692, containing extracts from Willis's first, third, fifth, and sixth books, the tenth publication, using the second of two titles, retaining one combination of earlier pagination errors, with the third issue of *A plain and easie method* [HJR Wing 62; and see also 7A3].

Title page: [1]. [within a double rule] The LONDON | Practife of Phyfick, | BEING THE | PRACTICAL PART | OF | PHYSICK | Contain'd in the | VVORKS | Of the FAMOUS | D^r. WILLIS; | Wherein are | His Definitions, Defcriptions, and Methods | Of Curing Difeafes, with all his RECEIPTS. | To which is now added | His plain and eafie METHOD for the Preventing | and Curing of the Plague, Publifhed by Mr. *Flemings*, Amanu- | enfis and Apothecary to the Doctor. | [rule] | *With the allowance of the College of* PHYSICIANS. | [rule] | *LONDON*: | Printed for *T. Baffett*, *T. Dring*, *C. Harper*, and *W. Crook*, and are | to be fold at the *Flower-de-Luce* in *Fleet-ftreet*, and at the | *Green-Dragon* without *Temple-Bar*. MDCXCII. | Dr. WILLIS's whole Works in *Fol.* With Forty Copper Plates are alfo to | be Sold at the Places above-mentioned.

[2]. [within a double rule] A | Plain and Eafie Method | FOR | Preserving [by God's Bleffing] | thofe that are WELL from the | Infection of the | PLAGUE, | OR | Any Contagious Diftemper in City, | Camp, Fleet, &c. | AND | For Curing fuch as are Infected | with it. | [rule] | Written in the Year 1666. | [rule] | By *Tho. Willis*, M.D. late Sidney Profef- | for in *Oxford*, and a Member of the | Royal Society and College of Phy- | ficians in *London*. | [rule] | With a Poem on the virtue of a Laurel | Leaf for curing of a Rheumatifm. | By *W. B.* | [rule] | Never before Printed. | [rule] | *LONDON*, Printed for *W. Crook*, at the *Green-* | *Dragon*, without *Temple-Bar*. 1691.

[1]. As in **10A1.c3**.

[2]. as in **7A3**.

Copy: DASC: this is the same book described as **7A3** (see chapter 11).

10A3.c2. THE LONDON PRACTICE OF PHYSICK; *with* A PLAIN AND EASIE METHOD FOR PRESERVING THOSE THAT ARE WELL FROM THE PLAGUE, London octavo 1692 [1691]

The third issue of the single edition, dated 1692, containing extracts from Willis's first, third, fifth, and sixth books, the tenth publication, using the second of two titles, retaining another combination of earlier pagination errors, with the third issue of *A plain and easie method* [not distinguished from HJR Wing 62; and see also 7A3].

Title page: [1]. and [2]., as in **10A3.c1**.

Then [1]. As in **10A2.c2**.

[2]. As in **7A3**.

Copy: Bodleian [Vet. A3 e.77 (1)]. Original calf with double-lined border, spine with five raised bands and double line at head and foot, lacking front and part of rear free endpapers. Leaves 180 × 112 millimetres, boards 185 × 117 × 50 millimetres. Inscribed: (1) Lett Pigott (unidentified); (2) John Williams Surgeon Corwen Gift of Mrs Lloyd Colomendy Corwen Decr 16th 1848 (×2, in part). Stamped: (1) Radcliffe Infirmary Oxford University Museum 17 OCT 1904 (×2); (2) Bodleian Library 22 JUN 1938.[6]

10A4. THE LONDON PRACTICE OF PHYSICK; *with* A PLAIN AND EASIE METHOD FOR PRESERVING THOSE THAT ARE WELL FROM THE PLAGUE. London octavo 1695

The fourth issue of the single edition, dated 1695, containing extracts from Willis's first, third, fifth, and sixth books, the tenth publication, using the second of two titles, retaining a combination of earlier pagination errors, correction of one headline, with *A plain and easie method* and the poem on a laurel leaf (**7A2**) [HJR Wing 63].

[6] John Williams (1801–1859) was a naturalist and physician born in the Conwy valley at Llansanffraid, north Wales. He was educated at Liverpool and apprenticed to his elder brother William, a physician and apothecary at Abergele. He studied at the Royal College of Surgeons in Dublin and practised as a physician at Corwen and Wrexham in Wales. He moved to California in 1849 during the gold rush, where he intended to combine work as a physician with gold prospecting, but he was robbed and suffered ill health, returning to Wrexham in 1853. He wrote *Faunula Grustensis: being an outline of the natural contents of the parish of Llanrwst*, Llanrwst (1830). His name appears in several books written in Welsh and published at Nantglyn and Bala, North Wales.

Title page: [1]. [within a double rule] THE | *LONDON PRACTICE* | OF | PHYSICK: | Or the whole | Practical Part of Phyſick | Contained in the Works of the Learned | Dr. WILLIS, | *Faithfully Engliſhed.* | [rule] | The Second Edition. | [rule] | To which is added a Treatiſe of the Plague, its Na- | ture and Cure: Alſo ſeveral Receipts to prevent | any Contagious Diſtemper in City, Camp, or | Fleet, and for Curing ſuch as are infected with it. | [rule] | *LONDON*, | Printed and are to be Sold by *Richard Wellington*, at | the ſign of the *Lute*, and *Edward Caſtle*, at the *Angel* | and *Crown* in St. *Paul's* Church-Yard. 1695. | *Price Bound Seven Shillings.* | [outside inner lower rule] Where are likewiſe to be had his Works in one Volume in Folio.

[2]. [within a double rule] A | Plain and Eaſie Method | FOR | Preserving [by **God's Bleſſing**] | thoſe that are WELL from the | Infection of the | PLAGUE, | Or | Any Contagious Diſtemper in City, | Camp, Fleet, &c. | AND | For Curing ſuch as are Infected | with it. | [rule] | Written in the Year 1666. | [rule] | By *Tho. Willis*, M. D. late Sidney Profeſ- | ſor in *Oxford*, and a Member of the | Royal Society and College of Phy- | ſicians in *London.* | [rule] | With a Poem on the virtue of a Laurel | Leaf for curing of a Rheumatiſm. | By *W. B.* | [rule] | Never before Printed. | [rule] | *LONDON*, Printed for *W. Crook*, at the *Green-* | *Dragon*, without *Temple-Bar*. 1691.

[3]. A | POEM | UPON A | Laurel-Leaf. | [rule] | Viris admodum Colendis, | PUBLICÆ SCHOLÆ, | Vulgò dictæ, | *Harrow ſuper Montem*, | GUBERNATORIBUS, | *VIZ.* | Dn° *CAROLO GERARD* Baronetto. | Dn° *EDVARDO WALDO* Militi. | *CHEEK GERARD*, | *DANIELO WALDO*, | *GULIELMO FEN*, | *EDWARDO WALDO*, | [the last four names bracketed] Armigeris. | Hoc qualecunque Poema, *Gulielmus Bolton* M.A. | & ejuſdem Scholæ Archi-didaſcalus, humil- | limè dedicat.

Then [1]., as in **10A1.c1** apart from:

Headlines: *Itch.* corrected to *running Scab.* at **Ff3r**, page 221.

[2]. and [3]., as in **7A2**.

Copy: Royal Society of Medicine; this is the same book described as **7A4** (see chapter 11).

10B. DR WILLIS'S RECEIPTS FOR THE CURE OF ALL DISTEMPERS, London duodecimo 1701

The only issue containing extracts from Willis's first, third, fifth, and second part of his sixth book, the tenth publication listing Willis's various medicines and therapies, published posthumously [HJR Wing 64].

Title page: [within a double rule] Dr. *Willis's* | RECEIPTS | FOR THE | CURE | OF ALL | DISTEMPERS: | Together with an | APPENDIX, | Containing the General Forms of Pre- | ſcription for Vomits, Purges, Diure- | ticks, Sudorificks, Cordials, and Opi- | ats. | [rule] | Collected out of the Writings of that Learned | and Eminent Phyſician, and Faithfully | Tranſlated into Engliſh. | [rule] | *LONDON*, Printed for *Thomas Leigh*, and *Da-* | *niel Midwinter*, at the *Roſe* and *Crown*, in | St. *Paul's* Church-yard, 1701.

Collation: duodecimo in 6s; 23 letter roman alphabet using I and U: A^4, B–U^6; \$1–3, signed apart from: -F3, -G3, -H3.

118 leaves: paginated as [8], 1–226, [2]. Mispaginated: 102 for 120, 145 for 144.

Type: 35 lines; height (20 lines) 71 millimetres, width 71 millimetres.

Contents: **A1r**, page [1], title; **A1v**, page [2], blank; **A2r–A3v**, pages [3–6], THE TRANSLATORS'S PREFACE.; **A4r–v**, pages [7–8], THE CONTENTS.

B1r–S3v, pages 1–198, [text] Dr. *WILLIS*'s RECEIPTS; **S4r–U5v**, pages 199–226, AN APPENDIX, containing the General Forms OF PRESCRIPTION FOR *Vomits, Purges, Diureticks, Sudoriticks, Cordials, and Opiats*; **U6r–v**, pages [1–2] *Books printed for, and Sold by* Thomas Leigh, *and* Daniel Midwinter, *at the* Rofe *and* Crown *in St.* Paul*'s* Churchyard, 1701.

Headlines and *Catchwords*: Sect. 24 for Sect. 34 at **Q3v**, page 174; Sect. 35 for Sect. 40 at **S1r**, page 193; **S2r**, page 195; Se3ct. 5 for Sect. 40 at **S1v**, page 194; Sect. 36 for Sect.41 at **S2v–S3v**, pages 196–7; Sect. 37 for Sect. 41 at **S3v**, page 198.

No catchword at **A4r** / **v**, pages [7] / [8]; **Q3r** / **v**, pages 173 / 174.

Frontispiece: none.

Portrait: none.

Printers' ornament: none.

No decorated initials.

Illustrations: none.

Copy: DASC (#1 of 2). Original sprinkled calf with blind stamped lines and borders, spine (restored) with five double rules, no lettering or label, original endpapers (no front or back pastedowns). Leaves 157 × 93 millimetres, boards 164 × 92 × 10 millimetres. Inscribed: (1) Sum E Libris Thomas Lilley (?) J^ary^ 19th 1702; (2) Wm Landys 1760; (3) Mr PA Saunders 4 Sarratt Vale Sarratt Rickmansworth Herts (all unidentified).

15

'The hearths and altars for the vital fire'

Medical chemistry and disease

***De fermentatione*; *De febribus*; *De urinis* (1659); *De scorbuto* (1667); *De sanguinis accensione* (1670).**

The principle of fermentation in the blood as the basis for how living systems work underlies all Thomas Willis's writings on the human body in health and disease. Fermentation was the subject on which he first wrote. The later treatises and Willis's many therapeutic recommendations make little sense without first considering his views on this fundamental process.[1] And yet the concept is seemingly so alien to the subsequent evolution of ideas on physiology and pathology that many commentators have dismissed his ideas as wild and speculative. Allowing for Willis's ready use of metaphor, and with only a rudimentary knowledge of biochemistry and molecular biology, his work can now easily be seen as coherent and revealing insights that earlier critics had denied this influential and stalwart advocate of iatrochemistry.[2]

When, in 1659, at the age of 38, Thomas Willis published his first three treatises it was against the background of having been taught as an undergraduate about earth, water, fire and air; and perturbation of the humours—blood, yellow bile, black bile, and phlegm—in disease. But with a fertile mind, and advantaged through being part of communities ripe for acquiring empirical knowledge, no longer shackled by the ancient doctrines, Willis was ready to think in novel ways about health and disease.[3]

Those working in the second half of the seventeenth century who committed to a better understanding of vitality needed to understand one main issue: where and in what way was the material substrate of animal life generated and sustained? By the end of their productive

[1] The narrative that follows leans heavily on a few main sources. Most prominent are the readings and analyses of Robert Frank as set out in *Harvey and the Oxford physiologists*, Berkeley (1980); and Robert G Frank, 'Thomas Willis and his circle: brain and mind in seventeenth century medicine'. In: Ed. GS Rousseau, *The languages of psyche. Mind and body in Enlightenment thought.* Clark Library lectures 1985–1986, Berkeley (1990): pages 107–46. The careful analyses of Hansruedi Isler, *Thomas Willis 1621–1675. Doctor and scientist*, London (1968) have also been used. The publications and unpublished manuscripts of Raymond Hierons (1921–2001) have provided many facts and insights that would otherwise have escaped attention. James Partington gives a concise summary of Willis's ideas on iatrochemistry in *A history of chemistry*, volume 2, London (1961): pages 304–10.

[2] See: Rebecca O'Neal, 'A love of "words as words": metaphor, analogy and the brain in the work of Thomas Willis (1621–1675)', PhD thesis, Queen Mary, University of London (2017) for a scholarly account of the clever use of language in conveying Willis's ideas on structure and function of the nervous system.

[3] It requires very little transference to see in Willis's writings the concepts of metabolism, biochemistry, and molecular and systems biology. However, it is a mistake retrospectively to transfer current ideas on science and medicine to the social and scientific climate of a different age in which knowledge was being gathered. Avoiding too much flow between the present and the past applies especially to the tendency for physicians who write history to hold retrospective diagnostic clinics and impose modern nosology on ancient accounts of disease.

lives, these scientists and physicians had resolved that a component of air interacts with dark venous blood in the capillaries of the lungs, thereby changing its colour and chemical composition; returned to the heart, the enriched blood circulates throughout the body where nutrients are extracted allowing the recipient structures to function; waste is removed and the darkened venous blood recirculates to the lungs where it is reenriched. Whilst others thought through the issue of respiration, Willis concentrated on understanding the change in blood that sustains life and which, when perturbed, is the generic mechanism of disease.

These physicians and scientists had begun with notions, loyal to Galen (AD 130–210), that were far removed from this formulation. They devised experiments using living animals to advance knowledge. Human disease was observed. And with speculation, reflection, and discussion, the emerging ideas were systematically honed. Encouraged and sustained by the intellectual environment in which they worked, this community of minds discussed and wrote periodically about their discoveries in books that served as repositories of ideas on natural philosophy rather than practical manuals rehearsing antiquated doctrines. Mostly written in Latin, the texts were aimed at the learned more than the general reader.[4] As they sought to articulate the new knowledge, these books were often shrouded in language that obscured the insights they gained, and the notions with which they grappled being misunderstood and dismissed. But by the time they were done, although knowing nothing of oxygen or haemoglobin and cell biology, the basics of how nutrition and respiration support life and deliver the substrate that keeps tissues healthy had been set down.

Natural philosophy and iatrochemistry

Physicians active in the 1640s had the option of remaining faithful to Galenic and Hippocratic teachings, or basing their medicine on the anatomical and physiological discoveries of Andreas Vesalius (1514–1564) and William Harvey (1578–1657), and the chemical doctrines of Paracelsus (born Theophrastus von Hohenheim: 1493–1541) and Jan Baptist van Helmont (1580–1644).[5] For Paracelsus, 'he who wishes to explore nature must tread her books with his feet'. Helmont and, in Willis's own time Franciscus Sylvius (born Franz de le Boë: 1614–1672), promoted 'palpable and visible evidence' in favour of the 'heathenish philosophy of Aristotle and Galen'. Paracelsus declared himself 'an iatrochemist: since I know both medicine and chemistry'. His school relied more on alchemy and chemical remedies than the botanical preparations used in Galenic medicine. The apothecaries and physicians who adopted the Paracelsian doctrine were described as 'chymists', 'spagyrists', or 'iatrochemists'. Later, as other people came to prominence, advocates of medical chemistry were dubbed 'Helmontians' or 'Willisians'.[6] The old and new ideas were contested. Battle lines

[4] See: John Fulton (1899–1960), *A bibliography of two Oxford physiologists: Richard Lower 1631–1691, John Mayow 1643–1679*, Oxford (1935): page 11 citing Kenneth Franklin (1897–1966) on the point that these authors thought in English but wrote in Latin since this sometimes provided a more eloquent means of expression.

[5] See: Antonio Clericuzio, 'From van Helmont to Boyle. A study of the transmission of Helmontian chemical and medical theories in seventeenth-century England', *The British Journal for the History of Science* 1993; 26: 303–34 for details of van Helmont's influence on iatrochemists in England, especially Robert Boyle, but without assigning particular significance to the contributions of Thomas Willis; and Antonio Clericuzio, *Elements, principles and corpuscles. A study of atomism and chemistry in the seventeenth century*, Dordrecht (2000): pages 75–101 for discussion of chemistry and atomism in England (1600–1660), and the work of Thomas Willis on corpuscular theory, at page 100.

[6] See: Isler (1968): pages 7–8 who makes the point that, as a student, Willis would have known and used the *Pharmacopoeia Londinensis*, London (1618) in which chemical remedies were promoted.

were drawn up between traditionalists within the Royal College of Physicians and these iatrochemists, to the extent that a splinter group of the latter formed a Society of Chymical Physitians. The exchanges were abusive. The Galenists dismissed the iatrochemists as a 'rabble of coal-burners ... whose mistress was chance'. The iatrochemists countered that the Galenists were driven by 'idleness and superstitious devotion to ... old heathenish Authors'. Henry Stubbe (1632–1676) argued that—with men like Willis and Richard Lower (1631–1691) promoting iatrochemistry and, in Robert Boyle's (1627–1691) case, iatromechanics—it was the unwelcome influence of the Royal Society that had promoted the 'Anti-Colledge of Pseudo-Chymists, encouraging Odowde and his ignorant Adherents in opposition to the Physicians'.[7] Thomas Willis seemed to please neither fraternity, being aligned with iatrochemistry, yet criticised by George Thomson (1619—1676), one of the founders of the Chemical Society, as being too accommodating in failing completely to discard humoral pathology and marooning himself as a 'Galeno-Chymist'.[8]

Willis summarized his incentive to study medicine by direct observation, and acknowledged the crucial importance of Harvey, in the preface to *De febribus* (1659). He pointed out that learned men had improved upon the false position of the ancients, especially with respect to the motion of the blood:[9]

> *For in truth, in the Medical Art, (and that deservedly) those things have not pleased the Men of our Age ... our most famous Harvy ... not only in removing the Rubbish of the former Building, but for the supplying this plentifully with Stone, Planks and other Matter.*

But any reading of his treatises makes clear that Willis was not able altogether to discard the ancient doctrines. His interplay of the four humours with activity of the five particles that were fundamental to his own thinking allowed confusion, and invited criticism that his ideas were muddled. Willis was clear that Hippocrates was to be admired. The problem lay with those who subsequently concocted 'almost out of their own Brain a deceitful pile of Speculative Science ... and unstable Doctrine'.

At least during the 1650s, Thomas Willis observed patients and studied chemistry but, unlike others, he was at that time rarely involved with human or animal experimentation. Rather, as he sets out in the preface to *De fermentatione*, his ideas were derived from reactions he had directly observed in chemical experiments that he himself had performed. However he did not intend to be unduly constrained by empirical observations and preferred to allow his imagination some freedom of manoeuvre:[10]

> No Man can blame me, if I should not here describe all things according to Rule, and Analytick Patterns; because in this Work, it chances me to wander without a Guide, or

[7] See: Henry Thomas, 'The Society of Chemycial Physitians. An echo of the great plague of London, 1665'. In: Ed. E Ashworth Underwood, *Science, medicine and history. Essays on the evolution of scientific thought written in honour of Charles Singer*, volume 2, Oxford (1953): pages 56–71 for a spirited account of this initiative and the role of Thomas O'Dowde (d.1665).

[8] See: Ed. Kenneth Dewhurst, *Richard Lower's Vindicatio. A defence of the experimental method*, Oxford (1983): page xv.

[9] See: Thomas Willis, *Of feavers* (1684): page 45.

[10] Most readers study the seventeenth-century translations of Thomas Willis works in English, but Frank (1980) emphasizes that caution must be used when using Samuel Pordage's texts which contain intercalated sentences or paragraphs and whole sections not present in the original editions. In the account that follows, the versions of Pordage's translations from 1684 have been used. The many brief quotes from *Dr Willis's practice of physick* (1684: **9F**) as printed are placed in '...', but not all are specifically cited.

> Companion, in solitary places, and as it were in a solitude trodden by no footsteps, where I make not only a Journey, but my way also: therefore, whenever I deviate, I cannot be said to err, among right Judges of our endeavours, who have no Path in which I should Walk, nor could find a Track, which I might fear to miss.

Willis was held in affection and remained close to the community that was providing critical new insights in natural philosophy. Many of these scientists and physicians had listened to his lectures and they deferred to a physician who was rooted in chemistry, prepared to change his mind, and nurtured their own careers.[11]

Willis's treatises list writers who failed to satisfy him, including not only the ancients but also many contemporaries, and the few that he admired.[12] He agreed that 'the sick should be the doctor's books', but he had to tread carefully. Publication was risky with restrictions imposed by religious doctrine and press censorship.[13] Whilst the danger of being burned at the stake for heresy may have passed, the Church applied censorship and, since introduction of the *Index librorum* (1559), controlled what came off the press.

Willis's opinions relating to medical chemistry are first described in the three treatises included in *Diatribæ duæ medico-philosophicæ* (1659), with further references in *Cerebri anatome* (1664), *Pathologiæ cerebri* and *De scorbuto* (1667), and as a last summary in *De sanguinis accensione* (1670).[14] That he shifted his position across this period merely reflects the rapid rate of change occurring around Willis, and his preparedness to rethink matters in the light of what was being learned. As an independent observer, Philip Fell (*c.*1632–1682) encapsulated the transition that Willis witnessed, and the stage that his ideas had reached by the late 1650s. Philip was a son of Samuel Fell (1584–1649), dean of Christ Church, younger brother of John Fell (1625–1686), and therefore also brother-in-law to Thomas Willis. Anthony Wood (1632–1695) wrote that 'no sufferer for the King's cause', Philip was 'turn'd out of Trinity College abruptly', where he had matriculated on 23 Aug 1660, without taking his degree but was subsequently made Master of Arts and Fellow of All Souls College, Oxford, from 31 Oct 1667, at the instigation of his older brother, vice-chancellor of the University. Later Philip moved to Eton College. Philip Fell died aged 49, in the house of Dr George Benson (1613–1692), canon of Hereford, who had married Philip's sister. He was buried in that cathedral.[15] It is significant that Wood describes him as an excellent Latin poet

[11] Others were less tolerant. See Frank (1980): page 179 and endnote 118 to chapter 7 for an account of scholars such as Samuel Sorbière (1615–1670) and Balthasar de Monconys (1611–1665) who came to Oxford during their grand tour. Sorbière could not understand Willis's Latin pronunciation, in return for which rebuke Willis declared Sorbière a 'poseur' who knew little of medicine and chemistry and flaunted 'the great names of DesCartes and Mersennas'.

[12] See chapter 2 for a summary of his favoured sources.

[13] For example, after 1669 all of Marcello Malpighi's (1628–1694) works were published and exported by the Royal Society of London through the initiative of Henry Oldenburg (1619–1677) and Robert Hooke (1635–1703). The Italian microscopist was nurtured in the interests of promoting science with the aim of 'bringing out the opinion of all the learned'. In the same spirit, the Royal Society launched the *Philosophical Transactions* in March 1665 such that the Fellows and other readers could 'wander freely within nature's realm' even though they were best advised to avoid politics and religion in their intellectual excursions.

[14] Willis's printers could never quite decide how best to name this treatise. Originally entitled *De sanguinis accensione*, it was also variously referred to as: *Exercitationis de accensione sanguinis*; *De sanguinis incalescentia*; *or De sanguinis incalescentia, sive accensione*.

[15] See: Anthony Wood, *Athenæ Oxoniensis*, 3rd edition, volume IV, part 2, London and Oxford (1820): pages 229–30; and Thomas Harwood, *Alumni Etonenses*, London, Cambridge, and Eton (1797): page 78. Philip Fell is described as being 'of Eaton Colledg' in Willis's will. Fell was a Fellow of Eton College from 24 June 1670 to 26 February 1682/3 where his letter of appointment is held (ECR 60 05 01 11). It seems that he was much in demand as an executor of wills. Fell attended the provost of Eton, Richard Allestree (1619–1681), in his last illness and Allestry bequeathed 'his Scrutore [writing desk] in his chamber at Eton to his dear friend Mr. Philip Fell, fellow of Eton, and his little regulator watch... [and] Mr. Philip Fell to see his burial. Dated June 23, 1680; proved Aug. 1681.

'as his copies of verses in several books occasionally published in the name of the university, and in others, do manifestly show'. This skill is apparent from his verse 'ON THE AUTHORS Medical-Philosophical Discourses' printed in the preliminaries to *Diatribæ duæ* (1659):

Carmen gratulatorium

ABſtruſas rerum cauſas quo ſemine litem,
Quo pacem natura paret, quis corpora motus
Urgeat, indomitos undis quid miſceat ignes,
Qui nexus elementa ligent, felicior ætas
Conſpexit tandem; cunctiſque ignota priorum
Abdita laxantur vaſti penetralia mundi.
 Progenies cœli, terræ defoſſa metalla
Viſeribus, quamvis Phœbo oſtentata parenti
Indiga lucis erant; radios obſcura premebat
Umbra, & lucenti ſplendor quæſitus in auro eſt.
Lumina præſtrinxit ferrum, ignotumque latebat
E damnis notum nimis; & ſimul agmina fudit
Ingeniumque una victor ſuperaverat enſis.
Sic olim curas, vanæque indaginis artes
Eluſit natura parens; ſic limine juſſit
Siſtere, & extremo defigere cortice lumen.
At nobis tentare adyta, atque inviſere rerum
Ultima conceſſit, mundique arcana tueri:
Nec nota eſt magis ipſa ſibi, quis montibus altis
Regnet amor, quæ flamma leves in Marmora ſuccos
Exquoquit, unde novi tellus rudimenta metalli[16]
Fæcundo fovet amplexu: cur vere tepenti
Pandit opes terra, & nativo fulgurat oſtro.
Qui Zephyri molles prægnanti ſemina Veſtæ
Inſpirent: nebularum arcu cælique relictis
Sedibus, in noſtris Iris quæ geſtiat undis.
Cur fluviis immerſa Ceres, comixtaque Nymphis
Intumeat: quæ bella movet, quas concitat iras
Fervidus, inque cadis celebraverit Orgia Bacchus.
Siciniæ quis deſertis fornacibus Ætnæ
Vulcanus, molles per corpora ſuſcitat ignes.
Quin etiam humanos agitet quis ſpiritus artus.
Unde hinc purpureus venas, hinc lacteus imber

[P.C.C., North, 115.]': see *Etoniana* 30 July 1935: page 140. Fell wrote to Dr Craddock (nd) in February 1681 when both were Fellows despairing at the state of the College register described by Fell as 'ill kept ... so short, and broken in time, so blotted ... and razed etc.', see: [Anon] *The appeal of King's College against the Fellows of Eton*, Cambridge (1817): page 27. Fell is considered to be the author of *Lex talionis: or the author of naked truth stript naked*, London (1676); see: the entry for Andrew Marvell (1621–1678), in: *Biographia Britannica*. Ed. Andrew Kippis with the assistance of Joseph Towers, volume V, London (1760): page 3056; and the entry for Herbert Croft (1603–1691) in volume 3 (1750): page 1529.

[16] In the second and later editions, two lines are amended and the verse reads: Ex quoquit, unde novi tellus connixa metalli / Cœca rudimenta, & duri primordia fœtus / Fæcundo fovet amplexu, etc.

Irrigat; in fontes quæ caufa recedere juffit
Sanguinis afsiduo remeantia flumina motu.
Qui cæci in venis ignes, quæ vifcere flamma
Deliteat, febremque ciet: quid mifceat æftu
Frigora, diverfæ cœant quo fœdere Zonæ.
Quæ Peftem Stygio furiarum emittit hiatu,
Graffarique jubet, ventofque armare veneno.
Quis fit fatidicus renes qui perluit humor
Qualis odor matulæ, quem nec faftidiit olim
Balfama cui victæ pelvis fpiravit Idumes.
Cuncta patent: nec cui furtivos impius ignes
Intulit, artifici melius fua cognita proles.
Artis circuimus mundum, indignataque Gades
Tranfiit extremos, veteremque fcientia Thulen.
Felix qui potuit rerum cognofcere caufas!
Naturæ Phœboque facer! Cui Delphica laurus
Amplecti frontem, radiataque tempora geftit
Flammæ illi parcent quem facris artibus Hermes
Imbuit, & doctos tenebris qui vindicat ignes.
Illum nulla dies rapiet, qui lumina Phœbi
Donavit radiis, lucifque fugaverat umbras.
Non illum afflato Peftis violare veneno
Audeat, aut tacita Febris torrere favilla,
Qui morbis vitam, & letho donaverit ævum.

Philippus Fell.
Med. Stud. Oxon.

This verse was translated by Samuel Pordage (1633–1691) for the first edition in English of *A medical-philosophical discourse* (1681):

ON THE AUTHORS Medical-Philofophical Difcourfes.

THE intricate and hidden caufe of things,
Both Peace and Strife by what means Nature brings,
What various motions Bodies do infpire;
What mixes with the Waters quenchlefs Fire?
What Bonds the Elements together tye,
Before this happier Age unfolded lye:
Things hid to former Ages, and unknown,
The Secrets of the world to all are fhown.
Metals dug from the Bowels of the Earth,
Tho they from Phoebus boaft their Heavenly birth,
We without light, dark and obfcure behold,
And Splendor's found only in burnifht Gold.
Iron unknown lay hidden without light,
By Slaves wrought from the Mine grows dazeling bright.
This to whole Troops confufion doth afford,
Wit, which firft fram'd, ftoops to, the Victor Sword.
We thus of old did Nature fearch in vain,

Our arts did only ith' outward bark remain,
But now we her hid myſteries unfold,
And the great ſecrets of the world behold.
Better than us, herſelf can hardly tell,
What Love doth far within high Mountains dwell.
What flame firſt gives the Marble Quarry birth;
To Metals forms blind Rudiments of Earth,
And the hard child doth to perfection bring:
Why Earth ſhows her rich Treaſures in the Spring;
And ſhines, made brave with her own Native flowers.
What gentle gales, and what ſweet moiſtening ſhowers,
Do on the pregnant Goddeſs Seed beſstow;
Whilſt Heavenly Iris *mounts the Cloudy Bow.*
Why Ceres *ſwells with watery Nymphs embrace,*
What Strife, what Wars ſpring from hot Bacchus *race:*
What Vulcan *doth th' Ætnean Fornace blow;*
What doth ſoft fires thorow all Bodies throw.
What Spirit nimbly moves the human frame:
Whence Milky juice here, there a Purple ſtream,
Watering the Body: when the Crimson flood;
And the quick Circulation of the blood.
What hidden fires in veins and intrals burn,
Which do the boyling Blood to Feavers turn.
What mixes freezing cold with parching heat,
And makes the different Zones together meet.
Whence comes the Peſtilence with Stygian breath,
Riding on blaſting Winds, and arm'd with death.
What Propheſying Humour through the Reins doth paſs,
What colour, and what odor in the Glaſs?
All things lie open now: He did not know
So much, to whom Prometheus did beſtow
His ſtollen fires: We now every part
Of the whole Earth compaſs about with art.
He's happy who Cauſes of things can ſhew;
Sacred to Nature and to Phoebus *too;*
About his Temples Delphic *Laurels ſpread,*
And flames of lightning ne'r ſhall blaſt his head.
Whom Hermes *doth with Sacred Arts imbue,*
Whoſe Labours, Learning out of Darkneſs drew,
May all's days happy be, may he ſhine bright,
And may he ſtill enjoy Celeſtial light:
May no Diſease infect with poyſonous breath,
Him, who gains Health from Sickneſs, Life from Death.

Particles and fermentation

Anyone studying medicine after 1628 was left in no doubt that the blood circulates. But as John Aubrey (1626–1697) reflected, Harvey 'did not care for Chymistry and was wont to speake against them with an undervalue'.[17] Everything was the blood. This was the first component to be formed in the foetus, the source of heat imparted to other parts, and essential for life. Harvey attributed the difference in colour of blood entering and leaving the lungs to physical properties of the arterial and venous circulation, rather than an alteration resulting from contact with air.[18] This explained why there was no need for the foetus to breathe. However, Harvey's discoveries formed the starting point for subsequent advances made in Oxford and London because the large community of chemists, physicists, and physicians gathered in those cities cooperated in solving issues relating to respiration, blood, and the circulation.

The first step was acceptance of the corpuscular theory of biological matter based on particles that form aggregates or 'moleculæ'. The theory was an elaboration of atomism proposed by Democritus (c460–370 BC) and Epicurus (341–270 BC), and developed in France by Rene Descartes (1596–1650) and Pierre Gassendi (1592–1655).[19] Differences between Descartes and Gassendi in terms of how atoms are arranged and interact did not undermine belief in the theory. Lacking an experimental basis, these French ideas were easily dismissed by William Petty (1623–1687) as 'witt and phancy'.[20] But they were appreciated by Nathanael Highmore (1613–1685) and Robert Boyle, and important for the doctrine of particles and iatrochemistry that was espoused in Oxford. Boyle used a microscope to study the limbs of a small insect and inferred that function arose from minute structures: 'what a multitude of Atomes must concurre to constitute the severall parts externall and internall necessary to make out this little Engine'. He concluded that atoms are the 'stopping point in the resolution of real bodies' even if they could not directly be visualized. But neither Boyle nor Willis abandoned divine influence. Willis wrote of 'Æthereal Particles of a more Divine Breathing, which our Parent Nature hath hid in this Sublunary World, as it were the Instruments of Life and Soul, of Motion and Sense'. For Boyle: 'God created matter in an innumerable multitude of variously configur'd Corpuscles ... and [caused creatures to act as if they had a] Design of Self-preservation'.[21]

Willis accepted Boyle's work in reaching his conclusion that all matter could be considered in terms of the properties of corpuscles made up of atoms and aggregated particles. But Boyle was not so attentive to Willis. Hierons noted that the only written reference Boyle makes to Willis is in the postscript to a discussion on the transmutability of chemical principles:[22]

[17] See: Frank (1980): page 19.

[18] In the debates that followed, two lines of reasoning should perhaps be distinguished: the iatrophysical notion in which the primary purpose of respiration and circulation was mechanical and needed to maintain matter in motion; and the iatrochemical in which the idea was that the critical events were chemical and related to the activity and state of corpuscles.

[19] See: Rene Descartes, *Principia philosophiæ*, Amsterdam (1644) and *De homine*, Lugduni Batavorum [Leiden] (1662, published posthumously); and Pierre Gassendi, *Animadversiones in decimum librum Diogenes Laërtii*, Lyons (1649).

[20] See: Frank (1980): page 92 and endnote 13, chapter 4.

[21] See: Frank (1980): page 94, and endnote 30, chapter 4; page 96; and page 123, endnote 50, chapter 4; and Malcolm Oster, 'The "Beame of Diuinity": Animal suffering in the early thought of Robert Boyle', *The British Journal for the History of Science* 1989; 22: 151–79.

[22] See: Robert Boyle, *The works of the Hon Robert Boyle*, volume 4, London (1772): page 503. This was added to Robert Boyle, *New experiments, and observations, made upon the icy noctiluca imparted in a letter to a friend living in the country: to which is annexed A chymical paradox*, London (1682). Hierons adds that Boyle does also refer to 'the writings of the famous Dr Willis (not being available to him) and 'the learned Dr Willis's notions about fevers' in the preface to Robert Boyle, *Of the reconcileableness of specifick medicines to the corpuscular philosophy to which is annexed a discourse about the advantages of the use of simple medicines*, London (1685).

> I do not take chymical principles in the strictest sense of that term, wherein it is confined to salt, sulphur, and mercury; but in the larger acceptance, wherein the learned Doctor Willis, and divers other chymists (that are not all his juniors) employ it, when they comprise under it two elementary bodies; as they do when they constitute five principles (which might be more clearly called familiar ingredients) in which number they comprise phlegm and earth, which other chymists, as well as the Aristotelians, would call elements (of the body that affords them). Taking then, in his whole writings, the word principles in the larger sense above declared (congruously whereunto I usually call them the chymical principles indefinitely, not the hypostatical principles, which are accounted but three) I proceed to the particular observations and reflections I was going to begin.

Willis was a reductionist but he did not altogether reject the humours: '[it is] almost the same thing, to say a house consists of Wood and Stone, as a Body of Four Elements'. He wanted to see beyond these vaguely conceived 'Elements of Bodies' and understand 'Knots of the Sciences and the Riddles of Nature' in terms of particles 'into which Physical things are resolved'. Acknowledging earlier concepts, Willis amended the Paracelsian belief in sulphur, mercury, and salt as the basis of all bodies and organs to five categories or 'principles'. Everything depended on their interactions and 'intestinal' (internal) motion. Three were active: sulphur, spirit (replacing mercury), and salt. Two were passive: water and earth:[23] Willis was generally credited with adding the two passive principles, but all five had already been proposed by Sebastian Basso (b.1573).[24] The five particles had colour, weight, taste, odour, consistency, form, and duration. The Galenic humours could be understood in terms of these five principles. Willis did not see atomism as contradictory to his own ideas:[25]

> If anyone shall object, That the Atomical and our Spagyric Principles are altogether subordinate, to wit, that these, tho at the last sensible, are resolved into those only to be signified by Conception; I shall not much gainsay him, so it shews that those Conceptions are real. I being dull and purblind, leave the more accurate to quick sights, being content to be so wise as to perform the business of the outward Sense with Reason: for I profess, it please me not, to devise or dream Philosophy.

He felt confident in his formulation: 'Because this Hypothesis determinates Bodies into sensible parts, and cuts open things as it were to the life, it pleases us before the rest'. The essential change in these particles which sustained life was fermentation. Whilst they might exist in isolation as the 'food' of life, critical to function of the five particles was that they were light and tended to 'fly away'. Motion generated heat, unless restrained by matter that was thick and able to 'intangle the subtile Particles, and detain them in their Embraces ... [from which] the wrestlings of these two twins, in one Womb, the motion of Fermentation chiefly proceeds'. Fermentation was a term borrowed from the chemistry of organic matter but also applicable to everything material. More than that, it was the analogy with fermentation, heat generated, and the sediments produced in the preparation of wine, beer and cider, bread, cheese and pickles, and the tastes of these foodstuffs, that provided the basis for Willis's

[23] See: Isler (1968): footnote page 49 for the point that Willis refers to 'spirit and spirits', 'salt and salts', but only to water, earth, and sulphur in the singular.

[24] See: Sebastian Basso *Philosophia naturalis adversus Aristotelem libri XII*, Geneva (1621)

[25] See: Thomas Willis, *Of fermentation* (1684): page 2.

adoption, partly as metaphor, of these reactions to his ideas on blood.[26] Where blood differed from wine and beer was in the need constantly to replenish its particles and dispose of waste, whereas the fermentation of liquors proceeded in a contained space. For Willis, the dynamic and cohesive properties of the five particles in their various states was fundamental to all living things and 'explicated . . . the bosom of the Earth', minerals and metals, meteors, and the 'Atmo-Sphear', and all animate and inanimate objects.[27] An organ or system such as brain or blood could be described, at any one time, in terms of the state and balance of the five particles, acting independently or as 'copula':[28]

> It is so certain that the Bodies of Animals, consist of the aforesaid Principles, that it wants no proof. For they so plentifully swell up, with spirit, salt and sulphur, that their Particles are obvious to the sense: wherefore they are moved with a more swift motion, and more excellent senses of Life, and functions of Heat, in the subjects, in which they are implanted, are enlarged.

Willis had studied chemistry in Peckewater Inne chamber in the 1640s[29] and, engaged in the preparation of chemical compounds with Ralph Bathurst (1620–1704), had tried to make the gold-based explosive *aurum fulminans*.[30] By the early 1650s, Willis was considering chemical explanations for the composition of blood and its active ingredients. In all of this he was deducing physiological principles from chemistry and his experience as a physician without the benefit of any original observations based on experiment. His formulation of corpusculean chemistry was refined in the interval between documenting case notes in 1650–1652 and the completion of *De fermentatione* in June 1656.[31] For Willis, sulphur was the most prominent particle and it became volatile unless restrained by salt, water, or earth. A major source of sulphur was fat in the diet. Sulphur made the blood red. Combined with spirit, sulphur became agitated imparting strength, maturation, 'sweetness', and 'sensible heat' on bodies. Under the most vigorous movement, sulphur induced flame and generated heat. In states of dissolution, when sulphur separated from other particles, bodies became putrefied, desiccated, and destroyed. Perhaps sulphur appealed so much to Willis because of its relevance to gunpowder and his focus on explosion in physiological processes. Spirit, established by divine instruction as the instrument of life and soul but nonetheless material and interacting with the others, was the most subtle particle. Even more active than sulphur, it was especially likely to move unless restrained by more inert particles. Salt resisted the flight of sulphur and spirit and so was less prone to 'inflameation'.[32] The main source

[26] See: *Of fermentation* (1684): pages 14–22 for Willis's description of the 'fermentation of art' by which he means the chemistry of natural substances such as beer and wine.

[27] See: *Of fermentation* (1684): page 9 for Willis's eloquent discussion of the life cycle and 'Herby state' of plants and trees, and ways in which the seasons follow 'the Dance of Natural Motions'. In pursuing the particulate nature of all matter, Willis allows himself the view: 'we have read of Men changed into Stones, yea a whole city to have been stiffened a stony substance, by the Air, or by some Vapour, brought forth out of the Earth: the Faith of which thing is left to the Authors'. See also: Frank (1990): page 117.

[28] See: *Of fermentation* (1684): page 11.

[29] The Bodleian Library copy of *The causes of the decay of Christian piety* (1668), thought to have been written by Richard Allestry, is annotated: 'Dr Allestree was author of this book, and wrote it in the very same year wherein he went thro' a course of chymistry with Dr Willis which is the reason why so many physical allusions are to be found in it'.

[30] Fulminating gold was a high explosive popular in western alchemy from the sixteenth century. It contained a yellow-orange amorphous mixture of gold, ammonia, and chlorine but of imprecise chemical constitution.

[31] See: Kenneth Dewhurst, *Thomas Willis's Oxford lectures*, Oxford (1980); Kenneth Dewhurst, *Willis's Oxford casebook (1650–52)*, Oxford (1981); Frank (1980): pages 165–9; and Frank (1990): pages 117–18.

[32] Used in everyday medical parlance, it does well to reflect that the term 'inflammation' has its origins in the iatrochemical notions of fermentation.

of salt was vegetables in the diet. Earth and water provided a matrix for the more mobile particles imparting solidity, structure, and stability on bodies. Willis assigned taste to these particles—bitter, sweet, sour, and salt—indicating that the physician might better understand the nature of disease using that sense. Particles bound in corpuscles were poised to 'ascend' and become enkindled,[33] as a result of which vital heat was distributed throughout the body: 'Fermentation is an intestine motion of Particles, or the Principles of every Body, either tending to the Perfection of the same Body, or because of its change into another'.[34]

Willis's primary concern was the fermentation that supports life. This occurred principally in four, perhaps five, locations. The place where aerial nitre from the lungs worked its effects on blood was the 'Chimny of the Heart'. Assigning fermentation and heating of the blood as its primary function modified the post-Harveian perception of the heart as a pump that propagated the circulation of blood and generated the pulse. Chyle fermented blood in the 'ventricle' (defined in the table of hard words, in this context, as 'that part of the stomach which receives the meat and drink, being swallowed down, and which hath in it self the virtue of digestion'). Here, fermentation was much influenced by the diet yielding sour, bitter, and acid chyle. Although it was not clear 'by what workman it is prepared, nor by what channels it is carried, at a distance, quicker than the twinkling of an eye', animal spirit was created in the brain where fermented blood was filtered. The spirituous, volatile, and subtle particles were absorbed as in a sponge and 'farther Perfected'. The more solid particles were hindered from passing and returned in the circulation thereby 'straining of the subtile from the thick'. The seminal vessels and genital parts were also a source of fermentation. This ferment not only flourished the foetus in the womb but was also able to:[35]

> Inspire through all the Body, the whole Mass of blood, that it may be more Volatile, and more sharply hot: Wherefore in Women who have the Ferment of the Womb in good order, their face is furnished with a curious and flourishing colour ... Also in men, from the seminal Ferment, happen abundance of heat, great strength, a sounding Voice, and a manly eruption of beard and hair; by reason of a defect of this, men grow womanish, to wit, a small Voice, weak Heat, and want of a beard are caused.

Willis was confident about these four (heart, stomach, brain, and genitals) but on fermentation in the spleen he was not so sure. Rejecting the opinions that this was either a source of blood or 'as it were the Sink or Jakes, into which the feculencies of the blood are cast', he considered the spleen a place where the blood is cleansed. The residue of its passage constituted a 'store-house of earthy and muddy parts of the blood', capable of being replenished and recirculated so that the 'crude juice of Melancholly' was removed and 'the same Juice concocted and exalted into the nature of a Ferment'.

Although in thinking about energy and fermentation, Willis began by considering the baker's oven and the brewer's furnace, he came to understand this process as the 'whole Provision and Dowry of all Nature ... those first forgotten Particles, by whose Orgasm or Heat, those vulgar preparations do Ferment, to beget the Causes of Motions, and Alterations, in whatever things they are mixed'.[36] His primary interest was the molecular processes that

[33] Almost invariably, Willis writes this as 'inkindled'.

[34] See: *Of fermentation* (1684): page 8.

[35] See: *Of fermentation* (1684): page 13. Either quoting a different passage, or possibly offering a much freer partial translation of the same text, Sir Charles Symonds, 'The circle of Willis' *British Medical Journal* 1955; i: 1–16, first drew attention to Willis's description anticipating the modern concept of hormones.

[36] See: *Of fermentation* (1684): preface, page [9].

invigorate the blood and he did not concern himself with chemical composition of the substance in air on which these changes depended. But others were giving this matter much consideration.

Respiration and circulation

The emphasis of intellectual effort in the interval between publication of Thomas Willis's treatise on fermentation (1659) and his final formulation in detail of the properties of blood (*De sanguinis accensione*: 1670) concerned the role of respiration in maintaining life. Although this was relevant to his interest in iatrochemistry and fermentation, Willis was increasingly preoccupied with work on the brain and made no original contributions to elucidating the interaction between blood and air.[37]

Nathanael Highmore practised medicine from the late 1630s becoming interested in anatomy from 1640 and carrying out dissections with Thomas Clayton (1612–1693). After entering medical practice in Sherborne, Dorsetshire, Highmore's reading led him to Harvey's work and they interacted after Harvey came to Oxford in 1642.[38] Highmore linked the beating of the heart to generation of the pulse and the circulation of heated blood. Fortified by spirits, this carried particles to all parts of the body but eventually the blood grew cold and needed replenishing. Whilst recognizing the need for respiration, Highmore dissociated air from properties of the vital spirits. Rather, respiration served the dual purpose of cooling the blood during inspiration and removing waste during expiration. Expansion of the thorax mechanically moved blood from the right to the left circulation. In this Highmore was perpetuating two false hypotheses that later had to be corrected. Although Willis did not enter much into that dispute, he and Highmore did come into conflict over the nature of hysteria.[39] Working with Willis and Richard Lydall (1621–1704), Bathurst thought about the mechanics of ventilation, the motion of the muscles of the ribcage and diaphragm, and the physiological purpose of respiration. He moved away from cooling and removal of waste towards the concept that inspiration provides the nitrous substance by which spirits in the blood are enriched. The material added is present in air, water, and earth and necessary for all forms of life. As to what the substance was, Bathurst veered towards a particulate corpuscular material. Given as lectures in Oxford, Bathurst's ideas were written in manuscript but he did not want them published: 'Mr Boyle knows one that hath an excellent Ms. De Respiratione which hee will not publish'. In possession of the script, and supported by John Wilkins (1614–1672), Boyle refused 'to have those jewells sent back to Oxford'; and, in passing, asked Bathurst to remember him 'to Dr Willis, Dr Ward, and the rest of those excellent acquaintances of yours, that have been pleased to tolerate me in their company'.[40]

Thomas Willis, Richard Lower, and even Highmore read and absorbed the implications of Bathurst's manuscript but it was Boyle who led the long path, never fully realized by this

[37] See: *Of feavers* (1684): page 54. Willis says very little about respiration although he was aware that impaired fermentation in the heart led to 'difficult respiration upon any motion', dropsy, cachexia, and yellow jaundice preceding the agonal gasps of death from poor fermentation or, in modern parlance, heart failure.

[38] See: Frank (1980): pages 27 and 97–101, for discussion of Nathanael Highmore, *Corporis humani disquisito anatomica*, The Hague (1651) which sets macroscopic anatomy in the context of Harvey's circulation of the blood. The book was dedicated to Harvey who, not surprisingly, approved of its focus on the heart as the 'king of the human realm', the origin of the heat that sustained life.

[39] Although ordained, by 1658 Bathurst was described (together with Willis) as a physician 'eminently known in the University': see Frank (1980): page 107 and endnote 129, chapter 4.

[40] See: Frank (1980): pages 106–13.

group of scientists, towards resolving the composition of the nitrous spirit that allowed it to nourish the blood.[41] In this Boyle was helped by Robert Hooke (1635–1703), on the recommendation of Willis, and their efforts culminated in construction of the vacuum air pump in 1659.[42] The experiments showed that animals were unaffected by breathing in a confined space but, despite maintaining respiratory movements, did not long survive if air was removed by suction, although they were soon resuscitated by letting in air.[43] The demonstration that air, deliberately or accidentally contaminated or rebreathed, no longer sustained life provided further argument in favour of an interaction between some expendable constituent and the circulating blood. In his considerations of the foetus surviving in the womb without breathing, and observations on fishes, Boyle realized that life could be sustained by air dissolved in liquids. Taken together, the evidence allowed Boyle finally to discard several pre-existing hypotheses: that the purpose of ventilation is to cool the blood; that the function of respiration is primarily to remove waste; and that air directly enters the ventricles of the heart. Rather, it followed that something essential is extracted from air which fills the lungs due to the negative pressure created by expansion of the chest during activity of the intercostal muscles and diaphragm. But before considering further the physiology of respiration, Boyle was deflected by his greater interest in the physical than the chemical properties of air.[44]

Others, including Christopher Wren (1632–1723), were also designing apparatus 'for cooling and percolating the Aire [and filtering out] the fulginous Vapours and Moisture, it was infected with in Expiration'. Although known to Thomas Sprat (1635–1713) and Christopher Wren the younger (1675–1747), who wrote on lives of the Wren family, the details are now lost.[45] As with Bathurst, Wren discarded the belief that the purpose of respiration is to cleanse the blood of impurities arguing that 'nitrous Fumes' must replenish those lost during circulation and suggesting experiments that mimicked respiration 'by placing some benign Chymical Spirits that by fumeing may infect the Air within the Vessel'.[46]

Thomas Willis followed these observations on the nature of respiration but the issue that concerned him was the next stage in the process. Understanding the mechanics of ventilation, and that air contained a factor necessary to support life, did not explain how the blood is heated. It was enough for him that nitro-sulphurous particles were in the earth, the air and, ever ready to explode during fermentation, in the body.[47] Willis maintained that the link between respiration and bodily heat was enkindling as the basis for fermentation. Boyle's

[41] Robert Boyle's 'Physico-chymical essay', subsequently included in *Physiological essays*, London (1661) on the corpuscular nature of saltpetre was later translated into Latin by Henry Stubbe.

[42] See: John Evelyn, *The diary of John Evelyn Esquire F.R.S.* Ed. William Bray, London (1818, printed *c.*1930): page 347 for details of how, on 7 May 1662, John Evelyn (1620–1706) commented on experiments using Boyle's vacuum pump: 'I waited on Prince Rupert to our Assembly, where were tried severall experiments in Mr. Boyle's vacuum. A man thrusting in his arm upon exhaustion of the aire had his flesh immediately swelled so as the bloud was near bursting the veines: he drawing it oute we found it all speckled'. See: Steven Shapin and Simon Schaffer, *Leviathan and the air pump*, Princeton (1985) for a recent analysis of this instrument and its inventors.

[43] See: Robert Boyle, *New experiments physico-mechanicall, touching the spring of the air*, Oxford (1660).

[44] It was left to Hooke to consider again the chemical constituents of air in *Micrographia*, London (1665).

[45] See: *Parentalia: Or, memoirs of the family of the Wrens; viz. of Mathew bishop of Ely, Christopher dean of Windsor, &c. but chiefly of Sir Christopher Wren, late surveyor-general of the royal buildings, president of the Royal Society, &c. &c. in which is contained, besides his works, a great number of original papers and records; on religion, politicks, anatomy, mathematicks, architecture, antiquities; and most branches of polite literature.* Compiled, by his Son Christopher, London (1750).

[46] See: Adrian Tinniswood, *His invention so fertile. A life of Sir Christopher Wren*, London (2001): page 244.

[47] Notwithstanding his acceptance that the same spirit maintained the vigour of the blood, Nathanael Hodges (1629–1688) believed that corruption of the nitro-aerial spirit as it arose from the earth was responsible for the plague, on which Willis was writing a manuscript at the time.

experiments had shown that combustion required a supply of air. For Willis it followed that flame, fuelled by nitrous particles derived from the air during respiration combined with corpuscles which fermented to produce the heat that maintained the body, must also sustain the *flammula vitalis* in the blood. All of Willis's writings are rich in metaphor[48] and whether he really thought that there were actual flames is unclear. Very often he inserts the phrase 'as it were' before mention of heat, ascension, or enkindling. He saw life as a lamp: the vessel was the heart; oil burned the blood; and air enabled combustion. Whilst his scheme can be aligned in modern terms with oxygenation, nutrition, and metabolism as the basis for physiology and vegetative functions, the insistence on flame as the underlying motor eventually invited ridicule and distanced Willis from matters with which many of his contemporaries were more productively employed.[49]

But the issue of respiration primarily exerting a mechanical effect on blood would not go away. Specifically, it was suggested that excursions of the heart mixed ingredients obtained from food and delivered as chyle through the thoracic duct to the lungs where the formation of nutrient blood was completed mechanically as it passed through the capillaries.[50] This debate culminated in experiments supervised by Hooke starting in 1664 under the auspices of the Royal Society, discussions of which were occasionally heated.[51] Initially Hooke showed that life was maintained for as long as air was used to inflate the lungs through the trachea, and that movements of the heart and lungs were not synchronized. Whereas Hooke drew no particular conclusions, Henry Oldenburg (1619–1677) saw that this prioritized a role for air mingling with blood in the lungs which was then returned to the left ventricle and, after it had become dull and torpid in the various organs, recycled to the place where it could again be revived, rather than the mechanics of thoracic movement sustaining the flame of life.[52]

Central to work on the effects of air was the reason for differences in the colour of venous and arterial blood. Lower observed that arterial blood darkened and cooled as it passed through capillaries before being returned to the veins and recirculated. Learning of this, Boyle tried manipulation with various chemicals to reproduce the changes in the colour of blood; and he proposed a series of experiments aimed at characterizing its chemical composition in various contexts. But, more interested in respiration than the colour

[48] The first words he wrote in the dedication to Gilbert Sheldon included in editions of *Diatribæ duæ* after 1660, and translated into English (1681) use metaphor: 'The Eagle will not acknowledge his suspected Chicken, by only one sign; for it is not enough that it can look against the Light, unless it be able to behold the Sun's Beams without Winking; and indeed although this our hasty Issue, whether by the help of its own blindness, or of that doubtful Light in which it hath liv'd, hath been able to come abroad, yet it hath not sufficiently given Marks of its true Race, until it might delight its Eye with your Brightness, as at the Sun's Beams'.

[49] The term 'explosio Willisiana', used in a slightly derogatory sense, is attributed to Johan Wepfer, *Observationes medico-practicæ de affectibus capitis internis et externis*, Schaffhausen (1727): Observatio CXXXIII, pages 629–30; '*Explosioni Willisianæ* hactenus assentire nequii, utcunque illam speciose proponat, imprimis *in hac Matrona*: me persuadet paroxysmorum duratio scil. ultra duas horas continuas: certe nervis graviter irritatis evenire hæc multis experimentis didici' [So far I have not been able to agree with the 'Willisian explosion', no matter how brilliantly he proposes it, especially *in this Housewife*: I am convinced by the duration of the paroxysms, that is, continuous for more than two hours; certainly many experiences have taught me that these paroxysms can occur by severely irritated nerves]. See: Owsei Temkin, *The falling sickness*, 2nd edition, Baltimore and London (1971): page 207, footnote 10 and page 442, endnote 1085.

[50] This was an idea implicit in Malpighi's description of the pulmonary capillary system set out in *De pulmonibus observatiationes anatomicæ*, Bologna (1661).

[51] See: Tinniswood (2001): page 244 for details of exchanges. Christopher Wren, for example, upset Hooke by suggesting 'that aether, which Mr Hooke had hypothetically proposed' was the solvent for 'the exhalations of vapours' which make up the atmosphere and hinted that he would be pleased to see an experiment that demonstrated its existence.

[52] See: Frank (1980): page 159.

of blood, Boyle and Hooke showed that air manipulated by chemical reactions often lost its life supporting properties. What emerged was consensus that respiration of natural air allowed extraction of a substance needed for fermentation and to support life. Specifically, John Locke (1632–1704) argued that during inspiration the particles of aerial nitre volatize and mix with blood in the lungs, changing the colour from dusky blue to bright red only for the hue to be lost as blood moves throughout the body. Expiration cleansed the blood of 'fulginous' waste as many others had proposed.[53] This theme was taken up by George Castle (*c.*1635–1673) who generalized the account, explaining that air supplies nitre, which mixes with food provided in the chyle enabling flame to heat, ferment, and change the colour and motion of blood.[54] Loyal to Willis, he located these events in the ventricles of the heart. But the debate between chemical exchange and the mechanical effects of ventilation was still not fully reconciled since these two events occurred in synchrony. Hooke was able to describe what needed to be done in order to make the distinction but he found the nature of the required experiment on a dog unpalatable, and his cooperation was needed in order for this to be done under the auspices of the Royal Society. For a while the matter again stalled.[55]

During the hiatus that followed, Walter Needham (*c.*1631–1691), inspired by Willis's 'immortal book on the brain' (*Cerebri anatome*: 1664) but not shy in taking his own position, made the point that the heart is a muscle that pumps but it is not responsible for the generation of vital spirits. Fermentation occurs elsewhere. In passing, he also rejected the notion that blood is inflammable and heats through enkindling, or that the pulse is the result of blood exploding.[56] For Needham, animal spirits were not derived from flame. Having taken several steps in the 'right' direction, Needham then stalled by rehearsing the old argument that air, whilst necessary, did not interact with blood and that the function of respiration is mechanical. Often an astute observer and commentator on evolving ideas relevant to respiration, Oldenburg recalled that, appended to a book published by Marcello Malpighi,[57] Carlo Fracassati (1630–1672) had described injecting various substances into the bloodstream of dogs, observing that both coagulation and excess fluidity were harmful and that blood left to stand remained red if continuously exposed to air. This added weight to the concept that a substance in air interacted directly with blood. Whilst agreeing with the claim, Boyle and Hooke felt that they, in principle, had already and independently made this observation.[58] Eventually the critical experiment was done by the reluctant Hooke who devised a system for keeping the lungs inflated but immobile whilst blood was exposed to a constant supply of fresh air. This confirmed that, for as long as air passed through the lungs, life was sustained even without the mechanical excursions that many had argued were necessary.

[53] See: Frank (1980): page 188.

[54] See: George Castle, *The chymical Galenist: a treatise wherein the practice of the ancients is reconcil'd to the new discoveries in the theory of physick*, London (1667).

[55] See: Frank (1980): pages 197–8; and Anita Guerrini, 'The ethics of animal experimentation in seventeenth century England. *Journal of the History of Ideas* 1989; 50: 391–407 for discussion of attitudes to research on animals relevant to Hooke's reticence, and emphasizing Willis's more enlightened view that the explanations of certain 'famous Philosophers' who 'suppose Brute Animals to be only certain Machines ... seem not to satisfie a Mind desirous of Truth'.

[56] See: Gualtero Needham, *Disquisitio anatomica de formato fœtu*, London (1667); and Frank (1980): pages 199–200.

[57] See: Marcelli Malpighi, *Tetras anatomicarum epistolarum*, Bologna (1665); and Carlo Fracassati, *Dissertatio epistoclica responsoria de cerebro*, Bologna (1665).

[58] See: Frank (1980): pages 205–8.

A flame in the blood

As these scientific discoveries unfolded during the 1660s, and despite the distractions of clinical practice and his work on the anatomy of the brain, Willis's interest in chemistry and fermentation were maintained.[59] His position that the process of fermentation occurred in the chambers of the heart was becoming increasingly insecure. Lower accepted that blood was the source of heat which was distributed to other parts but he distanced himself from the assumption that the difference in colour between arterial and venous blood had to do with fermentation in the heart. Nor was the heart involved in processes whereby the blood became foamy and effervescent thereby forcing its movement into the aorta. However, Lower was aware that these ideas needed to be approached with caution in order not to upstage his friend Willis:[60]

> But we are certainly warmed by a fire that is more than fictitious or metaphorical, and so it would be worth while in the next place to explain at somewhat greater length how the blood itself becomes heated and in its turn provides warmth for the whole of the body. However, since this would be outside the plan of the present work, and I also understand that the learned Dr Willis is giving the matter some thought in his book *On the soul*, and also *on the Heating of the Blood*, I should not like to depart so far from professional courtesy as to forestall him in this matter.

De sanguinis accensione (1670) was the product of eleven years listening and reformulating his ideas based on all that had been learned about respiration since he had published *De fermentatione* (1659). Willis was aware that his reshaped ideas might be 'laughed at by some as unusual things and Paradoxes' and that 'perhaps they may be found rough and strange to be applied to the animal œconomy'. He remained tolerant: 'it becomes me not to take ill, but to let everyone freely to enjoy his own sense'; and he asks his readers to 'weigh the Reasons and Arguments' anticipating that there would then 'be no one who will not give their assent, or easily pardon me mine'. He acknowledged that:[61]

> There are so many opinions concerning the growing hot of the Blood, for that some attribute it to an innate heat, others to a flame in the Heart, some also to a fermentation of the bloody mass, and others to its inkindling, therefore I shall endeavour more narrowly to introspect the matter, as much as I am able, to build upon a more certain Ratiocination, its genuine Cause, though very abstruse.

It is perhaps unfortunate that in describing the movement of particles and generation of heat, Willis used the terms fermentation, enkindling, and incalescence interchangeably in

[59] See: Frank (1980); page 240 and endnote 115, chapter 9 for details of how, in 1662, Seth Ward (1617–1689) had visited Nathanael Hodges, a physician who often turned to Willis for advice on cases, and observed that Hodges' bookshelf had a copy of Gunter Billichius' (1598–1640) chemical work with an appendix on fermentation 'from which Dr Willis doubtless had some of his notions of fermentation'.

[60] See: Frank (1980): pages 212 and endnote 110, chapter 8 citing Richard Lower, *Tractatus de corde*, London (1669): page 74; and Frank (1980): pages 217–20. Robert Frank admires the spirit of free transfer of technical and theoretical ideas amongst this group of close friends—in particular Lower, Hooke, Boyle, and Willis—who were less concerned with priorities and personal reputation than knowledge; and for whom 'innovation lay at the conjunction of men's talents' as the shift occurred gradually from Galenic doctrines, through Harvey's demonstration of the circulation, to agreement that air alters venous blood in the lungs and the heart pumps it round the body.

[61] See: Thomas Willis, *Of the accension of the blood* (1684): page 20.

a treatise entitled *Of the accension of the blood*.[62] However he soon made clear the sequence of events: the motion of particles determines enkindling which is the same as accension of the blood, and heat is a consequence of fermentation whereby, fuelled by fire or the flame of life, nutritious substances interact with air which, in turn, generates animal spirits in the solid organs.

Willis was on safe ground in asserting the central importance of blood. Harvey had shown that it is first formed and dies last: 'the undoubted testimony of the Sacred Scripture plainly asserts the animation of the blood ... the Blood is the Life or Soul'. The blood circulates in order to nourish the parts, reinvigorate itself, and 'separate all recrements and worn out Particles'. Without movement the blood stagnates and putrefies. Without heat, the blood can merely water the solid parts and prove insufficient for 'more perfect Animals'. Without fermentation the particles would be unable to fly away and serve their functions especially in the brain, nervous stock, and muscles. But from whence comes the fire? In a significant paragraph, having discoursed on the ways in which heat can be imparted or generated, Willis almost qualifies his former notion of a flame in the heart that heats the blood passing though it:[63]

> The Heart is a meer Muscle, nor doth contain in it self any tinder or matter for a flame or heat (I know not how) implanted, fit for their continuance. For though it be confessed, that on the continual motion of this Bowel, (which is only animal) the Circulation of the Blood doth depend, yet the Heart borrows heat from the blood, and not the blood from the Heart.

Having considered as one option the possibility that the corrosive effect of saline generates heat, Willis quickly rejected the notion of salt seeping into the blood and thereby stoking its furnace, since there is no such salt mine in the body. This left only fermentation of the blood as the source of heat. But here too, in restating his views, Willis nimbly adapted his earlier position incorporating knowledge gained by others during the 1660s. He wanted to make three points. The first, on which he expounds at some length, is that fermentation requires a free and continuous supply of air on which all fire depends. Willis had moved on but he avoided too much retrospective rehearsal of earlier views and rather let it be assumed that he had always known about the need for an external influence on blood in the form of aerial nitre in order to support its enkindling and generate heat. Intensity of the flame varies with the amount of nitrous material available to enkindle the sulphurous particles, just as a coal may glow or burst into flames depending on the wafts of air blowing across its embers. Equally, the fire is extinguished if either the nitrous air or sulphurous substrate are lacking. The 'more perfect' animals die quicker when deprived of air than others. This is not due to effects on the blood through failure to remove waste. Rather 'those that are hindred from respiration [die] because the vital flame of the blood is wanting of nitrous food of the Air'. Willis had clearly been following experiments at the Royal Society:[64]

> The illustrious Mr. *Robert Boyle* hath most clearly demonstrated that ... a Candle being lighted, and put into a capacious globe of Glass, and the Vessel stopped up: as soon as the

[62] 'Accension' is Latinized English (or perhaps derived from French) from 'accensio' meaning 'kindling' but now obsolete.

[63] See: *Of the accension of the blood* (1684): page 22.

[64] See: *Of the accension of the blood* (1684): pages 23–4.

> air was sucked out by a wind-instrument, the flame did expire . . . not so much that is suffocated by its own proper smoke, as because it is destitute of the nitrous food of the Air.

Willis then summarizes Boyle's experiments, 'the most famous Boyl also by his Experiments hath put it out of doubt'; and, unusually in any of his treatises, Willis inserts specific references to Boyle's work: '*Exper. Phys. Mec.* 50 *Exper.* 13; and *Exper.* 78, and *Experiment. Physicom.* 41, 42 and 43'. These last three experiments had convinced Willis that, unlike the fermentation of wine and beer, or the boiling of hot liquids, which proceed faster in the absence of air, hot living creatures expire rapidly in a chamber deprived of air even though there is 'more space left for the receiving the smoke, lest the retaining of it might constipate the blood'. It followed that the 'life of a living creature [is] either fire, or something analogical to it' and it required air to be sustained.

The second requirement was a constant supply of sulphurous food, the amount of which influences the intensity of fermentation and heating of the blood. Willis indicates that if food is denied, the blood 'consuming the solid parts, it snatches into its bosom their remnants, and other humours of the Body whereby it might be fed'. The third requirement was that the waste products of heating are removed in order for new supplies of sulphur to be enkindled and nourish the blood. The particles left behind from this process are either vapourized in expired air or form ashes of 'Earth, Salt, and stinking Sulphur'. Removal requires ventilation or the opening of pores through which sweat discharges the adust matter.[65]

As for how the flame is originally lit, it must either be kindled from an existing fire or generated from the internal motion of particles: 'we have largely shewed the Species of either, and the manner of their being made, in our Tract *of Fermentation* (only we omitted there, that the accession of nitrous food was necessary for the sustaining it)'.[66] Elaborating further, Willis considers the concept of parental fire being transmitted in the seed and smouldering in the foetus until ignited by the first breath of nitrous air after birth. Willis is now clear that the colour of blood changes from purple to bright crimson as it passes through the lungs and admixes with air before being returned to the heart in the pneumonick veins, darkening again in its passage through the body until refreshed 'as the most learned Doctor Lower hath observed'. The change in colour is due to the admixture of nitrous air with blood; and Willis rehearses the many experiments that involve exposing samples of venous blood to air and seeing its change in colour. But still Willis cannot quite let go of his earlier notion of the heart as the chimney of life:[67]

> It so much helps to moderate the accension of the Blood and its burning, according to the rage of the passions, and to direct other works and uses of the animated body, that we have thought the vital or flamy part of the Soul to have its chief, and as it were Imperial seat in the Heart and Lungs, in every distemper or affection, as of grief, Joy, fear, and the like; also in the Fits of Diseases.

The problem was that the flame that heats the blood, which the heart circulates like a 'Bannion or Bathing Engine' revealing the 'Divine handy-work of the Circulation of Blood, and what

[65] Adust is a term much used by medical writers of the middle ages. It was originally taken from the Latin verb 'aduro', past participle 'adustum' or 'singed'. Later it was adapted to the French 'aduste' describing a state of dryness of the body, heat, thirst, black or burned colour of the blood, and deficiency of its serum with an atrabilious or melancholic complexion.

[66] See: *Of the accension of the blood* (1684): page 25.

[67] See: *Of the accension of the blood* (1684): page 26.

burns in it, the Life-lamp', is not visible. Perhaps it flickered and flamed intermittently and in different places; or it could only be sensed as smoke, vapour, or breath. Alternatively:[68]

> Its shining ... may not be perceived by our sight, as in the clear light of the day we cannot behold a glowing red-hot iron, nor shining spark, nor false fires, nor rotten wood, nor many other things shining by night; why then may not the vital fire, even thinner than they, quite escape our sight?

Willis ends this account with text that comes close to a confession that his concept of flame is a metaphor. The key words are 'may be called' in the passage making the point that life in animate bodies requires blood that is:[69]

> Perpetually hot, and as it were inkindled; what should hinder, but that the act of Life, or of that corporeal Soul (consisting in the motion and agglomeration or heaping together of most subtil and agil Particles) may be called a certain Burning or perpetual Fire of the bloody Mass ... the form of fire is obscured, as being subjugated to a more noble form, viz of the corporeal Soul: not much unlike water, which being congealed into Ice or Snow, lays aside the species of water for a time, and may be applied to other uses far distant from fluidity.

Clearly Willis had been listening but, given his elevated position as teacher and mentor, it was hardly necessary for him to do more than move with the times and state the collective view of those with whom he interacted, and use their experiments and hypotheses to restate a position that others had already formulated with greater clarity.[70]

If anyone came close to identifying the component of air that lurked under the rubric of nitre, it was John Mayow (1640–1679). Expanding on his earlier publication and adding a long treatise on aerial nitre and two shorter ones on foetal respiration and muscular movement, respectively, Mayow started from the assumption that aerial nitre is the vital and fermentable spirit.[71] He concluded that the spirit is nitric acid which directly enters the blood and changes its colour during passage through the lungs. Fermentation occurs when nitric acid interacts with sulphurous and salt particles. This process was sufficient to heat the blood. Mayow had to differ from 'the learned Dr Willis' in the latter's emphasis on flame as the cauldron and his comments verged on the scathing:[72]

> From what has already been said, it is I think in some degree made out that the fermentation of the blood, and hence also its heat, arises from nitro-aërial particles fermenting with its salino-sulphureous particles; so that we do not need to have recourse to an imaginary Vital Flame that by its continual burning warms the mass of the blood, much less to affirm a degree of heat in the blood intense enough to produce light, from the rays of which, transmitted to the brain, the Sensitive Soul is supposed to be produced.

[68] See: *Of the accension of the blood* (1684): page 27.

[69] See: *Of the accension of the blood* (1684): page 27.

[70] See Frank (1980): pages 232–7.

[71] See: John Mayow, *Tractatus duo quorum prior agit de respiratione: alter de rachitide*, Oxford (1668); *Tractatus quinque medico-physici quorum primus agit De Sal-nitro, et spiritu nitro-aereo, Secundus De respiration, Tertius De respiratione foetus in utero, et ovo, Quartus De motu musculari, et spiritus animalibus, Ultimus De rachitide*, Oxford (1674).

[72] See: Frank (1980): page 270 and endnote 120, chapter 10, referring to the English version of Mayow's tracts, *Medico-physical works*, Edinburgh (1907): page 108.

He was reprimanding Willis for extravagant extrapolation of ideas but Mayow himself went too far in seeking to accommodate practically all phenomena of nature by placing nitric acid at the epicentre of the physical, physiological, and natural world. Willis had seen that the generation of heat was not innate and that respiration served a function other than cooling the blood. He had proposed flame as a mechanistic link between air, heat, and vitality or ascension of the blood. Mayow had it as fermentation due to the motion of interacting nitrous and sulphureous particles. The difference was not trivial and Mayow moved from deferential citation of Willis's views in the *Tractatus duo* (1668) to overt contradiction of Willis's works and criticism of his friend and mentor in the *Tractatus quinque* (1674).[73]

Fermentation and fever

Thomas Willis was interested in the physiological nature of enkindling, fermentation, flame, and heat; but, as a physician, he wanted to apply chemical theories to the study of disease. He concluded his first treatise by explaining:[74]

> And thus much for FERMENTATION in general ... Those hitherto brought, however chosen out of Natural Philosophy, were fit to wait upon the following Medical Dissertation, that we may more happily know the Original, Progress, and State, as also the Remedies and Cure of Motions and Mutations, in Causes, which variously happen to all kinds of Bodies, and somewhat respecting the Tumults, which from thence are begot in the human Body, from the Blood being irritated, and the rest of the humours; to which exercise, God willing, we will now proceed'.

Willis first applied his concept of vitality through 'observing the Accidents and Courses of Feavers'. This he did in the second treatise published in *Diatribæ duæ* on which it is clear that he continued to work up to late 1658. He mentions epidemics in Oxford that lasted until September of that year. Willis recognized that much had already been said, but he intended to 'receed from the Vulgar Opinion concerning feavers, as a way mightily worn out; and go on in a less trodden Path'.

In thinking about life and death, Willis formulated dissolution as a perturbation of fermentation.[75] Nature had endowed bodies with a finite amount of particles that ascend—'its height or *achme* is only an evolution'—through nutrition and ripening. As with fermentation in brewing, decomposition could be applied both to inanimate as well as living matter. Food becomes rotten and stale unless the particles are adjusted by salting, pickling, or spicing, as do 'humane bodies'. Death is reduction from a state of equilibrium through flying away or evaporation of the five principles. Spirit leaves first, then sulphur, salt, and finally water whereupon the whole crumbles into earth. Thus the sweet smell of life becomes the sourness and rank odour of rottenness and decomposition: 'the active Principles ... breaking forth in the Carcase produce Worms: at length when they are wholly exhaled from the subject, what remains falls into dust'. The more complex the particulate arrangements, the more vulnerable they are to putrefaction. On disease, Willis's position is clear: 'We are not only born and

[73] See chapter 16 for details of Mayow's explicit criticism of Willis, especially on muscular motion.
[74] See: *Of fermentation* (1684): page 44.
[75] See: *Of fermentation* (1684): pages 22–30, chapters VIII and IX for discussion of putrefaction and dissolution of bodies.

nourished by the means of Ferments; but we also Dye: Every Disease acts its Tragedies by the strength of some Ferment'.[76] From this it followed that Galenic medicines were shorter lasting and less useful over time than 'Chymical preparations'.

Because flame and fermentation result in heat, the focus of Willis's mechanistic interpretations focus on diseases characterized by fever. Blood is like the juice of grapes or milk and capable of abnormal fermentation in response to constitutional change or infection. Despite his adherence to corpuscular theory, Willis dutifully goes through the exercise of aligning Galenic humours with the various '*Phænomena's* of Disease' whilst arguing that these are now more accurately considered in terms of perturbed fermentation. He classifies fevers according to their temporal course and periodicity. Some are intermittent: 'every fit begins with cold or shaking, for the most part, and ends in sweat; that the accessions or coming of the fits, return at set Periods, and certain intervals of times, that a Clock is not more exact'.[77] Others are continuous. In the former, the disordered fermentation eventually corrects; in the latter it becomes 'outrageous'. Too much sulphur in the diet, or the addition of nutrients that cause excess agitation of the chemical particles in blood, result in intermittent fever. When spirit becomes too agitated and sulphur is more actively enkindled in the heart, 'fever burns forth with a long fire' and is continuous, over several days if not longer. The worst fevers are due to coagulation or coalescence of the blood. This interrupts the circulation, the ensuing effervescence of stagnation resulting in fever.

Willis also offers a classification based on severity. The most favourable are putrid fevers arising from altered fermentation within the affected individual, similar to the rotting of organic material. The malignant fevers are more severe and due to external forces, tending therefore to be contagious and seasonal, and sometimes localized to particular parts especially the 'Throat, Pleura, Lungs and Intestines'. The worst are pestilential. It was clear to Willis that contagion spread through contact between one infected person and another, either by lying in the same bed, from one household to another, or through handling a garment or 'Household-stuff' even including items left untouched for months or years. Apart from his awareness of susceptibility, contagion, and seasonal factors influencing the risk of fevers, Willis elaborated sophisticated concepts including the suggestion that the causative matter can survive between epidemics by transformation and (in modern terms) remain latent, altering its virulence and subsequently infecting vulnerable hosts. Without knowledge of infectious microbes, he used the analogy of envenoming by poisons, 'effluvia' vapourized from the bowels of the earth and 'either drawn in with the Infection of the commonly inspired Air ... or attracted through the Pores', and 'in an occult manner vehemently hurting the temper and actions of the parts'.

The many manifestations of fever are heat, weariness, anorexia, diarrhoea, burning pains, thirst, coating of the mouth and tongue, headache, disordered sleep (the 'Watchings'), swooning, convulsions, stupefaction, and phrensie—together reflecting disorder of the ventricle (stomach), blood, and brain. The pulse is nature's 'Thermometer or Weather-Glass' and its state is a harbinger of 'Death or Health'.[78] Through its colour, consistency, content, and sediment, the urine informs the choices of treatment and 'prognosticks'. As with so much of Willis's medicine, it is the brain and nervous stock which are especially at risk from 'very

[76] See *Of fermentation* (1684): page 14.

[77] See: *Of feavers* (1684): chapters III–VI, pages 56–73 which are devoted to the general properties of intermittent fevers of varying periodicity compared with a single account, chapter VII, pages 74–5 on continuous fevers. The lack of editing of Willis and Pordage's texts is illustrated by the last part of this sentence at page 56 being exactly repeated at page 58.

[78] See: *Of feavers* (1684): page 88.

rich provision in the nature of things ... [that] lie in wait for us'. More generally, it is clear that Willis had effects on the nervous system foremost in mind when writing on fevers:[79]

> The Juice with which the brain and Nervous Parts are watered, is wont often times to be in fault; for when this Liquor is seen to be carried back from the Blood, into the nervous stock by a constant motion, and certain Circulation, and from thence through the Lymphatick Vessels, into the bosom of the Blood, it is probable, if by reason of a Taint contracted from the Blood, that humour be depraved in its disposition, or is perverted from its equal motion, that from thence the Rigour, and Pain, Convulsion, Delirium, Phrensie, and many more Symptoms of the Nervous kind, usual in Feavers do arise.

Fever may resolve by 'fit' or crisis, for which Willis again turns to the nervous system in explaining the symptoms. The vital spirit is first suppressed, causing cold with headache, vertigo, sparkling before the eyes, and insomnia, but soon becomes disturbed by the awkwardly fermented blood and so responds with vomiting, trembling, and convulsions after which the vital spirits 'recollect themselves' and, for a while, the fever settles.[80] Fevers that last only twenty-four hours are 'an Ephemera, or feaver of a day'. Those that are more prolonged constitute 'an Ephemera of more days, or a Synochus not putrid'.[81] These transient fevers are often the consequence of a wound, ulcer, 'Squinancy' (sore throat), pleurisy, or 'Imposthume of the Lungs'. They may have an extrinsic cause, removal from which (when possible) terminates the condition, as does sweating or 'insensible breathing forth'. The fault lies with 'the vice of the blood' which becomes more acid, bitter, or harsh and unable to assimilate the nutrient chyle from the intestines.[82] Fermentation is disturbed, each bout developing when the diet provides a fresh supply of nutritious juice imperfectly associated with other particles and 'heterogenous', so that the blood repeatedly 'boils up' into a fever. It follows that 'if the sick are abstemious, and more sparingly take their food, the intermission is drawn out longer'.

Removal of waste is fundamental to Willis's iatrochemical concept of order in living bodies. Therefore partial or complete resolution of fever follows removal of the overfermenting principles by perspiration or compartmentalization in the cavities of the body. Ferments in the head may discharge through pores of the nostrils. These are often tinged with blood. Others are removed in the urine, stools, or vomit, or through buboes ridding the body of the adust matter. When the temper of the blood cannot be altered naturally, or through a 'change of air or place of abode', Willis's treatments are designed to improve fermentation, restore the chemical balance by attention to the diet, and suppress the paroxysms with antipyretics.[83]. These might include extracts of plants and herbs applied topically. Medicines that induce purging, vomiting, and sweating help by shaking apart the unruly particles. 'Cardiacks, Digestives, and especially Chalybeats or steeled medicines' invigorate 'depauperated' (impoverished) fermentation, as do dietary stimulants including yeast and beaten eggs. At odds

[79] See: *Of feavers* (1684): page 47. See also chapters 17 and 18 for examples cited by Willis of the bite of the tarantula causing 'dancing', the sting of the torpedo causing paralysis, the roots of wild parsnip or seeds of lolium temulentum making men mad, and opium, mandrake, and henbane causing deep sleep; and *Of feavers* (1684): page 101.

[80] See: *Of feavers* (1684): page 60.

[81] See: *Of feavers* (1684): pages 75–6.

[82] See: Frank (1980): page 179 and endnote 112, chapter 7 for the comment that, in 1661, the year after receiving his Doctorate of Medicine, Willis defended a thesis on the role of the blood in intermittent fever.

[83] Since fever encouraged removal of abnormal ferments in the sweat, urine, and other evacuations, some physicians, such as Lower, were reluctant to interfere in the cycle of fever and natural depuration by using an antipyretic.

with his own readiness to open veins, bleeding is not to be recommended: 'those who have their blood well filled with a Volatile Salt, are less obnoxious to feavers: also hence those who often are let blood, are more apt to Feavers'. With a swipe at the Galenists, Willis regards the empirical remedies advocated by 'Quack-salvers and old Women' as no less useful than the 'Prescriptions of Physicians administered after the exact method of Curing', which he likens to the use of a 'Sword in a blind man's hand'.[84] But Willis has some general principles that resonate with therapeutic medicine across the ages: early treatment is more likely to succeed than rescuing advanced disease; combination of remedies is often required; and medicines can do more harm than good.

Of the intermittent fever

Willis describes several disorders characterized by fever.[85] Intermittent fever has specific symptoms: jaundice, scurvy with ulcerated lips, widely distributed pustules and skin lesions, inflammation and swelling of various parts, and cachexia. It is seasonal, a disease of the autumn, and of sea coasts. The periodicity reflects the extent to which fermentation is perturbed. The blood is changed chemically under the influence of local climatic conditions (cœli constitutio) interacting with a diet too rich in wine and meat. Together these 'roast' the blood, perverting the nutritious juice and leading to an excess of salt and sulphur. Tertian fever describes a cycle with fever on the third day which, when the bouts recur ten or twelve times, may end in death. With excessively acid blood, the fever is quotidian, either following a tertian pattern or from onset. Although such frequent fever encourages obstructions and tumours of the liver, intestines, and spleen, the situation is not hopeless and, with intense treatments, some quotidian fevers may be cured. An excess of salt and earth encourages fever with a slightly longer periodicity. These quartan fevers are more persistent and less easy to treat but may be tolerated 'so that the fits are suffered out of bed, and sometimes in a Journey, or being about any business'.

Willis's intermittent fever would now be called malaria. Apart from indicating that the condition was common in seventeenth-century England, Willis's account stands out for the description of treatment using quinine in the form of Peruvian bark: 'the use of the Powder, of a certain Bark, brought of late from the *Indies*, seems to give some faith, and approbation; which is said, most certainly, to cure this Disease'.[86] He describes the preparation of Peruvian Bark and its conversion from powder to pills, the dose to be used, and effects observed on the frequency and periodicity of fever so that people affected have 'procured frequent truces of the Quartan … [and] … liv'd chearful, lively and ready for any business … scarce one of an hundred, hath tried this medicine in vain'. Nonetheless the bark is not a cure—'the Enemy still, tho asleep'—and recovery only occurs when 'Nature has recollected herself' and the condition settles spontaneously, usually in the spring. The subject is considerably expanded in the Amsterdam (1669) edition of *Diatribæ duæ*. Willis reaffirms the principles

[84] See: *Of feavers* (1684): page 92.

[85] In addition to sources quoted in the text that follows, the most detailed overall analysis of Willis on fevers is provided by Isler (1968): pages 69–86, who makes the point that Willis's treatise has generally been ignored.

[86] See: *Of feavers* (1684): page 71. In this respect Willis anticipated Thomas Sydenham (1624–1689) who also wrote on Peruvian bark in his essay attached to the Amsterdam (1667) edition of Edmund O'Meara's diatribe against Willis. See: Isler (1968): pages 83–6 for a detailed comparison of priority in the works of Willis and Sydenham in which the point is made that, although not guilty of plagiarism, Sydenham borrowed many ideas first expressed in Willis's *De febribus* (1659), including the assumption that Peruvian bark suppresses fermentation, although the material that causes fever remains in the system and can periodically renew its activity.

of restoring correct chemical balance of the blood and nutrient humour, inducing an alternative type of fermentation that suppresses, for a while, the 'heaping up of Excrementitious matter or ... the Feaverish turgencies'. He is not shy about the discovery:[87]

> Therefore I promise more willingly to this Age, or at least to the next, when being led by the Analogy of this Book, I have found out a medicine, for the profligating of Feavers, of use not contemptible, if not being long since variously tried, which also I am wont to give to the poorer sort, instead of something else, with good success.

Peruvian bark reached Spain in 1632 and was much used in continental Europe with varying results. It became available in London late in 1658 for sale by James Thompson from his lodgings at the Black Spotted Eagle in the Old Bailey or from Mr John Crook, bookseller at the sign of the ship in St Paul's Churchyard.[88]

Of a putrid fever

Typically, a putrid fever goes through four phases for each of which Willis has an iatrochemical explanation. Onset dates from the moment at which excess sulphur allows the blood to overheat. The phase of augmentation results from further enkindling as the sulphur interacts with other heated particles. At its height, the fever 'like a noble Wrestler, when his Adversary is a little yielding, recollecting all his strength, endeavours a bringing under' causes the 'adust matter (as it were ashes remaining after a Fire)' to separate and the fever gradually to abate by crisis, usually every fourth day but sometimes longer. Examination of the pulse and urine can predict success of the crisis: the illness concluding, further cycles ensuing or 'Nature overthrown at the first conflict ... and yielding her powers is precipitated into death'. The stage of declination is marked by cooling of the blood, dominance of vital spirits over the extraneous matter, and reassimilation of nourishing juice so that blood ascends in the heart and the lamp of life is sustained.[89]

One of Willis's fullest accounts of a 'putrid fever' is considered to be a description of typhoid. The initial manifestations are shivering, fever, sweats, lassitude, thirst, and pains in the head and loins. This is due to imbalance of juices in the stomach with excess of bile delivered from the 'choleduct'. At this stage, enkindling is modest and the flame reduced as if made wet. The urine has sediments and is discoloured. Vomits, purges, and gentle bleeding may stave off further developments. But in young people, the corpulent, or if the season is hot, matters advance over the next week and the blood ferments like wet hay or dung so that the heat results in headache, pertinacious wakings, delirium, phrensie, and convulsions. The 'flux of the belly' leads to irritation of the intestines and intense diarrhoea. The crisis follows when 'Judgment is discerned between Nature and the Disease, the strife ending in aequilibrium'. The fever abates once heating of the blood is exhausted and the 'adust material'

87 See: *Of feavers* (1684): page 73.

88 This is John Crook[e] (fl.1638–1669), uncle of William Crooke who printed several of Willis's books, see chapter 3.

89 See: *Of feavers* (1684): pages 80–1 where Willis makes clear that this resolution is due to 'Nature, being tired with the plenty of matter, tries to shake off part of its burthen' rather than, as some claim, the crisis being due to 'the influence of the Moon, and Stars, to follow their Aspects, Quadrations, or Conjunctions ... or the direction of the Planets'.

disaggregated and expelled. If this cycle stalls, or is impeded, fever may recur and become continuous so that 'rarely a perfect cure succeeds after that time'.[90] In discussing the dysentery, Willis considers that coagulation of the blood 'unlocks the little mouths of the Arteries, and makes there little Ulcers, and exudations or flowings forth … like as when … Pustules and Inflammations break forth outwardly'.

Willis observed cholera and dysentery in London but, living in the relatively affluent area of St Martin's Lane, was not exposed to the epidemics in children from the poorer parts. His account is of sudden onset with vomiting and watery diarrhoea: 'within twelve hours [cases are] so miserably cast down by the tyranny of this disease that they seemed ready to expire … their breath was short and gasping; and indeed many of them that wanted either fit remedies or the help of physicians, died quickly of it'. Willis concludes that the condition is not infectious because it 'seized those who kept out of the way of the sick and spared those who attended them'. More generally, dysentery is most common in camps and prisons 'by reason of the stench of the places and the evil diet'.

Willis returns to this distemper in his account of purgatives in part 1 of *Pharmaceutice rationalis* (1674), describing two epidemics in more detail. 'The Flux of the Belly (which is wont to be called the *Diarrhœa*, or Dystenterie)' is best exemplified by the annual autumn epidemic of the '*London* Disease' characterized by the 'Griping of the Gutts … in the one the Stools are watry, and as it were clear with a sudden failing of strength, but the other bloody'. Between the '*Autumnal Æquinox*' (21–23 September) and early November in 1670, within twelve hours diarrhoea and vomiting reduced affected individuals to a state of fever and 'the Tyranny of this Disease, that with a weak and small Pulse, cold Sweat, short and thick Breath, they seemed just ready to dye'. And many did. The disease did not spread beyond the City of London, nor were those close to the sick necessarily affected. A further epidemic occurred in 1671 after an unseasonably cold winter and dry summer. Associated with intermittent fever, now it spread throughout England, producing 'an unwonted *Languor*, watching, *Vertigo*, and frequently a cruel Headache'. Especially in London, after cases languished for several weeks with 'almost twenty times a day to stool … both full of blood and cruel', the disease 'greatly raging did precipitate very many to the grave'. Dismissing the popular belief that these distempers arose from injudicious eating of summer fruits, but allowing that the weather and 'smoaky, thick constitution of the Air' had predisposed some to the dysentery, Willis concludes that the rapid debility and languor indicated draining of nervous and nutritious juices from solid organs with loss of these particles through the urine, skin, and intestines, or in the bloody diarrhoea itself.[91]

Of the plague

Outbreaks of the plague had occurred in the British Isles on several occasions in the three centuries before Thomas Willis started work as a physician. Paradoxically the restrictions on foreign travel and importation during the early years of the Restoration may have limited

[90] See: *Of feavers* (1684): pages 78–80, and 87. Isler (1968) cites the entirety of chapters IX and X, pages 77–89; Ralph H Major, *Classic descriptions of disease*, Illinois (1932): pages 179–81 identifies page 93 but has mistaken *Dr Willis's practice of physick* (1684) for *The remaining medical works* (1681) and named Basset, who was only responsible for *The London practice of physick* (1685), as the publisher.

[91] See: Thomas Willis, *Pharmaceutice rationalis*, part 1 (1674): pages 56–65; and Charles Creighton, *A history of epidemics in Britain*, volume 2, Cambridge (1891): page 772.

the number of outbreaks.[92] Willis explains that plague is a pestilential fever resulting from envenomed infection, airborne in the first instance but propagated by contagion, its severity, and rate of dissemination varying between epidemics. It follows famine and natural disasters such as earthquakes; and is promoted by outbreaks of other illnesses, especially smallpox or measles. Apart from the usual symptoms of fever, plague is characterized by boils, buboes, carbuncles, whelks, inflammations, and malignant pustules. Sulphur is 'outrageous' and the blood 'coagulates between the narrow Windings of the Vessels'. The flesh falls away, buboes in the glandules suppurate, and the whelks blister into 'black, blue and purple spots'.[93] Willis gives a brief account of the plague in Oxford during 1645. The outbreak was not severe and the worthy Dr Henry Sayer (nk):[94]

> A very Learned Physician, and happy in his Practice, many others refusing this Province, boldly visited all the sick, poor, as well as rich, daily administered to them Physick, and handled with his own hands their Buboes and virulent Ulcers, and so cured very many sick, by his sedulous though dangerous Labour.

Wisely, Dr Sayer protected himself from the sick by taking a large draught of sack before perambulating 'about the Borders of Death and the very Jaws of the Grave' and another slug once his work was done. As to treatment, Sayer used a vomit (emetic) of *crocus metallorum* followed by a sudorific to increase excretion. But his luck did not last long because Sayer was summoned to Wallingford Castle where the disease was raging and 'being so bold, as to lie in the same Bed with a certain Captain (his intimate Companion), who was taken with the Plague, [Sayer] quickly received the Contagion of the same Disease'. His previous skills were now of no avail to Dr Sayer and 'with great sorrow of the Inhabitants, nor without great loss to the Medical Science, he died of that Disease'. In his magisterial account of the plague, John Shrewsbury (1898–1971) pauses before launching into the dreadful outbreak of 1665 to give an account of poor Dr Sayer concluding that the doctor was 'naturally antipathetic to fleas' and so remained immune to the plague, probably dying of 'the old Irish "bed-sickness", in other words typhus fever' brought upon him by sleeping naked with the friend in whom he had induced vomiting and sweating, thus spraying the bedroom with infected droplets.[95]

As Dr Sayer discovered, outcome from the plague 'is chiefly committed to Nature' and 'Physick is the Midwife'. Yet the doctor has a role in 'prevention of this malignant Disease' and, if Medicines are not stay'd for some hours, no nor minutes ... Remedies gathered from art' may effect a cure. Prevention is a matter for the 'Republick, and belong to the Magistrate' in cleaning the streets of 'Filths, Dunghills, and all stinking things', providing wholesome food at public expense, burning all sulphurous matter, isolating the sick from the sound, and rapidly removing dead 'Carcasses and Household-Stuff'. Apart from these civil measures, the individual can help by attention to 'Labour, Meat, Drink, Sleep ... [and] ...Venus should be taken moderately'. The 'passions of the mind' should be contained by eschewing

[92] See: JFC Shrewsbury, *A history of bubonic plague in the British Isles*, Cambridge (1970) for the definitive account; and in particular pages 433–541 for details of epidemics in the seventeenth century after 1650. John Shrewsbury was professor of bacteriology at the University of Birmingham (1937–1963).

[93] See: *Of feavers* (1684): pages 106–8.

[94] See: *Of feavers* (1684): page 111; and Creighton (1891): pages 559–60.

[95] See: Shrewsbury (1970): pages 444–5.

fear and sadness. Amulets containing 'Arsenic, Quicksilver and the Powder of Toads and other Poisons' are to be worn about the neck.

Matters changed with the London plague of 1665. The onset was stuttering with the first cases developing during the winter of 1664 in St Giles-in-the-Fields. The illness erupted in May 1665 and raged until October. Estimates of mortality are unreliable but between one-fifth and one-third of the population died of all causes over a period of seven months, the considerable excess over the number expected being attributable to plague: 32 332 of 38 195 deaths in the city during the month from mid-August. The mortality for infected individuals was around 85%. Once the availability of consecrated ground was exhausted, bodies were buried in large communal pits dug outside the city boundaries. In the parish where Willis subsequently lived, there were 2883 plague burials or 60% of all deaths in 1665, equating to 17% of the resident population. Numbers were deliberately underreported or made clandestine in order to avoid the deprivations of isolation and almost certain death for those confined to living with the sick. The authorities set up 'pest-houses' to which infected individuals were moved in order to protect the population. Infected premises were quarantined for 40 days after which the house was marked with a white cross for a further 20 days whilst fumigation and airing took place. Those who could left the city for their personal safety, and because trading was suspended, but returned to resume commerce in October after which a second peak of deaths occurred in November. Through death and desertion, the streets were largely empty. Amongst the measures that were thought to protect from the plague were smoking tobacco, and sniffing disinfectants and other pungent odours. Fires were lit in the streets to cleanse the air.

Cases were described both within and outside London throughout 1666. The plague spread along the Thames Valley by riverine portage and approached Oxford in the summer. But the city was spared by the autumn frosts, despite the Earl of Clarendon (1609–1674) warning: 'Wee have reason to complayne of the ill government of the citty of London which for want of shuttinge up infected houses, hath skattered the contagion over the kingdom … God knows how longer we shall continue free, many villages aboute us being infected.'[96] Eventually the epidemic disappeared, not as has been suggested from the incineration of rats during the great Fire of 1666, but through spontaneous loss of virulence of *Pasturella pestis* and restriction on travel from continental Europe and the Levant.

Although, in 1659, Willis already had views on medicines designed to evacuate the poisons through one orifice or another—vomits, cathartics, diuretics, or sudorifics—and reduce fever,[97] his pharmacopoeia was refined in the treatise written in 1666 but published posthumously. *A plain and easie method* (1691) adds little to Willis's experience of the plague. He offers a number of prescriptions made up either from sulphur, liquid mercury, or iron filings. Two which Willis says his patients much appreciated are 'aqua limacum' and 'aqua lumbricorum', the slimy liquors of slugs and worms. It appears, however, that Willis had little faith in his prescriptions for the plague. In 1659, he invoked 'the help of the Omnipotent God being requested through prayers'; and in 1666, his advice is that 'wine and confidence are a good preservation against the plague.'[98]

[96] See: Shrewsbury (1970: page 530 and end note 1, page 620, citing Historical Manuscripts Commission, *Verulam* (*Gorhambury*) MSS, page 67.

[97] See: *Of feavers* (1684): pages 108–10.

[98] See: *Of feavers* (1684): page 110 and Thomas Willis, *A plain and easie method for preserving those that are well from the plague* (1691): page 28.

Camp fever

Willis's account of the pestilential fever ('febres pestilenentes ac malignæ in specie') or camp fever describes typhus among the Oxford troops (1643).[99] War typhus was well known in continental Europe but England had previously been spared.[100] The outbreak in Berkshire and Oxfordshire, in which the pestilential fever 'spread with lesser diffusion and lower frequency of burials than the plague', was the first to be described by a physician.[101] Willis relates that in the spring of 1643, the Earl of Essex, with 15 000 foot soldiers and 3000 horses, besieged Reading then held by the King. On entering the town after eleven days, Essex found it infected and many of his men, discontented at lack of pay and plunder, became unwell. Essex decamped to Thame but, with the weather wet and hot, the epidemic increased so that Essex thought better of moving on Oxford and suggested to Parliament that peace be sought with the Royalists. Willis observed matters from the Royalist perspective. In the event, both armies were affected and the disease proved more deadly than their military foes so that both sides fought:[102]

> Not with the Enemy, but with the Disease; as if there had not been leisure to turn aside to another kind of Death, this deadly disease increasing, they being already overthrown by Fate, and as it were falling down before this one Death.

Essex retreated to the banks of the Thames where the majority of his men perished. The King moved to Oxford and, living in the fields or town and villages, his army fared no better:

> For his Foot [soldiers] being pack'd together in close Houses, when they had filled all things with filthiness, and unwholsom nastiness, and stinking Odors (that the very Air seemed to be infected) they fell sick by Troops and as it were by Squadrons.

Civilians were affected: 'the Entertainers of the Soldiers' began to perish and around the summer solstice the fever started 'to lay hold on the Husbandmen, and others inhabiting the Country'. The sphere of the contagion was at least ten miles around the City. No one was spared in each house it entered so that, without care, 'those who were sick of this Feaver, were avoided by those who were well, almost as much, as if they had been sick of the Plague'.[103] The elderly and children were especially vulnerable. In some villages all the older people died so that oral traditions and customs were, at one blow, lost. Writing after the event, Willis reflected that:

[99] See: *Of feavers* (1684): pages 111–18; and Major (1932): pages 169–71 who again confuses his texts (see earlier note); and Ralph H Major, *Disease and destiny*, New York (1936): pages 51–2.

[100] See: Friedrich Prinzing, *Epidemics resulting from wars*, Oxford (1916): pages 25–78, for an account of war typhus in Europe during the seventeenth century and later.

[101] See: Creighton (1891) volume I: page 547 where in footnote 1 he cites *Diatribæ duæ*, The Hague (1659), as the first issue. Notwithstanding Major's confusion (see earlier), unlike most commentators Creighton uses *The remaining medical works* (1681) not *Dr Willis's practice of physick* (1684) as his reference text.

[102] See: *Of feavers* (1684): pages 114–15.

[103] See: *Of feavers* (1684): page 115. There is no reason to think that Willis coined the term 'avoid like the plague'. Most sources cite Saint Jerome (AD 345–420): '*Avoid, as* you would the *plague*, a clergyman who is also a man of business'. Under 'avoid', the Oxford English Dictionary points to Daniel Defoe (1660–1731) *A journal of the plague year* (1722): page 131, which, although referring to 1665, clearly post-dates Willis.

> I remember in some Villages, that almost all the old men died this year, that there were [not] any left who were able to defend the Manners and Privileges of the Parish, by the more anciently received Traditions.

More poignantly, Willis's father had earlier been one of the victims. Anthony Wood recalled that others who died included 'some belonging to the king's and queen's Court, with a few scholars'. The early manifestations were typical of fever but the 'adust matter' moved to the brain, 'the Sick keeping to their beds with raging sometimes, but more often with a stupefaction, with great Weakness, and sometimes with Convulsive Motions'. By the summer, people were erupting in 'Whelks and Spots ... little Blisters or measles, now small and red, now broad and livid: in many, Buboes (as in the Plague) about the Glandulas'. Those who survived became 'furibundous' and suffered 'most horrid Distractions of the Animal Spirits ... [with] ... benummedness of the Senses, Tremblings, Vertigo, Debility of Members, Convulsive Motions ... and divers other Distempers of the Head'. As the dog-days of summer advanced, the disease was considered a lesser plague and treated by 'Poison-resisting Remedies', alexiteriums, and the induction of sweats. The Countess of Kent devised a remedy, and a courtier staying in Oxford did well for himself by selling a powder the colour of ashes 'at a great price', which produced a mighty sweat when half a dram was taken with liquor. It turned out to be made of powdered toads, purged with salt, washed in good wine, and calcined in an earthy pot. Coincidentally, the epidemic waned during the autumn of 1643 and was gone by the winter.

For Willis, the weak pulse, blisters, and buboes indicated disordered coagulation and corruptive disorder of the blood; and in iatrochemical terms the condition could be attributed to excess sulphur and reduction of saline in the body. The more proximate causes were the combination of 'the Souldiers Camps ... imputed ... to their Nastiness and stinking Smells, but in some sort to a common Vice of the Air' encouraged by climatic conditions, the spring of that year being moist and 'slabbery, almost with continual shours' followed by a hot summer.

Sir Edward Greaves (1608–1680) corroborated much that Willis wrote, emphasizing that the putrid fever was not the plague 'as the relations and hopes of your enemies, and the fears of others, have suggested'. Taking as evidence the insidious onset as the summer advanced and the presence of skin lesions, he concluded: 'but what need we any farther signs than the spots, which appear upon half the number, at least, of those that fall sick?'[104] Greaves argued that Oxford may have afforded some 'divine immunity from the spread of infection'. He and Willis agreed that filth, dung, and carcasses of horses and carrion encouraged the condition by rendering the air pestilential. As with Willis's advice on the plague, Greaves was of the view that cleaning the streets would have done much to abate the epidemic. The brewers might also have helped by drying their malt, boiling their beer for longer, and adding more hops. Lest anyone doubt that the condition was contagious, Greaves recommended that they chance their luck and enter an infected household.

[104] See: Creighton (1891) volume I: pages 550–2 for details of Greaves's observations on the putrid fever as described in *Morbus epidemicus anni 1643; or the new disease*, Oxford (1643).

Of the measles and smallpox

Considered as malignant and pestilential fevers, Willis makes the prescient point that unlike others 'it happens for every man only, and once to be distempered with the Small Pox or Measles'.[105] Although highly contagious and erupting in a particular place 'from the disposition of the Air', and spreading rapidly through households or regions, the individual is predisposed to smallpox by abnormal ferment originating in the foetal blood. Willis hints at concepts that would now be termed acquired immunity and the importance of age-at-infection through the hygiene hypothesis: 'there is less danger if it should happen in the age of Childhood or Infancy'. The most obvious manifestations of the disease are the skin lesions, initially like 'Flea-bites then growing into Whelks', red as the blood seeks to expel the poison by sweats, then white and crusty scabs which eventually 'fall away from the flesh or next Skin'. Much is to be gleaned from following the evolution of these lesions in terms of colour and crusting in predicting the outcome, especially if the omens suggest that extrusion of the poison has been reversed and 'the Venom driven outwardly, is again called back inwardly'. In discussing details of the abnormal fermentation, unusually (but in line with his concept of congenital predisposition) Willis places this first in the 'Spermatick parts' after which the animal spirits, especially of the spinal marrow and then the blood, are involved. The episode of smallpox in Oxford during 1641 was not extensive 'yet most died of it'. When it recurred in the city in the autumn of 1654, the spread was more rapid 'yet very many escaped with them'.[106]

The Stuart descendants of James I (1566–1625) were blighted by smallpox. The Duke of Gloucester (1640–1660) and the Princess of Orange (1631–1660), children of Charles I, died of the disease in the first year of the Restoration, and the offspring of the Duke of York (James II) fared no better. The latter were the children who occasioned Willis to remark that the family was tainted by 'mala stamina vitæ' for which implied insult he was ostracised by the Royal family.[107]

Willis had less to say on measles. It is a disease of children and more mild in those who have already survived smallpox. The mechanisms are broadly similar in terms of foetal origin, contagion, and 'the malignant constitution of the Air'. However the whelks are smaller and do not suppurate. Most cases recover. 'The Measles are so much akin to the Small Pox that with most authors they have not deserved to be handled apart from them'.[108]

Of feavers of childbearing women

Willis discusses puerperal fever in detail: 'Vulgar Experience abundantly testifies, that the Feavers of Women lying-in are very dangerous'.[109] The problem lies in the overly fermented blood usually discharged in the 'Monthly Flowers'. During pregnancy, this ferment is usefully diverted to the needs of the foetus, and discharged following delivery by the lochia and afterbirth, and then in the milk of the breasts. The problem is that the milk cannot always handle

[105] See: *Of feavers* (1684): page 119. Having made this valid point, Willis then contradicts himself by stating that sometimes 'the sick have fallen into this Disease twice or thrice'.

[106] See: *Of feavers* (1684): page 121.

[107] See: Bishop Burnet, *History of his own time: from restoration of King Charles the Second to the treaty of peace at Utrecht in the reign of Queen* Anne, London (1857): page 154; and chapter 1 for other details.

[108] See: *Of feavers* (1684): page 123.

[109] See: *Of feavers* (1684): page 125.

'the envenomed taint impressed on the mass of the blood'. If breast milk remains suppressed despite suckling, impurities, 'livid and green, and this very stinking', are concentrated and compressed through descent of the now empty womb and accumulate in the blood. The situation is far worse if the woman is torn during labour or 'part of the Secundine, or After-Birth, a Mole or piece of Flesh, Clodders of Blood etc.' are retained. From this nidus of disease, the whole mass of blood is 'restagnated' and fever results. Alternatively, the nerve endings in the womb convulse and secondarily affect the brain, which is 'pierced, and its functions to be as it were overwhelmed' compelling the whole nervous stock 'into irregularities of motion'.[110]

There are three conditions to be considered. None are contagious. First, the 'milky feaver' occurs when the filtrate of chyle from the intestines through which the foetus is nourished is diverted to the breasts but the milk retained and so spills throughout the body promoting a putrid or malignant fever. It is usually mild, self-limiting, and helped by suckling or, if that fails, binding the breasts to prevent entry of the ferment. Next is the putrid fever of women in childbed (designated 'Puerperarum febris' in the 1660 edition of *De febribus*) which spares:[111]

> Poor people, Labouring Women, Country Women, and others accustomed to hard Labour, as also Viragoes, and Whores, which are brought to Bed clandestinely, bring forth without any great difficulty, and then, after a little time, leaving their Beds, return to their wonted Labours. But more rich Women ... are subject to difficult and dangerous chances.

The reason is twofold. Exercise and effort in those who work 'agitate and eventilate' the blood, resulting in these women having their nervous parts more firm and so less prone to hysteria. Conversely, women of more delicate and idle disposition tend to have more agitated blood during pregnancy and with 'the system of the nerves, and the brain soft and weak ... suffer distractions of the animal spirits, and inordinate motions of the nervous parts'. Altogether a more serious condition than the milky fever, the putrid fever rarely resolves through an early crisis so that the adust matter swamps the brain and nervous stock; and with 'a phrensie, or, not seldom a stupefaction, and speechlessness ... the sick are suddenly precipitated to death'. Particularly ominous is the appearance of purple spots 'which argue no light Malignity'. As for treatment, 'the Physician having first made a prognostication of Death, may insist upon a few Remedies ... [but] ... such administrations beget only an odium or blame, that by so doing, we are esteemed by some Women, as wicked and cruel'.[112] Finally, the symptomatic feavers of women in childbed comprise those situations in which one or other of the regular putrid, malignant, or pestilential fevers occurs in, and is complicated by, the puerperium. Ferments which should be discharged from the womb are taken to 'nests of these [other] diseases' where the blood congeals rendering them 'more hard to be cured'.

Willis warns his readers that the recital of case histories will be mournful because these fevers are usually fatal due, most often, to disturbance of the animal spirits and affections of the brain and nervous stock. By way of example, soon after delivery of her sixth child, a 26-year-old gentlewoman develops fever with headache and confusion, 'phantasms in her head whenever her eyes were closed, clamped teeth, pricking and numbness in her whole body, palsy of the tongue and throat preventing speech and swallowing', so that increasingly breathless 'she knew not them about her [and] on the eighth day she died'.[113] In recounting

[110] See: *Of feavers* (1684): page 127.

[111] See: *Of feavers* (1684): page 129; and R Hierons, 'Willis's contributions to clinical medicine and neurology', *Journal of the neurological Sciences* 1967; 4: 5.

[112] See: *Of feavers* (1684): page 133.

[113] See: *Of feavers* (1684): page 135.

this and other cases and speculating on the cause, Willis attributes much to the diet: too much chicken, fruit, 'and any unwholesome trash' being particularly risky.

Of epidemical feavers

It will be clear to the modern reader that many of the conditions Willis described were restricted in time and place, although they may have recurred. They are contagious and therefore infectious. Willis described outbreaks of fever in the autumn of 1657 and the spring and autumn of 1658 that are considered to provide one of the earliest accounts of the epidemiology of infectious disease. As with other fevers, Willis attributed these epidemics to combination of the climate and predisposition of the people, with lesser influence from 'the particles of the Aire which we breathe'. The assumption is that he was describing influenza.[114]

The summer of 1657 was extremely hot and dry. From 1 July, a few cases of intermittent fever were noticed in villages and towns. Those affected sweated, vomited, and had diarrhoea. They remained languid and restless between bouts of fever which followed a tertian periodicity, although sometimes continuous, and associated with delirium, cramps, and convulsions. Called the 'new Disease', by August 'it became epidemial throughout all England ... [and] ... crept from house to house, infected with the same evil, most of the same Family, and especially those familiarily conversing with the sick; yea, old Men, and Men of ripe age, it ordinarily took away'.[115] However, even in those with persistent distemper and continuous fever, 'scarce one of a thousand died, which I scarce ever knew in an Epidemical Synochus'. Willis was not alone in observing this 'new disease', although other commentators including Sydenham and Samuel Pepys (1633–1703) put a different emphasis on their accounts. Consistent features were youth, a spotted fever, 'chiefly infestous of the brain and nervous stock', and significant mortality but with the possibility of recovery.[116]

By contrast, the winter of 1657 was cold with snow covering the ground from the ides of December (13) to the vernal equinox (between 19 and 21 March). The north wind blew mercilessly until June so that 'the Season was more like Winter than Spring'. Fever developed in April and 'in some Towns, in the space of a Week, above a thousand People fell sick together' with 'a troublesome Cough, with great spitting, also a Catarrh falling down on the Palate, Throat and Nostrils', fever, and lassitude. Although those 'indued with an infirm Body, or men of a more declining Age' died, the illness was often not so severe as to interrupt daily affairs, and most recovered. The epidemic settled after six weeks during which Willis estimated that a third of the population was affected. His view was that, in combination with a greater than usual 'effervescency of the blood' in the spring, the constant north wind had closed the pores and restricted sweating of the adust matter, like new wine shut up in closed bottles.[117]

[114] See: *Of feavers* (1684): pages 137–52; and Creighton (1891) volume I: pages 568–77.

[115] See: *Of feavers* (1684): page 138.

[116] Creighton, volume 2 (1891): page 7 offers a long list of diagnoses: 'as nearly as may be the signs of infantile remittent fever, or worm fever, or febris synochus puerorum, or hectica infantilis, or febris lenta infantum, or an acute fever with dumbness ... [later described by] Dr William Butter of Lower Grosvenor Street in 1782'. At page 9 and 13, Creighton quotes from Pepys: 'among others the famous Tom Fuller (1608–1661) [of the Worthies of England] is dead of it; and Dr (Mathew) Nichols [Nicholas] (fl 1660–61) Dean of St Paul's; and my Lord General Monk (1608–1670) is very dangerously ill'; and Pepys gives an account of the illness of Katherine of Portugal (Braganza: 1638–1705) married to Charles II who was affected, in October 1663, with spotted fever 'as of a leopard', raving and delirious with hallucinations of her unborn children but, after six weeks, 'the queen ... is become well again'.

[117] See: Willis, *Of feavers* (1684): pages 144–6.

The fever of autumn 1658 followed another hot summer and was broadly similar to the 1657 epidemic. 'It spread chiefly in the Villages, in lesser Towns, and the Country, when Cities and greater Towns, were less troubled' so that people moved to London in order to be spared.[118] Spots similar to measles were usual but most of the manifestations could be attributed to the overheated blood, rich in adust recrements and feaverish Matter ... continually poured on the Brain'. Starting with fever and severe headache:[119]

> Old men, melancholic or otherwise sickly persons ... became ... stupefied and for the most part vertiginous ... they were very unquiet, and still tossing about, oftentimes they talked idly and at random ... their strength became exceedingly cast down they were wholly fixt to their Beds, or rise only for a little while, could scarce stand or set a foot before another, to move from place to place, or able to walk; they laboured with a languishment, a difficult breathing, a nummeddness of the senses, and a great debility of the whole nervous stock ... to which also, contractures of the Tendons, and convulsive Motions of the wrists ... those who declined towards death ... lay for the most part without speaking, or knowing those about them, as it were stupid; and it rarely hapned in this Feaver that anyone about to die, was so perfect in their Memory and Intellect as to dispose of their Family-Affairs, or to take leave of their Friends. But it hapned to those that escaped ... not quickly or suddenly to recover ... but lying a long while wavering, stupefied and without strength, that Nature at length ... got indeed the better of the Disease, and then recovered ... by degrees, and health lingeringly and slowly.

The brain and nervous stock

As will already be clear, many of the conditions that Willis described were considered to have disturbed the animal spirits and affected 'the Brain and Nervous stock'.[120] The essential features were neurological symptoms, cough, and expectoration, and swollen glands. Willis devotes most of Chapter VIII of *Pathologiæ cerebri* (1667) to one such epidemic.[121] His account is reminiscent of that given for earlier periodic fevers with respect to the season and emergence of a 'new disease'. Again, the fever arose after a hot summer (1661), wet autumn, mild

118 Although not described by Willis, this tactic was of no avail to Oliver Cromwell (1599–1658) who became sick with the 'bastard tertian' fever at Hampton Court on 21 August and was taken to Whitehall where he languished for a few days and died on 3 September 1658.

119 See: Willis, *Of feavers* (1684): page 148.

120 The temptation retrospectively to diagnose these illnesses might best have been resisted. On somewhat insecure evidence, Dewhurst (1983): page viii accepts the opinion of Donald Bates, 'Thomas Willis and the epidemic fever of 1661: a commentary', *Bulletin of the History of Medicine* 1965: 39; pages 393–414, that the epidemic fever of 1661 was encephalitis lethargica. This is repeated by JD Spillane, *The doctrine of the nerves*, Oxford (1981): page 59 and endnote 43, chapter 3, in turn citing FG Crookshank *Influenza: essays by several authors*, London 1922: page 88 who describes this as epidemic encephalitis 'whereby men were grievously affected in their brains and nervous stock ... soporiferous epidemical fever in a ploughman taken ill at his plough who slept for days but recovered ... an Oxford gardener who drowsed for days and was foolish for two months but eventually recovered but never with the same vigour'. In his original edition, Leslie Morton, *A medical bibliography*, London (1943): page 256, #4013 (renumbered #4673, text unaltered, in the most recent printed edition, 1991), calls Willis's description of the 1661 'fever of the brain' the first description of cerebrospinal fever (meningococcal meningitis). If so, the recovery in a significant number of cases without specific therapy is remarkable. Hierons (1967): pages 1–2, citing cases from *De febribus*, *Cerebri anatome*, and *De anima brutorum* also attributes the epidemic described by Willis in autumn 1658 to meningitis.

121 See: Thomas Willis, *Pathologiæ cerebri, et nervosa generis specimen in quo agitur de morbis convulsivis, et de scorbuto* (1667): pages 95–113; and *An essay of the pathology of the brain and nervous stock: in which convulsive diseases are treated of* (1684): pages 46–54.

winter, and early spring in the following year. Most of the cases had continuous fever but sometimes this was intermittent. The individuals seen by Willis were mostly children or adolescents who presented insidiously with loss of appetite and lassitude followed within a few days by neurological symptoms. The children lapsed into 'deep stupidity or Insensibility', their 'knowledge and Speech failed' and, with incontinence, they remained ill for several weeks during which they were reduced 'to the highest *Atrophie*, or wasting of all parts'. When older people were affected the outlook for survival from the convulsions, diarrhoea, and dehydration, 'reduced to the leanness of a *Sceleton*', and severe catarrh with discharging swollen glands in the neck or weeping pustules elsewhere, was poor: 'those who were before obnoxious to cephalic distempers, as the *Lethargie*, *Apoplexie*, or Convulsion, it oftentimes kill'd them in a short space'. Several of the fatal cases underwent autopsy: [122]

> In one child the meninges were black and purple 'sprinkled in very many places with extravasated blood ... the rine or bark being taken off [the substance of the brain] was ... watered above measure with a watery humour ... [and] all the ventricles were full of a limpid or clear water ... more than half a pinte.

Treatments were usually not effective. Nor was this surprising: 'all distempers of the brain and nerves, as it were making a mock at medicines, are most difficulty cured'. Notwithstanding this wisdom, Willis proceeds to describe his use of catharticks, diureticks, sudorificks, cardiacks, clysters, and phlebotomy.

This epidemic reminded Willis of a family seen in 1653 with the pestilent feaver.[123] Five children were affected with an illness he recalls as starting with headache, sleepiness, 'mighty Stupefaction', and fever. The first child developed spots 'like Flea-bites', became incontinent, and by the fourteenth day could neither speak nor understand. At first 'what was put in his Mouth, though unknowingly' was swallowed but later he developed 'a Palsie of the Tongue and Throat'. Remarkably the child was fitted with 'an Instrument of a Pin of Chalk, put into a little pliant Wand, and on the top of it a little tuft of Silk ... and this being thrust down his throat, opened the closing for a time whereby the Food was taken in'. Although wasted and skeletal, by 'prudent Care of the Mother about his Diet, he recovered perfect Health, and is yet living, and well'. Meanwhile, on 14 January, his brother developed the same illness and, with 'his belly tumid like a Tympany, and mightily distended', died with convulsions on the fourteenth day. On 13 February, a third brother became ill and although at first apparently less severely affected, he bled from the nose and eventually 'fell into a Lethargy' and lay for three days 'as it were Apoplectick', dying on the thirteenth day. The family must have dreaded what came next when the only female child became ill with fever and 'a painful tension or stretching out of the Muscles of her Neck', heavy and somnolent, 'also petechial red spots (as in the rest) were conspicuous'. Mercifully, she recovered after Willis gave her spirit of hartshorn and a spoonful of cordial julep. The remaining brother was also affected but recovered as did 'many other Domesticks, and some strangers coming to help them' over the next four months, all of whom seem to have survived.

Three months after delivery, a woman, aged 30, developed a fever followed after six days by numbness and a sense of pricking in the extremities, especially the feet, legs, and thighs, associated with abdominal distension. The 'sense of bulk' rose across the abdomen and chest 'and thence to the Brain' so that she was 'weakened in her Intellectuals' and lay talking

[122] See: *Of convulsive diseases* (1684): page 51.
[123] See: *Of feavers* (1684): pages 116–18.

extravagantly and idly. The sense of pricking as if 'stung with Nettles' persisted and she became delirious, 'houling and crying out' then lying without speech or motion. This pattern lasted a further three days during which she was 'tormented with convulsive motions about the tendons of the muscles'. On the tenth day, she drew her breath deep and 'about the middle of the night died'.[124]

Other fevers

The chin-cough (now designated whooping cough) is described by Willis as preliminary to phthisis and as a convulsive or suffocating disorder of children and infants. It is seasonal, being most frequent in spring and autumn, and epidemic. Respiration is laboured, painful, and suspended for long periods so that the diaphragm convulses and, neither inspiring nor expiring, prevents the vital breath from being drawn. Coughing being strangled, the children hoop and, with blood stagnating, go black in the countenance and struggle until they faint.[125]

Scurvy

At first glance, *De scorbuto* might be considered the only treatise that Willis devotes to a single disease. Published in 1667 together with *De morbis convulsivis*, there are no internal clues exactly as to when this treatise was written. It may have been an older text that Willis wanted to make available during the decade in which he was mainly preoccupied with the nervous system. That 'On the scurvy' has much on the brain and nervous stock does not distinguish this treatise from the three published in 1659 on fermentation, fevers, and urines. Willis's citations to other authors omit mention of his contemporaries and developments made during the 1660s. The tract belongs more naturally to the earlier period of his professional life when Willis may have concluded that the scurvy was a suitable condition through which to illustrate his emerging formulation on fermentation in disease.

Not only the plethora of symptoms but also the case histories within the main text and those that form chapter XI make clear that Willis lumps many different conditions within his concept of the scurvy. It is a good example of the danger in applying modern medical nomenclature to the descriptions of an earlier period. But from the features described, some not mentioned in the context of any other condition, it is clear that within Willis's cluster of disorders described as the scurvy are examples of vitamin C deficiency.

Willis explains that the scurvy is not a new disease but one that is now increasingly well recognized, especially in children. Protean in its manifestations, any disorder 'never before heard of in an humane Body' which cannot be classified is often designated as scurvy: 'so that this Disease, like one condemned, and of an evil Name, suffers for others faults'.[126] The cause is multifactorial. Scurvy is linked to the sea and common in houses near any marine coast or surrounded by a moat or pond. This is explained by the 'humid Air, continually diffusing

[124] See: *Of feavers* (1684): pages 96–8.

[125] See: Thomas Willis, *Pharmaceutice rationalis*, part 2 (1679): page 40; and *Pharmaceutice rationalis*, part 2 (1684): page 38.

[126] See: Thomas Willis, *A tract of the scurvy* (1684): pages 169–70.

filthy ... stinking ... exhalations and infection'. The disease is hereditary in that the children of sickly parents are affected, just as are 'the Children of Parents touched with the venereal Disease ... obnoxious to the most grievous symptoms', in both cases the 'filthy taint being impressed on the genital humour'. Melancholy and sadness are predisposing factors. A diet rich in meat, especially if smok'd or cured, and shellfish encourages the scurvy as a result of those foods being depraved in the stomach, especially when mixed with the pancreatic juice. Conversely, milk, cheese, and fruit are protective.

The consensus is that scurvy starts with imperfect removal of waste from the bowel, the admixture with faeculencies interfering with fermentation of the blood. But Willis prefers an interpretation that accommodates respiration and circulation of the blood, the contagion occurring when the 'effluvia ... from an infected Body' enter through the pores or breath.[127] As to the mechanism, since scurvy is so difficult to eradicate it must involve chronic imbalance of the particles. Too much sulphur causes excess heat through deposition of its surplus. Too much salt 'stuffs the Viscera in its passages', silts the circulation, and interrupts fermentation and removal of waste. Scurvy may be the consequence of prolonged fever, the blood becoming 'lixivial' (alkaline) due the accumulation of sulphur and salt, thereby failing to be enkindled in the heart and circulated. Ultimately, dyscrasia of the blood corrupts the formation and function of the nervous juice so that the late manifestations of scurvy relate mainly to affections of the brain and nervous stock. Nonetheless, a regional tour of the body parts reveals other manifestations.[128]

At first there is weariness and heaviness in the limbs, fever, and night sweats, and bleeding from the 'Nose, the Fundament, Reins, Thorax, Gums and other places'. In the chest, dry cough and dyspnoea (with the breathing caught 'now of Systoles now of Diastoles like to asthmatick Paroxysms') results from the impoverished enkindling of the blood and its stagnation in the heart. Movements of the diaphragm and chest wall fail as the nervous spirit starts to degenerate. A rapid and irregular pulse occurs because of 'straightness' in the thorax and præcordium. Swoonings and 'fear of the same' are due to 'the cardiack Nerves ... beset with a morbifick matter'. In the abdomen, nausea, vomiting, and colic are associated with diarrhoea and, eventually, swelling of the stomach and hypochondrium leading to ascites and loss of weight. This is because the chyle is 'not rightly cook'd neither is it soon enough or sufficiently born through the milky Vessels'. Furthermore, 'the impurities admitted, from the bloody Mass, drop out from the little mouths of the Arteries, wherefore the things excreted are more copious than those put in'.

Typical of the scurvy is bleeding and ulceration of the gums, 'stinking in the Mouth', and loose teeth.[129] This is because, other routes of elimination being overcome, the salivary glands through which waste can be removed are overcome by the salty and mercurial (sulphurous) particles in the blood which coat the mouth with a 'whitish Scurf' and destroy the flesh of the gums. The skin suffers from excess waste in the sweat and this manifests as spots, whelks, tumours, pimples, and ulcers: 'pathognomick signs of the Scurvy'. The spots—'now Citron colour, now Dark, now Purple, and sometimes appear livid blewish or black'—are 'the bigness of a Penny, and often as big as a Shilling'. Caused by the impurities of the blood trying to escape, 'neither are they altogether forsaken by the Blood, but that the Blood

[127] See: *Of the scurvy* (1684): pages 173–4 for Willis's rehearsal of opinions held by the ancient authors who formulated their ideas before Harvey's demonstration of circulation of the blood.

[128] See: *Of the scurvy* (1684): page 179. As with all Willis's writings, there is much repetition within the eleven chapters of this treatise.

[129] See: *Of the scurvy* (1684): pages 182–3.

passing by adds to them others and new particles'. The sweats being unable to cope, sores form or noxious material returns to the blood, further contaminating it and seeking exit by other routes such as expired air. To these visible signs of the scurvy can be added examination of body fluids. In the absence of jaundice, the red or citron alkaline urine with sediments 'pronounce[s] a sign of scurvy'. At other times the urine is 'limpid, clear, and thin, and in abundance' because watery recrements pass directly from the lymph ducts to the kidneys, bypassing the circulating blood.

Willis devotes chapter IV to an account of the effects of scurvy on the brain and nervous stock: 'the locomotive power flags … the sick loving idleness and ease, shun exercises and labors of the Body, go about unwillingly any Task, and presently being weary give it off'.[130] There follow light spasms or twitches, cramps, and pains that anticipate 'horrid and grievous Affections'. There is weakness of the limbs because the nervous spirit no longer reaches the extreme parts: 'so I have known some, who have had a hand or foot wholly enfeebled … whilst the arm or thigh, with the rest of the Body was well'. Sensation is affected: 'a benummedness, and a sense of stinging, tingling or pricking'. These symptoms apart, severe pains in 'the Belly, Loyns, Thighs, Sternum, or Chest, and in the Head' are common. Discomfort in the legs occurs chiefly at night so that those with 'an inveterate Scurvy as soon as ever they are warm in their beds, are wont to endure intolerable torments … so that they cry out their flesh is gnawn, or torn in pieces like the biting of Dogs: these tortures if they leave their bed do somewhat abate'. Such a symptom is readily explained by the gravitational accumulation of excess recrements in dependent parts. The headache is due to:[131]

> Humours poured on the Meninx or Films in wrapping the Brain … for the Skulls of some of the dead being opened, I perceived both the membranes grown together, and every where set thick with little Whelks, and scirrhous tumors, which kind of tumors and concretions seem to have risen from the mutual coagulations of the two-fold painful humour.

Depending on which particular corpuscular particle is in excess at any one time, salt or sulphur, the effects on the brain are pain, palsy, vertigo, spasms, tremblings, and shaking or even 'outrageous assaults, like the falling sickness'. But this is not all. Later manifestations of scurvy include disorders of sleep, insomnia, or the wakings, 'stupidness', madness and moping, all culminating in stupor and coma: 'when I have opened such who were overwhelmed with perpetual sleep, I have found the Brain dry enough and altogether free from a Dropsie, or serous Colluvies … with which lethargic persons are wont for the most part to be affected'.[132] Even this catalogue of catastrophes is not the end. For when the abnormally fermented blood is combined with poverty of the nervous juice, there follows 'those great and Herculean Diseases, to wit, the assaults of the Apoplexie and Epilepsy, which sometimes happen to scorbutical Persons'.

The 'double Stock' (fermented blood and impoverished nervous juice) is also associated with marasmus, rheumatism, gout, and swollen joints, flitting from one to another or several at any time. The blood leaves its morbid deposits like the 'Eggs of Fishes, or as the feminine

[130] See: *Of the scurvy* (1684): pages 184–8.

[131] See: *Of the scurvy* (1684): page 186. Citing Thomas Willis, *Two discourses concerning the soul of brutes* (1683): page 123, Hierons (1967): at page 2 concludes that Willis described tuberculous meningitis, of which this case would appear to be one example. More generally, within the plethora of manifestations, any physician will recognize in Willis's description of scurvy the separate features of vitamin C deficiency, beriberi, restless legs syndrome and, perhaps, tuberculosis.

[132] See: *Of the scurvy* (1684): page 187.

Seed'; and arrival of the complementary nervous juice contributing 'the masculine Seed, rendering them fertil', is heralded by premonitory headache, restlessness, and pains. At this stage, and until the illness settles in the various body parts, scurvy is potentially treatable with antiscorbuticks. The condition carries a better prognosis than disorders in which the same symptoms occur for other reasons.[133]

When *De scorbuto* (1667) was translated as part of the project to make all his writings available in English, Samuel Pordage included *On the scurvy* with the two parts of *Pharmaceutice rationalis* (1679). This was logical since, after describing the symptoms, antecedent causes, and mechanisms of the blood dyscrasia, Willis devotes chapters VII–X (22 of 49 pages) to symptomatic treatments and cure of the scurvy.[134] The treating physician can proceed with cautious optimism because 'for very many (as have fallen under our observation) esteemed desperate have grown well'. The illness does not progress rapidly but, equally, cure takes time. However, scurvy following prolonged chronic fever, with involvement of the brain and nervous stock, or in patients who do not comply by moderating their diet, has a less favourable outlook; and when 'at length it induces a Dropsie or Consumption, the next passage then is to Death'. There are three strands to Willis's management: symptomatic therapies, surgical interventions, and alterations in diet.

The medicines used to effect a cure are purges, diaphoretics, diuretics, and digestives—given alone, in sequence, or in combination—as electuaries, confections, powders, pills, or lozenges. These increase the excretion of bilious and melancholy recrements forming in the lymph ducts, spleen, and gall bladder. The waste escapes through the pores, kidneys, and intestines, preventing their accumulation in the blood and brain. The respiratory and 'asthmatical paroxysms' require 'Cardiacks', foremost amongst which are Hartshorn (ammonium carbonate): but 'I never found a more ready Remedy than 10 or 12 drops of our tincture of opium, Laudanum'. This is also recommended for the dropsy. The use of opiates is a consistent theme running across Willis's symptomatic treatments. For the abdominal symptoms, a vomitary is used with rhubarb or cream of Tartar added, Epsom or Barnet waters,[135] topical application of foments, and the use of clysters. Chalybeate medicines are best for haemorrhages of the nose, 'menstrual flux', lungs or ventricle (stomach). For the 'vices of the Mouth', nothing other than washes and 'Gargarisms' are to be used with cleansing of the sockets using rags daubed in Egyptian ointment when the teeth fall out. Pain is treated with diaphoretics and diuretics, as is the rheumatism. The wandering gout is best managed by applying earthworms or their extracts as 'Sal Armoniack' (ammonium chloride) to offset the lixivial state with acid. In several of these situations, removal of the recrements by leeching, often best applied to the fundament, or repeated letting of small amounts of venous blood may help. For the vertigo, the treatment is unspecified 'Cephalick remedies'. On convulsions and paralysis, Willis is equally reticent and refers readers to the text of *Pathologiæ cerebri* but adding that 'we intend shortly to make publick some special

[133] See: *Of the scurvy* (1684): page 188.

[134] See: *Of the scurvy* (1684): pages 191–213.

[135] The Barnet Society website mentions that in 1586 William Camden (1551–1623) described the 'medicinal spring which is of great service to the sex where there is general languor, difficult respiration, febrile heat, and loss of appetite. In all colds and fevers and rheumatic complaints, the Barnet whey is much recommended'. In 1652, it was reported that 'There is lately found at Barnet ... an excellent purging water. It springs from a nitre mine and half the quantity works as effectively as that of Epsom. It is much approved of by several eminent physicians'. In 1664, Samuel Pepys rode from London 'to see the wells ... and drunk three glasses and went and walked, and came back and drunk two more. The woman would have had me drunk three more; but I could not, my belly being full—but this wrought me very well; and so we rode home ... and my waters working at least seven or eight times upon the road, which pleased me well'.

Disquisitions thereupon: In the meantime it is not fit, that we should in this place forestall the therapeutick Method'.[136]

As something of an afterthought, 'the cure and reason of which being omitted in the former Pathology', is the symptom of 'Cracking of the Bones'. This is assumed to result from the grating of joints on movement of the limbs or spine through loss of the interstitial 'Fat, Membranes and Ligaments' so that 'their junctures even as millstones, being altogether emptied by reason of their mutual rubbing together, make a noise'. But this is not so for the crackling is actually due to:[137]

> Dryness of the Bones or a defect of the medulla or marrow ... which [normally] thus moistened may become less brittle ... wherefore the heads of the Bones being destitute of this marrow, make a noise like to the wheel of a Cart that is seldom greas'd ... for the reason ... the Bones themselves ... cannot receive sufficiently the Balsam destinated for them.

On the futility of treatment for this manifestation of the scurvy, Willis has to confess that 'the same Distemper [is] altogether mocking and eluding the skill and pains of the Physician'. He describes a patient so inflicted with scorbutic affection of the bones that he lived miserably for several years but eventually 'he married, and as to the rest of the common Symptoms of the Scurvy became better'. Willis does not make the connection between this happy conjugal event and possible improvements in diet but it is significant that for each of the specific symptomatic remedies he usually adds the advice to give some 'anti-Scorbutick liquor'.

Thus the mainstay of Willis's strategy for curing the scurvy is a diet with 'Rinds of Oranges, Limons and Citrons' and nuts; or, preferably, infusions made from fruits, scurvygrass, or brooklime, watercress, or sorrel, used fresh since they lose their anti-scorbutical potency through boiling.[138] Fresh meat is good but flesh that is cured, pickled, candied, or preserved is to be shunned. As for sugar, it is:[139]

> So plentifully taken in ... it is very likely that from its daily use, the Blood and the Humours are rendered salt and sharp, and from thence Scorbutick. A very famous Author hath attributed the cause of the English Phthisick, or Consumption, to the immoderate use of Sugar among our country men, and I know no reason, but that I may rather think the increase of the Scurvy derives it self from this enkindling'.

Those accustomed to swilling a large morning draught of beer on waking should abstain until dinner, and plenty of exercise and labour are recommended, if the scurvy is effectively to be treated.

On individual cases,[140] Willis describes a gentlewoman, tall and handsome, aged 25 years who moves through the many scorbutic stages to a state of paralysis in which 'she could

[136] See: *Of the scurvy* (1684): page 208. This reference, presumably to *De anima brutorum* (1672), may place the writing of *De scorbuto* closer to its date of publication (1667) rather than being a text held over from the 1650s, although the brief promotion may have been added to an earlier work.

[137] See: *Of the scurvy* (1684): pages 210–11.

[138] See: *Of the scurvy* (1684): page 210. Scurvygrass is a brassica, *Cochlearia* species, also called spoonwort; brooklime or European speedwell, *Veronica beccabunga*, is a succulent herb which grows on the margins of streams and ditches.

[139] See: *Of the scurvy* (1684): page 212. Willis might well have been writing in 2021 of diabetes mellitus (type 2).

[140] See: *Of the scurvy* (1684): pages 213–18.

neither bend her hand or foot or any other part, nor move one jot from the place'. She is brought to Oxford and given every conceivable medicine for scurvy and paralysis, together with 'mercurial Medicine', after which 'she grew perfectly well and ... became the joyful Mother of several Children'. A man aged 40 has the typical manifestations of scurvy which respond to anti-scorbutick and anti-spasmodick remedies but relapses with dropsy spreading from the legs. He improves again with anti-scorbuticks, cathartics, and diuretics but returns a few months later with headache and many other symptoms indicating distemper of the brain, requiring prolonged treatment with anti-scorbutick medicines. Eventually he recovers. After childbirth, a lady of 25 years, of a fair skin and beautiful, develops scurvy and takes to her bed for a month. Later she develops acute pain in her left groin and calf and 'a hard tumour resisting the touch possessed all that space'. Finding her gasping for breath, Willis administers a clyster and laudanum despite which it seems as if she will expire for want of breath. She remains in this parlous state for some weeks and survives, despite developing identical pain and swelling of her right leg, Willis taking credit for having dispersed the stagnated blood in each limb and her lungs through treating the scurvy.[141] A noble gentleman, who lived immoderately, studied too much, and spent the whole night dancing, becomes unwell and gradually develops symptoms of the scurvy including perturbations of the head and nervous stock. There is little response to medicines including anti-Scorbuticks, nor is he helped by the 'Empiricks and Quacks'. The waters of Alstrop not suiting him, the gentleman is 'carried to the sulphureous waters at Knaresborough, but with what success I have not as yet learned'. This passage is printed on a page in *De scorbuto*, which is cancelled. Both versions of the variant text are available. Pordage's translation is closer to the cancellans than the cancellandum:[142]

> This Noble Person being often kept by business or more serious Studies even till Midnight, was wont to sup at that time, and presently to go to bed to sleep: Further, this Disease did partly arise from a sickly disposition of the Spleen, and perhaps other Viscera, supplying the Blood with a morbid ferment, neither is it altogether without reason, that we judge the Spleen should be accused.

Willis's purpose in relating the case is to show that lifestyle had rendered this fast-living scholar vulnerable to flooding of the brain with abnormal ferments, partly 'Narcotick, partly explosive'. Unable to escape through other pores, these cause 'Phlogosis or inflammation of the Face', after which there is falling down of the ferment to the 'Origin of the Nerves' and spinal marrow. Eventually the morbific material passed 'through into the anterior Brain or the regal Palace of the Soul ... the original of the nervous wandring pair, and the intercostal ... [and] being carried into the Brain itself, it possessed its more Noble cells'. Apart from waxing lyrical on the brain, Willis uses his analysis to argue that the abdominal symptoms of the scurvy are secondary to disordered function of nerves that move the stomach and related viscera (the wandring nerve) and not, as had been thought, a process starting with retained faeculent material that contaminates the blood and promotes abnormal fermentation. Willis concludes with a list of medicines to be avoided in managing the scurvy and those that he does recommend. Significantly, for each, 'with which Antiscorbuticks may be mixed'.

[141] Lest there should be confusion for those not trained in medicine, post-partum deep venous thrombosis, and pulmonary embolism are common after prolonged periods in bed and not infrequently prove fatal.

[142] See: *Of the scurvy* (1684): pages 216–17; and chapter 7 for further details.

It could be said that, in making the diagnosis of scurvy, Willis confused many different conditions, his remedies were no less inspired than any others favoured by countryfolk, and chance led him to favour fresh fruit and vegetables in curing some cases. But against that must be said that he emphasized disorder of the gums and teeth, and singled out both poor diet as a cause and citrus fruit as a solution to the problem.[143]

Fermentation and urine

Because excretion was fundamental to Willis's concept of fermentation in health and disease, it made sense that his treatise on urines was published as a third work alongside the *Diatribæ duæ* on fermentation and fevers. This is the least commented upon of all his writings but it is a pioneering work on biomarkers of disease.[144] Much has been made of the fact that Willis was the first to taste diabetic urine and note that it was sweet. But of that he makes no mention here.[145]

In his dedication to Ralph Bathurst, Willis admits that 'uromancy' is not a new subject. The ancients made judgments and evaluated their treatments by 'consulting the urinal'. This made sense since the liquor had washed all 'the parts and taken from many some little parcels'. Urine could reveal the many 'dyscrasies of our Bodies and their habitudes'. As a result 'The contemplation of this Excrement (as vile as it is) hath grown to a Science'. But in believing that inspection of the water can reveal the knowledge and prognostication of every disease, the 'Common People are egregiously deceived' and those who make this pronouncement 'deserve rather the name of a jugling Quack, than of a Physician'. The problem is that generalizations have been made based on the colour, consistency, and contents observed in one case or another; and, failing to address causation, the changes in urine merely denote the consequences of disease. It follows that Willis may not be capable of fulfilling 'the task which you have required of me, Worthy Sir, to wit, that the notions we have in time past discoursed together, and ... as it were collected notes, and what have since fallen under my own knowledge ... should be fram'd into a little treatise ... on Urinoscopy'. But nevertheless he will do his best for his old friend Bathurst.

Willis explains that, in the formation of urine, ingredients of the diet are 'boiled' in the ventricle (stomach) and become chyle in the intestines before being absorbed, circulated by the heart and washing the various bodily parts with nutritious juice, after which serous matter is separated from the rest by blood in the 'reins' and 'carried forth of doors' through the bladder. Willis is impressed by the rapidity with which drinking increases urinary flow and considers a route that bypasses the heart:[146]

> For of this opinion (though not very stubbornly) I always was that the chyme was in some measure immediately derived from the Ventricle, and Intestines by the branches of the

[143] Garrison and Morton make no mention of Willis's contribution to scurvy, listed in Norman (1991) under entries #3710–26. Priority is usually given to James Lind (1716–1794) for solving the problem as described in: *A treatise of the scurvy*, Edinburgh (1753): and see the many entries to scurvy and James Lind in RS Allison, *Sea diseases*, London (1943).

[144] The treatise was faithfully included in editions of *Diatribæ duæ*, the English translations and Latin *Opera omnia*, and published apart from the two other treatises, in Dutch and French.

[145] See: Thomas Willis, *Pharmaceutice rationalis*, part 2 (1684): page 74.

[146] See: Thomas Willis, *Of urines* (1684): page 2.

> Vena Porta, into the Mass of the Blood ... [and] ... rendered thin and clear ... continually sent away by the Reins.

Urine contains some sulphur and earth, salt aggregated with spirit carried 'as it were by the wings of others', but (self-evidently) mostly water. Sulphur, arising from the fat and particles of meat, adds to the colour and provides the 'stink' of urine. When urine is left to stand, the earthy threads or filaments that render the urine cloudy settle as a precipitate of 'muddy feculencies'. Because water is lost in bathing the bodily parts with the mass of blood, and in the sweats, the volume of urine is less than the daily intake of 'potations'. Drinking to excess makes the urine pale or, as Willis succinctly indicates, '*We drink thick beer, and Piss clear*'.[147]

Against this background, Willis is mostly concerned with the urines of sick people. His method is to note the volume and, after letting the urine stand, observe the sediment, colour, and smell. In general, excess production of urine 'signifies an evil disposition, with a tendency to wasting or Consumption'. In hydropic conditions, watery serum also accumulates in the abdomen, chest, and head, or swells the whole bodily habitus. Urine flow reduces with increased sweating or 'continual looseness' of the intestines. Stone in the bladder or urethra obstructs the flow of urine. As for the colour, when the absorption of food is defective, or fermentation insufficient, the particles are 'little dissolved in the mass of the blood, or rendered volatile' and the urine is pale. This appearance denotes many conditions: the green-sickness of virgins, dropsy, worms in children, gonorrhoea, and ulcers of the bladder and urinary passages. Urine that is deeper in colour than the usual citron has several causes. Flame-coloured urine occurs, often in the context of tertian fever, when yellow bile tinges the serum. More marked is the saffron coloured urine in which the 'Gall bag designed by Nature, for the separating [of yellow Bile] from the mass of the blood, its passages being rooted in the Liver' is impaired and admixed with salt and sulphur.[148] 'Where the Blood grows raging with a feverish heat, and is roasted, the Urine grows highly red' because the salt and sulphur are agitated and accumulate in the serum. Similar changes are seen in scurvy, arthritic disorders including gout, and consumption. Willis has not himself seen the urine described by others as black or green but he can imagine that these changes result from chemical reactions on the saffron urine in jaundice, 'the yellow carried forth to a worse state', especially in plague or after taking poisons.[149] And he is aware that pigments in various foodstuffs and potions may be carried over and both discolour the urine and alter its smell: examples are caffeine, rhubarb, turpentine, nutmeg and other spices, garlic, asparagus, cider, and rhenish wine.

The urine of the sick contains sediments and stains that reflect either the general 'habit of the whole Body' or the status of individual parts. In practice the reins and their dependencies are responsible for alterations in urine, 'the chief of which are sand, stones, blood, matter, bits of flesh, skins, branny or mealy sediments, corrupt seed which for the most part signify either the stony or an ulcerous distemper'.[150] Sometimes the urine remains normal in disease, the morbid ferments having been taken up by other bodily parts, not least the Brain and nervous stock. In these contexts: 'it is liar in the Plague and malignant fevers, and deceives ... scarce credit can be given to the Testimony of the urine'. Willis's conclusion is that those who claim to be able to 'know from the Urinal and divine a pain in the Head, an

[147] See: *Of urines* (1684): page 3. The use of italics by Pordage suggests that Willis may be quoting an unknown source.
[148] See: *Of urines* (1684): page 8.
[149] See: *Of urines* (1684): page 10.
[150] See: *Of urines* (1684): page 12.

Imposthume in the Throat, or any other Disease of any part ... shews rather his ignorance than the knowledge of any Disease'. And waxing somewhat lyrical in his pouring on of scorn, Willis adds:[151]

> I know there are ordinarily delivered by Medicasters and Old women almost an innumerable company of Rules and Directions of Urine-divination, that the urinal is no sooner inspected, but they will undertake to divine, whether it be a man or woman that is sick, how long they have been sick, what their disease is, and whether the distemper will end in health or death; whether the patient be subject to the passions of Love or Sadness, whether a Woman hath conceived with Child or not, or whether it shall be a Boy or Girl, and an hundred other the like, in which vain conjecture, they either impose by the confidence on the minds of the credulous, or (which is more frequently the custom) by a cunning craftiness they otherwise sift out the matter by inquiring, and falsly ascribe their knowledge in the inspection of Urine.

Although sceptical about the use of urinary assessment, Willis appears, by 1659, somewhat to have forgotten his habits of the early 1650s when the tasting of urine was part of his clinical assessment in the market at Abington. In the end, he acknowledges the limitations of this treatise written at the insistence of Ralph Bathurst: 'I desire you would be pleased not only to pardon the errors and barrenness of this Discourse, but also to excuse it in other things ... wherefore take care of this child hardly brought forth and almost an abortive, and as it were exposed and deservedly laid at your door, without portion. Farewell'.[152]

Responses and vindications of Willis on medical chemistry

Many welcomed Willis's advocacy of medical chemistry. Boyle acknowledged the teaching: 'how ordinary it is, especially since the learned Dr Willis's writings came to be applauded to look upon fevers as inordinate fermentations of the blood'.[153] Willis's occasional critic, Henry Stubbe wrote:[154]

> The suppositions I go upon depend so much upon the Doctrine of Fermentation, that I could not but think of you when I writ it: and who is a more competent judg of the Subject here debated, then the best of Philosophers, and Physicians? ... I have only time to tell you, that, without the noyse of much talk and frequent addresses and applications, I shall never cease to admire you, and to be Sir, your very humble servant, Henry Stubbe, Stratford upon Avon: Febr. 17. 1665.

[151] See: *Of urines* (1684): page 17.

[152] See: *Of urines* (1684): page 19.

[153] See: A Rupert Hall, 'Medicine and the Royal Society'. In: Ed. Allen G Debus, *Medicine in seventeenth century England. A symposium held at UCLA in honor of C.D. O'Malley*, Berkeley (1974): pages 421–52; citing, at pages 441–2, Robert Boyle, *Memoirs for the natural history of humane blood*, London (1684): page 102. Boyle also describes, at pages 189–91, 'a case of a memorable instance in a Patient of the very learned Dr. *Willis's*, ... being in the Fitt of an Apoplexy' who Boyle attended because Willis 'was necessitated to go ... out of the Town, and leave her in that Condition'.

[154] See: the dedication in Henry Stubbe, *The miraculous conformist of an account of several marvailous cures performed by the stroaking of the hands of Mr Valentine Greatarick with a physical discourse thereupon, in a letter to the honourable Robert Boyle esq; with a letter relating some other of his miraculous cures, attested by E. Foxcrroft M.A. and Fellow of King's College in Cambr:*, Oxford (1666).

Marchamont Nedham (1620–1678) advised universities to adopt Willis's ideas and not 'lie down ... under the shadow of a great name and make an Idol of it. We should rather reject what runs to superstition, and not pin the faith of mankind upon the sleeve of Hippocrates, because others have done so'.[155] Nedham considered Willis to provide 'an excellent example of Bacon's idea of raising a philosophy upon sensible experiments'. Prefacing his remarks with the qualification that 'Doctor Willis hath very excellently truss'd up all that is considerable in a narrow compass', Nedham rehearsed in some detail the chemical doctrine of disease and, more than others before, explained why this offered a sound basis for rational therapies.

He explained that, in recent years, men had come to suspect the Galenic school of physick and its opinion of the four humours because they are not constituents of blood but merely 'excrements of the cruentous gore'. Blood is one substance wherever it is distributed but its heat varies 'sometimes more effectually, sometimes more remissly' making men either 'Cholerick, Melancholick, or of some other Temper'. Moreover, as the blood circulates, some parts become stale and others are supplied anew so that from crudity or too much 'coction', particles that are somewhat 'excrementitious' are heaped together until separated by effervescence, as in the depuration of wine, leaving the blood free of 'Bile, Phlegme and Melancholie'. Nedham invited his 'ingenious readers to compare frivolous Galenic medicine with that of the noblest sect of philosophers and physicians who subscribe to the views of chymists and the five principles'. This knowledge was sufficiently secure for the vulgar acceptance of humours to be laid aside and the celebrated principles of the chemists in explaining the nature of blood and its distempers to be preferred.

Nedham recommends 'our learned Countriman Doctor Willis, in several places of his book *De Ferment. & Febr*.' for explaining that, especially after the heat of the summer, the blood passes from its 'sweet, spirituous and balsamick Nature' to acid, leading to seasonal outbreaks of scurvy and quartan fever similar to wine degenerating into vinegar, so that 'a physician may be compared to a wine merchant'. Pursuing the analogy with substances that ferment, Nedham explains Willis's view that coagulation of the blood, and failure of its circulation with stagnation in the heart and extremities, explains 'Scurvy and Quartan Agues ... all manner of Arthritick Diseases, the Scrophula, Nephritick Distempers, Leprous Dispositions, and almost all Chronick Diseases'. The great contribution of the iatrochemists is recognition that these conditions are amenable to remedies that restore the balance of the five principles. But caution is needed with vomits and purges which increase fermentation, for as Willis has indicated: 'Curatio Dogmatica [is] the common dogmatical way of curing Tertians, by which the Sick are miserably tormented, and its Disease seldom removed, so that this Disease is deservedly called Oppobrium medicorum, the shame and Reproach of physicians'. Worst of all is bleeding: 'I find Doctor Willis also (who hath had the honor of opening the eyes of the world, more than any before him, about the nature of Fevers) very positive against Bleeding'. Given that 'Maligne Fevers for the most part are seated in the Animal Spirits or in that Spiritous subtile liquor which is abounding in the Brain, the Nerves, and all the nervous parts; and their venom takes impression the more profoundly, if the Patients have been oppressed either with Fears or Griefs', it is not surprising that draining blood from a remote site does more harm than good.

[155] See: Marchamont Nedham, *Medela medicinæ. A plea for the free prosestion and renovation of the art of physick, out of the noblest and most authentick writers ...: Tending to the rescue of mankind from the tyranny of diseases, and of physicians themselves, from the pedansism of old authors and present dictators*, London (1665): pages 236–78 for a detailed assessment of Willis and the empirical method in medical science; and Isler (1968): page 36.

Willis must have been reassured by this advocacy of his medical chemistry and its therapeutic applications. But others were not so sure and, in one sense, he had invited criticism in the preface to *De febribus*: 'Doubting, I bring these thoughts into Publick, and submit them to the Examination and Emendation of the more Learned. That others before me have not spoken of all things truly concerning this thing, shall be an Argument that I may Err, yea (if you please) that I have Erred'. He was not to be disappointed.

In thanking Boyle for sending a copy, Samuel Hartlib (1600–1662) had mentioned the son of the London chemist Frederick Clodius (1625–*c.*1661): 'head and hands are much taken up with the animadversions on Dr Willis' book, he having very clear reason and experiences to dislike very many particulars in it'.[156] Martin Kerger (d.1691) considered Willis to be overly prescriptive in his insistence on just five chemical principles and too vague in his discussion of spirit. Behind all this was the general view that Willis was a theorist prone to opinion and hypothesis, much influenced by his rural youth surrounded by baking, brewing, and wine making, rather than reflecting the careful observations of a medical experimentalist. Addressing these farmyard processes directly, Martijn Schook (1614–1667), another critic, considered that Willis should have made a clearer distinction between fermentation, putrefaction, and effervescence.[157]

That these were not isolated views became clear when Edmund O'Meara (1614–1681) published *Examen diatribæ Thomæ Willisii doctoris medici, & professoris Oxoniensis, de febribus. Cui accesserunt historiæ aliquot medicæ rariores* (1665) dedicated to Sir Kenelm Digby (1603–1665). His critique was published with a treatise on hereditary diseases by O'Meara's father, Dermot (reprinted and dated 1665; see: Figure 159).[158] Whilst O'Meara's book might easily have been dismissed as sabre rattling by a disgruntled Galenist, it is important for having triggered a vitriolic defence of Willis from Richard Lower (see: Figure 160). Although hastily written, arguably Lower's *Diatribæ Thomæ Willisii doct. med. & profess. Oxon. De febribus vindicatio adversus Edmundum de Meara ormoniensum hibernum M.D.* (1665) offers a more accessible summary of ideas on fermentation and fevers than is to be found in *Diatribæ duæ*, and it includes the results of some new experiments. The book was dedicated to Boyle and published by John Martin and James Allestry, printers to the Royal Society. In turn Lower's vindication elicited a second diatribe against Willis written by Conlo Cassin, *Willisius male vindicatus* (1667). This was followed by an insulting last word from Lower in *Tractatus de corde* (1669). The story of O'Meara, Lower, and Cassin, together with a translation of Lower's book, is splendidly told by Kenneth Dewhurst.[159]

156 See: Frank (1990): footnote 35 page 116; and Frank (1980): page 122. Since Frederick Clodius was Hartlib's son-in-law, this son is presumably Hartlib's own grandson.

157 See: Kenneth Dewhurst, *Richard Lower's* Vindicatio. *A defence of the experimental method*, A facsimile edition, Oxford (1983): pages xv–xvi for discussion of Martin Kerger, *De fermentatione liber physico-medicus*, Wittenberg (1663): page 2; and Martijn Schook, *De fermento et fermentatione liber*, Wittenberg (1663): pages 435–8.

158 Between the text of *Examen diatribæ* and the 'Elenchus capitum examines' and 'Elenchus historiarum' is a list of twenty-two entries relating to nineteen cases collectively entitled *Historiæ aliquot medicæ rariores* seen between October 1653 and November 1662. One is written in English. Several are signed Edm. Meara, and others Joannes Bidgood (nd), both of Bristol. Reflecting the dogmatic views of the Spagyrists, the original title of Dermot Meara's book was *Pathologia hæreditaria generalis sive de morbis hæreditariis tractatus Spagyrico-dogmaticus. In quo generalis eorundem morborum radix, natura, & therapeutica indicatio ex utriumsque medicinæ fontibus investigatur*, Dublin (1619).

159 See: Dewhurst (1983), who points out that the 1665 edition of Lower's book is rare: Antoine Portal (1742–1832) who reviewed O'Meara's *Examen* in *Histoire de l'anatomie et de la chirurgie*, Paris (1770–1773): page 302 was unable to purchase a copy and John Fulton traced only eight examples, see: Fulton (1935): page 13, footnote 1, although that is known to be an underestimate. The example used for this bibliography was obtained through the antiquarian book trade in 2018. As with all other extant copies, it is state B with two stubs present before A7 and A8, which are both cancelled leaves. Fulton's copy, as shown in his Fig. 1 after page 14, is inscribed T Willoughby (1635–1672), the same as the copy of *Pharmaceutice rationalis* part 2 (1675) used for this bibliography (**6E**).

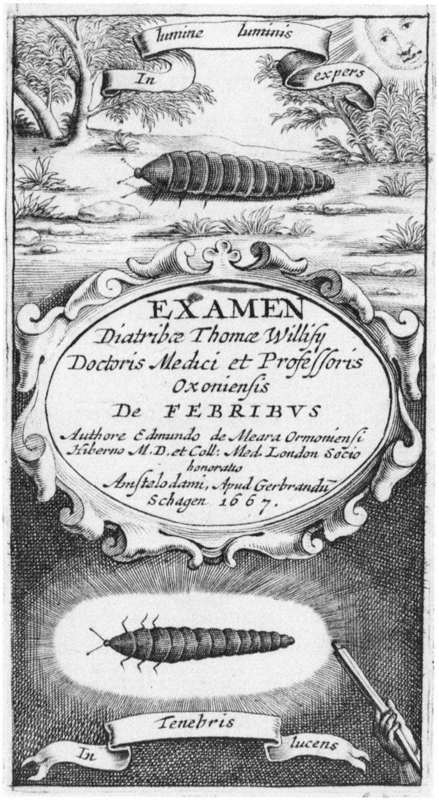

Figure 159 Engraved allegorical frontispiece: Edmund O'Meara *Examen diatribæ Thomae Willisii*, Amsterdam, 1667 (second edition).

Edmund O'Meara (1614–1681) was an Irish doctor working, during the 1660s, in Bristol from where, as a leading provincial physician, he was elected to honorary fellowship of the Royal College of Physicians in 1664.[160] He and Willis met when both attended the banquet at the College in December of that year. O'Meara had graduated at Rheims in 1636 and worked as physician to the Marquess of Clanricard (1604–1657). His Catholic contacts led to him aligning with the Royalists during the English Civil war but, on losing his land in County Wicklow, O'Meara came to England and settled in Bristol. He and Willis had a mutual friend in Dr John Malpet (nd); and O'Meara's patients included John Locke's father (d.1661). O'Meara became interested in fermentation after observing the effects of an acidic chalky material on the heating of water ('enough to boil an egg') and, whilst already at work preparing his attack on Willis, wrote an account of his chemical discovery.[161]

The tone of O'Meara's *Examen* (1665) is highly critical of Willis's views on fermentation and fevers as set out in *Diatribæ duæ* (1659). O'Meara explains that his book was written to prevent 'the lechery of the wanton mind and the mad itch for innovation [from causing] a dangerous chain of errors that will end in the ruin of the human race'. It was regrettable that an Oxford professor should lead students astray with erroneous and unorthodox concepts and treatments, and that men such as Harvey and Francis Glisson (1597–1677) had

[160] His father first published as 'Meara'; the son became 'O'Meara' and he then styled himself 'Edmund de Meara, Irishman of Ormond'.
[161] See: O'Meara (1661). In: John Childrey, *Britannia Baconia*, London (1661): pages 198–203.

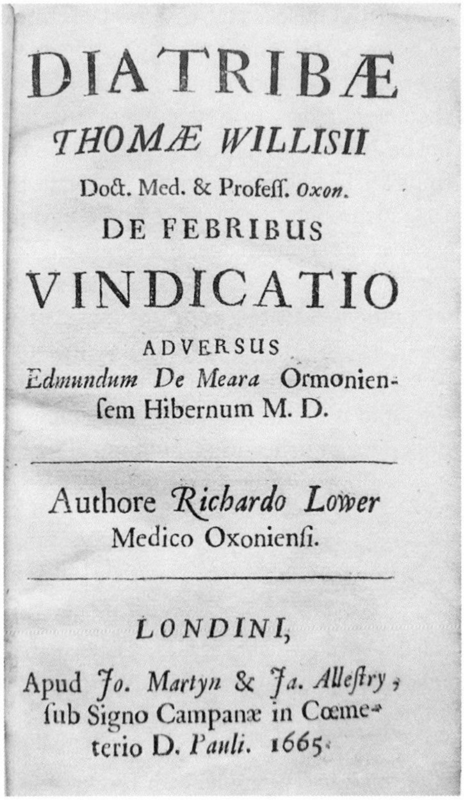
DIATRIBÆ

THOMÆ WILLISII

Doct. Med. & Profeſſ. *Oxon.*

DE FEBRIBUS

VINDICATIO

ADVERSUS

Edmundum De Meara Ormonien-
ſem Hibernum M. D.

Authore *Richardo Lower*
Medico Oxonienſi.

LONDINI,

Apud *Jo. Martyn* & *Ja. Alleſtry*,
ſub Signo Campanæ in Cœme-
terio D. *Pauli.* 1665.

Figure 160 Title page of Richard Lower's first book written in defence of Thomas Willis's views on fermentation and fevers, *Diatribæ Thomæ Willisii* etc., London, 1665.

spawned these views. In particular, Willis's monstrous opinion on the new mystery of fermentation should be placed 'out of human company'. O'Meara picked at Willis for describing rather than defining fever which could neither be caused by, nor located in, the blood; and for failing to consider certain types of fever, such as 'hectic', in his scheme. Agitation and perturbations of the blood might occur without fever. Some of Willis's terminology was inaccurate. Nor did O'Meara accept Willis's opinion on fire and ferment based on Descartes, who O'Meara considered to be nothing more than 'purveyor of a veneer of culture to the ladies and fops of the court'. Both concepts were unworthy, as surely a professor of natural philosophy would have known.

Any valid points that O'Meara might have offered were lost in a scholastic defence of the four humours. He insisted that the blood does not circulate, and nor is chyle delivered by the thoracic duct—two ideological strongholds of the iatrochemists. O'Meara did have a valid point in suggesting that fever is due to heat and putrid vapours emerging from febrile material in the viscera or other tissues rather than the blood. He was not slow in pointing out that Willis should have known this from his examination of patients. Had he carried out more autopsies, Willis would have seen tumours and abscesses in the abdomen and internal organs.[162] Moreover that evidence would have alerted him to the dire consequences of his

[162] See: *Of feavers* (1684): pages 57 and 65 for evidence that had O'Meara read Willis more diligently, he would have found a discussion of matter gathered as a tumour away from the circulating blood as the cause of intermittent fever.

empirical remedies borrowed from quacks and wise women. Instead Willis had spent his time 'sweating away at the bellows, and monotonously tasting one substance after another, but finding only earth, water, spirit, salt and sulphur'. Because Willis had no understanding of well tried and tested therapies used by orthodox physicians, his position was indefensible: 'a civil sword could not be drawn with more justice against murderers and highwaymen than against a plague of empirics'. Furthermore, Willis's acceptance of evidence from animal experiments had led him astray through the 'terrible tortures of vivisection', which were sufficiently unreliable to prove that 'the stomach does not digest, the eyes do not see, the feet do not walk, or the hands grasp'.[163]

Several commentators found O'Meara's book unsatisfactory. Henry More (1614–1687) told Lady Conway (1631–1679)[164] that he had 'sent Dr Hernshaw the book he spoke of, writ against Dr Willis, but I find it of no esteem at all'. Lower saw O'Meara's criticism not only as an insult to Willis but also a threat to the whole Harveian edifice of the circulation. Lower pulled no punches in responding. The literary style he adopted in the *Vindicatio* (1665) was more cutting than the dissector's knife. Lower described O'Meara as:

> A little frog from the swamps of Ireland, engendered against the will of nature and croaking against that of decency ... a market quack ... [more at] home in cookery than chemistry ... and [with a pen] born for stabbing flies ... far be it that you should prescribe for Willis or me ... or anyone not your intimate friend: for if a man is wont so to arm his pen with poison, I know not if he may also mix it with his medicines.

The burden of Lower's vindication was to argue, with Harvey and Willis, that blood is the inaugural material formed in the embryo. Because it is the vehicle of the soul, O'Meara was risking heresy in denying its supremacy over other bodily parts. Blood is in two states: homogenous in the arteries and heterogenous in the veins. This cannot be explained by Meara's reiteration of the four humours. Blood is heated in the left ventricle through ascension and fermentation. Disorder in that process gives rise to fever. Unlike combustion, the flame is invisible. In his recent lectures, Willis had established the chemical and physiological anatomy of the blood and the notion that it was made in the liver was untenable.[165] Lower included details of a further experiment carried out with Willis on 24 June 1664 and communicated to Boyle, which was designed to confirm that chyle enters the circulation through the thoracic duct.

Perhaps Lower risked overstating his case by aligning Willis with Harvey's work, since Willis had prioritized the process of fermentation involving salt, spirit, and sulphur held in a watery matrix which was something of a departure from Harvey and the circulation. In arguing that ascension of the blood involved commotion of particles in and by the heart, which then distributed this heat throughout the body, Lower was ignoring the change in colour effected by passage of blood through the lungs. He still argued that the main function of the lungs is to dispose of waste although he acknowledged that blood is impregnated with nitrous material during inspiration.

[163] For much of the account of O'Meara's text and the quotes, see Dewhurst (1983): pages xxi–xxviii.
[164] See chapter 17 for discussion of Lady Conway's headaches.
[165] See: Frank (1980): page 189 endnote 188, chapter 7.

This vindication was immediate and intemperate. Kenneth Dewhurst suggests that Lower, known later to have suffered from depression, may then have been in a manic mood.[166] However, the tone of Lower's response to O'Meara was ignored by Henry Oldenburg when reviewing the book.[167] Oldenburg saw 'this Curious piece' as a further account of modern physiology and a comprehensive rendering of contemporary 'medical and Anatomical inquiries' on fever and effervescence of the blood; the nature of the nervous and nutritious juice; where blood is made and whether it moves independently of the pulse; the nature of the maternal and foetal circulation; and the difference between arterial and venous blood. Altogether Oldenburg considered Lower's vindication to be 'a small, but very ingenious and Learned Treatise'. Much later, Thomas Willis's loyal grandson, Browne Willis made the point that:[168]

> *de Febribus* was attacked by Dr. Edmund de Meara, and defended by Dr. Richard Lower, who in the *Preface* to his *Vindicatio* tells the honourable Mr. Robert Boyle, that the reason of publishing that book was, because not only the name of Willis, but even of Philosophy itself, was injured: and that he does not attempt to affect the cause of Willis, as though he needed any assistance, but merely to ease him of the burthen of such attack, who was designed for nobler employments, than attending to the calumnies of his antagonist; and he adds, that he is extremely surprised, that Willis, equally celebrated for his writings and gentleness of manners, who neither by word or action had given offence to Meara, shou'd be persecuted with the most notorious falsities and reproaches; but this usage, continues Dr. Lower, may be expected from one, who has vilified the greatest names and persons, Des Cartes, Harvey and Glisson.

Lower did not go unanswered and the controversy continued with the publication by Conlon Cassin (1667)[169] for which the full title translates as 'Willis badly defended, or: an Oxford physician found guilty of lying and ignorance'. Hansruedi Isler (1934–2019) accepted that O'Meara and Conlon Cassin were the same person but this is corrected by Kenneth Dewhurst.[170] He concludes that Cassin, from a family of physicians in Ossory, was O'Meara's assistant. Since he offers no opinions of his own, Cassin drew his knowledge entirely from his teacher. Cassin was one of thirteen fellows elected to the proposed College of Physicians of Kilkenny, given a Royal charter by James II on 14 August 1687, and formed to govern doctors in the south of Ireland. It is worth quoting from Cassin's preface (as translated by Kenneth Dewhurst) in order to convey the flavour of unrestrained acrimony in exchanges between Dublin and Oxford:

> For some time I remained in doubt whether I should undertake to refute the book [Lower's vindication] or, shall I say, sewer of impurities that this person who describes himself as a physician from Oxford, and a vindicator of Willis's doctrine of fevers, has emptied

166 As a psychiatrist, the opinion of Dewhurst (1983): page xxviii that Lower suffered from manic depression should be respected.

167 See: Dewhurst (1983): page 291–2 citing Henry Oldenburg, *Philosophical Transactions* volume 1, issue 4 (5 June 1665): pages 75–6.

168 See: [John Bernard, Thomas Birch, John Locke, and other hands] *A general dictionary* Volume X (1741): pages 171–5. The authorship of this article is discussed in Chapter 1.

169 See: Conlone Cassinio, *Willisius male vindicatus, sive medicus Oxoniensis mendacitatis & inscitiæ detectus*, Dublin (1667).

170 See: Isler (1968): page 35; and Dewhurst (1983): pages 292–8.

shamelessly on the author of *Examen* throughout and in almost every sentence. For since there is nothing gentlemanly or scholarly to be found in it, nothing either elegant by the polish of its diction or solid by the strength of its reasoning, but there is to be found everywhere impudence more shameless than a harlot's, ignorance more arrogant than an alchemist's, a scurrilous abusiveness, ineptitude, fraudulence, mendacity, imposture, it will seem fairer, I think, to gentle readers that so vile a creature be smothered in contempt and silence than by the storming of so pestiferous a cesspit [lest] there be raised scandal for modest minds, and shame for honest ears. But since the rage of the Oxford physician has not vented itself on the author of *Examen* alone, I decided that a limit must be placed on such curbless licence, and the defence undertaken on truth and public decency. In attempting to do so, I chose to direct my principal labours to this end: that while subduing the wantonness of the adversary I myself might be found immune from his contagion; for what else that is arduous or difficult can be expected in so despicable an enemy, who has conducted Willis's cause so perfunctorily, that he may be seen, by badly defending it? Unless perhaps Willis himself is to be regarded as the betrayer no less of himself than of this vindicator, and having exposed to the laughter of the learned a discourse unsustainable by any advocacy with an even worse defence, prefixed to the work over him; and this conjecture seems to be supported by the continued consistency in both works of solecisms elementary schoolboys would blush at... But however it may be with the authorship, there is one thing of which I wish the reader to be informed, that this vindicator, who once acted the slanderer as *Terræ filius* at Oxford with indecency and malice but no wit, and was disappointed of the esteem he had sought by such a disgraceful effort was most deservedly appointed to plead Willis's cause, which had to be defended not by weight of reasons but by noise of insults.

Despite the vitriol, Cassin had some valid points. He reiterated O'Meara's position on fevers originating from vapourized humours in the viscera and rejected Willis's ideas on enkindling and fermentation of the blood. He turned around Lower's designation of O'Meara as a 'market quack' by reminding readers that Willis had plied his trade in the market towns around Oxford 'that with great profit and greater filth he should force into sale the secret treasure of his furnace-made imposture and bilk the purses of the country-folk'. Much of Cassin's book challenges Lower's reasoning on the change in colour between arterial and venous blood and details of the circulation but he makes the point that those who endorsed the suggestion that flame heated the blood—Harvey, George Ent (1604–1689), and Descartes—had not meant this literally but were writing metaphorically; and in any case Willis was not in the same league as these famous men. Not content with castigating Willis on fermentation and fevers, he added that time should not be wasted reading his 'doctoral drivel' on the brain (*Cerebri anatome*). As for remedies, Dr O'Meara had not infrequently had cause to rescue patients who had suffered from the therapeutic maladministration of Willis and other iatrochemists.

Clearly there was much sport here for impartial observers in reading these exchanges, and the audience broadened when Gerbrandt Schagen reprinted O'Meara's *Examen* from Amsterdam in 1667.[171] But Lower was determined to have the last word and, in the

[171] Schagen had access to several English texts. In the copy used for this bibliography, Edmund Meara's *Examen* (1667) in two parts, is in the original binding with Dermot O'Meara's *Pathologia hereditaria generalis*, as in the 1665 London edition. The Wellcome copy, in original binding, also has the sheets of Schagen's edition of Lower's *Vindicatio* (1666). The British Library has this edition of Lower's work bound as a single tract (1166 d 24). Dewhurst (1983) appears to have had access to a volume with these three and also the reprinting of Thomas Sydenham's *Methodus curandi febres* (1666), which leans heavily on Willis's treatise on fevers. He may have been quoting RT Gunther *Early medicine and biological* science, extracted from *Early science in Oxford*, London (1926): page 60, who agrees that 'the Willisian controversy was followed with such interest on the continent that Gerbrand Schagen

dedication of *Tractatus de corde* (1669) to Thomas Millington (1628–1704), he explains (mistakenly) that Conlonis Cassinii was a pseudonym used by O'Meara:[172]

> An Irishman, Meara, takes first prize for sheer perversity and stupidity. Himself unskilled he is pained that others know anything, as is clearly seen in his writings lately published under the pseudonym of Conlo Cassinius. But I pass over these personal passages because, if I had to contend with him in this matter, I should not have to go into the ring so much as into the cess-pit, and a victory in those regions would not compensate me for the filth I picked up in gaining it. On the other hand, the erroneous views he holds, especially about the function of the heart, the movement of the blood, the nature of the chyle and its passage into the blood (on these subjects he has written with so little skill that he might have been deep in sleep for the last forty years, and still imperfectly aroused from it), should not, in the interest of others, be passed over in like silence.

Lower did however distance himself somewhat from Willis by explaining that more careful consideration and further evidence made clear that arterial blood is red after admixing with air in the lungs and venous blood is dark through loss of that material. His former ambiguity expressed in the *Vindicatio* had arisen through not challenging the views expressed by Willis:[173]

> I relied more in the matter [of the colour of blood in the pulmonary veins] on the authority and preconceived opinion of the learned Dr Willis than on my own experience, and confused too far the torch of life with the torch bearer, as, too, the lapse of time has now taught me differently, I shall not be loath to exchange my former view for a better one.

In reflecting on this acerbic exchange of entrenched Galenic and iatrochemical positions, sides were taken, and various supportive opinions expressed. Oldenburg had acted as honest broker. He was adept at communicating matters of scientific interest, within and outside the Royal Society, which occurred during meetings or were discussed with him. As the first scientific journalist, telling Oldenburg something was a certain means of having the story brought to the attention of others. In turn, those wanting to learn about matters on which physicians and scientists were more reticent contacted Oldenburg to obtain the gossip. In correspondence with Oldenburg, Jean-Baptiste Duhamel (1634–1706) looked forward to 'a book from Mr Lower against a certain Irishman'. In June 1671, Philipp Jacob Sachs (1627–1672) asked 'under pledge of secrecy' for details of Willis' preparation that dissolved iron. Oldenburg stalled, explaining that Willis was too busy as a physician to be interrupted with the question, knowing that Willis had not divulged his secret in the past and would not do so now.[174] Marcello Malpighi was 'particularly pleased to find Richard Lower's reply to O'Meara

one of the most enterprising publishers of Amsterdam, brought out in [1663 and] 1667 an edition of all the papers which he stated on the title page to be 'the latest, far more correct and enlarged than the others'; or Dewhurst may have been copying the entry in Fulton (1935): page 13, item 3 which refers to this collection of reprinted works: 'The Schagen 1667 edition is embellished with a delightful frontispiece and title and to it is appended *Sydenham's Methodus curandi febres* (1666) and a most interesting treatise on the inheritance of diseases by Meara [Dermutio, not specified] entitled *Pathologia haereditaria*'.

[172] See: KJ Franklin, *De Corde By Richard Lower, London 1669*, with introduction and translation. In: Ed. RT Gunther, *Early science in Oxford*, volume IX, Oxford (1932): [Dedication, page 3], citing *De corde* (1669): pages vii–ix.

[173] See: Isler (1968): page 107, citing Fulton (1935): page 23, entry 18.

[174] See: A Rupert Hall (1974): pages 426–30.

which has stimulated my desire to see other works by this most polished intellect'. Battista Capucci (b.1614) praised the spirit of philosophical freedom in the face of the 'idolators of antiquity' but took a reserved position on some of the contradictions and Lower's tone of self-confidence; nor could he accept that enkindling and heating occurred in the heart or that respiration served the purpose of cooling the blood—concepts that Lower had faithfully rehearsed from Willis's writings.[175]

Posterity's views on fermentation and fevers

If Lower thought that he had finally disposed of O'Meara and his doppelganger, Conlo Cassin, he was to be disappointed. Other books soon appeared that rehearsed the arguments. In the same year as Lower published *Tractatus de corde*, the *Term Catalogue* advertised:[176]

> Αἱμάτωσις, or the True way of preserving the Blood in its integrity; and rectifying it, if at any time polluted and degenerate. Wherein Dr. Willis his Error of Bleeding is reprehended, and offered to be confuted by practice and frequent Experiments; and certain opinions of Dr. Betts proved dangerously false; and Phlebotomy declared to be destructive. By George Thomson, M.D. In Octavo. Price, bound, 1s. 6d. Printed for N. Crouch at the Cross keys in Bishopsgate street.

But with time, the opponents of medical chemistry fell away and by the mid-1680s, the *Term Catalogue* was announcing:[177]

> Michaelis Ettmulleri, Phil. Et M.D. Opera omnia Theoretica et Practica, in quibus Universa praxis Medica, sive omnium totius humani Corporis Morborum dilucida descriptio, eorumque causarum accurata explicatio, et curatio per selectissima et optima Medicamenta secundum Principia et Experimenta Chymica et Anatomica Helmontii, Willisii, Sylvii, Tackerii, etc. Accedit Chirurgia Medica pulcherima Methodo omnes affectus externos explicans, eorumque causas, restutionem et curam describens. Quarto. Sold by S. Smith at the Prince's Arms in St. Paul's Churchyard.[178] ... [and] ... Curious observations in that difficult part of Chirurgery relating to Teeth; shewing how to preserve the Teeth and Gums from all accidents they are subject to. To which is added, A Physical Discourse, wherein the reasons of the Beating of the Pulse, together with those of the Circulation of the Blood, are explained; and the Opinions of several Ancient and Modern Physicians and Philosophers as Galen, Gassendus, [Des] Cartes, Lower, Willis, etc. upon this subject are examined. Quarto. Printed at Dublin; and sold by W. Whitwood in Duck lane.

The translator of the English edition explains that Ettmuller combines theory, practice, and experience. He 'united the jarring Hypotheses of Willis, Sylvius and Helmont, and makes 'em conspire to illustrate and imbellish an uniform Practice'.[179] Ettmuller approaches

[175] For more detailed discussion, see: Dewhurst (1983): pages 297–300.

[176] See entry under *Term Catalogue* for Michaelmas 1669, November 22nd, I Numb. 5, I. 18 column 2, Physick.

[177] See: *Term Catalogue*, Michaelmas 1686 December 13th, IV Numb 24, II 177, column 2, Physick.

[178] See: *Term Catalogue*, Trinity 1685 June, IV numb 20, II 139, column 1, Lib. Lat.

[179] See: *Etmullerus Abridg'd: or, a compleat system of the theory and practice of physic. Being a description of all diseases incident to men, women and children. With an account of their causes, symptoms, and most approved methods of cure, both physical and chirurgical. To which is prefix'd a short view of the animal and vital functions; and the*

disease from the perspective that 'Whoever proceeds without Knowledge of Chymistry and Anatomy ... does but grope in the dark'. Chymistry is needed to understand 'the Vital Functions of the Body' and anatomy for 'the Animal Musculatory Motion'. There follows a faithful rendition of fermentation and the formation of vital and animal spirits in the functions of the brain and nervous stock, and in motion, taken from contemporary writings. The workings of the human body depend on minute particles combining and imposing the 'texture of parts'. Galenic humours are more imaginary than real. Flame is a convenient way of describing the force that promotes conjunction, separation, and transposition of particles which alter the constitution of bodies. By increasing excretion through one point of exit or another, with or without the additional use of blood-letting, medicines are chemical in their workings and rational in their usage. Readers will recognize much that is familiar in Ettmuller's advocacy of medicines that promote vomiting, purging, urination, and sweating, and those that act on the animal faculty.[180]

Section V acknowledges 'The choice of practical authors'. Paracelsus and Helmont are to be relied upon but Ettmuller explains that 'In pursuing my Design of gathering the whole Practice of Physic into one Body, I have proposed Sylvius and Willis for my Pattern ... Tho' if consider'd separately, either of them is liable to Censure'.[181] Sylvius overstates the role of fermentation between lymph and bile active in the right ventricle, and corresponding 'strife' in the 'first passages' (intestines). Writing in 1685, Ettmuller considers that Willis has usefully elucidated the nature of convulsions and the contraction of muscles but he has overstated matters in arguing that the elastic power of muscle is dependent on 'the prevalency of an Acid, or some such grating Substance, for their Cause'. Nonetheless, 'these two Authors join'd together are the Flower of our Modern Writers, and as such I recommend 'em to young Students'. There follow nearly six hundred pages of receipts in six 'Books' devoted, respectively, to the disorders of the various body parts, the brain and nervous stock ('performance of sense and motion'), diseases confined to men, those of women, and others in children, and on surgery for swellings, wounds, ulcers, dislocations, fractures, and gangrene. No conceivable symptom is omitted; no condition cannot be remedied; and no natural substance, mineral or animal extract is without use.

Willis's reputation suffered in the eighteenth and nineteenth centuries when, in the absence of information on molecules and medicine, too little allowance was made for his use of metaphor and analogy. John Bostock (1773–1846), for example, wrote:[182]

> One of the most respectable of the advocates of the chemical doctrines of medicine was our learned countryman Willis ... In the year 1659 he published his celebrated treatise on fermentation and on fever, the object of which is to prove that every organ of the body has its peculiar and inappropriate fermentation, and that a morbid state of these ferments is the cause of all diseases. The hypothesis is in itself totally false, but it is supported by considerable ingenuity, and his works are of real value, as containing an accurate account of the phenomena of disease.

several virtues and classes of medicines. Translated from the last edition of the works of Michael Etmullerus, late professor of physic in the University of Lipsic, London (1712): page [5].

[180] See chapter 18 for more detailed discussion of Willis's medical and surgical therapies.

[181] See: Ettmuller (1712): page 41.

[182] See: John Bostock, *Sketch of the history of medicine from its origin to the commencement of the nineteenth century*, London (1835): pages 158–9.

Pierre Victor Renouard (b.1798) was no less censorious in ridiculing Willis's ancient theories of fermentation and the excess or 'ebulliation' of the ferments in the context of diseases which settle only when the morbific matter has been expelled following the febrile agitation:[183]

> Thomas Willis … contributed more than any other to the propagation of the taste for chemical explanations among physicians … Willis concluded that there are five elements, namely: spirits, sulphur, salts, water and earth. He excluded air and fire … because they are neither visible nor palpable. 'For', he adds ironically, 'my intelligence is obtuse, and my reason cannot penetrate beyond the reach of my senses' … Could anyone so soon forget the philosophic maxim that he seemed to take for a motto? The 'spirits' according to him, are '… an emanation of the Divine breath, which a beneficent providence had placed in the sublunary world, to impress all things with vital action … All is equally fictitious and imaginary … Willis appears … more faulty than the ancients, for he puts himself in manifest contradiction with his philosophic principles … The system of Willis was more vast, complicated and subtile than the preceding, was less comprehensible to the vulgar, and, therefore, pleased better, minds accustomed to abstract speculation; but there are at bottom, the same defects, and it merits the same reproaches … he [did not] keep … the promise he made not to go beyond, in his speculations, the limits of sensible phenomena: he presents us … a series of deductions purely fictitious … I am compelled, in order to justify, in the eyes of posterity, the reputation of this great practitioner, to repeat what I have said in favour … of many others, namely: that they laid aside their fictitious theories when visiting the sick, and consulted their experience. I have the more reason to think that Willis acted in this way from what he says on the subject of Peruvian bark, whose effects contradict his theory – that it is better in every case to be guided by observation.

Others simply ignored Willis. For all his attention to farmyard matters and domestic science, Willis's name does not appear in Louis Pasteur's monograph on brewing.[184] Nor was the twentieth century much kinder. Osler, in his address at the 1916 Fenny Poppers celebration, pointed out that:[185]

> From time immemorial it had been one of the great mysteries how certain bodies undergo the extraordinary change known as fermentation … Willis studied this mystery and made it still greater in the pages he devoted to it. But he grasped one very important thing, the analogy between a fever and fermentation. He made the very interesting observation that there is no difference between the vintner and the physician; when the vat becomes too full in fermentation the vintner draws off some of the liquid, and he said; 'What is that but what we do with blood fermenting in a fever?' That was a good reason for phlebotomy.

Cecilia Mettler compared Willis unfavourably with Sydenham: 'Willis's writings are graceful, brilliant, but glib and airy without substance. There is something of the fencer about Willis,

[183] See: PV Renouard, *History of medicine from its origin to the nineteenth century*, translated by Cornelius G Comegys, London (1856): pages 516–20.

[184] See: L Pasteur, *Studies on fermentation. The diseases of beer, their causes, and the means of preventing them*, London (1879): page 1. In fact Pasteur pays scant attention to the history of his subject.

[185] See: Henry Viets, 'A patronal festival for Thomas Willis (1621–1675) with remarks by Sir William Osler, Bart., FRS', *Annals of Medical History* 1917: 3; 118–24.

a quality of artificiality and studied elegance which suffers by comparison with the dull solidity of Sydenham'.[186]

William Wightman (1899–1983) had it that Willis was 'debauched with chemistry, or with what passed for chemistry before his contemporaries—Boyle, Hooke, and Mayow—had brought more critical thought to bear on it. Yet I believe it is true that Willis had advanced beyond, for instance, Vesalius, not merely in detailed anatomical knowledge but in the possibility of detachment from a crude and sterile physiology'.[187]

In forming judgments, analysts from any period are constrained by contemporary opinion and knowledge. Adverse summaries of Willis's writings on fermentation treat the written word with rigidity, allowing little imagination in accommodating the concepts with which he was grappling. To the modern reader, accepting Willis's use of metaphor and the cautious tone in which he wrote, qualifying many statements with the phrase 'as it were', the reductionist approach of searching for one generic process on which the animate and material world depends was not so farfetched. For anyone versed in twenty-first century cell and molecular biology, biochemistry, and medical physiology, the resonance with fermentation and corpuscular theory is not difficult. Readers will easily manage the concept of flame energizing motile particles which ferment, generating heated blood that is circulated, used, and then cleansed. No writer likes endlessly to reuse the same word. The many synonyms for stages in this sequence that Willis offers can be taken as literary devices rather than implying subtleties of meaning.

That said, several charges can legitimately be brought against Willis's treatises on medical chemistry and disease. They are extremely repetitive and disordered, faults that would have benefited from judicious editing. Although his separation of putrid, malignant, and pestilential fevers is clearly stated, and the generic symptoms of fever set out, many of the conditions that he assigns to each class straddle his classification. Scurvy clearly includes a string of conditions apart from vitamin C deficiency including beriberi, tuberculous meningitis, osteoarthritis, and deep vein thrombosis with pulmonary embolism. Willis's explanations of mechanisms are limited: everything is overheating, too much sulphur, perturbation of the animal spirits and inadequate discharge of adust material through sweat, excretions, and expired air. With very few exceptions, most of his references are to writings of the ancients. Nor, for all his chemistry, does Willis altogether reject Galenic humoral analyses. Apart from the symptomatic quotidian fevers, prognosis is equally severe across the categories; and some remarkable recoveries occur from situations where, in the seventeenth century, death would have seemed inevitable. If his early treatises were intended as manuals for best practice, the therapeutics is ambiguous, especially for the role of bleeding early in disease. But despite these cavils, the reader cannot but admire the combination of observation, experience, and reasoning, and the logical progression of his ideas.

[186] See: Cecilia C Mettler, edited by Fred A Mettler, *History of medicine*, Philadelphia (1947): page 375.

[187] See: WPD Wightman, 'Wars of ideas in neurological science—from Willis to Bichat and from Locke to Condillac'. In: Ed. FNL Poynter, *The history and philosophy of knowledge of the brain and its functions*, Oxford (1958): page 136.

16

'Neurologie: the doctrine of the nerves'

The brain and nervous stock

Cerebri anatome, Nervorumque descriptio et usus (1664); *De motu musculari* (1670); *De anima brutorum* (1672).

Thomas Willis is remembered by physicians whose professional work relates to the nervous system for two reasons: his description of the anastomotic arterial arrangement at the base of the brain; and for promoting the term 'neurologie'. But the four treatises that deal with the 'brain and nervous stock' go much further. Willis returns repeatedly to several topics:

Function dependent on the cerebrum and cerebellum rather than the ventricles and cerebrospinal fluid
The role of the cortex in ideas and memory and, hence, the concept of cerebral localisation.
An account of the autonomic nervous system
The course and distribution of the cranial nerves within and outside the skull
Pathways for sensation and movement that converge on discrete ganglia
The duplication of brain structures and the concept of redundancy and plasticity
The interplay between complex and coordinated voluntary and involuntary movements
The flow of animal spirits and the nature of muscular movement
The arrangement of blood vessels supplying the brain and spinal cord.

Sir Charles Symonds (1890–1978) regarded *Cerebri anatome* as best known for the 'circle of Willis' but most distinguished for its description of the cranial nerves.[1] Mentioned at various places in the two treatises contained in this book, the most detailed and original parts of Willis's anatomy are the five chapters in *The description and use of the nerves* devoted to the wandring and intercostal nerves, and their courses from the medulla oblongata to the furthest reaches of the thorax and abdomen. Accepting the use of metaphor and speculation, and allowing for the discursive and repetitive narrative style, Willis's anatomical work reveals extraordinary originality and intuition at a time when the medieval cell doctrine had gone unchallenged for several centuries, methodology was largely confined to what the eye could see assisted by crude microscopy, experiment was primitive, and deviating from orthodoxy likely to excite religious and civil retribution.[2] Symonds was not the first to appreciate these

[1] See: Sir Charles Symonds, 'The circle of Willis' *British Medical Journal* 1955; i: 119–24.

[2] There are many analyses of Willis's contributions to structure of the brain and spinal cord. Several authors take as their authority Jules Soury (1842–1915), *Le système nerveux central. Structure et fonctions. Histoire critique des théories et des doctrines*, Paris (1899): pages 428–42, for a definitive and close reading. Edwin Clarke and CD O'Malley, *The human brain and spinal cord. A historical study illustrated by writings from antiquity to the twentieth century*, Berkeley and Los Angeles (1968) have read widely and translated from the original Latin. Hansruedi Isler,

two treatises. Their merits were set out in verse by Philip Fell (*c.*1632–1682) as part of preliminaries to the London 1664 quarto and octavo editions (**2A** and **2B**):[3]

AUTHORI In Cerebri Anatomen carmen

QUI terræ pelagíque vias, mundíque per omnes
Articulos ſpatiatur ovans, metáſque ſuorum
Herculeas audet ſupra poſuiſſe laborum,
Neglectus jacet uſque ſibi, dúmque omnia quærit,
Ipſe ſui quæſitor abeſt, incognita tellus
Solus nauta latet, propiórque ignotior orbis.
Tu melior Typhis, ſpreto jam Phaſidis auro,
In te vela paras, animatos detegis orbes,
Humanáſque aperis auſis ingentibus oras.
Jámque novos laxare ſinus, animæque latentis
Arcanas reſerare vias cæcóſque receſſus
Fas aperire tibi, totámque recludere mentem.
Humani quicquid ſuſpenſum eſt fornice cœli,
Quem teneant capitis laqueata palatia civem;
Altera cur foveat, cur protegat altera meninx;
Quos teſtes genuiſſe, animi quos utraque mater
Conceptus peperiſſe valent, quæ cella recondat,
Quis ſinus excipiat; quales mirabile nectit
Rete dolos, formas, rerum & phantaſmata captans:
Seu mens præteriti retinet ſimulachra laboris
Membranis deſcripta ſuis, ſeu provida ſatis
Imminet, & Lacheſi venturos præripit annos.
Quin ſpectare datum eſt tumidos quæ pectore fluctus
Suſcitet, & noſtrum tempeſtas miſceat æquor;
Unde Amor, atque arcum nervo quo tendere Natum
Idalium Cytheræa jubet; cur obice ſanguis
Siſtitur, & torto frænatur venula nodo.
Cernimus ut ſedeat Dolor & ſuſpiria ducat;
Ut Metus incertum condat caput, & ſibi fruſtrà
Conſulit, éque ſuis jam jámque evellitur umbris:
Ut nutans ægrè ſuſtentet corpora Somnus;
Ut Riſus dextrâ firmet latus; unde ſolutos
Gaudia dilatant animos, cùm gurgite pleno

Thomas Willis 1621–1675. Doctor and scientist, New York (1968) paraphrases Soury's text with further reading of the original Latin and use of Pordage's translation. As neuropathologists, Alfred Meyer, *Historical aspects of cerebral anatomy*, London (1971) and John Trevor Hughes, *Thomas Willis 1621–1675. His life and work*, London (1971) write from the advantage of expertise in dissection of the brain and spinal cord in health and disease, and readings of the seventeenth-century texts. In the tercentenary edition of *The anatomy of the brain and nerves*, Montreal (1965), William Feindel summarizes many aspects of Willis's anatomical discoveries as does John D Spillane, *The doctrine of the nerves. Chapters in the history of neurology*, Oxford (1981): pages 77–84. The present account leans on these authorities, various others as listed in the footnotes, and a diligent reading of Samuel Pordage's translations from 1681.

[3] See chapter 15 for details of Philip Fell, one of Willis's brothers-in-law.

Flumen abit, totóſque juvat laxare rudentes
Quâ Ratio ſublime ſedens per inane theatri
Nervorum dextrâ tenet & moderatur habenas.
 Exultat jam Diva, videt vultúſque laréſque
Agnoſcítque ſuos, & cui natura tueri
Indulsítque referre deos, jam vertice ſurgit
Lætior, & ſpectat cognata erectior aſtra.
Jámque neces & fata juvant. Stylus iſte nocentis
Expiat & toties crudelis vulnera ferri.
Ipſa novos ſtatuit de ſe Libitina triumphos,
Furca crucéſque placent, & bis ſpectacula latro.
 Sanguinis hic jactet primus moviſſe lacunas
 Sortitus famam vitæ cum fonte perennem:
 Hunc lymphæ, lactiſve latex, hunc glandula laudet.
 Diviſum vili ſectóque cadavere nomen
 Quæſierint alii: melior tua pagina geſtit
 Oſtendiſſe hominem ſpirantemque æthera mentem.

Philippus Fell, *A.M & Collegii Omnium Animarum in Acad.*
Oxon. *Socius.*

Song for the WRITER of Cerebri anatome[4]

WHO travels the lanes of land and sea, enjoying all
Corners of the world, and who daringly achieved
The higher than Herculean aims of his labours,
Rests unheeded as long as, while he searches all,
No one searches for him, the land unknown;
Alone the sailor hides, his route nearer but unknown.
You, better than Tiphys, having spurned the gold of Phasis,
You hoist sails homewards, discover animated worlds,
Find access to human shores with great daring.
Already able to unfasten folds, disclose the secret
Pathways of the hidden soul, open up
Blind nooks, and unveil the entire mind.
 What is suspended from the ridge of the human vault,
Whom the panelled palace holds as tenant;
Why one membrane warms, the other protects;

[4] Translated by Jan van Gijn, 2 May 2020, who points out that: Tiphys (not 'Typhis') is the helmsman of the 'Argo', the ship on which Jason searched for the Golden Fleece; Phasis is a river (later a town) in Colchis, at the Eastern shore of the Black Sea, the country of the Fleece; Lachesis, one of the three goddesses of fate, measures and cuts the thread of life; Libitina, twice mentioned, is the goddess of funerals and corpses; the references in the final six lines, set apart typographically, are to Harvey, those who described the lymph ducts, and Vesalius. Jan van Gijn joins Anthony Wood (1632–1695) in adding that the verse shows the splendid erudition expected from a Fellow of All Souls College, Oxford, in writing Latin verse in hexametric metre. Fell starts with the metaphor of a sailor who discovers unknown territories but dies on a faraway beach without having been able to share his discoveries with others. He then moves to the content of Willis's book, but the associations are loose and Fell may not have read or fully understood the text. He closes with six lines comparing Willis with the discoveries of a few illustrious predecessors.

Which testes were created, which products of the mind
Either membrane can beget, what the cavity hides,
Which sinus receives, what guiles the wonderful
Network knits, trapping forms and ideas of matter;
Or the mind retains images of past labours,
Inscribed on its membranes, or heralds what fate
Has in store, and wrenches future years from Lachesis.
One can even behold the swollen waves the tempest
Evokes in the chest, disturbing our tranquil water;
Then Love, and Venus commands her Son to draw
The bowstring; why blood is contained
By walls, and veins are slowed by twisted knots.
We discern where Grief resides and leads to sighs;
How Fear hides his doubtful head, and in vain
Seeks counsel, or is wrenched from its shadows:
How nodding Sleep hardly sustains bodies;
How Laughter adroitly strengthens the frame; then
Joys expand free minds, as when a river flows
With lively stream, the charm of ropes released,
Where Reason, perched high, holds and checks
The reins of nerves through the circus's void.
  The Goddess rejoices, sees faces, her homestead,
Descries her own; nature allowed her to protect
And bring back the gods; she rises with her crest
Happier, and prouder she beholds the kindred stars.
She rejoices in killings and ills. She atones for
The crook's knife and many wounds of cruel iron.
Libitina raised new triumphs on her own,
Pleased by gallows, crosses and criminal spectacles.
  Let this man boast to have first moved the pools of blood
  Having obtained eternal fame with the source of life:
  Let lymph, the juice of milk, let glands praise that man.
  Others again may have sought shared credit through
  Vile dissected corpses: your better writing achieves
  To have shown man, and mind breathing aether.

Philippus Fell, *A.M* and All Souls College, Oxford

Willis was not himself averse to purple prose. He ends the preface to *Cerebri anatome*: 'Minerva was born from the Brain, Vulcan with his Instruments playing the Midwife: For either by this way, *viz*. By Wounds and Death, by Anatomy, and a Caesarean Birth, Truth will be brought to Light, or for ever lye hid'.

'Neurologie'

The word Willis used to encapsulate his studies of the nervous system took -λογία as the body of knowledge on a given subject and prefaced this with νεῦρον (neuron), the Greek word for sinew, tendon, or bowstring based on observations made whilst dissecting the cranial nerves.[5] Consistent with the practice of learned physicians and scholars of all types from the Renaissance onwards, Willis's treatises, written in Latin, did occasionally include greek typography. The word is first printed in the 'Elenchus rerum' of the 1664 quarto edition of *Cerebri anatome* at c3r, page [29]: 'Νευρολογίας penſum, difficile licèt, utile ac iucundum eſt, 235.' (The task of neurology, though difficult, is useful and pleasing.) It refers the reader to page 235 where the text reads: 'Idcirco, etiamnum velis vento datis, procedere, & difficile νε υρολογίας penſum aggredi statuimus ...' In the English translation (1681), Samuel Pordage (1633–1691) has this (at page 125) as: 'Therefore although we know it is difficult to proceed with full Sail, we have resolved to undertake the task of the Doctrine of the Nerves ...' Although not listed in the 'Elenchus rerum', Willis first used νευρολογία at page 229: 'de quibus poſtea, cùm νευρολογίαν integram inſtituemus, erunt propria dicendi loca'.[6] Pordage translates this (at page 123) as: 'Of which there will be hereafter a proper place to speak, when we shall institute the whole Neurology or the Doctrine of the Nerves'. In his table of hard words, Pordage defines 'Nerves' as: '*the sinews which convey the spirits that serve for life and motion through the whole body*'; and 'Neurologie' as '*The doctrine of the Nerves*'.[7] As the name indicates, reference is to the cranial nerves not the anatomy of the brain or the study of disease affecting the nervous system. Having introduced νευρολογία, Willis calls it 'inſtitutum noſtrum' (our 'project' or 'creation') and speaks of a general and a special neurology.[8] He seemed pleased with the term and uses it liberally:[9]

At page 253, he writes: 'Interim methodi noſtræ ratio poſtulat ut Nervorum cenſu particulari facto, νευρολογίας (quantum tenuitas noſtra poteſt) exactum tradamus'; which Pordage has, at page 130, as: 'In the mean time, our Method demands of us, that (according to our weak skill) by the cense or numbering of the Nerves, being particularly made, we should deliver an exact Neurology or Doctrine of the Nerves'.

At page 273, he writes: 'Interim hâc ſpeculatione dimiſſâ, penſi noſtri Anatomici quod reſiduum eſt, νευρολογίας ſc[ientam] *ſpecialem*, aggrediemur.'; which Pordage has, at page 136, as: 'In the mean time, leaving this speculation, we shall proceed to the remaining Task of our *Anatomy*, to wit, the *Neurologie* or of the Nerves in particular'.

At page 306, he writes: 'quò diſcriminis ratio innoteſcat, libet hîc utriuſque νευρολογία diſtinctè & ſeorſim proſequi; ...'; which Pordage translates, at page 147, as: 'that the reason of the difference may be known, we will here prosecute apart and distinctly the *Neurologie* or Doctrine of the Nerves ...'

At page 410, he writes: 'Unaquæque Nervorum ſpinalium paria deſcribere, & ſingulorum divaricationes recenſere, eorúmque uſus & actiones explicare, eſſet opus immenſi laboris

[5] See: Mehta et al 'Etymology and the neuron(e)', *Brain* 2020: 143; 374–9; and 2021: 144: 1–2, e39.

[6] As an example of the looseness of Pordage's translations, Stephen Anderson, New College, Oxford suggests as more accurate: 'Therefore, even now spreading our sails to the wind, we have resolved to undertake the difficult task of neurologie'; and, on the variations of spelling, he explains that the printed word is in the accusative, νευρολ ογίαν, but when referring to it as a noun, it should appear in the nominative, νευρολογία, as in the sentence below.

[7] See: Thomas Willis, *The description and use of the nerves*, London (1681): pages 123 and [8]. Willis also used the term ψυχολογία (psychology: in *Cerebri anatome* (1664) at page 455; and first introduces the word ὁρμαί (hormones) at page 180 as substances made in one place that determine activity in remote parts.

[8] See: Isler (1968): page 101.

[9] Citations relate to page numbers in Thomas Willis, *Cerebri anatome*: *cui accessit nervorum descriptio et usus*, London (1664) in Latin and *Anatomy of the brain* (1681) in English.

ac tædii: cúmque hæc νευρολογία ſine exacta muſculorum notitia ſatìs intelligi aut addiſci nequit...'; which Pordage has, at page 178, as: 'To describe all the several pairs of the spinal Nerves, and to rehearse all their branchings, and to unfold the uses and actions of them, would be a work of an immense labour and trouble: and as the Neurologie cannot be learned nor understood without an exact knowledge of the Muscles, we may justly here forbear entering upon its particular institution'.

And he concludes at page 422 with: 'Interim ad inſtituti noſtri, νευρολογίας ſc[ientam] quod reſiduum eſt ut redeamus, non multa præterea circa Nervos obſervatu digna occurrunt'; which Pordage has, at page 182, as: 'In the mean time, that we may return to our purpose, to wit, what remains of *Neurologie*, there is not much more to be met with worthy of note concerning the Nerves'.

Explicating the anatomy of the brain

That people other than Willis contributed to his treatises is not disputed. Willis sought help with the dissections and their illustrations in his work on the anatomy of the brain and cranial nerves. With others, he studied animal and human material using macroscopic and microscopic techniques for delineating structure. The provenance of the anatomical work is made clear through correspondence between Richard Lower (1631–1691) and Robert Boyle (1627–1691):[10]

> The Doctor hath now perfected the anatomical part likewise, but being not satisfied in some things, I suppose he will hardly be induced to publish them yet a good while (26 November 1662)... I have been wholly diverted by Dr Willis whose desire it is, that I should be present at his operations, which now are very near finished, and I hope will make some apologies to you for my idleness before long; for the Doctor intends before midsummer, to put his book into the press (27 April 1663).

The debt that Willis owed to others was made explicit in the preface to *Cerebri anatome*:[11]

> I determined to ... believe Nature and ocular demonstrations ... I did chiefly inquire into the offices and uses of the Brain and its nervous Appendix ... I addicted my self to the opening of Heads ... on which not only a more certain Physiologie than I had gained in the Schools but what I had long thought upon, the Pathologie of the Brain and nervous stock, might be built ... But for the more accurate performing this work, as I had not leisure, and perhaps not wit enough of myself, I was not ashamed to require the help of others. And here I made use of the Labours of the most Learned Physician and highly skilful Anatomist Doctor Richard Lower ... the edge of whose Knife and Wit ... have been an help to me in searching out both the frame and offices of before hidden Bodies ... so that in a short space there was nothing of the Brain, and its Appendix within the Skull, that seemed not plainly detected, and intimately beheld by us. After this, when we entred upon a far more difficult task, *viz*, the Anatomy of the Nerves, then very much appeared the plainly to be admired skill of this Man.

[10] See: William Feindel, *The anatomy of the brain and nerves*, Montreal (1965): page 19.

[11] See: Hughes (1991): page 39 for the suggestion that Ralph Bathurst (1620–1704) helped revise the text of *Cerebri anatome* and may have written the preface which Pordage translated.

Apart from twenty-two lines in praise of Lower, Willis acknowledges Thomas Millington (1628–1714): 'a most Learned Man, to whom I from day to day proposed privately my Conjectures and Observations, often confirmed me by his Suffrage being uncertain in mind, and not trusting to my own opinion'. Christopher Wren (1632–1723) 'was pleased out of his singular humanity, wherewith he abounds, to delineate with his most skilful hands many Figures of the Brain and Skull, whereby the work might be more exact'.[12] Willis explains that 'both ... were wont frequently to be present at our Dissections, and to confer and reason about the uses of the Parts'.

Much of the early anatomical work on the brain was done in animals, perhaps not without some sense of impropriety on Willis's part although he sought exoneration from the church. In the dedication of *Cerebri anatome* to Gilbert Sheldon, Archbishop of Canterbury, Willis writes:

> After I had slain so many victims, whole Hecatombs almost of all Animals, in the Anatomical Court, I could not have thought them rightly offered, unless they had been brought to the most holy Altar of Your Grace.

John Ward's (1629–1681) commonplace book also makes clear that Lower and Willis were using animals in their work on blood in April 1665:[13]

> Dick Lower is answering ye fellow yt wrote against Willis: Dr Willis and Dick Lower opened a dogg and they first let him blood in ye jugulars to discover whether Arterial blood and venal blood did differ in colour and constitution. Mr ffrancis told mee yt hee and Dick Lower found much chyle extravasated.

They were also dissecting the victims of judicial hanging, such as Anne Greene, and carrying out autopsies on Willis's patients. Ward wrote: 'My lady Windsor is dead: her brain was good as Dr. Willis said, but her liver was rotten and corrupt much. Dr. Willis lays much store upon ye brain nowadays'. Methodology enabled Willis to realize his aim of advancing knowledge on the anatomy of the brain and cranial nerves: 'Dr Willis hath got a new way of opening ye Brains, as to cut them on all parts from what holds them and so to turn them upside down.'[14] He started by removing the top of the skull and cutting away the cranial bones with scissors or a penknife. Willis makes much of the fact that the meninges hold the brain together and he considers the hind part separate from the cerebrum except where held by the fornix. After inspecting the meninges, external carotid arteries and sinuses, and observing the richly vascularized surface of the brain 'like a curious quilted ball', he lifted the anterior part of the cerebrum, dissected away the membranes at the base of the skull and severed the vessels, cranial nerves, and lower medulla. This allowed him to take the brain out from the skull, whole and inverted, before splitting the corpus callosum and turning the occipital lobes forward.[15] Often examined fresh, Willis sometimes preserved tissue in wine or another alcohol.[16]

[12] See chapter 3 for more detailed discussion of the provenance of these and other illustrations.

[13] See: D'Arcy Power, 'John Ward and his diary', part I, *Transactions of the Medical Society of London* 1917: 40; 1–26, reprinted in D'Arcy Power, *Selected writings 1877–*1930, Oxford (1931): page 187; and Robert G Frank, *Harvey and the Oxford physiologists. A study of scientific ideas*, Berkeley (1980): page 187 and endnote 175, chapter 7 pointing out that D'Arcy Power misdated this as 1658.

[14] See: D'Arcy Power (1931): page 191. The technique had already been used by Constanzo Varolio (1543–1575) and others before Willis.

[15] See: *The anatomy of the brain* (1681): page 57; and Feindel (1965): page 49.

[16] His method of preservation in spirit of wine, on the chemical nature of which Willis had written in *De fermentatione* (1659) had been introduced to Oxford by Robert Boyle (1627–1691).

His observations were mainly macroscopic but he picked away at structures with a knife and occasionally refers to use of the microscope:[17]

> The passages of the Nerves are not bored through as the Veins or Arteries; for the substance of those are not only impervious to any Bodkin, but no cavity can be seen in them, no not by the help of Spectacles or a Microscope ... The Nerves themselves (as may be discovered by the help of a Microcosm or Perspective-glass) are furnished throughout with pores and passages as it were so many little holes in a Honey-comb.

Willis followed Nicolas Steno (1638–1686) in tracing individual nerve pathways, achieving a slightly more accurate anatomy of the brain:[18]

> To wit, by gently scraping with the point of a Pen-knife its parts, we removed every where the softer and brownish substance, a-Kin to the Cortex of the Brain and the Oblong Marrow, many Medullary Chords or Strings, as it were distinct Nerves, wonderfully communicating among themselves and, with other white or medullary Bodies, were brought into sight. For as much as this Anatomical Administration, render'd the more secret passages of the Spirits, and the motions belonging to the Arcana's of the animal Government, very Conspicuous.

Although not all are described in comparable detail, Willis discusses seven main structures: the cerebrum, especially the anterior cortex; the corpus callosum, comprising all deep white matter of the cerebrum; the cerebellum; the medulla oblongata, which includes the third and fourth ventricles, basal ganglia, thalamus, midbrain, and pons; the cranial nerves and related structures; the spinal cord and nerve roots; and the blood vessels of the brain and spinal cord.[19] He barely mentions the peripheral nerves, other than in passing reference to the brachial and sacral plexuses, and the nerve to the intercostal muscles and diaphragm. Willis was working at a time when the brain was sometimes considered to be an appendage of the spinal cord. He took the opposite view and emphasized the dominance of the brain and cerebellum: 'if the out-flowings of the Spirits from the Brain and Cerebel be shut up or hindred, the nervous System presently suffers an Eclipse; if [the oblong marrow] be primarily distempered, the Brain and Cerebel suffer not for its fault'.[20] Willis considered the cerebrum to be the locus for memory and ideas. The motor and sensory centres were in the corpus striatum. Involuntary movement originated in the cerebellum. Pathways for movement and sensation traversed the medulla and spinal cord. His metaphor, unsurprisingly, was a tree. The cortex and cerebellum were the roots; the medulla and spinal cord formed the trunk; and the branches, twigs, and leaves were the nerves of the face, internal organs, and extremities.[21]

[17] See: *The anatomy of the brain* (1681): page 127. Although Robert Hooke's (1635–1703) *Micrographia, or some physiological descriptions of minute bodies made by magnifying glasses with observations and inquiries thereupon*, London (1665) appeared the year after *Cerebri anatome* was published, Willis had known Hooke since the early 1650s. Christopher Wren had made drawings in Oxford which came to the attention of Charles II who asked the Royal Society for more; but Wren was busy with other projects and Hooke took on the work.

[18] See: Thomas Willis, *Two discourses concerning the soul of brutes* (1683): page 25; and Clarke and CD O'Malley (1968): pages 584, 819–20.

[19] See: Clarke and O'Malley (1968): pages 582–4 for their translation of Willis's own summary of these structures, citing *Cerebri anatome* (1664): pages 81–3.

[20] See: *The anatomy of the brain* (1681): page 91.

[21] See: Isler (1968): page 97.

As the title implies, *Cerebri anatome* is primarily about the anatomy of the brain and nerves. Here, Willis is less concerned with function. Nevertheless, in line with the doctrine of fermentation set out in 1659, he does argue that the brain works through the movement of animal spirits within nerve pathways. These pass outwards for movement and inwards for sensation. Animal spirits are produced in several locations from fermented blood and delivered through the medulla and spinal cord to the nerves: 'irradiating the medullary Rope, [they] are not produced in it but flow in from elsewhere; and why should not we think the same of the middle marrow ... this part is rather the Mart or Exchange of the Spirits than its Shop or Work-house'. Stored in 'the compartments and enclosures ... of their own accord, without a driver to direct or control their movements' they 'flow out in sequence and in proper and regular order'. The production of animal spirits mainly takes place during sleep, when activity is temporarily suppressed. Wakefulness occurs when production is sufficient.[22] The chemical basis of animal spirits is uniform throughout the brain and nervous stock. They move within preferred descending and ascending pathways seen as streaks on longitudinal section of the striatum. Protuberances and processes in these tracts provide places for the animal spirits to be 'parked' in order to avoid collision with those moving in opposite directions.

It is clear that, as early as 1663, Willis had planned three books that would explain anatomy and function of the brain in health, the diseases to which it was susceptible including their morbid anatomy, and the relationship between mind and brain. Although it was eight years before the project was finally completed, in the conclusion to *Cerebri anatome* he gives advance notice of the next two works, *Pathologiæ cerebri* (1667) and *De anima brutorum* (1672):[23]

> Thus much for the Anatomy of the Brain and Cerebel, and of their Appendix, both Medullar and Nervous, and of the Uses and Offices of all the several Parts ... There remains not only the outward Courts and Porches of this Fabrick, as it were of a certain Kingly Palace, but also its intimate Recesses and private Chambers, that we next inquire into, what the lady or Inhabitant of this Princely place may be, in what part she doth chiefly reside, and by what Rule and Government she disposes and orders her Family. Then we ought to take notice, what defects and irregularities happen to it, or to its parts and powers; then to what injuries or changes of Diseases this Building or House, to wit, the Brain and nervous Stock, may be obnoxious ... For the Crown of the Work, a certain theory of the Soul of Brutes should be added.

The meninges

Willis assigns several important properties to the meninges. Self-evidently the dura mater provides a covering for the brain. It also sleeves vessels and nerves that enter and exit the skull. The meninges delineate the main divisions of the brain. Less intuitively, they have 'nervous cords or strings', as in the ventricles of the heart. These form a network of cells which regulate the inflow and outflow of blood through the underlying brain 'according to the passions of the Soul, or the necessities of Nature, staying the blood sometimes longer near the

[22] See: Clarke and O'Malley (1968): pages 724–6 citing *Cerebri anatome* pages 73–5, 91–2.

[23] See: Willis, *The description and use of the nerves* (1681): page 192; and chapter 3 for comment on the architectural metaphor in this quote.

confines of the Brain, sometimes driving it forward from thence towards the Præcordia'. The dura mater heats the blood 'like a Balneum Mariæ' distilling a 'most subtil Liquor' and 'like an impervious Alembrick' prevents this from evaporation. The pia mater, much more intimately applied to the contours of the cerebrum, complements these functions.

Pursuing his theme that they provide both structure and function, Willis describes the meninges as one of the places where the nitro-aerial particles in arterial blood adapt to form animal spirit, the 'marriage ... as it were a masculine and feminine seed mixed together ... and so they impart to all parts both sense and motion, and all the powers of life and growth'. Movement implies function. Therefore on the basis that the dura mater pulsates, moves with respiration and contracts, it follows that the meninges also drive the newly synthesized nervous juice into the brain. But Willis has his doubts:[24]

> That it hath motion, it can hardly be thought, because it is tyed in very many place to the Skull; and yet it is probable, that the same may sometimes, in some parts at least, be contracted and wrinkled or drawn together: And certainly there is no doubt, that it is contracted and remitted in sneezing. In like manner, when from an hurt of this a Vomiting or Convulsive motions follow in the *Viscera* or Members, this Membrane is the cause, which being somewhere contracted or divided, infolds with it self the substance contained within the same Convulsion or Spasm.

The fact that they are sensitive argues in favour of the meninges having functional as well as anatomical properties:[25]

> As to sense, 'tis not to be doubted, but that it hath it exquisitely: For since all the Membranes have feeling, and owe that faculty to the afflux of the animal Spirits from the Brain, surely this Meninx, for that it is nearer and very much of kin to the Brain and its Appendix, so that it clothes very many Nerves going out of the Skull, it obtains a very accurate virtue of feeling: which thing also may be argued from the effect; because the pains of the Head often proceed from the breach of unity excited in this Membrane.

However, others assume that the dura mater merely stretches and contracts in response to movement of the underlying brain. And when it comes to his discussion of the pia mater, Willis himself finally backs away from the view that the meninges have motor and sensory properties even though they are clearly the seat of disease:[26]

> As to the motion of this Membrane, we wholly deny, that it hath in it self a perpetual Systole and Diastole; however, the Pulses in some Arteries, have seemed something like it, which have given occasion perchance to this vulgar Opinion. Yet in the meantime it may be lawful to believe, that this Meninx, for that it is very sensible, is rendred obnoxious to Cramps and convulsive motions: and that from its greater contraction the fits of the Falling sickness do arise, and from its lesser and more partial corrugation or wrinkling together, Head-aches, as hath been said, and also sometimes Scotomies, Vertigoes, and often Convulsions of the Members and Viscera, planted at a greater distance from the origine of the Nerves, being drawn into consent.

[24] See: *The anatomy of the brain* (1681): pages 79–80.
[25] See: *The anatomy of the brain* (1681): page 79.
[26] See: *The anatomy of the brain* (1681): page 90.

Eventually it was Humphry Ridley (1653–1708) who showed experimentally that the dura only moves as a result of pulsations in the brain. With that evidence, this slight diversion on brain function, from which Willis does not emerge with particular credit, came to an end.[27]

The ventricles

Willis explains that the cerebral ventricles are created by folding the 'exterior border of the brain' similar to 'the empty space contained within the cavity of the universe'. The fourth ventricle lies in the space below the connections of the cerebellum held by its peduncles to the medulla. The third and fourth ventricles communicate through the aqueduct.[28] He rejects a role for the ventricles and their contents in determining brain function. The animal spirits do not require these oceans in which to move but are sufficiently contained within the pores of the brain in order to serve the faculties of the soul. Rather 'almost all anatomists of more recent times have given to this more inward chamber of the brain the vile duty of a sewer'.[29] Even though the removal of recrements ultimately takes place through the veins and lymph channels, or by 'vaporization', those drains may become saturated and waste does then accumulate in the ventricles, 'the vile office of a Jakes or sink to this more inward chamber of the Brain'.[30] Made in the choroid plexuses, the cerebrospinal fluid not only provides a sump for the removal of waste but also acts as a hot spring that maintains the temperature of the distributed animal spirits.

Willis was uncertain how the ventricles themselves drain. The mammillary bodies, which he named 'glandulæ candicantes', pass recrements to the 'hollow' infundibulum and from there into the two parts of the pituitary, distinguished by colour, and thence to the nose: 'the root of the fornix ... tends towards the infundibulum as well as to the ventricle underlying the orbicular prominence'.[31] This analysis is close to the ancient doctrine that the ventricles discharge through passages in the 'Tunnel' (infundibulum) into the palate or through pores in the skull base to reach the nostrils. But Willis qualifies this dogma:[32]

> There is no body who presently will not easily think, that by neither of these ways the excretion of any humor can be made; for neither from the pituitary Glandula through the Wedge-like bone, nor from the mammillary processes through the holes of the Sieve-like bone, is there any manifest aperture or opening to be perceived.

His point is that the ventricles empty by seeping through the nervous tissue, as in a sponge or woollen cloth, not through holes in the bones. Having fumbled around the issue of how the ventricles drain, Willis ends chapter XII by explaining that it is not so much the route of exit

[27] See: Max Neuberger, *The historical development of experimental brain and spinal cord physiology before Flourens*, Baltimore (1981: translation of German edition from 1897 with additional notes): pages 71–92, citing H Ridley, *The anatomy of the brain*, London (1695); and H Ridley, 'Experimentum anatomicum ad veram duræ matris motus causam detegendam institutum', *Philosophical Transactions of the Royal Society* 1704: 23; 1480–4.

[28] See: AT Rasmussen, *Some trends in neuroanatomy*, Dubuque (1947): page 12.

[29] See: Clarke and O'Malley (1968): pages 723–6.

[30] In debunking issues such the primacy of the ventricles in brain function, Willis was also keen to explain that, well developed in species devoid of intellect and memory, the pineal is not the seat of the soul. Rather its function is to sift and return unwanted material from arterial blood towards the veins and lymphatics.

[31] See: Meyer (1971): pages 18, 20, footnotes 12, 75, and 76.

[32] See: *The anatomy of the brain* (1681): page 98.

of ventricular fluid through holes of the sieve-like bone that he doubts but, rather, the means of egress:[33]

> It is much more to be doubted, because these holes ... [are] covered over and fully stuffd, with the insertions of the *Dura Mater* and nervous Fibres; sent on either side from the mammillary Process, transmit nothing of humor ... Further, there is nothing more certain than that the serous humors are pressed out from the Glandula's and extremities of the Vessels ending within the Nostrils into their Caverns; so besides that 'tis scarce possible for the humors to descend from the brain, it is not absolutely needful to suppose this sort of means of Excretion. But that we may reason a little farther ... there is no reason that I may probably believe, that some humors also do shower down from the Brain into the cavities of the Nostrils ... creeping both through the Fibres and Membranes, as through the straining holes of a Filter or Strainer.

The cerebrum

The brain is composed of two hemispheres, each in two parts divided by the middle cerebral arteries: 'like a Bounding river to both, distinguishing them as it were into two provinces'. The most obvious feature of the cerebral cortex is that it is convoluted and with a twisted surface 'like intestines'. Willis makes the important point that folding much increases the amount of tissue but with preservation of the underlying structures which remain in continuity. The cortex is 'ploughed into furrows from which arise cliffs ... of uneven height ... in the bottom of each furrow a convolution arisen from the right side may be carried to the left'. Redundancy ensures that function continues when one part is injured or diseased: 'So the Brain, Like a Castle, divided into many Towers or places of Defence, is thereby made the stronger and harder to be taken'. More specifically, there are:[34]

> Banks or ridges of broken crevices, not in a direct series, but cross-wise; so that in the bottom of every furrow, a convolution arising from the right side, is carried to the left, then others following next, being sent to the left side, is drawn to the right, and so by turns the inequalities of the whole brain are variegated in this order.

This degree of complexity is needed to allow the animal spirits to roam freely within discrete pathways in recalling and acting upon memories. Furthermore, the convolutions, 'the anfractuous or crankling brain, like a plot of ground, planted everywhere with nooks and corners, and dauks and mole-hills', protect the blood vessels as they pass from the meninges and penetrate the cerebrum.[35] The size of the cerebrum and its convolutions reflects the relative requirement for animal spirits serving memory, imagination, and appetite in different species. Willis links his observations on the complexity of gyri (or 'plicae') directly to intelligence. Action by instinct requires no memory and therefore the cortex of beasts and fishes

[33] See: *The anatomy of the brain* (1681): page 100.
[34] See: *The anatomy of the brain* (1681): page 92.
[35] See: *The anatomy of the brain* (1681): page 92; and Clarke and O'Malley (1968): pages 388–90 citing *Cerebri anatome* (1664), pages 65–8.

is less developed or entirely flat, unlike the cerebellum which is relatively uniform across species:[36]

> For as the animal Spirits, for the various acts of Imagination and Memory, ought to be moved within certain and distinct limited or bounded places, and those motions to be often iterated or repeated through the same tracts or paths: for that reason these manifold convolutions and infoldings of the brain are required for these divers manners of ordinations of the animal Spirits, to wit, that in these Cells or Store-houses severally placed, might be kept the species of sensible things, as occasion serves, may be taken from thence. Hence these folds or rollings about are far more and greater in a man than in any other living Creature, to wit, for the various and manifold actings of the superior Faculties; but they are garnished with an uncertain, and as it were fortuitous series, that the exercises of the animal Function might be free and changeable, and not determined to one. Those Gyrations or Turnings about in four footed beasts are fewer and, in some, as in a Cat, they are found to be in a certain figure and order: wherefore this Brute thinks on, or scarce remembers any thing but what the instinct and needs of Nature suggest.

Tracts and pathways in the brain

Willis emphasized that the two halves of the brain are joined 'either by a contiguity, or by processes set forth [so that] every impression coming this or that way, becomes still one and the same'. The corpus callosum linking the two hemisphere acts as a 'market place' where the recently synthesized spirits are gathered. Willis describes 'a transverse medullary tract, resembling a larger nerve [which] extends from one striate body to the other, and, as it were, uniting these and effecting their mutual communication'. This is the anterior commissure.[37] Although drawn separately, the striae terminalis (named the 'tænia') and anterior commissure connect the amygdaloid nucleus to several anterior structures. Willis did not identify the hippocampus unless, as seems unlikely, this was his limbus posterior of the corpus callosum.

Andreas Vesalius (1514–1564) had described the corpus striatum and optic thalamus but Willis distinguished these structures in Tabula VIII of *De anima brutorum*, and gave a first hint at subdivisions, using 'prominentiæ lentiformes' as an alternative name. He understood the concept of a central ganglion in which there is a coming together of disparate pathways. Although Willis mentions structures that are integral to motor and sensory systems, he held that, in continuity with the cortex and the medulla oblongata, the striate body is both the head station for sensation and the centre for voluntary motor impulses. Willis conflated fibre tracts that make up the medial lemniscus (projecting to the ventrolateral nucleus of the thalamus) with the complex arrangement of descending motor fibres that pass through

[36] See: *The anatomy of the brain* (1681): page 92; and the flatter language of the translation by R Dow (1908–1995) in 'Thomas Willis (1621–1675) as a comparative neurologist', *Annals of Medical History* 1940; 2: 181–94, cited in Meyer (1971): page 122 footnote 2. Louis Gratiolet (1815–1865), *Mémoire sur les plis cérébraux de 'l'homme et des primates*, Paris (1854): pages 6 and 60, described these 'belles observations de Willis' as having inspired his own research.

[37] See: A Meyer and R Hierons, 'A note on Thomas Willis' views on the corpus striatum and the internal capsule', *Journal of the neurological Sciences* 1964: 1; 547–54, at page 548; and Meyer (1971): page 14 citing structure labelled G in *Cerebri anatome*, Figura VII, and discussion of prior accounts by Jean Riolan (1588–1657), 'Anthropographica' in *Opera omnia*, Paris (1649) and the contemporary observations of Marcelli Malpighi (1628–1694) 'De cerebri cortice', in *De viscerum structura exercitatio anatomica*, Amsterdam (1665).

the internal capsule and relay into the striate body.[38] He emphasized that the striate body is a paired structure but with the two halves united:[39]

> This joyning together of the chamfered bodies is made, that their actions and passions may not be double: but through the species of the sensible object or conceptions of the motions to be performed, coming from the Brain or Sensory being double, are carried also double to the first Sensory; yet for as much as either substance or frame of this, communicates with the other, every impression coming this or that way becomes one and the same. For it may be observed, in the whole Head, that though almost all things are double, yet each of them communicate among themselves, either by a contiguity, or by processes sent forth. And so by the duplication of it, care is taken against the absolute privation or defect of the act, so joyning together of its duplicature provides against the empty or contuse multiplication of the same species.

With some exceptions, Willis did not separately name structures within the hindbrain, collectively referring to these as the medulla. In commenting on *Cerebri anatome*, Raymond Vieussens (1641–1715) acknowledged that: 'it was without doubt ... that the famous Willis called the [anterior] processes of the medulla oblongata, corpora striata'.[40] In his discussion of voluntary movement, Willis described what is now called the internal capsule as the 'limbus posterior of the striatum' containing 'the optic striæ and indeed other medullary processes arising from the orbicular prominence'. He noticed that the internal capsule and striate body are sometimes atrophied in people who have been long paralysed.[41] Meyer points out that, in naming the thalamus, Willis confused the Galenic term Θαλάμη (a lurking place) for Θάλαμος (a bed chamber).[42] Willis traced the visual pathway from the optic nerves through the chiasm to the thalamus and corpora quadrigemina. On the naming of these significant parts, he declares: 'indeed the use of these (unless my conjecture deceives me) seems far more noble, than that they should deserve those vile names of *Nates* and *Testes* (Buttocks and Testicles)'. Willis regarded these prominences as a storehouse 'in which the animal Spirits go apart in their passage from the oblong marrow into the cerebral, and from this to that on the other side'.[43] He noticed the decussation of the motor tracts in the medulla and named the pyramids, stating that these carry ascending as well as descending pathways.[44]

For Willis, sensation involved a tier of linked structures which processed the crude impressions into increasingly refined perceptions. The incoming spirits are represented as instinct in the medulla and cerebellum and drive the reciprocal workings of the viscera and sexual function. Common sense is dependent on the corpora striata where animal spirits are sifted as if passing through a lens and projected onto the corpus callosum. From there

[38] See: Meyer and Hierons (1964): page 552.

[39] See: *The anatomy of the brain* (1681): page 103.

[40] See: Clarke and O'Malley (1968): page 588 citing Raymond Vieussens (1641–1715) *Neurographia universalis*, Lyons (1684). For Meyer (1971): page 14, Vieussens is more direct in his explanations whereas Willis gets distracted by theory; Vieussens puts right Willis's errors, amplifies some of his correct observations and has better and more detailed illustrations.

[41] See: Alfred Meyer and Raymond Hierons, 'On Thomas Willis's concepts of neurophysiology [part I]', *Medical History* 1965: 9; 1–15 at page 9; and Isler (1968): page 97.

[42] See: Meyer (1971): pages 8, footnote 6, 13, and 38 drawing attention to the structure labelled H in *De Anima Brutorum*, Tabula VIII, and pointing out that this was missed by Vesalius in *De fabrica* (1643) and usually attributed to Felix Vicq d'Azyr (1748–1794), *Œvres recueilles*, Paris (1805).

[43] See: *The anatomy of the brain* (1681): page 64, where Willis appears to have appreciated that some pathways in the hindbrain are crossed.

[44] See: Hughes (1991): pages 63–4.

they proceed as phantasies, passing through the fornix which evokes imagination. Once a sensory impression reaches the cortex it dissolves into recesses of the sulci and is stored as a retrievable memory. A newly arrived sensation may stir a stored element and evoke a reminiscence which has emotional content and, in turn, elicits voluntary movement. At any level, when charged with emotion, sensations may stall and be returned as an involuntary movement: 'Motus est reflexus qui a sensione prævia dependens illico retorquetur' (a movement is reflex if it depends upon a previous sensation, and is turned back at once).[45]

The cerebellum ('cerebel')

Considered by anatomists and neurologists working in and after the mid-nineteenth century as a centre that receives information on intended movement, reconciles this with sensory feedback on what has occurred, and smooths out the inaccuracies and oscillations, the cerebellum has since also been credited with planning, set changing, and cognition, thereby greatly elevating its status in brain sciences. Against this background, in a stroke of genius Willis understood that an essential property of the nervous system is to integrate reflex responses to the external and internal environments and orchestrate involuntary movement. Necessarily constrained by what he could observe, Willis emphasized that the nerves reaching the face and viscera that alter with emotion and involuntary responses originate in the cerebellum.[46] He attributed these vegetative functions to the generation of animal spirits, released rhythmically or in spurts, depending on demand, through the three peduncles that connect the cerebellum to the medulla and cranial nerves. The chapters that Willis devotes to the cerebellum (II, XV, and XVI) introducing the concept of involuntary movement serve as the basis for a more extensive discussion of the two cranial nerves that determine vegetative function: the 'wandring' and the 'intercostal' (the vagus and sympathetic chain, in modern classification). On 18 January 1661, Lower wrote to Boyle from Christ Church:[47]

> I ... should have wrote to you sooner, but that the doctor was not at leisure till of late to make those dissections of the brain, which he hoped; but at length we have had the opportunity of cutting up several, and the doctor, finding most parts of the brain imperfectly described, intends to make a whole new draught thereof, with the several uses of the distinct parts, according to his fancy, seeing few authors speak anything considerable of it; so that at present I shall suspend my thoughts which I had of sending you a relation of the discourse we had in the several dissections, and only tell you, that, according to his opinion of the use of the cerebellum for involuntary motion, he shewed me several times the nerves (which authors call the sixth conjugation) to proceed out of a stalk or stem, which comes down out of the cerebellum, and makes a great half circle under the medulla oblongata, and so returns and ends in that nerve on each side.

Willis's account of the gross anatomy of the cerebellum describes the orderly convolutions of gyri and twistings on the surface, 'thin lappets, or little rings or circles', similar to the

[45] See: Clarke and O'Malley (1968): pages 472–3 citing *De anima brutorum* (1672): pages 43–4, 47–8.

[46] See: Meyer and Hierons (1965): page 11 for a sympathetic plea that those who criticise Willis for placing the origin of the autonomic system in the cerebellum should be forgiving of the anatomical near miss and allow simple replacement of medulla for cerebellum and hypothalamus for corpora quadrigemina.

[47] See: Feindel (1965): page 15.

parallel lines on a sphere or globe. The surface is like an orderly cluster of grapes closely compacted and appearing as 'Tubercles or little Tad-stoles or Puffs which grow together on little stalks'.[48] The substance of the cerebellum converges on three distinct medullary processes which Willis illustrates, drawing the attention of readers to structures labelled Q, P, and R on Figura VII (Pl.8). In fact, Figura VII identifies only Q, the superior cerebellar peduncle, and P labels the testis of the quadrigeminal body. This is simply a misprint for it is Figura VIII (Pl.9) that depicts and correctly labels the three peduncles, designated by Willis as medullary processes.[49] The structure of the cerebellum 'is terminated in a process in form of a Worm' (the vermis).

Willis displaces the belief of the ancients that the function of the cerebellum is memory. Rather the cerebellum is responsible for the synthesis of animal spirits that flow out to the medulla and certain cranial nerves which: 'inhabiting the ... folds and lappets of the ... Cerebel perform unperceivedly and silently their works of Nature without our knowledge or care'. Although 'sometimes to contract, sometimes to extend its Systasis in the whole or in part', the flow of animal spirits from the cerebellum on which natural functions, instincts, passions, and impulses depend is continuous.[50] That outflow is responsible for alterations in 'the beating of the Heart, easie Respiration, the concoction of the Aliment, the protrusion of the Chyle, and many others';[51] and in response to fever or other warnings of 'the evil, by which they being incited to oppose the enemy, cause a motion of another kind'. Willis is aware that disconnections interfere with the flow of animal spirits. For this reason, diseases affecting the cerebellum produce 'cruel and horrid symptoms [that] seize upon the praecordia and the region of the thorax or abdomen'. He emphasizes that sudden movement of the head backwards might lead to altered respiration, heart rhythm, and consciousness.[52]

But Willis introduces one ambiguity. He is aware that there are reciprocal connections between the cerebrum and the cerebellum. Their animal spirits do not work in isolation. The cerebellum conveys natural impulses to the cortex changing emotions and allowing the internal organs to influence purposive movements. Conversely the flow of animal spirits from the cortex is diverted through the quadrigeminal bodies and pons to the cerebellum before reaching the medulla. In this way, voluntary acts are linked to involuntary visceral responses. In a fever, the pulse and respiration increase and the person reaches for a drink of water to cool the brow. And yet, for all this wisdom, it is unfortunate that Willis incorrectly suggests unilateral outflow from the cerebellum through the middle cerebral peduncle and waxes too lyrical on its function:[53]

> The [cerebellar] spirits are drawn from all the folds into the medullary tracts and thence into the two wide middle strips where they form a welling source or fountain, and there

[48] See: *The anatomy of the brain* (1681): page 123.

[49] See: *The anatomy of the brain* (1681): pages 67–8; and Clarke and O'Malley (1968): pages 637–8 pointing out that only Q is identified (in Figura VII). These bundles had been described by Bartolomeo Eustachius (*c.*1510–1574) and Costanzo Variola (1543–1575) but Willis gave the fullest account and named them peduncles.

[50] See: *The anatomy of the brain* (1681): page 114.

[51] See: *The anatomy of the brain* (1681): pages 110–11; and Clarke and O'Malley (1968): pages 636–40.

[52] Neurologists, failing to suppress the urge for retrospective diagnosis, may be tempted to suggest that this statement, somewhat out of context, refers to cerebellar ectopia.

[53] See: *The anatomy of the brain* (1681): page 113. As Vieussens (1684) correctly described, the cortex projects afferent fibres to the cerebellum through the middle cerebellar peduncles and those from the spinal cord enter the inferior cerebellar peduncle, whereas the main output to the cortex is via the red nucleus and other midbrain structures through the superior cerebellar peduncle.

like bubbling waters, with a constant whirling are circulated within, and then run forth into the appropriate parts of the nervous system.

Medulla oblongata and spinal cord

Willis knew that the parts of the brain influencing the spinal cord, and those receiving animal spirits from it, traverse the medulla oblongata. This structure therefore assumes special significance in his formulation on the anatomy and function of the brain and nervous stock as a whole. In describing its relationship to nearby parts, he wrote: 'The Tract of the oblong marrow, which as it were the King's High-Way, leads from the Brain, as the Metropolis, into many Provinces of the nervous stock, by private recesses and cross-ways'.[54] Willis describes the medulla as 'the Poets Parnassus ... like the letter Y' and he is clear that it is the structure through which the animal spirits emanating from the brain and cerebellum converge and flow into the nerves of the whole body. Here traffic is bidirectional: 'to wit, they are directed either outward towards the Nerves, when they exert the loco-motive Faculty, or they look inward towards their Fountains, when the acts of sense, or rather the apprehensions of sensible things are performed'.[55] Protuberances and processes provide recesses for the animal spirits so that these do not 'disturb one anothers offices'. These also allow animal spirits to be stored for specific functions and not swept on by the main torrent flowing towards the spinal cord. Willis has rather little to say about structure of the spinal cord itself other than that it conveys spirits from the brain to the nerves: 'from the bottom of the Brain even to the *Os sacrum*, seems like the Pneumatick Chest, or Bellows of a pair of Organs, which includes the blast or breath destinated to every Pipe'.[56] Where nerves are most abundant, its size increases. Willis describes the cervical and lumbar enlargements. He mentions the anterior and posterior nerve roots but, despite having the concept of reflex movement, does not speculate on their respective efferent and afferent connectivity.[57]

The cranial nerves

In describing structures that constitute the outflow of what would now be termed the autonomic nervous system, Willis's description of the cranial nerves is the monumental achievement of the two treatises published in 1664. He introduces these in *Cerebri anatome* but extends the account in *Nervorumque descriptio et usus*. The numbering of cranial nerves has been the topic of several historical reviews.[58] Willis was taught anatomy based on Galen's system of seven pairs starting with the optic nerve, the olfactory being considered part of the

[54] See: *The anatomy of the brain* (1681): page 110.

[55] See: *The anatomy of the brain* (1681): page 101.

[56] See: *The anatomy of the brain* (1681): page 124.

[57] There are many accounts of the Bell-Magendie disagreement played out early in the nineteenth century on who first correctly assigned motor function to the anterior and sensory input to the posterior nerve roots; but none better than Paul Cranefield, *The way in and the way out. François Magendie, Charles Bell and the roots of the spinal nerves*, Mount Cisco (1974).

[58] See for example: Raymond Hierons and Alfred Meyer, 'Some priority questions arising from Thomas Willis' work on the brain', *Proceedings of the Royal Society of Medicine* 1962; 55: 287–92 for a detailed account with original archival observations; and C Wilbur Rucker, 'History of the numbering of the cranial nerves, *Mayo Clinic Proceedings* (1966): 41; 453–61, who provides a slightly different perspective.

brain, and all movement of the eyes assigned to a single paired oculomotor nerve.[59] Three anatomists revised the Galenic scheme although their work was carried out in different periods. Eustachius made novel observations in 1563 but these were lost until 1714. By then Willis had independently described his own scheme. Twenty years after Willis, Vieussens provided further amendments which acknowledged and incorporated Willis's work. That system remained largely unchanged until 1778 when, aged 23, Samuel Thomas Soemmering (1755–1830) published his doctoral thesis proposing twelve paired cranial nerves—a system that, with some renumbering and transient attempts to add others and distinguish divisions, especially of the seventh and eighth, survives.[60]

There are difficulties in reconciling Willis's numbering, descriptions, and illustrations of the cranial nerves. Taken together he identifies ten pairs.[61] He describes eight in detail but several of these have independent branches. Mentioned much more briefly but illustrated in several figures are the ninth and tenth pair, the latter comprising the first or upper few cervical roots, and therefore not cranial nerves. In reordering and extending the Galenic system, Figura I (Pl.1) is important not only for its depiction of the vascular anastomosis at the base of the brain (see next) but also for showing Willis's classification of the cranial nerves, as described in the legend:[62]

> ... DD, *The smelling Nerves or first pair*; EE, *The Optick or seeing Nerves the second pair*; FF, *The moving Nerves of the Eyes the third pair*; GG, *The pathetick Nerves of the Eyes or the fourth pair*; HH, *The fifth pair of Nerves*; II, *The sixth pair of Nerves*; KKKK, *The auditory or hearing Nerves and their two processes on either side of them the seventh pair*; LLIIII, *The wandring pair, or the eighth pair consisting of many Fibres*; MM, *The Spinal Nerves coming from afar to the origins of the wandring pair*; NN, *The ninth pair consisting also of many Fibres (which tending downwards, grow together into one Trunk) which arises a little above the process of the hinder part of the Head*; OO, *The tenth pair tending downwards* ...

Willis's intercostal nerve (sympathetic trunk) is not included as one of the cranial nerves but it is highly relevant to his account of the function of the wandring nerve and extensively described in the text. In view of his focus on involuntary movements affecting structures within the thorax and abdomen, the ninth (Pl.11), tenth (Pl.12) and eleventh (Pl.13) tables which illustrate the wandring (vagus) and intercostal nerves (sympathetic) in man and brute beasts are of particular significance. The intercostal nerve is introduced and first depicted in Tabula IX (Pl.11):

> ... D. *The trunk of the intercostal Nerve consisting of the roots of the three aforesaid Roots about to pass into the Ganglioform infolding: which infolding of the intercostal Nerve, brought*

[59] See: John Evelyn, *The diary of John Evelyn Esquire F.R.S.* Ed. William Bray, London (1818, printed *c.*1930): pages 205, 414, and 737 for details of how, whilst attending the 'famous Anatomie Lecture' in Padua in January 1646, having purchased 'rare tables' of the nerves and veins from Dr Jo. Athelstenius Leonænas, Evelyn 'caus'd [him] to prepare a third of the Lungs, Liver and Nervi sexti par ... which I sent into England and afterwards presented to the Royal Society, being the first of that kind that had been seen there, and for aught I know in the world ...'. Evelyn did not make that gift until 31 October 1667, his birthday, when he 'receiv'd the public thanks of the Society; and they are hanging up in their Repository with an inscription'. On 21 January 1702, 'At the Royal Society there was read and approv'd the delineation and description of my Table of Veins and Arteries, by Mr Cooper the chirurgeon, in order to their being engrav'd'.

[60] See: ST Soemmering, *De basi encephali et originibus nervorum cranio egredientum libri quinque*, Gottingen (1778): pages 184; and Rucker (1966): pages 458–61.

[61] See: Rasmussen (1947): page 54; and Feindel (1965): page 52.

[62] See: *The anatomy of the brain* (1681): page 62.

> *without the Skull, seems to be the highest knot. . . . i. A shoot sent from the cervical Infolding of the intercostal Nerve into the trunk of the wandring Pair . . .*

Willis deals with the first four cranial nerves in a relatively perfunctory way. Precise in tracing its origin, the smelling nerve emerges from the 'shanks of the oblong Marrow within the chamfered bodies and chambers of the Optick Nerves' (the striate body and optic thalamus).[63] From there it passes along the base of the brain and, coated in dura mater, penetrates the 'Sieve-like bone' to reach the nostrils. Being purely sensory, the smelling nerve is soft and medullar allowing easy movement of the animal spirits. Its many strands pass through the cribriform plate preventing too sharp or painful an olfactory sensation. It is larger in herbivores than flesh-eating brutes and man who depends more on taste and sight than smell for discriminating food. The nose is supplied with a branch of the fifth nerve which also reaches the palate. The optic nerve receives visual impressions from the retina and its arrangements serve both to identify what is viewed but also:[64]

> That the visible species, received from either Eye, might appear still the same, and not double; for this conjunction of the twofold Organ frames the double image into one; which once united, when afterwards it is carried to either side of the common Sensory, for that it is on both sides alike, appears still the same.

Willis makes the point that the optic nerves come together close to the infundibulum and then diverge but he does not suggest a decussation of fibres at the chiasm. He shows most enthusiasm for cranial nerves which he considers to arise directly from the cerebellum. These are concerned with reflective, or involuntary, movements through which the animal spirits communicate the 'intestine commotions of the Affections'. These nerves pass through the corpora quadrigemina and Willis makes much of the comparative size of the nates and testes in species that differ in their dependence on instinct and wit, respectively. But, again, he is careful to emphasize the interplay between activities of the brain and cerebellum mediated through the cranial nerves:[65]

> Nerves . . . which owe their flock to the Cerebel, and seem to be designed for the offices of the involuntary Function . . . are compelled to obey the beck and government of the Brain . . . the Nerves of either Government communicate variously among themselves . . . so that the offices of one are drawn into parts of the other . . . This derogates nothing from the privileges of the Cerebel, that it may not be called a free and municipal City, and so Mistress of the involuntary Function . . . the Brain it self in many things is compelled to serve the Cerebel and its Government . . . the Brain owes much to the Cerebel . . . both these parts, though Principals, perform mutual offices, and as it were in a circle, require and accomplish services one for another.

The influence of animal spirits derived from the cerebellum is especially relevant to nerves reaching the eyes. This arrangement allows complex voluntary and involuntary movements such as, for example, those occurring in response to 'Fear, Shame, Anger, Sadness, yea and in all Affections of the Head and Heart, whether we will or no, the Eyes are respectively figured'.

[63] See: *The description and use of the nerves* (1681): page 137; and Meyer (1971): page 85, footnote 5 for the explanation that Willis's description of 'the peduncles of the medulla oblongata between the corpora striata and optic thalamus' merely refers to the entirety of the brain stem.

[64] See: *The anatomy of the brain* (1681): page 103.

[65] See: *The anatomy of the brain* (1681): pages 120–1.

Willis writes that in the Ox and other beasts, each ocular muscle is innervated by the third nerve with additional supply from branches of the fourth, fifth, and sixth nerves. But in man, the third nerve has a more restricted distribution:[66]

> Four branches, three of which are carried ... into three straight distinct Muscles, to wit, one for lifting up, the other bringing together, the third pressing close the Eye; the other branch of it goes forward further with a single trunk, and is implanted in the middle of the Muscle going about the Eye, turning obliquely to the inward corner downwards ... sufficient ... to perform most spontaneous motions of the Eye.

The fourth nerve, originating from the nates and testes, passes with others to the eye and is inserted 'wholly on the Muscle called the *Trochlear* Muscle'. Responding with involuntary movements in all species, it moves the eye 'pathetically' and is so named: 'we see the greater Pike gaping for his prey first of all to roll about the eyes, and to look sour; then with a swift shooting out of his body to invade the lesser fry of fish'.[67] With a branch of the carotid artery (ophthalmic vessel), Willis's sixth nerve enters the back of the eye with the third and fourth and one branch of the fifth cranial nerve, and reaches the muscle that 'draws back the Eye planed in its outward angle'. In brutes, a seventh muscle 'winks or twinkles' the eye (orbicularis orbis, in fact innervated by the facial nerve).

Unlike the first four, each of which is either sensory or motor, the fifth nerve 'serves for the exercise of either Faculty' and innervates the eyes, nose, mouth, and the rest of the parts of the face. It comprises a bundle of fibres that provide:[68]

> A certain Sympathy and consent of actions ... to wit, the communion of those nerves is the cause why the sight and smell move spittle and please the palate; nor by any other means are the Præcordia affected, according to the various conceptions of the Brain, and transmit their affections to the several parts of the Face.

In his more detailed description of the further course of the fifth nerve, Willis mentions a lower branch that reaches muscles concerned with chewing, sensation of the lips, and teeth, and (incorrectly but understandably) taste. In another near miss, he states that its superior branch joins the sixth nerve and, together, they unite to constitute a root of the intercostal nerve. Here he seems close to describing the sympathetic innervation of the eye. It is in the 'pathetick' functions of the fifth nerve that Willis describes the ophthalmic branch innervating structures around the eye, the sclera, and uvea and the lacrimal glands so that: 'wrinkling the Eye-brows, and by compressing the Glandula's produce those kinds of looks of the Eyes, and marks of sorrow and grief';[69] and through its innervation of the nostril, 'wherefore passing out of a dark place into the light, at the first beholding of the Sun, presently whether we will or no we shall sneez'. Taken with the remaining branches to the lower face, the involuntary responses mediated by this nerve:[70]

> Being disturbed by the imagination of an unseemly thing ... cause the blood to be more forced into the Cheeks and Face ... the mutual kisses of Lovers, impressed on the Lips, so

[66] See: *The description and use of the nerves* (1681): page 140.
[67] See: *The description and use of the nerves* (1681): page 141.
[68] See: *The description and use of the nerves* (1681): page 141.
[69] See chapter 17 for Willis's alternative and evocative naming of these muscles on the basis of the passions that their movements convey.
[70] See: *The description and use of the nerves* (1681): pages 142–3.

easily irritate love and lust by affecting both the Praecordia and Genitals; to wit, because the lower branching of the same fifth pair actuates these parts constituted in the middle and lower Belly, and draws them into the like affection with the Lips. The same reason holds of Love presently admitted by the eyes, that as the Poet says,

Mars videt hanc, visamq; cupit.
As soon as Mars *saw her, he desir'd her.*

The seventh or hearing nerve has two parts. One reaches the 'snail-like winding and Drum' in the inner ear. Four-footed animals respond to the movement of air and sound by pricking up the ears, raising the lid, and moving the eye. The other part moves the muscles of the lips, mouth, tongue, face, and nostrils enabling people to cry out through activity of the 'Organs for the framing the Voice'. From this, Willis speculates about language. Humans hear sounds and respond with utterances but, later, noise leaves an 'Idea in the Head, according to which afterwards, as occasion serves, the voice is formed, which bears the type and image of that, though some time before admitted'. In the context of hearing and sound, Willis speculates on the nature of musical ability:[71]

> Musick or melody is soon learnt by some men, which afterwards they bring forth with exact Symphony ... from the distinct accents of the heard harmony, the spirits moving within the Cerebel are disposed into peculiar Schemes ... which, when they flow on both sides into the vocal process of the auditory Nerve, they render as ... the measures or Tunes of the Instrument with which they had drunk in at the ears ... The reason may be sought, why some men learn Musick without any trouble, and others hardly or not at all ... some Children, before they can speak distinctly, quickly sing, and remember certain Tunes; whilst others, though very ingenious men and of excellent memory, are very Fools at Musick, and become uncapable, as an Ass for the Harp; wherefore 'tis commonly said, that some have musical ears, and others are wholly destitute of this faculty ... the genuine cause of this defect seems to consist in this ... when ... the audible Species go to the Cerebel ... being harder, and not easily yielding to the received impressions ... could impress nothing of themselves .. [and] being carried towards the common sensory, leave their Types or Ideas chiefly and almost wholly in the Brain ... which is less apt to keep distinctly the composures of the Harmony ... in others, the species of the Audible things ... affect the Cerebel ... [and] being disposed in convenient little places and cells ... flow out from thence, almost unthought of, without any endeavour or labour of remembrance ... [and] constitute sweet Tunes and vocal Musick.

With his description of the eighth nerve, Willis is able fully to link the dominant theme of his work on the anatomy of the brain. Through the cerebellum, the natural but largely involuntary movements of the viscera are driven by the wandring nerve. The eighth nerve is the union of at least twelve fibres emerging from the medulla oblongata. There are periodic swellings or discrete ganglia along its course. Together with the intercostal nerve, the eighth cranial nerve supplies the heart and vessels of the thorax, the oesophagus, trachea, and bronchi, and the

[71] See: *The anatomy of the brain* (1681): pages 118–19; and John Aubrey, *Brief lives with an apparatus for the lives of our English mathematical writers*, volume 2. Ed. Kate Bennett, Oxford (2015): page 1478 for reference by John Aubrey (1626–1697) to Willis's comments on the effect of music on the mind in 'his booke de cerebro'; Aubrey's copy of *Cerebri anatome* (1664) presented to Walter Charleton (1619–1707) is now in the University of Bristol Library.

pericardium before entering the abdomen. In places these two nerves even appear joined. One branch of the eighth, the returning nerve, supplies the larynx, arrangements differing on the left and right side of the thorax. Its function is 'as it were a Windlace ... [causing] the little rings of the *Trachea* or Weasand to be drawn hither and thither, like the folds of a pair of Bellows, both for breathing and making a sound'. Other branches end in the lungs and, with the nerve of the diaphragm, regulate respiration and cough: 'the Organs of respiration intimately conspire and agree among themselves, that although one of them do a thing inordinately, rather than there shall be a Schism, the rest do imitate or follow its irregularity'. Sometimes the activities end in convulsion, 'so that they cannot take in and send forth the Air after its due manner, as may be seen in Asthmatical Fits'. Others branches terminate in the 'Stomachial ... Mesenterick and Splenetick ... and Hepatick infoldings'.

The animal spirits move through discrete paths in the nerve, each of which can be separated back to its medullary origin by separation with a finger: 'otherwise how should it come to pass, that the Spirits to be carried for the performing the instincts of motion towards the Stomach, do not enter at the same time the Lungs or *Præcordia*, and actuate them with an inordinate influence?' Again, whilst the functions of the wandring pair are involuntary, there is connection with the vocal process of the seventh so that 'in every violent Passion ... the Tongue sends forth a voice, as an index of the excited affection; so that not only men, but some brute beasts, in their fleeing or rejoycing, wail, cry out, and make a noise'.[72] For Willis, this is a perfect reflex response to stimulation which, through involuntary movement driven by the cerebellum, governs many complex human behaviours.

Always concerned with linking structure to function, and in a rare account of experimental work, Willis writes that in order to determine whether the beating of the heart depends on activity of the animal spirits, 'we' (presumably he and Lower) ligated the wandring nerves in the dog and observed the animal to become 'silent, and seemed stunned, and suffered about the Hypochondria convulsive motions, with a great trembling of the Heart'. The dog survived, even after the nerves were cut until eventually, his 'strength and spirits worn out, he died. The carcass being opened, the blood within the Ventricles of the Heart ... being greatly coagulated, was gathered into clotters'. Willis concludes that the motion of the heart depends 'no less upon the inflowing of the blood, than upon that of the animal Spirit'. He leaves matters at the stage whereby the 'intercostal' nerve (sympathetic) and 'wandring nerve' (parasympathetic) are anatomically separate but part of one physiological system serving involuntary responses and bringing several organs and viscera into 'sympathy'.[73]

Willis is credited with having first described the spinal accessory: 'concerning this Nerve, because the beginning and distribution of it being very irregular, have not as yet been noted by other Anatomists, it may seem worth our labour to make a little more diligent inquiry'. His initial description makes the point that it is closely related to, but separate from, the bundle of fibres making up the wandring nerve:[74]

> To which is added a noted Fibre, or rather Nerve, much greater than the rest, from the spinal Marrow, which being joined with them, and wrapped about with the same Coat, taken from the *Dura Mater*, goes forth together out of the Skull, as if they all grew into

[72] See: *The description and use of the nerves* (1681): pages 146–57.

[73] See: *The description and use of the nerves* (1681): page 152; and Isler (1968): pages 100–1 referring to *Cerebri anatome* (1664): pages 323, 334.

[74] See: *The description and use of the nerves* (1681): page 146; and Hierons and Meyer (1962): page 289.

> one Trunk: but that accessory nerve, yea and many other fibres, do still remain distinct under that covering, and afterwards departing asunder, are carried into peculiar provinces. Because this spinal nerve having passed the Skull, leaving its Conjugation, is carried to the muscles of the Neck and Shoulders . . . and two other Fibres, having presently left the company of the rest, go into the muscles of the Throat and Neck.

In his further description, Willis describes the spinal origin of the accessory nerve at the level of the sixth or seventh vertebral body:[75]

> Arising up from the Neck after this manner, and being carried within the Skull, is joined to the Fibres of the wandring pair, and is ingraffed with them seeming to grow together into one Trunk, and goes out with them at the same hole from the Skull . . . This stranger or travelling nerve after a short commerce . . . is carried upon the Muscles of the Neck . . . till it comes to the Scapular Muscle, on which it is wholly bestowed . . . This nerve is found constantly, not only in Man and four-footed beasts, but also in Fowls and Fishes; and in these it seems to be destinated instead of Arms, and for the moving of their wings and fins.

Again Willis is most interested in the involuntary movement of muscles supplied by the accessory nerve, 'the pathetick and sudden motions, according to the force of the passions, the animal not being conscious of it' whereby the neck is turned in response to noise that might represent threat. Beasts respond by flying away 'their feet, wings, fins, or other parts . . . being set into a rapid motion'. In man the hands and arms are so responsive to 'almost all conceptions of the Brain' that they are:[76]

> Continually agitated ... with various gestures, whereof we are ignorant or not willing them: we scarcely think or speak any thing but at the same time the hands are flung out here and there; and whilst the Tongue hesitates . . . or the words as it were stick between the Jaws, the right hand is exercised, as if by its gesture it were endeavouring to draw out more swiftly the sense of the mind . . . these parts . . . do so nearly conspire with the Affections of the Brain and Heart . . . in all living Creatures, but more eminently in Man, the cause seems to be this nerve's coming from the spinal Marrow to the beginning of the wandring pair, and communicating with its nerves, and receiving from them as it were the note or private mark of the involuntary Function.

Having waxed lyrical on speech and music in his description of his seventh cranial nerve, Willis has not much to add on the ninth nerve which takes its origin from a prominence low in the medulla oblongata and is distributed entirely to perform 'the motions of the Tongue requisite for the articulation of Sounds'. He relates the inferior olives to speech because of their prominence in humans and relationship to the hypoglossal nerve.[77] Since he considers that it also receives impressions of taste through the fifth nerve, the tongue 'hath the virtue of a double Organ'. One branch of the ninth cranial nerve innervates the muscles of the hyoid bone and it contributes a twig to the tenth pair which also branches to the intercostal nerve but is otherwise 'destinated to the Sternothyroeidal muscle'.

[75] See: *The description and use of the nerves* (1681): page 173.
[76] See: *The description and use of the nerves* (1681): page 174.
[77] See: *The description and use of the nerves* (1681): pages 177–8; and Rasmussen (1947): page 11.

Another nerve originating from the spinal roots through the 'brachial nerves' is the nerve of the diaphragm (phrenic nerve). In supporting its function, the animal spirits are combined with a supply of sulphurous copula from the blood on which 'the action of this perpetual moveable depends' for synchrony with muscles of the thorax and the diastole and systole of the heart and lungs.[78] But the rhythms of the diaphragm can be interrupted and overruled in laughing, singing, and weeping and, illustrated by a further account of his favourite complex involuntary movement, sneezing. Of the remaining spinal nerves which innervate the many muscles of the body and limbs, Willis dismisses detailed description as 'a work of immense labour and trouble: and as this *Neurologie* cannot be learned nor understood without an exact knowledge of the Muscles, we may justly here forbear entering upon its particular institution'. But he does refer to the complexity of the brachial and crural plexuses formed from reorganization of the vertebral roots 'cross-ways after a curious manner'.[79]

In his account of the cranial and some spinal nerves, Willis has periodically mentioned one other important structure but has yet to deal with this in detail: 'Further out of the fifth pair two shoots, and another out of the Nerve of the sixth pair bending back, meet together; and what is wonderful, and not before taken notice of by Anatomists, the Intercostal Nerves, destined to the *Præcordia* and *Viscera*, do make a trunk'.[80] The intercostal nerve is so named because, although having its origin in the medulla oblongata and descending into the thorax with the wandring nerve, with which 'for most Anatomists, it is wrongfully taken for a branch', it also receives contributions from the interstices of the spinal marrow.[81] It has ganglia close to the spinal cord and sends branches to the thorax, many following the distribution of those from the wandring nerve.

The intercostal nerve reaches the abdomen sending branches to the ventricle (stomach), mesentery, spleen, liver, 'Gall-chest', pancreas, and kidneys. In a detailed exposition, each and every one of these branches is described, emphasizing their interaction with blood vessels. Willis speculates on the cooperation of these parts in health and disease, notably hypochondriacal and hysterical disorders and the 'Colical grief'. Unless subject to a convulsion of the animal spirits, perhaps interacting with nutritious juice contained in their walls, the intercostal nerve imposes on those hollow viscera 'almost no other thing than obscure Vermiculations or light Corrugations, so that in discharging the never resting 'Culinary work of Nutrition ... perpetual grinding in the Mill', there is required no greater preparation than for 'the slow progress of a Snail'. The intercostal nerve proceeds in its course into the pelvis reaching the colon, sphincter of the anus, and womb. Even in its terminal distribution the intercostal nerve still receives branches from the spinal marrow at the level of the *Os sacrum* through which the nerve enables:[82]

> Several Excretions, *viz.* of the Urine, Dung and Seed made in that place: for two Nerves enter into the end of the straight Intestine ... that the Excrements being carried towards the Arse-hole, may not slide out suddenly and unexpectedly ... and as many into the Womb or Prostates ... and into the Ureters ... to jog or shake those urinary Chanels, that the serum separated in the Reins, may be more readily drawn out towards the Bladder.

[78] See: *The description and use of the nerves* (1681): pages 173–6.
[79] See: *The description and use of the nerves* (1681): page 178.
[80] See: *The anatomy of the brain* (1681): page 116; and Hierons and Meyer (1962): page 289.
[81] See: *The description and use of the nerves* (1681): pages 157–73.
[82] See: *The description and use of the nerves* (1681): pages 159, 170, 171 for text relating to these various quotes.

Other terminal branches of the intercostal nerve reach the womb: 'without doubt, whatever of sense or motion is made about the Venereal acts, is owed to the influence of the Spirits through these Nerves'. Willis has traced the terminal branches of the intercostal nerve to the 'Womens testicles' but, curiously, 'we find scarce any nerve to belong to mens Testicles'; or in the fox, dog, calf, boar, or monkey other than to the cremaster muscle. Despite its limited innervation, 'in Men the delightful profusion of the Genital humor, and in Women the no less pleasant reception of the same depends on the action of those nerves'.[83]

Willis's description replaced the heart as the organ of emotions, with the cerebellum and its outputs through the cranial nerves governing involuntary response to the passions. Blood vessels are also influenced. By investing their walls with 'the thickset rows of processes', Willis argues that the arteries and veins receive a supply of spirits that enable them to 'imitate the movement of the heart ... and, constricted by this kind of nervous bridles, moderate the course of the blood according to the impulses of the passions, and the instincts'.

By any analysis, detailed study of the autonomic nervous system begins with Willis on the vagus as the 'wandring nerve' and the sympathetic chain as the 'intercostal nerve'.[84] He did not claim originality and Willis refers readers to the earlier notation of Gabriele Falloppio (1523–1562).[85] It has been suggested that the anatomical discoveries of Eustachius on the cranial nerves might have been available to Willis. Each described the sympathetic chain as separate from the vagus and with a cranial origin traced to the heart, lungs, and abdominal organs. But they both mistook the origin of these structures: Eustachius, with Galen, from the sixth cranial nerve; and Willis, as shown in Tabula IX, from the trigeminal nerve and abducens.[86] This common error allowed Donal Sheehan (*c.*1908–1964) to suggest that Willis had written with knowledge of Eustachius's work although each was mainly rehearsing the Galenic position.[87] Raymond Hierons (1921–2001) and Alfred Meyer (1895–1990) trace the provenance of Eustachius's thirty-eight plates from their production in 1552 to publication by Giovanni Maria Lancisi (1654–1720), indicating that they were retained by the artist Pier Matteo Pini (nd) at Eustachius's death and passed to his daughter. She married into the wealthy Rossi family, in whose possession the plates were eventually found at the suggestion of Pope Clement XI (1649–1721). Never previously seen, they remained in the Vatican until published in 1714.[88] That no anatomist contemporary to Willis mentions Eustachius's images and numbering of the cranial nerves attests to this analysis and refutes the charge of plagiarism against Willis.

[83] See: *The description and use of the nerves* (1681): page 171.

[84] See: Donal Sheehan, 'Discovery of the autonomic nervous system' *Archives of Neurology and Psychiatry Chicago* (1936): 35; 1081–115 on whom most subsequent accounts of Willis' contributions to the autonomic nervous system seem to lean; Spillane (1981): pages 89–94 also gives a full account.

[85] See: Gabrielle Falloppio, *Observationes anatomicae*, Venice (1561).

[86] As discussed earlier and in chapter 3, there is ambiguity on the provenance of these images. Hughes (1991) attributes Tabulæ IX and X to Lower and Willis, whereas Hierons and Meyer (1962): page 291, state that Tabulæ IX and X were drawn by Wren.

[87] See: Sheehan (1936). In their detailed account of descriptions and numbering of the cranial nerves, Hierons and Meyer (1962) go further and suggest that Lancisi could not have made a clear statement on Eustachius's anatomy of the accessory nerve and vagus without knowledge of the correct arrangement from Willis.

[88] See: Hierons and Meyer (1962), at page 288. Sheehan (1936) suggests that the notes to these plates had been included in Bartolomeo Eustachius, *Opuscula anatomica*, Venice (1564).

Comparative anatomy

As a comparative anatomist Willis can be accused of the uncritical transfer of concepts derived from the anatomy of one species to another by analogy but without following strict methodology.[89] In writing an analysis of Willis as a comparative neurologist, Robert Dow (1908–1995) mainly rehearses Willis's contributions to human anatomy and pharmacology. Dow lists some of the differences Willis observed in one or other of the 'fifteen' mammals and birds, fish, and invertebrates he studied, singling out comparative anatomy of the nervous system of the lobster and his account of the intercostal nerves.[90]

As Willis admits, his work with Edmund King (*c.*1630–1709) and John Masters (1627–*c.*1684) was that of a zootomist. Chapter V of *Cerebri anatome* is devoted to the brains of fowls and fishes on the basis that 'a compared Anatomy may yield us a more full and exact Physiology of the Use of the Parts'. Most of the treatise deals with man and domestic animals.[91] Figura II (Pl.2) depicts the base of a sheep's brain: 'Two Hemispheres of the Brain without lobes, different from that in a Man'. Figura VI (Pl.6) shows the base of the skull in a calf. Figuræ VII (Pl.8) and VIII (Pl.9) are of the sheep's brain unfolded to show the general arrangement of the white matter and structures of the hindbrain, respectively. Tabula XIII (Pl.15) includes the venous plexus of the spinal cord in a dog. Chapter VIII includes a description of the vascular anatomy of the horse and calf. Willis's illustration of muscle in *De motu musculari* (1670) is from the ox (Pl.17 and Pl.18). Against that background, most of his work on comparative anatomy appears in the first part of *De anima brutorum* (1672). In the preface, Willis explains that he:

> *Thought it necessary to describe the Vital Organs, both of all Kinds of living Creatures, by the Action of which the Lamp of Light is maintained; and also to show it plainly laid open, even to their intimate recesses, and least and secret Passages, the brains, both of the more perfect brutes and also of Man. The Anatomy of which being manifold; not being able to perform it only with my own hand, and Skill, being also almost continually interrupted by my Practice, the famous and Skilful Anatomist and Physician Dr* Edmond King *was much helpful to me, by his assiduous and notable assistance and labour. Also that learned Man, and my most intimate Friend, Dr* John Masters, *Skilful in Physick and Anatomy, imployed much of his Labour and Diligence in the same Business.*

Lessons could be learned because the beasts of the earth had been made on the fifth day of Creation and man not until the sixth. Willis studied the anatomy of many species other than the 'humane body' including the calf, horse, dog, cat, fox, stag, pig, goat, sheep, mouse, hare, rabbit, oyster, lobster, earthworm, and several species of birds and fish.[92] He

[89] See: FJ Cole, *A history of comparative anatomy*, London (1944): pages 23 and 47. Cole is amongst those who are grudging of Willis's contributions that are independent from those of his 'circle' who carried out work that Willis claims for himself and describes in elaborate and repetitive texts.

[90] See: Robert S Dow, 'Thomas Willis (1621–1675) as a comparative neurologist', *Annals of Medical History* 1940: 3rd series, volume 2; 181–94. There is nothing especially original in this article and Willis's work on the intercostal nerve was based on human not comparative anatomy.

[91] See: *The anatomy of the brain* (1681): pages 74–7; and *Concerning the soul of brutes* (1683): pages 15–18.

[92] See: *The description and use of the nerves* (1681): page 85 where Willis points out that he has not had the opportunity of examining the brains of a lion or monkey: however, at page 162 he does discuss the intercostal nerve of the monkey, arguing that this is prominent and innervates the diaphragm 'which is perhaps partly the reason, why this Animal is so crafty and mimical above other Beasts, and can so aptly shew and imitate, not only the gestures, but the passions and some manners of a Man'.

regarded invertebrates as bloodless creatures because the fluid in their vessels was not red. Comparative anatomy was also important since the availability of human brains was unpredictable and their size made manipulation difficult:[93]

> That the perfect knowledge of the Brain and its parts may be gained, it is necessary not only to dissect and look into mens Heads, but all other kinds of living Creatures heads: for besides, that the humane Heads or Bodies are not so readily to be had ... its most intricate frame and various recesses and Appendices ... reduced into an Epitomy, are plainly represented more commodiously in the dissection of Beasts ... from such a compared Anatomy not only the faculties and uses of every Organ, but the impressions, influences, and secret workings of the sensitive Soul will be discovered.

Notwithstanding these limitations, Willis did make several contributions to comparative anatomy. Especially praised is his illustration depicting the anatomy of the oyster.[94] He describes the two parts of the single adductor but incorrectly suggests that the anterior muscle opens rather than affects the rate at which the valves of the shell close.[95] His account of muscles around the mouth is considered accurate by assigning them the function of 'superior gills'. His description of the gut is correct but omits the caecum and crystalline style. He observed the foramina that connect the gut to the liver and the *typhlosole*, an internal fold of the intestinal inner wall, correctly concluding that this is not 'like a spinal cord'. The positions of the heart, its chambers and beating, and the arterial system to the various organs are accurate. The gills are described together with a chemical explanation on the extraction of 'nitrous particles' and removal of waste in the currents of water that wash through and interact with circulating blood, a topic that Willis also described in the pike, salmon, and cod.

There is no mention of a nervous system in the oyster but this is described for the lobster.[96] Here Willis seeks to assign structures with which he is already familiar in humans to this invertebrate: two cerebral hemispheres, the medulla oblongata, cerebellum, and optic nerves. The gut and genitalia are well described. The arteries and veins are confused and not anatomically accurate. Despite his account in the oyster and fishes, Cole concludes that Willis's attempt to explain the anatomy and circulation passing through the gills is 'unsound ... his ideas on respiration in the lobster do not readily commend themselves to the understanding, or call for exposition'.[97]

On the earthworm, Willis depicts and understands the mechanism of the setae in locomotion. Dissected from the ventral surface, Willis saw the nerve cord but mistook this for an artery and assumed that the pharynx was the brain. Again the beating hearts were observed but not the red blood circulating within. He saw structures relating to digestion and reproduction which required astute observation, but missed others.[98]

[93] See: *The anatomy of the brain* (1681): page 56; and Isler (1968): page 86.

[94] See: chapter 3 for discussion of Martini Lister *Conchyliorum Bivalvium utrisque aquae exercitatio anatomica tertia*, London (1696); Martini Lister *Historiæ conchyliorum* London (1685–1692); and Henry Oldenburg's (1619–1677) letter to Lorenzo Magalotti of 13 June 1672, extolling the plates in: *The Correspondence of Henry Oldenburg*, volume IX (1672–1673). Eds. A. Rupert Hall and Marie Boas Hall, Madison (1973): pages 106–8; Royal Society Library EL/O2/87.

[95] See: *Concerning the soul of brutes* (1683): pages 9–11; and more generally Cole (1944): pages 222–31 for the discussion that follows of Willis and the comparative anatomy of invertebrates.

[96] See: *Concerning the soul of brutes* (1683): pages 11–13.

[97] See: Cole (1944): page 351 for discussion Johann Conrad Peyer's (1653–1712) admiration for Willis's work on respiration in fishes.

[98] See: *Concerning the soul of brutes* (1683): pages 13–15.

In most species, Willis's primary interest is the brain. He emphasizes that the relative size of different regions varies between species. The pons is largest in man and more prominent in the dog and cat than other domestic animals. It is small in animals with a predominance of instinct and scarcity of emotions or passions such as sheep, cattle, goats, and swine, but their quadrigeminal bodies are large. Animals, including monkeys (ceropithecus), with intelligence capable of moderating instincts, show the reverse arrangement. Conversely the structure and size of the cerebellum and cortex are proportional in animals and man. In pups the normal streaked appearance of the striate body is underdeveloped: 'further, in Whelps newly littered, that want their sight, and hardly perform the other faculties of motion and sense, these streaks or chamferings, being scarce wholly formed, appear only rude'.[99]

The blood vessels of the brain and spinal cord

It was natural that, versed in the work of William Harvey and having the circulation of heated blood as essential for the function of bodily parts, Willis would want to understand how fermented materials reach the brain and nervous stock and are converted into animal spirits. He was not the first to describe the arterial network at the base of the brain, nor did he claim priority. But no one before him had combined an account of the anatomy and physiology, or explained the clinical significance of an anastomotic system for maintaining perfusion following partial failure of the circulation. In the event, his formulation on the vasculature of the brain and spinal cord combined evidence from embryology, human and comparative anatomy, physiology, pathology, animal experiment, and clinical observation.

Before Willis, the prevailing view was that the blood supply to the brain involved entry through a network, the rete mirabilis. Willis was clear that this is not the arrangement in man. Were that structure to be discovered in a human head it would follow that this must be in the brain of a person of 'slender wit or unmoved disposition, and destitute of all force and ardour of the mind ... little better than dull working beasts in fortitude and wisdom'.[100] In 1561, Falloppio had described union of the two vertebral arteries into the basilar and its subsequent division into the two posterior cerebral arteries.[101] He observed the termination of the internal carotid artery as the anterior and middle cerebral vessels and the anterior communicating artery. The posterior communicating artery was described although its significance in completing the circle was not appreciated. Johann Wepfer (1620–1695) provided an account of the anatomy but no illustration.[102] Willis had read Wepfer and it could be argued that he borrowed without attribution Wepfer's description of the carotid siphon, the anastomotic circle, and the further distribution of the carotid and vertebral arteries.[103] Writing on apoplexy, Wepfer described a patient who died of an abdominal condition but also had left sided headache and an occluded right internal carotid artery. In Willis's discussion of the meningeal vessels: 'these arteries perforate the hard Meninge in several places on the top of the Brain (as Wepfer observes) and impart some shoots to the Pia Mater'.[104]

[99] See: *The anatomy of the brain* (1681): page 102.

[100] See: *The anatomy of the brain* (1681): page 85.

[101] See: Falloppio (1561).

[102] See: Johann Wepfer, *Observationes anatomicae ex cadaveribus eorum quos sustulit apoplexia*, Schaffhausen (1658).

[103] See: Alfred Meyer and Raymond Hierons, 'Observations on the history of the "circle of Willis"', *Medical History* 1962: 6; 119–30 at page 120 for an extensive translation from Wepfer (1658): pages 106–114.

[104] See: *The anatomy of the brain* (1681): page 57.

In *Brief lives* (1898), John Aubrey suggested that the open book in the *c.*1652 portrait of William Petty (1623–1687) by Isaac Fuller (1606–1679) is Figure III on page 195 of the 1647 edition of Johann Vesling's (1598–1649) *Syntagma Anatomicum* (1647), which shows an arterial arrangement at the base of the brain. David Piper corrected this attribution to Tabula III, Liber II, drawn by Odoardo Fialetti (1573–1638) in Julius Casserius's (1552–1616) *Tabulæ anatomicæ*.[105] The image was also included by Adriaan van den Spigelius (1578–1625), together with several plates borrowed from Vesalius, in *Opera quæ extant* (1645).[106] Vesling depicted the basilar artery and its connection with the two carotids but omitted the posterior cerebrals and anterior communicating artery. The latter vessel was added when the illustration was again printed for Thomas Bartholin (1616–1680), who also copied Figure IV from *Cerebri anatome*, in *Anatomiæ quartum renovate* (1684, page 675). Meyer and Hierons conclude that:[107]

> The distinction of having opened the history ... should go to Fallopius ... save for the posterior communicating artery which he thought was only indirectly connected with the internal carotid through a network of small arteries. Casserio in his illustration corrected this mistake on one side ... Vesling illustrated a complete posterior communicating artery but failed to demonstrate ... union of the anterior cerebral arteries. Wepfer's description is superior ... but he did not give an illustration.

From this it is clear that each of the relevant vessels had been identified, and the community around Willis was well aware before 1664 of evolving ideas on the anastomosis of arteries at the base of the human brain. Willis's first concern was how blood vessels reach that site. He studied foramina within individual bones of the skull 'which transmit the Trunks of the Vessels like the hanging weights of a Clock'. The entry of the carotid arteries is through the 'Cuniform or Wedge-like Bone' which also houses the 'pituitary Glandula or knotty kernel'. Not previously well described is its double ascent and crookedness to the level of the 'Turky Chair' resembling 'in most the letter ~ inversed; but in man ... its site, by reason of the longer tract of the Vessel and its greater curvature, represents the same letter double after this manner ~ ~'.[108] This arrangement ensured that blood entering the skull did not stagnate in 'narrow Rivulets, which would scarce drive a Mill, but always with a broad and open chanel, such as might bear a Ship under Sail'.[109] It also allowed for the blood entering the brain to be separated from superfluous dregs of the serum, filtered to the pituitary, and with other waste diverted to veins for return to the heart.

In describing the 'fourfold Chariot' of vessels entering through the skull base, Willis makes several points. The carotid and basilar arteries are connected; the anterior and posterior communicating branches unite with those of the opposite side to complete the network; the carotids and basilar terminate in 'noteworthy' branches (the anterior, middle, and posterior cerebral arteries); the posterior circulation has other branches that nourish the cerebellum, medulla oblongata (that is, the hindbrain in its entirety) and the choroid plexus;

[105] See: David Piper, *Catalogue of seventeenth-century portraits in the National Portrait Gallery 1625–1714*, Cambridge (1963): pages 275–76, plate 8g.

[106] See: Feindel (1965): pages 39–40, with the quote from Harvey Cushing (1869–1939) 'I am somewhat confused about this one—Spigelius—Casserius—Bucretius et al.'; Hughes (1991): pages 66–7; and Meyer and Hierons (1964): pages 121–3 for clarification.

[107] See: Meyer and Hierons (1964): pages 124–5.

[108] See: *The anatomy of the brain* (1681): page 71.

[109] See: *The anatomy of the brain* (1681): page 84.

the anterior circulation 'gives off branches and shoots on all sides which creep through and, like vine shoots, tightly bind not only the external circumference of this sphere, but also its inner parts and recesses'; and the arteries eventually converge on four sinuses within the thinner membrane investing the surface and reaching veins within the brain. No less precise is Willis's description of the vertebral arteries which are more slender than the carotids and 'meeting as it were in a threefold way, are inoculated one with another'. They provide 'an innumerable series of shoots, which cover the oblong marrow, the Ceribel, and all their cavities and recesses, and water them with a plentiful flood of blood'.[110]

As for quality of the images, Trevor Hughes considers the artistry of illustrations depicting the base of the human (Figure I: Pl.1) and sheep's brain (Figure II: Pl.2) to be excellent but he has some misgivings concerning the anatomical arrangements:[111]

> The two carotid arteries are shown, right larger than left, and they divide into anterior and middle cerebral arteries. This division is acceptable on the left but on the right is shown as an implausible immediate division into four arteries of comparable size. The anterior cerebral arteries proceed medially and come together in a confluence, a possible but most unlikely anatomical variant. Consequently the normal short anterior communicating artery is not depicted. The posterior communicating arteries are both large, again an unusual variant, for commonly both are small, although in about 20% of cases one is large. The two vertebral arteries are well shown, but the anterior spinal artery is incorrect, and there are no posterior inferior cerebellar arteries. The vertebrals unite to form the basilar artery which lacks any sizeable branches preceding laterally over the surface of the pons. The division of the basilar artery into two posterior cerebral arteries is correct but after they receive the posterior communicating arteries, they dwindle in size into arteries smaller than could ever be normal ... The impression is of a drawing specially undertaken to show the arterial circle for its physiological importance, but with insufficient care to reproduce faithfully every detail of arterial anatomy.

Hierons and Meyer (1968) are amongst observers who point out that Willis, or Wren, omitted to illustrate the two posterior cerebral arteries in Figura I (Pl.1) and, with Symonds (1955), criticise joining of the two anterior cerebral arteries directly rather than through the anterior communicating artery. Feindel (1965) defends Willis by identifying two short stumps that represent the terminal branches of the basilar artery and, as a neurosurgeon, he was well familiar with the arrangement depicted by Willis at the anterior boundary of the circle.[112]

The time during which Willis and his close collaborators were dissecting and thinking about the vascular supply to the brain coincided with a busy period in physiology and the introduction of an innovative technology. Richard Lower explained in a letter to Boyle how the anatomical findings were studied experimentally:[113]

> And to confirm this, this week we took a young spaniel, and tied both carotid arteries in the neck very fast and close with silk, and the dog was not at all altered by it, but continued very lively and brisk, and was so far from taking unkindly what was done to him, that within a

[110] See: *The anatomy of the brain* (1681): pages 59, 69, 72–3 for this and the discussion that follows; and Clarke and O'Malley (1968): pages 775–9 citing the octavo issue of *Cerebri anatome* (1664): pages 7–8, 25, 32–3; and Feindel (1965): page 55.

[111] See: Hughes (1991): page 68.

[112] See: Hierons and Meyer (1962): at page 288; and Feindel (1965): page 55.

[113] See: Feindel (1965): pages 20–1.

> quarter of an hour after, he got loose and followed the doctor into the town, as he visited his patients. In this pleasant humour he continued two or three days, and then we opened his head, and found all the vessels of the brain as full of blood as usually they are in other dogs, who do not suffer the same experiment. But this I might have told you in a shorter time; for if one artery be syringed with any tinctured liquor, all the parts of the brain will be equally filled with it at the same time, as several times we have tried.

In his account of the vessels at the base of the brain, Willis explains that the arrangement has the appearance of 'bushy woodland' and, after injecting a black liquid in a large piston into the carotid artery, it was possible to trace the distribution of vessels.[114] Lower told Boyle in 1662 that Willis intended to inject 'some kinds of liquors, tinctured with saffron, or other colours', into the carotid arteries of an animal, recently killed, 'to try how the blood moves, and how the tincture may be separated into the brain'. Lower and Willis infused milk and ink successfully to disprove the claim of Franciscus Sylvius (1614–1672) that fluid moved from the brain through the infundibulum into the nasopharynx. They displayed the vessels of the meninges and rete mirabilis of animals in this way; and demonstrated the vascular anastomosis at the base of the human brain.

This was but one application in the long and complex history of intravenous injection and transfusion that evolved in Oxford and London after 1656.[115] In discussions with John Wilkins (1614–1672) and Robert Boyle, Wren suggested a method for injecting poisons into the blood stream of a dog with access using the great saphenous vein of the hind leg, writing to William Petty in a letter dated *c.*1656–1658:[116]

> Shall I trouble you with what we doe in Anatomy? ... the most considerable [Experiment] I have made of late is this. I have injected Wine and Ale in a living Dog into the Mass of Blood by a Veine, in good Quantities, till I have made him extremely drunk, but soon after he Pisseth it out: with 2 ounces of Infusion of Crocus metal: thus injected, the Dog immediately fell a Vomitting, & so vomited until he died. It will be too long to tell the Effects of

[114] Many accounts are given of the composition of this fluid. Sir Charles Symonds, 'Thomas Willis (1621–1675)', *Notes and records of the Royal Society of London* (1960): page 93 favours 'a compound of mercury with viscous substances'.

[115] See: Frank (1980): pages 169–78. The literature mainly documents the procedure in man. Most authorities cite *Philosophical Transactions* (23 November 1667): 2; 557–64 as the first account. The experiment is mentioned in [Robert Boyle] 'Tryals proposed by Mr Boyle to Dr Lower, to be made by him for the improvement of transfusing blood out of one live animal into another; promised Numb. 20. p. 357', *Philosophical Transactions*, 11 February 1666; Numb. 22: pages 385–88. This earlier paper and its preceding advertisement are also made clear by the table of contents for issues of '*THE PHILOSOPHICAL TRANSACTIONS* OF Two Years, 1665 and 1666, beginning *March* 6. 1665 and ending with *February* 1666; abbreviated in an ALPHABETICAL TABLE: and also afterwards Digested into a more *NATURAL METHOD*'. This index has the following headings: '*Animals*; one may live by the blood of another, the whole mass of his own blood being drawn out, and the blood of another infus'd in the meantime, [23 May 1665] 20. 353. See *Bloods Transfusion*'. Under that heading we read: '*Blood*. The new Operation of *Transfusing* blood into the veins, out of one Animal into another; with considerations upon it, [23 May 1665] 20. 353. The first rise of this invention, 7. 208 [something is wrong here: issue 7 contains pages 119–30; page 208 is in issue 12]. The success, 19. 352. Proposals and Queries, for the improvement of this Experiment, by Mr Boyle, 22. 385, 386'. Other papers on transfusion in animals appeared in the journal during 1667: volume 2: page 449 (calf into sheep); 1667: page 451 (mangy dog into a sound one); 1667: page 479 (account of the effects of transfusing blood, and of two monstrous births); 1667: page 489 (M Denis on ways of curing sundry diseases by transfusion of blood); the work of Lower and King, 1667: pages 557, 617; volume 3: pages 710, 731, and volume 4: pages 840, 1075 (transfusion practised on a man in London); and 1668: page 672 (Dr Clarck on the transfusion of blood). For these entries, see: [James Briggs], *An index to the anatomical, medical, chirurgical and physiological papers contained in the Transactions of the Royal Society of London from the commencement of that work to the end of the year 1817, chronically and alphabetically arranged*, London (1818): pages 2–3.

[116] See: Gunther *Early medical and biological science*, London (1926): pages 106–8.

Opium, Scammony, & other things that I have tried in this way: I am now in further pursuit of the Experiment, which I take to be of great concernment, and what will give great light both to the Theory and Practice of Physick.

Later, Boyle suggested that the procedure might be carried out in humans, 'especially those of Malefactors', a recommendation which seems to have been attempted, unsuccessfully, by a foreign ambassador who attempted to have *crocus metallorum* injected into one of his servants, 'an inferior Domestic ... that deserved to have been hanged'.[117] When the discussion turned to using this technique on patients in London hospitals, Willis suggested that the experiment 'might be proper to make use of in rotten sheep'. It is unclear whether this was intended as disparaging or a cautionary next step in moving towards human transfusions.[118] In 1667, King who had published an account of blood transfusion from a calf to a sheep, helped Mr Arthur Cogan transfuse himself with sheep's blood. Cogan survived but became a 'little cracked in the head'. Gideon Harvey (1635–1702), a staunch critic of Willis and other experimental philosophers, later concluded:[119]

They slay Dogs and Cats; take livers, lungs, calves-brains, or other entrails, dry, roast, parboil them, steep them in vinegar, etc., and afterwards gaze on little particles of them through a microscope: - then obtrude to the world in print whatever false appearances gleamed into their eyes; and all this to no other end, than to beget a belief in people that they who have so profoundly dived into the bottomless pores of the parts, must undeniably be skilled in curing their distempers.

As for Willis, the emerging experimental and anatomical work came together in a remarkable contribution to clinical science, although the basic ideas were already well formulated. After a long and repetitive passage on the role of the meningeal and cerebral vasculature that ensures distributed perfusion in the context of one or more feeding vessels being occluded, Willis describes the patient who died from carcinoma of the stomach:[120]

We dissected the body of a certain man, whom a great *Scirrhus* or hard Swelling within the *Mesentry*, growing at last ulcerous, had killed. When his Skull was opened, we beheld those things belonging to the Head, and found the right *Carotides*, rising within the Skull, plainly bony or rather stony, its cavity being almost wholly shut up, so that the influx of the blood being denied to this passage, it seemed wonderful, wherefore this sick person had not dyed before of an *Apoplexy*; which indeed he was so far from, that he enjoyed to the last moment of his life, the free exercise of his mind and animal function. For indeed, Nature had substituted a sufficient remedy against that danger of an *Apoplexy*, to wit, the *Vertebral* Artery of the same side in which the Carotidick was wanting, the bulk of the Pipe being enlarged, became thrice as big as both its Pipes on the other side: because the blood being excluded the Carotidick, adding it self to the wonted provision of the Vertebral Artery, and flowing with

[117] See: Adrian Tinniswood, *His invention so fertile. A life of Sir Christopher Wren*, London (2012): pages 36–8 and footnotes 3–6, referring to pages 285–6, in which Tinniswood rehearses the evidence for when this procedure was first carried out in humans and reported.

[118] See: frontispiece showing 'Christopher Wren making his first demonstration of a method of introducing drugs into a vein, before Dr Willis. 1667', painted by Ernest Board (1877–1934) as one in a series commissioned c1912 by Henry S Wellcome depicting important events in the history of science and medicine.

[119] See: Gideon Harvey, *The conclave of physicians*, London (1686): pages 55, 87.

[120] See: *Anatomy of the brain* (1681): pages 82–3.

> a double flood into the same belly, had so dilated the chanel of that Artery above measure. This Gentleman, about the beginning of his sickness, was tormented with a cruel pain of the Head towards the left side. The cause whereof cannot be more probably assigned, than that the blood excluded from right Carotidick Artery, when at first it rushed more impetuously in the left, had distended the Membrane; and therefore the same distemper did afterwards vanish of its own accord, to wit, the superfluous blood being derived through the Vertebral Artery.

In addition to maintaining perfusion despite occlusion of one main vessel, Willis suggested a related function for the arterial circle. Apart from using dye to trace the paths of the vessels, he injected more forcibly but, unable to permeate the brain and exit through the sinuses and veins, the dye crossed and descended through the opposite carotid into the chest:[121]

> Rather than the force should be carried to the Brain by the violent impulse of the liquor, it, returning from the injection, and otherwise threatening a flood to the Brain, finds the way of receding also by the opposite Arteries ... and here we cannot sufficiently admire so provident (and to be equalled by no mechanical art) a dispensation of the blood within the confines of the Brain. For in as much as the Carotidick Arteries do communicate between themselves in various places, and are mutually ingrafted; from thence a double benefit results, though of a contrary effect: because by this one and the same means care is taken, both lest the brain should be defrauded of its due watring of the blood, also lest it should be overwhelmed by the too impetuous flowing of the swelling stream or torrent.

Willis also describes regulation of flow out of the brain through the anatomical arrangements of the lateral sinuses and jugular vein. Each have furrows or cavities that serve as reservoirs of venous blood leaving the skull, the 'ample cavern [jugular bulb] ... so that the torrent of blood leaving the head does not burst into the veins with too rapid and dizzying an influx and besiege the heart'. Together 'nothing of greater ingenuity can be imagined, or can better demonstrate the providence of the Creator than this suitable disposition of the blood in the brain by its route of reflux in various animals, suited to the necessity of each'. Symonds adds a third function of the circle mentioned by Willis. This is thoroughly to mix the blood on arrival before distribution to the various parts of the brain.[122]

The vascular arrangement at the base of the brain was first designated the 'circulum qui dicitur Willisii [circle of Willis]' by Albrecht von Haller (1708–1777), who pointed out that Wepfer had provided the original description.[123] Medical works of the eighteenth and nineteenth centuries usually ignored Willis's contribution but posterity judges that he was responsible for formulating the physiological concepts. The architect of the injecting technique and the person who depicted the findings was Christopher Wren. Whether the role of Richard Lower was as observer or prosector is a moot point. But to whoever credit in resolving the anatomical and physiological arrangements at the base of the brain belongs, Willis neatly summarized the situation:[124]

[121] See: *The anatomy of the brain* (1681): pages 72–3; and Cole (1944): page 174, footnote 2 for discussion of how this experiment was repeated and described as original to himself by Samuel Collins (1618–1710), *A systeme of anatomy, treating of the body of man, beasts, birds, fish, insects, and plants*, London (1685).

[122] See: Symonds (1955): page 122.

[123] See: Albrecht von Haller, *Bibliotheca anatomica*, volume 1, Zurich (1774): page 476; and Feindel (1965): page 56, who argues that 'circle' is a misnomer based on the anatomical appearance; strictly it is nine-sided and would better be designated the 'polygon of Willis'.

[124] See: *The anatomy of the brain* (1681): page 82.

> Hence it plainly appears, that there is a communication between the Vessels watering the whole Head; and although every Artery is carried to one only Region, as its peculiar Province, and provides for it apart; yet, lest that any part should be deprived of the influence of the blood, more ways lie open to every part by the ingraftings of these vessels; so that if the proper vessels by chance should be wanting in their office, its defects may presently be compensated by others neighbouring.

Willis's main contribution to anatomy of the spinal cord was to demonstrate its vascular supply.[125] He distinguishes the arteries, sinuses, or 'bosoms', and the draining veins. Because the dissections were difficult and the fragile vessels easily damaged in breaking apart the vertebrae in adults, Willis used the human foetus, with softer bones, for much of his work on spinal arteries.[126] Using the technique of injection, 'we did cast in divers coloured Liquors. And we had our desired wish: for presently we found with much admiration, that those kinds of vessels, viz. arteries, Bosoms, and veins which respect the head, belong also to the spinal marrow with no less a noted disposition of provision'. This allowed him to see that 'the Vertebral Artery pays to the superior part of the Spine as great Tributes of Blood as to the Head itself', but also that:[127]

> The Arteries which carry the Blood toward the Spine, are disposed after one manner above the Heart, and after another below it. As to the first, whereas the Trunk of the *Aorta* being there cleft presently to many branches, departs from the Region of the Spine, therefore the Vertebral Artery is produced on both sides from its axillary branches, which ascending straight into the hinder part of the Head sends forth a branch into the meeting together of every *Vertebra*. But below the Heart, forasmuch as the *Aorta*, in its whole descent, lyeth on the Spine, two arteries are received into the Spine from its bottom nigh its *Internodia* or spaces between the knots of the *Vertebræ*; so that if the trunk of the *Aorta* be cut long-ways, there will appear a series of double holes through its whole tract.

The spinal vessels are depicted in *Cerebri anatome*, Tabula XII (Pl.14), where B identifies 'the Spinal Artery seen to descend through the whole marrow which however is made up of Arteries, brought into it from between several joyntings of the Vertebræ'. Tabula XIII Figure 1, D signifies 'The first jointing together of the Vertebral Artery above the spinal marrow, from which place the spinal Artery descends'; *g* represents 'Shoots sent in the Spinal Marrow which joyn together from either side in the Spinal Marrow nigh the several joynings of the Vertebrae'; and *f* indicates 'Two Arteries sent down from the Aorta into the Spine'. Tabula XIII Figure 2 (Pl.15) shows the spinal veins draining into jugulars. Figure 3 depicts the posterior aspect of the cord with its vascular arrangements. Figure 4 illustrates the venous plexuses of the cord. And Figure 5 shows a venous sinus in the dog.[128] These drain,

[125] See: *The anatomy of the brain* (1681): pages 179–82; and J Trevor Hughes, 'Spinal cord arteries described by Thomas Willis'. In: Ed.: F Clifford Rose and WF Bynum, *Historical aspects of the neurosciences. A festschrift for Macdonald Critchley*, New York (1982): pages 195–203.

[126] Hughes (1982) agrees that the particular dissections illustrated by Willis are indeed from a human foetus or an animal since the nerve roots enter transversely and not at angle; and all of the arrangements for the main arteries and their tributaries, and the veins, are unrealistically regular for an adult specimen.

[127] See: *The description and use of the nerves* (1681): page 179.

[128] See: Thomas Willis, *Of musculary motion* (1681): page 43 for Willis's description of ligating the anterior spinal artery in the dog and observing that the hind limbs were suddenly deprived of motion, being restored when the ligature was released, due either to depriving the spinal marrow or the muscles themselves of blood. Steno had carried out a similar experiment but by ligating the aorta: see Hierons and Meyer (1664): page 689 (offprint, page 3).

at the various levels, into the inferior and superior vena cavæ, and the azygous and jugular veins. Hughes (1982) considers that Vieussens (1684) perpetuated the unrealistic symmetry and regularity of Willis's illustrations of the vascular supply of the spinal cord, but provided images that were not bettered until the work of Albrecht von Haller.[129]

Muscle and movement

No less a preoccupation for those rethinking natural philosophy in the 1660s than the nature of respiration was the relationship between muscle and movement. Whereas structure of the brain, nerve, and muscle could be observed directly, function had to be inferred within the constraints of theory and crude experiment.[130] It was logical that Willis should seek to complement his ideas on the role of the cortex and cerebellum in voluntary and involuntary movement through an understanding of muscle contraction. Since all bodily processes were based on fermentation, and muscle unlikely to be different, it followed that Willis focused on chemical forces active within muscle orchestrated by the passage of spirit down the nerves. He had explored these ideas in *Cerebri anatome* (1664) and *Pathologiæ cerebri* (1667) but in 1670 Willis returned to 'our Myology or doctrine of the Muscles' in *De motu musculari*, one of the two treatises appended to *Affectionum quæ dicuntur hystericæ & hypochondriacæ*. He starts by rehearsing the sequence of events involved in muscle contraction:[131]

> First, the original of the Action, or the first designation of the Motion to be performed, which is always in the Brain or Cerebel. Secondly, its instinct or transmission of the thing begun to the motive parts, which is performed by the commerce of the Spirits lying within the Nerves. Thirdly, the motive force itself, or exertion of the Spirits implanted in the moving parts either into a contractive or elastick force. From this threefold Fountain, *viz.*, as the business is performed in every one of these in a various manner, very many kinds and differences of Motions are deduced.

In formulating his ideas, Willis inherited existing opinions. Two principles had been proposed, with neither of which he disagreed. Contraction requires substances provided by nerves but also from the blood. These constituent chemicals interact in muscle, contraction leading to an increase in breadth of the muscle belly as a result of which the distance between its head and tail shortens, bringing together the 'hanging' parts and thereby moving the joints.

Walter Charleton had described the rope-like properties of tendons but also recognized the importance of blood supply in muscle contraction.[132] Through no fault of his own, Willis

[129] See: Hughes (1982): page 203; and Albrecht von Haller, *Iconum anatomicarum, quibus præcipuæ partes corporis humani delineatæ continentur*, fasciculus VII, Goettingen (1754). The major feeder to the anterior spinal artery was eventually named after Albert Adamkiewicz (1882–1921).

[130] See: Alexander Wragge-Morley, 'Imagining the soul: Thomas Willis (1621–1675) on the anatomy of the brain and nerves', *Progress in Brain Research* 2018; 243: 55–73 for a persuasive defence of Willis's creative use of imagination as a means of understanding aspects of the nervous system that observation and experimentation could not address. Thus his intellectual approach to knowledge combined ideas that went beyond the evidence based upon the empiricism of dissection and clinical observation.

[131] See: *Of musculary motion* (1681): page 34.

[132] See: Walter Charleton, *Natural history of nutrition, life, and voluntary motion containing all the new discoveries of anatomist's and most probable opinions of physicians, concerning the œconomie of human nature: methodically delivered in exercitations physico-anatomical*, London (1659); and *Enquiries into human nature in VI anatomic praelections in the new theatre of the Royal College of Physicians in London*, London (1680).

was unwittingly confused with the work of William Croone (1633–1684) as a result of the anonymous reprinting of *De ratione motus musculorum* (1664) with the Dutch issues of *Cerebri anatome* (1664). This suited his emerging ideas since Croone, who was not identified as the author until 1667, suggested that the spirits from nerve and arterial blood expand the space between muscle fibres, transmitting to them the chemical force that results in contraction.[133] Moreover, expansion of the muscle belly further increases the arterial supply by offering less resistance to the inflowing blood and so encourages the process. Croone considered that nerves are in a state of tension and the impulse consists of transmitted vibrations like the tightened string of a musical instrument.[134] Willis readily endorsed the views of Charleton and Croone that the blood supplies particles that interact with animal spirits leading to the explosion of contraction. He incorporated these principles in his first iteration of a chemical theory of muscle contraction in *Cerebri anatome* (1664). Movement is a 'systasis' (setting together) partly of animal spirits generated in the cerebrum and cerebellum which flow from the spinal cord and seep down the nerves:[135]

> The subtil humor, which is the Vehicle of the Spirits, may pass through their frames or substances, even as the spirits of Wine, the extended strings of a Lute, only by creeping leisurely through ... as it were so many little holes in a Honey-comb ... like an *Indian* cane, is every where porous and pervious.

On reaching the muscle fibres, these animal Spirits gather 'so many distinct Troops or Companies of Souldiers, all which being set as it were in a Watch-tower, are ordained, as a new impression is carried to them by the Nerves ... for the performing of motion'. Willis had already articulated a general principle of function in healthy organs that depended on nerve and blood supply and assumed that this applied equally to muscle contraction:[136]

> The nourishing matter of the whole Body is distributed into all parts from the blood through the Arteries; yet it may be lawfully thought, that the conversion of this matter into nutriment, and the assimilation of it into the substance of the part to be nourished, is performed by the influence and help of the nervous Juyce, as it were of a certain spiritous Ferment ... the nervous juice (which we have said is like the male seed) is poured out with the nutritious humor copiously suggested from the Arteries, as it were the genitive or seed

[133] See: William Croone, *De ratione motus musculorum*, London (1664); LG Wilson, 'William Croone's theory of muscular contraction', *Notes and Records of the Royal Society of London* 1961: 16; 158–78 for an analysis of the work; and A Rupert Hall, 'Medicine and the Royal Society'. In. Ed. Allen G Debus, *Medicine in seventeenth century England. A symposium held at UCLA in honor of C.D. O'Malley*, Berkeley (1974): page 433 for the suggestion that Croone's essay 'may have been attributed to Willis himself'. It is unlikely that this is a reference to the previously unrecorded 1667 Dutch issue of *De ratione motus musculorum* naming Willis as the author (**2G**). See also chapter 6 for details of Croone's eventual clarification of the matter in 1667 (**2E1**), and Wilson (1961), page 177 footnote 38 for discussion of the authorship being unknown to other writers including Christiaan Huygens (1629–1695) and Giovanni Borrelli (1608–1679).

[134] This anticipated the work of David Hartley (1705–1757) on vibratiuncles as the basis for propagation of the nerve impulse: see David Hartley, *Observations on man, his frame, his duty, and his expectations*, 2 volumes, London (1749). Croone had planned to inaugurate a series of annual lectures on muscular motion; and in her will dated 25 September 1701, his widow, by now Lady Sadlier, bequeathed to the Royal Society one fifth of the rent of the King's head Tavern, Old Fish Street, London, for the purpose of a lecture on local motion or a related subject that the president considered useful in promoting the objects for which the Royal Society was instituted. The Croonian lecture remains the most prestigious award to a Fellow of the Royal Society working on biological sciences. The residue of Lady Sadlier's bequest went to the Royal College of Physicians for the support of a similar lecture.

[135] See: *The anatomy of the brain* (1681): pages 128–9.

[136] See: *The anatomy of the brain* (1681): pages 134–5.

> of another Sex, every where upon all the parts; and that this former, being induced with active Elements imbues the more thick matter, as with a certain Ferment, and impregnates it with the animal Spirit.

As to what happens next, Gassendi (1658) had previously proposed the concept of an explosion within muscle. This was readily acknowledged when Willis next wrote on muscular contraction in *Pathologiæ cerebri* (1667):[137]

> This Rational man, weighing in his minde, how much that force or strength might be, with which ... the whole animal Machine is moved ... who can easily comprehend that small thing, whatsoever it is, within the body of an Elephant ... that it should be able to agitate such a bulk, and cause it to perform a swift, and regular dance? ... The same fiery nature of the soul ... is able to perform within the body, by its own mobility, the same thing that a little flame of Gun-powder does in a Cannon ... it not only drives forth the Bullet, with so much force, but also drives back the whole machine with so great strength.

In fact Willis had already adopted Gassendi's work in *Cerebri anatome* (1664) stating that muscle contraction: 'seems like the explosion of Gun-powder ... by reason of this copula, highly flatuous and apt to be rarified, the spirits become more active, whereby the muscle is suddenly intumified, they, as if inkindled, are exploded'.[138] In line with his doctrine of fermentation, Willis's theory of contraction acknowledged that muscle activity generates heat, but, as a chemist, he needed to understand the nature of the underlying explosion. He favoured highly volatile nitro-aerial derived animal spirits in the nerves and saline-sulphurous particles in arterial blood which combined to form the copula capable of breaking apart in the explosion, causing muscle to swell and shorten its length. He gave a vivid account:[139]

> If anyone shall be displeased at the word Explosion, not yet used in *Philosophy* or *Medicine*, so that this spasmodick Pathology, standing on this basis, may seem only ... an explication of unknown things, it will be easy to shew the effect of this kinde of notion ... the mixtures of *Nitre* with *Sulphur*, with *Tartar*, and with *Antimony*, all which are fired with a thundering noise; also *Aurum fulminans* or *fulminous Gold*, and a Composition of salt of *Tartar*, with *Nitre* and *Sulphur*, without any actual fire, being only thoroughly heated, are exploded with a vehement Crash ... being powred on one another, or either of them thrown upon the filings of Iron, cause a great *Ebullition*, with heat and black smoke ... which without doubt, if they were restrained within the space of any body, as the *fibres* of a Muscle, they would suddenly intumify it, and so would constitute an instrument of Local motion.

Those who studied in Oxford during the 1660s had already heard Willis lecture on muscle fibres and their explosion resulting in contraction.[140]

[137] See: Thomas Willis, *An essay of the pathology of the brain and nervous stock in which convulsive diseases are treated of* (1681): page 3; and Raymond Hierons and Alfred Meyer, 'Willis's place in the history of muscle physiology', *Proceedings of the Royal Society of Medicine* 1964: 57; 687–92 (section of the History of Medicine, pages 31–6; and authors' offprint pages 1–6) citing P Gassendi, *Opera* omnia, *Lyon* (1658).

[138] See: *The anatomy of the brain* (1681): page 129.

[139] See: *Of convulsive diseases* (1681): page 2.

[140] See: Kenneth Dewhurst, *Thomas Willis's Oxford lectures*, Oxford (1980): page 151.

> These are not extensions or offshoots of the nerves as they are far too numerous ... although the animal spirits continuously flow through the tubules of the nerves, they do not perpetually glow into and inflate the fibres ... the humour hidden in these fibres does not ... consist of succus nervosus and animal spirits but partly of the vital spirits carried through the arteries. The fibres seem to be replenished with this spirituous matter as much from the nerves as from the arteries, and seems to be the *humidum primegenium*. The spirits lying in these fibres are quiet until aroused by a command from the brain brought through the nerves, when they perform their functions. The nerves therefore are a kind of channel through which animal spirits continuously flow whereas the fibres are lakes where they stagnate and are at rest.

One student in particular took the ideas further. In his treatise on respiration, originally published as part of *Tractatus duo* (1668) and later as the first of five tracts in *Tractatus quinque medico-physici* (1674), John Mayow (1640–1679) argued that aerial niter is directly needed for all forms of muscle contraction, including that of the heart, without which life ceases.[141] Although confessing initially to having been uncertain, Mayow came to share Willis's position that the blood delivered sulphurous particles and the nerves nitro-aerial animal spirits. But Mayow differed from Willis on one matter of detail:[142]

> As to the nature of the animal spirits, the authority of the learned Dr Willis had no small weight with me; he supposes that the animal spirits are of the volatile salt. For this learned man in his *Diseases of the Brain*, chapter xi, speaks as follows: *And indeed the Animal Spirits when in a healthy and regular condition seem to behave to some extent as a spirituous liquor full of volatile salt which distils from the blood*. But, indeed, with all respect to so eminent a man, since muscular contraction is produced by particles of diverse kinds mixed together and mutually moving themselves (as is the view of the learned author, and as also seems most consonant with reason), if the animal spirits consist of volatile salt, then the other motive particles supplied by the blood must be acid salt.

In dismissing the notion of acid blood, Mayow was mainly concerned to emphasize that, for him, the nitro-aerial particles were the animal spirits and sufficient to interact with sulphurous blood in muscle and cause contraction of its fibres. But he had another point to make and again took Willis to task, perhaps unfairly, for adhering to the issue of expansion: 'I cannot admit that muscles are contracted by the inflation of the fibres, a view approved by some ... the fibrils, which in our opinion primarily undergo contraction, seem to be solid bodies; so that they are quite incapable of being inflated.'[143] Others had also challenged this view in seeking to understand the basic principles of vitality in the animal and vegetable world. Written in 1662 but not published until 1677, and admitting that his views lacked evidence ('let me hope that the Royal Society and other inquirers after truth will be moved to furnish it'), Francis Glisson (1597–1677) developed a concept (initially around the periodic discharge of bile into the intestines) that all tissues respond to 'irritability'. He challenged

[141] See: John Mayow, *Tractatus quinque medico-physici quorum primus agit De Sal-nitro, et spiritu nitro-aereo. Secundus De respiratione. Tertius De respiratione foetus in utero, et ovo. Quartus De motu musculari, et spiritus animalibus. Ultimus De rachitide*, Oxford (1674).

[142] See: John Mayow, *Medico-physical works being a translation of tractatus quinque medico-physici*, Edinburgh (1907): pages 250–1.

[143] See: Mayow (1907): page 282.

the prevailing view that muscle expands on contraction.[144] Glisson was quoting Jonathan Goddard's (1617–1675) evidence that, using plethysmography, paradoxically the level of water in the funnel of a sack of fluid in which a man's arm is encased oscillates with the arterial pulse but falls with contraction and rises with relaxation of the forearm muscles:[145]

> From which it is clear that muscles are not inflated or swollen at the time they are contracting, but on the contrary are lessened, shrunk and subsided ... we may infer that the fibres are shortened by an intrinsic vital movement and have no need of any abundant afflux of spirits, either animal or vital, by which they are inflated, and being so shortened carry out the movements ordered by the brain.

The sequence of events at the Royal Society was described by Thomas Birch:[146]

> On 21 January 1669 Dr Croune brought in his hypothesis of motion, which was read, and ordered to be registered, and to be compared by those members, who were formerly nominated for that purpose, with the other theories already given in Register 4: 44
>
> On 28 October 1669, it being mentioned, that Dr Goddard had been formerly desired to give in writing his experiment about the manner of the motion of the muscles, whether they in their contraction grow bigger upon the whole or not; and this not being yet done, the doctor was again desired to do it, that it might be entered in the Register-Book
>
> On 16 December 1669 Dr Goddard's account was read of an experiment formerly made by him before the Society, to shew, whether the muscles of an animal, in their motion, are bigger or less in their sum of dimensions? This account was ordered to be registered, as follows: Register, Vol iv, p 95
>
> Upon reading this paper, it was suggested by Mr Hooke, that it would be worth considering what it is, by its influx makes the muscles act by contraction; and then how the muscles are again relaxed by nature's discharging that liquor or spirit, which contracted them. To illustrate this, he mentioned, that the spirit of wine (for example) poured upon gut-strings contracts and shortens them, and being thence evaporated relaxes and lengthens them again. So that, he said, there must be a very subtle volatile spirit that enters into the muscles; and the same must very quickly be discharged again to cause the contraction and expansion of the muscles. He likewise intimated, that if he could communicate the force of gun-powder to a spring, he might then command as much strength as he would.

Goddard's evidence meant that by the time *De motu musculari* (1670) was published Willis was out of touch with contemporary views. But, unaware or unconvinced, he did not altogether abandon his earlier position on explosion and expansion:[147]

[144] See: Sir M. Foster, *Lectures on the history of physiology during the sixteenth, seventeenth and eighteenth centuries*, Cambridge (1901): page 288; and Francis Glisson, *Tractatus de natura substantiæ enegetica seu de vita naturæ eiusque tribis primis facultatibus, I. Perceptiva, II. Appetitiva, III. Motiva*, London (1672); and Francis Glisson, *Tractatus de ventriculo et intestinis cui præmittitur alius, de partibus continentibus in genere; & in specie de iis abdominis*, London (1677). The concept of irritability then rested until taken up by Albrecht von Haller in (English translation) *A dissertation on the sensible and irritable parts of animals*, London (1755). However, Hierons and Meyer (1964): page 690 (authors' offprint page 4) emphasize that Glisson's account of the key experiment refers to Goddard, not his own work.

[145] See: Foster (1901): pages 290–1.

[146] See: Thomas Birch, *The history of the Royal Society of London for improving of natural knowledge*, volume 2, London (1756): pages 340, 399, 411–12.

[147] See: *Of muscular motion* (1681): page 42.

> But that the fleshy belly of the Muscle, whilst it is contracted, doth swell up, is not all to be doubted, because this is evidently beheld by the sight and touch in the dissection of living Creatures: to wit, all the fleshy fibres being wrinkled together, are made more tumid and sharper, and so shorten the Muscle, and make it also thicker and broader: For the more certain belief of this, when I had bound some of the fleshy fibres, separated from the knitting of the rest, and had left others near them loose, there appeared a notable difference between those flaccid or not swelled, and these intumified or swelled up in every contraction of the Muscle.

In his final iteration of the chemical principles of muscle contraction, Willis focused on the distribution of combustible materials delivered in blood and the nervous juice, and the dynamics of their combination. Despite steady delivery of animal spirits from the nerves to the muscles, 'night and day . . . waking and sleeping . . . [in] work or idleness', muscles avoid a constant state of contraction because the active particles are temporarily stored. Nonetheless, this store cannot always be contained and unwanted muscle contraction may occur 'bringing forth a long and very painful contraction of the Muscle, Which kind of Spasm, sufficiently known, we vulgarly term the Cramp'.[148] Willis pauses to remember that in considering convulsive disorders, he had omitted to mention the nature of 'tetanism' and contraction of an antagonist when a muscle is palsied which, unlike spasm, is usually painless.[149] As to where the animal spirits are stored, Willis argues that material originating from the brain is placed in the tendons and returned there after contraction:[150]

> Spirit or subtil matter doth flow from the Tendons into the flesh or fleshy fibres, which entering them on either side, blows them up, and at the same time draws them together nearer within themselves, that presently all the Fibres are made shorter and intumified; then when the matter recedes from the flesh or fleshy Fibres into the Tendons, the Fibres being emptied and loosned from their corrugation or wrinkling, are restored to their former longitude, and so by turns: whether this in truth be so done or no, shall be discoursed anon.

Conversely Willis shows, using infusions of ink in spirit of wine, that arterial blood suffuses throughout the muscle but does not stain the tendons. And whereas the animal spirits are recirculated, the explosive copulae in muscle must be replenished by a fresh supply from arterial blood.

The most original parts of *Of musculary motion* concern muscle mechanics. Muscles are either simple, although variously shaped (rhomboid, trapezoid, pyramidal, spiral, or semilunar), or complex with several bellies lying parallel between the tendons of origin and insertion. Nicolas Steno had suggested that muscle is arranged as a parallelogram with two individual components, and that these parts contract independently rather than requiring integrity of the entire muscle belly.[151] In *Tractatus de corde* (1669), Lower took this concept

[148] See: *Of musculary motion* (1681): page 45.

[149] In this context, Willis ends *Of musculary motion* (1681): pages 46–7 with an account of spasticity from spinal cord disease: a Noble Woman developed paralysis of the lower limbs which became stiff and extended with spasms so that 'the Tendons under either Ham, being made tumid and shorter, were so contracted, that she could not stretch out her Legs straight' due to simultaneous contraction of agonists and antagonists. In her case, the spasms were helped by her nose being wafted with tobacco smoke.

[150] See: *Of musculary motion* (1681): page 38.

[151] See: N Steno, *De musculis et glandulis observationum specimen*, Copenhagen (1664); and N Steno, *Elementorum myologiae specimen*, Florence (1667).

further by proposing that with contraction the two bellies slide together so that muscle hardens and shrinks rather than swelling and enlarging during contraction. As Henry Oldenburg explained, this refuted 'the way of movement in the muscles taught by Mr Willis, exploding his explosion'.[152] Quoting from Steno, Willis agreed that muscle is '*a Collection of moving Fibres, so framed together, that the middle flesh constitute an oblique angular Parallelopipedum* [a three dimensional figure formed by six parallelograms] *but the opposite Tendons compose two quadrangular Prisms or Figures*'.[153]

Willis explains that the angle made by the insertion of the tendon and the greatest width of the muscle belly increases with contraction as the muscle expands and its length shortens, and vice versa with relaxation. Conversely, the tendons change neither their length nor breadth when the muscle contracts. Willis wonders why the 'motive force doth in the muscles so far exceed the force transmitted from the Brain through the Nerves' by the simple action of animal spirits. The principle of levers and forces acting remotely from the centre of gravity of the muscle belly is one explanation. Additive effects of the explosive force, as in compacted air escaping or the activity of gunpowder, offers another. Willis's position is that contraction starts at either end of the muscle belly and proceeds towards the centre. He is satisfied on this point by applying ligatures at each end of the muscle, or cutting the muscle belly into sections, and observing that the central parts remain flaccid whereas those in continuity with the tendons continue to contract. Any residual flickers of movement in the isolated parts can be attributed to unused animal spirits present when the dissections were made.

But here too, Willis did not escape criticism. John Mayow disagreed that tendons are the repository of the combustible material and on the mechanics of contraction. He made the point that if one end of a muscle is fixed to an immovable part, as is the case with those that serve for local motion, the contraction will be towards the fixed point with all parts moving in that direction. The same is true of the individual fibres or fibrils. Somewhat labouring his point, Mayow wrote:[154]

> I am aware that the learned Dr Willis has expressed a contrary view in his treatise *On musculary motion*, for that distinguished man altogether denies that the fibres contract from the termination towards the origin; and indeed affirms that when they are shortened, both of their ends are drawn towards the middle. But with all respect to such a man, when one end of a fibre is fixed to immovable tendon, it seems to me necessary that the more movable end of the contracted fibre, as also its middle should be moved towards the immovable end, as is evident from the premises.

Of musculary motion (1670) is additionally important for a further version of Willis's concept of reflexes, and the integration of activity of the brain and nervous stock in complex behaviours:[155]

[152] See: Frank (1980): page 233 and endnote 60; and Hall and Hall *Correspondence of Oldenburg volume V: 1668–1669* (1968): pages 435, 451, and footnote 21 for the comment that: 'Richard Lower's criticism of the theory that muscles swell in contracting and of explosion as the cause of the swelling contradicts both Willis and Croone and may indicate that Willis's hypothesis was well known before its appearance in print'.

[153] See: *Of musculary motion* (1681): page 37 for Willis's explanation that 'I had designed Figures, almost of every kind of Muscles, to be engraved according to the natural appearances: but the printer making haste, I had not the opportunity to dissect an humane Body, having only taken from some few Muscles from the leg of an Ox, we have caused them to be delineated to the life, which are to be seen at the end, although the famous Steno hath already accurately performed this task'.

[154] See: Mayow (1907): pages 285–6.

[155] See: Franklin Fearing, *Reflex action. A study in the history of physiological psychology*, Baltimore (1930): page 57, citing *Of musculary motion* (1681): page 34; and Alfred Meyer and Raymond Hierons, 'On

> When the ordinary offices of the natural and vital Function are performed, according to the solemn Rite of Nature; or the motion of either kind is reflected, to wit, which depending on a previous sense more immediately, as an evident cause or occasion, is presently retorted, so a gentle titillation of the Skin causes rubbing of it, and the more intense heats of the Præcordia stir up the Pulse and Respiration.

Impressions of sensation are interpreted as good or evil. Movement is directed to grasp or move away from an object. Thus, for example, the nerves that move the limbs are in connection with those that activate the diaphragm so that respiration is adjusted to allow running and flight. In *Cerebri anatome* (1664) Willis had already applied the concept of the reflective movement to voluntary and well as involuntary responses:[156]

> After that the sensible Species, having past from the common Sensory to the *callous Body*, hath stirred up the Imagination, the Spirits, reflecting from thence, and flowing back towards the nervous Appendix, raise up the Appetite and Local Motions, the Executors or Performers of the same.

Willis understood that integrative action involves the coordinated involvement of agonist and antagonist muscles. This he thought was achieved by gating the main nerve trunk with doors, like those found in musical Organs, so that networks of individual nervulets, 'little nerves like hairs', were selectively activated as the nerve reaches the muscles of a particular part:[157]

> Although there be singular passages or channels of the animal Spirits of most Nerves, distinct amongst themselves; yet some do variously communicate with others through the branches and shoots sent on either side; which indeed ought to be so made, that when many Nerves together, are required to some motion of a Muscle equally, all these, by reason of the commerce mutually had between themselves, might conspire in the same action; hence, in some motions of the members, as in the striking of a Harp or Lute and other complicated actions, many Muscles cooperate with admirable celerity; so that, although many be imployed at once, they perform their task severally without any confusion.

The interest in muscle and movement at the Royal Society did not end with Willis. On 5 April 1682 the president, Sir Christopher Wren reported on the work of Giovanni Borelli (1608–1679: incorrectly designated *De motu musculorum*):[158]

> The author had been very elaborate and ingenious in his inquiries into that subject, but seemed much mistaken in several things that he asserted; particularly as to the motion of the horse, and in the strength of the motion of a muscle; for that, according to his

Thomas Willis's concepts of neurophysiology' [part II], *Medical History* 1965; 9: 142–55 for discussion of Willis's originality in use of the term 'reflexi', and contributions the concept of neurophysiology.

[156] See: *The anatomy of the brain* (1681): page 96; and Neuberger (1981): page 241, citing *Cerebri anatome* octavo (1664): page 73.

[157] See: *Of musculary motion* (1681): page 48.

[158] See: Giovanni Alfonso Borelli, *De motu animalium*, 2 volumes, Rome (1680–1681); and William Carleton Gibson, 'The bio-medical pursuits of Christopher Wren'. The Monkton Copeman lecture of the Worshipful Society of Apothecaries read at the Wellcome Institute of the History of Medicine on 4 March 1970, *Medical History* 1970: 14; 331–41, at page 339.

> calculation of the strength, it was impossible that the tensions of several muscles could sustain such a force, though they be as strong as a piece of iron of the same dimensions.

Borelli argued that the succus nerveus is not a breath of air but a fluid that moves in one direction or another through the spongy matrix of nerves like 'elderpith'. Being saturated with succus nerveus, a jolt or perturbation at one end of the nerve is rapidly transmitted through the sponge to the muscle 'whence the ebullition and explosion follow by which the muscle is contracted and rendered tense'. And the same process allows sensation to be registered when the 'skin, nose, ears or eyes are compressed or struck or titillated'. The succus nerveus does not act remotely but only by agitating the spongy matrix of nerves.

Willis on the brain, nerves, and muscle: contemporary and subsequent opinions

It did not take long for contemporary satirists to taint Willis's work on voluntary and involuntary movement with the usual accusation of doctors more interested in their purse than their patients. In Samuel Garth (1661–1719), we read:[159]

> How sick'ning Physick hangs her pensive Head,
> And what was once a Science, now's a Trade.
> Her Son's ne'er rifle her Mysterious Store,
> But study Nature less, and Lucre more.
>
> I show'd of old, how vital Currents glide,
> And the *Meanders* of their refluent Tide.
> Then, *Willis*, why spontaneous Actions here,
> And whence involuntary Motions there:
> And how the Spirits by mechanick Laws,
> In wild Careers, tumultuous Riots cause.
> Nor wou'd our *Wharton*, *Ent* and *Glisson* lie
> In the Abyss of blind Obscurity.
> But now such wondrous Searches are forborn,
> And *Pæn*'s Art is by Divisions torn.
> Then let your *Charge* attend, and I'll explain
> How Physick her lost Lustre may regain.

But the concerns went further. Willis had presented the Royal Society with a copy of the quarto edition of *Cerebri anatome* via Dr Bathurst.[160] Some of his claims appeared to cause awkwardness not least through having been written by a Fellow of the Society. With residual

[159] See: Samuel Garth, *The dispensary. A poem in six cantos. Quod licet, libet*, London (1699): canto VI, lines 241–56. Garth became involved in dispute between the apothecaries and physicians on the dispensing of medicines and taking fees. A turf war followed in which the Royal College of Physicians decided to use its laboratory to prepare and dispense medicines at cost price to patients. The House of Lords opined that the physicians seemed more concerned with upholding their privileges than welfare of the sick. Garth promoted the stance of the Dispensarians. The poem was successful and went into several editions. It is considered to have been influential in the development of eighteenth century literary style.

[160] It was not reviewed since *Philosophical Transactions of the Royal Society* did not start until 1665. A notice did appear in the year of publication in the *Journal des Sçavans*.

belief in the rete mirabilis, Charleton was asked to confirm the observations on the vasculature of the brain. He reported on 4 May and 8 June 1664 identifying differences between man and animals. It was suggested that these discrepancies be communicated discretely to Willis:[161]

> On 20 April 1664 Dr Charleton proposed an anatomical administration to examine Dr Willis's observations of the brain, and to fit a skeleton, in order to consider articulation and motion of the bones. It was ordered that the operator take care to demand a body; and that reference to it, the amanuensis draw up the copy of the warrant for such a demand, and attend the president to sign it.
>
> On 8 June 1664 Dr Charleton's discourse concerning certain differences observable betwixt the brain of a man and the brains of other animals, was read, and ordered to be transcribed, and kept for the comparison of the particulars thereof with the autopsia in anatomical administration; and also to be communicated to Dr Willis, several of whose opinions, delivered in his *Anatome cerebri*, and therein impugned. It was ordered likewise, that what shall pass between those two doctors upon this occasion, shall not be made public without their consent.
>
> On 29 June 1664 Dr Willis caused his book *De anatome cerebri* to be presented to the Society by the hands of Dr Bathurst; by whom also he excused himself for not having presented it sooner, as also for not having owned himself a member of the Society in his book, alledging his want of confidence for the one, and that of an example for the other. The Society desired Dr Bathurst to return their thanks to Dr Willis, both for the present, and for the civility of his excuse; and ordered that Dr Charleton's discourse concerning the difference between the brain of man and the brains of other animals, should be communicated to Dr Willis by the care of Dr Bathurst.

Others also were not fully persuaded. Nicolas Steno wrote a detailed analysis:[162]

> *Willis* is the Author of a very singular Hypothesis. He lodges common Sense in the *Corpora Striata*, the Imagination in the *Corpus Callosum*, and the Memory in the cortical Substance; But without being at pains to enter into details of his whole Hypothesis, we need only make the following Remarks upon it. He describes the *Corpus Striatum*, as having two sorts of Striæ, one ascending the other descending; and yet if you separate the cortical from the white Substance, you will perceive that these Striæ are all of the same Nature, that is, they are part of the Substance of the *Corpus Callosum* which runs towards the Medulla Spinalis, parted into different Lamellæ by the Intervention of the ash-coloured Substance.

[161] The discussion that follows is based on Raymond Hierons' transcription of entries in Birch, volume 1 (1756): pages 416, 436, and 444.

[162] Nicolas Steno's views on Willis are in a dissertation read to the assembly held in the house of Melchisédech Thévenot (1620–1692). That group became the Academie Royale des Sciences in 1666. The manuscript of Steno's lecture was left in Paris and printed by Robert Ninville (d.1688) in 1669. James Benignus Winslow (1669–1760), who was related to Steno, incorporated the dissertation in his work on anatomy published in 1732; and this was translated into English by George Douglas (nd: but elected FRS on 15 March 1732) in 1733. Winslow gives the date of the lecture as 1668; the edition edited by Edvard Gotfredsen in 1950 indicates 1665, and the title page of an early French edition is dated 1669. In order therefore, see: [Anon] *Discours de Monsieur Stenon sur l'anatomie du cerveau a Messieurs de l'assemblée, qui se fait chez Monsieur Thevenot*, Paris (1669) with 4 plates; Jacques-Beninge Winslow *Exposition anatomique de la structure du corps humain*, Paris (1732) without the plates; G Douglas, *Mr Steno's lecture on the anatomy of the brain.* In: *An anatomical exposition of the structure of the human body*, volume 2, London (1733–1734); and reprinting of the 1669 issue in facsimile with Douglas's translation: [Nicolas Steno] *A dissertation on the anatomy of the brain by Nicolaus Steno read in the assembly held in M. Thevenot's house in the year 1665*, Ed. Edvard Gotfredsen, Copenhagen (1950): pages 11–12, 23–6 in French; and 8–9, 17–18 in English.

> How can he then be sure that these three Operations are performed in the three Bodies which he pitches upon? Who is able to tell us whether the nervous Fibres begin in the Corpora Striata, or if they pass through the Corpus Callosum all the way to the cortical Substance? We know so little of the Structure of the Corpus Callosum that a Man of a tolerable Genius may say about it, whatever he pleases.
>
> The best Figures of the Brain are those of *Willis*; but even these contain a great number of important Mistakes, and they want many things to perfect them. In the third Figure he represents the Superior or Pineal Gland like a round Ball; and consequently according to this Figure, the Apex of that Gland cannot be said to be turned either forward or backward. Besides, we see here nothing of the Substance of the Brain on the foreside of the Gland, and which goes from one side to the other; all which the Figure would make us believe to be annihilated. Behind the Gland, a Space appears on the Basis of the Brain between the two Tubercles of the third Pair, which in the natural state, has a quite different appearance. The thin Expansion of the white Substance of the Cerebrum, which is continued to the middle of the Cerebellum where it is very thick, is quite wanting; as also the Origin of the Nervi Pathetici [trochlear] which go out from this Expansion. He likewise represents the second Pair of Tubercles as distinct, which commonly adhere to each other. The underside of the Fornix appears to be uniform, which is of an uneven and very elegant Structure. When we cut the Corpus Striatum transversely, we see Radii very different from what they are exhibited in *Willis's* eighth Figure. The white Radii appear there to be continuous with the forepart of the Corpus Striatum, which nevertheless is of an Ash-coloured Substance, and as it runs in between the white Radii, does not appear in that method of Dissecting, to adhere to any other Body whatever.
>
> In the third Figure the Infundibulum has no resemblance to Nature. The Nervi Motores Oculorum are streight, and not oblique as they ought to be; neither do we see the true Origin of the Filaments of which these Nerves are composed, from the Basis of the Brain. The Pons Varolii might have been better and more distinctly expressed; and the anterior Roots of the Fornix are not separated as in the seventh and eighth Figures, but touch each other at the upper part, and form an acute Angle. The Line marked G. G. G. in the seventh Figure appears to be a continued Line though the part between the Roots of the Fornix which is represented, has no Connexion with the Extremities; and in the same Figure the Glandula Pinealis is connected to the Substance of the Brain by two Funiculi.

Surprisingly, Willis did not take these criticisms unkindly and spoke of Steno as 'the most learned' and 'famous'. Or perhaps, written in French and published in Paris, the criticisms never came to his attention. Robert Plot summarized the achievements much more generously but, again, made the point with respect to whom credit was due:[163]

> His placing the *Spirits* to serve the voluntary actions in the *Cerebrum*, and those that serve the *Involuntary* in the *Cerebellum*, is a noble and useful *discovery* ... His assigning the *cortical* part for generating *Spirits*, and the feat of *Memory*; the *Medullary*, or *Corpus callosum*, for the operations of the *Phantasie*; the *Corpus striatum* for the *common sense*; the *Medulla oblongata*, a *promptuary* for the *Spirits*, for performing the office of *Sensation*, and *spontaneous* motion; and the *Prominentiæ orbiculares*, and their *Epiphyses*, for conveying the

[163] See: Robert Plot, *Natural history of Oxfordshire, being an essay toward the natural history of England*, Oxford (1677): page 301.

> *impresses* of the *passions*, and *natural instinct*, between the *Cerebrum* and the *Cerebellum*, are highly ingenious and his own; and so is his, and Dr. *Lowers* joint discovery of the curious *plexus*, of the *Vertebral* and *spinal* Veins and Arteries; their *Neurologia* is also most elaborate and no less admirable, tracing the *Nerves* from their very source, and following them through all the *Meanders* of the Body, and thence shewing us the reason of the secret *sympathies* of the parts.

The three treatises published by Willis in 1670 were reviewed by the Royal Society, presumably by Oldenburg. The final paragraph provides a neat summary of the ideas that Willis expounded on muscular motion:[164]

> Having declared that Dr *Steno* hath been the first that hath delivered aright the Structure of Muscles, and that the Figures described by him are visible in them; and also made out the motions of their Fibres by divers Anatomical Experiments; besides many other considerable particulars: He asserts that the Motion of the Muscles depends from a constant Influx both of the Bloud and the Animal spirits; and that the latter alone, without being associated by the former, cannot perform that moving function; maintaining, that as the Spirits (or Springy particles) in the contraction of a Muscle rush out of the Tendons into the Fleshy parts of it, and in the relaxation, skip back from these into those, so those Spirits lying quiet within the Tendons, do swell the Fleshy fibres by conflicting and struggling there with the particles of Bloud. To which he adds the manner, how the Instinct (as he pleaseth to call it) of performing or stopping the Muscular Motion, is imprinted by the Nerves in the Muscles: Subjoyning also divers important particulars concerning two sorts of Spasms or Convulsions proceeding from the Muscles, with an illustration of the same by a very remarkable case. All which he concludeth with solving the Objections which this his Doctrine of the Muscles may be lyable, and annexing some Figures, very lively representing some Muscles, together with an explanation of the same.

Willis's ideas on physiology were promoted in continental Europe by Daniel Duncan (1650–1735) who drew on the work to propose a mechanistic neurophysiology of movement and perception.[165] This was more sophisticated than that of René Descartes while still based on the concept of animal spirits moving through the nervous system. Rejecting Descartes's localization of the soul in the pineal gland and arguing that no activity took place in the cerebral ventricles, Duncan attributed the most highly developed cerebral activity to the *corps canelés* (basal ganglia) and to the *substance cendrée* (cerebral cortex). With Willis, he also localized memory and imagination in the brain. Using this physiological framework, Duncan applied his derivative ideas on physiology to explain cases of paralysis, anaesthesia, and epilepsy, as well as frenzy and somnambulism. He is credited with having described the Duncan ventricle, or the cavum septi pellucidi.[166]

[164] See: [Anon] 'Affectionum quæ dicuntur hysterica & hypochondriaca', *Philosophical Transactions of the Royal Society* 1st January 1670, volume 5, issue 57: page 1178.

[165] See: M. Duncan *Explication nouvelle et mechanique des actions animals. Où il est traitédes fonctions de l'ame. Avec une method facile pour démontrer exactement toutes les parties du cerveau, sans couper sa proper substance. Et un discours sur la formation*, Paris (1678). Born in southwest France, his work on the brain was written shortly before he spent two years in London studying the great plague of 1666. He led an itinerant life between 1685 and 1714, eventually settling in England where he died on 30 April 1735.

[166] See: Oliver Walusinski 'Daniel Duncan (1650–1735) ou le cerveau machine. Un aperçu des neurosciences au XVIIe siècle en France', *Histoire des Sciences Médicales* 2018; 52: 427–39.

Another near contemporary opinion was provided by Humphry Ridley. In his preface, explaining that 'there has yet escap'd undiscover'd a great deal of the Materials which Nature is wont to furnish for the framing of Parts', Ridley wrote:[167]

> That Reason which, upon first thoughts, seemed most force to diswade me from engaging my self upon the Subject I have made choice of in these few following Sheets, (which was, its having been already undertaken by two so eminent Persons, as the late *Willis*, and the present *Vieussens*) upon second became the greatest motives to it.

In his account of the ten pairs of cranial nerves, Ridley takes Willis to task in describing the third, 'par oculorum motorium', which Ridley traces to an origin in the cerebellum 'affording us no weak argument against the Hypothesis of Dr Willis, who hath reserv'd that part in Nerves subservient to involuntary motions only'. Others also made a point of drawing attention to Willis's mistakes. Benjamin Hutchinson (nd) cited Dr Wotton who had observed that in *Cerebri anatome* Dr Willis:[168]

> Was so very exact, that he traced the medullary substance of the brain thro' all its insertions into the cortical, and the medulla oblongata; and examined the rise of all the nerves; and went along with them into every part of the body with wonderful curiosity . . . and though Vieussens and du Verney have in many things corrected the Anatomy of the Nerves of Dr WIILIS, yet they have strengthened his general hypothesis, even at the time when they discovered his mistakes.

In his comments on Willis, John Freind (1665–1728) wrote:[169]

> On the topic of the cranial nerves and the writings of Hildanus that the 6th and 7th serve voluntary motion whereas the others are for the natural or vital motion: I take notice of this, because it is exactly the notion of the famous Dr Willis, the first inventor of the nervous system: who wou'd have the difference between the Cerebrum and the Cerebellum, as to their several uses, to consist in this, that the former is concern'd in animal or voluntary motion, and the latter in vital or involuntary. But this notion is entirely overthrown by what we may observe of the nerves: for we see a great many parts, which are subject only to voluntary motion, as the tongue, mouth, eyes, and all the face, receive branches from the 5th, 6th, 7th and 6th pair of nerves, all arising from the Medulla Oblongata, which by him is reckon'd to belong to the Cerebellum.

Freind goes on to explain that involuntary, i.e. autonomic, functions continue after the cerebrum is removed in a dog as long as the cerebellum is intact. Respiratory and circulatory functions may continue after apoplexy, despite complete paralysis, whereas wounds of the cerebellum are usually fatal. But having made these astute neurological observations, Freind weakens his argument by explaining that this is not because of innervation of the viscera when the cerebellum and medulla oblongata are intact but because the heart and lungs are muscles

[167] See: Ridley (1695): pages [1], 146.

[168] See: Benjamin Hutchinson, *Biographia medicia*, volume 2, London (1799): pages 481–5. Dr William Wotton (1666–1727) was a linguist and theologian with whom Browne Willis (1682–1760) lived and was trained for three years in Middleton Keynes after Browne Willis left Oxford.

[169] See: John Freind, *The history of physick from the time of Galen to the beginning of the sixteenth century*, part 2, London (1725, 2nd edition): pages 315–16.

that can function with a lesser direct supply of animal spirits than those needed for voluntary motion. Much later, William Stirling (1851–1932) was dismissive of Willis's contributions:[170]

> He gave accurate descriptions of the brain, but, perhaps, the chief merit in this regard belongs to Lower, rather than to Willis. His views about the physiology of the brain in particular were vague to a degree. There are some indications in his works that he had some glimmering of what are known now as reflex actions.

Cecilia Mettler (1909–1943) was equally uncharitable. She considered that the '13 small plates' (*sic*) in *Cerebri anatome* are stiff and unnatural and the text lacks sequential development. The discovery of the accessory nerve belongs to Eustachius; and the 'circle of Willis' was described by Wepfer. All Willis's ideas are Cartesian modifications of Galenic opinions. The ophthalmic division of the trigeminal is sometimes absurdly called by his name. He makes no statement on the crossed relationship of the cerebrum but considers the division of the cerebrum into two parts of protective value. His philosophical and physiologic opinions are imaginative but lack any proof and are of very poor quality.[171] If Willis's reputation for having made contributions to anatomy did not invariably prove persuasive after his death, Michael Foster was no less ready to credit the physiology:[172]

> Love of truth was in him less potent than love of fame … mixing with … the band of exact inquirers … who were striving to advance by experiment natural knowledge, Willis caught up their phrases and thinking himself one of them, attempted to expound in their fashion the physiology of the nervous system … Willis loved words as words, looked upon an illustration as an argument, and when he discovered analogy thought he had found a proof … Willis … had no great critical power in judging the value of evidence.

But for all his disparagement, Foster had to admit that Willis's account of afferent and efferent impulses and the transition from sensory impression to perception in passages through the cord, striatum and cortex was imaginative and that Willis 'dimly laid hold of the modern doctrine of reflex action':[173]

> The impression of an object, driving the animal spirits inwards, and modifying them in a certain peculiar manner, gives rise to sensation, and that the same animal spirits in that they rebound from within outwards in a reflected wave as it were, call forth local movements.

But just as Sir Charles Symonds had rehabilitated Willis's work on the cerebral blood vessels and restored his uncertain reputation on that point, so too did Sir Charles Sherrington (1857–1952) understand Willis's ideas on reflexes and the integrative action of the nervous system:[174]

> Willis … gave numerous instances of automatic acts, where stimulus was promptly followed by movement without conscious participation of the 'will'. He spoke of this as being

[170] William Stirling, *Some apostles of physiology*, London (1902): page 38.
[171] Cecilia C Mettler, edited by Fred A Mettler, *History of medicine*, Philadelphia (1947): pages 66–7.
[172] See: Foster (1901): page 270.
[173] See: Foster (1901): pages 278–9.
[174] Sir Charles Sherrington, *Man on his nature*, Cambridge (1940): pages 189, 245.

'reflex'. The 'animal spirits' ran up a sensory nerve, reached the nervous organ, and thence ran down the motor nerve. These acts were all of them simple. The lifting of the touched foot in sleep. The closing of the touched eyelid ... Willis put the brain and nervous system on their modern footing, so far as that could then be done ... *Willis was struck by the* greater richness of blood supply to the grey than the white nervous matter. He argued from it that the place of generation of the spirits was the grey matter, and that white matter merely formed their paths of travel. He held that there was a long causeway from the grey crust of the brain down to all the nerves of the body, and that the grey matter scattered along that route provided further generating stations threaded along the pathway of conduction. These points proved to be well taken.

17

'A great and difficult thing, and full of hazard'

The discourse of the soul

Pathologiæ cerebri **(1667),** ***Affectionum quæ dicuntur hystericæ et hypochondriacæ*** **(1670),** ***De anima brutorum*** **(1672)**

In the conclusion to *Cerebri anatome* (1664) Willis explained that he was already planning two other books on the brain and nervous stock. One was intended to show how diseases could be understood on the basis of disordered structure and function; and the other, 'the Crown of the Work', would be an account of mind in health and disease.[1] Here, Willis necessarily wrote more from a theoretical perspective than in his two earlier treatises on anatomy of the brain and nerves. He understood the limitations:[2]

> *I must confess, that in delivering the Theory of Diseases, leaving the old way, I have almost everywhere brought forth new Hypotheses: but what being founded upon Anatomical Observations, and firmly established, better solve all the Phenomena of the Sick,* (viz.) … *althô we follow not exactly, after the manner of others, the Ancients, we have nevertheless rejected nothing verified by grave Authority, or approved by daily Experience; and besides, we have added many things found out Empirically and Analogically by the Moderns.*

Pathologiæ cerebri et nervosi generis specimen: *in quo agitur de morbis convulsivis* (1667) is primarily an account of convulsive diseases. As used by Willis, the term includes epilepsy in adults and children; movement disorders, several of which bring to mind conditions 'first described' two or three centuries later; hysteria and hypochondriasis; and pulmonary conditions manifesting as cough. Willis's concept is that physiological interaction of the blood and animal spirits becomes perverted so that chemical activity of the particles converts ordered movement into convulsion. Logically, this has three explanations: delivery to the brain of noxious material, reduction in the passage of nutritious juice from the arteries, or faulty interaction with animal spirits present in the brain.[3] In chapter XII of *Pathologiæ cerebri* Willis includes as a convulsive disorder his clinical description of asthma, probably the first

[1] In the account that follows, the texts used are: Thomas Willis *An essay of the pathology of the brain and nervous stock: in which convulsive diseases are treated of* (1681), hereafter referred to as Of convulsive diseases, printed as part of *The remaining medical works* (1681); and *Two discourses concerning the soul of brutes* (1683), referred to throughout as *Concerning the soul of brutes. Affectionum quæ dicuntur hystericæ et hypochondriacæ* (1670) has not been translated into English.

[2] See: *Concerning the soul of brutes* (1683): page [8]; and R Hierons, 'Willis's contributions to clinical medicine and neurology', *Journal of the neurological Sciences* 1967: 4; 1–13.

[3] See: Hansruedi Isler, *Thomas Willis 1621–1675. Doctor and scientist*, New York (1968) for reference to Willis's concept of the blood-brain barrier, often inferred but never described as such in the various treatises.

statement that bronchial spasm is the cause of the attack.[4] The short treatise *Affectionum quæ dicuntur hystericæ et hypochondriacæ* (1670) rehearses chapters X and XI of *Pathologiæ cerebri* and restates Willis's concept of hysterical and hypochondriacal passions as disorders of the brain. Prefaced by description of the nervous system in brutes, the first part of *De anima brutorum* (1672) tidies up some aspects of human cerebral anatomy and introduces 'the nature, parts, powers and affections of the soul'. Whereas Willis's real interest relates to mind, the rational soul of man, the text plays safe with ecclesiastical doctrine of the time by focusing on the corporeal or sensitive soul of brutes since this can safely be described in materialist terms. In the second part of *De anima brutorum*, Willis describes a variety of disorders 'unfolding the diseases which affect the soul and its primary seat, namely, the brain and nervous stock'. These come within his concept of 'neurologie', the doctrine of the nerves; and 'we search into what part powers, and affections she [the soul of brutes] has, which shall be the chief Members of our Psycheology or Discourse of the Soul'.[5]

Pathologiæ cerebri (1667) was slow to appear. Richard Lower (1631–1691) wrote to Robert Boyle (1627–1691) on 24 June 1664: 'Dr Willis will send his book of the Diseases of the head to the press this winter, if he be not hindered or forced to defend his last. There is not a disease of the head, which he doth not excellently illustrate with very rare observations and cases; so that it is a pity that the world should be any longer deprived of them'.[6] In the dedication to Archbishop Sheldon, Willis makes clear that his sensitivity to the business of the Church is consistent with his subject matter and that the patients he describes have as much to gain from the 'Communion of Saints' as they have from physicians:

> Those Epilepticks which are to be met with here precipitating themselves into the water or the fire, and those whose members variously Contracted and distorted with Spasms or Convulsions, and those whose whole Bodies so bent, that they could not stand upright, by and by, as if by Inspiration of the Devill, they are agitated with Stupendious leapings, and other wonderfull gesticulations. These I say, and many other Sick men whom I here everywhere describe, seem not so much to differ from those whom we read in the Evangelists, to be cured by our Lord Jesus Christ.

Willis presented his book to the Royal Society on 30 November 1667 and this was reviewed, presumably by Henry Oldenburg (1619–1677):[7]

> WHat this excellent *Author* formerly promised of the whole *Pathology* of *Brain* and *Nerves*, he gives us in this *Book* a very considerable *Specimen* of. The knowledge of the Diseases which use to affect these parts, is esteemed very difficult and intricate, and particularly the true Causes of *Convulsions* are of a very deep research. For the clearing them up, this Author Philosophiseth after this manner. He teacheth, that there are indeed *Animal* Spirits, that they constitute the *Being* of the *Corporeal* Soul, and are also the *next* and *immediate* Instruments of all Animal motions, producing them by a kind of *Explosion* or Shooting;

[4] See also: Thomas Willis, *The description and use of the nerves* (1681): page 156 for mention of asthma in the context of disorders of the wandring nerve.

[5] See: *Concerning the soul of brutes* (1683): page 18. Having settled on the usage 'doctrine of the . . .' Pordage uses this term repeatedly to describe Willis's study of the brain and nerves, muscle, and psychology.

[6] See: William Feindel, *The anatomy of the brain and nerves*, Montreal (1965): page 22.

[7] See: [Anon], I. PATHOLOGIÆ CEREBRI ET NERVOSI GENERIS SPECIMEN; in quo agitur de MORBIS CONVULSIVIS & SCORBUTO, studio THOMÆ WILLIS, M.D., *Philosophical Transactions of the Royal Society* (1668), Volume 2, number 31: pages 600–2.

> upon which *Elastick*, or *Explosive* power he establish's his whole *Doctrine* of *Convulsions*. To which he annexes a Disquisition of the *Scurvey*, as being near of kin to the same Doctrine, and grounded upon the same *Hypothesis*.

The reviewer painstakingly summarizes the twelve chapters: (I) convulsive motions in general; (II) the epilepsy or falling sickness; (III) the different types and causes of epilepsy; (IV) convulsions in children; (V) convulsions in adults and the aged; (VI) convulsions arising from extremities of the nerve plexuses; (VII) convulsions attributable to liquors and poisons, and cramps; (VIII) convulsions in the context of fevers especially 'that *Epidemical* Feaver, which raged *An.* 1661 in *England*, and did principally affect the Brain and Nerves'; (IX) convulsions due to '*Scorbutick* Disposition of the Nervous Juyce'; (X) 'Of *Hysterick* passions, where he maketh the *Womb* plead *Not Guilty*'; (XI) hypochondriacal passions that are convulsive and treatable with '*Chalybeat* Remedies'; and (XII) convulsive coughs and asthma.

Written 'after the death of my dear wife ... that I might the less think on my grief', *De anima brutorum* (1672) is the work that Willis regarded as his greatest. For its analysis of brain and behaviour in animals and man and the clinical descriptions, few would disagree. In the preface Willis pays tribute to Dr Edmund King (1630–1709) and Dr John Masters (1637–*c.*1680) for their valuable assistance as he was 'being almost continually interrupted by my practice'. *De anima brutorum* is the first significant medical work from the Sheldonian Press and it is dedicated to Gilbert Sheldon (1598–1577), Archbishop of Canterbury:

> All the Schools partake of what is imputed to your Theatre; and moreover all the professors, whils't every one of their private Patrons acknowledged, Celebrate Sheldon; who exceeds, by your gifts that of other Mecænatuses, and Crowns the whole.

Willis addresses the vice-chancellor, doctors, and masters of the University of Oxford and urges readers not to rescind previous acceptance of his ideas communicated verbally, in lectures, and in conversation, with criticism of his written word reminding them that he has 'a place of Safety, in that the Arguments and Reasons fight on my Side'. Paul Cranefield points out that the title of the book is borrowed from Pierre Gassendi (1592–1655) who had argued that animals must have souls since they show evidence for memory and reason:[8]

> Anima is the specific difference which distinguishes the animal from the inaminate and from plants: for as little as we may know about it, the soul of the animal is assuredly something very distinct from that soul which we may concede to plants ... [Gassendi] feels moreover the danger of dealing with the Anima in a way that might bring him into collision with ecclesiastical authority: he chooses therefore to express himself *de anima brutorum*, though it is not the anima but the animus which makes the crucial distinction and superiority of man.

[8] See: Paul F Cranefield, 'A seventeenth century view of mental deficiency and schizophrenia: Thomas Willis on "stupidity or foolishness"' *Bulletin of the History of Medicine*, 1961: 35; 291–316, citing page 306; and page 292, footnote 6 citing Pierre Bayle, *Dictionnaire historique et critique*, Rotterdam, volume 3 (1702): pages 2699–2703 for discussion of the lively dispute that arose early in the seventeenth century about the soul of brutes following charges of heresy brought against Daniel Sennert (1572–1637) accused of having attributed to animals a soul that was too close to the immortal soul of man; and Alfred Meyer and Raymond Hierons, 'On Thomas Willis's concepts of neurophysiology [part I]', *Medical History* 1965: 9; 1–15 at pages 4–6 for a detailed assessment of Gassendi's views and their influence on Willis.

By reference to the soul of brutes in his dedicatory epistle, Willis once more hoped to steer clear of conflict with the ecclesiastical bodies on the material basis of the human mind:[9]

> Concerning the Soul, I have enter'd upon a great and difficult thing, and full of hazard; where we may equally fear the Censures of the Church, as the Schools. For that I assert a Man (as the Mad-man in the Gospel posses't with a legion) to be induced with many distinct Souls, and design sometimes a legitimate Subordination of them, and sometimes wicked Combinations, troublesome Contests, and more than Civil Wars.

Willis presented this work to the Royal Society on 1 May 1672 and it was reviewed in *Philosophical Transactions* on 30 May, the notice being largely paraphrased from Willis's preface. The writer, again presumably Oldenburg, reminds readers that Willis had promised this 'difficult Argument' in the '*Pathology of the Brain*, and *the Nervous kind*, explicating the Diseases that affect it ... together with some previous Physiological Considerations of the *Soule of Brutes*'. Sensing the potential controversy, the writer points out that Willis makes it his business first of all to free readers from what may seem offensive by explaining that the vital or sensitive, and subordinate, soul 'whereby both Brutes and Men have life, sense, and local motion ... but also peculiar diseases' is distinguished from the Rational and so 'maketh man a Double-soul'd Animal'. Dancing, as it were on the head of a pin, and aware that *De anima brutorum* is dedicated to Archbishop Sheldon of Canterbury, the reviewer writes that Willis has previously argued that the corporeal soul of brutes:[10]

> Is embodied in the *Flammeous* Life of the *Bloud*, and the *lucid* or Æthereal substance of the *Animal Spirits*; both which he hath formerly asserted, and endeavoured to prove. For, if it be granted him, that the *Vital* portion of this Soul, lodging in the Bloud, be a kind of Fire and the *Sensitive* part be nothing but an Aggregate of Animal Spirits, diffused all over in the Brain and Nerves; he draws this consequence, That the Soul of a Brute, co-extended to the whole Body, hath not only many and distinct but also somewhat dissimilar, parts. And if it be objected, that the Soul of a Brute is immaterial, because it perceiveth, or is aware that it feels, Matter seeming incapable of Perception, he answers, That would be very probable, if that Perception did exceed the bounds of things material, and were of a higher pitch, than what is generally ascribed to Natural Instinct, or *Idiosyncrasis*: Adding, that none is like to undertake to prove, that the Omnipotent Maker, and First Mover, and Constant Governor of all things should not be able to impress such powers upon Matter, as might be proper and sufficient to perform the functions of the Sensitive life.

The reviewer attributes to Willis the hope that 'so far from being Heretical or pernicious' his views will 'prove altogether Orthodox, and conducive to a good life, and a powerful confutation of Atheism'. The important point is also made that although physicians usually refer the seats of disease to the solid parts, humours and vital spirits, some people are 'rather sick in their Soul, than in their Body'; and 'since that that Soul hath a material Being co-extended to the Body, and peculiar parts, powers and affections, [Willis] rationally concludeth, that it

[9] See: *Concerning the soul of brutes* (1683): page [4].

[10] See: [Anon], I. De ANIMA BRUTORUM Exercitationes duæ. Prior PHYSIOLOGICA, altera PATHOLOGICA. Auth. Thoma Willis M.D. Philos. Natur. Prof. Sidlej. Oxon nec non Med. Coll. Lond. & Soc. Reg. Socii. Oxonii, A. 1672 in 4°. *Philosophical Transactions of the Royal Society* (1672), Volume VII, number 83: pages 4071–8. Isler (1968) reprints this in full at pages 149–52 on the basis that it is easier to follow than the original preface (1672) or Samuel Pordage's translation (1683).

is subject also to preternatural affections, and frequently needs the Physitians aid'. Thus, in addition to the many descriptions of neurological disease, *De anima brutorum* is a manifesto for organic psychiatry:

> Besides, he esteems to have made it out in his *Pathology*, That the Corporeal Soul extends her Diseases not only to the Body, but also to the *Mind,* or Rational Soul, and often involves the same in her defects and perturbations.

In order to pursue his arguments, Willis describes the vital organs of animals 'by whose operation the Lamp of Life is maintained', the comparative anatomy speaking to the 'manifold and wonderful wisdom of the Creatour'. The reviewer indicates that the reader will learn about the silkworm, oyster, lobster, earthworm and the sheep, prior to a further but brief account of the human brain beyond that of *Cerebri anatome* (1664) 'where a Section being made through the *falx*, the *Corpus callosum* and the *Fornix*, and their parts displayed and orderly laid open, are exhibited the streaked bodies, as also the Optick and Orbicular prominences, &c' in order better to show 'the vast difference of the Soul of a Brute and that of a Man'. For all Willis's special pleading, the reviewer could be construed as attributing to Willis an unashamedly materialist insistence on the anatomical localization of the human soul.

On the part based upon pathology, the reviewer ends by asserting that Willis's theory of disease 'will prove useful both for improving medical knowledge, and the happier curing the Diseases of the Head; which he enumerates, and discourses upon, both as a Naturalist and a Physitian'. Another contemporary, Robert Plot (1640–1696), summarizes Willis' contributions to clinical neurology and, as set out in *De anima brutorum*, the improvements he made to ancient doctrines:[11]

> 218 ... He further obliges *Mankind* with a most rational account of the *diseases* seated in it, and the *Nervous Juice*, according to the different parts of the *Brain*, and the *Systema nervosum*; placing the *Cephalagies* in the *Meninges*; *Lethargies*, *somnolentia continua*, *Coma*, *Carus*, *Pervigilium*, and *Coma vigil*, in the *Anfractus* and *Cortical* part of the *Brain*; the *Incubus* in the *Cerebellum*: then descending to the *Corpus callosum*, he finds the *Spirits* there sometimes hurled round into *Vertigo's*, sometimes exploded in *Spasms*, *Convulsions*, *Epilepsies*, sometimes eclypsed in *Apoplexies*.
>
> 219. In the *Corpora striata*, and *Medulla oblongata*, if the *spirits* that serve to *motion* be disturbed, thence he shews some like-wise *Spasms* and *Convulsions*; if those that serve to *sensation*, *dolor*; if either, or both, are impeded or destroyed, the *Palsie*: And as the *sensitive Soul* is the seat and organ of the *Rational*, so the ill constitution of *that* (he observes) proves oftentimes the disorder of the *other*: For the *Animal spirits* being *spirituo-saline*, if they are inflamed, they produce a *Phrensie*; if acid, *Melancholy*; if *acrous*, like *Aqua stygia*, *Madness*; if *vapid*, *Stupidity*. In discoursing of which distempers, his *Aetiologies* of the various *symptoms*, his *methods* of *cure*, and forms of *prescriptions*, are founded upon far more rational *principles*, than ever *Greece* taught us. And how far *Antiquity*, and later *Ages* too, were mistaken in their *notions* of divers other *diseases*; his evincing *Hysterical* and *Hypochondriacal affections*, the *Colic*, *Gout*, *Scurvy*, some sort of *Asthma's*, the *Tympanitis*, with *others*; either wholly, or in part to be *Nervous*, does plainly demonstrate.

[11] See: Robert Plot, *Natural history of Oxfordshire*, Oxford (1670): paragraphs 218 and 219, page 302.

Epilepsy and convulsive movements

In using the term in the title of the first treatise published in *Pathologiæ cerebri*, Willis considered 'convulsion' to be a generic expression of disorder in the brain and nervous stock. The best example of a convulsive distemper is 'the epilepsie'. In a prescient move from existing orthodoxy, Willis proposes that epilepsy is not an affection of the part that is seen to move but a remote consequence of disordered activity in the brain.[12] He distinguishes the spasm, or stiffness, from the convulsive or rhythmic movement that follows. In order to make this point clear, he prefers the term '*Cardan*' or 'tetanon' for the initial stiffness, followed by 'convulsive motion in generall'.[13]

For Willis, 'epilepsie' has a specific connotation: convulsion with insensibility. His description cannot be bettered for its account of the repetitive episodes of sudden falling, with incidental injury from earth, fire, or water (more violent that the falling of 'the Syncope and Apoplexie'), gnashing of the teeth, foaming at the mouth, shaking of the head with tetanic posturing of the trunk, thrashing of the limbs, disturbances of the bowels and breathing, and slow recovery followed by headache and a period of lassitude. He describes the aura: especially in young people, sometimes 'a spasm or cramp proceeds … [from] the back, or Hypochondria, which ascending from thence, like a Cold air, and creeping towards the head, seems to bring on their falling down'.[14]

As a general principle, epilepsy involves an explosion of spirits in those parts of the brain concerned with imagination and striving or appetite, the unstable 'copula' (corpuscles) then spreading like gunpowder. First, 'scorbutick or cacochymick' (having the humours corrupted) blood suffused with 'morbifick matter' enters the brain and interacts with animal spirits. The consequences of this union may be offset by storing particles in recesses of the brain, or rapid drainage through the lymphatics and veins. In these situations the symptoms, visual and vertiginous, are transient. Epilepsy ensues when the explosive copula flood throughout the brain, enter the nerves and pour down towards the muscles leading to movements no longer constrained by the will. Leaning much on his assessment of muscle contraction, Willis explains that ultimately the movement results from animal spirits derived from the nerves interacting with sulphur delivered in the blood, heaped up and 'intumefeing' the parts that move. The involuntary muscle contraction moves the limbs with great force, as in a pulley or windlace.[15] In the viscera this process leads to intestinal movement or vermification. In addition to these physical manifestations, 'every internal function of the soul, to wit, the sense and Imagination [are] obscured, and its external locomotive faculty perverted … the interior powers of the Soul suffer an Eclipse'.

Willis's account of a typical epileptic fit is comprehensive and needs little improvement:[16]

> The Spasm begun at first in the bottom of the belly, or some intumescency or rising up in the *Abdomen*, then, the same spreading higher, with the same effect, through the pipes of the Nerves, the Ventricle, and by and by the *Præcordia* are drawn together, and at length, the Spasm forceably rushing to the head, the patients fall down, and all Knowledge is taken

[12] Allowing for some retrospective analysis, Willis describes what would now be classified as generalized epilepsy, complex partial seizures, symptomatic epilepsy, focal epilepsy, and pseudo-seizures.

[13] See: *Of convulsive diseases* (1681): page 1.

[14] See: *Of convulsive diseases* (1681): page 13. As is often his style, Willis is sufficiently pleased with this description of the aura to repeat and elaborate the account, with other details, at page 16.

[15] See: *Of convulsive diseases* (1681): page 2.

[16] See: *Of convulsive diseases* (1681): page 11.

> from them, and lastly, the Disease being reflected into other nerves, Convulsive motions of the exterior members succeed.

Details of the paths and direction taken as the explosive copula diffuse through the brain and its appendages are important. Which nerves are most affected varies between children, those 'of riper years', and others 'more tender' accounting for variations in the parts affected by convulsions. In children, the most susceptible nerves are the third, fifth and sixth (cranial nerves) leading to convulsions affecting the face and mouth. In adults, the intercostal and wandring pair (autonomic nerves) are involved resulting in manifestations affecting the abdomen and thorax.[17] However the process may reverse. When he observes focal epilepsy starting in an extremity before becoming generalized, not unreasonably Willis identifies the part that first moves, the finger or toe, as the seat of the precursory phenomena before the convulsive process spreads centripetally from the nerve to involve the brain.[18] And in the same context, 'in some respect also from the extremities of the Nerves', epilepsy may be a response within the head to a peripheral stimulus. However, Willis suggests that the direction of spread is reversed in the hysterical fits of women and the hypochondriacal disorders of men:[19]

> The Spasmodick Disease, doth most often arise, by reason of the evill first fixed in the Brain, and from thence it is transmitted, into various parts of the Nervous system: for it happens from hence, that a vehement Passion, as of fear, or Anger, or of Sadness of spirit, affecting the inhabitants of the Encephalon, the passion called Hysteric, and Hypochondriac, doth so often arise.

Ambiguity may be detected in these accounts that undermines Willis's concept of epilepsy. Rather than describing a centrally generated process, he might be read as also arguing that the explosive copula move from nerves in the extremities towards the brain. Sensing this criticism his repeatedly stated position is that from wherever it first manifests, ultimately epilepsy is a disorder of the brain: 'To wit that the spirits inhabiting [the head] being disposed to explosions, and there being exploded, bring on or cause every Falling Evil'. Although favouring origin from the 'middle of the brain', Willis debates the seat of epilepsy in the meninges but discards this hypothesis other than in the context of 'the membrans so contracted and the globe of the brain to be more straitly thrust together'.

Willis is aware that epilepsy may be hereditary or congenital, especially in those prone to recurrent seizures. The 'procatartick' diathesis occurs when the passages and pores are too lax: 'or the door-keeping Spirits leave or are called off from their watches . . . morbifick matter creeps in together with the nervous juice, and unfolds its malignity'.[20] However the majority of cases follow accidents, intemperance, malignant fevers, poisons, and chronic diseases creating a constitution that increases the tendency for the morbifick interaction of blood and nervous juice to act as the 'proæmium' (introduction) of spasms. Not unreasonably, he considers that the tendency for epilepsy to reduce in frequency or stop at the time of puberty relates to the diversion of morbific matter away from the brain to the genital organs. But old ideas are not easily dislodged and, reverting to an outdated doctrine of magic and medicine,

[17] See: *Of convulsive diseases* (1681): page 7.
[18] For more detailed discussion, see Isler (1968): pages 122–6.
[19] See: *Of convulsive diseases* (1681): page 5.
[20] See: *Of convulsive diseases* (1681): page 6.

Willis allows the possibility of demoniacal possession in cases of epilepsy and nervous diseases. Epilepsy affects:[21]

> The whole *Encephalon*, but ... in all parts of the nervous Sistem at once, wherefore by the Ancients, it was called *Morbus Herculeus* ... *morbus Sacer*, or, the holy disease, to which may be added, the conjecture of a certain Divine of our own Country ... that many, who were taken to be *Dæmonicks*, or possessed with the devil in the New Testament, were only Epilepticks ... we may have deservedly suspected it, to be an inspiration of an evill spirit, at least it is probably, that as often as the Devill is permitted to affect miserable Mortals, with his delusions, he is not able to draw more Cruel Arrows, from any other quiver, or to shew miracles by any better witch, than by the assaults of this monstrous Disease.

Epilepsy may cause sudden death or be followed by 'the Palsie, stupiditie, or melancholy, for the most part incureable'. In a description of what would now be termed status epilepticus, Willis recognizes that 'whenas the fits are often repeated and every time grow more cruell' vital function is compromised 'till at length, the whole body languishing, and the pulse being loosned, and at length ceasing, at last the vital flame is extinguished'.[22] Always the therapeutic optimist, Willis has a strategy: to ensure that the enkindled matter supplied by the 'vicious blood' derived from the viscera and first passages be cut off, and 'the evill disposition of the Brain, and the spirits its inhabitants, which is peculiar to the Epilepsie, be taken away'. His remedies, summarized and then specified in three pages of receipts on 'The Therapeutic and Curatory Method', assemble the usual array of purges, clysters, bleedings and extracts of plants—'Pæony, Misseltow, Rue, the lily of the vally'—but not sparing his patients 'the claws of an Elk [and] preparations of a dead mans Skull'.[23]

Willis illustrates his discussion of epilepsy with case histories. At the time of puberty, a fair maid develops episodes of vertigo during which 'she is wont to talke idlely and to forget whatever she had just done'. After six months these symptoms are followed by epilepsy with 'Insensibility and horrid convulsions', always falling to the same side and, on one occasion when not supervised by the 'Domesticks', burning her face on hot coals. Since various kinds of medicine 'availed nothing', she preferred 'every Empirick and outlandish Mountebanks' to the advice of physicians but eventually 'a Cautery accidentally, and by chance ... freed her from the fits of the Disease'. About the age of 14, the daughter of a brewer in Oxford develops epileptic fits coinciding with the phases of the moon. Willis prescribes a vomit of precipitate Solar to be taken three days before the full moon followed by a dram of male-Pæonie root in powder with a draught of black Cherry water, as a result of which she seems to be cured.[24]

Willis's views on epilepsy were generally well received. A book on diseases of children was published in 1742 which, as the title page indicates, included a careful abridgement of 'WILLIS on the Epilepsy'.[25] The nineteen pages of text are taken from chapters

[21] See: *Of convulsive diseases* (1681): page 12.

[22] See: *Of convulsive diseases* (1681): page 18.

[23] See: *Of convulsive diseases* (1681): pages 23–4; and chapter 18 for more detailed discussion of Willis's medicines.

[24] See: *Of convulsive diseases* (1681): pages 21–2.

[25] See: [Anon], *A full view of all the diseases incident to children, containing a translation of Dr. Harris's book upon the acute diseases of infants, and of the eminent Dr Boerhaave's treatise upon all their diseases, as well acute as chronical. Together with a careful abridgement of the best authors who have wrote upon their particular diseases, viz. Sylvius on the thrush, Willis on the epilepsy, Sydenham on the small pox, ------ on the measles, Andry on werms, Burton on the chin-cough, Glisson on the rickets, Wiseman on the King's-evil. Teething with all the various accidents which attend that critical stage of childhood, and the most effectual methods to prevent or remove them, are fully laid down by Boerhaave and Harris, as contained in this collection*, London (1742).

II, III, and IV in *Of convulsive diseases* (pages 1–31). These are rewritten and reordered even though in the first person, but with occasional passages that do faithfully reproduce Willis's wording.

Other types of convulsion

Willis's theory of corpuscular explosion can be applied to other types of convulsion. The distinction from epilepsy depends upon the preservation of sensibility. A further difference lies in the fact that epilepsy arises from excitation in the brain with spread through the nerves to muscle, whereas the spasms of convulsion depend upon the local accumulation of explosive copula in the 'beginnings, middle processes, and foldings, or ends of the Nerves'.[26] The distinction may seem overly precise but Willis is grappling with the realization that within his concept of convulsion are disorders that have a local cause and in which the sensorium is unaffected. Anticipating ideas formulated in more detail by Robert Whytt (1714–1766) and Albrecht von Haller (1708–1777) in the eighteenth century, Willis observed that stimulating an exposed spinal nerve with a knife causes irritation leading to involuntary movement of the dependent part. This led him to consider that, in some situations, convulsive spasms are exaggerated regional reflex involuntary movements:[27]

> When the sense of a very grievous Trouble torments any part, and from that is communicated to the chief Sensorie, presently from thence, an involuntary and irregular motion, is wont to be reflected on the spirits in that part irritated ... but sometimes also the Convulsion is reciprocated, by others, either neighbouring, or altogether extraneous.

But before making the differences explicit, Willis explains that the cause and effects of convulsions differ in children and (to use a favourite phrase) those 'of riper age'. Especially in children born prematurely, spasms may affect the head and face, the limbs and organs of the abdomen and thorax. The 'procatartick' disposition is exposed by events such as teething, infestation by worms and a variety of other hazards of childhood.[28] These children sometimes dying, Willis has 'opened the dead bodies' and found no abnormality in the viscera but 'in the heads of many, a serous water being heaped up, within the cavity under the Cerebel, and distending the Membrane which cloaths the oblong pith or marrow'. Much more than in the previous treatises, Willis illustrates his ideas with a large number of case histories.[29] It has been suggested that one example of convulsions in childhood described by Willis refers to non-accidental injury:[30]

> Sometime past, in this City, many children of a certain Woman dyed of this Disease, at length, the fourth, as the others, dyed within the month; we dissected the Head, and here no serous Colluvies or water did overflow the ventricles, but only the substance of the

[26] See: *Of convulsive diseases* (1681): page 25.
[27] See: *Of convulsive diseases* (1681): page 42.
[28] See: *Of convulsive diseases* (1681): page 25.
[29] In the narrative that follows, it is not always possible to decide whether Willis is describing epilepsy or convulsions without alteration of sensibility. Many of the disorders characterized as convulsions would now be designated movement disorders, upon which those keen on retrospective diagnostics will feast.
[30] See: *Of convulsive diseases* (1681): page 27; and AN Williams and L Bermingham, 'The art of making ineffective treatments effective', *Lancet* 2002: 359; 1937–9.

> Brain, and its appendix, was moister than ordinary, and looser; what was most worthy of observation was, that in the Cavity, which lies under the Cerebel, upon the trunk of the oblong pith, we found a remarkable heap of clotter'd, and as it were concreted blood.

Another man dwelling in the neighbourhood lost all his children in turn from convulsions. He sought advice from Willis in advance of the birth of his wife's next child. Leachings, powders, and syrups given to the child and its' wet nurse staved off the convulsions for a while but eventually they emerged together with a painful tumour at the lower part of the spine with distortion of the vertebrae, weakness of the legs and 'at length a Palsie'. For Willis the logic here is that the obnoxious copula first affected the brain, entered the spinal marrow, and 'thrust out at its further end, it wholly stopt up the heads of the appending nerves, and shut out the passage of the Spirits'.[31] Knowing that there is a 'procatartick' phase, Willis is keen on prophylaxis and recommends spooning 'purest hony ... Canary sweetned with Sugar, and some oyl of Sweet Almonds fresh drawn' into the mouths of newborn infants from families with a history of childhood convulsions. Nor should the wet nurse be spared since it may be her milk that precipitates the convulsions.

Convulsions in adults may arise from the accumulation of morbific matter in the cranial nerves supplying the muscles of the head leading to distortions of the face, eyes, and mouth. If the wandring nerve is involved there follows disorder of the viscera especially palpitation and irregularities of the pulse. When the spinal marrow is flooded, the manifestations are in the limbs. In all cases, damming back the explosive matter into the brain causes focal 'convulsion' manifesting as vertigo, giddiness, and scotomie (by which Willis means swooning or, as he uses elsewhere, 'Leipothymy'). Examples follow of persistent vertigos, considered by Willis to be symptoms of impending convulsion that, in one example, are resolved by discharge of copious yellow matter from an 'Imposthume' (abscess) in the ear. A 16-year-old 'fine maid' injures her breast in falling from a horse and develops a persistent swelling. Three years later, the 'Tumour about to degenerate into a Cancer', she develops local 'prickings, also convulsions and contractions' followed by disturbances of the abdomen and, later, insensibility and 'Convulsive motions ... in the whole Body, so strongly, that the Sick party could scarce be held, by three or four strong men'. Recurrent convulsions and vertigo persist until she is married and 'brought to bed', after which by degrees she grows well.[32]

Ingestion of poisons that act directly on animal spirits in the nervous juice rather than the blood causes convulsions. Willis explains that 'the eating of *Hemlock*, the *laughing-Parsly* (Ranunculus sardous), *man-drakes*, the furious *nightshade*, *wild Parsnips*' and the biting of a mad dog lead rapidly to 'horrid Contractions of the *Ventricle*, *numbness*, *delirium*, Convulsions, twitches of the *tendons*, in the whole body'. Most characteristic is the bite of the Tarantula and 'a numbness, and Trembling, also Convulsions, and loosning of the members ... with a great loss of strength'. But, as Willis relates based on writings of the ancients, most remarkable is that those stung 'as soon as they hear musical Instruments, presently they are eased of their pains, and leaping into the middle of the room, they begin to dance and jump about' until the fiddlers cease their play, at which point those 'Tarantulasized' fall to the ground and resume their former pains. As a result, musicians are hired to play and keep the victims quiet. But 'they are not excited indifferently with any musick, but with certain

[31] See: *Of convulsive diseases* (1681): page 28. Others may prefer the interpretation that the family had tuberculosis and this child suffered from Pott's disease.

[32] See: *Of convulsive diseases* (1681): pages 42–3.

kinds of Tune, and that they dance to some measures, before others'. Willis describes men and women 'tormented with ... inquietude of their members ... that they have been forc'd to walk, till they were tyred, as also to dance, leap, and run about ... that by this means they might shun the grievous trouble'. From here, not surprisingly, Willis strays again into witches and 'the delusions of the Devill' concluding that no sooner is a child or well-connected adult affected by convulsions than 'the next old woman is accused of witchcraft, she is made guilty, and very hardly, or not at all, the wretch escapes the flames, or an halter', whether or not the convulsions are cured through the efforts of physicians. But the point is made that witchcraft or the devil are suspected when the contortions or gesticulations are such that 'no sound man, nor mimick, or any tumbler can imitate'; and when the strength of the contractions exceeds 'all humane force', or strange matter is passed by vomiting 'or a live Eel ... voided by stool'. Wisely, Willis deigns not to elaborate relevant case histories since he considers these invariably to be subject to exaggeration.[33]

Malignant fevers are a potent cause of convulsion, delirium, and madness. These carry an ill omen. When the morbific matter after being 'lay'd up in the Brain, from the Blood' is 'slidden down into the nervous stock' there follows 'a remarkable Prognostification, of Death or peril ... Contractions and twitches of the muscles, and tendons; also sudden shakings of the members, and Limbs; and sometimes most horrid stiffnesses, in the whole body succeed'. Often manifesting without many premonitory symptoms, these distempers are best designated a '*malignant hectick feavour*' or, even better, the '*Convulsive nervous pestilence*'.[34] Against this background, Willis pauses, in chapter VIII of *Pathologiæ cerebri*, to consider the epidemic of 'populary or childish feavour, very much infecting the Brain, and nervous stock, exceedingly spread in this country, yea almost thorow all *England*: the History of which Disease, being described in that time, in which it raged, *viz.* in the year 1661'.[35]

Another type of convulsion, described by Willis as 'universal', is associated with palsy: 'the muscles and tendons, are perpetually urged with Convulsive motions, notwithstanding, the sick being made weak, they are not able strongly to move any of their members ... pains equally diffused thorow all the Limbs, are adjoyned'. In 1656, a 'very fine and religious maid', aged 20, developed headache, vertigo, neck stiffness and convulsions of the limbs which were so 'wonderfully turned about, that no juggler or tumbler could imitate their bendings, and rollings about' and 'her strength was grown so feeble, that she could not stand or walk' but her 'memory, understanding and phantasie' were unimpaired 'nor said any thing madly, or foolishly'. Finding her father also sick 'with the most grievous Convulsive passions', Willis resists attributing the family illness to 'the delusions of witches' and interprets the condition in terms of morbific matter. He prescribes natural remedies, clysters, and 'various antispasmodic oyntments' applied topically with warm woollen cloths. Eventually, violent convulsions of the limbs are replaced by palsy so that she lay in her bed 'immovable like a stone'. Despite some respite, the maid eventually died of cough and pthisis.[36]

[33] See: *Of convulsive diseases* (1681): pages 47–8 for these accounts of the tarantula, St Vitus dance and witchcraft. As is well known, the Tarantella is a fast and light folk dance in 6/8 time from Taranto, southern Italy, characterized by teasing and flirtatious behaviour between one or two couples and often accompanied by tambourines. Its origin is connected with the appearance of tarantism seemingly associated with the bite of the tarantula spider whose victims were cured by frenzied dancing. Amongst others, Tarantellas were written for the piano by Frédéric Chopin (1810–1849), Franz Liszt (1811–1886), and Carl Maria von Weber (1786–1826).

[34] See: *Of convulsive diseases* (1681): page 50.

[35] See: *Of convulsive diseases* (1681): pages 51–8; and chapter 15.

[36] See: *Of convulsive diseases* (1681): pages 66–8; and Hierons (1967): page 8 who describes this case as an example of torsion dystonia. The analogy of a juggler or tumbler is clearly well liked by Willis or Pordage and used several times in *Of convulsive diseases*.

A noble virgin developed convulsions of the diaphragm and respiratory muscles so that her chest jerked repeatedly with head movements and repetitive utterances of the same word interspersed with moments of ease from the 'throttling, and noisie distemper'. It followed that the explosive particles had enter'd into ... passages of the nerves ... dedicated for the office of breathing, and also by fits, into those designed for the motion of the Tongue, and almost perpetually tormenting the Spirits abounding in them, with Rage and fury'.[37] In other cases, in which mostly young women take fright of illness or other unpleasantness in their surroundings and suffer palpitations, panic, and thrashing of the limbs, Willis faithfully describes events but concludes that this distemper arises from a vehement fear disturbing the spirits in the brain and thorax. There follows an account of mechanisms in the brain that are not dissimilar to those underlying other forms of convulsion where fear is not implicated. One such 'illustrious virgin aged about 18 years' is exposed to a raft of remedies that includes shaving her head and the application of 'an Hysterical plaister mixed with *Galbanum* (an aromatic gum resin extracted from the Persian *Ferula gummosa*)' on her abdomen, and drinking of Astrop waters, after which 'she was perfectly well'.[38]

So rich are these descriptions that it is easy for any neurologist to read into Willis's account of movements that are not intentional affecting the trunk and limbs, conditions that are now part of the nosology of movement disorders. The temptation has not always been resisted:[39]

> I have known some, who have had all the muscles and tendons through their whole body, afflicted with Contractions and leapings without intermission; I have known others whose thighs, arms and other members, were perpetually forced into various bendings and distortions.

Never one to avoid repetition, much the same description is later repeated by Willis:[40]

> I have known some sick people, who have had all the muscles and tendons, all at once in their whole body, perpetually to leap forth, with so many distinct Convulsions ... inordinate motions, almost of all the members, ... being risen in one part, presently passe over to others ... *Horstius* relates of a maid ... whose members and Limbs not only were forced into divers manner of flections and distortions ... not being able to stand in a place, she was necessitated to run up and down ... and to dance.

In a case of involuntary movements with ascites, Raymond Hierons sees 'Wilson's disease'.[41] A patient with generalized writhing movements and contractions of the respiratory muscles together with vocalization, 'she would repeat the same word very often, yea sometimes twenty times at least', may have had 'Gilles de la Tourette' disease; but for Hierons this is a description of palilalia and, because she recovers, his diagnosis is acute encephalitis.[42]

[37] See: *Of convulsive diseases* (1681): pages 68–70.

[38] See: *Of convulsive diseases* (1681): pages 72–5; and chapter 1 for details of Willis's discovery in about 1657 of the medicinal value of water at Astrop, near King's Sutton, where he noticed that stones in the stream were discoloured by the presence of iron.

[39] See: *Of convulsive diseases* (1681): page 8; cited by Spillane (1981) page 67 as another example of torsion dystonia, but with the incorrect page number (as page 7).

[40] See: *Of convulsive diseases* (1681): page 61; or *Dr Willis's practice of physick* (1684): page 55, cited by Hierons (1967): page 8 but with the incorrect page number (as page 66).

[41] See: R Hierons and A Meyer, 'Willis's place in the history of muscle physiology', *Proceedings of the Royal Society of Medicine* 1964; 57: 31–6, at page 36. Unusually the authors provide no guide to which of many cases with convulsions and abdominal swelling, some of whom recovered and others died, they refer.

[42] See: *Of convulsive diseases* (1681): pages 68–9; and Hierons (1967): page 8.

A stronger case can be made for Hierons's suggestion that Willis described the symptoms of paralysis agitans, including sweating and salivation, one hundred and fifty years before James Parkinson (1755–1824). Willis attributed the condition to poisoning with mercury and the patient's symptoms increased when 'sitting near the Chimney'. Hierons was particularly influenced by the description that:[43]

> Sometimes, when his mind was carried forth by some sudden occasion of Joy, he would be able, his spirits being raised with a wonderful strength suddenly to rise out of his chair, and without the help of another, to stand upright, and to jump, which interval however lasted scarce a minute or an hour, but that his members flagg'd, and were affected with wonted langor and trembling.

At autopsy, Willis 'could find but very few footsteps of these kind of most grievous symptoms ... the bulk of the brain was less than it should be'. Hansruedi Isler (1934–2019) emphasizes Willis's further description of this patient with a history of slowly increasing coarse tremors, akinesia, painful muscle tension, laboured gait with bent body and propulsion, hypersalivation, and death from pneumonia.[44] But the dangers of retrospective diagnosis are well illustrated by the early part of Willis's description of this honourable gentleman, aged 36, with recourse to a chair 'set upon bow-fashion'd feet, such as are Childrens Cradles', who was worse in hot weather, warm Bathes', and 'abhor'd the very sight of the fire afterwards becoming weaker'.[45] In another case, Macdonald Critchley diagnoses restless legs:[46]

> Wherefore to some, when being a bed, they betake themselves to sleep, presently in the arms and leggs, leapings and contractions of the tendons, and so great a restlessness and Tossings of their members ensue, that the diseased are no more able to sleep, than if they were in a Place of the greatest Torture.

Willis concludes *Pathologiæ cerebri* (1667) with an account 'Of the Convulsive cough and Asthma'. Cough is symptomatic of alteration in the rhythm of respiration, its systole and diastole, and, for Willis, a disorder of the brain and nervous stock. Not for the first time, he makes a distinction between conditions and then merges these in his mechanistic explanation.

The convulsive cough is more a disorder of children than 'persons of ripe years'. The diaphragm rises up and is held 'in a long systole' leaving the victim 'choaked, and often [with] a livid, or dead countenance'. Apart from cough, there is vomiting and, as the breathlessness persists, convulsive motions of the face, eyes, and limbs. In some years, the distemper appears to be epidemic amongst children. Asthma, continual or periodical, also arises from the

[43] See: *Of convulsive diseases* (1681): page 61–2; and Hierons (1967) pages 7–8, and footnote 1 page 7 supporting his case by pointing out that John Aubrey (1626–1697) described the philosopher Thomas Hobbes having 'the shaking Palsey in his hands; which began in France before the year 1650, and haz growne upon him by degrees, ever since, so that he haz not been able to write very legibly since 1665 or 1666, as I find by some letters he hath honoured me withal. MR. HOBBES was for severall yeares before he died so Paralyticall that he was scarce able to write his name'.

[44] See: Hansruedi Isler, 'The development of neurology and the neurological sciences in the seventeenth century'. In: Eds. Stanley Finger, Francois Boller, and Kenneth L Tyler. *History of neurology*. Handbook of neurology, volume 95. Amsterdam (2010): page 99, citing *Pathologiæ cerebri* caput IX (1667): page 115.

[45] The urge to point out that it is a description of the phenomenon named after Wilhelm Uhthoff (1853–1927) that characterizes demyelinating disease is too great to resist.

[46] See: *Concerning the soul of brutes* (1683): page 139, cited by Macdonald Critchley, 'The pre-dormium', *Revue Neurologique* 1955: 93; 101–6.

lungs being inflated, 'into a violent Systole', and unable to 'fall down as they should do' so that expiration is laboured and 'fresh aire' cannot be 'induced'.[47]

Faithful to his belief in fermentation, Willis argues that the cough is due to blood being held up in its circuit through the lungs and, overheated, leading to 'the more cruel fruits of the *Dyspnœa*'. It is 'sometimes excited, by reason of the bronchia of the Trachea ... being too much streightned, and often almost drawn together ... and in some places wholly shut up'.[48] But Willis makes the important and prescient point that the convulsive particles in the blood may enter and slide down the pneumonic nerves without any 'great fault of the Lungs' causing '*Asthma* of the *Thorax*, at first simple and moderate, to become periodically vehement, and Convulsive'.

In support of his belief that the brain and nervous stock are partly or wholly responsible for convulsive dyspnoea, Willis describes cases in which autopsy was carried out. One communicated to him by Walter Needham (*c.*1631–1691) concerned a butcher of Wallsallen in the county of Stafford, who died in an asthmatic fit. All that was found was gall stones 'but (added he [i.e. Needham]) the causes unknown to us, certainly not Conspicuous to our eyes, were to be attributed to the nervous stock being affected'. And an infant, dead with convulsive epileptic fits and 'a cruel sobbing, or hooping Cough', in whom the lungs being normal 'it clearly appeared that this cough meerly Convulsive, was excited by reason of the Distemper of the nervous stock'. On the evidence given, at least in these two examples, the neurogenic cough and putative pathology in the brain appear to have been mostly in the eyes of the beholders.

Hysteria and hypochondria

Factitious movements as manifestations of disease were well known to Willis. In 1374, at Aix-la-Chapelle, men and women arriving from Germany formed circles in the street and danced for hours on end, blind and deaf to others, haunted by visions, shrieking out the names of spirits, and often seeing into the heavens where the Saviour sat enthroned alongside the Virgin Mary. Eventually those afflicted with the dancing mania fell to the ground, groaning and convulsing, until restrained by cloth bands. The condition, designated St John's dance and St Vitus dance, spread to the Netherlands, Belgium, and Germany.[49] Even though Thomas Sydenham (1624–1689) dignified the St Vitus variant of the dancing mania as acute post-infectious chorea in *Schedula monitoria de novæ febris ingressu* (1686: 'A pamphlet warning against the advent of a new fever'), he was otherwise not persuaded by the organic nature of uncontrolled dancing in groups. Sydenham's notion of hysteria as anything he could not understand generally survives, whereas Willis's formulations have gradually been accommodated within the spectrum of organic neurological and psychiatric disease.[50] Although Thomas Willis is often credited with having written the first treatise on hysteria as a neurological disease, it was preceded by Edward Jorden's (1569–1633) *A briefe discourse*

47 See: *Of convulsive diseases* (1681): page 103.

48 See: *Of convulsive diseases* (1681): pages 104–5.

49 For more lurid details, see 'The Dancing Mania': in Justus Hecker, *The epidemics of the middle ages*, London (1844): pages 81–174.

50 Sydenham had already published *Dissertatio epistolaris ad Guliemum Cole MD ... de affectione hysterica* [Discourse in the form of a letter to William Cole MD ... on the hysterical condition], London (1682) in which symptoms designated as hysterical were those 'which cannot be accounted for on the common principle of investigating diseases'.

of a disease called the suffocation of the mother (1603) describing the case of Mary Glover. These writings on hysteria did not go unnoticed. John Purcell (1674–1730) paid homage to Sydenham and the combination of theory and practical experience in his writings and offered a grudging compliment to Willis and others who had taught physicians of Purcell's own day. Twenty-five years after Willis's death, he praised:[51]

> The method the Learn'd in Physick now take of reasoning upon Matter of Fact. 'Tis true, *Riverius, Sylvius, Willis*, and many others of the last age seem to have follow'd the same method [as Sydenham]; but they wanted those great Lights into Nature, which Anatomical and Philosophical Discoveries, in these our days, have given us; whereby, together with the benefit of their writings, we may hope to give more satisfactory reasons, than they could for what shall be advanc'd.

Willis includes an account in *Pathologiæ cerebri* (1667) on the 'Passions Commonly called Hystericall' (chapter X) and 'Of the Distempers commonly called Hypochondriack' (chapter XI), subjects to which he returned three years later in *Affectionum quæ dicuntur hystericæ et hypochondriacæ* (1670). In 1667, his position is that:[52]

> When at any time, a sickness happens in a womans body, of an unusual manner, or more occult original, so that its Cause lies hid ... presently we accrue the evill influence of the womb (which for the most part is innocent) and in every unusual Symptom, we declare it to be something hysterical, and so to this Scope, which oftentimes is only the subterfuge of Ignorance, the medical Intentions, and use of Remedies are directed.

The usual sequence of events is 'from a sudden fear, great sadnesse, or anger, or other violent passion', a rising sensation from the abdomen, belching and the urge to vomit with 'breaking forth of blasts of winde', irregular breathing and a sense of choking, vertigo, rolling of the eyes, ringing in the ears, emotional lability, and 'sometimes Convulsive motions, in the face and Limbs ... but universal Convulsions rarely happen'. The condition affects 'Rich and poor, Virgins, wives, and widdows' and spares neither 'maids before ripe age, also in old women after their flowers have left them'. Rarely 'sometimes the same kinde of Passions infest men'. Willis easily dismisses the ancient doctrine that the fits are due to rising of the uterus and the discharge of its vapours:

> For that the body of a womb is of so small bulk in virgins, and widows, and is so strictly tyed by the neighbouring parts round about, that it cannot of itself be moved, or ascend from its place, nor could its motion be felt, if there were any.

Significantly for what follows, Willis mentions that Nathanael Highmore (1613–1685) also discards the womb as the seat of the condition, preferring a mechanism involving 'blood, most impetuously rushing on the Lungs' that interferes with respiration and the circulation; whereas Carolus Piso (also known as Charles Lepois: 1563–1633) favours 'serous

[51] See: John Purcell, *A treatise of vapours or hysterick fits*, London (1707): pages 2–7; and Richard Hunter and Ida Macalpine, *Three hundred years of psychiatry 1535–1860*, London (1963): pages 288–91 citing the first edition (1702).

[52] For the quotes that follow, see: *Of convulsive diseases* (1681): page 76–7; and citations by Isler (1968): pages 127–9, and Spillane (1981): page 72.

colluvies heaped together near the *origin* of the Nerves'. On Highmore, to whom Willis returned later:[53]

> Tho it be far from our Custom to contradict any ones opinion, and that it is almost unlawfull for me, to dissent from this famous man; yet, because our Pathologie standing on a contrary *basis*, (viz. the cause of the hystericall distemper being imputed more immediately to the nervous stock, than to the blood) will seem to be only asserted, unless we shew the Reasons, which combat against that *hypothesis*, and for ours, therefore taking leave, here we will try more exactly either opinion, put as it were in a balance.

Willis politely points out that, ingenious at it may be, this 'Doctrine of the suffocation of the womb' will not do and he proceeds to a detailed and critical analysis. It makes no sense that too much blood in the lungs should result in hysteria since the patient may have no symptoms referable to the thorax and the fit starts elsewhere. Rather, 'we are persuaded to that opinion, that the distemper named from the womb, is chiefly and primarily convulsive, and chiefly depends on the brain and nervous stock being affected', the respiratory and abdominal symptoms being a consequence of the tainted animal spirits entering the wandring and intercostal (autonomic) nerves. This does not exclude predisposing uterine contexts for hysterical passions including situations in which normal evacuation of the nervous liquor is impaired: 'in maids and widows, to wit, the untimely restraint of the seminall humour, which ought to be bestowed about the pleasure of Venus; at least, if they receive help from the state of a conjugal Life ... the restagnations of the nervous humour, which often fix a taint to the brain and nervous stock, by this means are prevented'.[54] In one of his longest case reports, taking the opportunity of an autopsy in 'a very noble Lady of a most curious shape' who died insensible and speechless in an *Apoplexie* after a prolonged illness characterized by obstetric and gynaecological disorders, colic and recurrent convulsions, Willis found the womb to be faultless but the brain with excess 'clear water' seeping into all the crevices and insinuating itself into the oblong marrow and origins of the nerves.[55]

As for hypochondriacal distempers, mainly disorders of lean men of a melancholy temperament, the prevailing view is that they originate from vapours emitted by the spleen. But although he argues back and forth, for Willis these also are primarily convulsions of the nervous parts. Much less stereotyped than those of hysteria, the symptoms variously affect the abdomen, chest, and head but not in any predictable sequence. Perhaps most prevalent are indigestion, asthmatic breathlessness on exertion, palpitations, sweats, and facial flushing, a sense of impending death, and 'an Iliad of evills' in the head. These include: 'Vertigoes, long watchings, a Sea, and most troublesome fluctuation of thoughts, an uncertainty of minde, a disturbed fancy, a fear and suspicion of everything, an imaginary possession of diseases, from which they are free; also very many distractions of Spirits, yea sometimes Melancholly, and madness accompany this sickness ... wandring pains, also Convulsions, and numbness, with a sense of pricking, invade almost all the outward parts'. Again:[56]

> The famous *Highmore*, affording relief, as well to the Spleen, as to the Womb, hath cast the chief Cause of this Disease, wholly on the vitious Constitution of the ventricle ... the tone

[53] See: *Of convulsive diseases* (1681): page 77.
[54] See: *Of convulsive diseases* (1681): page 81.
[55] See: *Of convulsive diseases* (1681): pages 83–7.
[56] See: *Of convulsive diseases* (1681): page 91.

> of the stomach to become too loose, and weak, that ... it very imperfectly Concocts the aliments ... then the residue of the food ... degenerates into a ponderous, and viscous or clammy Phlegme.

Willis writes that 'this famous Author ... cannot draw me into that opinion, that the ventricle [stomach] is always chiefly in the fault'. He makes clear that many of his most troubled patients with hypochondriasis enjoy a healthy appetite and excellent digestion. Conversely, others who have led debauched lives with ill digestion and 'windiness' remain untroubled by hypochondriasis. Furthermore, in assuming that this is merely a recipient of digested material from the ventricle, Highmore has misunderstood the function of the spleen and ignored its essential property of fermenting the blood. For Willis, the spleen and the brain have a reciprocal relationship in orchestrating the mechanisms and symptoms of hypochondriasis. The spleen is rich in branches of the wandring and intercostal nerves, and so interacts with the brain and nervous stock. 'Black bile or melanchollic tumour' chokes the nerve endings causing a cascade of local explosions that eventually reach the brain. Thus, as a result of abnormalities of the spleen in people with 'sickly distemper of the left hyopchondrium':[57]

> Heterogenous and Convulsive Particles ... are poured frequently into the brain ... and nervous stock ... by reason of the evill being impressed on the head, hypochondriacks use to be troubled with ... frequent *Vertigoes*, Scotomies, headaches, and often paralytical Distempers ... as the morbific matter, slides down from the head, into the nervous stock, Convulsive Diseases are excited ... chiefly about the *Præcordia*, and *Viscera* of the lower belly.

Conversely, 'a grievous distemper of the minde ... excited within the brain' carried to the origins of the wandring and intercostal nerves reaches the spleen and causes convulsions in the abdominal viscera and local 'fibres and membranes'. Thus, 'from this kinde of reciprocal affection of the brain and Spleen, it comes to pass, that hypochondriacks are so unquiet, unstable, and fluctuating, at every thing thats proposed, as if, according to the Poet, Ten minds strove in them at once'.[58]

Given the contributions of the spleen and brain, the treatment of hypochondriacal convulsions requires attention to four principles: purging the abdominal organs in order to prepare the ground for curative remedies; correcting the obstructions in the spleen; cleansing the blood of the abnormal recrements; and amending the 'enormities of the brain and nervous stock' of 'the inhabiting Spirits contracted by the fault of the blood'. Against the background of this rather generic and platitudinous advice, there follow six pages of receipts of which the recurring theme is various 'Chalibeat or steel medicins'.

Perhaps in the rush to distance himself from Highmore's views on hypochondriasis, Willis allowed some ambiguity on whether the affection is primarily of the spleen or brain. In setting out a description that highlights emotional states as the precursor but then provides a mechanism merging with that assumed for all other convulsions, Willis can be said to have formulated an organic position of these disorders, justifying the view of Sir Charles Sherrington (1857–1952) that 'It was Willis who said of hysteria, thought then, as its name implies, to be a uterine affection, "it is not; it is an affection of the brain"'.[59]

57 See: *Of convulsive diseases* (1681): page 95.
58 See: *Of convulsive diseases* (1681): page 95. This refers to the verse of Titus Maccius Plautus (*c*.254–184 BC).
59 See: Charles Sherrington, *Man on his nature*. Cambridge (1940): page 246.

Highmore had set out his view on the pulmonary basis for hysterical symptoms, and hypochondria as a disorder of the stomach, in *Exercitationes duæ quaram prior de passione hysterica: altera de affectione hypochondriaca* (1660: 'Two exercises of which the first is On hysterical disease, the other On the hypochondriac state'). His theories did not go unchallenged. The dispute with Willis began through private correspondence after Willis published *Pathologiæ cerebri* seven years later. The fragment of a letter from Highmore to Willis reads:[60]

> I read your Pathology of the Brain with the greatest pleasure, in which you assigned to certain dread and grievous afflictions a cause at once terrible and fulminating. Among the graver symptoms I find enumerated hysterical and hypochondriac passions and there with great candour and in your accustomed manner, you destroy my hypothesis about the causes while at the same time you set out in a workmanlike manner the reasons for your dissenting from my theory. Your first argument [is] against my theory about hysterical women, who being of a frigid temperament often suffer from Pica and Malacia, and whose blood, being weak and prone to stagnation does not easily boil over into the lungs without any noticeable signs of its effervescence.

And in another letter, Dr Highmore writes:

> I find enumerated Hysteric and Hypochondriac passions; and there you tear to pieces our hypothesis about the cause of these passions, though quite sincerely and according to your usual manner.

As a result of the challenge to his ideas, Highmore then published *De hysterica et hypochondriaca passione responsio epistolaris ad Doctorem Willis medicum Londinensem celeberrimum* (1670: 'Written defence on the hysterical and hypochondrial condition, to Doctor Willis, the very famous London physician'). He did not mince his words: hysteria is not a convulsion, the nervous juice does not necessarily exist, and the concept of an explosion is untenable since, if correct, not only the muscles and nerves but also the blood ought to explode. His book was reviewed by the Royal Society. The writer, once more presumably Oldenburg, explained that Highmore had 'thought himself obliged to write a defence of his 1660 treatise on "the Causes of the Hysterick and Hypochondriack Passions"' in response to *Pathologiæ cerebri* (1667). The reviewer sets out the controversy: whether hysteria is primarily a convulsive disorder referable to the '*Genus Nervorum*', or 'the Blood rushing too impetuously into and stuffing up the Lungs'. Highmore's position is based on the analysis that:[61]

> 1. The Hysterick Passion is not always accompanied with Convulsions; where also the existence of the *Succus nutritius* (on which Dr. *Willis* his Doctrine seems to depend) is called in question and several Arguments alledged to the contrary. 2. That, if the *Succus nutritius* in the *Nerves*, be by a violent explosion dilated, and by that means of *Fixed salts* mixed in the *Nerves* with *Acid* ones (according to Dr. *Willis*) the same may happen upon the

[60] See: Hierons archive: Sloane MS548 f23b–8b: translated for Raymond Hierons by Elizabeth Palmer in 1961 for the two letters cited from Highmore to Willis.

[61] See: [Anon], II. NATHAN. HIGHMORI de HYSTERICA & HYPOCHONDRIACA PASSIONE, Responsio epistolaris ad Doct. Willis Med. Londinensi. Londini, 1670. In quarto, *Philosophical Transactions of the Royal Society*, December 1669, Vol IV, number 54, pages 1089–91.

> Concurrence and Conflict of the like Salts in the Blood. Concerning the *Hypochondriack Passion*, the Question between these two Physitians, is Whether the first and chief cause of that distemper, be the Weakness and Laxeness of the tone of the Stomach and its Fibres, whereby a vicious Chyle and Blood is generated that causes such a Fermentation, upon which do ensue Trembling and Palpitations of the heart, Swoundings, Fear, Sadness? &c... the Reader will finde the best satisfaction in resolving the matter by perusing the writings of each author. In the mean time he may please to take notice here, that Dr. *Highmore* in this *Epistle*, intersperses some not inconsiderable remarks concerning the *Use* of the *Spleen*, which part he endeavors to free from those imputations it is commonly charged with, being of the opinion, That the Blood is originally depraved not by the *Spleen*, but its matter by the *Stomack*.

Willis responded to Highmore with *Affectionum quæ dicuntur hystericæ et hypochondriacæ pathologia spasmodica vindicata contra responsionem epistolarem Nathanael Highmori* (1670: 'The spasmodic pathology of conditions called hysterical and hypochondriac vindicated against the written defence of Nathanael Highmore').[62] His short treatise was also reviewed by the Royal Society. The notice is indexed: 'The Learned and Ingenious Author of this Book, lately come to the Publishers hands, though not yet (which is much disliked by the curious) into our Stationers Shops'. In his first paragraph, the reviewer comments:[63]

> THe Learned Author of this Book makes it his chief business therein, to vindicate his Doctrine, which maketh the two Affections, expressed in the *Title*, to belong to the *Brain* and the *Nerves*, from the Arguments alledged by the other Learned Physician Dr *Highmore*, who makes the one to be a distemper of the Bloud and Lungs, and the other of the Stomach. In the doing of which, our Author *first* undertakes to shew, by several considerable Arguments, that the affections called *Hysterical*, cannot proceed from the Lungs stuffed up to a great degree of stiffness with flatulent Bloud; seconding them by some Histories and Observations, which seem very pertinent to his purpose: Which done, he proceeds to remove the difficulties and Objections, alledged by Dr Highmore in his Epistle, formerly printed, and taken notice of in N. 54 of these Transactions.

The corporeal compared with the rational soul

Preceded by work on comparative anatomy and further contributions to structure of the human nervous system, the main aim of the first part of *De anima brutorum* was to consider the nature of mind in animals and man. Willis's position is that there are two souls. This was not an original concept.[64] Brutes have only a corporeal soul which consists of flame in the blood interacting with a sensitive component diffused throughout the nervous system.

[62] Since it was not translated into English, this treatise is omitted from *The remaining medical works* (1681) and *Dr Willis's practice of physick* (1684).

[63] See: [Anon], III. *Affectionum quæ dicuntur hysterica & hypochondriacæ pathalogia spasmodica vindicata, contra responsion. epistol. Nathanaelis Highmori M. D. cui accessere exercitat. Medico-physicæ duæ, I. De Sanguinis Accension. 2. De Motu Musculari*, Auth. Tho. Willis M. D. Nat. Philos. Prof. Oxon, nec non med. Coll. Londini & Soc. Regiæ Sodalis. Londini apud Jac. Allestry In 4°, *Philosophical Transactions of the Royal Society*, December 1670, Vol V, number 57, page 1178.

[64] See: Carl Zimmer, *Soul made flesh*, London (2004): pages 9–23, 25–42, 209–35, 261–96, and elsewhere, for a lively and wide ranging popular account of Willis and the many others who considered and wrote about the soul of man in and before the seventeenth century.

Man has this corporeal soul but also a rational soul gifted as 'a particle of divine breath' (divinæ particulam auræ) responsible for judgement and reasoning. Willis's concept of the corporeal soul is closely aligned with his ideas on reflected (reflex) or involuntary response to the senses. He locates this 'inferior Chamber of the Soul, glased with dioptric Looking-Glasses' to the middle part or 'meditullia' of the brain. Throughout, Willis refers to 'hypostasis' of the corporeal soul as the medium that connects the material world to the rational soul: 'nothing is in the brain or heart which has not been in the senses first'.[65] But his intentions for *De anima brutorum* go further. In order to discriminate the 'Dignity, Order, and Immortality of the Rational Soul', Willis intends to deliver a 'certain or Doctrine of the Soul, previous to shewing the Doctrine of the Diseases of those Parts'.[66] The task is not easy. As he points out: 'Truly 'tis no unjust Complaint of the Soul, that she understands all things but her Self'.

Aware that he needs to be careful, the corporeal soul of brutes serves as a smokescreen for explaining workings of the brain and spinal cord in man without committing too much on the exact nature of the rational soul, since this is the province of religion. The corporeal soul is the basis for 'Ingenuity, Temperament and Manners of every Man ... as also the Causes, and formal Reasons of many Diseases, as of the Phrensie, Lethargy, Vertigo, Madness, Melancholy, and others, belonging rather to the Soul than to the Body'. Focusing on the corporeal soul of brutes allows Willis, directly or by implication, to consider human psychology, physiology, and psychiatry. But for all the clarity of his distinction, Willis is having to juggle two very different functions, one material and the other not:[67]

> The animal spirits being procreated wholly in the Cortical or Barky substances of the Brain and Cerebel, do descend by and by into the middle or marrowy parts, and there are kept in great plenty, for the businesses of the Superior Soul; in the mean time, a sufficient stock of these, gently flowing from this highest Province into the oblong and Spinal Marrow, and thence into the Nerves and Nervous Shoots, actuates all these passages, and blows them up into a certain Tensity.

It follows that disorder of the rational soul may manifest as human disease. This implies that these disorders are the result of perturbation affecting the material substance of the brain and nerves. There is no means of knowing whether Willis believed absolutely the position he felt obliged to take on the corporeal and rational souls of man. Careful not to risk censure, his materialist views are sometimes thinly disguised. Whilst his position on divine intervention is clearly stated, what he writes may not be what he thinks. Willis was a man of faith and comfortable with the doctrines of the church. He hints that a person writing at one time in history knows that discoveries may lay ahead which make it necessary to qualify contemporary opinion. Little wonder that occasionally he blurs the distinction and allows too much reasoning in brutes and too much material basis for the rational soul of man.

The ancients had veered between material and immaterial, mortal and immortal, concepts of the soul: 'the Animal is as it were the Loom, in which the Yarn is the Body, and the Woof the Soul'.[68] In considering contemporary views, Willis debates the position that

[65] Self-evidently, his use of 'hypostasis' is in the philosophical not the medical sense: i.e. the underlying state or substance and the fundamental reality that supports all else rather than the accumulation of fluid under the effects of gravity.

[66] See: *Concerning the soul of brutes* (1683): pages 1–2.

[67] See: *Concerning the soul of brutes* (1683): page 24; and Cranefield (1961): page 307.

[68] The metaphor of the 'Enchanted loom' is usually attributed to Sherrington who wrote 'The brain is waking and with it the mind is returning. It is as if the Milky Way entered upon some cosmic dance. Swiftly the head mass becomes an enchanted loom where millions of flashing shuttles weave a dissolving pattern': see *Man on his nature*

brutes act through 'an artificial Motion of a Mechanical Engine ... a reflected undulation or wavering ... [of] certain Nerves and Muscles ... performing the respective motion of the Member'. This leads him to the rhetorical position that: 'if Cognition be granted to the Brutes, you must yield to them also Conscience, yea and deliberation and Election, and a Knowledge of universal things, and lastly an incorporeal and rational soul'.[69] Current opinion was divided, René Descartes (1596–1650) and Kenelm Digby (1603–1665) taking different positions on the material basis of animal cognition. Willis felt instinctively that the soul of brutes, in its entirety, is material and not part of the ethereal Platonic 'Soul of the World'. It seemed probable that the souls of the many fishes and insects, which serve only as food for other creatures, 'preserve them only for a little time, and as it were to pickle them to keep them from putrification ... the Souls of those, may be said to be born and dye with their Bodies, and to be altogether Corporeal'.[70] Because it is embodied in the vital and animal spirits, this sensitive or corporeal soul, 'a-Kin to Flame', is distributed throughout the body to which end 'Worms, Eeles and Vipers, being cut into pieces, move themselves for a time, and being pricked will wrinkle themselves together'. For Willis, the corporeal soul is based on nimble and spirituous particles: 'the Specter, or the shadowy hag of the Body ... but of a most slender third, it cannot be perceived by our Senses, but only is known by its Effects, or Operation'.[71]

As background to his 'Psychelogie or the Doctrine of the Soul', Willis starts by considering the anatomy of several species of living creatures.[72] Whilst this consideration of comparative anatomy may seem like a diversion, it allows Willis to define more precisely structure and function and inform his ideas on the soul of brutes and those of man. He classifies creatures on the basis of respiration—branchiæ, or gills in insects and fishes, or those with lungs; whether they are bloodless; and, if not, whether they are hot or cold blooded. In explaining respiration in insects, Willis describes at length the findings of Malpighi on the silkworm and borrows the figures of Tabulæ III and IV from that work. He emphasizes that the cavity of its skull is mostly filled with ocular muscles whereas the spinal cord is more prominent. Respiration occurs through widely distributed pores, 'very many Lungs gaping every where outwardly, and dispersed every where inwardly [so that] the Heart ... ventricle, Genitals, spinal marrow and all other parts of the Soul dispersed ... are inspired with the admitted Air'.[73] But because they have flame and fermentation from the consumption of crops and leaves and are dependent on air, dying rapidly in Robert Boyle's vacuum chamber, insects have 'great Souls'.

These beasts of the earth correspond to the cuttlefish, sea wolf, oyster, cockle, lobster, and crab in water. Here, Willis's account of digestion and respiration through gills in the oyster, lobster, and crab is less derivative. Crustacea are protected from the buffeting of the sea and tides through having their bones placed outermost, as armour. So also the contents of their

Cambridge (1940): pages 224–5. It seems likely that Sherrington borrowed his usage from Thomas Willis, whom he greatly admired.

[69] See: *Concerning the soul of brutes* (1683): page 3.
[70] See: *Concerning the soul of brutes* (1683): pages 4–5.
[71] See: *Concerning the soul of brutes* (1683): page 6.
[72] See: Claire Crignon, 'How animals may help us understand men'. In: Eds Roberto Lo Presti and Stefanie Buchenau, *Human and animal cognition in early modern philosophy and medicine*, Pittsburgh (2017): pages 173–85, for discussion of Willis's use of comparative anatomy and observations of behaviour in reaching a position on the relationship and hierarchy of the corporeal and rational souls of brutes and man, set in the context of contemporary ideas; and see chapter 16 for further discussion of Willis's contributions to comparative anatomy.
[73] See: *Concerning the soul of brutes* (1683): page 9.

thorax and viscera are 'Histeron Proteron, topsie-turvie'.[74] The lobster brain, 'of a greenish colour' has mammillary processes and optic nerves, 'two shanks of the oblong marrow [which] descend into the spinal marrow … sometimes divided, and sometimes placed together, now united, and then again separated one from another'.[75] Willis ponders the apparent ambiguity of whether souls dependent on fire can be assigned to these creatures of the sea 'because they rejoice in the element that is deadly to fire itself'.

The same problem arises with the earthworm, which survives below the surface of the earth. Although Willis has explained 'in a late Tract' (*De fermentatione*) that life, 'fire and flame', require a supply of 'Sulphurous food [and] … something nitrous from the Air', he evades the problem of creatures that do not respire by arguing that: [76]

> Much of sulphur thick and Earthy, with little of Nitre, and very little only of spirit and volatile Salt, may be so temper'd that it being inkindled into Life, may burn with a silent and almost suppressed fire … but as it hath a certain intestine task, its burning is more securely performed in the Earth or Waters, than in the open Air.

The excess of sulphur is apparent from the 'most stinking smell' emitted when these creatures putrefy. Independent of air, they have 'Organs of respiration' that allow access to nitre 'for as long as it pleases'. This function is served in fishes by the arterial supply and venous drainage through gills. No inventiveness is needed in considering the anatomy of fowls and four-footed beasts in whom the arrangements of the heart and lungs, brain, and nervous appendages make for easy comparison with the anatomy of man.

Having described invertebrates, fishes, and cold-blooded beasts, Willis expands upon the basis of the corporeal soul in more perfect brutes: circulation of the vital liquor and 'the Animal Liquor or Nervous Juyce, flowing gently within the Brain and its Appendages'; and the fire and the light, respectively, being independent but jointly active.[77] Now his interest moves away from respiration and the circulation towards the brain and nervous stock: 'the more noble part of the Corporeal Soul, commonly called the Sensitive, or by us the Lucid or Etherial'. With this change in emphasis, Willis is again intolerant of those who insist that the perceptions and faculties of brutes are due to the presence of an immaterial substance and he cannot accept anything other than a mechanical basis, ridiculing the concept of an immortal soul in 'Fleas, Flys, and other, more vile Insects'. But not for the first time, he encounters difficulties in taking a strictly materialist line on the corporeal soul. Despite his iatrochemical stance and training in chemistry, it is self-evident that chemical liquors such as 'Spirits of Wine, Turpentine, and Harts-Horn' cannot be made to represent the images of objects and, in their permanence, chemicals differ from spirits which vanish once life is extinct:[78]

> The Animal Spirits, according to this *Analogy* … instilled from the inkindled Blood into the Brain, and its Appendix … partly from the agreeable furniture of the Organs, for that they are shut up within Passages, as it were Pipes and other Machines, abound with both an

[74] A rhetorical device designed for emphasis by placing items in reverse order: from the Greek ὕστερον πρότερον, *hýsteron próteron*, or 'later earlier'.

[75] See: *Concerning the soul of brutes* (1683): page 11.

[76] See: *Concerning the soul of brutes* (1683): page 15.

[77] See: *Concerning the soul of brutes* (1683): page 22 where Willis refers readers to his treatise *Of the accension of the blood* (1670) for details of his most recent views on the vital flame in blood.

[78] See: *Concerning the soul of brutes* (1683): page 24.

> objective Virtue, by which many rays of Light promptly meet together in the Images of all sensible things, and effect the sension of every Kind, and also ... by which the loco-motive powers, and also the acts of the Spasmodic Affections, are performed, beyond the forces or Instincts of wind, or any blast shut up in machines.

Apart from the blood and brain, a third element of the corporeal soul lies in the 'spermatick Bodies' needed for 'the formatrix of a new animated Body'. This comprises 'a certain heap of animal spirits, or most subtil Atoms, or a little Soul not yet inkindled'. It precedes the 'Foundations, or first ground-work of the body' and, with a nod to religious doctrines, develops according to the 'Law of creation ... from divine providence'. This component of the corporeal soul is independently generated in the genital organs. However its excess demands divert material away from the brain and other tissues: 'the strength of the whole Soul and Body is consumed, on the mad insatiate fulfilling of Lust or Venus; and in these desires ... it is known to burn up the Flesh, Inwards, and Bones, and to reduce them to rottenness'. But lest he seem unduly prudish, Willis explains that:[79]

> The Venerian imagination Causes presently an insurrection in these parts, and on the other side a swelling up of the seminal humor ... the Act of Generation, greatly necessary, and formed with a most vehement Affection ... the incentives of Lust are most swiftly powred forth thorow the universal parts of the Soul, fiery of themselves, and Extreamly perclive or apt for such fires.

Willis tidies up the anatomy of certain structures of the human brain in the first part of *Two discourses concerning the soul of brutes*. Because the medullary pathways were not adequately described in *Cerebri anatome* (1664), Willis and his associates have since adopted a method for gently scraping away the softer and brownish cortex of the brain with the point of a penknife to reveal 'many Medullary Chords or Strings ... wonderfully communicating among themselves'.[80] Indeed, the medulla seems to be made entirely of 'strings compacted together; as if they were so many distinct paths'. Willis draws attention to Tabula VI in *De anima brutorum* (1672: Pl.24), in which he depicts connections between the brain and cerebellum through the oblong medulla and corpora striata involving the orbicular prominences close to the testes and nates. His improved method has shown more clearly that the pathways for vision reach the middle of the brain, allowing Willis to make the point that disturbances of sight may arise not only from the 'Eye and Optick Nerve' but also the brain. This more sophisticated anatomy has also shown the central connectivity of the olfactory nerve with the mammillary bodies. And it has improved his description of the 'chamfer'd or streaked Bodyes', their vascular supply and reciprocal relationship to the corpus callosum. Everything reenforces Willis's conclusion that all sensory traffic reaches the cortex through the striate bodies, which also transmit the 'Force and Instincts of all spontaneous motions begun in the Brain'. From this, returning to his theme, he concludes that 'the Sensitive Soul, as to all Powers and Exercises of them, is truly within the Head, as well as in the nervous System, merely Organical, and so extended, and after a manner Corporeal'.[81]

[79] See: *Concerning the soul of brutes* (1683): page 31. Willis returns to the issue of lust temporarily defrauding the brain and nerves of their 'due Pension' by diverting the corporeal soul to the genital organs at page 55 but, although rich in language, the ideas are largely repetitive.

[80] See: *Concerning the soul of brutes* (1683): page 25; and chapter 16.

[81] See: *Concerning the soul of brutes* (1683): pages 26–7.

Life and the corporeal soul are mutually dependent. If the soul is extinguished and the kindling and motion of the 'subtil particles' ceases, the frame of the body begins to be 'dissolved and loosned'. It follows that the salt or pickle of the Soul preserves the fleshy bulk of the Body from putrefaction'. Conversely, like 'Oyl to a Lamp', the animal spirits require circulation of the blood 'chylifyed' by nourishing juice and the nitrous air of respiration.[82] The experiences of the senses alter not only the workings of animal spirits but also enkindle the vital flame in the blood, and activity of organs in the chest and abdomen. Anger and indignation, joy and sadness, depend both on sudden impulses of the passions and the state of the flame: weak in the cold, dropsie and the longing of maids; hot and overkindled in those with a choleric complexion or intemperate fever. Metamorphoses and strange species of the corporeal Soul occur in 'Melancholy diseases or to mad men'.

But the corporeal soul of brutes has to be more than a mute recipient of sensation and a machine for reflective movement. It must have the capacity for perception and intention, properties that are more easily assigned to the rational soul of man. Persistently troubled by the dichotomy of material and immaterial souls, Willis asks himself somewhat frivolously why, if brutes have immaterial souls that manage these matters, using the same organs as man, 'should not Four-footed Beats … learn Sciences and Arts'?[83] His answer, predictably, lies in the difference of state imposed by enkindling through the innate restlessness of atoms, just as inert substances such as oil, wood, and resin are altered and consumed by fire. Once again, he is crossing the divide between the material and immaterial, the corporeal and rational souls.

Brutes have 'Natural Instinct' that preserves and reproduces their existence through various patterns of behaviour, seen individually or in groups. They learn from experience but this skill varies between species:[84]

> The strokes of sensible things, being not deeply fixed, are presently obliterated, and in them local motions hardly follow: yea in some Beasts, in whom the Blood being continually and habitually thick, and who have a less Clear Brain, tho through their whole Life some acts of the Exterior senses and Motions are performed, yet few Characters are left, of any interior Knowledg.

Willis argues that, beyond instinct and sensory experience, perception may occur in 'more perfect Brutes'. Anatomically this depends on animal spirits passing to the striate body and from there to the corpus callosum and localized parts of the brain. He follows this with a comparison of 'other reflected Species of the same Object' assessing whether they are 'Congruous or Incongruous' before the response, or 'Appetite', is executed through motion and 'the habits of things to be done … are little by little produced'. In time these learned patterns leave 'Marks or Vestigia' as phantasies, memories, and 'Store-houses full of Notions … as so many tracts or Ways … engraven in the Brain'. Thereafter these can be activated without the original stimulus resulting in spontaneous behaviour 'as it were drawn forth from an inward Principle'. Moreover, these habits which act to the advantage of individual brutes, can be copied by others of the same or different species 'to perform more excellent Actions'. From this follows Willis's admiration for the complex 'Subtilties and Craft of the Fox' coaxing a Turkie Cock out of its roost in a tree by giddily circling around the trunk: the 'most intricate

[82] See: *Concerning the soul of brutes* (1683): pages 30.
[83] See: *Concerning the soul of brutes* (1683): pages 32.
[84] See: *Concerning the soul of brutes* (1683): pages 34–5.

Actions of brutes, which seem to contain Ratiocination ... [are] reduced into Competent notions of the sensitive Soul'.[85]

Not for the first time in this account of perception and learned behaviour Willis is moving dangerously close to describing a rational soul in brutes. Aware that he has blurred the distinction between instinct and reasoning, Willis qualifies his position by making the point that the 'manifold and divers' complexity of sensible things cannot be appreciated in one small part of the brain. His analogy is the pinhole through which a complex scene is projected onto paper in a dark chamber, 'as if done by the Pencil of an artist: Why then, may not also the Spirits, even as Rays of light, frame by a swift Configuration, the Images or Forms of things, and exhibit them without any Confusion or Obscuring of the Species?' This leads him to propose that localized functions of the brain are communicated amongst themselves to create a more complex perception. In formulating this hypothesis, Willis uses his creative imagination to provide an insight that goes far beyond the evidence of his anatomical observations. But, drawing back and in order to play safe, Willis cannot suggest any process of integration leading to purposeful behaviour in response to perception other than 'Excellent and truly Divine Workmanship... the Institution of the most great God, that from the Soul and Body mixed together, the same Kind of Confluence of the Faculties doth result, by which it is needful for every Animal, to the Ends and Uses destinated of it'.[86]

This self-reassurance allows Willis to move on and explain the superiority of the rational soul of man over the corporeal soul of brutes: in abstracting 'universal things from singulars'; in the ability to contemplate 'God, Angels, It Self, Infinity, Eternity, and many other Notions remote from Sense and Imagination'; and in resisting slavish adherence to sensory experience and consequential behaviour and habits. The rational soul can exercise judgement and restraint; be aware of what it has not necessarily sensed; devise the methods of algebra, geometry, and astronomy; resolve natural philosophy from its causes; and contemplate metaphysics and the supernatural—'the whole *Encyclopædia* or Circle of Arts and Sciences (excepting Divinity)'. It follows that because the rational soul can 'make things almost wholly naked of matter, or carry it self beyond every sensible Species ... beholding them wholly immaterial, this argues that the Substance or Nature of the Rational Soul is Immaterial and Immortal'.[87]

Pausing to dismiss ancient and more recent doctrines, Willis returns to his hierarchical concept of a rational superimposed on a corporeal soul, poised to monitor and amend faults as it carries out its brutish activities. The point of contact is localized to the middle of the brain, there being 'no necessity for a King, to be in his whole Kingdom, but only in his Palace'. This bond is important. Despite differences whereby 'the mind of one Man understands more, and reasoneth better, than that of another, it does not thence follow, that Rational Souls are inequal, but that every disparity ... proceeds immediately from the Phantasie, but mediately and principally from the Brain, being variously disposed'.[88] In situations where functions of the rational soul are imperfect, the fault lies not in its intrinsic properties but 'in some hurt coming to the Brain' disturbing the 'Phantasms ... and the Faults or Vices of these infecting the Intellect'. Recognizing that in protecting the virtue of the rational soul and assigning all faults to inadequacies of the animal spirits or of the corporeal soul there are nevertheless potential grounds for confusion on their respective roles, Willis restates the ancient doctrine:[89]

[85] See: *Concerning the soul of brutes* (1683): pages 37–8.
[86] See: *Concerning the soul of brutes* (1683): page 33.
[87] See: *Concerning the soul of brutes* (1683): pages 39–40.
[88] See: *Concerning the soul of brutes* (1683): page 41.
[89] See: *Concerning the soul of brutes* (1683): page 42.

> There is said to be in Man, a twofold Knowing Power, viz. The Intellect and the Imagination, so it is commonly affirmed, that there is a twofold Appetite, viz. The Will, which proceeding from the Intellect, is the Handmaid of the Rational Soul; and the Sensitive Appetite, which cleaving to the Imagination, is the Hand or Procuress of the Corporeal Soul.

His purpose is to emphasize that the rational soul is not remote from appetites. The 'doing of good Works, in the knowledge of things by their Causes ... the Love of God, of Virtue, and of all that is good, and the detestation of Vices, and of wicked Men ... belong to the Rational Soul' whereas the 'vehement Affections or Perturbations of the Mind, by which it is wont to be moved, and inclined hither and thither, for the Protecting of Good, or shunning Evil, belong wholly to the Corporeal Soul'.[90] Although subject to the benign governance of the rational soul, the corporeal soul is more closely aligned with the body and so serves its needs and urges. 'Deaf to Reason ... [and] growing weary of the yoak of the Other ... [it] frees itself from its Bonds' and may mutiny. Having regained his footing on distinctions between the corporeal and rational souls, Willis offers a favourite military metaphor that reflects his service with the Royalist cause in order to illustrate their interplay and occasional struggle for dominance:[91]

> *Infestis obvia signis signa pares aquilas, & vota minantia votis*

> Where Ensigns Ensigns meet / And where with Arms, they one another threat;

The outcome of this civil conflict is not always predictable: morality and sacred religion may be displaced by the blandishments of the flesh 'seducing the Mind or Chief Soul ... to the Mud of Sensual Pleasures: So that Man becomes the Beast, or rather worse', unless and until conscience allows the rational soul to reassert its authority. It sometimes happens that quiet and undisturbed activities of the corporeal soul, 'confined to a certain Chest or Cabbinet ... are snatched hither and thither'. The passions perturb many parts of the body and contaminate the rational soul. The animal spirits are contracted and flag so that 'their Acts are sluggishly or perversely performed'. Like the sea, calm or 'waving by the blasts of the Wind', passions dictated by the corporeal soul vary under different physical, metaphysical, and moral conditions.

On the physical passions, Willis writes of the irrational behaviour of those disappointed in love, 'drawn as it were by Witchcraft', and of people with phobias concerning particular animals, foods, or smells proceeding from the 'occult Enmities of the Sensitive Soul'. Metaphysical passions are those that exercise a superior appetite of the will, replacing conceptions of the mind with sacred affections inspired by God. These are enacted through the corporeal soul and directed from the brain and its appendages to the præcordium and viscera: 'worship of God, Piety and Devotion ... Repentance, Love of God, and Hate of Sin, Hope of Salvation, Fear of Divine Vengeance ... are wont to be ascribed to the work and endeavour

[90] See: *Concerning the soul of brutes* (1683): page 43.

[91] See: *De anima brutorum* (1672): page 123 lines 3–4; and *Concerning the soul of brutes* (1683): page 43. Willis elides the two lines in Latin to become a couplet in his transcription. A literal translation is: 'Ensigns opposed to enemy ensigns, eagles similar, & pledges threatening pledges'. See: Allison Muri, *The enlightenment cyborg. A history of communications and control in the human machine. 1660–1830*, Toronto (2007): pages 138–140 for the origin of this line borrowed from Lucan's (39–65 AD) *Pharsalia* or *De bello civili* (On the civil war) describing the wars between Julius Caesar (100–40 BC) and Pompey (106–48 BC), who criticised the Roman emperor for overseeing the demise rather than the dawn of a nation. She quotes a translation (by S Braund) of the relevant extract from Lucan as: 'and of standards ranged in enmity against standards, of eagles matched and javelins threatening javelins'.

of the Heart ... as it were an *Holocaust* to be offered to God'. Conversely 'Drinking of Wine, Banquetting, and every kind of Dissolute Life ... render the Blood lawless and ... make hard the heart'.[92]

The moral passions amount to the forces of good and evil. The sensitive soul, although bound by 'obsequiousness to the Rational Soul as part of their Conjugal Contract', tends by default to expand into pleasure but may contract into the grief of 'Fear, Hatred, Anger, Desperation, Shame [and] Pusillanimity'. With pleasure, the animal spirits enliven the nerves, eyes and face causing 'all Members to shine'. In grief, the spirits retreat into a more narrow space within the brain so that 'the Countenance is cast down, the Limbs grow feeble ... bring[ing] a troublesome oppression of the Heart ... the Exterior Parts being deprived of its wonted afflux, languish and Contract a paleness'.[93] As with other habits of the corporeal soul in which the imprinted imagination is summoned, over time states of pleasure and grief may be experienced without external stimulus. A wise and strong man easily moderates the moral passions of pleasure and grief. Some bear torture or cutting off a member with 'Stoical Patience'. Others swoon or faint with 'the skin scarce wounded'. Some are seduced by 'softness and Luxury'. Others eschew 'Pomp of Delights, or Exquisite Blandishments of Pleasures'. And on the matter of morality, Willis argues that, difficult as it may be, there is a need for reason so that the animal spirits are 'called away from their Carnal Genius' and 'changed into Sacred and Moral meditations'.[94]

The passions

Against this background of a symbiotic but sometimes volatile relationship between the corporeal and rational souls, Willis discusses the individual passions. This represents his first direct excursion into human psychology and a prelude to Willis's consideration of psychiatry. The number of passions has long been counted as eleven. The first six are 'concupiscible [greatly to be desired or lusted after] and irascible' states: 'Pleasure and Grief, Desire and Aversion, Love and Hatred'. The five others are 'Anger, Boldness, Fear, Hope and Desperation'. For Willis, this seems illogical. Hope is not irascible whereas hatred and aversion are; and 'Shame, Pity, Emulation, Envy' and others ought also to be included. Rather, his position is highly reductionist. The extremes of passion belonging to the corporeal soul are pleasure ('the greatest height of its felicity) and grief ('the sickness of the sensitive soul') within which boundaries the others can be accommodated. The passions are either sensory experiences or matters of judgement. 'The Good exciting Love' is a shared response to the various senses. It has its substrate in activity of the animal spirits. But love may also be a matter of opinion and more individual as when considering an idol or thing of beauty. Building upon prior sensation, or awareness, a 'Passion of Love brought in, either Metaphysical, or merely Sensitive, or mixt', primarily inspires activity in the organs of the præcordium with the 'Love of this imaginary Good'.[95] Hatred also is driven by

[92] See: *Concerning the soul of brutes* (1683): page 47. Pordage's translation from Willis is literal: see: *De anima brutorum* (1672): page 132 for 'eumque illic velut holocauftum Deo immolandum'. The word 'holocaust' is not original to Willis. William Tyndale's (1494–1536) translation of the Gospel according to Mark chapter XII, verse 33 as '... all holocausts and sacrifices' (1526) was later altered for the King James Bible (1611) to '... burnt offerings and sacrifices'. John Milton (1608–1674) also preceded Willis, entitling Sonnet 18 (1655) 'A holocaust' to denote complete destruction by fire.

[93] See: *Concerning the soul of brutes* (1683): page 48.

[94] See: *Concerning the soul of brutes* (1683): page 49.

[95] See: *Concerning the soul of brutes* (1683): page 50.

sense—offensive smell, sight or hearing—or opinion in which there is 'Detestation of the Imaginary Spectre, from hence the Brows are contracted, the Teeth gnash together, and the Face is writhed'.[96] Desire and aversion are very much the business of the corporeal soul. As with the other passions, some are purely sensory, such as hunger and thirst, coldness, and the seeking of clothing. These are easily assuaged, familiarity tending to quieten the movement of the spirits and novelty being needed again to excite them. Desires 'got by Custom' change constantly so that 'the Palate being accustomed to delicate Victuals, loaths every thing unless spiced Aliments and prepared with most exquisite Sawce ... the Appetite, proper to any [sense], (for as much as it once exceeded what sufficed Nature) is always carried to more excellent Objects'. Desires based on opinion are more fragile, for Willis asserts that man is never satisfied with his lot: 'there is an immense Company of Concupiscible things, yet as most Men place their felicity in Riches or Honours, hence the Chief Species of Desires arising from Opinion; and therefore not to be satisfied, are Covetousness and Ambition'. Again, aversion is the inverse of desire and equally subject to sensation and opinion. States of desire and aversion both manifest as 'Gesticulations or Gestures'; and 'Men betray their passions by the Countenance'. But the spirits are fickle: 'the blood, entring inequally and impetuously the Confines of the Brain ... sometimes they will do this, anon that, as *if ten Minds were together by the Ears in one Man*'.[97]

Hope is driven by opinion. Willis waxes lyrical with a domestic metaphor of events leading up to the arrival of a welcome and distinguished guest: 'the Spirits inhabiting every sensory, are prepared to go forth to salute this approaching ... conferring on it Adornments and Splendour, borrowed from the Phantasie'. The organs of the præcordium participate in the reception, unless events prove disappointing in which case the process reverses and 'a sinking of the whole Soul, ensues'. Fear contracts the spirits:[98]

> Greatly binding up ... the Pores and Passages, as it were fastning its Doors, to shut out the Enemy ... from this constriction, the Pores of the Skin being drawn inward, oftentimes succeeds an erection of the Hairs ... the Locomotive Faculties fail, yea by a resolution or by a loos'ning of the Nerves, made in the Bowels, oftentimes the Excrements involuntarily flow out.

From fear may follow hope and 'audaciousness' but more often the passions of desperation 'presently being carried into Confusion, all things being turned upside down, she Contracts [into] Melancholy, or Madness'. Perturbations of spirits and the blood, expansion and contraction and variations in their distribution throughout the brain and præcordium, are also the explanation for pallor, flushing, wrinkling of the forehead, trembling of the lips, and murmuring of the tongue seen with the passions of anger and sadness.

Readers now familiar with Willis's style of making contrasts—voluntary or involuntary, corporeal or rational, accidental or habitual—will readily appreciate his analysis of the passions as based either on sensation or opinion.

[96] See: *Concerning the soul of brutes* (1683): page 51.

[97] See: *Concerning the soul of brutes* (1683): page 53. Printed in italics with a marginal note, 'Plaut' in the Latin text, Willis indicates that this aphorism is taken from Titus Plautus. Willis liked this quote and used it twice: see above referring to *Of convulsive diseases* (1681): page 95.

[98] See: *Concerning the soul of brutes* (1683): page 53.

The senses

The first part of *Two discourses concerning the soul of brutes* emphasizes the importance to Willis of sensation and reflective responses in the workings of the corporeal and rational souls. The brain is a system for sensing the external and internal environment, integrating responses through voluntary and involuntary actions, and learning from these experiences to initiate behaviour and interact socially with other nervous systems. It is necessary therefore that Willis should deal next with the five senses and consciousness or, in his formulation, sleep as a state in which these are each suppressed.[99]

'The faculty of perceiving Sensible objects' is dependent on particles or 'Effluvia's falling' from many organs so that the corporeal soul 'hath many Sensories'. As the ancients had it, 'All knowledge is made by the Sense'. Although the mechanism of stimulation is broadly similar, it is important that the corporeal soul can distinguish the various sensations. Willis resolves in several ways the problem of whether, for example, particles emanating from the eye are the same as those that respond to smells and sounds. He argues that pores in the sensory organs are gated in a way that only admits material in response to a specific sensation: 'the Particles ... which are proportionate to one Sensory, are incommunicable to the rest'. Through the complexity of their formation, the animal spirits which move through the streaked body to the corpus callosum and cortex are heterogenous. Some are more 'moveable, these Naked, those smered with Humor' and thereby better suited to transmission of sight (more crystalline), hearing (more moveable) or taste and smell (more viscous). Further discrimination also occurs in the striate body based on wavelike motion and relative activity of the spirits: 'the images of things to be perceived ... are not distinctly painted ... as on a Table; but every Impression there shown, depends on the Motion, as it were by a certain waving, of some Spirits separate from others, and within these or those peculiar Tracts of them ... [whilst] others lye quiet'. The work of those spirits that pass from the sense organs, 'like Darts', is done once the appropriate waves have reached the streaked body. At this point other spirits, stored locally, take up the onward process of sensation and perception. And it is in this upward passage of the sensory percept that the rational soul of man 'beholds the Image of the thing there painted ... represented as upon a white wall.[100]

Although it might be considered 'of a more gross Nature' than other sensations, touch is 'excellent by far than the rest' because it judges and integrates 'Heat and Cold, Moisture and Dryness, Hardness, and Softness, and other Modifications of Bodies, their Make, Motions, Influences and Types, or Figures of Appearance'. Willis argues that there are no organs of touch other than the nerve endings 'stuffed, and as it were distended with a Company of Animal Spirits; which as the strings of a Lute, as often as they are struck by the strokes of Tangible things, propagate the Impulse ... forthwith to the Common Sensory'. Repeating his point about individual sensations eliciting 'divers ways of Contractions or wrinklings', Willis likens touch to the separate sounds from the playing of a multi-stringed harp. And in line with his distinction between the voluntary and involuntary, eventually touch registers in the cortex; or, if the impulse is stronger, elicits `by nature in every Animal' a reflected response consistent with 'the Common Proverb, *Where the Pain is, there the Finger will be.*[101]

[99] As will be clear from what follows, Willis's ideas are so sophisticated that it is hard to understand why his writings were discarded by many contemporary and subsequent commentators. Rather than discrediting Thomas Willis, their superficial analyses are more revealing of the impoverished imagination of the commentators than the target of their waspish pens.

[100] See: *Concerning the soul of brutes* (1683): pages 58–9.

[101] See: *Concerning the soul of brutes* (1683): page 61.

The fibres of nerves distributed to the tongue, palate and upper throat are the organs of taste. Food 'reduced into bits, by Chawing, the Tongue, and other parts of the Mouth, and Throat, pour forth as it were a certain Menstruum, which washing ... the savory little Bodies ... insinuates them into the Pores of the Tongue'. As a result, by occupying these pores, one taste tends to counteract another, until the palate is cleansed. Whilst the status of the fifth nerve is certain, Willis is not so sure that his ninth cranial nerve (hypoglossal) subserves taste in addition to moving the tongue. But he makes an important point about cooperation of the senses: 'nothing pleases the Palate unless the Sight, and hearing, Smell, and Touch approve it'. Nine simple individual tastes can be discriminated which may be compounded into more complex gustatory sensations: sharp, bitter, salt, acid or tart, astringent or biting, sour, sweet, oily, and insipid or tasteless. Willis lays out in several pages a catalogue of each, drawn from natural foodstuffs, chemicals, and concoctions.[102]

Smell serves the purpose of distinguishing whereby 'wholsom Aliments may be known, and discerned from disagreeable and hurtful'. Willis makes the point that 'this Kind of Primary use is seen more excellently in brute Animals, than in Man'. Smell is more closely related to taste than other senses. Acknowledging that the loss of one may compromise the other, Willis takes a strictly anatomical stance on the observation that anosmia and ageusia may be dissociated because each is dependent on different cranial nerves: taste by both the fifth and ninth nerves, and olfaction through the smelling nerve and mammillary body.[103]

Perhaps reflecting the relative importance of oral communication in preference to reading in his lifetime, Willis states that hearing is 'far more Excellent than the other senses; for as much as by its help chiefly, Sciences and Learning are acquired'. Sound is a wave created by the shaking or vibration of 'Sonorifick Particles' which spreads through the air like the ripple of waves, and with echoes or 'leaps back from a solid body'. The pinna and outer ear focus sound on the 'den of the Ear' and its sensory nerve fibres, in the way that a pipe or trumpet 'supplies the defect of Hearing'. Sound is amplified through 'the turning and winding passages' as in a cornet or wreathed instrument to agitate the drum, protected and supported by three bones—the hammer, anvil and stirrup. From there, the fibres of the seventh nerve transmit the sensation of sound to the streaked body. On the 'open passage [from the middle ear] to the Palate',[104] Willis assumes a double purpose: to remove the sonorific particles of sound reaching the inner ear, and to provide an alternative portal of entry in the context of deafness. Ever the keen observer, Willis points out that the ears of beasts can be moved and directed towards a sound, a skill that he considers to be present in infants but subjugated in adults by 'continual use of Head-bands'. Here Willis pauses to describe paracusis:[105]

> For we meet with a certain kind of Deafness, in which those affected, seem wholly to want the Sense of Hearing, yet as soon as a great noise, as of great Guns, Bells, or Drums, is made near to the Ears, they distinctly understand the speeches of the by-standers, but this great noise ceasing, they presently grow deaf again. I heard from a Credible Person, that he once knew a Woman, thô she were Deaf, yet so long as a Drum was beaten within her Chamber, she heard every word perfectly; wherefore her Husband kept a Drummer on purpose for

[102] See: *Concerning the soul of brutes* (1683): pages 63–[88], that is 68.

[103] See: *Concerning the soul of brutes* (1683): page [89], i.e. 69; and Meyer and Hierons (1965), part I.

[104] Unlike most of Eustachius's descriptions relating to the nervous system, Willis might have known of his descriptions on the anatomy of the ear in Bartholomæi Eustachii, *Opuscula anatomica*, Venice (1564): pages 148–64.

[105] See: *Concerning the soul of brutes* (1683): page 73.

his Servant, that by that means he might have some converse with his Wife. Also I was told of another Deaf Person, who living near a Ring of Bells, as often as they all rung out, he could easily hear any word, and not else.

Browne Willis accepted that criticisms of his grandfather's work had 'not escaped the censure even of some persons of real merit'. He quotes eight lines of text in Latin from *De anima brutorum* (1672) relating to the drum of the ear. On this passage, Hutchinson[106] refers to Dr Wotton (1666–1727) who had observed that 'a Dutch physician, named [Günther Christoph] Schelhammer [1649–1716] in a book, *De auditu*, printed at Leyden in 1684, took occasion to animadvert upon a passage in Dr Willis's book *De anima brutorum*, printed in 1672; and in such a manner, as reflected not only upon his skill, but also upon his integrity'.[107] The offending passage on the style of theorists rather than those who respect scientific evidence, translated by Meyer and Hierons, castigates Willis for being amongst those who are:[108]

> Unaware that similarities do not prove anything, unless it is previously known from other reasons, that what is alleged to be similar is similar; nor consider that similarity is merely an incentive for obtaining evidence which in science, and thus also in physiology alone has a place ... for these reasons we cannot differ more from the opinion of this famous and, in Medicine, so well-merited man; although I admire his ingenuity whenever he explains the effect of medicaments or the causes of diseases, when he goes beyond his field, and takes on the role of philosopher, and ponders over the uses of organs or the nature of chemical events, I hardly ever desire his judgment nor would I have any confidence: for I have myself recently and publicly shown that the experimental results on which he relies are often different from reality.

Hutchinson follows Browne Willis in qualifying this criticism with the riposte from Dr William Derham (1657–1735) discrediting Schelhammer:[109]

> And then faith, *Ob has rationes à clariss. Viri, ac de re Medicâ præclare meriti, sententiâ non possumus non esse alienores; in quo uti ingenium admiror, quoties medicamentorum vires, aut morborum causas explicat, sic ubi forum suum egressus, Philosophum agit, ac vel Partium usum, vel Chymicarum rerum naturam scrutatur, eius haud semel non modo judicium desidero, verùm aliquando etiam fidem.*
>
> [For these reasons I cannot be more different in opinion from this highly illustrious Man, deservedly famous in Medical matters; while I admire in him the talent with which he so often explains the properties of medicines or the causes of illnesses, yet where he leaves his territory, acts the part of Philosopher and investigates the nature of body parts or the nature of Chemical matters, I lack not only any wish for his opinion but even the trust.]

[106] See: Benjamin Hutchinson, *Biographia medicia*, volume 2, London (1799): pages 481–5, relating to *De anima brutorum* (1672): page 195, translated in *Concerning the soul of brutes* (1683): page 72.

[107] See: William Wotton, *Reflections upon ancient and modern learning*, London (1694): pages 196–7. In fact, Dr Schelhammer was born in Jena and died in Kiel, Germany.

[108] See: Alfred Meyer and Raymond Hierons, 'On Thomas Willis's concepts of neurophysiology [part II]', *Medical History* 1965: 9; 142–55 at page 147.

[109] See: William Derham, 'On the sense of hearing'. In: *Physico-Theology: or a demonstration of the being and attributes of God from his works of creation being the substance of sixteen sermons*, book IV, 5th edition, London (1720): pages 124–8.

For Hutchinson, taking his own position in support of Willis:

> This is so severe and unjust a Censure of our truly famous Countryman, (a man of known Probity) that might deserve a better Answer; but I have only time to Say, that although Dr. *Schelhammer* hath out-done all that wrote before him, in his Book *de Auditu*, and shewed himself a Man of Learning and Industry; yet as our Countryman wrote more than he, (though perhaps not free from Errors too) so he hath manifested himself to be as curious and sagacious an Anatomist, and as great a Philosopher, and as learned and skilful a Physician, as any of his Censurers; and his Reputation for Veracity and Integrity was no less than any of theirs too. But after all this Clamour, Dr. *Schelhammer* prejudicately mistakes Dr. *Willis*'s Meaning, to say no worse.

Whether or not Dr Schelhammer had a valid general point, Willis did fail to appreciate the dual function of the labyrinth. He assigns only the amplification, clarification, and orderly processing of sound, but no contribution to balance even though he has discerned that in each ear there is a twofold organ of hearing. This is a missed opportunity since, in the pathological part of *De anima brutorum* (1672), Willis describes the physiology of vertigo and disorders in which the labyrinth is a symptom of disease. Its seat is the middle part of the brain and, returning to his favoured military metaphor, vertigo may involve 'troops or rather mighty armies of Spirits ... and sometimes also small handfuls or bands'. Physiological vertigo 'or a turning round in the Head' is an example of the latter in which the spirits are 'partly perverted, and partly suppressed'. Occurring 'with a long turning of the body, looking down from high places, passing over Bridges, Sailing, and by Drunkenness', the imagination is deceived into believing that objects are moving even though judgement remains rational 'for we understand our error'. Despite not having appreciated the nature of the semicircular canals, Willis gets close to a more modern interpretation in arguing that, being fluid, the animal spirits continue to move after cessation of motion, as in a phial or vessel. This stimulates the nerves with intermittent influx leading to 'a Scotomy or dizzyness, and a failing of the feet, together with a rotation or whirling about of visible objects'. The vertigo induced by sailing or riding in a coach may be associated with vomiting. Wine, strong ale, and tobacco generate 'fierce particles, and untameable' which drive the animal spirits from their 'wonted tracks of flowing and reflowing or ebbing, and so move them into whirlings, and turnings about'.[110]

Vertigo may happen when 'the flowing of Blood [is] suddenly called away from the Brain' following haemorrhage, fasting, 'passions of violent sadness and fear ... failure in the heart', by distraction through disease of the viscera, or with pain and inflammation from ulcers in the limbs. In all these situations, there is '*Syncope* or Swooning' due to withdrawal of animal spirits from the nerves 'for when their spring is cut off, those that remain ... wander about confusedly ... and stir up the Vertiginous Distemper'. But sometimes vertigo 'is a disease of it self ... within the middle part of the Brain ... often terrible, and very hard to be cured'. Instead of the animal spirits normally radiating from the 'Callous and streaked bodies' so as to represent 'pleasant imaginations and phantasies ... notions of memory ... [and] the instincts of motions', the perverted 'rays of light seem to be intercepted' and 'whirled about ... or cross one another' and 'a dizziness and failing of the motive function follows'. This unprovoked type of vertigo is likely precipitated by extraneous morbific particles contaminating

[110] See: *Concerning the soul of brutes* (1683): page 146.

the animal spirits and acting on 'Procatartick' disposition, 'the crime of the Brain' being its 'Pores too much open and gapeing' and so admitting the unhealthy recrements.[111] Whereas symptomatic vertigo resolves spontaneously, or with the help of 'a Cephalick', the habitual form 'admits of only a difficult and long Cure, it tires out both Patient and Physician, that before the Disease can be Cured, they both become weary of one another'.[112] Willis's strategy is to prevent morbific matter entering the brain by alterations in diet, blood-letting, purging, cutting issues in the leg or arm, and the use of tea and coffee; and to deal with the predisposition using antiscorbuticks, cephalicks, vomits, and spaw-waters. Willis gives three examples of individual cases, not always immediately successful so that in a difficult case 'however I did not desist from my curator work, the most skilful Physician Doctor [Thomas] Wharton [1614–1673] being called to my assistance'. But always the therapeutic optimist, Willis eventually tries powder made from the roots of the male peony, the dung of the peacock, and white sugar downed with a decoction of sage or rosemary impregnated with the tincture of coffee:[113]

> It is scarce credible how much help he received from this Remedy; visiting me after a month, he seem'd a new and another man; being freed of the Vertigo, he not only confidently walked about, but was able to take care of his household affairs, and to meddle with any hard business, which he was not able to do before.

Despite having already handed out the laurels, when it comes to sight Willis declares that 'if there be any strife for Dignity among the senses, the Palm is given … as the most noble Power'. The many aspects of vision—images, colours, and movement—are all properties of the rays of light. It seems improbable to Willis that light depends on the emission of particles, 'fiery little bodies' in the case of the glowworm, for how would 'these Effluvia streaming from a small Light, presently possess the whole Hemishear?'[114] Taking a more iatrochemical stance, he prefers the explanation that light is particulate and like a flame emitted from a fire. It consists of sulphurous particles that leave the viewed object meeting with nitrous matter in air and enkindling 'a thin white Flame'. Unlike the dark flame emitted from a fire which is fat and thick, 'made crooked by the blasts of the Wind, yea to be carried within tubes or hollow Pipes very crooked', the flame of light is carried in straight lines and capable of passing through glass and all clear bodies: 'thô they are wont ordinarily to be broken or reflected, yet they cannot be made crooked'. Speculating on the sun, the stars and other coelestials, Willis comes down to earth by concluding that vision requires emitted light to be in direct line or reflected on to the eye.[115] On colour and images, no one has written with more sense than Pierre Gassendi and Willis intends to summarize his views, 'to Plow with his heifer'. Colours change when the beams of white light are mixed with 'Particles, not lucid, interspersed within its Body … so when Soot or Smoke stream forth with inkindled Light, the Light becomes more red or darkish'. The evidence for admixture lies in the spectrum of colours observed when light enters a prism.[116]

[111] See: *Concerning the soul of brutes* (1683): page 148.

[112] See: *Concerning the soul of brutes* (1683): page 149. This confession of the experienced neurologist brings to mind the words of the late Bryan Matthews (1920–2001). See: WB Matthews, *Practical neurology*, Oxford and Edinburgh (1963): page 69; 'There can be few physicians so dedicated to their art that they do not experience a slight decline in spirits on learning that their patient's complaint is dizziness'.

[113] See: *Concerning the soul of brutes* (1683): page 152–3.

[114] See: *Concerning the soul of brutes* (1683): page 75.

[115] See: *Concerning the soul of brutes* (1683): page 75.

[116] See: *Concerning the soul of brutes* (1683): page 77.

Initially distracted by light rather than sight, Willis returns to the anatomy and physiology of vision. Images penetrate the narrow pupil, are refracted 'according to the best Dioptrick Rules', and projected onto the retina. Many have written on the anatomy of the eye and although Willis prefers his own description made, at the risk of a feeble pun, 'by our own ocular inspection', his account of the globe, eyelids, lacrimal glands ('Kirnels'), and other nearby structures has nothing much novel to add on the macroscopic appearance or innervation that has not already been made in *On the description and use of the nerves* (1664). An exception might be his account of weeping, peculiar to man and not seen in brutes, since this relates to the 'Doctrine of the Passions' and the associated changes in the face and præcordium. His example is 'sobbing ... for as much as the Air is hardly blown into the Windpipe' that accompanies laughter and crying, the mechanism of the tears being diversion of turbulent liquor to the lacrimal glands in order to protect the brain from 'all things upside down ... in danger to be either overturned, or drowned'.[117]

In a lyrical passage, Willis refers to colloquial names of the muscles that move the eye and keep it aligned for vision. The elevator is called 'Superb or Proud' because of the appearance of pride, although 'the Name of Holy or Devout' might be preferable in reflecting the upward rolling of the globe in states of religious ecstasy. The depressor muscle is 'Pious'. The one that draws the eye in 'may not improperly be called Drunken'.[118] The muscle moving the eye out is the 'Indicator'.[119] The two oblique muscles 'may be called Amatory, because Lovers behold one another side-ways, and as it were fearing the sight of one another, they role their Eyes like those of Cattel, hither and thither'. The optic pole, or visual axis, passing through the pupil 'or Apple of the Eye', falls on different parts of the retina (the fovea) away from insertion of the optic nerve in man and other sagacious creatures compared to cattle, swine, birds, and fishes in which the nerve head lies on the visual axis. Willis considers that the difference allows man to see more complex scenes than lesser brutes, albeit with less sharpness of the image. Much the same explanation, the trade-off between complexity and clarity, is offered for the difference in shape of the pupil—round in man but oblique in many four-footed beasts. Willis makes much of this variation in shape and also of colour in the pupilla (iris) of brutes, 'grey, or blewish, like the Sky, or of a shining red', and its unvarying black appearance in man so as to explain, as best he can, how these differences enable brutes to see in the dark, 'wherefore it is very shining in a Cat'.[120] Willis's anatomy of the globe, its coatings and crystalline and glassy humours is detailed. He lays particular emphasis on the vascular supply derived from the carotid supplying the optic nerve; the six terminal branches and draining veins in the retina; and the cranial nerves that innervate the muscles and ciliary processes which adjust the pupil size.

Sleep and waking

Aware that an account of movement should logically follow his discussion of the senses, but having already written on that topic and not wishing to be repetitive, Willis ends the first part of *De anima brutorum* with a discussion of 'certain Affections, belonging to the Corporeal

[117] See: *Concerning the soul of brutes* (1683): page 80.

[118] See: *Concerning the soul of brutes* (1683): page 81 where, somewhat out of context, Willis tells us that he once knew a young man, 'obnoxious to the palsie', with eye indrawn 'in whom every object appeared double'.

[119] This designation does not add to the suggestion in chapter 3 that portraits of Willis show exotropia resulting from unrestrained activity of the lateral rectus muscle.

[120] See: *Concerning the soul of brutes* (1683): page 84.

Soul, as to the Exercise of the Motions and the Senses, to wit, Sleeping and Waking'. He does not accept the view of Conrad [Konrad] Schneider (1614–1680) that sleep and waking are innate properties of the corporeal soul, 'wholly inorganical', which 'sometimes withdraws, and as it were hides itself; and sometimes puts forth, and expunds it self'. This would not explain why organs of the præcordium and the abdominal viscera do not sleep when the external senses, internal powers such as phantasy and memory, and spontaneous motions are at rest. Part of the difference lies in how arduous are the tasks imposed on the relevant animal spirits. Those emanating from the brain (cortex) and serving the spontaneous acts of sense and motion are hard worked and not tied to continual performance, so can rest. Conversely those generated in the cerebel performing the 'more assiduous Offices of the Vital and Nutritious Function ... absolutely necessary for the preserving of Life, that they ought not almost at any time to lye still ... are not suffered to keep Holy-day long, and to indulge themselves with Sleep'. That is not to say they do not pause. The resting phase of these organs is apparent from the rhythmicity of respiration and the pulse: 'condemned to the stone of Sisyphus; to wit, that they still lift up the same burthen. Then resting whil'st it slides down again, they presently, and so perpetually, repeat their Labour'.[121]

Sleep follows certain predictable events: the nightly patterns of custom; 'hard labour of the Body, or too serious intention of the Mind'; 'Meditation, and when employed with Hearing (chiefly of Sacred things)'; 'after Eating, reading or Philosophical Lectures being attended to, they shall sleep sooner than an Opiat'; in response to the soft harmony of voice or music, the murmur of water or the breeze, or pleasant fantasies of the imagination; but also in the various 'Soporiferous or Sleepy Diseases'.[122] Natural waking occurs once the animal spirits are refreshed, usually at a set time. Sleep may also end when a troublesome external sensation, touch, or sound, occurs or an internal stimulus rouses the subject, whether or not the spirits are ready, yawning and stretching indicating attempts to shake off 'the Dewie Humor'.[123]

The immediate mechanism of sleep is straightforward. A flood of serous humour moves from the outside parts of the brain to the middle, suppresses expansion of the spirits responsible for phantasy and memory which 'grow stupefied ... [and] slothful', and prevents others from moving into the nerves thereby also soliciting them to idleness. In this quiescent state, through nightly access to rest and food, the spirits are prevented from becoming 'wholly loosned and perishing'. The brain is refreshed 'like a dry sponge, imbibing most greedily the nutritious Liquor'.[124] Sleep also allows the brain to dispose of 'veteran' particles and refresh the animal spirits. Those active in waking states as the 'Executors of every Spontaneous Function' are drawn to the cerebel which 'performs its [automatic] tasks better in the rest and silence of the others'. Organs other than the brain participate in the preparation for sleep. The stomach being full, the eyes close 'that the Windows being presently shut, the meeting with External Objects may be hindred'. Blood is withdrawn from the extremities, which cool and need to be covered in bedclothes, so that it can more intensely be enkindled in the præcordium and lungs. No longer committed to its hectic passage through active and moving parts: 'yea whil'st the Animal Spirits lie quiet, like allayed winds, the Sea of the Blood presently becomes Calm'.[125]

[121] See: *Concerning the soul of brutes* (1683): page 87.
[122] See: *Concerning the soul of brutes* (1683): pages 89–90.
[123] See: *Concerning the soul of brutes* (1683): pages 95–6.
[124] See: *Concerning the soul of brutes* (1683): page 88.
[125] See: *Concerning the soul of brutes* (1683): pages 91–2.

Encouraged by wine, tobacco, too much exercise or study, and the passions, sleep does not necessarily stifle the senses and motions. The consequence is dreaming and sleep walking. In introducing this topic, Willis does not intend to consider the meaning of dreams or whether they are 'fatidical, as if they were inspired by a *Dæmon*, and are affirmed to Prophesie things to come'.[126] His interest is more mechanistic. Dreams and adventitious movements during sleep occur when the animal spirits, normally bound 'with Embraces as it were with Chains that they may not enter into Motion', break free and 'wander about without any Guide or Ruler'. Movements are repeated 'as it were Dances before learnt ... and the Cogitations of things, though after a very confused manner'. Free from the bondage of sleep: 'all of them will not be bound or restrained, but that some of them will walk about the Sepulchers of the rest, like Spectres in a Church-yard, and cause stupendous Apparitions of things'.

The character of dreams implicates stimulation of specific organs. One analysis is that, as a result, rogue spirits enter the brain and engage the Phantasie rehearsing 'the Series of things before acted, or only *Chimera's*, or Notions altogether incongruous and disagreeing'. Pausing to mention that 'Immodest Dreams' occur when the stimulus comes from the genital organs, Willis's main interest is the '*Incubus* or Nightmare'. These 'Terrible and frightful Phantasies' are experienced when the stomach is loaded with undigested meats, and people sleep lying on the back. This disturbs sleep 'as if with some Animal or heavy weight lying upon the Breast, stops our breathing' until the victim wakes with trembling of the heart and violent beating of the diaphragm: 'the fit being over, the deception of the phantasie, conceiving the horrid image of the *Incubus* or spectre, is perceived'.[127]

Nightmares are discussed by Willis in both parts of *De anima brutorum*. At first, perhaps in deference to popular lore, he is tolerant of the view that they are the business of 'Witches ... whilst they lye Buried in a profound Sleep ... imaging things wholly unknown to them, which without doubt is, because the Devil brings the Idea's of these things before the Phantasie'. Later he prefers the explanation that nightmares arise from natural causes rather than devilry. But Willis questions his earlier assumption of the nightmare as a secondary disturbance of the brain that follows stimulation of individual organs during sleep. Focusing on the heart and thorax, he asks himself why the typical symptoms are confined to sleep and do not occur more frequently in people with diseases of the chest. Eventually, his discursive and contorted reasoning prefers the interpretation that the problem is primarily of the brain with discharge of incongruous matter generated in the cerebel through the cranial nerves to the præcordium.[128]

This leads him to a consideration of sleep walking: 'the Animal Spirits, being agitated by this means, within the Brain ... do often leap back, into the Nervous Stock, and there stirring up other Spirits, produce divers sorts of local Motions'. Here, Willis has in mind complex behaviours not merely slight thrashing around the bed. In their most complicated manifestations these include dressing, carrying out household activities, conversing with those they meet, 'taking them by the hand and often-times striking them', moving aside obstacles, and hearing, seeing and responding to 'Impressions made from sensible things'. Eventually the sleep walker returns to bed. Because the rampant spirits have passed from the middle part of the brain down the nerves without reciprocal traffic up to the streaked body and corpus callosum, somnambulists neither perceive nor remember their actions. Their automatic actions are like those of a musician playing a harp in which the strings are plucked: 'whilst he

126 See: *Concerning the soul of brutes* (1683): page 93.
127 See: *Concerning the soul of brutes* (1683): page 142.
128 See: *Concerning the soul of brutes* (1683): pages 94 and 143.

is thinking of some other thing, his fingers being before taught the Numbers of the Tune, exactly strike the Strings, with wonderful agility and discretion'. Willis adds that sleep walking is like one or two rogue dogs starting out obediently but who then leave the pack 'and fall to Hunting'. Movement is encouraged by the fact that there is more freedom in the spinal cord and nerves for these agitated spirits to roam than in the brain itself.[129]

Willis resumes his discussion, with emphasis on sleepy distempers, in the second part of *De anima brutorum*. Morbid sleep occurs with disruption of the sequence in which animal spirits rest and the nervous juice is replenished by nutrients in the bloodstream seeping through the pores and passages of the brain. The type and severity of sleep disorder depend on where in the brain this perturbation occurs. His first category is 'the Lethargie'. This is of two types. The more severe occurs in the context of another disease, especially fever: 'as the proverb says, *None dyes without a Feavour*'.[130] Lethargy is associated with loss of memory and impairment of reasoning, sensation, and motive powers commensurate with the degree of sleepiness. Willis bases his analysis on examinations of the brain where he finds the cortex swollen and softened with fluid in the sulci, the 'whole frame of the Brain overflowed with a Dropsie, or rather a flood'. Several mechanisms can be proposed. Lethargy may result from excess delivery of serum that drowns the nervous spirits; morbific matter in the bloodstream; 'tasteless water . . . instead of the subtil and spirituous nervous Juice, that is the parent of forgetfulness, and of sleepiness'; and the pores of entry 'too lax or open'.

Of the many remote causes of morbid sleepiness, Willis highlights 'Surfeits, Drunkenness . . . Spaw-waters being drunk in a larger quantity, and not again render'd . . . by Urine . . . acute Feavours . . . and other Chronical Diseases . . . especially the Headach, Frenzie, *Empyema*, or collection of gross Humors upon the Lungs and the *Colick*'. Because the muscles of the thorax contract 'laboriously . . . and with repeated tryals or forces', according to the ancients 'Lethargy [is] not the disease of the Head, but of the Breast'. But they are wrong: 'the symptom . . . depends on the cerebel, participating the hurt of the Brain, grievously distemper'd'. Willis recalls his earlier experience in Oxford and asks:[131]

> But wherefore are all these subterfuges? When it often happens that the Morbific matter, at first fixed in the head, and stirring up a continual sleepiness, or Lethargy; the same being thence supped up by the Blood, and deposited in the breast, doth produce an *Empyema*, or a spitting like those whose Lungs are wasted. In the description of a Soperiferous Epidemical Feavour, which raged in the year 1661, we noted the same to have happened to many'.

More direct as a cause of lethargy is the use of opiates which act both on the ventricle (stomach) and animal spirits in the brain. Immoderate use may prove fatal.[132] Willis allows the possibility that there are narcotic particles, the 'Lethean Copula', that creep into the brain and extinguish the animal spirits: 'the sum of all which is, That the Animal Spirits, the inhabitants of the exterior Brain, being hindred from their wonted motion and emanation, lye down in a profound and inextricable sleep'. The prognosis is best in cases where one or other

[129] See: *Concerning the soul of brutes* (1683): pages 94–5.

[130] See: *Concerning the soul of brutes* (1683): page 130.

[131] See: *Concerning the soul of brutes* (1683): page 131.

[132] See: *Concerning the soul of brutes* (1683): page 128 where Willis mentions that 'we have already discoursed of these things in a particular Tract, *Of the Operations of Medicines on the Humane Body*', a reference to *Pharmaceutice rationalis* (1674): part I, pages 285–303. This is not an intrusion by Pordage since Willis writes in *De anima brutorum* (1672): page 312, 'Super his in peculiari tractatu, *de operationibus medicamentorum in corpus humanum fuse* disseruimus'. It follows that the first part of *Pharmaceutice rationalis* was ready for publication in 1672 or earlier.

of the evident causes listed by Willis can be identified. Treatment over several days is needed, as Willis reports in the case of 'a country-man, of a Phlegmatic Complexion ... [who] whilst he was following the Plow in the Fields, lying down on the ground, fell into a profound sleep ... [from which] he could not be awakened by pulling, thumping, noise, and other means'. He was revived over several days by Willis's administration of cephalicks, purges, blood-letting, blisters, and clysters. Less immediately successful was 'an Oxford Gardiner being sick of a Feavour' who 'remained like a Bruit ... for two months, and still very sleepy'; or a father and his son who had eaten henbane (*Hyoscyamus niger*, commonly known as stinking nightshade) mistaking this for parsnips but were revived by 'Oyl or Oxymel poured down the thoat, and a Feather thrust down ... that made them vomit ... [so that they] ... should be set free from the sleepy poison afflicting them'.[133]

These cases differ from the 'Lethargick' predisposition which, in a somewhat rambling account, Willis also describes as the condition of 'Continual Sleepiness' in his category of 'the Coma'. Those affected are constantly drowsy 'so that in the midst of a journey, yea at dinner, or though busied about any thing, they presently fall into a drousiness'. Due to involvement only of the superficial part of the brain, this is not a dangerous condition although the narcotic particles may pass to the cerebellum and convert into 'tremblings of the Heart, the *Asthma*, loss of spirits, and other troublesome Symptoms, commonly taken for the *Hypochondriacal*'. Although lacking any mention of the three associated symptoms—cataplexy, sleep paralysis and hypnogogic or hypnopompic hallucinations—not unreasonably it has been suggested that this is a description of narcolepsy. Willis explains:[134]

> Most authors call this not a Disease, but an evil habit, or a sleepy disposition, for the distemper'd, as to other things, are well enough; they eat and drink well, go abroad, take care well enough of their domestick affairs, yet whilst talking, or walking, or eating, yea their mouths being full of meat, they shall nod, and unless rouzed up by others, fall fast asleep: and thus they sleep continually almost, not only some days or months, but (as it is said of *Epemenides*) many years; wherefore we ought to believe this a Disease, and worthy of Cure, which defrauds one of more than half his life.

Treatment combines the usual natural remedies, including 'Coffee, or the liquor prepared of that Berry, first boiling in it, the leaves of Sage or Rosemary, till it has got a greenish Tincture'; together with holding the nose over a pot of urine, or wearing a 'quilted thing of Cephalicks and Spices' under a cap over the shaven skull. Willis adds a case history:[135]

> A certain Gentleman of a Sanguine Complexion, and when he was young, of a sharp and cunning wit, but afterwards growing aged, being given to idleness and drunkenness, became dull and stupid, and also Dropsical, with a great paunch, and his thighs and legs swelled. Yet from these Diseases (which he frequently fell into) when he abstained at any time from drinking, and took Physick, he oftentimes quickly grew well. But at length,

[133] See: *Concerning the soul of brutes* (1683): page 132–3.

[134] See: *Concerning the soul of brutes* (1683): pages 126, 134; and William G Lennox, 'Thomas Willis on narcolepsy' *Archives of Neurology and Psychiatry* 1939: 41; 348–51. Epimenides (fl.600 BC) was a Cretan poet of the seventh century BC who slept in a cave for 57 years. He is remembered for the paradox 'all Cretans are liars' which turns back and forth around the fact that as a Cretan himself he might be lying in which case 'All Cretans are honest', and so on.

[135] See: *Concerning the soul of brutes* (1683): page 135. The modern reader would probably prefer a number of explanations other than narcolepsy, as presently understood, not least because the bouts of sleepiness ceased when he discontinued wine and beer and drank coffee until, after many years, he died with cough, asthma, and cachexia.

> though he was freed from the Dropsie, he was oppressed with so heavy a sleepiness, and that almost perpetually, that in what place soever he was, or what ever he was doing he would sleep; then being awakened by his Servants or Friends, his mind appeared well enough, and for a few minutes he would discourse of any thing well enough, then immediately fall again to sleep.

Lethargy is a less severe condition than the 'sleepy coma' which results from more diffuse penetration of the morbific matter throughout the brain and confines victims to their chair or bed. Yet more severe is *carus* in which the process affects the corpus callosum interfering with imagination and memory. 'A Palsie or dead-Palsie' on one side follows if the morbific matter moves from the corpus callosum to the streaked body. Apoplexy occurs when a 'malignant or ill handled Feavour ... Headach ... convulsive Distemper ... blow on the Head ... an Imposthume broken in the Meninges ... or on a Woman in Childbed' complicates the carus with involvement of the 'middle Marrow' of the brain leading to 'tracts or paths of the Spirits ... obliterated or blotted out'.[136]

Willis contrasts sleep disorders with morbid waking, the 'preternatural Watchings'. Sleeplessness may be symptomatic of another distemper such as 'Feavour, Phrensie, Madness, the Colick, Gout or such like'; an isolated disorder in which those affected 'are forced to fly to *Opiates*'; or due to the 'drinking of coffee also (in use formerly among the *Arabians* and *Turks*) which is drunk by our Country-Men' in order to study late into the night.[137] Inability to sleep is due to the animal spirits 'being grown too outrageous, and as it were struck with a fury'; or failure to fill and stop up the pores so that they are constantly disturbed by matter delivered in the serum and cannot rest. As a result, these spirits: 'tumultuating within the middle part of the brain, raise up many, and often most horrid phantasies ... and break off Sleep, though it seems ready to creep upon them'. If these unruly spirits reach the origins of the (cranial) nerves innervating the præcordium, there follow various symptoms 'commonly taken to be *Hysterical*'. If the spinal marrow is swamped, the patients experience convulsions of the limbs 'with Cramps, and such unquietness and flying about ... that the sick can no more sleep, than those on the Rack'. Individuals affected by 'the Waking *Coma*' crave sleep but it eludes them and leads to 'a *Delirium*' in which the sick lie with their eyes closed, rambling in their talk, the limbs restless, and 'being raised up, they look about them doggedly'. Living 'like those ... under the Pole, who only see (when the Sun is in the Equinox) the light on the Horizon, and neither have perfect night, nor perfect day; so those afflicted enjoy only a kind of twilight betwixt sleep and waking'. Treatment lies in dealing with the underlying provocative disorder.[138]

Headache

Returning to his military metaphor, Willis opens the second part of *De anima brutorum* by telling readers that headache is 'the chiefist of the Diseases of the Head, and as it were to lead the troops of the other Affections of that part'. So common is headache, with no 'temperament, constitution or manner of living' spared, that 'it is become a Proverb, as a sign of a more rare and admirable thing, *That his head did never ake*'.[139] Willis has points to make

[136] See: *Concerning the soul of brutes* (1683): page 136.
[137] See: *Concerning the soul of brutes* (1683): pages 138 and 140.
[138] See: *Concerning the soul of brutes* (1683): pages 138–41.
[139] See: *Concerning the soul of brutes* (1683): page 105.

about the site and mechanism of headache, the different clinical types and their provocative causes, and both medical and surgical treatments. Not for the first time, his narrative is repetitive, somewhat contradictory, and needs editing.

Maintaining his central belief in the circulation of fermented blood, its local modification and use, and the removal of recrements, Willis argues that ultimately headache can be attributed to local accumulation, agitation, and disordered motion of the animal spirits. Because particles contributing to these 'painful corrugations or wrinklings' are delivered in the blood, disorder of the meninges with their rich arterial network is a recurring theme. Other pain sensitive structures are the coatings of nerves, the pericranium, and tissues of the scalp but not the brain, cerebellum, or medulla.

Willis attributes headaches to overheating of blood which is 'sulphureous, saline, sharp, acid, bilous, or melancholic' by reason of which 'remote cause' they occur 'in the Winter time, in a moist Air, and in a Southern Wind: Moreover, *Catarrhs* of the Face, Mouth, *Larynx*, and of other parts, oftentimes accompany this Disease'. Other causes are abnormalities of the nourishing juice, 'fresh *Chyme*', so that sufferers soon learn to avoid 'drinking of Wine, Exercise, Baths, &c'. Those affected time their eating and attend to the quality and quantity imbibed in order to limit the otherwise predictable post-prandial headache. More often, fault lies with stagnation of the nervous juice itself, 'without any errors of dyet or living', these headaches typically occur in the morning after oversleeping through allowing the nervous fibres to 'drink in this humor more largely'.[140] Headaches due to one or other of these mechanisms are usually mild. More severe are those that result from two humours, the nervous liquor and the nutritious, combining to produce 'Morbifick matter'. But for all his rehearsal of different putative mechanisms and causes, Willis attributes most headache to the climate, seasons, overeating, or drinking, 'Sharp and thin Wines, Cyder, yea and Beer', excess bathing or, a recurring theme, 'immoderate Venus, violent passions'.[141]

Willis classifies headaches on the basis of their periodicity. The account is repetitive and not always consistent with his views on mechanisms. Occasional headache may arise from closure of the vascular pores preventing dispersal of humours. This is caused by exposure to 'the Northern winds, Snow, or Rain'. Habitual headache usually lasts twelve hours and has a predictable periodicity measured in days, weeks, or months. Its relationship to eating and sleeping, sometimes preceding and sometimes following each, and especially in those with an hereditary predisposition, indicates interaction of the nutritious and nervous juices. The causes include 'drinking of Wine, Surfetting, lying in the Sun, or vehement exercise, also in the fits of Feavours . . . also by a blow, wound, or contusion of the Head'. Headache that is continual for many days or weeks occurs in various contexts: 'Yea, I have known Inflammations, Imposthumes, Whelks, Scirrhous tumors growing to the meninges . . . and other Diseases of an evil conformation, excited in the Membranes of the Brain'.[142]

Willis writes very little on tumours. Most are meningeal, being primary lesions or secondary deposits, abscesses or (presumably) tuberculomas. He seldom mentions specific intraparenchymal swellings although the process of compression is described. Amongst the cases described in the Oxford lectures is that of a scholar who died rapidly with lethargy and in whom autopsy showed a gelatinous mass in the pituitary gland 'not unlike that of the pelvis of the kidney' which had obstructed the passage of fluid from the ventricles and

140 See: *Concerning the soul of brutes* (1683): page 108.
141 See: *Concerning the soul of brutes* (1683): page 109–10.
142 See: *Concerning the soul of brutes* (1683): page 107; and page 121 for description in detail including a case with autopsy.

led to distortion of the medulla oblongata.[143] Willis observes that swellings of the meninges tend to end 'in sleepy Distempers, and at length deadly; for when I have opened the Heads of many dead of these diseases, the signs or footsteps, declaring the aforesaid kinds of Morbific causes, have appeared'.[144]

There is a further category of 'evident' headaches but Willis's account mainly rehearses details of the 'occasional or habitual' distemper. However, within this category, he provides one additional description. Headache that creeps forward from the 'Stomach, Mesentery, Womb, yea sometimes from the members or outward parts, to the Head', commonly called 'Sympathetic', is usually severe and prolonged, and associated with vertigo and vomiting:[145]

> Degenerate Matter … heaped up to … a Fermentative *Miasm* or Infection is fixed to the Blood; from which, that, being as it were imbued with rage, impetuously grows hot … and partly by transferring what is incongruous into the Membranes of the Head, stirs up fierce and cruel fits of pains.

Those afflicted grow weary of 'a noted sourness, and ravenous hunger' which precedes the vomiting and headache: 'in striving to Vomit, the Gallish or Pancreatick humor, either one or both of them, being thrust forth into the *Duodenum*, and cast forth by Vomit, is ignorantly taken for the Cephalick matter'.[146] Increased flow in the carotids or vertebral arteries 'produces a Meagrim on the side, sometimes in the forepart, and sometimes in the hinder part of the Head'. Allowing that morbific material may reach the brain through 'the passages of the nerves of the wandring and Intercostal pair', Willis has no time for 'the voice of the people' that this type of headache is a disorder of the spleen typical of 'Hypochondriacks'.

Willis declares that cure of the headache is 'sometimes easie, sometimes difficult or scarce possible; so that from thence it may be lawful to declare the event of the Disease, either safe, or very dangerous, or wholely uncertain'. Best for 'Prognostick of the Headach' are cases of evident headache for which lifestyle can be blamed and habits altered. Persistent intermittent headache lasting years is not dangerous but unlikely to be cured. Continuous headache due to altered structure—inflammation, tumour, abscess, or 'Worms'—carries 'very little hope of Cure especially because the sick will refuse great remedies, as Salivation, or opening of the Skull'. The same is true of headache associated with vertigo, vomiting and 'Convulsive or Soporific Distempers … which often passes into a deadly Apoplexie, and not seldom into an Epilepsie, Palsie, Blindness, Deafness, and other funestous [calamitous or fatal] and incurable Diseases'.[147] In all of this, physicians from any age will read much good sense.

Less persuasive in its wisdom is the advice that, where the natural history is known to be favourable, temporary improvement follows diverting the morbific matter away from the head by letting blood from the arm or jugular vein, and the use of plaisters applied to the head or abdomen together with medicines that induce sweating and diuresis.[148] In the case of headache following convulsion of a remote part, preventing propagation to the brain is

[143] See: Kenneth Dewhurst, *Thomas Willis's Oxford lectures*, Oxford (1980): page 109, endnote 5 referring to communication between Richard Lower and Robert Boyle on 24 June 1664 documented in Thomas Birch, *The works of the honourable Robert Boyle*, volume 6, London (1772): page 471. Also described in AN Williams et al, 'A case of pituitary adenoma: Thomas Willis revisited', *European Journal of Paediatric Neurology* 2003: 7; 183–5.

[144] See: *Concerning the soul of brutes* (1683): page 112, the same point having already been made at page 107.

[145] See: *Concerning the soul of brutes* (1683): page 111.

[146] See: *Concerning the soul of brutes* (1683): page 112.

[147] See: *Concerning the soul of brutes* (1683): page 114.

[148] See: Thomas Willis, *Pharmaceutice rationalis*, part 1, (1679) and chapter 18 where Willis sets out his logic for increasing excretion as one means of curing disease.

effective. Once this has been achieved, the predisposition to headache can be tempered and with success: 'which kind of Indication, though it be very seldom suddenly or wholely performed, yet sometimes the Cure is by degrees laboured out ... however fixed and rooted the Morbid matter may be'.

There follow several pages of receipts amongst which is the cure for the periodical headache characterized by redness or flushing of the face, headache, and facial pain which, failing blood-letting and a gentle purge, responds to 'Antiscorbuticks and Chalybeates'.[149] Willis also suggests coffee as a specific remedy.[150] More generally, he makes the point that cutting off 'the nest, or feeding of the Disease' allows the brain time to adjust: but 'in this case the helps of the Medical Art, are rather to be sought from the Chirgurgical part, than from Physick'. These surgical interventions include blistering the shaven scalp through application of hot plaisters of Red-Lead or mustard; cauterizing the sutures of the scalp but with the caution that 'if we should measure this practice by the fruit or success, it will appear to be rarely beneficial, but more often unlucky'; cutting 'issues' in the limbs or neck to draw away the recrements; inserting the root of hellebores into a cavity bored in the ear; and, as recommended by William Harvey (1578–1657: who also advised lancing an artery close to a painful place) in the case of a most noble lady 'opening of the Skull, near the grieved place, with a *Trypaning* Iron'.[151] Generally dismissive of these radical approaches. Willis is equally sceptical about salivation induced with mercury, unless the headache is venereal, which in the case of Doctor G.D. led to blindness. Resisting a detailed catalogue of ill effects from use of mercury in the treatment of headache, Willis refers his readers to a forthcoming account of salivation by 'the learned Physician Doctor *Needham* ... as to its measures and effects, and its benefits and hurt'.[152] Even Willis's most dedicated readers may be relieved by his concession that after 'delivering the Aetiology, or the reason of this Disease so confusedly shown, and its Therapeutic or Curatory part sufficiently shadowed' he intends for the more clear illustrating of these things to 'add some more rare cases of sick persons'.

Willis' most famous patient with headache was Anne, countess of Conway (1631–1679). Anne (née Finch) lived at Kensington Palace until, aged 19, she married Edward, Earl of Conway (1623–1683). Lady Conway was a scholar who published, anonymously and posthumously, *Principles of the most ancient and modern philosophy* (1690). Willis wrote:[153]

> Some years since, I was sent for to visit a most noble Lady, for above twenty years sick with almost a continual Headach, at first intermitting: She was of a most beautiful form, and a great wit, so that she was skilled in the Liberal Arts, and in all sorts of Literature, beyond the condition of her sex, and if it were thought too much by Nature, for her to enjoy so great endowments, without some detriment, she was extremely punished with this Disease. Growing well of a Feavour before she was twelve years old, she became obnoxious to pains in the Head, which were wont to arise, sometimes of their own accord, and more often

[149] See: *Concerning the soul of brutes* (1683): page 125; and Hierons (1967): page 6. Not unreasonably, modern commentators conclude that Willis is describing migrainous neuralgia, or cluster headache; and this is also the preferred explanation for 'a venerable matron—of a lean habit of Body, and imbued with a Cholerick temper, after she had lived for a long time obnoxious to Headaches, wont to be caused occasionally' who began to suffer every afternoon at about 4 pm from severe recurrent daily headache for a period of five weeks.

[150] See: *Concerning the soul of brutes* (1683): page 115; and Isler (2010): page 102.

[151] See: *Concerning the soul of brutes* (1683): page 119. Although the remedy was refused, and Willis remained highly sceptical, this is his first reference to Lady Conway and her headaches (see next).

[152] This work has not been traced in any of the library catalogues consulted or ESTC.

[153] See: *Concerning the soul of brutes* (1683): pages 121–2 where, after the earlier oblique reference, the case is fully described.

> upon very light occasion. This sickness being limited to no one place of the Head, troubled her sometimes on one side, sometimes on the other, and often thorow the whole compass of her Head. During the fit (which rarely ended under a day and a nights space, and often held for two, three, or four days) she was impatient of light, speaking, noise, or of any motion, sitting upright in her Bed, the Chamber made dark, she would talk to no body, nor take any sleep, or sustenance. At length about the declination of the fit, she was wont to lye down with an heavy and disturbed sleep, from which awaking, she found herself better, and so by degrees grew well, and continued indifferently well till the time of the intermission. Formerly, the fits came not but occasionally, and seldom under twenty days of a month but afterwards they came more often: and lately she was seldom free. Moreover, upon sundry occasions, or evident causes (such as the change of the Air, or the year, the great Aspects of the Sun and Moon, violent passions, and errors in diet) she was more cruelly tormented with them. But although this Distemper most grievously afflicting this noble Lady, above twenty years (when I saw her) having pitched its tents near the confines of the Brain, had so long besieged its regal tower, yet it had not taken it: for the sick Lady, being free from a Vertigo, swimming in the Head, Convulsive Distempers, and any Soporiferous symptom, found the chief faculties of her soul sound enough.

The case of Lady Conway, her doctors and their recommendations are fully assessed by Macdonald Critchley (1900–1997).[154] Anne had sought advice from the most distinguished and fashionable physicians: Harvey was 'much commended, and they say he knows very many secrets in physicke unknown to other physicians'. His recommendation was for 'opening of the skull with a Trypaning Iron ... cry'd up by many for a pertinacious Headache' carried out by surgeons in France, advice which Lady Conway rejected. Théodore de Mayerne (1573–1655) advised mercurial salivation using the powders of Charles Hues (nd). Robert Boyle advised the use of 'Ens Veneris ... a calcined and dulcified colcothar of Dantzic vitriol elevated with sal-aramoniac with the form of reddish sublimate'. Lady Conway also saw Kenelm Digby, the charlatan Valentine Greatrakes (1628–1683: the 'Irish Stroker', whose art delivered in the presence of a large entourage was of no avail), and Franciscus Mercurius van Helmont (1614–1699), who attended Lady Conway in her terminal illness. Willis summarized the many remedies, to date, given without success and not free from risk:[155]

> Some years before, she had endured from an ointment of Quicksilver, a long and troublesome Salivation, so that she ran the hazards of her life. Afterwards twice a Cure was attempted (though in vain) by a Flux at the Mouth, from a Mercurial Powder, which the noted Empirick *Charles Hues* ordinarily gave: with the like success with the rest she tried the Baths, and the Spaw-waters, almost of every kind and nature: she admitted of frequent Blood-letting, and also once the opening of an Artery; she had also made about her several Issues, sometimes in the hinder part of her Head, and sometimes in the forepart,

[154] See: Macdonald Critchley, 'The malady of Anne, Countess Conway: a case for commentary', *King's College Hospital Gazette* 1937: 17: 44–9; reprinted in Macdonald Critchley, *The black hole and other essays*, London (1964): pages 91–7. In his interleaved and annotated copy, Critchley has added that Edward was the first and last Earl of Conway. In the last part of his essay which deals with erudite female migraineurs, Critchley has added the names of Mrs Wordsworth (presumably Mary Hutchinson, 1770–1859), Dr Elizabeth Garrett Anderson (1836–1917) and Pamela Handford Johnson (1912–1981, Baroness Snow). Opposite a comment on the printed page describing Ursula Bloom's (1892–1984: British novelist) article in the *Daily Mirror* for 16 December 1936, indicating that she consulted twenty-six Harley Street specialists concluding that 'The cold in the head, headache, they leave them slightly ga-ga', Critchley adds on the interleaf, 'before seeing me!'

[155] See: *Concerning the soul of brutes* (1683): page 122.

> and in other parts. She also took the Air of several Countries besides her own native Air, she went into *Ireland* and into *France*: there was no kind of Medicines both *Cephalicks, Antiscorbuticks, Hysterical*, all famous *Specificks*, which she took not, both from the Learned and the unlearned, from *Quacks*, and old Women; and yet notwithstanding she professed, that she had received from no remedy, or method of Curing, any thing of Cure or Ease, but that the contumacious and rebellious Disease, refused to be tamed, being deaf to the charms of every Medicine. Further, this so long possessing the out-parts of the Head, though it could not invade the cloysters of the Brain; yet, when I visited her, unfolding its ends in some other parts of the nervous kind, it had begun to stir up most cruel pains in her members, and also in her Loins, and bottom of her Belly, as is wont to be in *Rheumatism*, and in the *Scorbutick Colick*.

Speculating on the aetiology, Willis concludes that a fever had delivered morbific matter to the meninges which thereafter became the seat of recurrent and recalcitrant accumulation of overheated matter so much so that 'small scirrhous tumours developed on the *Dura mater*, the *Pia mater* being in the meantime safe'. Lady Conway gave her own account of the ailment in letters. Writing to her husband:[156]

> Dearest Deare, – I have been exceedingly ill ever since Saturday night in a terrible fit, which have left me so ill still that it hath been as much as I could doe to keep off my bed this day to entertain Dr. Taylor ... [and later] ... I have been so extremely ill all this week and the last, that I have scarce enjoyed any respite from my fits.

Lady Conway also corresponded with a fellow philosopher, Henry More (1614–1687):

> I have formerly given you some intimation of the great increase of my distemper and other indispositions since this last winter, which doeth not yet quite abate upon me, but contrarily I have been so much worse than I was when I writ last that since good fryday I have not been able to go abroad, and am very little off my bed. I find myself very faint and weak, but yet as little strength as I seeme to have, I still endure those violent paines (which I always thought would be accounted intolerable by a stronger body than I ever had), and that most frequently than ever. I cannot dissemble so much as to profess myself very weary of this condition.

The last decade of her life was spent increasingly as an invalid with the headaches unabated. As her steward Charles Coke (nd) reported to the absent Earl of Conway:[157]

> Night and day two persons are constantly with her to support her, her violent paines having taken away her rest and stomach, which makes her groane and crye continually ... Her Honour continues very painefull and weak, taking nothing but now and then a spoonefull of small-beer ... M. v. Helmont ... tell me that my Lady is grown so weak, that she has lost all motion in her armes, but her excessive paines continues still, causing her continuall cryes and groanes, so that he judges her Ladyship cannot last long ... [until] ... My Ladyship parted this life, having her perfect understanding and senses to the last minute, giving up

[156] See: Critchley (1937): page 45–6, citing Ed. Marjorie Hope Nicholson, *The Conway letters*, New Haven (1930).

[157] See: Critchley (1937): page 47.

> her Spirit very peaceably without any perceivable motion and keeping a very sweet face, her pains have held her to the last, about Saturday at noone her legs began to swell.

Of the other cases described by Willis,[158] one had rapidly progressive headache, with 'knotty Concretions in the Neck ... stiffness of the Tendons, and at length convulsions and convulsive motions in the Brain' followed by delirium and death. 'Though we had not leave for the dissecting the dead body', another case, 'a young man of the University' had an equally rapid course to death with 'the membranes ... distempered thorow the whole, with a fiery Tumor'. After a long headache, a second 'Academick' with localized pain under the temporal suture fell into a deadly 'Apoplexie', and was found at autopsy to have 'a fiery swelling ... in the Meninges ... from which, being ripened and broke, the filthy bloody matter falling on the Brain, had distemper'd its substance with a rottenness and blackness'. These examples of continual headache are contrasted with intermittent cases including a 'venerable Matron' aged 40 years who, over a period of three weeks, had daily headache for several hours starting promptly at 4pm cured by blood-letting, a gentle purge, and an electuary of natural substances. In this case the cause lay in overheating of the nourishing juice flooding the otherwise normal meninges. Much the same outcome was achieved in 'a very comely Woman, tall and slender' with daily headaches on waking that last until noon. Other women have intermittent headache that is timed around 'the Monthly Flowers'. A 'beautiful and young Woman, indued with a slender habit of body, and an hot Blood' had morning headache always preceded by 'a most plentiful Supper, with an hungry, I may say greedy appetite ... and the event never failed this Augury'. Headache might be associated with cerebrospinal rhinorrhoea:[159]

> Not long since, a Virgin living in this City, was afflicted with a most cruel headache, and in the midst of her pain much thin and yellow Serum daily flowed out from her Nostrils; the last Winter this excretion stopped for some time, and then the sick party growing worse in her Head, fell into cruel convulsions, with a stupidity; and within three days dyed Apoplectical. Her Head being opened, that kind of yellow Latex overflowed the deeper turnings and windings of the Brain, and its interior Cavities or Ventricles ... [and] ... I knew a Gentlewoman that was wont to be infested with a most cruel headache, also with a Vertigo, and a frequent melting of the animal spirits, or swooning away; who when she began to feel better, after a grievous Fit, felt at first a creeping motion in the top of her Brain, as it were sliding down of water; then that motion passing a little more forwards and downwards, at length many drops of clear water distilled from her Nostrils. This symptom she used to have so ordinarily, that the sick Gentlewoman did not doubt that this water stilled out from the brain itself.

All commentators acknowledge that Willis's account of the headache is most notable for the description of migraine. The most diligent analysis comes from the monograph on that disorder by Edward Liveing (1832–1919), who read Willis's three books on the brain and nervous stock with great care and much admiration:[160]

> Headache, however, and especially megrim, was sometimes referred to 'cold humours' as well as hot, to black bile as well as yellow bile, to the spleen as well as the liver, and

[158] See: *Concerning the soul of brutes* (1683): pages 122–25.
[159] See: *Anatomy of the brain* (1681): page 100; and Spillane (1981): pages 64–5.
[160] See: Edward Liveing, *On megrim, sick-headache, and some allied disorders: a contribution to the pathology of nerve-storms*, London (1873): page 227, citing Latin text from *De anima brutorum*, 'De cephalalgia' ... Works, quarto, 1680, Geneva, vol ii, page 155.

> hence it came to be regarded as one expression of the malady known as Hypochondriasis, which was supposed to be due to 'Atra bilis' or 'melancholia'. 'Headaches', says old Willis, 'are wont to be imputed no less to the *spleen* than the stomach; and indeed it is a common observation that in hypochondriacal subjects when a pain, inflation, rumbling, or other disturbance arises in the left side from the distempered spleen, that a headache frequently succeeds as if excited by it.

Liveing emphasizes that, against this background, Willis took an insightful position on predisposing factors and mechanisms:[161]

> The frequent existence of an inherited tendency to the more severe forms of Headache did not escape the notice of our countryman Willis. In a chapter on headache, including megrim, he refers to a 'vicious or weak constitution of the affected part' as the chief predisposing cause of the malady, and this, he adds 'is sometimes innate and hereditary, as appears from hence, that the disease is often handed down from parents to children'.

Incorporating the term in the title of his monograph, Liveing likens the paroxysm of migraine to a nerve-storm, after which equilibrium is temporarily restored. In footnotes supporting this statement, he writes:[162]

> If apology be needed for thus introducing the illustration of a storm or explosion, we may offer that of Willis ... [who] ... in treating of convulsive diseases, observes – 'These kind of paroxysms are periodical, and return at stated times; this arises from the morbid material being daily supplied to the nervous system in about the same amount, and consequently accumulating there to an explosive extent, in about the same space of time'.

Liveing defers to Willis in his account of gastrointestinal symptoms and migraine: 'Cases of this kind appear to have attracted the notice of medical men in all ages'.[163] Migraine may be anticipated by a craving for food as the inaugural symptom of the neuronal paroxysm: 'Willis records a case of hereditary megrim where the attacks were always ushered in in this way'.[164] On vomiting: 'The cerebral nature ... in headaches of this class was distinctly pointed out two centuries ago by our countryman Willis'.[165] Liveing acknowledges that Willis considered migraine to be dependent on irritation in the stomach as well as morbid susceptibility of the nerves:[166]

[161] See: Liveing (1873): page 27 citing in the footnote 'De cepalalgia', caput I, page 247, ed. 12mo' (1674), and transcribing: 'Ex his priorem quandoque innatum et hæreditaram esse inde constat, quia morbus a parentibus sæpe ad liberos traducitur' [Given these, it is thus a fact that it is sometimes innate and hereditary, since the disease is often transmitted from parents to children].

[162] See: Liveing (1873): page 336, footnote * citing *De morbis convulsivis*, caput I, Ed. Amstel, 1670, page 4; and Liveing (1873): page 338, footnote † citing *Path. Cerebri, De morb. convul.* Caput i. Ed. Amstel. 1670, page 117. Each footnote includes transcription of the relevant Latin text.

[163] See: Liveing (1873): page 216 with an extensive quote from *De anima brutorum*, 'De colica, page 550, edit. duodecimo Amstel' (1674).

[164] See: Liveing (1873): pages 363–4 citing *De anima brutorum*, 'De Cephalalg. Curat, Cap. ii p. 289. 12mo Amstel' (1674).

[165] See: Liveing (1873): page 139 where the Latin text is cited from *De anima brutorum*, 'De cephalalgia, cap. i. p. 259', Amsterdam (1674).

[166] See: Liveing (1873): pages 42–3. In the footnote marked †, Liveing cites 'Thos. Willis, M.D., De anima brutorum, Cephalalgia curatio Caput I, p 247. 12mo Amstel., 1674'; in * he transcribes text from *De anima*

> The same essential facts with regard to the nature and influence of such causes were long since set forth by old Willis in his treatise on Cephalalgia, which includes megrim. After having stated 'an evil or weak constitution of the parts ... sometimes innate and hereditary' to be the chief predisposing cause of the malady, he adds – 'But further, an irritation in some distant member or viscera is sometimes the occasion, and in a sense the cause of the headache'. This he afterwards illustrates by reference to cases where the attacks were determined by gastric disorder and by the catamenial period; the latter, he says, 'recur monthly at the commencement or termination of the menstrual discharge'. In the case of a lady which he has recorded at length, who had suffered from childhood, generally every three weeks or month for twenty years, from headache of the true megrim type, he observes that the seizures would sometimes occur spontaneously, but more often on some trivial occasion; and he afterwards mentions as accessory causes, 'changes of season, atmospheric states, the great aspects of the sun and moon, violent passions, and errors in diet'.
>
> [adding in a footnote] What Willis may mean by the 'great aspects of the sun and moon' is not very clear; but exposure to a hot sun has been frequently mentioned as an exciting cause of Megrim, and the idea of the moon as determining the recurrence of periodical complaints, however absurd, is barely yet an exploded doctrine.

Liveing accepts Willis's pessimism about curing patients, especially those with an hereditary predisposition: 'With well-marked hereditary migraine, which has commenced in early life, and recurred with great regularity for a number of years, I know of nothing which will certainly free him from this constitutional infirmity'.[167]

Isler (1986) subsequently analysed the two chapters on headache, based on his reading of *De anima brutorum* (1672) rather than Pordage's English text, summarizing the contents as: constitutional factors, inferences from therapy, the nature and mechanism of the pain, the types of headache including occasional and habitual, the immediate precipitants, and the role of the blood and various spirits with emphasis on serum or chyle interacting with nerve fluid.[168] Isler speculates on the mechanisms and contexts of intermittent headache described by Willis: 'it is common for the attacks to increase around equinoxes and solstices often in "subordinate periods" during which they usually infest at certain fixed hours within the space of every day and night, the pathogenic material "surging into fullness at fixed hours"'. He points out that Willis returns to Galenic concepts of disease in *De anima brutorum*, substituting blood, serum, chyle and nerve juice for yellow and black bile, blood, and phlegm. The sequence of events leading to headache and vomiting involves black bile from the spleen, entering the blood and carried to the meninges through the vagus and intercostal nerves, causing painful corrugations or spasms. Fluid then accumulates in the meninges before being excreted through the kidneys: 'I have observed in several cases that limpid and very copious urine preceded or accompanied the paroxysms of this disease'. Isler is not dismissive of Willis's revisionist Galenic position and he sees in the text several concepts

brutorum, Amsterdam (1674): page 282 and further refers the reader to 'Sieveking's Epilepsy, p. 42'. However, this page in Edward Sieveking *On epilepsy and epileptiform seizures. Their causes, pathology and treatment*, London (1868) has no relevant passages.

[167] See: Liveing (1873): page 428 citing *De anima brutorum* (1672–1674) 'Cephalalgia curatio, cap. II'.

[168] See: Hansruedi Isler, 'Thomas Willis, two chapters on headache of 1672: a first attempt to apply the "new science" to this topic', *Headache Journal* 1986: 26; 95–8.

that were further developed in the twentieth century. These include anticipation of Harold Wolff's (1898–1962) hypothesis of cluster headache, quoting (in Isler's translation):[169]

> Sometimes the blood itself is incited to move more rapidly and, boiling up towards the head, is constricted or stopped, in its passage at predisposed sites; then it soon gathers there in greater abundance and distends the vessels, strongly inflating the membranes, tearing the nerve fibres apart from each other, and thus inducing painful corrugations in them. For this reason, those who are subject to headache are compelled to avoid all occasions that cause the blood to effervesce immoderately, such as drinking wine, exercising and bathing.

On the slowly spreading spasm, 'quasi perreptando ascenderet', Isler sees an anticipation of the concept of cortical spreading depression, quoting (in his own translation):

> A spasm, beginning at the end some nerve, which creeps ahead up towards its origin ... having shown, indeed, that when pathogenic matter occupies the origins of the nerves, or the nearest parts in the head, the spasm begins often at the ends of these nerves, and ascends from there, transferred upwards to the places that were first affected, as if creeping through.

Apoplexy

Willis on apoplexy is impressive. Without wavering from his theory of disease as a process determined by perturbations of the heated blood and the animal spirits, here is summarized for the modern reader all that is known of cerebrovascular disease: infarction and haemorrhage, thrombosis and embolism, local atheroma, large and small vessel disease, occlusion and compression of vessels in the neck, cardiac causes, transient episodes as harbingers of fatal apoplexy, and the ominous manifestations of haemorrhage compressing the medulla.

Denoting percussion, 'a Sideration or Blasting', apoplexy results from a 'full eclipse' of spirits affecting the inward cloister of the brain. Those affected lose every spontaneous and knowing function 'being as it were Planet struck, or with an invisible *Numen*, falling suddenly to the ground ... they lye a long time as if dead, and sometimes yield to death; But if they revive, oftentimes they are taken with an universal Palsie, or else of one side'.[170] Willis uses the term apoplexy to describe any sudden or extreme event in the context of several underlying conditions including convulsions, headache, and sleep disorders. Opinions are divided on the seat of the disease: is this of the heart or the brain, the cavities or the pores, the inward flow of the blood or the outward passage of the animal spirits? 'The famous Wepferus' has resolved the matter by showing that in those dying of the apoplexy he found 'the blood extravasated ... out of the vessels here and there in great clodders, and had largely marked the substance of the Brain'. Willis quotes directly from (Johann) Wepfer (1620–1695):[171]

> The whole cause of every *Apoplexy* doth consist ... either because the flowing of blood thorow the Arteries to the Brain is deny'd ... by reason of the obstruction of the inner

[169] See: Isler (1986): page 97 for transcription of Willis's Latin text; and Harold George Wolff, *Headache: and other head pain*, Oxford (1948).
[170] See: *Concerning the soul of brutes* (1683): page 153.
[171] See: *Concerning the soul of brutes* (1683): page 154.

> *Carotid* Arteries, and of the *Vertebrals*, to wit, which happens in the greater Vessels and chiefly about the ascent of the Brain from the blood concreted into cloddery pieces; or in the lesser Vessels, which pass thorow the Brain from a Viscous matter planted in them: Or, Secondly, the flowing in of the blood is detained from the brain by reason of the compression of those Vessels, which sometimes happens, because the *Paristhmia*, or Kirnels of the hinder part of the Neck, do so swell up, from a Serous heap of watry Humors, that by pressing together the Arteries passing thorow, shuts forth the passage of blood to the Head. Or, Thirdly, the Bloody flood may be hindred, because a Vessel being preternaturally opened within the Skull, great quantity of blood is poured forth, which should otherwise go to the benefit of the brain. As to the other cause of the astonishing Disease, *viz.* from the flowing forth of the Spirits being hindred, he affirms that may be caused by two ways; to wit, either by reason of the obstruction of the beginning of all the Nerves, caused by a serous inundation, or by a sudden compression of the same; which is caused either by an heaping up of too much blood in the *Meninges*, or in some parts of the brain it self, or in its Ventricles; or else by a disposition of the *Phlegmonodes*.

Even though minor refinements can usefully be made, with unqualified admiration Willis concludes: 'his most ingenious reasons seem to challenge our assent so that more probable or more likely are not easily to be brought'. In pursuing Wepfer's principles, Willis refers to the anastomosis at the base of the brain which should offset occlusion of the individual great vessels. Of course this famous observation has already been made but Willis mentions another example in which, despite one carotid and one vertebral being 'bony and impervious ... the sick person was not troubled by the astonishing Disease'.[172] He has an important point to make in referring to the apoplexy that occurs when blood flow is impaired through failed motion of the heart leading to '*Syncopy*, or Swooning away, or the *Hysterical* passion', and also in nightmares.

Willis considers haemorrhage to be the usual cause of apoplexy. This occurs after an extrinsic blow on the head or when sharp and thin overheated blood ruptures through the overly porous 'little mouths of the Vessels', compressing the underlying marrow by 'intumifying the distemper'd places'. Blood may leak from an 'Imposthum or Ulcer' in the meninges, initially causing headache and then 'the filthy stuff flowing ... into the shelly part of the Brain, gnaws and putrefies it ... and raises up at last the fit of the astonishing disease'. And 'the Serous heap or deluge being poured forth from the blood' may reproduce the features of apoplexy, as in a long and total suppression of the urine, or fever (suggesting that Willis is referring to cerebral oedema rather than haemorrhage).[173]

In all types of apoplexy, the pulse and respiration are maintained if spirits are still produced by the cerebellum. But the situation is fragile. In writing on lethargy, Willis has already made the point that when the morbid process extends to the cerebel, 'the respiration and Pulse are altered: for that become unequal and slow, sometimes drawing the breath deep and long, sometimes short, repeated, and as it were double'.[174] Given the prescience of this clinical observation, Willis can be forgiven for thrice repeating himself in the chapter on apoplexy. He provides an almost identical description in the context of haemorrhage in the

[172] See: *Concerning the soul of brutes* (1683): page 154.

[173] See: *Concerning the soul of brutes* (1683): page 156.

[174] See: *Concerning the soul of brutes* (1683): page 129. This description anticipates that of John Cheyne (1777–1836) and William Stokes (1808–1878) by almost one hundred and fifty years: see J. Cheyne: 'A case of apoplexy in which the fleshy part of the heart was converted into fat'. *Dublin Hospital Reports*, 1818: 2; 216–23; and William Stokes (1854), 'Fatty degeneration of the heart', in *The diseases of the heart and aorta*, Dublin (1854).

brainstem when 'with a foam at the mouth, and snorting; upon which comes a sweat, which is often like melted greace, and indicates a very sudden death to be at hand'.[175] Then there are cases that: 'follow upon a great weight in the hinder-part of the head, in which the sick become senseless and immoveable, with the pulse and breathing very much lessened, and scarce perceivable, and lye quite cold ... more like dead than living persons'. Some sufferers have been put in their coffin but subsequently revived even without the palsy on one side that characterizes most cases of apoplexy.[176] And, finally, the prognosis is always ominous: 'for the Apoplexy is never without present or future danger' especially when the pulse and respiration slow.[177]

Willis has observed cases in whom 'the astonishing disease', at first transient, eventually becomes habitual 'by reason of which, at first they are exercised only with little skirmishes, but after some time they become more grievous, and of which at last for the most part they dye'. Here, Willis assumes that the transient episodes, affecting one or other of the streaked bodies causing 'the *Hemiplegia*', or rendering his patients speechless with 'Scotomies ... mists before the eyes, and the Distemper of the *Vertigo*' are due to partial penetration of the brain by morbific matter; or that spirits in the middle of the brain made 'numb' have been driven away to lie suppressed until the malignant matter 'is dissipated or supped up into the blood'. Later, new matter descending from the Callous body brings on another fit and the patients 'perish by degrees'. Despite his endorsement of Wepfer's opinion, in seeking a mechanistic explanation for transient episodes characterized by weakness on one side, Willis settles on the chemical nature of morbific matter in the thin acid blood and overly accommodating pores of the vessels rather than flow or extravasation of blood: 'their *Copula*'s have divers sorts of adjuncts, some of which induce an *Elastick* and very *explosive* virtue, as in the Convulsive Distempers, and others a stupor, numness, or immobility, as in the sleepy Diseases, and also in the *Apoplexy* and *Palsie*'.[178]

When the presence of transient episodes indicates a propensity to apoplexy, prophylaxis with purging, vomiting, and bleeding, supplemented by cephalicks, should be given in the spring and autumn. That said, the treatment of established apoplexy is no different apart from the additional advice not to put the patient to bed, since this will cause the blood to grow hot and deliver yet more morbific matter to the brain. If possible, the patient should be nursed in a chair awaiting phlebotomy, clysters, blistering plaisters, vomits, and comforters. These are repeated with the addition of purges, sneezing powders, and cupping. Should these measures fail, the head is shaved and glowing iron placed on the scalp, leeches applied, and spirits of Harts-horn 'poured down the throat ... till you see death at hand; which (as *Celsus* saith) these sort of Remedies only defer, but sometimes hasten life'.[179]

Amongst the histories upon which Willis was able to draw in order to illustrate his account, none is more apposite than that of his patron and supporter in appointment to the Sedleian professorship in 1660. Willis attended Archbishop Sheldon who, despite suffering from apoplexy, outlived Willis himself:[180]

[175] See: *Concerning the soul of brutes* (1683): page 158.
[176] See: *Concerning the soul of brutes* (1683): page 155.
[177] See: *Concerning the soul of brutes* (1683): page 158. In repeating this astute clinical observation, Willis recommends that, although seemingly dead and cold, these individuals should not be buried for three days since spontaneous recovery sometimes occurs.
[178] See: *Concerning the soul of brutes* (1683): page 157.
[179] See: *Concerning the soul of brutes* (1683): page 159.
[180] See: *Concerning the soul of brutes* (1683): page 160.

> The most Reverend Father in God the Lord *Gilbert* Archbishop of Canterbury, recovered of a grievous *Apoplectical* Fit, six years ago, (God prospering our medicinal help, to whom we render eternal thanks) and from that time, though he sometimes suffer'd some light skirmishes of the Disease, yet he never fell, or became speechless or senseless.

Although Willis carried out autopsies in cases of apoplexy following a blow on the head, in other situations his interest in the morbid anatomy was frustrated: 'we have been prohibited often by their Friends, from opening those dying of an habitual *Apoplexy*, who expecting to have them revive again, held it as deadly thing, and so wholly forbid *Anatomy*'. An exception made in Oxford five years before publication, relates to an ancient Divine so obese and unfit that he could do no more than move laboriously between his chamber and chapel, where one morning he was suddenly rendered speechless and senseless, and carried to bed. Willis found him cold, stiff, not breathing, and pulseless. Carrying out an autopsy the next day, and expecting to find extravasation of blood in the head, Willis was surprised to find the brain normal and, with the lungs stuffed with a frothy matter, concluded that 'the Heart presently failing, like the first moving wheel in a Clock or Watch, immediately all other functions, their impulses being taken away, wholly ceased'.[181]

Palsie

Willis has mentioned in passing the palsy but this topic requires special attention since it so closely relates to his concept of a discrete pathway for voluntary movement from the cortex, through the 'Streaked Bodies, Oblong Marrow, and also to the Nerves, and nervous Fibres'. Whereas minor alteration results in cramps and convulsions, hindrance or abolition of the spirits in these places through obstruction of their passage, 'impotency' or reduction in number, leads to palsie: '*That it is a resolution, loosening, or relaxation of the nervous parts, from their due tensity of stiffness; by which means motion and sense, to wit, either one only, or both together, in the whole body, or in some parts, cannot be exercised after their due manner*'.[182] The immediate causes are blockage of the pathways by extraneous matter; pressure from blood flowing out from the vessels; or discontinuity of the tracts 'as by a stroke, or wound, or bruise, also by excess of cold or heat'.[183] In some cases 'whilst not able to perform the more strong motive endeavours', crude movements so that 'they could extend, bend, yea and move their members hither and thither' are retained. Those with the palsie sometimes tremble with repeated attempts to move, 'the nervous Fibres flagging or growing weak, they are not able to sustain the Tonick endeavour, or the stiffness in the Animal regiment'. Palsie may be the consequence of lethargy, the carus, or apoplexy. The weakness is often preceded by dullness of mind and forgetfulness, and afterwards with 'a stupidity and foolishness'.

When one side is affected, 'such a distemper … is wont to excite a sense of numbness, or pricking or tingling, such as in members lean'd or lain upon'. As to why sense is not always lost in the palsie, Willis explains the dissociation by reverting to his metaphor of light that can pass through glass, whereas wind does not. Also, sense is less demanding on the spirits

181 See: *Concerning the soul of brutes* (1683): page 161.

182 See: *Concerning the soul of brutes* (1683): page 161. The use of italics suggests that Willis is quoting; but, if so, the source is unidentified,

183 See: *Concerning the soul of brutes* (1683): page 162.

than the more laborious business of motion and so less vulnerable to their perturbations. The muscles of the eyes, mouth, and face may be spared because they depend on spirits generated in the cerebel not the streaked bodies. But in other cases:[184]

> The oppilative or stopping Particles being fallen down, from the Brain, and carried forward into the oblong Marrow, enter into the Nerves, destinated to the Muscles of some parts of the Face, and by obstructing the ways of the Spirits in them, bring forth the *Palsie* in the Tongue, and sometimes a loosening of these or those Muscles of the Eyes, Eyelids, Lips and other parts.

This observation is preceded by a description that has been interpreted as an example of general paralysis of the insane:[185]

> I have observed in many, that when, the Brain being first indisposed, they have been distemper'd with a dullness of mind, and forgetfulness, and afterwards with a stupidity and foolishness, after that, have fallen into a Palsie, which I often did predict; to wit, the Morbific matter being by degrees fallen down, and at length being heaped up some where within the Medullar Trunk, (where the Marrowy Tracts are more strained than in the Streaked Body) to a stopping fullness. For according as the places obstructed are more or less large, so either an universal *Palsie*, or an half *Palsie* of one side, or else some partial resolutions of members happen.

Willis offers tabes dorsalis as the explanation for 'a Gentleman who was much disordered in his body, and troubled with nocturnal pains which proceeded from the Pox—to whom I prescribed many things, but all in vain'.[186] Discussing cachexia in his final treatise, *Pharmaceutice rationalis* (1675), he argues that degeneration of the nervous juice may impoverish the nutritive state so that 'certain members ... affected with a Palsie, at length they wither away ... languish, and in a short time become much emaciated'. His example is '*Tabes Dorsalis* ... although it hath almost lost its name in this our Age, or perhaps changed it into a Gonorrhœa ... from a distillation into the Spine of the Back'. Here, the morbific matter descends through openings of the vertebral nerves in the spinal marrow causing pain in the loins and back followed by lameness and 'an Atrophy in ... the lower parts'. In this sense, tabes refers to emaciation or wasting through chronic disease. Willis is aware that 'another kind of *Tabes Dorsalis*' follows immoderate use of Venery, the efflux of seed 'defrauding the Brain of its due share' of nervous juice in order constantly to replenish the genital humour, diverting blood 'destined to nourish the Back' towards the testicles. Ever the realist, Willis explains that whereas 'our furious Whoremongers are sensible of a great debility about the Loins ... and the Thighs and legs do chiefly wither away', the efflux of seminal fluid may be involuntary 'by dreams or obscene phantasms'.[187] William Shakespeare (1564–1616) had

[184] See: *Concerning the soul of brutes* (1683): page 164.

[185] See: *Concerning the soul of brutes* (1683): page 163; and Jeremy M Norman, *Morton's medical bibliography*, fifth edition, Aldershot (1991): page 738, entry 4793 referring to *De anima brutorum* (1672): page 397. The identification appears originally in Leslie T Morton, *A medical bibliography*, London (1943): page 262, entry 4105. But, commenting as neurologists, Hierons (1967): page 8 citing EH Hare, 'The origin and spread of dementia paralytica', *Journal of Mental Science* 1959; 105: 594–626, and Spillane (1981): page 71, rightly consider more probable the diagnosis of cerebral arteriosclerosis.

[186] See: Hierons (1967): page 8 citing *Pharmaceutice rationalis* part 1 (1684): page 132, which corresponds to *Pharmaceutice rationalis* part 1 (1679): page 143 where the text is less florid.

[187] See: *Pharmaceutice rationalis* part 2 (1679): pages 28–9; and chapter 18.

already allowed Timon of Athens, addressing rapacious courtesans, to list amongst manifestations of the pox the secondary effects of venereal disease:[188]

> Consumptions sow | In hollow bones of man: strike their sharp shins, | And mar men's sparring ... | And let the unscarr'd braggarts of the war | Derive some pain from you: Plague all; | That your activity may defeat and quell | The source of all erection ....

In dealing with palsy attributable to disease of the medulla and spinal cord, Willis emphasizes compression explaining that, compared to the brain and cerebel, 'either Marrow, and especially the Spinal' are more easily damaged by 'extravasated Blood; or the Corruption flowing from the broken Imposthum, and perhaps a Serous deluge being deposited within the hollowness of the Back-bone; yea also an hard Tumor, being risen somewhere in it, by pressing together the marrowy rope'. He makes the further point that 'either a stroke, wound, or bruise of the Head, or spine; yea a distortion of this latter, do often prevent or break off the Marrowy Tracts'. Willis is making an astute observation about spinal damage secondary to brain disease through herniation from a supraspinal lesion. The medulla and spinal cord are also more likely to suffer from accumulation of deadly particles, 'not only oppilative or stopping, but sometimes *Narcotick* or *Stupefactive* ... and as it were of a *Vitriolock* nature', because the morbific matter must pass through narrower passages than the more tolerant architecture of the brain and streaked bodies. Furthermore, Willis observed isolated peripheral nerve palsies, or possibly conditions in which restricted parts of the spinal cord degenerate before the process becomes more generalized. He writes that, at first, the particles traverse the spinal marrow and selectively disrupt the nerves in their 'beginnings, middle processes, or utmost ends' so that 'the muscles of one side of the Neck are loosened, the other opposite being too much contracted, render the Neck twisted or awry'; or 'some fingers of the Hand, or Toes to the feet' are loosened prior to 'a *Palsie* in the whole Arm or Thigh'.[189]

As with most of his clinical neurology, Willis classifies cases as either accidental, by which he means acute, or habitual, that is chronic and reflecting the cumulative burden of events in the context of a 'Procatartick' disposition. The mechanism, as usual, is the combination of faulty blood and increased transport across the pores of vessels in the brain. Some cases are secondary to another distemper: prolonged fever, long and immoderate sadness, consumption, the scurvy, and old age. Many of these conditions have been addressed in earlier treatises, but Willis expands upon convulsions and colic as harbingers of the palsie. Convulsion and epilepsy may lead 'the motive function being abolished or inhibited, in this or that part, to become at first lame, and then Bed-rid'. Those with 'pains about the Viscera of the Abdomen, cruel and almost continual, at length have wandring pains in their Body and Members, and afterwards stupors or numbness, and lastly resolutions or want of motion'.[190] Other cases follow gout. In all these situations, it is erratic living that precipitates events in those predisposed:[191]

> Drinking thin clear Wine, or strong hot liquors, too much sleep, or too untimely, and idle and sedentary life, immoderate *Venus*, too much loss of blood, a moist Air or Marshie

[188] See: *Timon of Athens*, Act iv, Scene 3, discussed in John Charles Bucknill, *The medical knowledge of Shakespeare*, London (1860): page 250; also cited by Hierons (1967): page 8.

[189] See: *Concerning the soul of brutes* (1683): page 164.

[190] The temptation retrospectively to diagnose porphyria in the case with colick and palsy should be resisted. Spillane (1981): page 71 prefers lead poisoning.

[191] See: *Concerning the soul of brutes* (1683): page 166.

> dwelling, an House new Plastered, Metalick fumes and vapours, frequent use of Narcoticks, or stupefying medicines, or too much taking Tobacco, excess cold, heat, or moisture, vehement and long passions of sadness or fear.

Lest anyone might hope to escape this censure, Willis adds 'with many others, all which wc have not here leisure to recite'. Willis is aware that recovery from palsy may occur in distempers of the brain and nervous stock, but it is bound to be prolonged and probably incomplete. He discusses convalescence from 'Chronical Disease'. In view of what follows, the first ten lines of the paragraph are significant:[192]

> Not only *Scorbutical* persons, but also many others, hardly and long growing well from some *Chronical* Disease, are distemper'd with Members very much loosened from their due vigour and strength, and with a languishing of their Limbs; that though they are well in their stomach, and have a good and laudable Pulse and Urine, yet they are as if they were enervated, and cannot stand upright, and dare scarce enter upon local motions, or if they do, cannot perform them long: yea, some without any notable sickness, are for a long time fixed in their Bed, as if they were everyday about to dye; whilst they lie undisturbed, talk with their Friends, and are chearful, but they will not, nor dare not move or walk; yea, they shun all motion as a most horrid thing.

It is in this context of rehabilitation from illness that Willis describes in the text that follows what has been interpreted as a description of myasthenia gravis. This suggestion was first made by Leonard Guthrie (1858–1918) quoting from *The London practice of physick* (1685). His interpretation was endorsed by Geoffrey Keynes (1887–1982) who, assessing Willis's writings as 'packed with shrewd observations–along with much nonsense', cites the corresponding passages from *Two discourses concerning the soul of brutes* (1683).[193] Appearing to transcribe continuous text, undue emphasis may have been achieved by adding words to link the sections and through judicious reordering of key sentences (as has been done extensively throughout the present book in order to achieve coherence of repetitive and redundant text). Taking Guthrie's sentences in order, the correct sequence (in both English translations), as listed next, is (1), (4), (5), (2), and (3). Context is important and the effect of this marginal sophistry is to remove the point made by Willis that this type of palsy characterizes recovery from chronic illness, or time spent in bed, rather than necessarily constituting the description of a specific palsy. From Guthrie:[194]

> (1) There is another kind [of this Disease] depending on the scarcity of the Spirits in which the motion falls wholly in no Part or Member, yet it is performed but weakly only, or depravedly by any: ... (2) [but] those who being troubled with a scarcity of Spirits, will [force] them as much as they may to local Motions, are able at first rising in the

[192] See: *Concerning the soul of brutes* (1683): page 167, para 3, lines 1–10.

[193] See: Leonard G Guthrie, '"Myasthenia gravis" in the seventeenth century', *Lancet* 1903; i: 330–1; and Sir Geoffrey Keynes, 'The history of myasthenia gravis', *Medical History* 1961: 5; 313–26, reprinted with some modifications as Geoffrey Keynes, 'The history of myasthenia gravis'. In: *Myasthenia gravis*. Ed: Raymond Greene, London (1969): pages 1–13; and also Trevor Hughes. 'The early history of myasthenia gravis, *Neuromuscular Disorders* 2005: 15; 878–86. For a celebrated bibliophile, Keynes is curiously sloppy in referring to Willis's 'three folio volumes from 1683'.

[194] See: Thomas Willis, *The London practice of physick*, London (1685): pages 431–2. This corresponds to *Concerning the soul of brutes* (1683): pages 166–7 where the passages are at: (1) page 166, para 5; lines 4–7; (2) page 267, para 3, lines 7–10; (3) page 267, para 3, lines 14–18; (4) page 267, para 3, lines 18–22; and (5) page 267, para 3, lines 22–4.

> Morning to walk, move their Arms this way and that, or to lift up a weight with strength; but before Noon, the stores of the Spirits which influenc'd the Muscles being almost spent, they are scarce able to move Hand or Foot. (3) I have now a prudent and honest Woman patient who for many years has been obnoxious to this kind of bastard Palsey not only in the Limbs but likewise in her Tongue: This person for some time speaks freely and readily enough, but after long, hasty or laborious speaking presently she becomes mute as a fish, and cannot bring forth a word, and does not recover the use of her Voice till after an hour or two ... (4) Without any considerable sickness, keep their Beds for a long time, as Persons ready to dye; whilst they lye undisturbed they discourse with their Friends, and are chearful, but they neither will, nor dare be raised up, or walk about, nay they abhor all motion as some dreadful thing. (5) The Spirits residing in the Brain are conscious of the Weakness of the others placed in the Members, they refuse to impose local motion on their Companions, as being a task too difficult for them: for which cause the affected are scarce led by any persuasion to try whether they are able to go or not.

There is no reason to think that the case for a description of myasthenia gravis has been enhanced by inaccurate English translation since identical conclusions are reached by consideration of the Latin text:[195]

> Curo iam nunc *fœminam* prudentem, & probam, quæ per plures annos huiuſmodi *ſpuriæ paralyſi* non tantum in *membris* ſed etiam in *linguâ* obnoxia fuit; hæc per tempus quoddam liberè, & expeditè ſatis loquitur, poſt ſermones tamen longos, aut illos feſtinanter, & laborioſè prolatos, illico ſicut piſcis obmuteſcens, amplius *ne gry quidem proloqui* poteſt, porrò nec niſi poſt horam unam, aut alteram vocis uſuram ullam recuperat
>
> [At this moment I am treating a sensible and proper *woman,* who was for several years prone to *pseudo-paralysis* of this kind not only in the *limbs* but also in the *tongue*; for some time she speaks freely and without difficulty, yet after conversations that are long, or hesitatingly and laboriously produced, she is suddenly mute like a fish and can no longer utter even a syllable; next, after not more than one or two hours she regains some control of her voice]

Willis's final comment on this type of palsy restates his concept of the general mechanism of palsy:[196]

> In this kind of spurious *Palsie* arising from the defect, or rather, the weakness of the Animal Spirits, than their obstruction, it may be suspected, that not only the Spirits themselves, as to their first numbers of them, and particular originals, are in fault; but besides, that sometimes the imbecillity and impotency of local motion doth in some measure also depend upon the fault of the explosive Copula suffused everywhere from the blood, into the moving Fibres.

[195] See: *De anima brutorum* (1672): page 406; and Ludo van Bogaert and J Radermecker, 'L evolution de nos connaissances sur la myasthénia de Thomas Willis à Walker', *Acta Neurologica et Psychiatrica Belgica* 1955: 4; 287–308 drawing attention to *De anima brutorum*, Amsterdam (1672): page 288.

[196] See: *Concerning the soul of brutes* (1683): page 167, para 4, lines 1–6.

Taken in isolation, quote (3) here strongly supports Guthrie's interpretation. But without wishing to spoil a good story, if the order is restored as written the account can equally be read as muscular fatigue and weariness developing during the day in those with a recent debilitating disease that is starting to recover. The hazards of retrospective diagnostics are evident. The charge of overly imaginative diagnosis can legitimately be directed at Raymond Hierons who sees in this passage about individuals strong in the morning but weak by noon, not myasthenia gravis but hypokalaemic periodic paralysis.[197] Keynes does not challenge Guthrie's interpretation but does restore order to the quote and points out that this comes within a section on the 'habitual and spurious palsies'.[198] He also mentions a case considered to be ocular myasthenia in the chapter on seeing:[199]

> I knew a young Man, obnoxious to the Palsie, when the drawing in Muscle was strongly drawn, the other Muscles of the left Eye being loose, by reason of the Eye being thus distorted, every object appeared double, nor could he distinguish the true one.

It is instructive that Willis includes sensation in his account of the palsie. He makes the point that, by comparison with disorders affecting structures within the skull, spinal cord disease usually combines motor and sensory deficits:[200]

> Such an hurt of both [motion and sense] together ... sometimes happens, though rarely from the Morbific matter fallen down from the brain into the oblong Marrow, but more often by reason of a grievous hurt of the Spine or Back-bone ... by compressing the marrow cord, or by too much distending or writhing it, all the tracts of the Spirits are blotted out.

On the nerves, Willis writes that loss of sense with preserved motion is seen in 'Lepers, those distemper'd with the *Elephantiasis*, and some Mad-men, who are wont to go naked ... whose skin and musculous flesh are so benumned ... that they feel not the gashes made in their flesh with a Pen-knife, nor needles any where thrust into them'. He concludes that this dissociation is due to the motive and sensory functions being carried in different fibres within the nerve.

Management of the palsie is determined by predictions on prognosis in the various accidental cases, those secondary to another distemper, or patients in whom it is a habitual disease. In accidental and secondary cases, the outcome may improve with bleeding, clysters of horse dung and plaisters applied to weak members, sweats, a suitable diet, and natural remedies. Willis's approach to habitual cases resonates with the generality of his therapeutics for distempers affecting the brain and nervous stock: improve the blood and its nutritious juice, and reduce the entry of morbific matter through the pores of vessels by prophylactic measures especially in the spring and autumn. Bleeding is generally to be avoided. A purge is given 'about the *Æquinox*' and repeated three or four times, together with vomits, cephalicks, and antiscorbuticks. Issues are cut in the arm or leg, especially in obese people, or between the shoulders. 'Wine and Women ought to be forbidden, or but moderately to be used'. But the state of fermentation needs to be assessed and Willis concludes that 'it seems convenient

[197] See: Hierons (1967): page 9

[198] See: *Concerning the soul of brutes* (1683): page 167, para 3, lines 2–10, 14–22, and 22–7.

[199] See: *Concerning the soul of brutes* (1683): page 81; and Keynes (1969): page 2, and Hughes (1991): page 82 for mention of the case but without details of the citation.

[200] See: *Concerning the soul of brutes* (1683): pages 167–8.

that we institute here a double Method of Cure, and two classes of medicine [are needed] of which these may be given to cold Paralyticks, and those to the hot', by which he means the habitual and the accidental cases. Readers who study the double method will detect little difference.[201]

There follow several case histories. These include a man 'beyond the tenth lustre of his age' who became sedentary and with the tendency 'to break forth into weeping and tears, without any manifest occasion. This man a little after ... was distemper'd with an imbecility and trembling of all his members, and then with a resolution [weakness] of the lower parts ... to which Disease ... he dyed within six months'. A young man 'sitting ... after a large supper, and immoderate drinking of wine, was ... distemper'd with ... stupidity in his right hand ... then getting up, and endeavouring to walk, he felt a resolution or loosening in his Thigh and Leg of the same side'. He became dull and confused, lost the vision of that eye,[202] and deteriorated with delirium and convulsions to his death on the eighth day. 'His Head being opened, the anterior cavity of the brain was filled, partly with Ichorous Blood, partly concreted and in clodders or gobbets'. Soon after childbirth, 'a young and handsome Woman' developed fever and abdominal pains with vomiting and a sense of stupefaction followed by tingling and 'the palsie' affecting every member, so 'that she could not move hand nor foot, or the fingers or toes of either'. Brought to Oxford and attended by Willis and 'the noted *Physician* Dr. *Lydell* being also called to our assistance', she developed 'grievous Headach, and *Vertigo* ... with Convulsive Motions' but recovered with mercurial salivation and 'temperate Bathes'. Not so fortunate was the 'mournful catastrophe [which] happened whilst we were writing this': a merchant of London putting his foot out of joint tried the 'temperate Bathes' and persisted despite advice to cease as a result of which he became weak 'from the *Os sacrum* to his Feet [which] withered away' together with abdominal distension and progressively weak respiratory muscles causing dyspnoea from which he died.[203]

Delirium and phrensie

In the final chapters of *De anima brutorum* (1672), Willis considers distempers of the head in which the fault is with the rational soul. Imagination and memory are 'deformed, distracted one from another, and very confused'. The brain, 'evilly affected', represents to itself, by reflection, 'monsters from a multiplying or distorted Glass'.

Delirium is a symptom likened to 'going crooked' as in drunkenness. The animal spirits becoming tumultuous in the Callous body or middle of the brain, the parts responsible for intellect and imagination, pass 'incongruous and absurd *phantasies* to the Rational Soul ... all the spirits leap forth at once ... like mad *Bacchanals*'. Carried into openings of the nerves, this contagious chaos of the spirits leads to 'incongruous speeches, absurd gestures of the body, and members'.[204] The mechanism of delirium is the now familiar immoderate heating of the blood or presence of morbific matter, and opening of pores in the vessels. Delirium may also arise from a primary deficiency of animal spirits without abnormality of the blood. But Willis's logic is confused for, in this context, he adds the use of emeticks, colic, ulcer, and

201 See: *Concerning the soul of brutes* (1683): pages 169–74.

202 This presumably was a right homonymous hemianopia.

203 See: *Concerning the soul of brutes* (1683): pages 174–8. These two cases provide an adventure playground for retrospective diagnosis by any competent neurologist.

204 See: *Concerning the soul of brutes* (1683): page 179.

gangrene amongst causes arising from the brain. More easily understood is that delirium occurs in diseases such as plague or smallpox, and others resulting in fever, and from poisons especially 'the furious night-shade, *Mandrakes*, and some other plants'. Willis relates the case of a family in which entering the house of a gentleman, an acquaintance found the 'Mistress of the Family, her Daughters, and all her maids (except one) ... Delirious' after eating roots of wild Parsnips.[205]

The discussion of delirium allows Willis to make an important point on the evolution of disease. He has developed the general concept, applied in several other contexts and to which he often returns, that transient events are tolerated whereas those that are habitual leave permanent architectural traces. In the case of delirium, because 'none of their wandring tracts are imprinted in the Brain, the Delirium soon passes'. Whilst the prognosis from a first episode is good, recurrent bouts, whatever their cause, may lead to '*Carus, Apoplexy*, or *Palsie*'.[206]

Not to be confused with paraphrensie, a disorder of the diaphragm which may occur with or without cerebral symptoms, the phrensie is a primary disorder of the animal spirits. Agitated and unruly, these allow:[207]

> Ideas of things raised up out of the Memory, the old confounded with the new, and some evilly joined, or wonderfully divided, are confounded with others, the imagination suggests manifold Phantasms ... the common sensory represents the images of sensible things distorted, double or incongruent ... the mind and will ... pick out nothing but ridiculous and impertinent conceptions.

The phrensie has long since been considered to arise from inflammation of the meninges. For Willis, this is not logical since he has opened the heads of those with meningeal swellings who had no phrensie in life; and compression of the brain from inflamed meninges would act to compress, not liberate, the unruly animal spirits in the callous body and midriff of the brain. Since spirits in the cerebellum are also affected, contaminating the openings of their dependent nerves, 'Frantick people not only talk idly, but breathe unequally, speak aloud, strike with their fists, fling about their hands and feet'. In short, the phrensie is a 'burning or inflammation of the whole sensitive soul'. The animal spirits receive sulphurous incendiary matter from the blood, providing constant fuel if the brain is receptive through being loose and its pores opened up. Constituents of the blood, sulphur to burn and salt to increase access through the vessels, and a brain too hot and dry, create the procatartick state in which episodes are precipitated by fevers, excess eating and drinking, and 'violent passions, as of Love, hatred, envie, indignation, or sadness; or immoderate studies'. The prognosis is generally good unless the animal spirits 'contract a vicious nature' or the pores of the brain are unduly perverted, in which case:[208]

> A perpetual raving succeeds ... passing into Madness, or Melancholy, or foolishness or stupidity. Wherefore it is vulgarly said of those that are Frantick, and not soon cured, that their Brains are crack'd or broken, so that after that, they are always mad or raving.

[205] *Pastinaca sativa* is a member of the *Apiaceae* family related to carrot and parsley. It is not usually toxic but the sap contains furanocoumarins which can blister skin exposed to sunlight.

[206] See: *Concerning the soul of brutes* (1683): page 181.

[207] See: *Concerning the soul of brutes* (1683): page 182.

[208] See: *Concerning the soul of brutes* (1683): page 185.

Treatment is with phlebotomy, leeches, cupping, clysters and emetics, purges, hypnoticks, narcoticks, and much else besides, selected from Willis's rich pharmacopoeia. One case history suffices to illustrate his concept of the inflamed soul. A maid, confined to bed by fever and 'highly raging', is given clysters and emeticks but continues for several days 'furious perpetually calling and bauling for cold drink'. This does not help so that, it being summer time, Willis suggests:[209]

> In the middle of the Night, she should be carried by Women forth of doors, and put into a Boat, and her Cloths being pull'd off, and she tyed fast with a Cord, should be drenched into the depth of a River, the Rope being tyed only about her middle, that she might not be stifled in the Water; but there was no need of that, for the Maid of her own accord, fell to swimming, that scarce any Man could do better who had learned the art: After about a quarter of an hour, she came forth of the Water sound, and sober, and then being had to Bed, she slept, and sweat very much, and afterwards, without any other remedy she grew well.

Attributing this to the water having cooled her blood, Willis offers no further comment on whether this was an example of the phrensie following fever, or an hysterical passion.

Melancholy

Melancholy is 'a raving without Feavour or fury, joined with fear and sadness'. Amongst the melancholic, Willis includes people who bark or howl, thinking themselves dogs, wolves 'or some Monster'; others who imagine themselves dead, asking to be buried; and those who conclude that their bodies are made of glass and so afraid to be touched 'lest they should be broke to pieces'. Willis distinguishes universal melancholy from the special type in which fear of an event or loss of 'some good before obtained' leads to a morbid preoccupation, so that the activities of the corporeal soul are neglected and the affected person 'omits all domestick care either of itself, or of the Body, or of the Rational Soul'. Amongst the circumstances which provoke melancholy are 'chiefly *furious Love*, *Jealousie*, *Superstition*, *despair of Eternal Salvation*, and lastly *imaginary metamorphosis* of the Body or its parts'. The minds of the melancholic are never at rest, always ruminating on the same topic, and taking their deformed 'hobgoblins' out of proportion 'so that all things seem to them great and difficult'.[210]

Willis cannot agree with those who regard melancholy as primarily a splenetic or choleric disorder of the viscera, or uterine in origin. Rather, it is a condition both of the brain and heart: 'for as Melancholick people talk idly ... but as they become very sad and tearful, this is deservedly attributed to the Passion of the Heart'. Sadness and fear depend upon stagnation and agitation, respectively, of blood in the præcordium and failure of its fermentation in the heart. As a result of the heat being 'blown out with every blast of wind ... *Melancholicks* rarely have a Feavour'. Ultimately, the fault lies with animal spirits in the brain becoming obscure, thick and dark through excess acidity, rather than maintaining the transparent, subtle and lucid properties of spirits rich in sulphur and saline. Willis takes the opportunity of once more stating his concept of the alterations in brain structure that characterize chronic brain disease. The rogue spirits are in a state of perpetual motion and their vices are 'not only to be

[209] See: *Concerning the soul of brutes* (1683): page 187.
[210] See: *Concerning the soul of brutes* (1683): page 188.

carried in open ways, but to cut new Porosities in the neighbouring bodies, and to insinuate themselves into them'. Once more the carving of aberrant pathways is the basis for many habitual distempers of the brain, of which the melancholick distemper is but one example:[211]

> Beginning ... from the Acetous disposition of the Spirits, yet afterwards, the conformation of the Brain it self is often brought to be part of the cause; to wit, forasmuch as the Recrements of the *Melancholick* Blood, being perpetually poured forth, renders its substance more thick and dark, and the primary Tracts or paths of the Animal Function being near blotted out, new, oblique, and by-paths are made; insomuch, that the Spirits, though better should be forgotten, could not easily irradiate the Brain, or presently recover their former passages.

It follows from Willis's analysis that, being of the brain and heart, melancholy has very many antecedent causes within the framework of 'Sacred, or, Magical, or, Humane' conditions, of which those impinging on the practice of medicine are the 'Religious, Amorous, and Jealous *Melancholy*'. It is self-evident that melancholy often starts with assaults on the 'Animal Government' from 'destroying Love, vehement sadness, panick fears, envy, shame, care and immoderate study'. Less obvious is the influence of lack of exercise, reduction in 'usual evacuations, as of the Menstrual Blood ... also the Seed being suddenly suppressed', and bleeding haemorrhoids. Willis also points out that 'some are made obnoxious to this Disease from their Parents'.[212]

Only in prefacing his remarks on treatment does Willis give any hint that the melancholy is anything other than a material disturbance of the blood and brain: 'There is scarce any better thing to be expected from them who lying sick with only imaginary Diseases, take all Remedies, and require still more, and of diverse kinds to be given them'. But not for the first time, in his consideration of melancholy, does Willis straddle the boundary between the material and the immaterial, the corporeal and the rational souls. Whereas the nature of love and jealousy require no special consideration, it is significant that despair of salvation must represent a defect of the rational, and hence immaterial, soul. This enforces material manifestations on the corporeal soul setting up a continual skirmish, the animal spirits 'drawn hither and thither' eventually succumbing to delirium or idle raving, as the corporeal soul 'assumes a new image, either Angelical or Diabolical'; and the intellect 'because the Imagination furnishes it only with undecent and monstrous notions, is wholly perverted from the right use of reason'.[213]

Whilst acute episodes may resolve, recurrent cases of melancholy pass into 'Stupidity, or Foolishness, and sometimes also into Madness; further, sometimes it brings on Convulsive Distempers, or the *Palsie*, or *Apoplexy*, yea sometimes a violent Death'.[214] Management is by replacing troublesome passions with those composed to 'chearfulness and joy'; and in place of 'mad Love, Jealousie, Sorrow, Pity, Hatred, fear and the like ... pleasant talk, or jesting, Singing, Musick, Pictures, Dancing, Hunting, Fishing, and other pleasant exercises'. Should these diversions not suit the temperament of the melancholic person, there is always 'Mathematicks and Chymical Studies, also travelling ... [and] Those who will stay at home ... should build Houses, plant and order Gardens, Orchards, or Till the ground'. In

[211] See: *Concerning the soul of brutes* (1683): page 191.
[212] See: *Concerning the soul of brutes* (1683): page 192.
[213] See: *Concerning the soul of brutes* (1683): page 200.
[214] See: *Concerning the soul of brutes* (1683): page 193.

short, anything that distracts the mind and 'at last deserts more easily, vain and mad cogitations ... [and] the Animal Spirits, being called outwards, may be solicited from their diversions, into their former and accustomed tracts'. These practical measures failing, recourse is to bleeding, purging, and emetics taken as concoctions, syrups, pills, powders or boluses, hypnoticks, and the use of spaw-waters or bathing in sweet water 'to wipe away the filth in the Pores of the skin'.[215]

Madness

Madness is an extension of melancholy: 'These two, like smoke and flame, mutually receive and give place one to another.' The distemper is characterized by phantasies constantly busied with impetuous thoughts so that 'night and day they are muttering to themselves various things, or declare them by ... bauling out loud'. Their notions and conceptions are incongruous 'or represented to them under a false or erroneous image'. And madmen have 'Audaciousness and Fury, contrary to melancholicks, who are always infected with fear and sadnesses'.[216] The mad shun no dangers, and attempt the most improbable and difficult tasks. They are strong 'so that they can break chains and cords, break down doors or walls'. Mad men never tire 'although playing mad pranks ... without sleep or eating'. They 'bear cold, heat, watching, fasting, strokes, and wounds, without any sensible hurt'.

As always, the blood is at fault, both for hereditary and acquired reasons: 'men born of Parents that used sometimes to be mad, are obnoxious to the same disease, and though they have lived above thirty or forty years prudent and sober ... the morbid seeds do ripen into fruit ... *Hereditary Madness* is sometime continual, and sometimes intermitting'. Poor diet may convert those 'at first sad ... and after a little Mad'. Other causes include 'the biting of Mad animals, or by the taking of some poisons'. We read of a certain Gentleman who ate leaves of Wolfs-bane [aconite], in a Sallad with other herbs' and feared madness which duly came to pass for 'he fell into Madness, and dyed in a night's space'.[217] The animal spirits may be thrown into confusion following a violent passion after a solitary event: those 'seeing a true or an imaginary Spectre or Ghost, afterwards fall into a perpetual Madness'. Others 'being first highly troubled in mind, anon become Mad' after breaking oaths or vows, 'some notable disgrace or repulse', through despair or guilty conscience, and 'Ambition, Pride, and Emulation have made some mad'.

The morbid influence of blood on the brain is clear from the overly saline and sulphurous nature of the animal spirits, likened to the '*Stygian*-Water', in madness. As with melancholy, the particles carve out new passages in the brain, 'new little spaces or walks, and plainly devious ... quickly passing thorow the frame of the Brain and its Appendix, cause the distemper'd not only to be furious but, as it were Demoniacks and possessed with the Devil'. The acidic nature of the spirits is evident from the case of 'a certain Noble Man, grievously obnoxious to distempers of the Brain and Nerves, whose sweat (when he was in a fit [of madness]) presently eat thorow his shirt ... as if it had been dipped in *Aqua sortis*'.[218]

[215] See: *Concerning the soul of brutes* (1683): page 194.

[216] See: *Concerning the soul of brutes* (1683): page 201. Spillane (1981): pages 73–4 summarizes these as Willis's description of anxiety.

[217] See: *Concerning the soul of brutes* (1683): page 204.

[218] See: *Concerning the soul of brutes* (1683): pages 202–3. Having launched on acid spirits and Stygian water, Willis is then distracted into an account of how '*Scirrhous*, *strumous* or *Cancrous* Tumors' are formed.

Whereas cases that follow some event or concurrent illness improve, hereditary madness and that following the bite of a mad dog are 'not at all to be cured'; and those with recurrent episodes, 'about Midsummer, or when the Dog Star arises, are in great danger'. More than physick, management requires the mad man being placed in 'a House convenient for the business' and restrained by 'warnings, chidings, punishments' in a 'strait room' so that they 'stand in awe of such as they think their Tormentors'. Should this fail, blood-letting, cupping, clysters, blisters, purges and emetics are to be used, together with specific remedies including the purple flower of the pimpernel and the tops of St John's wort. Willis dutifully mentions that others have advocated opening an artery, trepanning, and applying 'the hot Lungs of a Lamb' to the shaven head. Rather than describing individual cases, he recommends the curious to visit:[219]

> *Hospitals* of Mad people . . . where they may behold . . . a new and monstrous nation of men, contrary to rational people, and as it were our Antipodes; all which, if they were gathered together in one place, and that all, Madmen and Fools were joined to them; I know not whether the world would not be equally divided between them and the sober and prudent.

Stupidity or foolishness

In writing on foolishness and stupidity, Willis uses terms that might be considered synonymous but, although repeatedly careless in maintaining the differences and often blurring the distinction, his intention is to distinguish two quite separate conditions:[220]

> Those afflicted with *Foolishness* apprehend simple things well enough, dextrously and swiftly, and retain them firm in their memory, but by reason of a defect of judgment, they compose or divide their notions evilly, and very badly infer one thing from another; moreover, by their folly, and acting sinistrously and ridiculously, they move laughter in the bystanders. On the contrary, those who are *Stupid*, by reason of the defect of the Imagination and Memory, as well as the Judgment, do neither apprehend well, or quickly, nor argue well; besides they behave themselves not as the others by toying and gesticulation, but sottishly, foolishly, or like a dull Ass; so that the simplicity of these is the more miserable, who shew so the Disease in their countenance and behaviour.

Stupidity can be gauged in terms of the ability, or not, to engage with certain activities. The reference to letters indicates that even in an age that did not aspire to universal education, inability to read and write was considered abnormal and one level of stupidity:[221]

> Fools in the learning of letters or the liberal Sciences, are yet able enough for the *Mechanical Arts*. Others of either of these incapable, yet easily comprehend *Agriculture*, or Husbandry and Country business. Others unfit almost for all affairs are able only to learn what belongs to eating or the common means of living; Others merely *Dolts* or drivling Fools, scarce understand any thing at all, or do any thing knowingly.

[219] See: *Concerning the soul of brutes* (1683): page 208.
[220] See: *Concerning the soul of brutes* (1683): page 212.
[221] See: *Concerning the soul of brutes* (1683): page 212.

Taking the view that Willis's contributions to psychiatry in *De anima brutorum* had not been fully appreciated, Paul Cranefield (1925–2003) considered the chapter '*Of stupidity, or Foolishness*' a treasury of clinical astuteness. He transcribed Pordage's translation in its entirety including the marginal notes.[222] Cranefield summarizes Willis's analysis of foolishness, 'stultitia', as characterizing individuals with preserved comprehension and memory but defective judgement, poor reasoning, and inferences, and awkward social behaviour inciting ridicule. Conversely stupidity, 'stupiditas', comprises defective apprehension and judgement, poor memory, and simplicity in appearance and behaviour. Cranefield sees in Willis's account of foolishness a description of schizophrenia, whereas stupidity equates to mental deficiency.[223] This formulation distinguishes the social disruption of foolishness with preserved intellect from the defective memory and simple behaviour of stupidity; but for all the superficial clarity of this distinction it is unfortunate that Willis uses the terms interchangeably. Although *Cerebri anatome* (1664) is primarily an account of normal brain anatomy, in Figura IV (Pl.4) Willis included the depiction and description in the legend of a child with hydrocephalus, described as foolish but who would more neatly match the features of stupidity:[224]

> The Effigies of an humane Brain of a certain Youth that was foolish from his birth, and of that sort which are commonly called Changelings; the bulk of whose brain, as it was thinner and lesser than is usual, its border could be farther lifted up and turned back, that all the more interior parts might be more deeply beheld together.

Willis mentions that a disturbance of the passions, unexpected fright or vehement sadness, may cause 'Sottishness or Foolishness'; and foolishness may accompany the many diseases of the head described in the earlier chapters of *De anima brutorum*. But most of his comments on causation relate to stupidity. Despite temperate living, this may first affect with age those 'at first crafty and ingenious'. Injuries to the head in falling from a high place lead to stupidity, as do drunkenness, overeating and the use of opiates. At whatever age it develops and whatever the cause, stupidity is almost never healed. But Willis soon forgets the distinctions and, once again, the categories of foolishness and stupidity are merged.

Hereditary influences are important. Willis explains that 'wise men and highly ingenious may beget fools or changelings because, given too much to study, reading and meditation, the animal spirits place the supply from blood in such high demand that 'but few only, and small, are permitted to descend to the *Spermatick* Bodies'. Equally, parents who have dissipated themselves with intemperance, luxury, and evil manners' may beget 'languishing and unhealthy Children', as are often those born of 'Parents broken of old age, or of such as are not yet ripe or too young, or of drunkards, soft, and effeminate men', and those that have a weakened brain from '*Palsie, Epilepsie, Carus, Convulsions*, and the like'. In short 'to be born of Parents who have a sound mind in a sound body, is far beyond a large patrimony'.[225]

[222] See: Paul Cranefield, 'A seventeenth century view of mental deficiency and schizophrenia; Thomas Willis on stupidity or foolishness', *Bulletin of the History of Medicine* 1961: 35; 291–316, with reprinting of chapter XIII from *Concerning the soul of brutes* (1683). Cranefield acknowledges as the only survey of the entire book, J Vinchon and J Vie, 'Un maître de la neuropsychiatrie au XVIIe siècle: Thomas Willis (1662 [*sic*]–1675), *Annales Médico-Psychologiques* 1928: 2; 108–44.

[223] See: Cranefield (1961): page 313. Here Cranefield compares word for word Willis and Paul Eugen Bleuler (1857–1939), who coined the term 'schizophrenia'. Cranefield finds too close a similarity for comfort in the Swiss psychiatrist and eugenicist's phraseology questioning the priority of this 'original' description.

[224] See chapters 3 and 16 for further details.

[225] See: *Concerning the soul of brutes* (1683): page 211.

That said, Willis emphasizes how some children who are dull and slow to learn later become young men of great wit; and sagacious children who 'by their literature and discourse have caused admiration' may became dull and heavy young men. Offering somewhat risky stereotypes, Willis explains that:[226]

> Those that are born of Plowmen and Rusticks ... hence in some Families, reckoning many descents backwards, there is scarce one witty man or wife found. In some places, the influences of the Heaven and Air incline ... the Inhabitants to Stupidity; so to be born in *Batavia*, is proverbially, as much as to say, a Fool.

'*Stupidity* or *Morosis*, or Foolishness' is a disorder of animal spirits in the brain: 'although it chiefly belongs to the Rational Soul, and signifies a defect of the Intellect and Judgment, yet it is not improperly reckoned among the Diseases of the Head or Brain; for as much as this *Eclipse* of the superior soul, proceeds from the Imagination and the Memory being hurt, and the failing of these depends upon the faults of the Animal Spirits, and the Brain it self'.[227] In stupidity, 'being obtuse and dull of their own proper nature', encountering a brain that is also hostile to movement the spirits 'cannot exercise themselves rightly, for the performing the offices of the Animal regiment'. The sulphurous animal spirits are depressed and 'almost drowned and overwhelmed with the watery and terrestrial' particles. Alternatively, the structure of the brain may be primarily at fault both in stupidity and foolishness, as is apparent from the size and shape of the head: 'for as to its bulk, it is a Proverb, that it argues little of Brain or too much Foolishness ... in a little Brain but a few spirits are begotten and exercised; but in a greater, consisting for the most part of a vile or base texture or frame, it is less fitted for the quickness or sharpness of the mind'.[228] The flow of spirits is impeded in those with a flat head, 'or otherwise improportionate'; and when the texture of the brain is moist and cold, 'too thick, and Earthy', limiting the ability of the spirits to 'cut tracts for themselves'.

As for treatment: 'it must be the work both of a *Physician* and *Teacher*, that the wit of such that are so affected, may be somewhat trimmed, and they being at least brought to the use of reason in a little measure, may be accounted out of the number of *Brutes*'. The frequent care of a Master is needed 'because dull or senseless Beetles, or the more dull Loggerheads or Blockheads, do not readily learn the common notion of things, no more than Children the first element of letters ... and the same things are again and again to be inculcated in them' in order to sharpen the spirits by 'perpetual exercise', so that they can cut tracts and passages in the brain.[229] Education apart, treatment is phlebotomy, purges and trepanning. As for diet, a morning draught of coffee with boiled sage leaves, or chocolate is recommended.

Pain

De anima brutorum (1672) concludes with chapters on gout and colic on the basis that, because these are painful conditions, their seats are in the brain. Perhaps a disorder of the periostea, tendons, or ligaments, Willis argues that gout cannot result from distemper of the blood, for there is no fever; or of the nerves supplying the affected parts because the pain is

[226] See: *Concerning the soul of brutes* (1683): page 210.
[227] See: *Concerning the soul of brutes* (1683): page 209.
[228] See: *Concerning the soul of brutes* (1683): page 209.
[229] See: *Concerning the soul of brutes* (1683): page 213.

only felt locally in the joints. Rather it is the meeting of several aberrant humours, some from the blood and others of the brain (as in the mechanism of muscular motion), which excite pricking and provocation, the 'Vellications [twitchings] or pullings of the nervous Fibres'.[230] Not for the first time, Willis's imagery is of the feminine seed of disease planted by the blood, 'like an Egg without a Cock; until the nervous liquor growing turgent . . . as it were the masculine seed, renders the other prolifick'.

There follows a detailed consideration of the unsatisfactory balance of particles in the blood and nervous juice generating the 'Morbific Mine' that gathers in the pores of the joints. Either hereditary or the result of an 'evil manner of living' in those who indulge in 'inordinate eating and drinking . . . on salt and spiced meats, and guzzle down great plenty of Wine . . . and sleep at noon', gout is precipitated by combination of the morbific matter with the overly acidic nervous juice. This much is evident from the premonitory symptoms of headache and vertigo. Gout is seasonal and related to the weather, thereby explaining the 'Proverb, That *Gouty* persons carry their *Almanack* in their joints'.[231]

Treatments are as expected—blood-letting, purges, emetics and botanical extracts, bathing the affected part in saltwater—but with some less usual remedies: 'the poultice of the fresh dung of a Cow applied warm'; and 'to drink every Morning their own Urine; which I know has been beneficial to some'. This did prove helpful for 'A very learned and Pious Man of this Nation, and also the glory of learned Men, Dr. *H.H*' until he suffered 'a total suppression of Urine [so that] in about a fortnights time this reverend Gentleman dyed', autopsy being consistent with the interpretation that, through imbibing urine, 'the Disease of the *Gout* was changed into the mortal Disease of the *Stone*'.[232]

The pain of colick, arising from the 'hauling or notable pulling of some parts of the *Abdomen*', is often preceded by 'a *Vertiginous* Distemper of the Head . . . and at length ends in the *Palsie*'. As the name indicates, the condition is assumed to originate in the colon irritated by 'wind, medicines, Choler, and perhaps other humors, contained within their cavities'. Yet it may increase despite 'those things which loosen the Belly, and draw forth plentifully the wind, and the dregs or *Feces*'. To Willis, it seems improbable that the various places in which pains of the colic are experienced can all be attributed to the large intestine or the effects of a single humor. Although not primarily a disorder due to stopping up the origins of the wandring nerve, rather it is a distemper in which 'the dolorifick matter', fixed in the part experiencing discomfort, arises from the heaping up of particles from the brain discharged through the wandring nerve or spinal marrow. Therefore, much as with the gout:[233]

> We shall suppose, that for a Seed-plot or Mine of the *Colick* Distemper, some Recrements of the nervous humor fallen from the Brain, thorow the Nerves, and slid down into the *Mesentery*, and other infoldings of the *Abdomen*, are there heaped up . . . [and] grows hot or ferments with a *Saline fixed* humor, poured forth thither, from the Blood . . . till the hot or Fermentative matter being shaken off, or pressed forth into the cavities of the *Intestines*, is at length overcome.

Having come this far, readers of *De anima brutorum* will not be surprised by Willis's account of causes, accidental and habitual; prognosis, dependent on resolving the underlying

[230] See: *Concerning the soul of brutes* (1683): page 215.
[231] See: *Concerning the soul of brutes* (1683): page 219.
[232] See: *Concerning the soul of brutes* (1683): page 224.
[233] See: *Concerning the soul of brutes* (1683): page 227.

provocative condition, abdominal organ affected, or procatartick disposition; and treatment with clysters, fomentations, 'the Caul of a Lamb or the Lungs, or the Inwards of any other Beast, being laid warm to the Belly', hypnoticks, purges (given in small doses), emetics, mercurial salivations, sudorificks, opiates, and baths.[234] These principles are set out in the account of three cases of whom two were cured. But a 'Reverend old Man' accustomed to the colick:[235]

> Suffer'd about his throat a resolution of loosning in the Muscles serving for swallowing, which troubled him oftentimes, so that he was in danger to be choaked by food, and chiefly by liquid things sticking in that place ... the Recrements of the nervous liquor, that were wont to be deposed about the nervous Infoldings of the *Abdomen* ... getting another nest for themselves about the *Ganglioform* nervous Infoldings of the Throat, brought in the resolution or short Palsie of the *Oesophagus*; and lastly, by reason of the same matter restagnating in too great a plenty in the middle part of the Brain, that deadly senselessness followed.

A Victorian perspective on Willis's contributions to the nature of brain and mind

There are many admirers of Willis's contributions to diseases of the brain and nervous stock but, as with all of his works, the most severe criticism of *De anima brutorum* came from Michael Foster (1836–1907).[236] Pedantic in the extreme, Foster distorts Willis's account of the relationship between the corporeal and rational souls of man and attributes to him the belief that all 'the nervous as well as other phenomena both of animals and man may be regarded as the phenomena of a corporeal machine'. Willis may have been less of a dualist than Descartes, who Foster praises, but blinkered materialist he was not. For Foster:

> Willis's mind was of that sort which when it has hit on an illustration or discovered an analogy, thinks it has found a proof. And the great discovery was simply this, that the part of the soul residing in the blood was of the nature of 'flame', and the part residing in the brain and nervous system was of the nature of 'light'.

Foster reproduces several passages from Willis. But in condemning these, he is obtuse in reading the text as literal and seems resistant to the use of metaphor or the qualifiers, 'as it were', 'as', 'like' which Willis inserts throughout all his texts when trying to explain his iatrochemical concepts. As printed by Foster (adopting modern typesetting practices and paraphrasing from the original):[237]

> The corporeal soul common to man and higher animals while it extends over the whole organic body and vivifies, actuates and irradiates every part, both tissues and humours, yet seems more eminently to subsist in two of these, and to hold them as its imperial seats as it were. These subjects of the soul are on the one hand the vital fluid, the blood, circulated in

[234] See: *Concerning the soul of brutes* (1683): page 229–33.
[235] See: *Concerning the soul of brutes* (1683): page 233.
[236] See: Michael Foster, *Lectures on the History of Physiology*, Cambridge (1901): pages 268–80.
[237] See: Foster (1901): page 272.

> a perpetual round in the heart, arteries and veins, and on the other the animal fluid or nervous juice streaming gently through the brain and its belongings. Both these provinces the soul inhabits and adorns with its presence, but since the whole soul cannot be in both provinces at the same time, it is as it were divided, it actuates each province by its appropriate half. One of its halves, since it is as we have shewn of the nature of fire, glides into the blood after the fashion of a heated flame, while the other half seems diffused through the animal after the manner of light, like the rays of light emanating from that flame, rays which taken up by the brain and the nerves as by dioptic glasses and manifoldly reflected or refracted, form various figures according to the workings of the animal faculties. The animal soul therefore, corresponding to its dual chief functions in the animal body, consists of two distinct parts, namely, flame and light; for as regards the functions called natural, these are in truth only involuntary animal functions and are carried out by the aid of animal spirits.

Foster then supports his case by an analysis of Willis's treatise on fermentation in which, unlike the rigid position taken on the corporeal soul, he allows some freedom and agreement that Willis had in mind 'many sound physiological views': on the diverse functions of the blood, the supply of nutrients to the brain, the transport of particles from one organ to 'appropriate emunctories', access to air and food in order to maintain life, and excretion including in sweat through the skin. Foster even relaxes his position on the problem that the flame in the blood is not visible. Nevertheless, 'Willis had no great critical power in judging the value of evidence, and he was led to this idea of the flame in the blood, more by the force of simile than by reasoning on facts'. But on the matter of light in the brain, Foster is less easily reconciled, quoting Willis (again, somewhat inaccurately):[238]

> The animal spirits, vanishing directly that life is extinct, leave no trace of themselves behind. Wherefore we may far more rightly, according to our hypothesis, say that these spirits emitted from the flame of the blood, are like rays of light, at least these joined with those of wind and air. For just as light is moulded to the impressions of all visible things, and air is moulded to the impressions of all audible things, so the animal spirits receive the images impressed on them, not only of the above, but also the odours and all tangible qualities, and deposit them in the common sensorium.

Acknowledging that Willis knew nothing of electricity and nerve conduction, Foster reprimands him for explaining the functions of the brain, including the sensitive soul, on the basis of light and optical images:

> It seems allowable to conceive of the middle regions of the brain as constituting an inner chamber of this soul fitted with dioptric mirrors, as with windows. The pictures or images of all sensible things admitted into these secret places by means of the ducts of the nerves, as by means of tubes or narrow openings, first pass through the corpora striata, which serves the purpose of an objective glass, and then are represented on the corpus callosum as on a whitened wall. And so the things which give rise to sensation induce perception and a certain imagination. These images or pictures thus formed there very often produce nothing but the mere knowledge or sensation of the object, but presently or at times having passed on, as it were by a second undulation from the corpus callosum towards the cortex

[238] See: Foster (1901): page 274; and *Concerning the soul of brutes* (1683): pages 22, 24 for the correct quotes.

of the brain, and being stored in its folds, give rise to the memory of the thing, though the mere image vanishes.

Eventually Foster expresses some sympathy with Willis in trying to explain all the phenomena of brute beasts, lacking the rational soul of man, on the basis of reflex function and the corporeal soul. After quoting the passage explaining that sensation may rebound and initiate a reflected movement:

> We have not, however, as yet stated how this soul or some part of it *perceives that it feels*, and in accordance with that *perception* is driven into various *passions* and *actions*, is turned to the *desire* of this or that object, and sometimes, as we may at times observe in certain beasts, in following up the thing sought for, enters upon and carries out acts which seem to have no other source than *judgment* and a *certain deliberation*. Of course in man we can readily understand that the *rational soul*, the governor as it were, looks upon the images and impressions presented to the rational soul as to a mirror, and according to the conceptions and notions thus derived exercises the acts of *reason*, *judgment* and *will*. In what way however in brute beasts, perception, the discrimination of objects, desire, memory and other forms of so to speak lower reason, are carried out seems very difficult of explanation.

Foster ends his critique by turning to John Mayow (1640–1679) for support of the criticism that light serves as a metaphor for the workings of the brain and the souls of brutes and man:

> Much less are we to suppose that such an intense heating of the blood takes place as to be strong enough to give rise to light, the rays of which, transmitted to the brain, are to be thought to form the sensitive soul ... I ask how it comes about that the light which is supposed to illuminate the whole brain and all the nerves can never be seen by the eye? Assuredly Fires of this kind and New Lights no less in Anatomy than in Religion appear to me things wholly vain and fanatic.

With time, this harsh Victorian insistence on literal interpretation of what was intended as a metaphor has softened. Fire in the blood and light in the brain have evolved into the concepts of metabolism and nerve conduction. Willis's description of involuntary reflective movement is accepted as an early account of the brain as a reflex organ that learns and adapts. Reconciling within a unifying analysis the material and explicable with the immaterial and mysterious, whilst avoiding censure and not undermining his belief in the brain as the organ of mind, was indeed hazardous but makes *De anima brutorum* a foundational work in medicine. Despite ambiguities and the occasional blurring of definitions and distinctions, Willis's writings on psychology and the phenomenology of neurological and psychiatric disease are original, insightful and wise. In drawing together the many threads from his earlier treatises, justifiably this book can be considered the 'crown of the work'.

18

'To practice medicine with a safe conscience'

Rational therapeutics

***Pharmaceutice rationalis* part 1 (1674) and part 2 (1675); *The London practice of physick* (1685); *A plain and easie method* (1691); and *Dr Willis's receipts for the cure of all distempers* (1701).**

Of all Willis's writings, that which seems most remote from present day medicine is his treatise on rational therapeutics. And yet, no clearer account of the therapeutic strategies and combination of medicines and management used routinely in seventeenth-century England could be given. Sceptical readers learning of Willis's claims for the success of his remedies and the survival of his tolerant patients may reasonably conclude that nature is a wonderful healer. The theme that runs through these treatises is Willis's concept that vitality is dependent on healthy nutrition, respiration, fermentation, circulation, and excretion. It follows that mechanism-based therapeutics of disease must address one or other of these disordered processes, usually in combination. Willis's pharmacopoeia is entirely rational in the context of the ideas he held. It incorporates advice on lifestyle together with the use of botanical remedies and the products of chemical laboratories. In detailing his ideas, Willis uses numerical classification. He lists 'first, second, thirdly' in advance of more detailed exposition within each category, often further separating each section into several more divisions. For all this sense of organization, Willis has not edited or reworked his text. Once more, it is repetitive and sometimes contradictory. But if most of the specific remedies are no longer used, the two parts of *Pharmaceutice rationalis* (1674 and 1675: in English, 1679) are important for setting out principles of therapeutics, not all of which are now merely of historical interest. Furthermore, he makes several contributions to knowledge on anatomy of the lungs, arteries, and stomach; and provides original descriptions of disease affecting structures other than the brain and nervous stock.

As before, Willis has not worked alone. He has been assisted by 'the sedulous labour of my most learned friend Dr. *Edmund King*, and to his most dexterous Dissections'; and 'also my Friend Doctor *Masters* hath set to his helping Hand, in the finishing of this Task'. Conscious that he has previously not been systematic when making reference to treatments and their effects in individual cases, Willis explains that he now intends to explain matters in a logical sequence. But he needs to proceed cautiously:[1]

> When I consider that I must Sail in a dangerous Sea, everywhere full of Rocks of censures and Contumelies, I think it no Wisdom to venture my whole Cargo at once in this weak

[1] See: Thomas Willis, *Pharmaceutice rationalis or an exercitation of the operations of medicines in humane bodies shewing the signs, causes, and cures of most distempers incident thereunto*, part 1, London (1679): preface, page [8]. Throughout this chapter, the English translation from 1679 has been used rather than Pordage's later version from 1681.

> Bottom, but first of all with these few to try my Fortune, which if it be prosperous, I may perhaps be less afraid to expose the rest of this Nature hereafter.

Willis's overall aim is to bring physick to the same level of precision as 'a true Science … not inferior to Mathematicks'. He admits that 'it is more than the task of one Man or Generation, to exhibit a compleat Curatory Method and absolute in all points'. He starts by dismissing treatments based on irrational beliefs and folklore as 'empiricks' and nothing more than the work of 'quacking Jugglers and old women'. And he advises against being beguiled by 'those Pseudochymists with notable danger and abuse of the humane Body … who bragg that they have framed their Furnaces … [as] a great Elixir, a certain Panacea, or an universal Medicine'.[2] But despite these protestations, Willis explains that his medicines are 'Simple and Compound, both Old and New, both Dogmatical and Empirical, gathered out of the Physick-books of every Age, as also those chiefly celebrated by Quacks and Nurses'.[3] This turns out to be a correct summary.

Willis had time to complete the text and write his preface to the reader before the second part of *Pharmaceutice rationalis* (1675) went to press, but he did not live see the published work. There is a palpable sense of urgency in finding time away from his busy practice in order to speculate upon the 'Operations of medicines in Humane Bodies', replacing the use of empirick medicines governed more by 'Chance or Fortune than by Advice' with physick 'practiced with a safe conscience'. Whereas the first part of the treatise is about classes of medicine and their formularies, Willis's focus in the second part of *Pharmaceutice rationalis* (1675) is on regional disease. He combines knowledge as taught by the ancients, advanced 'further by the Knife or Microscope', with the observations of physick and hypotheses on disease mechanisms: the 'Disposition of Blood and Humours, from what Affection of Animal Spirits, from what habitude of Fibres, and other solid parts, every disease proceeds'. Willis views his work as not so much a treatise, as a collection of essays. He appeals to 'Physicians … intent only on their Practice and Gain … but to the genuine Sons of Art' to improve upon his work. And in a valedictory premonition, he reflects that 'when I shall be well conscious to my self, that I have not suffer'd my Faculties although small (as the Talent entrusted with me by God Almighty) to perish through sloth, nor suffered them to be buryed in the earth … I shall seriously rejoice and triumph'. That anticipated period of satisfaction proved to be brief.

Throughout, Willis sets out the mechanism of each symptom or condition of interest as the basis for treatment. Because disease is usually a disorder of the heated blood, his first aim is to rebalance fermentation. He also proposes cleansing the system by increased excretion of toxic recrements through normal channels: the bowel, urine, expired air, sweat, vomit, saliva, and nasal secretions. His preparations are mainly ingested or given as clysters (enemas). Some are applied topically as poultices and foments so as to draw out unhealthy material. Willis uses surgical procedures including phlebotomy to remove aberrantly fermented circulating blood, and local manoeuvres including ligatures around the limbs or incisions in the skin and underlying tissues to contain the blood and prevent wider distribution of the

[2] See: *Pharmaceutice rationalis*, part 1 (1679): preface, page [5].

[3] It follows that Willis's use of 'empiric' is both a term of use and abuse. Readers can be forgiven for pausing to work out whether he is in favour or disapproves of empiricism; but will conclude that he favours logic and evidence rather than whimsy and folklore in prescribing for his patients.

morbific matter. More elaborate procedures include stenting a stricture of the oesophagus, and drainage with lavage of purulent collections within the thorax. In order to make surgery more tolerable, Willis offers the patient an alcoholic julep.

Symptomatic treatment is required for conditions that are 'accidental' (acute and unpredictable) whereas prophylaxis is used for individuals predisposed to diseases that are habitual (chronic). Although Willis distinguishes remedies that cure, preserve, and save life, much overlap is apparent and his segregation of medicines into these three categories is rarely consistent. His analysis of success is anecdotal with no attempt at objective evaluation. But it is characteristic of his approach to rational therapeutics, and to his credit, that Willis writes as much on the hazards of his medicines and management as their benefits.

Listing the many ingredients in Willis's pharmacy would be an onerous task from which little might be gleaned other than admiration for the extensive scavenging of animal, vegetable, and mineral sources; the chemical ingenuity; and the preparedness of his patients to sample so many concoctions and to endure so stoically the invasion of their orifices and integument. By way of mitigation for skirting over encyclopaedic documentation of the medicines, Willis's own dictum when faced with too much information was to point out that: 'of which to give an account would fill many volumes ... to unfold them with Commentaries added to them, we have neither leisure, nor doth it seem worth our endeavours ... to enumerate would be a vast and tedious work'.[4] The reader does not learn enough from the two parts of *Pharmaceutice rationalis* to set up his or her own pharmacy. Prepared to divulge some details of his therapeutics, Willis holds back on too explicit an account of the chemistry 'because it contains Secrets easily violated by those rash Quacksalvers, who not without danger to the sick make experiments dayly of every medicinal Precept they find written, without any Controul'.[5]

Most of Willis's medicines require chemical liberation of the active therapeutic particles from a variety of starting materials: the leaves, flowers, seeds, or roots of plants and fruits; animal material such as horn, shell, tooth, or bone and occasionally fresh organs; and metals or minerals. Willis describes several therapeutic classes in detail: vomits and antiemeticks; purges and stopping medicines; cathearticks, deoppilatives, and carminatives; diuretics and antidiuretic (ischurial) remedies; diaphoreticks (hydrogogues and sudorificks) and antidiaphoreticks; opiates (narcoticks, hypnoticks and anodynes) and coffee as a stimulant; cardiacks (cordials); hepaticks; and phlegmagogues and errhines (acting on respiratory and nasal secretions). Other medicines are mentioned in passing but not further described: antiscorbuticks, cephalicks, and alexipharmicks (antidotes to poison). Medicines varying in potency are chosen deliberately, but not infrequently the effects are overdone and correctives needed. These remedies are usually given together with changes in diet and fluid intake, including the use of chalybeates (iron containing) and other healing waters. Almost invariably Willis's regimen offers a cascade of medicines taken in combination and sequentially so that, as time passes and the distemper continues, his patients are exposed to a vast pharmacopoeia. Despite confident explanation of the different mechanisms, Willis's claims for specificity of the regimens offered with confidence for each distemper take on rather

[4] See: amongst many other such disclaimers, *Pharmaceutice rationalis*, part 2 (1679): pages 68, 97, and 163.
[5] See: *Pharmaceutice rationalis*, part 1 (1679): page 3.

a familiar ring as the same medicines are enthusiastically listed for each newly described condition.

The many solutes and solvents making up each medicine represent a giddy mixture of ingredients combined into various formularies.[6] A few are described in the text that follows in order to illustrate their complexity, diversity, chemistry, and variety of source materials but with no attempt to be comprehensive. The leading apothecaries who made up Willis's prescriptions in Oxford were (John) Hazlewood (nd), (John) Crosse (1627–1698), and Stephen Toone (1636–1681).[7] The London pharmacists are not identified. Electuaries—juleps, tinctures, liquors, elixirs, apozemes, and potions—were made palatable with liquorish, spices, and sweeteners. Other decoctions were used as powders, boles, pills, morsels, tablets, troches, and lozenges; linctuses, lohochs, eclegmas, and lambitives (material licked on the tongue); or fumigations and balsams. Almost never are Willis's patients spared topical application of irritants or liniments soaked in soothing or astringent substances: blisters, vesicatories, scarification, cupping glasses, cataplasms, poultices, foments, and leeches applied to the affected part. Many of his patients are subjected to surgical procedures including phlebotomy, the cutting of issues, or cauterization to produce 'fontinels'.

A quarter of a century after his death, a practical manual of Willis's medicines was published in a single edition, with no further issues: *Dr. Willis's receipts for the cure of all distempers* (1701: **10C**).[8] The translator, assumed to be John Hemming (nd) is at pains to extol the virtues 'both to the English and Foreign World'. Willis's name is synonymous with excellence in his knowledge of 'Chymistry and Pharmacy'. These receipts are of general use and 'fitted for the meanest Capacities'. Conversely, his 'other Speculations' are 'only proper for the Learned ... some, with whom his Speculative Advances will not go down' but who nevertheless 'Approve and Imitate his Receipts'. The translator has organized the material into classes of medicines arranged under the headings of the diseases to which they relate, further distinguishing the particular circumstances in which one or another are best used with respect to temperament and other factors. He is also sensitive to the cost of these medicines, singling out those that are affordable for the 'Poor, who cannot go to the Charge of Costly Chymical Preparations'. He goes further by 'throwing ... into an Appendix, because they are not Calculated for any particular Distemper', all 'Vomits, Purges, Diureticks, Sudorificks, Cordials and Opiats'. He is confident that the book will be well received since it has the imprimatur of the best Physician of his Age, supported by the Remotest Mysteries of Chymistry ... and backed by the Experience, not only of the Author, but of most Physicians'.

[6] See: JR Partington, *A history of chemistry*, volume 2, London (1961): page 309–10 where James Partington (1886–1965) provides a summary of Willis's methods of preparation for many of his medicines, pointing out that although the pharmacopoeia is described as 'rational', Willis was not averse to using human skull, powdered toads, and waters of snails and earthworms, to which many other curious ingredients might have been added. But Partington acknowledges Willis's effective use of Peruvian bark for intermittent fever and the preparations containing iron.

[7] See: TD Whittet (1915–1987), 'Some Oxford apothecaries', *Journal of the Royal Society of Medicine* 1979: 72; 940–5 for a detailed account of John Cross but no mention of John Hazlewood. Cross-matriculated as a 'pharmacopola' and is remembered as such on an inscription in the University Church of St Mary the Virgin. Stephen Toone matriculated as 'apothecary' on 14 September 1666, aged 30 and also has a monument in St Mary the Virgin; see: http://www.oxfordhistory.org.uk/doctors/apothecaries/index.html.

[8] See chapter 14 for bibliographic details.

Contemporary opinion on Willis's medicines

The Royal Society wrote at length when each of the two parts of *Pharmaceutice rationalis* was published. The first notice mistakenly dates the appearance of the book as 1673.[9] It is a dutiful and close sequential reading on a topic 'which, he faith, hath been hitherto one of the *Desiderata* in Physick, *viz.* In what manner, and by what kinds of impression upon the parts of an Human Body, Medicaments perform their operations'. Willis writes to 'satisfie intelligent Readers' in a structured way: first where the medicines act, 'the Mass of Blood ... or the Brain and the Nervous Systeme'; then on what they act, 'the *Animal Spirits*, or the *Humors* ... they either provoke them to excretory motions, *or* enlarge and refresh them, *or* allay their disorders, *or* asswage their fury'. There follows a series of long paragraphs, one each dedicated to '*Vomitives* ... *Purgatives* ... *Diureticks* ... *Sudorificks* ... *Cordials* and *Alexiterials* ... and *Opiates*'. Clearly the reviewer has read carefully but chooses at no point to analyse or criticise. When the second part was reviewed, the author lamented:

> This Learned and Worthy Author (whose Death may certainly be reputed a publick loss, and a detriment to the very Faculty of Physick) saw but a very few dayes before his decease this book of his finished in the Press; to which, if Heaven had thought good to have sparred him longer amongst us, he would doubtless have added many other Philosophical and Useful pieces for the improvement of Knowledge and the Art of Physick.

Again, the account is faithful to Willis's narrative on the anatomy of the lungs and singles out the illustrations: 'the matter for these Figures is furnish'd by the Ingenious and Diligent Dr. *Edmund King*, with great skill and dexterity'. Hinting at the debate played out within the Royal Society on the purpose of respiration, the writer confirms that 'the Use of the Lungs seems to him to be; That the Blood may ... meet with the Nitrous particles of the Air, and be inspired with Vitality from the same'. He pauses to emphasize that respiration depends on 'Animal Spirits that are dispens'd by the *Cerebrum* ... [and] those that are furnish'd by the *Cerebellum*; proving withal, that respiration is, as t'were, a mix't work partaking of ... the spontaneous and natural'. In describing 'the ways and accidents, by which that manifold apparatus of organs may be vitiated', the author develops one of Willis's many analogies, this time the clock: 'that this Pneumonique Engin ... is exceedingly subject to depravation; as a Watch that is with great Art composed of a spring, balance, wheels, strings, &c. is very liable to disorder'. Leaning much on 'Sylvian' iatrochemical doctrines of failed 'crasis' of the blood and the presence of impurities, 'miasmata', the reviewer rehearses Willis's pathology of the chest and abdominal viscera and of the various dropsies and their 'Sylvian' remedies. A paragraph on the surgical treatments and cutaneous disease, with which the book ends, is followed by the author's summary in which, whilst praising the 'great care and exactness' with which Willis has laid out his 'solid and genuine *hypotheses*', he hints at reservation on whether Willis has succeeded in his endeavour to 'shew from what disposition of Blood and Humors, from what affection of Animal Spirits ... every sickness he treats of proceeds', and how valuable are 'the abundance of Medicaments all which he subjoyns their respective Reasons'.[10]

[9] See: *Transactions of the Philosophical Proceedings of the Royal Society*, 31 December 1673, volume 8, issue 99: pages 6166–71.

[10] See: *Transactions of the Philosophical Proceedings of the Royal Society*, 16 March 1675, volume 10, issue 121: pages 505–9.

Within a few years, Robert Plot (1640–1696) credited Willis's 'Pharmacea' with the introduction of:[11]

> 220. *Spiritus Salis Armoniaci succinatus, Syrup of Sulphur, preparation of Steel* without *acids*, and from thence of his *artificial Acidulæ* ... that what was formerly *Empirical*, and but lucky hits, is now become most rational, by his making the *operations* of *Cathartic, Emetic, Diaphoretic, Cardiac*, and *Opiat Medicines*, intelligible by *Mechanical Explanations*; having subjoined to each most neat and artificial *Formula's*, as well *Chymical* as *others* ... And where nature is exorbitant in any of these *Evacuations*, he has likewise taught us how to check, and reduce *her*; adding a new *Anatomy* of the *Stomach, Intestines, Gula, Veins* and *Arteries*.
>
> 221. Which he has seconded with a further discovery and rational account of *Thoracic* and *Epatic Medicines*, and of the *Diseases* belonging to those *parts*; discoursing also of *Venesection*, stopping of *Haemorraghies*, of *Issues* and *cutaneous Distempers*. In all which it may be observed, what is almost peculiar to him; that there is nothing *trivial*, most *new*, and almost all *ingenious* ... But it is too difficult a task to give a just account how far *Physick, Anatomy, Chymistry*, and *Philosophy*, stand indebted to him for their *Improvements*. Let it suffice to say, that he has introduced a new Body of *Physick*, almost universally embraced before all *others*, and a new *Sect* of *Philosophers* at home and abroad called *Willisians*; so that *England* (for ought I know) may have as much reason to boast of her learned *Willis*, as *Coos* [Chios], and *Pergamus* of old, of their great *Masters* in *Physick*.

John Ward (1629–1681) emphasized the novelty of Willis's spirit of sulphur:[12]

> Hee hath a syrup of sulphur wch hee makes much use of. Itt is his owne composition and no Apothecarie hath itt or knows itt but y two forementioned [Hazlewood and Crosse]. Itt may be taken and is so usually with a Liquorish stick. It is a compound not above 4d an ounce, but itt is most used in Colds and distempers of the Lungs ... [On mercurial quicksilver] ... Two ounces and a half of quicksilver given by Dr Conyers to a patient yt was troubled with ye Iliack passion. Itt is very good for yt distemper. Dr Willis uses to give more: ye more ye give ye less is ye danger. Itt does by its own weight passe quickly. Doe but mix itt with a plaister and heat itt a little and presently it flies away, but boyling hurts itt not at all.

But after Willis's death the critics emerged. Frederic Slare (1647–1727) had a double gripe against Willis and the medicines he had both favoured and scorned. The evidence showed that bezoar stones, much used by Willis, were of no therapeutic use in physick. And Slare refuted the charge by Willis 'and others with prejudices' that sugars are harmful. Addressed to the Royal Society, of which he was a Fellow, and reminding them that he had often published in the *Transactions*, Slare's aim was to show that 'the celebrated BEZOAR, a medicine of the first Rank ... [does] not deserve the great Encomiums which were given it'.[13]

[11] See: Robert Plot, *The natural history of Oxford*-shire, Oxford and London (1677): pages 303–4; and RT Gunther *Early medicine and biological science* (extracted from *Early science in Oxford*), London (1926): page 59 for an alternative transcription of these paragraphs.

[12] See: Sir D'Arcy Power, 'John Ward and his diary'. Presidential address, 9 October 1916, *Transactions of the Medical Society of London* 1917; xl: 1–46, reprinted in *Selected writings*, Oxford (1931): page 190; also cited by Gunther (1926): pages 62–3.

[13] See: Frederick Slare, *Experiments and observations upon oriental and other Bezoar stones ... to which is annex'd a vindication of sugars against the charge of Dr Willis, other physicians, and common predujices. Dedicated*

Slare's presentation at a lecture to the Society in *c.*1700 had been well received other than by Dr (Edward) Tyson (1651–1708) and the apothecary Mr (John) Houghton (1645–1705). Despite encouragement from Dr (Hans) Sloane (1660–1753) to publish in *Philosophical Transactions*, Slare waited for additional evidence on bezoar stone from colleagues who had spent time in India at the Fort of St George, Madras, and the endorsement of friends who shared his view that 'they also found just cause to suspect its Vertue, and others to condemn it'. To the reader, Slare explains that the oriental bezoar with which he is concerned is a 'concreted' laminated stone said to be found exclusively in the stomach of she-goats and formed of dietary residues. Slare places Bezoar even below Hart's-horn, another medicine favoured by Willis: '*this being so poor and insipid a Part of Physic, as deserves to be exploded out of the* Materia Medica'. It is a material so inert that one may take '50 or 60 Grains in a Mess of Broth ... without being in any respect Philosophically or Physically benefited or hurt by it'.

Printing letters from Dr Robert Griffith (1663–1719), professor of Physick and Chymistry in Dublin, dated 18 October 1714, from Chester, and Dr John Cooke (nd) of Bristol, dated 5 January 1714,[14] in support of his case, Slare laid out evidence from chemical decoction that bezoar is made of earth not animal or vegetable material and best designated 'dry'd Mud'. Incapable of exciting any reaction in the contents of the stomach, it is better to lift the 'spirits' with a 'glass of good Ale, or Beer, or of generous Wine'. Having previously used bezoar stone over many years, no one patient of Slare's acquaintance had benefitted from a medicine costing two or three shillings that a dose of '*Venice* Treacle ... scarce valued at two Farthings' would not have helped. Feeling faint and weak, his own experience of taking fifteen grains of bezoar stone on 3 May 1699 had been unrewarding. Bezoar was big business. It cost 'Three Pounds and Ten Shillings, the finest Four Pounds, equal ... with Gold' on the London market. Slare relates that a dealer of his acquaintance traded five hundred ounces annually, each requiring stones from a minimum of twelve animals representing an outlay of twelve hundred pounds, an investment that '*Indian* Travellers and Natives' sourcing the dubious material 'do laugh at our *European* Credulity, to see us so easily put upon'.[15] Eventually through his researches, Slare concludes that the material is: 'a downright Piece of Sophistry, only Goats Hair beat up with some bitter juices ... I know nothing that can recommend it but its vast price'. Indeed Slare was told by Dr (Robert) Boyle (1627–1691) a little before Boyle's death 'that one of the Poisons us'd in the Indies, where they intended a slow and lingering Death, was Minc'd Hair'. In short, were the bezoar stone to disappear 'Mankind would suffer [no] Loss or Injury ... [one of] many others ... [that] deserve to be garbled and cast upon

to the Ladies. Together with further discoveries and remarks, London (1715). The book is cited in Norman Moore, WILLIS, Thomas, MD (1621–1675). *Dictionary of National Biography* 1900: 62; 25–6; and see also, Norman Moore *The history of the study of medicine in the British Isles. The Fitz-Patrick lectures for 1905–6 delivered before the Royal College of Physicians of London*, Oxford (1908): pages 119–20.

[14] Details of Dr Cooke are not known but his library was sold at auction in 1722. See: *A catalogue of the library of the late learned Dr. John Cooke sen. of the city of Bristol. Containing many scarce and valuable books in divinity, physick, history, &c. With a Curious Collection of the Best Editions of the classicks, cum Notis Variorum, in usum Delph. &c. which will begin to be sold by auction, on Monday the twelfth of February, 1721-2. at the dwelling-house of Mrs. Cooke, the relict of the said Dr. Cooke, in Corn-Street, Bristol; beginning every Evening at Five of the Clock. Catalogues will be deliver'd gratis at any of the Coffee-Houses in Bristol, and at the Place of Sale*, Bristol (1722). Works in the sale by Thomas Willis, but with erratic transcription and formatting, are: Item 36, duodecimo: *Pharmaceutice rationalis*, 2 volumes 1674; item 94, octavo, *Pharmaceutice rationalis*. 1679; item 166, octavo, *Pathologiæ cerebri* 1668; item 70, duodecimo, *Willius historie contra Highmorum*; item 98, duodecimo, *De anima brutorum* 1672; item 101, duodecimo, *Cerebri anatomia* 16[1]2.

[15] See: Slare (1715): [1] page 35.

the Dunghil, and may in time be expos'd in their true Colours and Nakedness'.[16] The finger is pointed even more directly at Willis's criticism of sugar:[17]

> Thus we see a * [* footnote: 'Willis de Scorbut'] Great Physician highly condemning it; whereas in the same Book, and many others of his writing, he uses it in Syrups and Electuaries, and other Confections. To me it seems a more grateful Employment to write Encomiums, and celebrate the just and deserv'd Praises of an Subject, than to offer Violence to an innocent Reputation.

Willis had written that sugar being added to almost every aliment was likely the cause of scurvy; nor had he disagreed with the opinion of others that it was responsible for consumption.[18] Slare appealed for support from women with palates accustomed to take refined sugar in 'Tea, Coffee *and* Chocolate … at the Morning Repasts, called Break-fasts'. He argued that it was less of a contaminant than men who drink 'sowre and uncouth Wines' and smoke tobacco and Indian Henbane.[19] Slare's only caution for these women was that 'sugar being very high a Nourisher, may dispose them to be fatter than they desire to be, who are afraid of their shapes'. Ever one to consider commerce, Slare mentions merchants who have 'gain'd such Wealth' from their plantations in the West Indies that they 'do daily purchase great Estates' on their return, and the grocers who have also made their fortunes through the sale of sugar.

Arguing that sugar is soothing when applied topically to the skin, not irritant to the eyes, pleasant to the palate, and as 'Sugar-Candy' a linctus for children with the 'hawk and cough', Slare disputes that sugar might do 'mischief to the Gums … [and] spoil the Teeth'. As a sweetener in various natural and prepared foodstuffs, sugar is favoured not only for pleasure and nourishment, but as 'a good pectoral healing Balsamic Medicine, taken inwardly' or as a vulnerary foment applied to ulcers which is no less effective than red lead and mercury.[20] In order to make his case, Slare needed to 'take off the Censure which the Famous *Willis* has left upon Record against Sugar'. Extending his condemnation directed at Mr (John) Ray (1627–1705), who has endorsed Willis's erroneous criticism of sugar, Slare adds 'yet the Celebrated Dr. *Willis* is not fully content with this venomous Character; He exasperates it much more in the following Account'. Slare transcribes Willis's Latin text and provides his own English translation:[21]

> I DO so much condemn those Things that are season'd with Sugar … to have contributed very much to the vast Increase of the Scurvey: For it plainly appears by the Chymical Analysis … That this Concrete contains a sharp and corrosive Salt, but is little touch'd with Sulphur; for Sugar being distill'd by it self, gives a Liquor scarce at all inferior to *Aqua Fortis*: Should you also distil Sugar in an Alembec … there will come up a Liquor like the most sharpest *Aqua Vitæ*, burning, and very pungent. Now since it is mix't with most of

[16] See: Slare (1715): [1] page 45.

[17] See: Slare (1715): [2] page [4].

[18] See chapter 15; and Thomas Willis, *Of the scurvy* (1679): page 50.

[19] In passing, Slare (1715): [2] page [6], mentions that he suffered 'Paralytic Affections' in his youth from too much coffee, restoring with abstinence for thirty years 'the good Tone of my Nerves, which continue steddy to this Day', the fault lying with the 'Exotic Plants' not the sugar added to sweeten 'these Entertaining liquids'.

[20] See: Slare (1715): [2] pages 44–9.

[21] See: Slare (1715): [2] pages 22–4; and Thomas Willis, *De scorbuto* (1667): pages 303–4 for the original text. The English is Slare's translation and does not exactly match that in *Of the scurvy* (1679): page 50, or (1684): page [4] 212 which differ slightly from each other.

our Food, and taken in great Quantity, how likely is it, from its daily use that our Blood and Humors should be render'd sharp, and by consequence scorbutical.

Acknowledging Willis's reputation, but aware that the 'horrid Charge upon Sugar has been taken for granted', Slare sets out to 'examine this Satyrical Treatment of Sugar very fairly, with due respect to the Author; but yet with much more regard to the Truth, and to the Good of Mankind'. The satire is on Slare's side in arguing that the disturbance of particles proposed by Willis would result in 'all Sorts of Cholicks, Vomitings, and convulsive Diseases, and ruin the whole Animal System, and make short Work with Human Kind. I am well assur'd, that no such Mischief has happen'd since the Author first printed this Arraignment of Sugar at *Oxford,* Anno 1667'.[22] Slare has conducted his own experiments and finds Willis's chemistry to be unsound. Postulating that all vegetable and animal foodstuffs would be noxious if sugar was so corrosive, Slare concludes that: 'we see what unjust, nay dangerous Prejudices may be stamp'd upon People's Minds ... against so wholesome a Concrete as Sugar'. But just in case his readers are not yet persuaded, Slare ends with two case reports. Dying in his 70th year of a fever, (Henry Somerset) the Duke of Beaufort (1629–1700) was opened and his viscera and teeth found to be in perfect order despite the duke having consumed a pound of sugar daily in his sherry, chocolate, and sweetmeats, for 'near 40 years', the duke pointing out to his housekeeper, Mrs Grymes (nd):[23]

> That which preserves Apples and Plumbs,
> Will also preserve Liver and Lungs.

And Mr Malory of Shelton in Bedfordshire, Slare's maternal grandfather, remained fit and active until he died of apoplexy aged 100 years, despite indulging in sugar at every meal and losing all his teeth at 80 at which point, happily, another set erupted.

The plague

Willis had been writing on medicines for many years before *Pharmaceutice rationalis* was published. John Hemming (nd) found amongst Willis's papers the manuscript of an unpublished treatise on management of the plague.[24] Hemming explains that he had transcribed the text 'from the Doctor's papers in the Year 1666, being then his *Amanuensis*' but was reluctant to publish 'any of Dr. *Willis's* Posthumous Works'. He was prevailed upon by a third party to make an exception with this treatise, on behalf of an acquaintance who was going in 'the late Embassie to *Constantinople* where that distemper then was, and did frequently rage'. The suggestion is that Hemming may have access to other unpublished manuscripts. If so, these are long since lost. In the event, after making a copy available to his correspondent, a further outbreak of plague in 'their Majesties Army in Ireland' prompted Hemming to publish the work. Several prominent physicians who were consulted approved of the decision. Writing on 1 September 1690 from St. Martin's Lane, Hemming expressed concern that, in choosing not to publish the treatise which 'want[ed] his last Hand to compleat', Willis would have disapproved. Hemming hoped that: 'The regard I have always had, and shall still have for the

[22] See: Slare (1715): page [2] page 24.
[23] See: Slare (1715): [2] page 59.
[24] See chapter 11.

Reputation and Memory of my dear Master, and best Friend, will not, I presume, be thought to lessen, by my giving way'.[25] Perhaps the reason why Willis had sat on the work was because it was intended as a manual for public use. It did not pretend to be a scholarly treatise written for physicians which might be compared with his other writings. Willis's aim was simply to show 'how to preserve the Whole from taking Infection; And how to cure the Sick that are infected'.

Willis argues that the best tactic for avoidance of the plague is to get away from the distemper, conforming to the 'Publick Magistrate's [orders]' or through personal initiative. Protection requires that 'our Houses, and Streets [are] kept clean; removing all Filth . . . and noisom smells, be taken away . . . and the smell of Sope-Suds, and Lye, in the washing of Clothes, be avoided'. The air should be kept pure by lighting fires; and rooms, entrance doors and roofs fumigated with '*Sulphur*, *Nitre*, *Frankincense*, *Pitch*, *Resin*, *Tarr*, and the like'. In addition, Willis recommends fumigation with a mixture of '*green* Vitriol *calcin'd*, Saltpeter, *and* Sulphur' or 'Vinegar with Rue, or Wormwood, chopt small, and evapourated in a Perfuming Pot . . . [with] Myrrh' poured on 'Coals in a Chafing-dish'.[26]

In order to increase resistance, he advises a diet free from salt meats and shellfish, with a moderate portion of wine to 'keep the Spirits lively and cheerful, and endeavour to compose [the] Mind and Affection against fear and sadness'.[27] Recognizing that this positive attitude could not always be sustained, Willis has many recipes as preservatives against the plague for those at risk. Often he takes as his authority the Dutch physician Isbrand van Diemerbroeck (1609–1674). Most of Willis's preferred remedies are concoctions of plants, vegetables, and fruits with wormwood added as an alexipharmical and given, depending on preference or constitution, as an electuary or tablet. As his later treatises on rational therapeutics expand in greater detail, these are best used together with sudorificks, the patient remaining in his chamber until the pores are again closed. So as to keep out the unwholesome vapours and prevent the contagion from entering the brain, lungs, and stomach, Willis recommends smoking tobacco in a pipe: 'Amongst us in England, 'tis reported, That in the last great Plague, no Tobacco-Shop was infected'.[28] Also useful are medicines to 'hold in the Mouth, and chew on . . . [amongst others] *Myrrh* is very excellent: Some commend Tobacco, and chew it almost continually'. Willis also recommends releasing the contagion by cutting issues. Measures to be avoided are 'strong and hot Cordials', purges and phlebotomy.

Cures for those who already have the plague are quite different. These involve cycles of vomitives and sudorificks given every eighteen hours, induction of sleep, and plaisters applied behind the ears, under the armpits and in the groins, the patient supported in the intervals by broth and cordials. Writing in 1666, Willis places most faith in the sweating medicines and gives more than twenty formulations to be taken as potions, boluses, or powders.[29] In time the symptoms usually abate or the malignity is driven 'out in Boyls or Carbuncles' and suppurating 'Bubo's'. These skin lesions are best managed with poultices made from 'the Fundament of some living Fowl, or else a *Colewort-leaf* dip't in scalding Water, dried and smeared over with *Oyl of Lillies* or *Scorpions*'. It may be necessary to lance the swollen glandules and dress the wounds with a pledget or liniment soaked in turpentine or the yolk of an

[25] See: Thomas Willis, *A plain and easie method for preserving [by God's blessing] those that are well from the infection of the plague, or any contagious distemper, in city, camp, fleet &c. and for curing such as are infected with it*, London (1691): page [9].

[26] See: *A plain and easie method* (1691): pages 3–5.

[27] See: *A plain and easie method* (1691): page 8.

[28] See: *A plain and easie method* (1691): pages 20–1.

[29] See: *A plain and easie method* (1691): pages 32–48.

egg.[30] And the plague may be complicated by haemorrhages from any orifice for which specific medicines are needed. The most useful ingredient is root of tormentil.[31]

It must be said that this manual written 'for such as cannot procure the attendance of Physicians' seems to go beyond what a citizen threatened by the plague might reasonably be expected to organize for him or herself.

Digestion and anatomy of the gastrointestinal tract

When he wrote his treatise on rational therapeutics several years later, Willis first considered treatments that 'act their Comedie' in the 'first passages'. His medicines target the 'innumerable Glandulas incrusting the Back of the interior Coat from the Mouth even to the Anum'. It follows that Willis's regimens almost invariably include lifestyle advice related to diet and drinking habits.

Willis begins by describing the anatomy of the upper gastrointestinal tract. The four coats of the ventricle (stomach) are illustrated with explanatory legends in Tabulæ I–V of *Pharmaceutice rationalis* part 1 (1679: Pl.27–Pl.31). The stomach is a source of much distemper: 'the Ventricle is oftentimes disturbed, and after divers manners moved by the Phantasie, by the Appetite, yea and by divers affections either of the Soul, or every part of the Body'.

The inner lining 'with an hairy Crust as it were a certain Down' holds the ingested material which is converted to chyle and enters the pores of blood vessels so that 'rich Food is given to the vital Flame'. In order rapidly to pass ingested material to the circulation, the coeliac vessels 'lay up some humour ... and the veins ... carry away thence perpetually some other, so that there may be made ... an immediate and constant commerce [from the stomach] backward and forward between the Chyle and the Blood', bypassing 'the long wanderings of the Intestines, and of the Chyliferous Vessels'.[32] This transfer of nutritious juice is aided by 'wrinklings' which expand the surface area. The stomach may lose these rugae: 'In Gluttons and great Drinkers, in whom by the too often, and too much filling of the Ventricle the fleshy Coat is very much extended ... all its wrinkles vanishing, it seems plain like a blown Bladder'.

The inner coat is surrounded by a dense network of sensory nerve fibres responsible for conveying the pleasure of eating, 'Satiety and Complacency', or conversely the sense of nausea which initiates the process of vomiting. The nervous layer receives branches of the wandring pair and intercostal nerves (autonomic system). This coat is surrounded by muscle with the fibres arranged obliquely so that they 'knit together, which make four parallel Lines with the Opposite Fibres, and cutting one another across', moving the parts involved in 'Swallowing, Spitting, Vomiting, Yauning, and other affections ... troublesome and unhandsom'. This arrangement enables the muscle coat to contract in order to mix the chyle, 'cooking for nourishment, what is there more strictly compressed and rolled together'. Directed both to the oesophageal inlet and the 'Orifice of the *Pylorus*', the matter 'in the Stomach ... [is] conveyed forth either by Vomit, or by Siege'. Willis has 'known some by reason of a vehement Palsie in this fleshie (muscle) Coat of the *Oesophagus*, to have swallow'd with very great difficulty, and others by reason that these Fibres were wholly loosned, to dye with Famine'.[33]

30 See: *A plain and easie method* (1691): pages 65–74.
31 See: *A plain and easie method* (1691): pages 53–4.
32 See: *Pharmaceutice rationalis* part 1 (1679): page 11.
33 See: *Pharmaceutice rationalis* part 1 (1679): page 6.

The muscle is surrounded by a thin membranous outer layer which prevents overdistension of the ventricle: but 'Dryness, or Saltness, or Heat, or Spiced Meats, or Wine' and 'Winds begot within the cavity of the Stomach' distend the viscus like a bladder, as happens 'in Hysterical Passions, and Colicks, and very often in the Hypochondriack passion'. Furthermore 'deadly and venomous Medicines … often induce horrid Inflations and Distensions … of the Ventricle'.[34]

The pylorus delivers well digested chyle to the duodenum, 'little by little and by very small portions thrusts it forth' or 'in purges and Diarrhæas'. Although vomiting medicines usually act on the orifice between the oesophagus and stomach, they also 'draw from within, and upwards the *Pylorus* it self with the *Duodenum* hanging to it, so as to make an Evacuation of the forc'd *Bilis* into the Ventricle'. Moving down the gastrointestinal tract, details of the intestines and their conformation are well known 'not only to Anatomists, but to every Butcher'. Their function is to elaborate and further ferment the chyle, mixing this with 'Choler and the Pancreatick juice' in the 'Jejune or empty Gut', converting the sour chyle to 'greater volatileness' and reaching the 'Ileon' where it is transmitted to the 'milkie Vessels and Mesaraick Veins' from where the 'Fæces … are moved forward to the thick Intestines'.[35] It is remarkable to Willis that, attached to the mesentery, every part of the intestine, 'about six Ells long',[36] is arranged in folds from the centre each holding 'twelve handfuls on the Intestines'. These folds of intestine are rich in arteries and veins. The coats and blood vessels follow much the same arrangement as those of the ventricle. However the orientation of the muscle fibres, circular and longitudinal, is such as to move 'by a slow and successive motion, and as it were creepingly [the contents] from one end to the other … performing this peristaltick motion of the Intestines'.[37] This orderly process is vulnerable to convulsions from 'sharp Humors, and hurtful Suffusions from within the Arteries … from disagreeing and disproportionate Ailments, also from Medicines and Poysons'. Furthermore violent passions of the mind or body originating from the encephalon[38] may induce a '*Diarrhæa*'. The muscular coat of the large intestine is necessarily strong, as a result of which 'if there be an Inflammation or Sphacelisimus' so the fleshy fibres cannot function at the origins of the colon, 'the '*fæces* … flowing back towards the Ileon, do cause the incurable Iliack Passion'. It is 'Among these Intestines [that] Cathartick Medicines do chiefly perform their operations'.[39] Willis illustrates the various coats of the intestines in Tabula VI of *Pharmaceutice rationalis* part 1 (1679: Pl.32).

Enhancing excretion: vomitory medicines

Having dealt with the anatomy and physiology, and touched on some of the distempers, Willis considers in more detail the symptoms and treatment of disorder in the abdomen. He regards vomiting as a physiological process in which actions of the stomach 'may shut up the Throat behind for the casting forth of its Balast … [but] for as much as it is a violent motion of the Stomach, and very often involuntary, it is not undeservedly called Convulsive … contrary or at least opposite to the ordinary and natural Action of the Stomach'. Willis's emetic metaphor is that: 'as it were a Tower, as often as an external Enemie shall invade, or that

34 See: *Pharmaceutice rationalis* part 1 (1679): page 7.

35 See: *Pharmaceutice rationalis* part 1 (1679): page 11.

36 An 'Ell' is a cubit, or the combined length of the forearm and extended hand.

37 See: *Pharmaceutice rationalis* part 1 (1679): page 13.

38 Throughout, Pordage retains Willis's use of greek type for encephalon: 'ἐγκέφαλος' usually corrupted to 'ἐγκέφαλον'.

39 See: *Pharmaceutice rationalis* part 1 (1679): page 15.

a sedition shall arise among the proper Inhabitants, forthwith, whatsoever Guests, as persons suspected, are cast forth at the nearest Passage, to wit, the Gate of the Ventricle'.[40] Vomiting occurs when disagreeable matter is generated in the chyle, agitating animal spirits in the muscle coat but also, as in the plague and distempers of the brain and nervous stock, from morbid matter delivered to the stomach through the arteries or nerves causing the 'Convulsions or ἀταξίας'. Amongst the cases with which Willis illustrates pathological vomiting is one that has been much quoted for its therapeutic ingenuity:[41]

> A strong Man ... labouring for a long time with often Vomiting, he was wont, very often, though not allways, presently to cast up whatsoever he had eaten ... growing hungry he would eat until the *Oesophagus* was filled up to the Throat, in the mean time nothing sliding down into the Ventricle ... when that no Medicines could help and he languished away ... and was in danger of Death, I prepared an Instrument for him like a Rod, of a whale Bone, with a little round Button of Spunge fixed to the top of it ... by this means he hath daily taken his sustenance for sixteen Years and doth yet use the same Machine.

Vomiting has local causes: the presence of 'ingrateful Meat or Drink, almost as soon as tasted in the Mouth, also by a feather put down the Throat', violent coughing, or disorder below the pylorus in the 'Cholerick Disease, Iliack Passion and other Torments of the Intestines'. But it also follows stimulation from 'the Passage or Commerce of the [wandring] Nerves', agitation of the animal spirits following head injury, and the motion of 'being in a Ship, or riding in a Coach':[42]

> The more dangerous Convulsions of the Ventricle, to wit, a yexing or hickcock: and truly by reason of the animal Spirits being disturbed in their whole *Systasit*, and sometimes too much dissipated or excited, frequent Swoonings, cold Sweats, and not seldom deadly Convulsions of the Members or of the whole Body happen.

In considering 'Emetologie', Willis explains that vomiting is induced by orderly irritation of the inner 'hairy Crust' transmitted to the nervous coat which wrinkles and causes violent contractions in the muscle layer. This is more likely to happen when the inner lining is worn flat 'in Gluttons, and great Drinkers'. Vomiting may continue due to the overly provoked spirits expelling 'nourishing and cordial Drink' until appeased by sleep. Indeed, with bile in the stomach 'that yellow Poyson [is] not less troublesome than the emetic Tincture'. The severity of induced vomiting also depends on whether the medicine is ingested or delivered remotely through the application of poultices, including 'a Liniment or Fomentation of the Juice or decoction of Tobacco applied to the Head'. Using the recently introduced technique, Willis (and presumably King) have:[43]

> Injected into the Jugular vein of a strong Dog about six ounces of Wine impregnated with an infusion of Antimony; about five or six minutes after he began to reel, and faulter in

[40] See: *Pharmaceutice rationalis* part 1 (1679): pages 19–20.

[41] See: *Pharmaceutice rationalis* part 1 (1679): page 23; and R Hierons, 'Willis's contributions to clinical medicine and neurology', *Journal of the neurological Sciences* 1967, 4: 5 for an account of how Walter Rumsey (1584–1660), a Welsh judge and politician, made an instrument from whale bone and wrote a short account of cleansing the stomach in this way. See: *Organon salutis an instrument to cleanse the stomach: as also divers new experiments of the virtue of tobacco and coffee, how much they conduce to preserve humane health*, London (1657).

[42] See: *Pharmaceutice rationalis* part 1 (1679): page 25.

[43] See: *Pharmaceutice rationalis* part 1 (1679): page 27.

his going and afterwards to vomit extreamly. But we may suppose this effect to have been caused from the medicine assaulting the Brain rather than the Stomach.

There are many indications for the use of emetics: 'the long disease of Maids, and in Men after ... inordinate Eating'; in the 'Gout, Asthma, Epilepsie, Madness, and very many other diseases'; in those with 'a more short Breast and Neck, and whose Mouth and Ventricle are not far distant'; and in 'a consumptive disposition, with an Ulcer of the Lungs, or spitting of Blood ... a great Cachexie ... [and] in the Paroxysms of feavours'.[44]

In describing his 'chymical emetick' medicines, Willis focuses attention on those '*prepared first out of Vitriol, secondly out of Antimony, thirdly out of Mercurie*'.[45] Salt of vitriol makes available saline and sulphurous particles. It is slow-acting and may need to be taken with a hot drink and mixture of honey and vinegar, a 'Carduus Posset-drink or Oxymel of Squills', together with a feather down the throat to induce vomiting. The source of antimony needs to be free of lead. The medicinal properties are released by exposing the sulphur and saline content. '*Glass of Antimony*' is made by decocting the element on glass, the dried powder being taken with wine. The '*Flowers of Antimony*' is made by roasting stibnite (antimonite) and separating the white residue from the 'Yellow, Citron Colour' saline and sulphur residue. Antimony heated with pure nitre 'by flinging in a live Coal' produces the 'Liver of Antimony' which, known as the 'Crocus metallorum', is the 'most used Emetick'. It is effective unless the process has rendered the material 'with less Sulphur ... no more red, but yellow or citron Colour, and less Vomitive'. '*Sulphur of Antimony*' is made by mixing the element with salt of tartar (potassium carbonate) or wormwood, after which the saffron or yellow matter is 'edulcorated' with wine.

Mercurial emetic involves heating a source of that element with antimony: it 'is commonly called the Mercury of Life and *Mercurius Vitæ*, but not truly, when as it contains nothing at all of Mercurie in it, and unless it be cautiously given, it is oftner the Author of death than Life'. In fact it is no different from the flowers of antimony unless the mercurial content is revived by boiling the mixture with iron, whereupon it is a 'most cruel vomitory' until 'brused with calcined Sea Salt, and sweetned by often washings ... [it] becomes much gentler, and safe enough'.[46] Mercurial vomitories can be precipitated with other metals or salts: *Aurum vitæ* with gold; *Aqua fortis* with spirit of nitre; and *Aqua regis* with nitric and hydrochloric acid or with oil of vitriol and sulphuric acid, each of which may 'stir up most violent Vomiting'. The 'Hercules of Bovius' is made by judicious heating of vitriol and nitre, sea salt, mercury, and gold which, by repeated distilling or 'Cohobations', forms a powder sweetened with spring water that acts on the ventricle. Distributed in the blood, this may cure 'cutaneous Diseases, leprosies, and Gouts'. More generally, the mercurial medicines increase 'evacuation by Urine, Sweat, and sometimes Salivation ... wherefore in inveterate and contumacious Diseases they run to the use of these as to the last refuge'.

Willis is aware that there may be a need for 'Antiemetick Medicines' when nature 'goes beyond its bounds' and the animal spirits are 'irritated beyond measure and grow angry' sometimes 'with manifest danger of Life'; or when emetics have been overused. Simple measures such as the application of a warm foment of wormwood, mint, or spiced wine and 'a piece of bread tosted, and dipped in Claret Wine warmed' may help. Also useful is a clyster of

[44] See: *Pharmaceutice rationalis* part 1 (1679): page 28.

[45] See: *Pharmaceutice rationalis* part 1 (1679): pages 29–36 for details of prescriptions for vomiting medicines.

[46] See: *Pharmaceutice rationalis* part 1 (1679): page 32.

milk and treacle, massage of the limbs, and ligatures placed above the knees to retain the animal spirits and keep the legs free from convulsions. Failing these measures, Willis resorts to 'Treacle Andromick, or *Diascordium*, also sometimes a solution of *Laudanum* or Opiatick Tinctures'.

Applying somewhat contorted logic, Willis asks why not dispose of the morbific matter using a vomitory when vomiting is itself a symptom of disease and due to inappropriate agitation by spirits of the ventricle and oesophagus. Dispersal of the vomitus may also be increased by 'Whey, the drinking of medicinal Waters, the juice of Herbs, *Sal Prunellæ*'. Once everything is settled, it is time for a 'Digestive'. Wavering further from the precision and logic of his earlier narrative, Willis offers an encyclopaedia of remedies for belching and acid regurgitation, within which can be traced the recurring mention of wormwood and a remedy made from powder of ivory, the eyes of crabs, and red coral. This is to be taken with rhubarb, cinnamon, lemon juice, and extracts of various other fruits and flowers, further supplemented with steel-based substances and chalybeates. It is a typically complex Willisian regimen. Finally, if all else fails, 'I have known this Disease [lack of appetite and acid vomiting] sometimes happily cured by bathing in our Baths of *Bathe*'.[47] The pun is feeble and, taken together, the exposition on vomiting and vomitories is not Willis's most persuasive passage.

Enhancing excretion: purging medicines

Willis has made much of the contraction of the stomach at its 'left end' (oesophageal junction) in vomiting. Now he identifies the 'right end' (pylorus) as the place at which 'thorow the intestinal Pipes, as it were through a sink, the whole impurity of the Body is ... purged forth' of the 'chyle and *Fæces*'. Purges are necessary because digestion leads to many effluvia which 'being ... within a membrane ... constitute an heap of Vapours as it were wind ... which shut up creates torments, and not rarely an inflation of the belly'. Willis relates that 'when I have opened the dead bodies of many dying of an inflammation in the *Colon*; I found in all of them their whole Intestines distended to the utmost and as it were blown up with wind'. Continuing his scatological theme, he points out that sulphur generated as a consequence of the need for repeated nourishment 'contracts a most grievous stink', making it desirable that the intestines conduct 'an almost constant ... solemn excretory motion ... this Vermicular ... as in a creeping Worm' motion being achieved through coordinated contractions of the circular and longitudinal muscle fibres until 'the *Sphincter* of the Arse-hole being opened ... the Excrements are cast forth'.[48] This natural process is prone to overactivity and therefore a symptom of certain ailments. Excess flow from the gall bladder and pancreas leads to frequent and watery stools, and distempers of the blood result in a 'dysentery or bloody Flux'.

Because the salt and sulphur in purging medicines act less forcibly than emetics, these are able to pass through the stomach and stimulate nerves and muscles of the intestines. This forces the 'unloading of the Belly with wringing pains and with a noyse', sometimes with material from the mouths of the vessels so that 'meer Blood flowing out causes the Stools to be bloody'. The salt and sulphur particles within purgatives act not only on the abdominal

[47] See: *Pharmaceutice rationalis* part 1 (1679): page 40.
[48] See: *Pharmaceutice rationalis* part 1 (1679): page 43.

viscera but also enter the blood influencing the 'smell and colour' of the urine. This explains why 'the Milk of a Nurse taking Physick purges the Infant'. Moreover, and justifying their widespread use in a variety of distempers, circulation of purgatives enables the abdomen, præcordium, and brain to be washed, and their recrements discharged through the colon with other 'exempted Matter'. But the use of purgatives is not without its dangers, especially if vegetable or mineral derived tinctures fail to exert the desired effect and accumulate. Willis tells of two sons of an Oxfordian given mercury purges, one of whom had a hundred evacuations in forty-eight hours and was cured, whereas the other had none after which his hair fell out, his nails blackened and he developed pustules and scabs that lasted for two years.[49] Given the nature of his own encyclopaedic pharmacopoeia, an eyebrow may rise when Willis writes: 'the more ancient Physicians . . . as often as cathartick Evacuation is prescribed, a long series of destinated preparations for every humour, in a solemn manner as it were with a certain pomp is proposed; the use of which though specious enough seems not to be profitable'.[50] And, repeating admonishments from his preface, Willis concludes the general account of purges with the advice: 'Wherefore they who have a care of their health or life, must shun Empiricks, using for the most part only mercurial or Elaterian evacuation, more than a Dog or a Snake'.[51]

Willis provides the formularies for a variety of gentle, moderate, or strong purgatives. Of these, he specifies *Mercurius Dulcis* made from quicksilver and *Aqua fortis* (nitre); *Jalap* roots with spirit of wine; refined Scammony (bindweed) made in the same way; and *Extract of Black Hellebore* made medicinal with salt of tartar, lignum aloes and cloves. As with vomitories, cathartics may be given to excess, 'a Bridle as well as Spurs', and medicines are then needed to stop '*too great Purgation*'. In describing 'the Flux of the Belly', he goes on to advise against the use of phlebotomy, vomitories, and purges, preferring for immediate relief various hot and strong cordials based on Treacle Andromach and other opiates, especially 'a good dose of *Laudanum*', and St John's wort with diluents and very many other ingredients.[52] More generally, since 'the Flux of the Belly' is primarily the result of morbific particles present in the blood, treatment is by increasing their excretion with diaphoreticks and '*Alexipharmicks*' to break up the morbid 'Coagulations'. Willis interrupts his narrative with a chapter on the outbreaks that occurred in London during 1670 and 1671.[53] He illustrates the success of his combination therapy—'Alexiterick or preservative, Styptick or binding, Diaphoretick or evaporating & Opiatick or causing sleep or stupifying'—in cases treated during 1671 'when this disease Cruelly raged'. With some satisfaction, Willis relates how he cured an illustrious young man aged twenty-five with 'Caruncles, Gobbets of the membranes, and bloody phlegm or Gelly in his excrements' from the bloody dysentery using:[54]

> Tops of the Cypress Tree . . . the leaves of Periwinkle, and of Mouse-ear [chickweed] . . . Red Rose Flowers . . . boyled in broth made of a Sheeps Gathers . . . add to it the Oyl of St *John's*-wort . . . honey of Roses . . . mingle them for two Clysters, one of which he took in the morning, and the other at five a Clock in the afternoon. A plaister of red Lead and

[49] See: *Pharmaceutice rationalis* part 1 (1679): page 48.
[50] See: *Pharmaceutice rationalis* part 1 (1679): page 49.
[51] See: *Pharmaceutice rationalis* part 1 (1679): page 51.
[52] See: *Pharmaceutice rationalis* part 1 (1679): pages 61–5: mithridate and theriac andromache (Venice Treacle) consisted of opiates, sometimes also containing viper flesh, combined with up to a hundred other ingredients, many of which are listed by Willis.
[53] See chapter 15.
[54] See: *Pharmaceutice rationalis* part 1 (1679): page 64.

Paracelsus ... laid upon his belly ... he took besides twice a day of the juice of Plantan with water of *Scordium* or Germander, and Plague water ... also he eat every day a Quince rosted in the Ashes ... filled with the powder of *Olibanum*, Mastick, and Tolutan Balsom. By the constant use of these Remedies, he grew perfectly well within a Month.

Enhancing excretion: diuretick medicines; the Pissing evil

Since increased removal of recrements through natural passages is fundamental to Willis's rational therapeutics, methods of increasing the flow of urine are prominent in his regimens. As Willis has previously set out, the amount, odour, and colour of the urine, formed 'by a certain percolation in the Reins', naturally depends on the nature of products carried in the blood. In sustaining the vital flame and supply of animal spirits in the brain and other organs, the particles of enkindled blood are suspended in watery serum which must constantly be removed and replenished. But sometimes 'the old doth not always so readily ... go away ... the *Serum* sticks more unseasonably to the Blood as in Feavours evilly ... the phlegmatic Dropsie, and Cacochymy or ill digestion'.[55] Conversely, too easy separation occurs 'in the *Diabetes* or Pissing Evil, and in great floods of Urine which sometimes happen, and by and by cease again'. Rather than being excreted, the excess watery material may be deposited as in 'Cephalick Diseases or Thoracious, now an *Ascites* or *Anasarca*'.

Willis distinguishes diuretics that act through one of three putative and, as he argues, different mechanisms. Some release the watery humour from tenacious particles; others dissolve coagulations in the blood which have 'put away the Serum ... in divers places'; and some 'sup up again the Serum any where gone out of the vessels ... and deliver it to be sent away by the Reins'. Persuasive as the logic seems, the many remedies mostly share the same ingredients; and, for several, Willis has to admit 'but yet the reason ... doth not so clearly appear'. He lists liquors which induce diuresis based on spirit of nitre (saltpetre or potassium nitrate) or distilled from sea salt, human urine itself, tartar (potassium bitartrate), and the salt of amber.[56] Perhaps in his discussion of diuretics, more than can reasonably be argued for other topics, the writings of Thomas Willis justify the censure of writing 'nonsense' levelled at him by critics down the centuries. Altogether different is the unambiguous acclaim attached to his account of 'too much evacuation by Urine ... the *Diabetes* or Pissing Evil'.

Known to the Ancients, but rare in their experience, the diabetes is now met with daily 'in our Age given to good fellowship and gusling down chiefly of unalloyed Wine', as a result of which 'those labouring with this Disease, piss a great deal more than they drink ... joined with it continual thirst'. And in a famous statement, Willis adds 'the Urine in all (that I have known who hath hapned to have it, and I believe to be so in all) ... was wonderfully sweet as it were imbued with Honey or Sugar'.[57] Disagreeing with those who consider the quantity of fluid intake to be excessive, or the kidneys primarily at fault, Willis has it that 'the Chamber-pot Dropsy' is 'an affection of the Blood than of the Reins'. The problem is that serum too easily separates from the other constituents of blood: 'watry Particles cannot be contained by the more thick, but ... quickly sliding from their embraces ... do run thorow the most open Passages of the Reins' leaving the blood ready to coagulate and humours 'supped from the solid organs'. As a result the pulse quickens and patients 'quickly grow lean'.[58] The evident

[55] See: *Pharmaceutice rationalis* part 1 (1679): page 68.
[56] See: *Pharmaceutice rationalis* part 1 (1679): pages 72–9.
[57] See: *Pharmaceutice rationalis* part 1 (1679): page 79.
[58] See: *Pharmaceutice rationalis* part 1 (1679): page 80.

causes are dietary but also depressions of the animal spirits. Being primarily interested in the brain and nervous stock, Willis considers that this loosening of the watery from other particles in the blood is encouraged in diabetes when 'the nervous Juice is depraved … [so that] the animal Spirits do very much languish, and presently all nutrition is frustrated'. That the urine loses its normal salt taste is unsurprising; but why it should be sweet is less easy to explain. Perhaps it is the effect of sulphurous particles in the undigested chyle and 'meltings of the solid parts … these fat juices being mixed with Stale'. Willis is aware that polyuria may also occur in 'the *Nephritis* or Gravel' although that is more likely to result in 'a bloody than a copious water', and with abnormality of the '*Tubuli* being too ample, and open'.

As for treatment of the diabetes, vulgar opinion favours 'a solution of quick Lime with shavings of Sassaphras, Anis seeds, Raisins and Liquorish'. Willis has a better strategy. First, it is necessary to increase binding of serum to other particles in the blood using 'thickners … viscous and glutinous Particles … Rice, white Starch, also Gums, and some Resins'. Then the concretions need to be dissolved in an orderly way, restoring the '*Crasis* of the Blood' using 'nitrous Salts, also spirits of Harts horn, of Sal Armoniack and such like'. As for his successes: 'A certain noble Earl … in the space of a day and a night, he voided almost a gallon and a half of limpid Urine, wonderfully sweet, and as it were honied … with huge thirst, and a feavour as it were hectick, with great languor of the Spirits, the failing of Strength, and Consumption of the whole Body'. Sent for by the 'famous Physitians Doctor [John] *Mickelthwait* [1612–1682] and Doctor [Thomas] *Witherly* [1618–1694]', the three doctors prescribed liquors and powders containing many and familiar ingredients from Willis's pharmacopoeia, and a diet of milk and barley water. The Earl grew well but was not cured. Relapses occurred whenever his former habits were resumed. Eventually he 'suffered great enormities and defects in the nervous Stock; *viz.* a numbness or torpor and vertigo in the Brain, sudden convulsions in the Members, little leaping of the tendons, and felt various runnings about as it were of a wind creeping here and there'. But 'the aforesaid Physitians being called to Council, they advised the same method, and the patient was again restored to health'.[59]

Enhancing excretion: diophoreticks

Sweating increases when urine volume decreases, and *vice versa*, so that 'Diophoretick and Diuretick medicines, are of a very near alike use, and sometimes reciprocal'.[60] Sweating, '*Ephidrosis*', depends on the heat and rapidity of the circulating blood and 'animal spirits flowing from the Cerebell or little Brain' removing surplus serum through the 'Pores of the whole Body … sufficiently unlocked and lying open'. The sweat, containing serum with some particles of salt and sulphur, may appear 'like … vapours sent forth from boyling water, make wet the cover of the Pot that lies over them'.[61]

Profuse sweating in healthy people renders 'the Bodies of some … so cribrose or full of holes that they are not able to suffer the least breath of air, who also by every more quick motion … would be forthwith dissolved into moisture'.[62] Of particular interest to Willis, and on which he speculates at some length, are individuals who shun the outside air because,

[59] See: *Pharmaceutice rationalis* part 1 (1679): pages 84–5.
[60] See: *Pharmaceutice rationalis* part 1 (1679): page 66.
[61] See: *Pharmaceutice rationalis* part 1 (1679): page 90.
[62] See: *Pharmaceutice rationalis* part 1 (1679): page 92.

more through mechanical effects of its blasts than ambient temperature, it triggers intense sweating.[63] This also occurs with 'running, leaping, carrying of burdens, pulling or drawing forth and such like'. As a result, the contracted muscles squeeze and agitate blood in the nearby veins: 'and as of the Body, so also the immoderate exercises of the Mind move sweats'. Also, the ambient heat of the 'Sun, Fire, a Bath, Hot house' or 'lying in Bed . . . covered with many bed-cloaths' heat the blood and open the pores. Hot aliments, such as spices and 'strong Beer', swamp the blood with 'active Particles and provokatives' and 'as it were oyl to a Lamp, they stir up a more plentiful *Diapneon* of halituous or breathy matter, and for that cause greater sweatings forth of the abounding *Serum*'. Cold sweats occur with 'panick fear, a very acute grief, swooning, and in every sudden failing of the Spirits, and the agony of Death' like dew forming when a fire is extinguished.

So much for normal sweating. Hot sweats occur in fevers when the blood is overloaded with crude juices from undigested chyle and the pores are opened: 'In times past, it was a custom of the Irish, if any one were sick of a Fevour, to roll him up in woollen cloths wetted with cold water, by which means a plentiful sweat succeeding the disease was often broken'.[64] Referred to variously as Hydrocticks or sweating medicines, diaphoreticks given by mouth need to enter the blood unaltered, thereby acting to increase enkindling, liberating the water from other particles and, through animal spirits reaching the præcordium, increasing circulation of the blood. Their active ingredients, spirit, or saline without too much sulphur and 'loosened by Chymistry', are mainly derived from the fleshy and bony parts of vegetables and animals. Diophoreticks work best when given together with substances applied topically in order to open the pores of the skin; and with the patient kept warm in 'Bed, or a Bath, or in the heat of a hot-house, or else exercised with a more quick or hard motion of the Body' to encourage the sweating.

Once more, readers face a giddy list of Willis's preferred medicines. 'Bezoarticum minerale' is an extract of the rectified butter of antimony made by adding nitre and with repeated decoction in a crucible. It is free from sulphur as is 'Antimonium diaphoreticum' made from antimony thrice calcined with nitre. 'The Flowers of Sal Armoniack' is made by distilling ammonium sulphate obtained from soot, urine, or sea salt with iron filings; or from salt of tartar mixed with steel or copper. Tartar calcined with nitre and mixed with a source of ammonium sulphate is one of several methods for preparing 'Spirits of Sal Armoniack'. In this way, the saline is released and captured and the sulphur driven away so that the distilled spirit 'hath no stinking smell as the *Stagma* of Soot or Urine'. Some of these ingredients will already be familiar to those carefully following Willis's therapeutic recommendations. Perhaps new to his pharmacopoeia in the context of diophoreticks is the soot of burned wood heated in a retort with the distillate forming a volatile salt and 'a yellow Oyl and black'. This is obtained from '*Resinous Extracts of* Guaicum, *Box, and other ponderous Woods*', including the roots of scammony or jalap (Ipomoea purga). Alternative sources for the 'Spirit of Soot' are 'little pieces of Harts Horn . . . Skulls, Bones and Blood'. Spirit and oil that form the basis for diophoreticks can also be distilled from white tartaric acid.[65] Despite having introduced the topic, Willis omits to tell his readers anything of topical measures designed to open the pores and increase sweating.

[63] Willis identifies cold air as the cause of toothache, headache, and 'the Pose or stuffing of the head', albeit in a list of so many conditions that he cannot be said to have had in mind conditions such as trigeminal neuralgia; see: *Pharmaceutice rationalis* part 1 (1679): page 108.

[64] See: *Pharmaceutice rationalis* part 1 (1679): page 93.

[65] See: *Pharmaceutice rationalis* part 1 (1679): pages 101–4.

As with diuresis, medicines may be needed in order to reduce excess sweating: 'Nature oftentimes knows not a measure' leading, in this context, to '*depraved* Diaphoresis'. Excess '*Ephidrosis*' may also persist beyond successful treatment for a disease manifesting fever, from the accumulation of acid excrements and water with too little sulphur, or from overkindling of the blood. A young man recovered from a quartan fever but after ten months 'was necessitated to change his Shirt and Sheets all wetted ... thrice every night'. Although 'almost reduced to the dryness of a Skeleton', he was cured at length by drinking 'Asses milk'. Willis also knew of a noble Lady 'famous ... for that she does not only every night, moysten or thoroughly wet ye Linnen and bedcloaths, but besides distils into a basin put under her thighs many ... pounds of mere Sweat'. Since she deigned not to consult Willis, he huffed and puffed that 'I know not whether any Remedy, or any Method of curing would be profitable. And certainly nothing would be proposed by me if I should by chance speak to her about it'.[66]

Treatment of excess diaphoresis is by reequilibrating the aberrant salts with 'Antiscorbutes' or 'Chalibeates' and a meadow full of botanical preparations. Topical measures involve binding the open pores with linen soaked in ointments made from almonds and orange flowers. Even more plausible and equally soothing is bathing in cold water or a river. Finally, Willis advocates driving the excess serum away from the skin and towards the kidneys. He omits to tell his readers how this might best be achieved but he has a more urgent point to make. He provides an historical account of the 'English Sweat' and 'the bloody, black, bluish, stinking, or sweet smelling Sweat'. The absence of 'Spots, Pimples, Buboes and other marks of an envenomed or very much fermenting Blood' indicates that these sweats resulted from nervous Liquor flooding the blood stream producing premonitory symptoms of 'Langour, a defection of the Mind, an utter overthrow of strength, pain of the Head'. Willis proposes a similar mechanism for contemporary cases of persistent sweating in which 'the nervous Liquor scarce ever agrees with the Blood'.[67] He has already offered this explanation for the 'unbloody Dysentery', diabetes and some 'Tumours of an evil kind'. But, in sweating, the nervous liquor continually flowing into the blood is so malignant and pestilential that it is immediately cast 'adoors' from pores in the skin. This prevents circulation of the morbific material which, were it 'permitted to stay in the bloody Mass for a few Hours and to circulate and be thoroughly mixed with it, would wholly corrupt, and plainly mortifie it'.

Fermentation and the circulation: cardiacks

Although familiar to 'ancient Medicine, and also in our yet Vulgar and Empirical, which old Women and Quacksalvers exercise', there is no satisfactory explanation for the mechanism of action of the many medicines that act on the heart. But since it is assumed that in many diseases the heart is 'corrupted or beset with Venom or malignity ... [its] Remedies ... are not only called simple Cordials but *Alexiterions* and *Alexipharmacas*, that is preservatives or Antidotes against Poisons'.[68] In line with his doctrine of 'psychologie', Willis points out that much importance was formerly attached to cardiac medicines on the basis that these sustained vitality whereas, in truth, life is maintained by the corporeal soul, and manifest in

[66] See: *Pharmaceutice rationalis* part 1 (1679): pages 110–11.

[67] See: *Pharmaceutice rationalis* part 1 (1679): pages 111–13. For other accounts of the sweating sickness, see John Caius, *A boke, or counseill against the disease commonly called the sweate, or sweating sicknesse*, London (1552); and Charles Creighton, *A history of epidemics in Britain*, volume 1, Cambridge (1891): pages 237–81.

[68] See: *Pharmaceutice rationalis* part 1 (1679): page 114.

circulation of the blood and the work of animal spirits, whereas the heart is 'a mere muscle consisting only of Flesh and Tendons, after the manner of the rest, serving for the driving about of the Blood'.

Cardiacks 'unlock and open this joynting together of the Blood' when the particles are 'complicated within themselves' and will not separate for normal excretion of the recrements. Most of the medicines are similar to those that induce diuresis and diaphoresis. They act by increasing salinity of the blood. Having distanced himself from the life-preserving properties of cardiacks, Willis pays lip service to some popular remedies. 'The Salt of Vipers, powder of Toads' are also used; and the 'only and universal medicine of a late Doctor, a Physician going over to the empirical Sect, [was] the spirits of dead mens Sculls dug out of their Graves … These sorts of remedies have called back many from the very jaws of Death'.[69] Better favoured by Willis (but, as explained, deprecated by Slare) are the powdered extracts of solid materials, 'the Alchalisate or petrifying Salts of bezoar, *Bolus armenius* and Lemnian sealed earth (clays from Armenia and Lemnos)', shells, bones, horns, and teeth. And for different reasons, nitre taken in substances by mouth may encourage an enkindling flame when the blood is 'vitiated with Smoak and Soot … [or] fumes forth with a suffocating heat … rather than openly flames forth'. Conversely, the union of blood particles may be too lax through the presence of poisons, 'all its functions by degrees to flag, and lastly, Life to be destroyed', in which case the cardiacks prescribed are '*Alexiterions* and *Alexipharmacas*', to deal with the 'hurtful *miasmata*' and restore the normal particulate constitution of fermented blood.

The other class of Cardiacks is medicines that draw the animal spirits of the corporeal soul into the blood through the cranial nerves and in this way influence the heart and circulation. As for the details, Willis lists many familiar ingredients: 'Sage, Betony, Rosemary, Vervain and others'. He does allow one additional means of stimulating the heart:[70]

> Breathing forth a grateful scent or odor: hence also sweet smells, and pleasant sights for as much as they … delight the Spirits presiding in every Sensory, doth by and by raise up and amplifie the whole Soul … Cardiacks of this Rank … are perceived to operate first within the compass of the Head.

Animal spirits stagnated in the præcordium, or 'the animal motion of the Heart being stopped' as in 'swooning, Syncopes, Oppression or Convulsion of the Heart; yea almost in all other Irregularities, Langours, and Faintings away' can be stimulated by practical manoeuvres such as 'Chymical Oyls … put to the Nose … sprinkle cold water on the Face, to shake very much the Body, to pull the Nose, and sometimes to Strike or buffet the Body'.[71]

For all their logic and rationale, the ingredients recommended by Thomas Willis do not sit comfortably within the three mechanisms he proposes: suppression of enkindling, breakup of inactive coagulations of particles, and tempering the excess of animal spirits in the blood. Readers will be bedazzled by the display of familiar ingredients wheeled out for yet another set of indications. It is therefore with some relief that, as with diuresis and the 'pissing evil', Willis pauses to consider the various 'Cardiack Passions' for which his remedies may be used. But first he has a warning. There is an inherent danger in undisciplined use of readily available medicines that can have diametrically opposite actions and 'for which many people

[69] See: *Pharmaceutice rationalis* part 1 (1679): page 117.
[70] See: *Pharmaceutice rationalis* part 1 (1679): pages 119–20.
[71] See: *Pharmaceutice rationalis* part 1 (1679): page 120.

are brought into this most evil custom of sipping', not only gluttons but also 'learned men and very fair and ingenious Women'. The cardiac stimulants are particularly troublesome in this respect: 'by reason of stretching forth the Sails of the Soul to no purpose, the fabric of the Body as of a Ship, perishes and decays'.[72]

Against this cautionary background, two conditions do require 'cordial remedies'. These are the 'trembling of the Heart and its Palpitation', representing abnormalities of the frequency and force of the beat, respectively.[73] Not only can the palpitation or rapid heartbeat be felt by touch, it can be seen and heard from a distance: 'by the more vehement vibration of the Heart and percussion of the Ribs they have sometimes been broken or in younger people driven forth and continued protruberous or sticking out'. Willis doubts that it is the normal activity of the heart which displaces the chest wall. Rather it is the violent filling of the great vessels during systole, when the heart reduces in volume, which is responsible. For all the pounding in the chest, 'the Artery in the wrist for the most part beats languidly and weakly, as it were containing but a small River of Blood'. The fault may lie in the blood being too 'watry' and slow to enkindle or circulate because of sluggish particles, as in 'Virgins labouring with the green Sickness or cachectical men or women'. In hysteria and hypochondria, the palpitation is associated with 'a *Dyspnœa* or shortness of breath'. But, in other cases, the heart or great vessels are diseased: 'an old man ... was wont to suffer frequent assaults of the aforesaid disease ... who afterwards dying ... I found the Trunk of the great Artery ... to be bony or rather stony and its sides to be greatly compressed that a chink only be left, not that half the torrent of the Blood could flow'.[74] Sometimes Willis has found clotting in the 'bosom of the Heart, and the adjoining Vessels, and being concreted as it were into a fleshy Crust'.

The brain and nervous stock are never far from Willis's thoughts. At first, he had thought that palpitation of the heart is the result of local convulsion but 'the Neurology being more fully understood I presently fell from this opinion'. His account of this insight shows uncertainty. At one level the 'Heats, Fluxes and Refluxes, yea sometimes Stagnations of the Blood' are influenced by the rich supply of nerves to the heart and præcordium in response to the passions: 'the Splanchnick and Cardiack Nerves ... wont often to be beset with a morbifick matter ... subsisting either in the Head or neer to the Nervous beginning ... and are carried into Convulsions or Cramps of divers Kinds'.[75] But it is also the case that the 'constant turns of Systoles and Diastoles' and circulation of the blood are intrinsic properties of the heart and vessels, not forces imposed on them by the nervous spirit. Willis's difficulty is as much perceived as real, for that the heart beats intrinsically but is also influenced by its nervous supply and the emotions is not so controversial a position for him to have adopted. Treatment of the palpitation is with Cardiack cordials. These are unlikely to work if the arteries are primarily diseased, in which case: 'the life of the sick though miserable may be a little longer prolonged by some ease being procured by means of Hypnoticks'.

The 'Trembling of the Heart' is a disorder in which the 'moving Fibres ... being but half contracted, quick, but broken and as it were but half turns of Systoles and Diastoles; so that the Blood can both be brought into, and also carried out ... but only by very little Portions'.[76]

[72] See: *Pharmaceutice rationalis* part 1 (1679): page 121.

[73] At the risk of making retrospective diagnoses, it is remarkable that, in his account of the cardiac passions, Willis identifies and distinguishes tachycardias from local and remote causes, heart block and atrial fibrillation, heart failure to due muscle disease, ventricular aneurysm, aortic stenosis, and arteriosclerosis of the aorta and great vessels.

[74] See: *Pharmaceutice rationalis* part 1 (1679): page 126.

[75] See: *Pharmaceutice rationalis* part 1 (1679): page 127.

[76] See: *Pharmaceutice rationalis* part 1 (1679): page 129.

Here, the problem is very much a disorder of muscular motion. Returning to principles set out in *De motu musculari* (1670), Willis aligns palpitation with any other disorder of muscle, qualifying his position by specifying that it is a form of tetany or cramp rather than spasm resulting from the spirits conveyed by 'the Nerves from the Brain or the Cerebel or little Brain (in the hinder part of the Head) ... being compelled into irregularities'. Through the influence of the nerves and their juices, spirits present in the tendons and driving contraction of the muscle belly move in a disorderly way:[77]

> To this latter kind of convulsive motion properly belongs the Passion, or trembling of the Heart. Further to this Cense ought to be referred an affection commonly enough known and familiar to many, to wit, that sometimes they suffer a leaping, or very frequent and equal trepidations of some private Muscle, to wit, in the Lips, Cheeks, Eyes, or other Members.

Willis relates that 'I was advised with by Letters from *France* concerning a certain Gentleman, all whose Muscles thorow his whole Body, did almost perpetually use such leapings ... so that his outward Flesh ... imitated exactly the Vibrations of Pulses of the Heart itself'. Emphasizing that, for the reasons given, treatment is with cephalicks rather than cardiacks, Willis offers as remedies a now familiar list of extracts from bezoar, shells, ivory, coral and Harts horn, and fruits and flowers, together with chalybeates.

In the context of the cardiac passions, Willis has observed dysrhythmias: 'in these as to its motion it is amiss and irregular, in the other, as to its rest; for it is sometimes twice as long as it uses to be according to its ordinary course ... the Pulse being felt sometimes seems to intermit at the Wrist, whilst the Heart is perceived to shake ... most swiftly and incessantly in the Breast'.[78] One reason is poor output from the heart so that the great vessels are incompletely filled and do not always pass on their contents. In these chapters, Willis repeatedly uses a nautical metaphor: 'lest it should act so often in vain, it sometimes intermits its contraction, and seems even as in the unloading of a Ship when the wares are ... let for a time, staid in drawing them forth of the hold, the Porters ... pretermit some turns of going and coming'. Sometimes the heart regularly fails to contract, the strength of each beat lessening until the gap occurs: 'to a certain change of the Pulse, to wit, the third, fourth, fifth, or some other more often or more rare, now they are uncertain and wandring, as a cessation happens after a few Pulses, by and by after more'. Noticing that abnormalities of the pulse may precede severe headache, Willis favours intermittent reduction in supply of animal spirits in the cardiac nerves as the mechanism, the pulse resuming when sufficient have accumulated, like a mill ceasing until the flow of water in the wheel secures its rotation. Willis also indicates that the intermittent pulse may predispose to 'the Incubus and sometimes the Apoplexy'.[79]

Because he has emphasized the role of the arteries, Willis supplements his account of the cardiac passions with an anatomical description of the aorta.[80] This has four coats. The outer is rich in a network of nerve branches and 'little shoots of every kind of Vessels, shoot forth into the other underlying Coats of the Artery' (the vasa vasorum). This surrounds a 'glandulous' coat which, unlike the stomach, is placed outside the muscle layer. Willis

[77] See: *Pharmaceutice rationalis* part 1 (1679): page 130.

[78] See: *Pharmaceutice rationalis* part 1 (1679): page 132.

[79] Since 'apoplexy' is not used here in the context of cerebrovascular disease, this does not necessarily imply cardiac embolus. Why the intermittent pulse should encourage the sense of male demons threatening during sleep is unclear.

[80] See: *Pharmaceutice rationalis* part 1 (1679): pages 133–5.

suggests that this arrangement serves to distance this coat from the heat of blood in the lumen, whereas in the stomach and intestines, where it lies closer to the inner lining, 'there is need of the former fire of the Blood'. The 'transverse or annulary fibres' of the muscle layer enable the rapid contraction and constriction that drives forward the 'River of Blood'. Close to the heart for about two inches, the muscle coat is thicker in order to accommodate the impulse from the heart. The inner membranous layer has a further supply of nerves that, affected by the passing blood, ensure that contractions of the vessels are synchronized with systole and diastole of the heart and propagation of the pulse. This short section attracted attention:[81]

> On 18 December 1673, Mr Oldenburg presented to the Society from Dr Thomas Willis his new book, entitled, *Pharmaceutice rationalis, sive Diatriba de Medicamentorum Operationibus in humano Corpore*, printed at Oxford, 1673. Dr King having already perused this book, gave some account of it to the Society, and mentioned particularly the author's description of an artery and of its muscular motion like that of the heart, promising, that he would bring in the scheme of an artery not added to Dr Willis's book.
>
> On 5 February 1674 Dr King, according to his promise, produced a piece of an artery of a bullock, as it is described by Dr Willis, in his late book *De Medicamentorum Operationibus in humano Corpore*, shewing the four several membranes, of which it consists, *viz.* the vasculous, glandulous, muscular, and that which is contiguous to the blood; Asserting withal the doctrine of Dr Willis, that the motion of an artery is muscular, and the same with that of the heart.

Sleep and analgesia: opiates

Although sleep and waking, like '*Castor* and *Pollux*', are natural states that have their turns one after the other, 'the dominion of either of them being too long continued ... the faculties both of the natural and animal Function, become very much stupefied, and from hence one becomes more fit for the Grave than for Society'. To which end 'the most wise Creator hath abundantly provided opiates ... that it should be in our power to procure or repel Sleep or Waking'.[82] Opiates act by destroying selected animal spirits in the brain and nervous stock so that the 'rest as being amazed, or compelled more inwardly ... do relinquish or remit for a little while their Tasks'. But as 'extinguishers and poysoners' of the animal spirits, 'Narcoticks ... taken in too great a Dose ... cause death'. Opiates reach the brain in the circulating blood and act first on the shell or '*Cortex* of the Brain'. Returning to his favoured military metaphor, Willis writes:[83]

> They meet within this place the first forces of the animal spirits and ... extinguish wholly many of these placed in the fore part of the Battle; then, by reason that the other spirits of this Troop being made thinner ... withdraw themselves from the Battel, and rejoice

[81] See: Thomas Birch, *The History of the Royal Society of London for Improving of Natural Knowledge*, volume III, London (1757): pages 116, 122. This brief section is also included by Le Clerc and Manget, *Bibliotheca anatomica*, volume 2, Geneva (1685): pages 633–4; see chapter 3.

[82] See: *Pharmaceutice rationalis* part 1 (1679): page 136.

[83] See: *Pharmaceutice rationalis* part 1 (1679): page 138.

for their retreat, all the rest within ... so many watch-towers ... follow and leaving their watches recede, and give way to idleness.

'Intimate Sympathy' between the spirits of the stomach and brain indicates that opiates act directly on the stomach accounting for the rapidity of action after oral administration: people 'having eaten more gross and undigested meats ... become presently sleepy'. Opiates induce sleep when applied to the forehead, given as an enema, or by nasal solution. Effective in the 'watchings and *Delirium*', the condition 'chiefly requiring this Medicine is pain ... for which *Opium* ... it deservedly is wont to be called *Nepenthe*, and is truly a divine Remedie'. Pain relief is independent of sleep, often arriving before and persisting after narcosis. Whether analgesia results from direct action on the injured part, or on the 'common sensorie or ... whole sensitive Soul', is unclear. This is not easily resolved because, as Willis mentions in a sentence that has been recognized as an original and important observation, pain 'being excited in one place is felt in another'. This referral is because the 'excandelscency, distraction, and mutual allusion or beating of the tumultuating Spirits one against another' reach the sensorium by converging on the 'chamfered Bodies' from where they 'diffuse a certain trouble or inquietude'.[84] The pains for which Willis advises opiates include the colick, gout and stone, and 'in Arthritick Pains that Anodyne has been an egregious and as it were a divine Succor'. These are situations in which he has 'persuaded some to the constant and daily use of *Laudanum* or *Diacodium*'. But Willis is aware that use may become habitual: although 'the Impressions ... made deaf only to the approaches made from the paining part' produce 'an *Analesia* or Cessation from pain' for a while the dose must be repeated, 'the strength of the Medicine being spent, presently the same Tragedy returns, this Knot certainly deserved to be loosed'.[85]

Opiates also act on convulsions such that a 'many and divers cases in which ... the animal Spirits like fierce and furious Horses run about ... they ought to be reduced ... by Opiates as it were with Bridles'.[86] In this context, they are especially useful in settling disorders of the præcordium and viscera. By disconnecting the spirits flowing between the 'Cavities of the Viscera ... and [those] within the Cerebel', they affect the pulse and respiration, cough and asthma; and in the abdomen 'horrid Vomiting and ... the Dysenterick Affections can scarce be cured without *Opium*'. Opiates directly influence the humours of the blood allowing the 'Serum and other superfluidities or malignities ... to go forth, yea drive ... them out adoors' as is needed in the plague, smallpox, and malignant fevers. Willis describes a gentleman with nightly pains from venereal disease, ascites, and anasarca, who close to death pleads for Laudanum to ease his suffering so that Willis, 'granting it with a certain admonition ... left ... and gave him as I thought the last farewel' but the patient, daily increasing the dose and taking 'an incredible quantity', recovered so that he 'got a Stomach and went abroad' free from pain, thirst, and sweats.

Aware that the effects of opium are not always 'its Angelical Face', Willis considers the other side of this medicine when 'as of a turned piece of Coyn ... it will appear plainly Diabolical'. Physicians should remember 'as with a Sea Voyage; that the less danger and difficulty be met with, 'tis that both the Ports they may run into, and the Rocks to be shunned, be well known'.[87] Many examples can be given of people who through 'Quacksalvers and

[84] See: *Pharmaceutice rationalis* part 1 (1679): page 140.
[85] See: *Pharmaceutice rationalis* part 1 (1679): page 140.
[86] See: *Pharmaceutice rationalis* part 1 (1679): page 139.
[87] See: *Pharmaceutice rationalis* part 1 (1679): page 144.

Empiricks' have 'fallen into so profound a sleep that they could never be awakned'. The ultimate cause is cutting off the flow of animal spirits to the præcordium with consequent suppression of the pulse and respiration. Less immediately catastrophic are 'the want of Appetite and slothfulness of the Belly'. There is an effect on 'Memory, Discourse, and sharpness of Wit', or even the provocation of madness.

There are psychotropic substances other than opiates: 'Mandrake, Henbane, Cynogloss or Dog's Tongue'. Not all are necessarily harmful and some may be taken to advantage. Tobacco is 'not only necessary but profitable for Soldiers and Mariners', making them fearless and tolerant of physical discomfort. Taken at the mouth 'in the vulgar way', the animal spirits 'astonished' by this '*Enthymiama* or inflamed smoak, and as it were provoked into certain dances, they are wholly deaf to the approaches of any troubelsome thing'. But there is rite of passage before these soothing effects are noticed. The initial exposure to tobacco involves:[88]

> Great perturbations of the Brain and nervous Stock ... dizziness in the head, then a cruel vomiting ... the feet grow weak and stagger, the hands tremble, the tongue falters ... [as] the animal spirits ... intoxicated by the narcotic Sulphur ... are agitated into *Ataxias* ... oftentimes, 'tis for a very long while after their first taking it before they can ... take the fume of Tobacco without great confusion ... this smoaking gently awaking the animal spirits ... and as it were tickling them ... into ... expansive motions, with which they are wonderfully recreated, as with the drinking of Wine.

Willis equates the use of tobacco 'in our Countrymen as *Opium* with the Turks'. No less than tobacco, opium 'as we have observed concerning the taking of Tobacco in a Pipe ... 'tis wont at first ... to cause a Vertigo or dizziness, and oftentimes vomiting or purging, yea a cold Sweat with a trembling ... yet afterward we take it without any disturbance, yea at length with great delight'.[89] With increasing tolerance comes 'a boldness of Mind, so that they go to fight undauntedly and with notable confidence'. Noting the view held by some that 'Opiates provoke to Venery', and suggesting rather that they ought to reduce libido, Willis argues that this might be because opiates suppress animal spirits in the brain and so divert them to the 'genital members'.

Given this balance between benefit and risk, Willis advises that the decision to prescribe opiates should take into account the constitution of the patient and the prior state of the animal and vital spirits and humours in the blood. He avoids their use in the context of fever when the blood is 'turging with plenty and boyling up' and where giving a narcotic would be the 'work rather of a poysoner than of a Physician'. Opiates are not indicated in situations where diminishing circulation of the 'River of Blood' after haemorrhage would be inadvisable. By reducing excretory convulsions of the intestines, opiates allow recrements to 'stick more pertinaciously'; from which follows 'the old Precept, if that there be any thing to be evacuated, let it be evacuated before the Narcotick Pharmacy'. Opiates are to be given sparingly 'in the cough with much spittle and thick in the *Asthma*, and in all other thoracious Affections with an oppression of the Lungs, and in the Hysterick and other convulsive Passions'. That said, and with some apparent contradiction, Willis offers a list of situations in which opiates can be given with relative impunity:[90]

[88] See: *Pharmaceutice rationalis* part 1 (1679): pages 152–3.
[89] See: *Pharmaceutice rationalis* part 1 (1679): page 146.
[90] See: *Pharmaceutice rationalis* part 1 (1679): page 147.

> In the Palsie, *Vertigo*, *Incubus*, or Night-mare, Apoplexy, also in the *Orthopnoea* or straightness of the Lights, in the Dropsie of the Breast or *Abdomen*, in the *Stupor* or trembling of the Members, in very malignant Fevers, or in the *Crises* of others, Narcoticks are most often interdicted ... But yet in the cruel Headache, Catarrhs, Colicks, Plurisie, ordinary Fevers, in Vomiting, Dysentery, in Nephritic Paroxysms, in Gouts and all kinds of Pains, the opiatick Pharmacy is not only allowed, but is sought for as the only, and as it were divine *Panacea*.

Sensitivity to opiates varies, Turks and dogs being resistant and cats unduly susceptible. Based on common observation, this opinion is endorsed by an experiment in which Willis and others transfused three ounces of the tincture of opium into the jugular vein of a small dog which, making the animal drowsy, sleep was prevented by 'beating, terrifying, and coursing him about so that he soon became lively'.[91] Although described as having been done 'many years ago', this is probably not the occasion, in March 1656, when Christopher Wren (1632–1723) suggested he could 'easily contrive a way to convey any liquid Poison into the mass of Blood', whereupon Boyle obliged by providing a large dog on which to open the crural vein of the beast's hind leg and infuse 'opium in sack', which made the dog transiently sleepy 'by the circular motion of That, carry'd to the Brain'.[92] (Nor is it the experiment in which a dog was made to vomit after infusion of antimony dissolved in wine: see earlier.)

Having discussed the merits and demerits of opium and tobacco, Willis mentions that there are many unorthodox narcoticks. He advises that these pharmaceutical mavericks be prevented from entering practice since there 'is no need of new ones daily to be devised':[93]

> Among our Countrymen there is not only a company but a swarm rather of false Chymists and Quacksalvers; every one of which boasts of his peculiar *Laudanum*, which they rashly give in every Disease and Condition, and if by chance it happens for the sick to sleep and wake again, presently they sing and are Cock a hoop, when rather they merit the gallows ... wherefore it behoves you to be warned whoever hath any regard to his Life, that you diligently be aware of these Laudanists.

His own 'Opiology' consists of extracts of white and wild poppy, seeds of henbane, the roots and juice of hound's tongue, and oil of tobacco. Each is rich in sulphur and saline giving them a familiar odour. These are less hypnotic and easier to prepare than the juice of opium. His preferred method for 'Meconology or Poppyology' is to extract tincture of opium from the white poppy in spirit of wine or lemons with salt of tartar coloured and flavoured with 'Saffron, *Castor*, Cloves and *Lignum Aloes*'. He has no time for the claims that narcoticks can be extracted from mineral, or for anodynes that act without also 'stupyfying'.

Finally, Willis considers antihypnoticks which 'driving away sleep too much troublesome do render us wakeful'. His focus is 'a certain Liquor called Coffee, highly efficacious for the driving away the Narcosis or stupifyingness'. Introduced 'among the Turks, and ... Arabians and other Eastern People ... this drink also of late years is brought into custom by our own Countrymen, and that there is almost none but understands well enough by experience its efficacy and virtue for the driving away of sleep'. Coffee acts by diverting serum to the 'Reins and habit of the Body', inducing a diuresis, opening the pores of the brain, and

[91] See: *Pharmaceutice rationalis* part 1 (1679): pages 149–50.
[92] See: Robert Frank, *Harvey and the Oxford physiologists*, Berkeley (1980): page 171 and endnote 40, page 332.
[93] See: *Pharmaceutice rationalis* part 1 (1679): page 150.

preventing the displacement of animal spirits to the middle of the brain by incoming nutritious and serous particles, thereby 'laying aside their *torpor* or drowsiness'. Willis warns habitual imbibers of coffee that through the 'old veterane spirits rendred more agil and nimble [and] the supplies of the new ones ... diminished' they may become 'lean, and oftentimes paralytick and obnoxious to an impotency to Venus'. Nonetheless in certain disorders of the brain and nervous stock, he indicates that 'I frequently prescribe this drink sooner than any thing else for their cure, and therefore am wont to send the sick to the Coffee houses sooner than to the Apothecaries shops'.[94] As with all his medicines, coffee may stimulate 'an humid brain ... [with] slothfulness of the animal Spirits' but pervert the spirits and humours and makes worse those obnoxious to the 'Headach, *Vertigo*, the Palpitation of the Heart, the trembling or numbness of the joynts producing an unwonted Languor in their whole Body'.

The lungs and mechanism of breathing

In moving at the start of *Pharmaceutice rationalis* part 2 from discussion of medicines that exert general effects through increasing excretion or restoring 'the fainting Spirits' to regional disorders and their therapies, Willis starts with the lungs. First he must explain the anatomy and physiology of breathing in health, as the basis for considering 'Cough, Phthisic, Catarrh, Asthma, Dyspnoea, and other Diseases of the Brest'. Benefiting from the experiments and reasoning of his colleagues during the 1660s, Willis is aware that life depends on blood and air coming into contact, even though the nature of what may be exchanged is unknown.

Willis defers to Marcello Malpighi (1628–1694) and his experiment of first washing out the blood and then expanding the lungs with clear fluid to show that they consist of a network of bladders. When inflated, these appear as a 'Polypody-leaf' richly supplied by arteries and veins, 'Lymphæducts' and nerves. These structures are organized into lobes surrounded by a membrane, all connected to the '*Aspera Arteria*' (trachea) on a stem 'not much unlike to a bunch of Grapes'. The text is illustrated with eight plates depicting the gross and microscopic features of the trachea, lungs, nerves, blood vessels, and pleural membranes (Pl.33–Pl.40). Willis describes the cartilaginous and membranous structure of the larynx, trachea, and airways. The two main bronchi branch extensively into sprigs, making 'as it were a certain private Grove' where the blood can mix with the inhaled nitrous particles. Their cartilages are arranged like a 'Coat of Mail' so that they can stretch and contract with movement of the lungs much as 'the shelly Coat of a Lobster'. Willis assumes that air does not enter all the little bladders with every breath, being normally confined to the 'threshold and dens ... lest the external air is too sharp, or otherwise disagreeable to the Lungs'. The extremities of the lungs are held in reserve and called upon 'as in running, singing, or much speaking, also in some crazy dispositions ... the inward air ... supplying in a manner the defect of the outward'.[95] Equally, the smaller bladders of the lungs do not empty with each 'Systole of the Breast', or expiration, unless the muscle coat contracts to exhale fully or cough out matter in the air.

Inspiration and expiration, the diastole and systole of the lungs, are partly aided by the outer (pleural) membrane, patterned 'like a Hive of Bees' and acting as an elastic restriction on movement. But more important is the 'cunning artifice of the Divine Creator, evidently

[94] See: *Pharmaceutice rationalis* part 1 (1679): pages 154–5.
[95] See: *Pharmaceutice rationalis* part 2 (1679): page 6.

adapted into Mathematical rules' in the arrangement of muscles acting on the chest wall, 'three ... to the shoulder, one belonging to the loyns, and eleven intercostal'. During inspiration these change the shape of the ribcage from a cylinder to a square, enlarging the space within, at the same time as the diaphragm contracts downwards to the abdomen.[96] The mechanics of inspiration are perfected by cartilages which give rigidity to the ribcage. The reversal of these movements with systole or expiration is not a passive process resulting from cessation of contraction in the muscles of inspiration, but due to the action of antagonists assisted by the abdominal muscles allowing the force of expiration to increase during exercise.[97] Willis draws attention to a muscle well developed in the dog, but vestigial in man, inserted into the lower sternum which 'Divine Providence touching the Fabrick of Animals' serves the purpose of rapid respiration in animals 'for that fresh air may be more freely suckt in ... [and] the old be strongly cast out and exploded'.[98]

Whilst the reciprocal activities of agonist and antagonist muscles of respiration 'have their conveyance through the Nerves', less intuitive is whether these rhythmic activities are voluntary or involuntary, and therefore either 'of the Brain or Cerebellum'.[99] Respiration continues during sleep for the preservation of life but can be interrupted at will when awake. Therefore animal spirits in the pneumonic nerves and wandring pair must each exert an effect on the muscles. These nerves also drive the 'instinct' of respiration in 'breathing, coughing, laughing and other actions ... according to the several exigencies of Nature'. In these 'singular offices of the lungs and wind-pipe' the intercostal muscles are supported by involuntary accessory movements of the neck and abdomen, unless the 'nerves of the Diaphragma do warn the other nerves of the arms, plucking them and as it were admonishing of their duty to desist from an over intense motion'.[100]

The anatomy of the pulmonary artery is much as already described for the aorta. The pulmonary vein, lacking valves, is structured so as to allow it to dilate and carry back the 'Blood now hot and boiling' and changed in colour from black-purple to scarlet. No better evidence than this vascular arrangement could be offered in favour of the view that the function of the lungs is not to mix the blood but to replenish it with the nitrous 'Particles of the Air'.[101] The anatomical arrangement of the vessels and bladders favours separation, not mixture, of particles leaving dregs as found in persons with the 'Green-sickness, Cachexy, and that sort of Dropsie called *Leucophlegmatia*'.

Anticipating the text that is about to follow, Willis concludes his account of the anatomy and physiology of breathing by explaining that cough occurs when the upper part of the 'Wind-pipe ... is so much provoked by the smallest prejudice ... [and] wonderfully forced into a convulsive motion ... as a sense of annoyance'. This forcible expulsion of air in the

96 See: [Samuel Mihles], *Medical essays and observations relating to the practice of physic and surgery: abridg'd from the Philosophical Transactions, from their first publication down to the present time. The Latin papers are English'd, some occasional remarks are made, and the whole illustrated with necessary copper-plates*, two volumes, London (1745) for an account of Richard Lower, 'The manner of respiration', *Philosophical Transcations*, 11 November 1666, number 29: page 544. Here 'the doctor' sectioned the [phrenic] nerves in a dog in order to show that the diaphragm is the 'chief organ' of respiration. The dog was observed to 'draw his Breath like a Wind-broken Horse'. Lower makes the observation, still used in neurological practice, of observing the normal outward movement of the abdominal wall on inspiration due to downward motion of the intact diaphragm, and its reversal on expiration. Lower also concludes that the diaphragm is more important for comfortable respiration than movements of the intercostal muscles.

97 See: *Pharmaceutice rationalis* part 2 (1679): page 10.

98 See: *Pharmaceutice rationalis* part 2 (1679): page 12.

99 Until this point, Samuel Pordage has translated Willis's text as 'Cerebel' and this is the first use of 'Cerebellum': the Latin in *Pharmaceutice rationalis* part 2 (1674): page 30 is 'Cerebello'.

100 See: *Pharmaceutice rationalis* part 2 (1679): page 13.

101 For discussion, see chapter 15.

'inward Pipe of the Wezand' (windpipe) is 'depraved or hindred ... [in] an Asthma, a Dyspnoea, and some other diseases about breathing'. Washed with blood and spirits and drained by veins and lymphatics,[102] 'when too much filled ... a humour distilling from the Glandules as well as from the Arteries into the hollowness of the Wind-pipe brings a Catarrh'.

Sundry kinds of breathing hurt

In introducing the distempers to which structures of the chest are vulnerable, Willis reuses an old metaphor: even a watch with its spring and wheels 'plain and toothed, with chain and balance ... is not more prone or easie to be obnoxious' than the lung, its vessels, muscles, nerves, and the substances contained therein. He points out that diseases of the chest arise either from impairment of the circulation in the 'right *Sinus* of the heart', the pulmonary artery or vein; or through failure to move air during inspiration and expiration.[103]

On the first point, rejecting (Franciscus) Sylvius's (1614–1673) theory of inadequate mixture of chyme and lymphatic humour leading to impoverished heating of blood in the right ventricle, Willis argues that, in addition to the cardiac disorders already discussed in the first part of *Pharmaceutice rationalis*, it is usually failure of the moving fibres of the heart to contract that 'drives out the blood either infirmly or irregularly' and impairs the pulmonary circulation. That is not to say that inadequate enkindling of blood in the pulmonary circulation, or a deficiency of sulphur and spirit with too much saline and water, does not make the pulmonary vessels 'heavy and muddy', obstructing the forward propulsion of blood from the right ventricle. As a result, 'grumous or fleshy concretions called the Polypi of the Heart' accumulate and cause 'painful breathing' and 'very troublesom Cough'. Furthermore the vessels may be compressed by 'some humor from without' when 'the little Cells or bronchial Pipes ... are filled with a viscous phlegm, purulent matter, or blood extravasated'; or by 'tumors, little swellings, worms, also stony, sandy, and curdly concretions'. Sometimes the artery or veins are made bony, so that a very 'small chink remains for the blood to pass'.[104] When the passage of blood is impaired and forced by the beating of the heart, it may rupture the vessels into spaces between the lobes causing a 'Peripneumony, or falling ... into the cavity of the Chest ... an Empyema'. Opening of the mouths of vessels into the trachea results in spitting and coughing of the extravasated blood. More generally, the lungs are particularly prone to suffer from the 'corruption and putrefaction of the blood ... toucht with an infection or a pestilent or venomous contagion', as in the measles, smallpox, plague, and malignant fevers. And with cough, difficult breathing and bloody spittle, death may result from the 'blood clodding in the vessels of the Heart or Lungs'. Taken together, here is an intuitive and comprehensive account of circulatory disorders of the thorax leading to breathlessness.

Under other circumstances, the 'Pleurise and Peripneumony' result from blood reaching the lungs being so overheated, its particles rich in sulphur and salt but deficient in serum, that the heart beats inordinately in order to mix with air. An excess of water in the blood, through closure of the skin pores and failure of perspiration when cold, causes the blood

[102] See Hierons (1967), at page 2 mentioning Willis's claim to have first described the superficial lymphatics of the lungs; citing WS Miller, 'Thomas Willis and his De phthisi pulmonari', *American Review of Tuberculosis*, 1922; 5: 934–49.

[103] See: *Pharmaceutice rationalis* part 2 (1679): page 17.

[104] See: *Pharmaceutice rationalis* part 2 (1679): page 21.

'presently to boil up, and cast off the serous superfluities in the Lungs'. Pursuing this logic, more than once in his text Willis attributes cough to ambient temperature: 'wherefore in our Idiom the cause being put for the effect, a Cough is called Catching of cold'.[105] Much the same follows drinking sharp liquors, and Willis tells of his own experience:[106]

> I have experimented this upon myself yearly, when in the summer season (when the blood abounds with Sulphur) I have drunk Cider with tartish Wines safely, yea frequently to advantage, the same in winter (when the blood is prone to but moderately tasted of), do presently provoke a Cough.

Willis adds to his account of respiratory disease a description of suffocation through want of air, so that the blood is not nourished, the pulse ceases, the vital spirit is 'subtracted from the brain', and life is lost. This serves to introduce his discussion of less immediately catastrophic situations in which disease results from various impairments in the entry or expulsion of air. Experience shows that breathlessness results from a deficiency in Nitre, as in 'a low-rooft Chamber ... places crowded with an assembly of men, or made hot with the ardour of the Sun ... on the tops of those mountains exceeding the top of the Atmosphere'. Less obvious is that nitrous particles are corrupted 'as often as the South-wind blows' whereas with 'the North-wind ... most nipping particles are adjoined to the Nitrous'. Difficulty in drawing breath occurs with lungs stiff through a 'phlegmon ... and other concretions' and therefore not able to expand passively with movements of the chest wall and diaphragm. Not infrequently these muscles fail due to pain or are weakened through loss of animal spirits in the 'passages of the nerves', affected individuals being 'surprised with horrid fits of an Asthma'. But the commonest reason is obstruction of the trachea with 'a Catarrhal distillation of the Serum' thickened by digestion, or from extravasation of 'blood, also of *Pus* or ichorous matter out of the Lympheducts'. And ever the advocate of plain living, once again 'a plentiful meal, or abundant drinking of Wine or strong Ale' may make the blood turgid, compress the trachea, and fill the lungs 'rather than from a cram'd stomach hindering the Systole of the Diaphragma'. Convulsive contraction of the tracheal muscle fibres also results in 'dreadfull fits of an Asthma'. Equally, again rehearsing one of his favoured nautical metaphors, difficult breathing may arise from '*Polypus* in the Nose, the Quinzy in the Throat, of inflammation of the Tonsils ... as a heap of sand about a Haven, obstructs the ingress and regress of Ships'.

Disorders of breathing may result from impaired expiration, especially when this needs to be vigorous as 'in a cough, in sneezing, in laughing, in crying and in Hiccough'. Although aware that cough usually results from local irritation, Willis also describes sharp humour lodged in the brain stimulating the pectoral muscles, and a discharge of serum from the arteries in the nostrils, palate, '*Gula*' (throat), or larynx as additional causes of cough. Equally, 'an inflammation, a tumour, a little swelling ... gravelly, stony, or polypose Concretions, worms and many other preternatural things ... inasmuch as they almost perpetually provoke the nervous fibres' may trigger dry cough.[107] Moist and productive cough, the disorder next to be discussed, is 'either white or yellow, or somewhat greenish ... blewish, or black', or bloody and purulent, as in consumption.

[105] See: *Pharmaceutice rationalis* part 2 (1679): page 33.
[106] See: *Pharmaceutice rationalis* part 2 (1679): page 19.
[107] See: *Pharmaceutice rationalis* part 2 (1679): page 25.

Phthisis or consumption

Most, if not all, disorders of the thorax, like lesser streams into a greater lake 'losing their natures and ancient names', lead to the 'Phthisis or Consumption'. This has first place of 'all diseases of the Breast'. Although a 'private' pulmonary disorder, the symptoms of phthisis affect the 'œconomy of the whole natural and animal function'. Sometimes without cough or any apparent fault in the lungs, phthisis leaches particles from many solid organs in order to replenish those defective in the blood through poorly assimilated nutritious juice: 'persons so affected seldom pine away to death, yet they grow old sooner, and end their life in a shorter space'. For Willis, phthisis is indistinguishable from the many other causes of chronic wasting. Although wary not 'to put our sickle . . . into another mans harvest', he pauses briefly to give a general account of cachexia, especially in disorders of the abdomen:[108]

> How often do we see a Schirrus happening in the Spleen, Liver, Pancreas or Mesentery . . . an Ulcer or cancrous Tumour of some Gout, also of a Kidney, Womb, or Bladder, or otherwise malignant Sore, a deadly Atrophy to have succeeded without any notable fault of the Breast or Lungs?'

This leads to an account of tabes dorsalis. By this Willis means the generic symptom of wasting but he also recognizes tabes as a specific disorder of the brain and nervous stock.[109] On '*Phthisis* or *Tabes*' in the context of disease affecting the lung, where 'the threads of life are spun', Willis explains that he has opened the dead bodies of many and found 'little swellings, or stones, or sandy matter'. For the reasons given, he prefers '*a withering away of the whole body arising from an ill formation of the Lungs*' to the standard definition of phthisis as 'A pining away of the whole body, taking its rise from an Ulcer in the Lungs'. The 'enemy to the Lungs' must enter through the trachea, the pulmonary artery or the nerves. When the trachea is at fault, the material is 'moist air . . . replete with fumes, or abounding with malignant vapours' supplemented by spittle and catarrh formed from secretions seeping through its various coats. This is removed 'every morning by expectoration then more copiously'. Eventually, material fills the lungs causing the little bladders to rupture and form a lake within which the 'consumptive matter petrifies, clefts or ulcers are formed . . . in many places, and all the other hollownesses are stufft with frothy quitter'.[110] The blood passing through is defiled and the 'pining of the whole body' follows.

When the phthisis results from dyscrasias of the blood, material deposited through the vessels 'among other parts, so . . . often into the lungs' can be removed by coughing 'spittle like black Ink', thereby 'purging the lungs of melancholy fæculencies from the blood'. Alternatively the lungs act as a receptacle for any matter that is dammed back from its normal passage of evacuation: 'the menstruous flux or the Haemorrhoids . . . bleeding at the Nose if by chance it ceases, Issues closed up, Pustles, Scabs and Wheals driven back, do frequently affix a taint in the *Thorax*'. So too does impairment of insensible perspiration. When degenerate nervous juice settles in the lungs, the 'more grievous passions of the brain and nervous kind frequently call on a troublesome Cough'.

[108] See: *Pharmaceutice rationalis* part 2 (1679): page 27.

[109] See: *Pharmaceutice rationalis* part 2 (1679): pages 28–9, and chapter 17 for Willis's account of tabes dorsalis as a disorder of the nervous system.

[110] See: *Pharmaceutice rationalis* part 2 (1679): page 31.

One cause of the phthisis is immobility of the thorax through 'crookedness or shoulders like wings', meaning that 'the Lungs do neither injoy a space so free and ample, nor can the moving Muscles be so strongly contracted as in a square breast'. Peculiarities of shape affecting the thorax, such as a narrow chest with a neck somewhat long, may explain hereditary disposition to consumption. Here Willis makes an important distinction between nature and nurture pointing out that within the family, individual members are related but also exposed to the same climatic conditions and 'polluted thick and smoaky City air'.[111] Any previous distemper of the lungs predisposes to phthisis: empyema, pleurisy, peripneumony, and imposthume; or smallpox, measles, and irregular fever. Common to all these situations is the nature of inspired air. As a result, people troubled with consumption often flock to the southern parts of France, 'mountainous places exposed to the Sun' or, if unable to go abroad, leave the City for villages.[112] But this is often in vain. Many 'in those places rather find their graves than health'. As for London, 'some avoid this City as Hell, others fly to it as to an *Asylum*'. Also protective is living in places where domestic fires are nourished by turf and 'a suffumigation of Sulphur and Arsenic'.

Although a new cough may be innocent, 'as in a strong man, and one who hath often before endured a Cough Scot-free', more ominous is cough protracted and with discoloured phlegm, breathlessness, loss of appetite, and languishing of the whole body. When to these are added 'hectic Feaver with a continual thirst, night Sweats, an Hippocratical face, an utter decay of the flesh almost to the driness of a Skeleton', the phthisis is confirmed and 'all hope of Cure being waved, we must insist upon Anodynes, whereby an easie death may be procured'. In the early stages, overheating of the blood with release of serum needs to be reduced by use of a thin diet and promotion of sweating through wearing thick garments, staying in bed, and taking a posset drink boiled with rosemary or sage. If these fail, phlebotomy and hypnoticks are to be used together with a pectoral decoction (linctus) containing 'Root of Chervile, Butchers-broom, Elicampane ... Hog-lice, volatile salt of Amber ... and Powders of Shells'. When other symptoms develop, the need is to drive the recrements from the lungs to other routes of excretion using diuretics, diaphoretics, and purges. Lastly, the lungs are strengthened to prevent 'the reception of serum and other humours', again with linctus and soothing lohochs made with liquorish, sweet almonds and syrup of jujubes to close the pores and moisten the lining of the trachea. Willis describes the ingredients of 'some choice receipts': mixtures, linctuses, lohochs, tinctures, balsams, troches, lozenges, powders, pills, decoctions, and distilled waters.[113]

Never one to dismiss an idle thought, Willis's discussion of phthisis brings to mind 'the suffocating Cough of children, and in our idiome called the *Chin-cough*' which is seasonal and often epidemic.[114] The infants or young children convulse with coughing and respiration is suspended either in 'the Systole, or Diastole, that Inspiration, or Expiration being suppres'd for a space, the vital breath can scarcely be drawn'. Coughing being almost strangled, 'they hoop' and 'contract a blackness in their countenance'. This arises from the lungs being constantly irritated by serum soaking out of the mass of the blood, and the nerves disposing the motive parts of the thorax to convulsions from 'heterogene and elastic matter falling from the brain through the nervous passages'. Because the condition

[111] See: *Pharmaceutice rationalis* part 2 (1679): page 33.

[112] See: *Pharmaceutice rationalis* part 2 (1679): page 34; and chapter 1 for details of Willis sending his son, Thomas, to Montpellier, France, when the young man developed consumption whilst at Westminster School.

[113] See: *Pharmaceutice rationalis* part 2 (1679): pages 37–40.

[114] See: *Pharmaceutice rationalis* part 2 (1679): pages 40–1. See also chapter 15.

improves and the usual remedies are unhelpful, 'old women and Empiricks are oftener consulted than Physitians'. They advise 'Cup-moss, or Chin-moss or Chin-cups', a remedy of which Willis does not disapprove believing that it both fixes serum in the blood and volatilizes the nervous juice, so settling the convulsive disposition. Also popular, and logical in terms of distracting the animal spirits and forcing them into other nerves where they are less troublesome, is giving children with chin-cough a great fright: 'while a great Mill is driven about with a screeching noise, and a dreadful aspect of the wheels, the distempered be put into the Trough or receiver of the Grain or Corn, and from thence the sudden cure of this disease sometimes happens'.[115] If this seems somewhat drastic, a more conventional approach is a purge, blisters raised on the nape of the neck behind the ears and in the axillae, and a draught of china root with shavings of ivory or Hart's-horn, raisins, and liquorish.

A different approach to treatment is needed once it is clear that cough is a manifestation of well-developed phthisis with matter from the blood, 'superfluous Serum, but also the nutritive Juice, and perhaps the nervous, the Lympha', deposited in the passages of the lungs and putrefied in the distended pulmonary bladders. It follows that now the strategy is to stabilize the dissolute blood, clear the passages by expectorating the purulent material, and allow the bladders to dry out. Dealing with dyscrasia in the blood is achieved by improving the nutritive juice through a diet restricted to ass's, cow's or goat's milk rather than flesh, eggs, and gelly broths or strong drink; medicines prepared with brimstone (sulphur); and deploying the full panoply of bleeding, purges, diuretics, hot baths, 'frictions of the extreme parts', issues and blisters with, new to his regimens thus far, 'Depilatories, Errhines (medicine that promote nasal discharge), Gargles, and other private or public sluices either of humors or vapors'. The lungs are cleared with linctuses, fumigations, lohochs and 'Eclegmas' (electuaties sweetened with honey) and other concoctions, described in more detail, that act both on the trachea and blood delivered through the pulmonary arteries.[116] The lungs are dried by sulphurous inhalations 'suckt through a Pipe or Funnel'. Mountebanks and vulgar opinion have it that inhalation of arsenic smoked like tobacco is preferable. In its later stages, once phthisis enters the phase of thirst, watchings, 'hectick feaver and an Atrophie', little can be done as 'daily weakening precipitates them to the grave', other than support with asses milk and broths strengthened with snails, application of pectoral herbal remedies, and hypnoticks all aimed at helping towards 'light toleration and an easie death'. As usual, Willis illustrates 'a stubborn and tedious Cough' with two case histories showing to advantage his skills as a treating physician so that, after prolonged ill health, the one 'now lives altogether exempt from that distemper' and the other, a child of ten, 'praise be to God he enjoys his perfect health'.

Willis used the term phthisis to describe progressive wasting diseases, although no doubt some of his patients had pulmonary tuberculosis. There is much in his account that physicians will recognize in terms of seasonal risk, poor air quality, shape, and impaired excursion of the chest wall, adequate movement of air through the respiratory passages during inhalation and exhalation, and the ill effects of copious secretions. His treatments may appear to lack specificity but he understood the need for systemic remedies and local measures that clear and maintain the upper and lower airways.

[115] See: *Pharmaceutice rationalis* part 2 (1679): pages 41.
[116] See: *Pharmaceutice rationalis* part 2 (1679): pages 44–6.

Of spitting blood

Given the rich supply of blood to the lungs, Willis finds it surprising that 'an Hæmoptyis or spitting blood' is not more frequent. Other than in wounds or other forms of violence when the veins are punctured, when it does occur the bleeding is usually arterial and due to opening of the mouths of the vessels through distempers of the blood. Bleeding often originates from vessels near the larynx and trachea, but sometimes from the pneumonic arteries pouring out 'a dreadful quantity of blood; the spitting out whereof proves plentiful and violent'. Coughing clears the extravasated blood unless material accumulates between the lobes or outer membrane as 'an Empyema, and frequently an Imposthume'. The predisposing causes are familiar: diet and climate (the North wind again blamed), and dyscrasia of the blood. Newly added are poisons (unspecified), nosebleeds and, 'according to [Johannes] *Heurinius* [1543–1601], the Lunar beams (the reason whereof doth not easily appear, neither doth there remain any credit thereto)'.[117] Logically, Willis's therapeutic strategy is to reduce the flow of blood to the site of bleeding through phlebotomy, ligatures, and frictions. Juleps, herbal syrups, linctuses, and diacodiate (opiate) hypnotics also help close pores of the offending vessels. Much the same list of remedies is offered for the secondary aim of 'healing ... the hurt of the lungs', together with fresh air, reduced physical activity and abstaining from 'grosser foods, from Noon-sleeps, from plentiful suppers, and other errors in diet'. After a long and detailed formulary, Willis threatens that it would 'be easie to reckon up very many other remedies ... notwithstanding the harvest of these already gathered together doth at present seem rich enough'. Sparing his readers a long discourse, the 'pectoral Decoction' brought to Willis's attention by a noble young man who suffered from the palsie, consumption and copious spitting of blood and for whom all other remedies had not been effective, does deserve mention:[118]

> Take of all the Sanders of each six drams, infuse them for twelve hours in seven pints of Spring-water, then boil them to a consumption of a third part, after add leaves of Colt's-foot, Maidenhair, Mouse-ear, Speedwel, flowers of St. Johns-wort, each two handfuls; sweet Fennel seeds six drams, Liquorish half an ounce, Raisins stoned half a pound: boil them to four pints, afterwards strain it, and keep it for an ordinary drink.

Another case described by Willis is 'that Reverend person Dr. *Berwick* S.T.P. and lately Dean of St. *Pauls* Church', the details communicated to him by the patient and 'from his brother that most skilful Physician Dr. Berwick my most dear Friend'.[119] The dean suffered many years of intermittent 'bloody and salt spittle, with a grievous breath stinking like Hell'. But finding himself in prison for being a Royalist during the Civil War, Dr Berwick was forced to drink water instead of his usual tipple, and recovered for the next ten years. When he relapsed, perhaps due to inclement weather and resuming his former dietary indiscretions, 'his spittle remitted much of the usual stench' and he died. Opening the body, Willis found one lobe of the left lung 'hardned from a scirrhous Tumor', the

[117] See: *Pharmaceutice rationalis* part 2 (1679): page 52.
[118] See: *Pharmaceutice rationalis* part 2 (1679): page 58.
[119] Pordage takes Willis's lead in misspelling John Barwick (1612–1664), dean of St Paul's from 1661 to 1664, attended in his final illness by Peter Gunning (nd) who preached the funeral sermon, and with Humphrey Henchman (1592–1675) performing the obsequies.

blood bursting out from vessels 'which were joined together, or suffered not a circulation by reason of the Schirrosity'. Mystified by the source of the vile stench of his breath, Willis offers a brief account of halitosis concluding, not unexpectedly, that this is due to excess release of sulphur from blood perfusing the lungs through the local action of salt and acid.

Of peripneumony or inflammation of the lungs

The peripneumony (pneumonia) is usually defined as 'an inflammation of the Lungs with an acute Feaver, a Cough, and difficult breathing'. The mechanism is stagnation of the overheated blood leading to obstruction, inflammation and a 'Phlegmon in the frame of the Lungs'. As with most disorders of the breast, impurities of the air and diet are the evident (immediate) causes. After a detailed iatrochemical consideration, Willis concludes that 'the liquor containing ... recrements and impurities, grows clammy as glue ... and contracts an inflammable disposition'.[120] From here the process may spill over to the outer membranes causing pleurisy or a squinancy (tonsillar abscess). As expected, the fault lies not primarily in the lungs but with the blood distributing 'a Phlegman hither and thither'. This explains why Willis has observed 'a Delirium, a Frenzy, convulsive motions, or a Palsie on one side' due to the clammy blood 'stuffing ... the vessels of the Carotides'. As for the prognosis, 'common experience doth attest, that ... many people die of it, or very difficultly recover health'. It is no surprise that, given the turgid and stagnant blood, the mainstay of treatment for improving circulation through the lungs is phlebotomy. This also has the effect of removing the tendency, which Willis has observed, for the drained blood when cold to develop an unusually viscous and discoloured film separate from the coagulum. That this serum may disappear in sequential samples provides a means of judging when sufficient blood has been drained of the morbific matter. Medicines to be taken by mouth are the familiar remedies aimed at loosening the clammy blood and increasing expectoration. Although syrup of red poppies may be given for the want of sleep, Willis makes the valid point that 'Opiates, because they do further prejudice the breathing, which in this disease is already hindred, are scarce safely administred, nay sometimes may become mortal'.[121]

In his treatise on acute diseases, John Pechey (1655–1718) reproduced text from *Pharmaceutice rationalis* part 2.[122] His book was issued in parts and is poorly organized. In the epistle dedicatory included in part V, Pechey explains that 'the chapter of a peripneumony was taken from Willis'. This is in part IV which has independent signatures and pagination but no title page. The contents list only the first of four chapters: 'A peripneumony' closely paraphrases the English translations of Willis's text but does not precisely follow the wording from 1679 or 1684.

[120] See: *Pharmaceutice rationalis* part 2 (1679): page 61.

[121] See: *Pharmaceutice rationalis* part 2 (1679): page 64.

[122] See: John Pechey, *Collections of acute diseases, in five parts. I. Of the small pox and measles. II. Of the plague and pestilential fevers. III. Of continual fevers. IV. Of agues, a pleurisy, peripneumonia, quinsey, and the cholera morbus. V. And last, of the bloody-flux, miscarriage, of acute diseases of women with child, a rheumatism, bleeding at nose, apoplexy, lethargy, and of several other diseases*, London (1691). The imprimatur from Rob. Mingley is dated 22 September 1686: the book has a collective title page (1686), subsidiary titles for parts II and III (1688) and part V (1691) which contains the preliminaries, and ends with part IV.

Of pleurisie

Other than the part affected, there is no difference in mechanism between pneumonia and inflammation of 'the membrane ... environing the inside of the ribs ... taking its motion through the vertebral Arteries' causing the pleurisie. Apart from 'a pricking pain of the side', which may be confused with a more innocent disorder of the intercostal muscles producing 'most fierce tortures', the symptoms—cough and shortness of breath—are much the same. Treatment of the pleurisy is traditionally by generous 'phlebotomie in every Age by all physitians (excepting some Fanatick or false Chymists)'. In one of his rather infrequent historical diversions, Willis considers the particular vein selected for opening favoured by the Greeks, Arabians, Italians, and French. Whether this should be on the same or opposite side has excited vitriolic dispute with advocates for each location. But the debate is now largely resolved:[123]

> Damning the phlebotomy of the same side by Bell, Book and Candle ... one side judged the others of the opposite persuasion as it were guilty of murder [until] ... at length the Doctrine of the Circulation of the Blood held out like a new Light by the most renowned Harvey, discuss'd all the clouds of this Controversie; so that immediately it clearly appeared to be almost the same thing.

Nonetheless Willis does have a preference. Although the effect of phlebotomy is indirect, the delivery of morbific matter to the pleura may be reduced by diverting arterial blood towards the arm in order to compensate for withdrawal from the basilic vein on the affected side. Much the same can be achieved with cupping glasses over the painful part. Anodynes, 'powder of red Poppies ... [or] they may lawfully drink Diacodiates' are given 'both inwardly, to provoke sleep in case it be very much wanting, or externally, to alleviate the pain of the side'. Other local treatments include the 'hot bowels of Animals newly slain'. For all his logic and therapeutic rationale, Willis wheels out a mostly familiar and internally repetitive list of medicines to be taken in order to loosen the thick particles of the blood:[124]

> The eyes or claws of Crabs, the tooth of a Boar, the Stone of Carps, the jaw of a Pike Fish, the Bone in the heart of a Stag, the Priapus of a Hart, Sal Prunella, Salt of Coral, Salt of Urine, or volatile salt of Hart's-horn, powder of Goats-blood, infusion of Horse-dung, Spirit of Harts-horn, of salt Armoniack, Spirit of Tartar, the simple mixture, mineral Bezoar, Diaphoretick Antimony, flowers of salt Armoniack are very famous Remedies in a Pleurisie.

Empyema is 'a Collection of rotten matter within the cavity of the Thorax'. It is disputed whether the material is purulent matter derived from degenerate blood, or an imposthume (abscess) complicating pneumonia comprising 'pure and meer pus'. Observations that the physician might make in the form of physical signs can help. Each type of matter is sulphurous but a simple empyema, incised and yielding 'white pus to ... skip out with ease', is kinder on the nose than matter originating from an imposthume. Abscess confined to the lung remains silent initially, with 'no pathognomical Signs', but eventually discharges pus into the blood and trachea. Although the prognosis is now 'treacherous', management is with expectorants, diet, purges, cordials, anodynes, and preparations of sulphur. If Willis judges

[123] See: *Pharmaceutice rationalis* part 2 (1679): page 69.
[124] See: *Pharmaceutice rationalis* part 2 (1679): page 70.

that the outlook for empyema is favourable, he places his patients in the care of an 'expert Chirurgeon' for drainage and lavage. Time is not wasted with medicines but the patient prepared for opening with cautery applied close to the sixth and seventh vertebrae:[125]

> The Eschar [dead tissue] rais'd, the incision knife be obliquely forced ... towards the hinder and upper part, until it penetrate into the very Cavity of the Thorax; afterwards a little silver Pipe be put in, let the contained matter be sent out by degrees ... a portion thereof being left within, often contracts a hideous stench ... which evil, that it may be provided against ... a vulnerary and abstersive liquor [made from Myrrh and bitter herbs] is to be cast in twice or thrice a day by a Syphon or Syringe.

The patient receives a julep to ward against 'fainting of the Spirits, and swoonings which happen in that operation'. Amongst his autopsies Willis includes description of an imposthume that with 'a most horrid stench, exceeding any Jakes' eroded the lung, diaphragm, stomach and viscera of the lower belly as far as the 'intestinum rectum', the foul material emerging 'through the fundament together with his excretions'.[126] But he has had some success, apparently as surgeon himself from the case histories that follow, with an incision into the thorax followed by drainage and lavage when the 'stinking pus and Corruption' are localized in the periphery of the lung.

Asthma

Not mincing his words, Willis describes the asthma: 'sometimes denominated likewise an Orthopnoea' which, 'for tyranny and cruelty' amongst diseases of the breast, 'does not deserve the last place ... the organs of breathing ... the foundations and Pillars of Life, are shaken by this disease, as by an Earthquake, and so totter'. The term asthma is from the Greek 'to breathe pursie, or [with] difficulty'.[127] The problem is difficulty in 'moving the Lungs' because the passages bringing air are obstructed by catarrh and other material or compressed by the arteries and veins resulting in 'straitness of the Bronchia', individual attacks being provoked by overheating of the blood. Alternatively, asthma results from a defect of the intercostal muscles or diaphragm due to morbific matter interfering with the flow or content of animal spirits in 'the origin of those Nerves planted within the Brain', provoking the 'inmate Spirits' of the muscles into a 'convulsive asthma'. In support of this mechanism, Willis recalls that he has found 'a huge collection of sharp serum ... gathered within the cavities of the brain' in patients with asthma who had been unable to lie down without becoming breathless and therefore held their heads erect.

Of the many precipitating factors, 'the diseased find themselves better in Summer, when they breath more freely, than in Winter; likewise better in hot countries than in cold, the South or West wind blowing, than the North or East'.[128] It follows that symptomatic treatment

[125] See: *Pharmaceutice rationalis* part 2 (1679): page 76.

[126] See: *Pharmaceutice rationalis* part 2 (1679): page 77.

[127] See: *Pharmaceutice rationalis* part 2 (1679): page 82. Presumably taken from 'pursick', an obsolete word for shortness of wind in a horse. See: Hierons (1967): page 3 for the suggestion that, within the account of asthma, Willis describes emphysema: 'We have known some to have died Asthmatic or short winded ... have swelled so much, that they wanted room for their motion within the cavity of the Chest', citing *Pharmaceutice rationalis* part 2 (1684): page 20; or (1679): page 21.

[128] See: *Pharmaceutice rationalis* part 2 (1679): page 85.

is by placing the patient in fresh air away from smoke and the 'breath of bystanders' with the clothing loosened, any pressure from the abdomen relieved by a clyster, and the tracheal passage cleared with 'Lambatives, Lohochs, pectoral Decoctions and suffumigations'. Dealing with the convulsive component requires Willis's usual armamentarium of sulphurous medicines, narcotics, and opiates, notwithstanding the danger of further compromising breathing with Diacodium and Laudanum. The morbific matter is diverted away from the lungs with vesicatories, cupping glasses, friction, and ligatures applied to other parts. Preventive measures between attacks rely upon pectorals taken with anticonvulsives. Amongst the many medicines specified, Willis mentions a broth favoured by physicians, ancient and modern, in one version of which plants, liquorish, and raisins are 'sewed into the belly of an old Cock, which boyl in fifteen pounds of water until the flesh depart from the bones', the clear liquor being mixed with fresh Caffia and Manna and six ounces 'taken for many days together, and sometimes for a whole month'.[129]

Of the cases described, 'a very Honourable old Gentleman dignified by many great Titles, himself being greater than them all' and obnoxious to the asthma with nocturnal attacks 'that almost kill'd him' suffered all and sundry medications at the hands of other physicians but to no avail so that he 'was not able to walk fast or ascend steep places without danger of choking . . . and now (while I am writing this) not so much an Asthma or Consumption, as a Dropsie is feared'.[130]

Dropsie in the lung

Considered by Willis a worse devil than the asthma itself, the 'Dropsie of the Breast', occurs when accumulation of water affects the lungs in isolation. It may result from condensation of vapour, a process that must frequently occur in health with the fluid, 'even as shut within a Still', normally seeping out through the walls of the thorax or in the exhaled air. More likely as a cause of the dropsy is selective accumulation of serum in the lungs. Although this might in other distempers localize to the abdomen, brain, or limbs, perhaps it is the 'Lymphaducts' that chose the lungs to be flooded with watery chyle. In a case known to Willis in which 'the left side of his Lungs seem'd to begin to swell, and his heart to be thrust out of its place to the right side; for that he perceived the pulsation thereof to be on that side chiefly', due to 'fluctuation of water gathered within', a gentleman consulted Dr Lower who proposed 'opening of the Thorax for his only remedy'. Willis and Dr Micklethwait concurred with this decision so that a 'Chirurgeaon' incised through the vertebrae and milky fluid was drained. Thereafter, for several months the patient 'wears a silver pipe in the orifice with a tap . . . opened once in a day and a nights space . . . being well in stomach, visage, and strength, he walks abroad, rides, and performs all exercises he was formerly accustomed to, vigorously enough'. When, later, the fluid reaccumulated, 'Nature by chance discharging the function of a Chirurgeon', it drained through the old wound, the patient being careful to keep 'that orifice constantly open like a sink'.[131] Other than surgical drainage, treatment of the dropsie in the breast is, as expected, by removing serum from the blood with purges, diuretics, and diaphoretics.

[129] See: *Pharmaceutice rationalis* part 2 (1679): page 87.
[130] See: *Pharmaceutice rationalis* part 2 (1679): page 89.
[131] See: *Pharmaceutice rationalis* part 2 (1679): pages 91–2.

The viscera of the abdomen

As in the preceding sections, Willis writes on diseases and their treatments as a physician for whom physiological speculation rooted in fermentation is accommodated within his knowledge of anatomy. This means that he is reluctant to consider diseases attributed to disorder of organs which he has not previously studied through the opening of bodies.

Perhaps for that reason he avoids a detailed account of the small and large intestines or spleen: 'What relates to the Spleen we have finished in the Hypochondriac Pathologie; and what to the Womb in the Hysterical. As to what appertains to the Genital parts and their Diseases, and help, I reserve for another time and place'.[132] Willis has dealt in part 1 with the stomach and medicines active in the abdomen but now considers the chief diseases of the liver. Because this organ acts to filter 'excrements and feculencies whatsoever of the depraved Blood', disease of the liver involves enlargement through 'obstruction, inflammation, induration, and schirrus'. As a result, the nutritious juice is diverted as 'in Children affected with the Rickets', all of which are to be treated with 'remedies commonly called Hepaticks'. What is remarkable about his account of 'the Jaundies' is the classification into disorders either of biliary drainage or of the blood. In obstructive jaundice, 'the yellow choler ... overflows into the mass of blood and pollutes it with its greenness, whereby also the very skin is discolour'd'. This may result from compression of the '*vena porta*, and the *porus biliarius*' in the liver, or from sand and stony matter in the gall bladder and bile duct. The treatment of obstruction is to invigorate movement of the bile with vomits and sieges (purges), and further aid excretion of the green choler in the sweat and urine.

The jaundice that follows abnormalities of the blood occurs when excess sulphur and salt produce choler faster than it can be discharged by ordinary means. The causes include poison, 'chiefly the biting of Vipers, and the dayly use of more generous drinks', and 'a tertian intermitting Feaver'. In this situation, adjustment of the 'ragings of the Sulphur and fixt salt' is with chalybeats and spirit of Harts-horn but also 'dung of Sheep, and Geese'. Willis provides the details, now familiar in principle, of how to prepare his preferred medicines in each type of jaundice. One novel approach, 'often tried by the vulgar' but disappointing to Willis, is:[133]

> A living Tench-fish, whose Scales and outer superficies do resemble a yellow colour, applied to the right Hypochondria, or Stomach according to some (to the soles of the feet, according to others) whence a sudden flight of this disease is expected; hence although many promise themselves a cure, it hath often deceived me.

Another cure of the jaundice, 'at a distance ... by I know not what sympathy or manner of working', is a paste made from fresh urine of the jaundiced patient with the ashes from an ash tree: 'after this course, I have known this inveterate disease happily cured, although resisting many other remedies; the practice thereof is very familiar with the Vulgar'. Prevention of the 'jaundies' is easier than cure and the mainstay is medicines that either reduce the nutritive load on the liver or break up coagulations and concretions in the blood for dispatch through the usual routes of excretion before these are deposited in that organ. Here, perhaps more than at any other point in his narrative, Willis makes a persuasive case for diet. For the rickets he advocates the importance of milk and exercise, advocating that the children 'suck thin

[132] See: *Pharmaceutice rationalis* part 2 (1679): page 133. In the event, Willis died soon after making this summary and the intended treatise on genital diseases and their treatment was never written.

[133] See: *Pharmaceutice rationalis* part 2 (1679): page 100.

and serous milk, that they be shaken or tossed in their Nurses arms, and tumbled quickly to and fro, or carried swiftly in a Chair or Coach, and as soon as may be, learned to go and use their feet'.[134] Listing many plants and vegetable extracts and offering a somewhat obscure analogy, Willis mentions that 'if I omit Chalybeates, most Chymists will censure me very unjust to the Liver; for truly as the prerogative of *Venus* is vulgarly attributed to this bowel, so as to constrain to Love, we may expect that *Mars* will be perpetually kinde unto it. And really it is manifest by reason, as well as by Experience, that preparations of Steel are convenient in hepatical affects'. Willis is generally reticent on the use of chalybeates and merely reminds the curious reader that he has explained this treatment 'in another place, so that here is no need for repetition'.[135] AC Wootton (1843–1910) is more helpful:[136]

> Thomas Willis had a secret preparation of iron of which Dr. Walter Harris, physician in ordinary to Charles II, in 'Pharmacologia anti-empirica' (1683) writes:– 'The best preparation of any that iron can yield us is a secret of Dr. Willis. It has hitherto been a great secret and sold at a great price. It was known as Dr. Willis's Preparation of Steel'. Dr Harris thinks it will not be an unacceptable service to the public to communicate this masterpiece of that eminent and ever famous man. 'It was no strained stately magistery, no sublimation or salification, no calcined crocus, and no chemical mystery; but an easy and a natural way of opening this hard body that it may open ours'. It was given particularly for the removal of obstructions. The formula was equal parts of iron filings and crude tartar powdered and mixed with water in a damp mass in a glazed earthen vessel. This was to be dried over a slow fire or in the sun; wetted and dried again; and this process repeated four or five times. It might be given in white wine, or made into a syrup, or into pills, electuary, or lozenges. Dr. Willis preferred the crude tartar because the cream of tartar sold by the druggists was generally a cheat, often combined with alum. The crude could be bought at 6d. to 8d. per lb. In the apothecaries shops cream of tartar was sold at 3s. to 3s. 6d. per lb.

Ascites, tympany, and anasarca

Willis's descriptions of abdominal distension and generalized oedema are insightful, especially for the account of ascites in liver disease and conditions in which fluid accumulates due either to exudate or transudate. Mentioning a few of his preferred deoppilatives for liver disease, Willis goes on to explain that once the blood has been filled with cholerick excrements for a while, 'the Dropsie called Ascites ... a waterish tumour' of the abdomen follows 'the fault of the Liver ... and the Jaundies'. The amount accumulated in the abdomen may be considerable: 'I have once seen a Tub would hold 15 gallons filled with water taken out of the Abdomen of a Woman dead of a Dropsie'.[137] Willis rejects suggestions that the fluid descends from the liver or spleen, and that it results from vapourized air or distillation of a nervous humour. Rather, the water is serum derived from blood and delivered through the open mouths of the coeliac and mesenteric vessels, sometimes in association with 'secret tumours gathered in the lower belly'. The fluid may also be derived from the 'milkie

[134] See: *Pharmaceutice rationalis* part 2 (1679): page 103.

[135] Willis mentions chalybeates in the treatises *De fermentatione* (1659) and *De anima brutorum* (1672) but in neither are these expounded in detail.

[136] See: AC Wootton *Chronicles of pharmacy*, volume 1, London (1910): pages 400–2.

[137] See: *Pharmaceutice rationalis* part 2 (1679): page 105.

Vessels' obstructed by a vicious chyle. Whatever the origin, Willis points out that, removed by 'a Paracentesis ... with a hollow Needle', ascitic fluid thickens with heat 'and grows white, like the white of an Egge'. The prognosis is so predictably poor when ascites is 'coming from tumours about the bowels' that the vulgar do not bother with medicines but 'with them presently the next question is, Who shall be his heir?' Willis is less despairing, especially if ascites is the manifestation of more generalized dropsy, advising paracentesis and his usual approach of increasing excretion using strategies with which his readers are now well familiar. Foremost are cathartic purges and vomits but, as Willis explains, diuretics ought also to be capable of 'draining waters out of every place or cavity of the body'. The problem is that the ascitic fluid is not easily sucked up by the mesenteric veins in order to reach the kidneys. Through their effect directly on the blood, some diuretics may divert serum towards, not away from, the abdomen 'and so augment rather than remove the inundation of the belly'. In imitation of an empirical medicine introduced by Dr John English (nd) and endorsed by Dr Theodore Mayern (1573–1635), Willis has met with success using, for him, a surprisingly simple medicine:[138]

> Take of green Plantane-leaves four handfuls, Liverwort, Brookline, of each two handfuls, bruise them together, and pour upon them half a pound of small compound Radish-water, or other appropriate Magistral, express it strongly, the dose three ounces three times in a day.

Diaphoreticks are not helpful because they do not attract the ascites back into the veins and merely add to the problem, overheating the belly and causing vapours to precipitate and the blood to boil, thereby accentuating the accumulation of fluid. The same applies to the use of foments and liniments placed on the 'Paunch of the Belly'; whereas 'Remedies that are chiefly wont to be administered with success near the places affected (when a Cure is intended without Paracentesis) are Clysters and Plaisters'. The most effective clyster is made from 'a pint of Urine of a sound man that drinks Wine, Venice turpentine dissolved with the yolk of an Egge ... [and] Sal Prunella ... which repeat dayly'. An obvious treatment is to pierce the paunch and drain the ascites. But caution is needed: 'a Paracentesis being made; which administration however doth not oftner cure the disease, than kill the patient' especially when 'Quacks and Empiricks rashly and unluckily essay it, Artists not being consulted'.

Willis describes one case. Whilst nursing her infant, 'a young Woman wife to a Merchant ... to increase her milk day and night did immoderately guzzle one while plain Ale, another while Posset-drink'. After a fortnight this led to ascites, 'her Abdomen being great with water fluctuating within, did much swell up, and its bulk when she turned from one side to the other fell without the Ileon and borders of the rest of the body: when in the mean while the flesh of all her Members was very much consumed'. But once the child was weaned, Willis instituted a better diet and together with Hydragogues, Dr Mayern's empirical remedy, and his own preferred urine based clyster and a plaister on her belly, eventually she settled after moving to the Countryside and drinking asses milk 'and lives yet in health'.[139]

The 'tympanie' is altogether more mysterious. It results from an abdomen full of 'winde', yet on opening the bodies of the dead nothing other than ascites may be found. Pricking the distended belly in life, as in paracentesis, may discharge 'a stinking wind' but usually leads to death. As to where the wind accumulates, Willis does not accept uncritically the

[138] See: *Pharmaceutice rationalis* part 2 (1679): page 112.
[139] See: *Pharmaceutice rationalis* part 2 (1679): pages 112–13.

prevailing view that it is within the bowels of the lower belly, the closed space within the mesentery, or in the 'Peritonæum'. As an anatomist his approach is methodical. Swelling of the abdomen may occur with inward tumours of the bowels, '*viz.* scirrhous, strumous, cancrous, glandulous, and some perhaps of another kind'; temporary distension of the gut from digestion and fermentation of foodstuffs; or ascites 'as at large set down'. Somehow, no one of these seems right and, as a neurologist, Willis 'loosens the knot by reasoning', as explanation for the tympanie, that 'delinquent' animal spirits 'cramm'd thick' in the nervous fibres of these parts collide with viscid and tenacious juice delivered by the wandring pair (vagus). As a result, the swelling 'which before was a wandring Symptom ... at length grows to be a fixt and permanent disease'. The peritonæum, mesentery, and guts all 'blown up and enlarged ... being turgid with an impetuous Spirit', the putrefied humours eventually vaporize and turn to wind. Perhaps not entirely sure of his reasoning, and admitting that 'we may suspect, that the true cause of the disease lyes as yet conceal'd', Willis restates his neurological formulation:[140]

> This Pathologie although it may seem to some a Paradox, and uncouth, I doubt not but it will serve assent from many, if it be thoroughly weighed, that those who have been a long time obnoxious to Hypochondriack, Colick, and other convulsive distempers of the nether Belly, do at length become sick of a Tympany ... It is a fixt and constant Tumour of the Abdomen, hard, stiff, and yielding a noise upon striking, taking its origin from a convulsive inflation of the parts and membranous bowels, by reason of the Animal Spirits being driven into those fibres in too great abundance, and through the fault of the nervous juice obstructing, being hindred from their return back; to which disease consequently an accumulation of winds in the empty places, accrues as a complement.

Once it is established, the prognosis from the tympanie is poor. It will not surprise readers that treatment is with purges that discharge phlegm, melancholy, choler, and water, 'although with small or no success', despite 'abundant watery and flatulent stools'. Taking his usual approach, Willis advocates diuretics and clysters with foments and a plaister of 'Cow-dung, with the powder of Dogs-turd' applied to the abdomen. Chalybeates are given to prevent further incursion of the animal spirits and improve the nervous juice, as preservatory remedies. Cardiacks and hypnoticks are required as vital treatments to ward 'against fainting of the Spirits, and difficult breathing, and against Watching and Thirst'.

Dropsie affecting the whole body is 'the Anasarca ... a white soft Tumour of the whole outward Body, or of some of its parts, yielding to the touch, and leaving a dent upon compression' due to accumulation of water 'within the pores of the flesh and skin'.[141] It results from imbalance between outpouring from the extremities of the arteries and supping by the veins and lymphaducts, the surplus accumulating because it is not excreted in the sweat or urine. Once again, primarily at fault is the blood and a defect in assimilation of the various particles, in this instance water, during fermentation of the chyle and nitrous spirit. This leads to the serum being discharged upon the tissues so as not to stifle and extinguish enkindling of the blood. Since dropsy, and hence anasarca, is more frequent in persons 'inhabiting Maritime or Moorish places', and others recover their health by 'removing their residence into Sunny and Mountainous places', a proximate cause may be unwholesome air failing to heat the blood. But there are more immediate causes. Loss of particles needed for fermentation through

[140] See: *Pharmaceutice rationalis* part 2 (1679): pages 117–18.
[141] See: *Pharmaceutice rationalis* part 2 (1679): page 123.

against a Plethora ... Rusticks and Countrey-men for healths sake, once or twice a year cause blood to be drawn from themselves and their Beasts'.[149] Others are more reticent to the point of refusal. Willis veers towards their cautious position on the basis that excess bleeding encourages 'a pinguifying and more fiery' sulphur with less salt in the blood, predisposing 'all men to be feaverish and ... fat'. Too much trivial bleeding compromises the advantages of opening a vein when phlebotomy is really needed. But Willis forgets his judicious reasoning in allowing that the diseases in which phlebotomy is needed:[150]

> Rehearse almost the whole Pathologie of the humane Body. An aching Head, a Brain oppres'd with blood, or over-flowed with Serum (whence spring a world of evils) burning of the eyes, inflammation of the face, mouth and throat, all the diseases of the Breast and Præcordia ... affections of the Liver, Spleen, and other Bowels; moreover as a Plethors, and Athletick habit of the whole body, so also the tumours of each member, painful and convulsive passions, seem to accrue blood as Author of all the evil, and require its sending out, as a certain kind of revenge.

Faced with negotiating text designated 'first, secondly, thirdly', each with its own 'first, secondly, thirdly', forming an apparently unedited flow that merges theories of fermentation with indications for phlebotomy, it is with some relief that readers reach Willis's practical account of where, how, when, and for how long a vein should be opened. For general purposes, the median vein of the forearm is best, whereas the foot is preferred for stemming the flow of 'menstrual flux or Haemorrhoids'. Diseases of the head require bleeding from the temples or throat. For tumours or pain in the joints, blood is taken from a nearby vessel. There are even more specific relationships: the outer brachial vein (the 'Cephalick') respects the head, the inner (the 'Jecorary') the liver, and the vessel on the fourth finger (the 'Salvatella') is best for the spleen. Willis wonders why the jugular is not more often opened in disorders of the head, although the drainage of blood from that vessel can be prodigious and leach the whole body as in the slaughter of beasts. But these distinctions are specious, 'vulgar errors', and other than avoiding a nearby artery, nerve or tendon, any large vein will do.

Each of the methods used for drawing out blood from a vein—the lancet, suction by leeches, or cupping glasses after scarification—is 'in familiar use by Quacks, Barbers and Women, and all things relating to them commonly known, as a man his own house'. Because it is now established that the blood circulates, the preference of the ancients for draining bright red arterial rather than black-purple venous blood is immaterial. Moreover, Willis is aware that mistaking an artery for a vein leads to unstoppable bleeding due to the 'perpetual turns of Systole and Diastole', whence 'either death or loss of the member sometimes ensues'.[151] Bleeding needs to be carried out early in the course of disease and not at its height when the healing of blood by 'crisis ... ought not to be disturbed'. Bleeding should not be carried out in infants and children, old men, and pregnant women. Ideally it is confined to the spring and autumn, avoiding the solstices, although timing phlebotomy by observing 'the position of the Heavens, and the Aspects of the Moon and Stars ... appears altogether frivolous ... absurd ... and frequently malevolent'. Bleeding is best done in the morning on a fasting stomach. The amount of blood removed should be enough to avoid the space created being filled by morbific matter regurgitated from recesses, and thus intensifying

[149] See: *Pharmaceutice rationalis* part 2 (1679): page 137.
[150] See: *Pharmaceutice rationalis* part 2 (1679): page 139.
[151] See: *Pharmaceutice rationalis* part 2 (1679): page 140.

inflammation and heating of the blood. Draining too much so that 'strength languishes, or the body labours under a notorious Cachexia' is equally hazardous. The prudent physician must judge the 'strength of the Disease and the ability of the Patient', and not allow the 'Quacks, Empiricks and Barbers to play with humane life'.[152]

Remedies are required to stop 'immoderate Haemorrhages, whether engenderd by Nature or by accident'. Willis is not here concerned with bleeding from the lungs, kidneys, or bowels, although each is mentioned, but with staunching the excesses of menstruation, haemorrhoids, and nosebleeds. In fact he deals only with epistaxis. The nostrils are supplied by a branch of the carotid artery which, according to Willis, reaches the nose from the cranium through the cribriform plate with the 'smelling nerves', the serum in blood normally separating to form the nasal secretions. If excessive, their discharge is promoted by sneezing medicines or 'Errhines'. Nosebleeds constitute a disease rather than a means for physiological cleansing of the brain. They occur when the mouths of nasal vessels open further in order to release blood destined for the head that has become turgid and needing to break out. This happens in many situations, and Willis has many therapeutic suggestions, 'first … tenthly'. The flow of blood can be staunched with ligatures retaining blood in the limbs, or by diverting the flow using phlebotomy, cupping glasses, and friction applied to various parts. These measures restrict flow in the carotid and vertebral circulation. Less drastic as a means to the same end is cooling or splashing water on the face, immersing the patient in cold water, and applying vinegar to the 'Pubes and Testicles'. Swooning induced by physical means or the patient 'suddenly affrighted with some feigned rumour' may also abruptly stop the bleeding through reduction in strength of the pulse. Those affected are exposed to a whole host of occult remedies, including 'a silk bag with a dry Toad … worn on the pit of the Stomach' or carrying the 'moss of a humane Skull'. On the suggestion of cauterizing the foot, 'we advise not since any benefit is unlikely to compensate for the pain and lameness'. Willis is surprisingly uncritical of the advice offered by '*Crato* [Johannes Crato von Krafftheim: 1519–1585] to bend the little finger on the affected side which 'because done with no trouble we may try'. The nostrils can be treated directly with a pledget dipped in Roman Vitriol (copper sulphate) or the application of a styptic powder, but also famous amongst Practitioners is 'Hogs-dung, thrust into the Nostrils, which by the meer ill favour is thought to repell the blood'. All of these remedies are used with the patient sat upright, sustained with a slender diet, given medicines for cooling the overheated blood, and slowing the heart rate with hypnotics and opiates.[153] The specific strategy of converting nasal haemorrhage into sweats in managing nosebleeds associated with 'the Spotted Feaver, Small-pox, Measles, or the Plague', turns out merely to use many familiar botanical powders and concoctions taken for 'twenty or thirty dayes' by mouth together with purges and chalybeates. Lest his readers are mistaken in concluding that Willis condones all these various means of staunching nosebleeds, periodically he distances himself by explaining that: 'the reasons of effects of this kind are concealed from me'.

'Called by the Ancients *Phænigms* or *Sinapismus*', which take away the 'Scarf-skin' and expose the vessels so that they 'spue out the serous humours', vesicatories are similar in principle to phlebotomy as a means of allowing recrements to escape without being deposited in 'parts and places where they shall offend'. Made of 'Mustard, Pidgeons dung, Squills masht, Garlick, Milk of Figs', or stronger astringents based on Cantharides,[154] they raise caustic

[152] See: *Pharmaceutice rationalis*, part 2 (1679): page 142.

[153] See: *Pharmaceutice rationalis* part 2 (1679): pages 145–7.

[154] Derived from the male blister beetle and given to the female as a copulatory gift during mating so also used as an aphrodisiac.

blisters that both redden the skin and leach fluid. Willis uses the analogy of fire to explain how the particles mediating chemical burns also convulse the union of blood vessels and nerves under the skin, dissolving the humours and venomous particles, and allowing serum to be squeezed out close to the application. Even though applied topically, vesicatories may enter the circulation and be deposited in some weak or tender channel. Willis makes the point no less than five times in a few paragraphs that, in this way, vesicatories injure the neck of the bladder causing strangury. Avoiding their use in nephritick disorders, Willis has not himself encountered these complications and believes that the medicines can usefully unlock morbific recrements throughout the body, enabling these to be removed in sweat, urine, vomits, and stools. Nonetheless he is careful to avoid excoriation and inflammation of skin under the blister, not to 'infect and impoyson the blood passing through', and to avoid formation of cicatrices. Willis recounts the case of 'a famous Doctor of Physick in *London*' recovering from a malignant feaver who sweated out ichor daily from blisters but found them 'troublesome and tedious'. They were stopped whereupon the disease revived with swooning, a cold sweat and weak pulse with which he soon died, the cause being that the malignant matter had evidently fallen 'into the Cardiac Nerves, whose action being hindred, the vital function quickly failed'.[155]

Useful in any regional disorder, because they act close to the termination of nerve fibres, vesicatories are especially beneficial in convulsive distempers of the brain and nervous stock: 'the heterogenous particles ... agitated and derived from the Brain, slide towards their newly opened Emissary, by degrees, and at length are removed wholly forth'. Thus, Willis advocates their use in soporific, convulsive, and painful distempers; and he asks: 'Was ever any surprized with a Lethergy, Apoplexie, or Epilepsie, but that immediately Friends and Attendants however unexpert, have tormented his Hide with the application of Cantharides?'[156] But, not for the first time, having argued persuasively on the basis of mechanisms for specific indications, Willis cannot resist a long and comprehensive list of the many conditions in which vesicatories are used with success. Twenty-six pages away from the last words that Willis was to write (in the English translations) before his death from pleurisy and pneumonia, he makes a poignant point:[157]

> I confess, when I have often been surprised with a great Cough, with abundant and thick Spittle (whereto I am originally obnoxious) I have received relief from no other Remedies more than Vesicatories; wherefore I am wont, while that distemper doth urge, to apply medicines drawing blisters first upon the Vertebra's of the neck, then those little ulcers being healed, beneath the ears, and afterwards if need require it upon the Scapula's.

By their nature, vesicatories are temporary measures designed to cure 'acute or other Diseases', whereas surgical 'Issues' placed deeper and seeping more slowly drain the ichor or serous humour 'with a constant spring'. Flow is maintained by a 'pease', which Willis does not describe but presumably he means packing the wound with an irritant.[158] Issues attract and remove humours derived from blood vessels and nerve fibres, and material fixed in the pores of the skin or the interspaces of muscles and membranes.

[155] See: *Pharmaceutice rationalis* part 2 (1679): page 155.
[156] See: *Pharmaceutice rationalis* part 2 (1679): page 154.
[157] See: *Pharmaceutice rationalis* part 2 (1679): pages 153–4; and, for the original text, *Pharmaceutice rationalis* (1675): page 360.
[158] See: *Pharmaceutice rationalis* part 2 (1679): page 160.

Whilst 'there is scarce any disease happens, wherein this remedy is either hurtful or unprofitable', issues are particularly useful in 'the Convulsions of Infants, or Youths, for sore-Eyes, Kings-evil, as also for head-ache in persons adult or ancient, for drousie, vertiginous or Cramp-like distempers'.[159] Care is needed in placement of the surgical issue. It needs to be done by a surgeon, not 'Quacks, and others ignorant of Anatomy' and, avoiding arteries and tendons, ideally lies between the bellies of muscles. For diseases of the brain and its outer coverings, some practitioners create a wound through which morbific matter may discharge by burning a fontanel with a cautery over the coronal suture on the top of the head, over the sagittal suture on the forehead, or at the back over the lambdoid. Others recommend holes cut or burned behind the ears, or 'a Seton with a skane of Silk drawn through the Lobes thereof'. But Willis has found that these close rapidly from 'the Cuticula, or skin growing under' and are rarely successful. These procedures are not necessarily safe: 'for it is a common observation that many from an Issue raised near the head, have been presently surprized with a certain defect, and weakness of sight' due to excess removal of the animal spirits. Willis prefers an issue placed in the nape of the neck for 'painfull distempers of the brain, and Meninges' in children and youths, or between the shoulder blades in adults and old men, these also being useful in a variety of other disorders. Avoiding fontinels in the abdomen, he has cured the sciatica by one inserted in the groin.[160]

As with any therapy, the cutting of issues has its complications. Although much used by others, those in the thigh tend to dry up and become inflamed and painful. Willis is also aware that the wound may develop into 'a filthy and malignant Ulcer', the 'putrefying pollution ... [of] the streaming Ichor doth so stink, and black the Covering' and this gangrene soon contaminating the whole mass of blood. Less catastrophically, issues often become inflamed raising a tumour with redness and heat that may resolve spontaneously but can also lead to a 'Sphacela' (gangrene), as 'a Pus, to be evacuated by an abscesse', or spilling into the mass of the blood constituting 'a fiercer Phlogosie with a Feaver, and sometimes other dreadful symptomes'. In order to prevent this unwelcome accumulation, the cutting of issues is often preceded by phlebotomy, purging, and the topical application of foments and emollients.[161]

When discharge from the issue is excessive, 'thin and stinking' as may happen in order to strengthen the blood and preserve 'the tone of the place ulcerated by the Fontinel', Willis's approach, unsurprisingly, is diet and purging with frequent change of dressings soaked in 'St. *John's* wort' and other plant extracts. If too dry and leaking insufficient serum, the issue is challenged with 'Pease made of Ivy-wood, or Box, or the roots of Gentian or Hermadactyls'. If it closes too soon, or develops a cavity and overgrowth of spongy flesh about the edges, the excess is best reduced with escharotick powders; or the wound abandoned and moved to another site.[162] Finally, Willis reminds his readers of a 'contumacious opinion' that one or more fontinels lead to barrenness and so should be avoided in women desirous of having children. On this his view is clear, anticipating epidemiological distinctions between association and causation, and the need for evidence other than:[163]

[159] See: *Pharmaceutice rationalis* part 2 (1679): page 156.
[160] See: *Pharmaceutice rationalis* part 2 (1679): pages 157–8.
[161] See: *Pharmaceutice rationalis* part 2 (1679): page 159.
[162] See: *Pharmaceutice rationalis* part 2 (1679): page 160.
[163] See: *Pharmaceutice rationalis* part 2 (1679): page 161.

> Stories of certain women that have been barren having Issues, when it were as easie to enumerate more barren women without issues, and many others that have been fruitfull with them; and truly I used to retort (whenas there is no need of any other refuting), this as a chief Argument against that opinion.

Diseases of the skin

The cutting of issues and the complications thereof, and the place of sweating for the increase of excretion as a major part of his therapeutic rationale, brings Willis to the last topic on which he ever wrote: disorders of the skin. On the anatomy, Willis defers to Malpighi's description of the microscopic structure of the various layers, sweat glands, hair follicles, and arterial, nervous, and lymphatic networks. He considers variations in texture of the integument dependent on occupation, the use of emollients and soaps, or the cold north wind likened to the 'skin of a Goose new pull'd', these variations being due to the amount of humour present in the glands and pores.

The deeper layers and subcutaneous tissues are involved in skin disease due to tumours and fever, 'Small-pox, measles, or other malignant wheals ... [and] the fleeting pushes of Infants'. Many of these conditions have been discussed in *De febribus* (1659) although Willis does have more to say: 'perhaps, an opportunity may happen, when I may treat more specifically of Tumours of every kind'. But, as with his proposed treatise on genital diseases, this was not to be. Rather his account is confined to superficial lesions of the outer layer, 'Scarf-skin', which is insensitive and so rarely gives rise to symptoms other than a change in appearance. Sunspots, 'Ephelides', are seasonal and affect exposed parts 'in the more beautifull persons, and of a thinner skin ... [and] a fair Complexion'. These are the size of a fleabite and no different from freckles, or lentil-sized lesions known as 'Lentignes'. They are harmless and arise because cholerick humour drawn out by the sun is caught in the pores of the cuticle. Liver spots, larger and often pigmented, are so named because they are due to 'feculencies and excrements' inadequately separated from blood in the liver and spleen discolouring the skin on the back and breast. They also are innocent but, pandering to the 'importunate, craving for Medicines', Willis applies cosmetics and offers 'hepatical Remedies'. There is a 'plentiful harvest' of remedies for 'the Art of Beautifying' amongst 'curious Ladies' that either open the pores of the skin or drive back the 'spotty matter' into the blood. Somewhat dutifully, Willis provides his formulary for cleaning the skin—astringents, vitriol, and mercurial preparations included. Always one to advise caution, in discussing the management of blackheads on the nose 'which little Insects being squeezed out of the pores, and exposed to the sun, are easily seen to live, and to move themselves', Willis explains that 'to this Hony there is a Thorn at hand' and the peccant material driven back in the blood may be deposited in the brain so that 'women or men that have long used Mercurial Cosmeticks, are troubled with a Vertigo, and convulsive Distempers, or are obnoxious to paralytical, and their Teeth grow black, and sometimes fall out'.[164] We can agree that this is a heavy price to pay for squeezing a black spot on the nose.

Willis describes 'the Psora or Scab' (psoriasis) which manifests as scaly lesions, dry or sometimes moist and prone to ulceration. Acid and salty humour, 'every atome let in by holes and pores', delivered in the blood is caught in the glandules of the skin causing swellings and pustules. This glandulous humour may become 'Lousie' (as in lice) in those held

[164] See: *Pharmaceutice rationalis* part 2 (1679): pages 163–5.

'long in prison ... and those being of a sedentary life ... used to nastiness and sluttishness'. From this it follows that even those who live decent lives may develop the itch if they 'lye in the same bed either with a scabby person, or where he hath lately lain ... [or] with the Linnen of the Scabby, oftentimes washed ... [so that] surely, the taint of no disease (the Plague only excepted) is more easily or certainly propagated than this of the Mange'.[165]

The particular feature of the psora is 'the sense of that troubelsome itch'. (In passing Willis also mentions that the same itch and eruptions occur is some who 'daily and often eating of Shell-fish ... salted meats hung in the Sun or Smoak ... disagreeing Drinks, and venemous Medicines'). Ever ready to propose a neurological explanation, Willis expands upon his assumption that itch results from animal spirits entering the nervous fibres. Given the satisfaction of scratching, he wonders whether the stimulation is of fibres in the nerve endings concerned with pain or with pleasure. Apologizing in advance, 'Let the reader pardon me, if I should by way of digression expound this at large, and even to tediousness', he sets out his views on the physiology of touch concluding that sensory pleasure is merely release from pain.[166] But since it is the stagnation of spirits in the nerve ends in the psora that are 'neither put to flight, nor repulsed', itch cannot be either pain or pleasure but a middle state and therefore its own passion. The aim of treatment is straightforward: to disperse the morbific matter rendering the glandules and pores freed from the 'Ichorous congealings'. The mainstay is purging without which the condition 'can scarce ever be cured', supplemented with phlebotomy, vomitories, diureticks, and diaphoreticks, and by dietary prudence and abstemiousness from drink. Much is also to be gained from topical remedies with liniments soaked in oyntments prepared from brimstone or mercury. These are to be used sparingly to avoid 'a salivation, also sometimes dimness of the eyes, or drowsie or convulsive Affections' and adverse effects on the viscera of the præcordium and abdomen.[167] The smoke of cinnabar heated over coals, sulphur baths, and wearing a shirt washed in brimstone each has its place.

Similar to 'the Scab with Itch' is a distemper characterized by pustules known as 'the *Impetigo*, by some a Tetter or Morphew, and by others the leprosie of the *Greeks*'; and described by Willis not 'according to Books, but from the proper observation of the Patients themselves'. The wheals and red pustules, starting on the arms or thighs but spreading elsewhere, round or irregular, and being in size between 'a Penny ... [and] a Silver Crown', itch and are scratched leaking liquor and healing in a 'shelly scale'. Unlike the psora, the lesions of the impetigo often coalesce. The condition is not propagated by contagion in that 'the Miasma from the Husband doth not pass to the wife, or from her to him, though they lye together'. This distinction from the psora is not readily explained by Willis's account of tartarous concretions from the blood being increasingly heaped up in the skin, since this mechanism is much as proposed for both conditions. Nor does causation based on a diet rich in smoked meat and fish help to explain the differences. Using epidemiological arguments in favour of the dietary hypothesis, Willis points out that the people 'of Cornwal for the most part dwelling on the Sea-coast ... fed with fish, became very obnoxious to the leprous Distempers; insomuch that for their relief many Hospitals were erected in that Countrey'. The reason is that such food is rancid and conveys heterogenous nutritive particles, oversalted, to the blood so that tartarous coagulations are deposited in the skin as the 'seeds of the Leprosie or of the Impetiginous Evil'.[168]

[165] See: *Pharmaceutice rationalis* part 2 (1679): page 167.
[166] See chapter 17 for a fuller discussion of Willis's views on touch and the other senses.
[167] See: *Pharmaceutice rationalis* part 2 (1679): page 171.
[168] See: *Pharmaceutice rationalis* part 2 (1679): pages 173–4.

More generally, the impetigo may follow the taint of 'an inveterate Pox ... although none distempered ... wants the suspicion of that Shamefull disease'. The prognosis seldom threatens death or imminent danger and, as always, early treatment is most useful through a diet lacking the offending foodstuffs, drink free from 'thick and foggy Ale', and moving from the 'Sea-coast and Fenny places; to dry and clean air'. The skin lesions settle if the morbific matter is driven back into the blood through purging and the use of 'Cathartícks, Phlebotomy, Whey, Chalybeate Waters, Juicy expressions of Herbs, Decoctions of Woods, steel'd Medicines and Salivation'. Although chalybeates and steel medicines, and extracts of wholesome wood, have often featured in his pharmacopoeia, Willis has seldom emphasized the drinking of whey thrice daily for at least one month, 'if the Stomach will bear it' as a means of 'sweetning the Blood and washing of the Salts thereof'. These various remedies described, 'sixthly' Willis gets to salivation 'as the stoutest Wrestler and only match for such an Enemy'. His experience is evidently based on the pox rather than impetigo and limited to two patients in whom nothing helped and everyone:[169]

> Despaired of Cure: Whence it is manifest that the Venereal Distemper, although highly malignant, and raising most filthy Ulcers consuming the flesh and bones is more easily and certainly cured than the Impetigo.

The situation is no better when impetigo follows scurvy. Most antiscorbuticals, 'Garden Scurvy-grass, Water-cresses, the Horse-radish, Pepperwort and others' do more harm than good. Willis prefers juices of herbs rich in nitrous salt of which a diet of cucumbers 'in lieu of a Sallad ... three or four ... cut into slices ... infused in Spring-water the dose is half a pint thrice or oftener a day' is recommended. Even better are spawaters rich in vitriolic salt 'of which kind ... the *S P A W*, and *Tunbridge*, and *Astrope* Wells, do far excel those Nitrous, and all other Remedies'.[170] Mentioned periodically as a rational therapy, Willis adds tissue of the viper as another remedy, taking his authority from Galen:[171]

> That drink being pour'd out of a Bottle wherein a Viper was put to poyson one labouring with an Elephantiasis, and so given him to free him from his misery, prov'd his remedy, and what was destined for his murder, dispatched an incurable Disease.

Willis does not subscribe to the view that extract of viper 'and other Oviparous Snakes' is effective because annually they throw off their scaly coats, as has been suggested. Rather, the active ingredient is volatile salt in 'broths from their flesh boyl'd' and powders from dried flesh. Better than sulphur baths, the most useful external treatment for removing the scales of impetigo is liniment impregnated with 'water out of Tubs wherein Tarre hath long stood', or bathing in tarwater.

When all else fails, mercurial remedies may be used but with caution. That message is made clear by the account of two cases with the impetigo described in the last paragraph that Willis wrote. These are unusually revealing of Willis's style in not disguising his failures. So covered was a 'Virgin of a Noble Family' with scabs of the impetigo, from head to foot, that

[169] See: *Pharmaceutice rationalis* part 2 (1679): page 175. At page 177, Willis refers to an appendix in which he has written on the pathology of the venereal distemper but this was either never written or lost from the published edition of *Pharmaceutice rationalis* part 2 (1675), perhaps as one of the manuscripts that John Hemming inherited at Willis's death.

[170] See: *Pharmaceutice rationalis* part 2 (1679): page 176.

[171] See: *Pharmaceutice rationalis* part 2 (1679): page 177.

she was 'ashamed to appear abroad or converse with others of her rank'. After the requisite purging and phlebotomy, Willis prescribed salivation and a mercurial ointment applied to 'bending of the Joynts'. Optimistic when the eruptions resolved, and maintaining purges, sweats and diet, hopes were later dashed. The young woman's friends persuaded Willis to try another mercurial salivation which he did, but with recurrent cycles of scaly eruption after each apparent relief so that 'the Pustules and Clusters ... encreasing daily in number and bulk at length grew fouler than before, insomuch that like an *Hydra*, after the loss of one head this disease received sevenfold'. A young man had impetigo 'so that every night the Scales fell off like bran in great plenty in his bed'. He obtained temporary but no lasting relief from salivation so that 'it exercis'd its Tyranny during the Patient's life'.

'Valete'

With these cases, Willis concludes his contributions to medicine. In one sense he has ended where he began with an account of distempers affecting those organs which provide nourishment and aerate the blood. Fermented and enriched, this circulates to body parts, especially the brain and nervous stock, and is the basis for vitality. His story is one of movement: agitation of the five particles, diffusion of animal spirits through the brain and nerves, contraction of muscle and the mechanics of motion, the arrival of sensation and the traces it leaves, rhythms of the viscera, the tracking of waste to points of exit. His story is one of contrasts: the orderly assembly of molecules in health and their agitation in disease, voluntary and involuntary movement, the corporeal and rational souls, our `neurologie' and `psychologie'. Undoubtedly Willis had more to say and his last printed words are a message of hope and expectation, perhaps tinged with weariness and a sense of his impending mortality.[172]

> I confess I am scarce able to contain my self, but that I should enter upon that pleasant Field of Speculation. But this seems as irrational and unusual, as for one wearyed with a long Course, and breathless at the end, running beyond his Post, presently to begin a new Race.

[172] See: *Pharmaceutice rationalis* part 2 (1679): page 179.

Index

Footnotes are indicated by n. and illustrations by locators in italics. Variant spellings of names are given in parentheses. Throughout the index, Dr Thomas Willis is referred to as TW.